International Association of Fire Chiefs

National Fire Protection Association

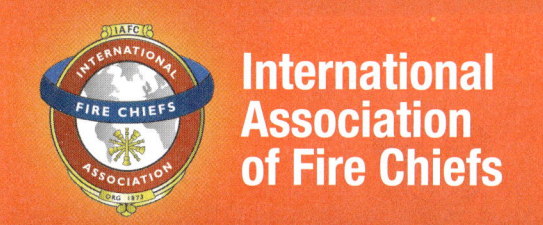

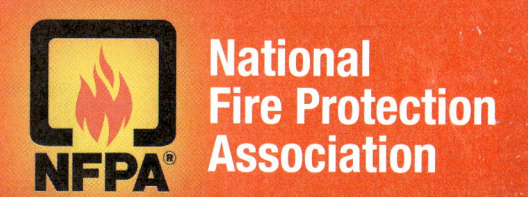

Fire Apparatus Driver/Operator

Pump, Aerial, Tiller, and Mobile Water Supply

SECOND EDITION

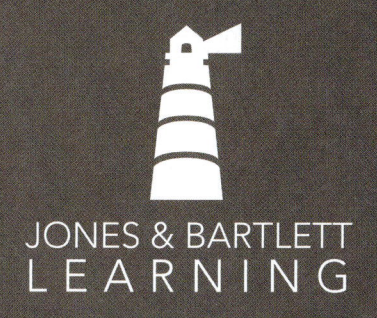

JONES & BARTLETT LEARNING

Jones & Bartlett Learning
World Headquarters
5 Wall Street
Burlington, MA 01803
978-443-5000
info@jblearning.com
www.jblearning.com

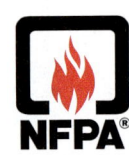

National Fire Protection Association
1 Batterymarch Park
Quincy, MA 02169-7471
www.NFPA.org

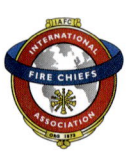

International Association of Fire Chiefs
4025 Fair Ridge Drive
Fairfax, VA 22033
www.IAFC.org

Jones & Bartlett Learning books and products are available through most bookstores and online booksellers. To contact Jones & Bartlett Learning directly, call 800-832-0034, fax 978-443-8000, or visit our website, www.jblearning.com.

Substantial discounts on bulk quantities of Jones & Bartlett Learning publications are available to corporations, professional associations, and other qualified organizations. For details and specific discount information, contact the special sales department at Jones & Bartlett Learning via the above contact information or send an email to specialsales@jblearning.com.

Copyright © 2016 by Jones & Bartlett Learning, LLC, an Ascend Learning Company and the National Fire Protection Association®.

All rights reserved. No part of the material protected by this copyright may be reproduced or utilized in any form, electronic or mechanical, including photocopying, recording, or by any information storage and retrieval system, without written permission from the copyright owner.

The content, statements, views, and opinions herein are the sole expression of the respective authors and not that of Jones & Bartlett Learning, LLC. Reference herein to any specific commercial product, process, or service by trade name, trademark, manufacturer, or otherwise does not constitute or imply its endorsement or recommendation by Jones & Bartlett Learning, LLC and such reference shall not be used for advertising or product endorsement purposes. All trademarks displayed are the trademarks of the parties noted herein. *Fire Apparatus Driver/Operator: Pump, Aerial, Tiller, and Mobile Water Supply, Second Edition* is an independent publication and has not been authorized, sponsored, or otherwise approved by the owners of the trademarks or service marks referenced in this product.

There may be images in this book that feature models; these models do not necessarily endorse, represent, or participate in the activities represented in the images. Any screenshots in this product are for educational and instructive purposes only. Any individuals and scenarios featured in the case studies throughout this product may be real or fictitious, but are used for instructional purposes only.

The procedures and protocols in this book are based on the most current recommendations of responsible sources. The National Fire Protection Association (NFPA), the International Association of Fire Chiefs (IAFC), and the publisher, however, make no guarantee as to, and assume no responsibility for, the correctness, sufficiency, or completeness of such information or recommendations. Other or additional safety measures may be required under particular circumstances.

05717-1

Production Credits
Chief Executive Officer: Ty Field
President: James Homer
Chief Product Officer: Eduardo Moura
Vice President, Publisher: Kimberly Brophy
Vice President of Sales, Public Safety Group: Matthew Maniscalco
Director of Sales, Public Safety Group: Patricia Einstein
Executive Editor: William Larkin
Senior Acquisitions Editor: Janet Maker
Senior Development Editor: Alison Lozeau
Production Editor: Cindie Bryan
Senior Marketing Manager: Brian Rooney
VP, Manufacturing and Inventory Control: Therese Connell
Composition: Cenveo Publisher Services
Cover Design: Kristin E. Parker
Rights & Media Manager: Joanna Lundeen
Rights & Media Research Coordinator: Ashley Dos Santos
Rights & Media Research Assistant: Robert Boder
Media Development Editor: Shannon Sheehan
Cover Image: © Keith Muratori/ShutterStock, Inc
Printing and Binding: LSC Communications
Cover Printing: LSC Communications

Library of Congress Cataloging-in-Publication Data
Fire apparatus driver/operator : pump, aerial, tiller, and mobile water supply / National Fire Protection Association.—Second edition.
    pages cm
Includes bibliographical references and index.
ISBN 978-1-284-02691-7 (pbk.)
1. Fire extinction—United States—Equipment and supplies. 2. Fire engine driving. 3. Fire pumps. I. National Fire Protection Association.
TH9360.F525 2016
629.28'45—dc23
                        2014033499

6048
Printed in the United States of America
22 21 20 19 18   10 9 8 7 6 5

Brief Contents

CHAPTER 1 Evolution of the Fire Apparatus... 2

CHAPTER 2 Driver Training and Selection ... 16

CHAPTER 3 Types of Fire Apparatus 34

CHAPTER 4 Water 50

CHAPTER 5 The Fire Pump 74

CHAPTER 6 Fire Hose, Appliances, and Nozzles................. 100

CHAPTER 7 Mathematics for the Driver/Operator 118

CHAPTER 8 Performing Fire Apparatus Check-Out and Maintenance... 166

CHAPTER 9 Driving Fire Apparatus 190

CHAPTER 10 Emergency Vehicle Driving 214

CHAPTER 11 Fireground Operations........244

CHAPTER 12 Drafting and Water Shuttle Operations 278

CHAPTER 13 Relay Pump Operations....... 310

CHAPTER 14 Foam 324

CHAPTER 15 Apparatus Equipped with an Aerial Device 354

CHAPTER 16 Driving Apparatus Equipped with a Tiller 398

CHAPTER 17 Operating Apparatus Equipped with a Tiller 420

CHAPTER 18 Testing, Maintaining, and Troubleshooting Aerial and Tiller Apparatus..........432

CHAPTER 19 Performance Testing 464

Appendix A: Daily/Weekly Inspection Check Sheet............................508
Appendix B: An Extract from NFPA 1002, *Standard for Fire Apparatus Driver/Operator Professional Qualifications*, 2014 Edition 512
Appendix C: NFPA 1002 Correlation Guide 516
Appendix D: Pro Board Assessment Methodology Matrices for NFPA 1002 520
Glossary 524
Index.......................................536

Contents

CHAPTER 1 Evolution of the Fire Apparatus 2

Introduction 4
Early Fire Equipment 4
   Fire Protection in Early Cities 5
   Hand Pumps and Hose Carts 5
   Fire Apparatus Evolution 5
   Ladder Wagons Pulled by Horses 6
   Elevated Streams 6
   Gasoline-Powered Fire Apparatus 6
   Adding a Pump 7
   Triple-Combination Pumper 7
   Improvements in Aerial Devices 7
   Other Uses for Motorized Apparatus .. 8
   Diesel-Powered Fire Apparatus 8
Today's Fire Apparatus 8
   Protecting the Driver/Operator at the Scene 11
   Visibility for the Driver/Operator 12
   The Driver/Operator's Role in Safety .. 12
Modern Fire Apparatus 12

CHAPTER 2 Driver Training and Selection 16

Introduction 18
The Many Roles of the Driver/Operator . 18
   Promoting Safety 19
   Educating Crew Members 20
   Trust and Team Building 21
Maintaining a Safe Work Environment .. 21
   Lead by Example 22
Fire Apparatus and Equipment: Functions and Limitations 24
   Fire Apparatus and Equipment Inspections 25
   Safety Across the Board 26
NFPA 1002 Requirements 26
   NFPA 1002: General Requirements of a Driver/Operator 27
   NFPA 1002: Medical and Physical Requirements of a Driver/Operator 28
Driver/Operator Training 28
Driver/Operator Selection 29

CHAPTER 3 Types of Fire Apparatus 34

Introduction 36
Fire Apparatus Requirements 36
   Working with a Manufacturer 36
Fire Department Pumper 37
Initial Attack Fire Apparatus 38
Mobile Water Supply Apparatus 41
Aerial Fire Apparatus 42
Quint Fire Apparatus 44
Special Service Fire Apparatus 44
Mobile Foam Fire Apparatus 46

CHAPTER 4 Water 50

Introduction 52
Chemical Properties of Water 53
   Physical Properties of Water 53
   Harmful Characteristics of Water ... 54
Municipal Water Systems 54
   Water Sources 54
   Water Treatment Facilities 55
   Water Distribution System 55
Fluid Dynamics 56
Fire Hydrants 59
   Dry-Barrel Hydrants 61
   Wet-Barrel Hydrants 61
Operation of Fire Hydrants 61
Shutting Down a Hydrant 62
Locations of Fire Hydrants 62
Inspecting and Maintaining Fire Hydrants 62
Testing Fire Hydrants 66
   Fire Hydrant Testing Procedure 66
Rural Water Supplies 68
   Static Sources of Water 68

CHAPTER 5 The Fire Pump 74

Introduction 76
Exterior of the Fire Department Pumper 76
Interior of the Fire Department Pumper: The Cab 76

Fire Pumps 77
Types of Fire Pumps 79
   Positive-Displacement Pumps 79
   Centrifugal Pump. 81
Fire Pump Anatomy 86
   Pump Intake Connections 86
   Pump Discharge Outlet Connections . 87
The Pump Panel 88
   Master Pump Intake Pressure Gauge . 89
   Master Pump Discharge Gauge. 89
   Pressure Gauges. 89
   Flow Meters. 90
   Engine Tachometer 91
   Engine Coolant Temperature Gauge
      and Engine Cooling Devices 91
   Engine Oil Pressure Gauge. 91
   Voltmeter 92
   Water Tank Level Indicator 92
   Fuel Level Indicator 92
   Primer Control. 92
   Pump Pressure Control Systems. 92
   Pumping Engine Throttle. 93
Power Supplies for Pumps. 94

CHAPTER 6 Fire Hose, Appliances,
and Nozzles 100

Fire Hose, Appliances, and Nozzles
     Overview 102
   Sizes of Hose 102
   Attack Hose 103
   Supply Hose 104
   Fire Hose Appliances 105
   Nozzles 111
   Other Types of Nozzles 114
   Nozzle Maintenance and Inspection. 114

CHAPTER 7 Mathematics for the
Driver/Operator 118

Introduction 121
Pump Discharge Pressure 122
   Nozzle Pressures 122
   Nozzle Reaction. 124
   Determining Nozzle Flow 125

Friction Loss 127
Calculating Friction Loss 127
Multiple Hoselines of Different
    Sizes and Lengths 128
Elevation Pressure 129
Appliance Loss 131
   Determining Friction Loss in
      Appliances. 136
   Total Pressure Loss. 139
Wyed Hoselines 140
   Siamese Hoselines 143
   Calculating Elevated Master Streams . . 145
Standpipe Systems 147
   Pressure-Regulating Valves. 151
   Net Pump Discharge Pressure 155
Fire Service Hydraulic Calculations. . . .156
   Charts 157
   Hydraulic Calculators 158
   Hand Method. 158
Subtract 10 Method (gpm Flowing
    Method) 160
Condensed Q Method 160
   The Condensed Q Method in
      a Relay Operation 161
   Preincident Plan. 161
   Determining Additional Water
      from a Hydrant 161

CHAPTER 8 Performing Fire Apparatus
Check-Out and Maintenance 166

Introduction 168
Inspection 169
Inspection Process 171
Fire Apparatus Sections. 172
   Exterior Inspection 173
   Engine Compartment. 174
   Cab Interior 176
   Brake Inspection 178
   General Tools/Equipment
      Inspection 179
   Pump Inspection 180
   Aerial Device Inspection. 184
Safety 185

Weekly, Monthly, or Other
  Periodic Inspection Items 187
    Completing Forms. 187
    Removing Vehicles from Service. . . . 187

CHAPTER 9 Driving Fire Apparatus 190

Introduction 192
Preparing to Drive. 192
  360-Degree Inspection. 192
  Starting the Apparatus 194
  Seat Belt Safety. 196
  Getting Underway 196
Driving Exercises 200
  Performing a Serpentine Maneuver. . . 200
  Performing a Confined-Space
    Turnaround 201
  Performing a Diminishing Clearance
    Exercise. 203
Returning to the Station 204
  Reversing the Fire Apparatus 205
  Shutting Down the Fire Apparatus. . 207

CHAPTER 10 Emergency Vehicle Driving 214

Introduction 217
Pre-Emergency Vehicle Response 217
  Dispatch 217
  Maps 218
Emergency Vehicle Laws 219
Emergency Vehicle Driving 220
  Level of Response. 220
  Passing Vehicles 220
  Defensive Driving Practices 221
  Maintaining Control on Hills,
    Turns, and Curves. 222
  Night Driving. 223
  Bridges and Overpasses 223
  Intersections 223
  Railroad Crossings 225
Approaching the Scene of
  an Emergency 225
  Slow Down 225
  Identify the Address/Location 225
  Recognize Potential Hazards 226

Fire Scene Positioning 226
  Proper Positioning 226
  Working Fire 227
  Staging. 227
  Engines and Ladders 229
  Positioning of Other Fire Scene
    Apparatus 232
Positioning at an Intersection or on a
  Highway 232
  Never Trust Traffic 233
  Engage in Proper Protective
    Parking 233
  Reduce Motorist Vision Impairment . . 233
  Wear High-Visibility Reflective Vests. . 233
Manual on Uniform Traffic
  Control Devices 234
  Motor Vehicle Accidents. 236
Positioning at the Emergency
  Medical Scene 238
Special Emergency Scene
  Positioning. 238

CHAPTER 11 Fireground Operations 244

Introduction 246
Fire Pump Operations 246
  In-Cab Procedures 246
  Exiting the Cab 248
Internal Water Tank 249
Pressurized Sources. 249
  Supply Line Evolutions 249
  Connecting a Fire Department
    Engine to a Water Supply 252
Securing a Water Source 253
  Hand Lays 254
Standpipe/Sprinkler Connecting 255
  Connecting Supply Hoselines
    to Standpipe and Sprinkler
    Systems. 255
Performing a Changeover 259
Monitor the Fire Pump 261
Operating Other Fixed Systems
  and Equipment 263
  Apparatus-Mounted Equipment. . . . 264

CHAPTER 12 Drafting and Water Shuttle Operations 278

Introduction 280
The Mechanics of Drafting.......... 280
Inspections, Routine Maintenance,
    and Operational Testing 281
    Inspecting the Priming System..... 281
    Performing a Vacuum Test 284
    Finding a Vacuum Leak 284
Water Supply Management in the
    Incident Management System 284
Selecting a Drafting Site 284
    Determining the Reliability of Static
        Water Sources 284
    Estimating the Quantity of Water
        Available 286
    Accessibility of the Static
        Water Source................ 287
    Special Accessibility
        Considerations 287
    Operational Considerations
        for Site Selection 289
Pumping from a Draft.............. 289
    Making the Connection 289
Preparing to Operate at Draft by
    Priming the Pump 291
Drafting Operations 293
Producing the Flow of Water 294
Complications During Drafting
    Operations..................... 294
Uninterrupted Water Supply 297
Water Shuttle 297
    Fill Sites...................... 298
    Filling Tankers................. 301
    Safety for Water Shuttle
        Operations................. 301
Establishing Dump Site Operations .. 302
    Using Portable Tanks 302
    Offloading Tankers.............. 303
    Use of Multiple Portable Tanks..... 303
    Source Pumper Considerations for
        Portable Tank Operations 304
    Traffic Flow Within a Dump Site ... 305

Nurse Tanker Operations........... 306
    Communication for Tanker
        Operations 306
Water Shuttle Operations in the
    Incident Management System 306

CHAPTER 13 Relay Pump Operations 310

Introduction 312
Relay Pumping Operations 312
    Components of a Relay Pumping
        Operation 312
    Equipment for Relay Pumping
        Operations 314
    Personnel for Relay Pumping
        Operations 314
    Preparing for a Relay Pumping
        Operation 314
    Calculating Friction Loss 315
    Relay Pumping Operations........ 316
    Operating the Source Pumper 316
    Operating the Attack Pumper 316
    Operating the Relay Pumper 317
    Water Relay Delivery Options 319
    Joining an Existing Relay
        Pumping Operation........... 319
    Pressure Fluctuations in a
        Relay Pumping Operation 320
    Shutting Down a Relay Pumping
        Operation 320
    Safety for Relay Pumping
        Operations 321

CHAPTER 14 Foam........................324

Introduction 326
History........................... 326
Overview......................... 327
    What Is Foam?................. 327
    Foam Tetrahedron 328
    Foam Characteristics 328
Foam Classifications 329
    Class A Foams 329
    Class B Foams 330
    Synthetic Foams................ 331

Alcohol-Resistant Aqueous
  Film-Forming Foams. 332
Synthetic Detergent Foams
  (High-Expansion Foams). 332
Foam Concentrates. 333
Foam Expansion Rates. 333
  Low-Expansion Foam 334
  Medium-Expansion Foam 334
  High-Expansion Foam 334
Foam Proportioning 334
  Proportioning Foam Concentrate. . . 334
  Foam Proportioning Systems 334
  Around-the-Pump Proportioning System 337
  Balanced-Pressure Proportioning
    Systems. 340
  Injection Systems. 340
  Compressed-Air Foam System 341
Nozzles 342
  Medium- and High-Expansion Foam
    Generators. 342
  Master Stream Foam Nozzles 345
  Air-Aspirating Foam Nozzles 345
  Smooth-Bore Nozzles. 345
  Fog Nozzles 345
Foam Supplies 345
Foam Application 345
  Applying Foam 345
Foam Compatibility 349

CHAPTER 15 Apparatus Equipped with an Aerial Device 354

Introduction 356
History of Aerial Apparatus 356
Tactical Priorities 356
  Rescue 357
  Aerial Deployment Priorities 357
Aerial Apparatus Types and Features . 358
  Three Main Types of Aerial
    Devices 358
Aerial Ladder Construction 359
  Aerial Ladders and Platforms 359
  Hydraulic and Electrical Systems . . . 359
  Stabilizers (Jacks, Outriggers,
    and Downriggers) 360
  Aerial Reach. 362
Inspection of Aerial Apparatus 363
Aerial Apparatus Positioning. 363
  Residential Structures. 363
  Commercial/Industrial Structures. . . 364
  Positioning and Spotting
    Considerations 364
  Building Type and Height. 365
  Approach to the Scene 366
  Collapse Zone 366
  Turntable Positioning for Rescue
    Sweep/Scrub Area 366
  Rescue Profile. 367
  Making Up for Poor Placement 367
Setup and Stabilization of
  Aerial Apparatus 367
  In-Cab Procedures 367
  Setting Stabilizers. 368
  Compensating for Uneven
    Grades. 370
Operation of Aerial Ladder or
  Platform Controls. 371
Safe Aerial Practices. 372
  Operation in Supported Versus
    Unsupported Positions 372
  Load Placed on the Aerial. 373
  Improper Aerial Operations 375
  Personal Protective Equipment
    Needed 375
  Fall Protection 375
  Climbing or Riding a Moving
    Aerial Ladder. 377
  Allow Space for Deflection. 378
  Maneuvering Aerial Device 378
Using the Aerial to Effect a Rescue . . . 378
  Tip Positioning. 380
  Rescue Priorities. 381
Ventilation Positioning. 382
  Horizontal Ventilation via
    Windows. 382
Elevated Streams 384
  Elevated Stream Positioning. 384

Operating Under Adverse
  Environmental Conditions 384
Stream Types 385
Water Supply 386
Stream Application 386
Exposure Protection 387
Other Considerations 388
Use of the Aerial to Deploy an
  Elevated Stream 388
Use of the Aerial Device's
  Emergency Power or Operations
  Feature 388
Key Points for the Driver/Operator . . . 390
Skill Building 390
Positioning and Setup 390
Stabilizing the Apparatus 390
Operation of Aerial Controls 390
Maneuver to Multiple
  Windows/Targets 391
Maneuver to the Roof 391
Flow Water into a Training Tower . . 391
Combining Multiple Skills 391
An Example of Skills in Action 391

CHAPTER 16 Driving Apparatus Equipped With a Tiller 398

Introduction 400
Safe Driving 400
En Route 401
Turning at Intersections 401
Communications 401
Vehicle Control 403
Traveling Forward 403
Procedures for Negotiating
  Intersections 404
Backing Up 404
Braking 405
Night Driving 405
Principles of Tiller Operation 406
Manufacturer Limitations 406
Maneuvering in Adverse Weather . . . 406
Responsibilities 406
New Driver/Operators 407

Practical Driving Exercises 407
Alley Dock 407
Serpentine Course 407
Confined-Space Turnaround 407
Diminishing Clearance 409
Straight-Line Drive 409
Lane Change 410
Straight-In Parking 410
Crossover Backing 412
The Learning Curve 412
When the Alarm Sounds 413
Approaching the Incident 413
Maneuvering and Positioning a
  Tiller Apparatus 414
Benefit of the Aerial Ladder 414
Tactics May Determine the
  Placement 415
Conditions Are Never Ideal 415

CHAPTER 17 Operating Apparatus Equipped With a Tiller 420

Introduction 422
Safety Tips Before Aerial Deployment 422
Positioning the Tiller 422
Transferring Power 422
Stabilization Requirements 422
Raise, Rotate, Extend, and More 423
Raising the Aerial 423
Placing the Aerial 424
Climbing the Aerial 424
Ladder in Place 425
Aerial Ladder Supporting Weight . . . 425
Using the Aerial in a Defensive
  Strategy 427
Operating the Aerial Under
  Adverse Conditions 428
Lowering the Aerial 428
Aerial Rescue Strategies and
  Tactics 428
Positioning the Aerial for Rescue . . . 428
Shift Change 429
Aerial Ladder Testing 429
Summary 429

CHAPTER 18 Testing, Maintaining, and Troubleshooting Aerial and Tiller Apparatus 432

Visual Inspection 434
   The 360-Degree Walk-Around 434
Operational and Equipment Checklists..................... 435
   Aerial Device Hydraulic Fluid 435
   Stabilizer Systems 436
   Extension Retraction and Hoist Cables 436
   The Turntable and Its Components . 437
   Turntable Control Pedestal........ 438
Ladder Components and Classifications 440
   Ladder Sections 440
   Lift Cylinders................... 440
   Rotation Controls............... 441
   Waterway and Associated Plumbing. 441
   The Hydroelectric Swivel 441
   The Ladder Section 442
   Platform Controls............... 442
Tiller Trucks...................... 442
   The Tillerman 442
Aerial Device Operations........... 443
   Placement and Foundation 443
   Cab and Predeployment Procedures. 444
   Outrigger Types and Deployment... 444
   Fast Idle Control 445
   Deploying the Outriggers......... 446
   Outrigger Safety Devices 446
Operating the Aerial Device......... 447
   Aerial Device Working Height 447
   Angles of Operation............. 447
   Load Charts 448
Raising the Device 448
   Rotation...................... 449
   Extension and Retraction......... 449
Discharging Water and Waterway Safeties 450
Cradling Up and Going Home 451
   Storing Outriggers 452
Apparatus Testing................. 452

Magnetic Particle Testing........... 455
Acoustic Testing 455
   Ultrasonic Testing 455
   Dye Penetrant Testing 455
   Additional Testing 455
   Testing of Structural Components .. 456
   Testing Throttle Controls and Communication Systems........ 457
   Stabilizer Inspections and Tests 457
   Stability and Load Test........... 457
   Time Trial Test 458
   Water System Inspection and Test .. 458
Troubleshooting Aerial Problems During Tests and Checkouts...... 458
   Visual Cues to Alert the Driver/Operator to Problems.... 458

CHAPTER 19 Performance Testing.............464

Introduction 467
Performance Testing............... 467
   Weight Verification Test 467
   Road Test..................... 468
Testing Low-Voltage Electrical Systems 468
   Batteries...................... 468
   Starter System 469
   Charging System 470
   Regulator Test 470
   Battery Charger/Conditioner Test... 471
Total Continuous Electrical Load Test ..471
   Solenoid and Relay Test 471
   Foam Proportioning Systems 471
   Performance Testing of Compressed-Air Foam Systems .. 473
   Performance Testing of Line Voltage Electrical Systems 474
   Performance Testing of Breathing-Air Compressor Systems 475
Fire Apparatus Requirements 476
   Environmental Requirements...... 476
   Test Site 477
   Equipment Requirements......... 478
No-Load Governed Engine Speed Test 480

Intake Relief Valve System Test........481
Pump Shift Indicator Test.............481
Pump Engine Control Interlock Test .. 482
Gauge and Flow Meter Test.......... 483
Tank-to-Pump Flow Test............. 488
Vacuum Test 488
Priming System Test.................491
Pumping Test Requirements 491
Pump Performance Test..............491
    Capacity Test/150 psi (1000 kPa)
       Test (100 Percent Test) 497
    Overload Test/165 psi (1150 kPa)
       Test 497
    200 psi (1350 kPa) Test (70 Percent
       Test) 499
    250 psi (1700 kPa) Test (50 Percent
       Test) 499

Pressure Control Test............... 500
Post Performance Testing 501
    Final Test Results................ 501
    Problem Solving................. 503
Rerating Fire Pumps................ 504

Appendix A: Daily/Weekly Inspection Check Sheet ... 508
Appendix B: An Extract from NFPA 1002,
    Standard for Fire Apparatus Driver/Operator
    Professional Qualifications, 2014 Edition 512
Appendix C: NFPA 1002 Correlation Guide 516
Appendix D: Pro Board Assessment Methodology
    Matrices for NFPA 1002 520
Glossary 524
Index 536

Skill Drills

CHAPTER 4	Water
Skill Drill 4-1	Operating a Fire Hydrant 63
Skill Drill 4-2	Shutting Down a Hydrant............64
Skill Drill 4-3	Obtaining the Static Pressure 67
Skill Drill 4-4	Operating a Pitot Gauge 69

CHAPTER 6	Fire Hose, Appliances, and Nozzles
Skill Drill 6-1	Connecting a Coupling for a Soft Sleeve Hose from a Hydrant to a Pump 106
Skill Drill 6-2	Inspecting a Solid-Stream Nozzle.....113
Skill Drill 6-3	Inspecting a Fog-Stream Nozzle 115

CHAPTER 7	Mathematics for the Driver/Operator
Skill Drill 7-1	Calculating the Nozzle Reaction from a Smooth-Bore Nozzle 124
Skill Drill 7-2	Calculating the Nozzle Reaction from a Fog Nozzle..................124
Skill Drill 7-3	[Standard] Calculating the Flow of a 1¼-Inch Smooth-Bore Nozzle on a 2½-Inch Handline..................126
Skill Drill 7-3	[Metric] Calculating the Flow of a 32-mm Smooth-Bore Nozzle on a 65-mm Handline 126
Skill Drill 7-4	[Standard] Calculating Friction Loss in a Single Hoseline....................130
Skill Drill 7-4	[Metric] Calculating Friction Loss in a Single Hoseline....................131
Skill Drill 7-5	[Standard] Calculating Friction Loss in Multiple Hoselines of Different Sizes and Lengths..................132
Skill Drill 7-5	[Metric] Calculating Friction Loss in Multiple Hoselines of Different Sizes and Lengths..................133
Skill Drill 7-6	[Standard] Calculating the Elevation Pressure (Loss and Gain)...........134
Skill Drill 7-6	[Metric] Calculating the Elevation Pressure (Loss and Gain)...........134
Skill Drill 7-7	Determining the Friction Loss in Appliances 137
Skill Drill 7-8	Using a Pitot Gauge 138
Skill Drill 7-9	Using In-Line Gauges to Test Friction Loss 139
Skill Drill 7-10	[Standard] Determining the Pump Discharge Pressure in a Wye Scenario with Equal Lines 140
Skill Drill 7-10	[Metric] Determining the Pump Discharge Pressure in a Wye Scenario with Equal Lines 141
Skill Drill 7-11	[Standard] Determining the Pump Discharge Pressure in a Wye Scenario with Unequal Lines................142
Skill Drill 7-11	[Metric] Determining the Pump Discharge Pressure in a Wye Scenario with Unequal Lines................143
Skill Drill 7-12	[Standard] Determining the Pump Pressure for a Siamese Line by the Split Flow Method 144
Skill Drill 7-12	[Metric] Determining the Pump Pressure for a Siamese Line by the Split Flow Method 144
Skill Drill 7-13	[Standard] Calculating Friction Loss in Siamese Lines by the Coefficient Method 145
Skill Drill 7-13	[Metric] Calculating Friction Loss in Siamese Lines by the Coefficient Method 145
Skill Drill 7-14	[Standard] Calculating Friction Loss in Siamese Lines by the Percentage Method 146
Skill Drill 7-14	[Metric] Calculating Friction Loss in Siamese Lines by the Percentage Method 147
Skill Drill 7-15	[Standard] Calculating the Pump Discharge Pressure for a Prepiped Elevated Master Stream Device 150
Skill Drill 7-15	[Metric] Calculating the Pump Discharge Pressure for a Prepiped Elevated Master Stream Device 151
Skill Drill 7-16	[Standard] Calculating the Pump Discharge Pressure for an Elevated Master Stream 152
Skill Drill 7-17	[Standard] Calculating the Discharge Pressure for a Standpipe During Preplanning......................152
Skill Drill 7-16	[Metric] Calculating the Pump Discharge Pressure for an Elevated Master Stream . 153
Skill Drill 7-17	[Metric] Calculating the Discharge Pressure for a Standpipe During Preplanning 153
Skill Drill 7-18	[Standard] Calculating Pump Discharge Pressure for a Standpipe ...154
Skill Drill 7-18	[Metric] Calculating Pump Discharge Pressure for a Standpipe 155

Skill Drill 7-21	Performing the Hand Method Calculation . 159
Skill Drill 7-22	Performing the Hand Method Calculation for 2½-Inch Hose 159
Skill Drill 7-23	Using the Hand Method Calculation for 1¾-Inch Hose...........159
Skill Drill 7-24	Using the Subtract 10 Method (gpm Flowing Method)...........160

CHAPTER 8 — Performing Fire Apparatus Check-Out and Maintenance

Skill Drill 8-1	Performing an Apparatus Inspection ..186

CHAPTER 9 — Driving Fire Apparatus

Skill Drill 9-1	Performing a 360-Degree Inspection ..193
Skill Drill 9-2	Starting a Fire Apparatus...........198
Skill Drill 9-3	Performing the Serpentine Exercise ...201
Skill Drill 9-4	Performing a Confined-Space Turnaround .202
Skill Drill 9-5	Performing a Diminishing Clearance Exercise........................204
Skill Drill 9-6	Backing a Fire Apparatus into a Fire Station Bay 208
Skill Drill 9-7	Shutting Down and Securing a Fire Apparatus 210

CHAPTER 10 — Emergency Vehicle Driving

Skill Drill 10-2	Performing the Alley Dock Exercise .. 239

CHAPTER 11 — Fireground Operations

Skill Drill 11-1	Engaging the Fire Pump with an Automatic Transmission 250
Skill Drill 11-2	Hand Laying a Supply Line 257
Skill Drill 11-3	Connecting Hose to a Fire Department Connection............ 260
Skill Drill 11-4	Performing a Changeover Operation .. 262
Skill Drill 11-6	Disengaging the Fire Pump with an Automatic Transmission 264
Skill Drill 11-7	Engaging the PTO Generator 267
Skill Drill 11-8	Disengaging the PTO Generator 268
Skill Drill 11-9	Engaging the PTO-Driven Hydraulic System 273
Skill Drill 11-10	Disengaging the PTO-Driven Hydraulic System 274

CHAPTER 12 — Drafting and Water Shuttle Operations

Skill Drill 12-1	Performing an Annual Vacuum Test .. 285
Skill Drill 12-2	Positioning the Fire Apparatus for Drafting Operations 292
Skill Drill 12-3	Drafting from a Static Water Source .. 295
Skill Drill 12-4	Providing Water Flow for Handlines and Master Streams................ 296

CHAPTER 14 — Foam

Skill Drill 14-1	Batch Mixing Foam................. 335
Skill Drill 14-2	Operating an In-Line Eductor 338
Skill Drill 14-3	Operating an Around-the-Pump Proportioning System 339
Skill Drill 14-6	Operating a Compressed-Air Foam System........................ 343
Skill Drill 14-7	Applying Class A Foam on a Fire 347
Skill Drill 14-8	Applying Foam with the Roll-On Method 348
Skill Drill 14-9	Applying Foam with the Bankdown Method (FF2) 349
Skill Drill 14-10	Applying Foam with the Raindown Method 350

CHAPTER 15 — Apparatus Equipped with an Aerial Device

Skill Drill 15-1	Positioning and Stabilizing an Apparatus on a Level Surface..... 369
Skill Drill 15-2	Compensating for Uneven Grades ... 371
Skill Drill 15-3	Maneuvering the Aerial Device...... 379
Skill Drill 15-5	Using the Aerial Device for Ventilation . 383
Skill Drill 15-6	Using the Aerial Device to Deploy an Elevated Stream 389

CHAPTER 19 — Performance Testing

Skill Drill 19-4	Conducting the No-Load Governed Engine Speed Test 481
Skill Drill 19-5	Performing the Pump Shift Indicator Test 483
Skill Drill 19-6	Performing the Pump Engine Control Interlock Test............... 484
Skill Drill 19-7	Performing a Gauge Test 486
Skill Drill 19-8	Performing a Flow Meter Test 487
Skill Drill 19-9	Testing the Tank-to-Pump Rate 489
Skill Drill 19-10	Performing a Vacuum Test.......... 490
Skill Drill 19-11	Performing a Priming System Test ... 492
Skill Drill 19-12	Performing a Capacity Test [150 psi (1000 kPa) Test] 498
Skill Drill 19-16	Performing a Pressure Control Test... 502

Acknowledgments

Jones & Bartlett Learning, the National Fire Protection Association, and the International Association of Fire Chiefs would like to thank all the authors, contributors, and reviewers of *Fire Apparatus Driver/Operator: Pump, Aerial, Tiller, and Mobile Water Supply, Second Edition*.

Contributing Authors

Alan Conkle
Al Conkle's Fire Tech Support
Millbury, Ohio

Paul Dow
Battalion Commander, Albuquerque Fire Department
Albuquerque, New Mexico

Jimmy Faulkner
Dallas Fire Rescue, Dallas Fire Department
Dallas, Texas

Al Hom
San Francisco Fire Department
San Francisco, California

Tim McIntyre
Fire Fighter Specialist, Los Angeles County Fire Department
Los Angeles, California

Drew Smith
Deputy Chief, Prospect Heights Fire Protection District
Prospect Heights, Illinois

Contributors and Reviewers

Tim Baker
Lansing Community College
Lansing, Michigan

Robert M. Barron
TEEX & Prairie View Fire Department
College Station, Texas

Doug Bolthouse
Department of Public Safety, Standards & Training
Salem, Oregon

W. Parker Browne
Fire Protection Specialist
Akron, Ohio

Dr. Harry R. Carter
Howell Township Board of Fire Commissioner's Fire District #2
Adelphia, New Jersey

Steven Colburn
New Hampshire Fire Academy
Concord, New Hampshire

Aaron Dean
Sacramento Fire Department
Sacramento, California

Christopher Drake
Muskegon Fire Department
Muskegon, Michigan

Brent S. Elliott
Green Bay Metro Fire Department
Green Bay, Wisconsin

Bret Gervasoni
San José Fire Department
San José, California

Bryan Goustos
Brampton Fire and Emergency Services
Brampton, Ontario, Canada

James A. Graves
Maine Fire Service Institute
Brunswick, Maine

Robert Matthew Hinkle
Mississippi State Fire Academy
Jackson, Mississippi

Mark S. Huetter, Jr.
Kennedy Space Center/NASA
Kennedy Space Center, Florida

Shawn Kelley
International Association of Fire Chiefs
Fairfax, Virginia

Dave LaFountain
Waterville-Winslow Fire Department
Waterville, Maine

Ron Lindroth
Central Valley Fire District
Belgrade, Montana

Victor Loesche III
San José Fire Department
San José, California

Acknowledgments

Tom McGowan
Public Fire Protection Division, National Fire Protection Association
Quincy, Massachusetts

James Mendoza
San José Fire Department
San José, California

Mario Minoia
San José Fire Department
San José, California

Andrew J. Murtagh
San Francisco Fire Department
San Francisco, California

Mark Romer
California State Fire Marshal's Office, Training Division
Sacramento, California

Don Tryon
Los Angeles County Fire Department
Los Angeles, California

Eric Uitts
New Hampshire Fire Academy
Concord, New Hampshire

John West
Department of Public Safety, Standards & Training
Salem, Oregon

Photographic Contributors

We would like to extend a huge *thank you* to Glen E. Ellman, the photographer for this project. Glen is a commercial photographer and fire fighter based in Forth Worth, Texas. His expertise and professionalism are unmatched!

We would like to thank Alan Conkle, Paul Dow, Jimmy Faulkner, Al Hom, Tim McIntyre, and Drew Smith, who provided many of the photographs that are new to this edition.

We would also like to thank the following departments that opened up their facilities for these photo shoots:

Burleson Fire Department, Burleson, Texas
Gary A. Wisdom—Fire Chief
Tom E. Foster—Battalion Chief
Mike Jones—Lieutenant
Shane Mobley—Fire Fighter
Casey Davis—Fire Fighter
Shelby Stone—Fire Fighter
Juliet Knight—Fire Fighter
Rob Moore—Fire Fighter
Jake Hopps—Fire Fighter

Crowly Fire Department, Crowley, Texas
Robert Loftin—Fire Chief
Larry Swartz—Division Chief
Christopher Young—Lieutenant
Scott Calhoun—Driver/Operator
Bud Hardin—Fire Fighter

Fort Worth Fire Department, Fort Worth, Texas
Rudy Jackson—Fire Chief
Homer Robertson—Captain, Apparatus Officer
Frank Becerra—Fire Fighter
Larry Manasco—Captain

A special thanks to the Training Facility, Maintenance Shop, and Stations #1, #2, #5, #10, and #26.

Granbury Volunteer Fire Department, Granbury, Texas
Darrell Grober—Fire Chief
Kurt Brown—Fire Fighter

Houston Fire Department, Houston, Texas
Terry Garrison—Fire Chief
Kevin J. Alexander, Jr.—Assistant Fire Chief
Josef Gregory—District Chief
Charles Ortiz—Captain
Jason Noland
Brandon Knepprath
Dwayne Wyble
Gerard Taylor
Michael Dixon
Danielle Van Berschot Wilson
Humberto Trevino

Evolution of the Fire Apparatus

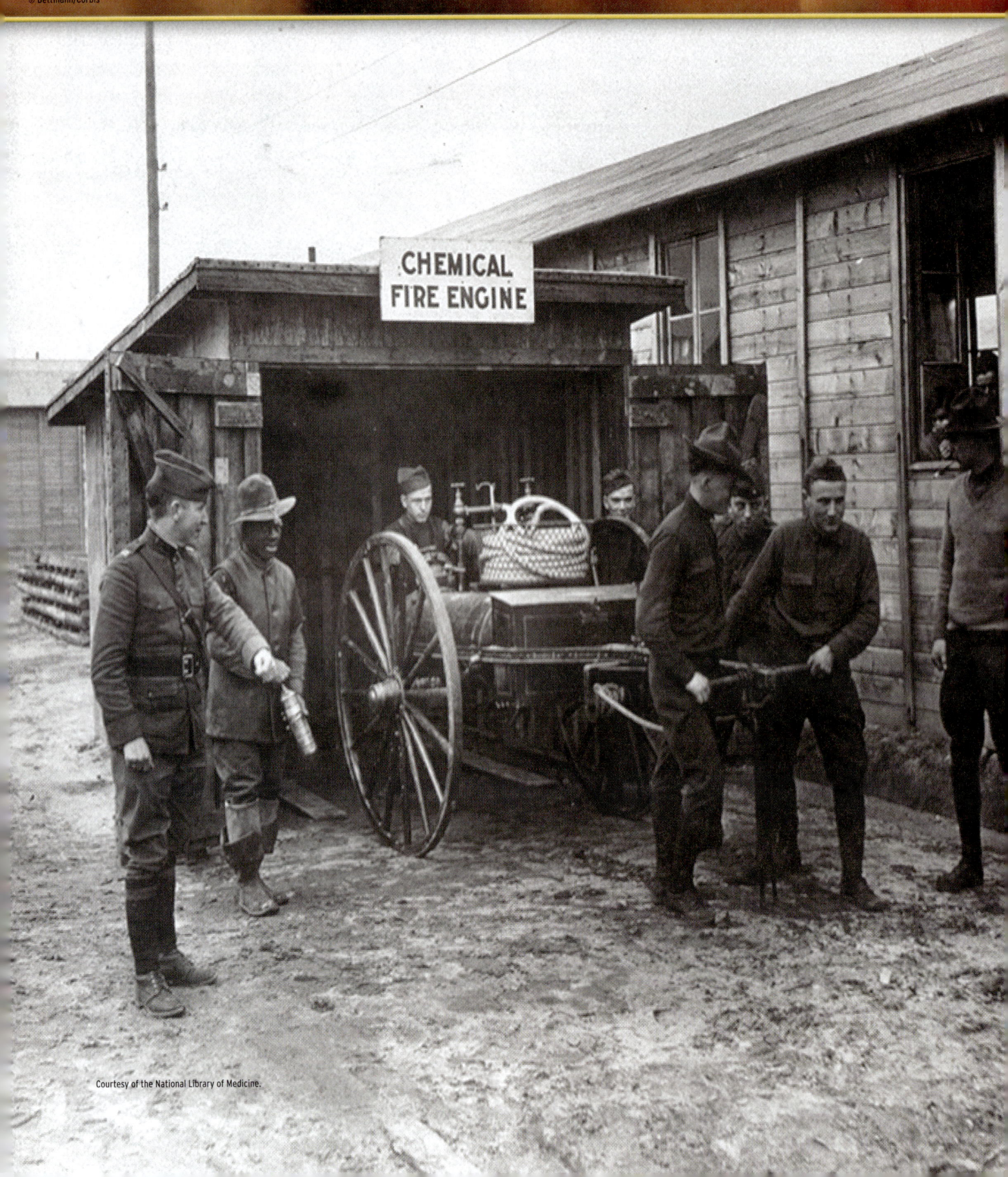

CHAPTER 1

Knowledge Objectives

After studying this chapter, you will be able to:
- Describe how the fire service has progressed from the colonial period to the present day. (p 4–13)
- Describe the major changes in transport equipment and personnel from the colonial period to the present day. (p 4–13)
- Identify the role of the driver/operator in the safe operation of fire apparatus. (NFPA 1002, 4.1, 5.1 ; p 8–13)

Skills Objectives

There are no skill objectives for driver/operator candidates. NFPA 1002 contains no driver/operator Job Performance Requirements for this chapter.

Additional NFPA Standards

- NFPA 1500, *Standard on Fire Department Occupational Safety and Health Program*
- NFPA 1901, *Standards for Automotive Fire Apparatus*

You Are the Driver/Operator

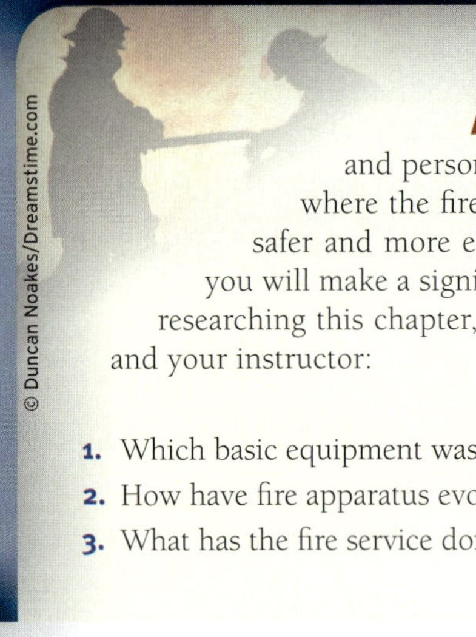

As a driver/operator candidate, it is important for you to understand the history of the position for which you are training. The fire apparatus that you will drive is very different from the type of equipment that was once used to transport tools, equipment, and personnel to fires. Understanding the equipment that was used in the past will help you appreciate where the fire service has been and where it will go in the future. Fire apparatus will continue to become safer and more efficient throughout your career in the fire service. Perhaps during the course of that career, you will make a significant contribution to the fire service by improving the safe operation of fire apparatus. While researching this chapter, you come up with the following questions to discuss with the other members of your class and your instructor:

1. Which basic equipment was used to fight fires in early cities?
2. How have fire apparatus evolved over the years?
3. What has the fire service done to make it safer to operate fire apparatus?

Introduction

The fire apparatus and equipment in use today have evolved over a number of centuries as new inventions have emerged and been adapted to the needs of the fire service. In this chapter we cover this progression from the early colonial days of the fire service, when firefighting equipment was limited to a few simple tools, to the present day, when apparatus feature advanced firefighting equipment and technologies. It is important for new drivers to understand that the apparatus they are now trained to operate has changed in ways intended to make fire fighters more efficient and to provide a higher level of safety to fire service members. Without these innovations, we would not be capable of protecting the public with the incredible firefighting force that the fire service has established.

Early Fire Equipment

Colonial-era fire fighters had only buckets, ladders, and fire hooks at their disposal. Because early settlements featured buildings with thatch roofs and wooden chimneys, firefighting with these limited tools posed a serious challenge. Fire protection was limited to the use of water relays with leather buckets passed from person to person, a system called a **bucket brigade** **FIGURE 1-1**. These buckets were made from leather, which was either secured by rivets or sewn together. In many communities, residents were required to place a bucket filled with water on their front steps at night in case of a fire in the community. Any fire would require all residents to help stop the progress of the fire and save the settlement. Water would be dipped from a well and passed from one person to another until the bucket reached the fire. A second line would return the bucket to the water supply. Compared to today's fire suppression capabilities, this method of firefighting seems archaic and time consuming.

Some towns also required that ladders be available so that fire fighters could access the roof to extinguish small fires. If all else failed, the **fire hook** would be used to pull down a burning building and prevent the fire from spreading to nearby

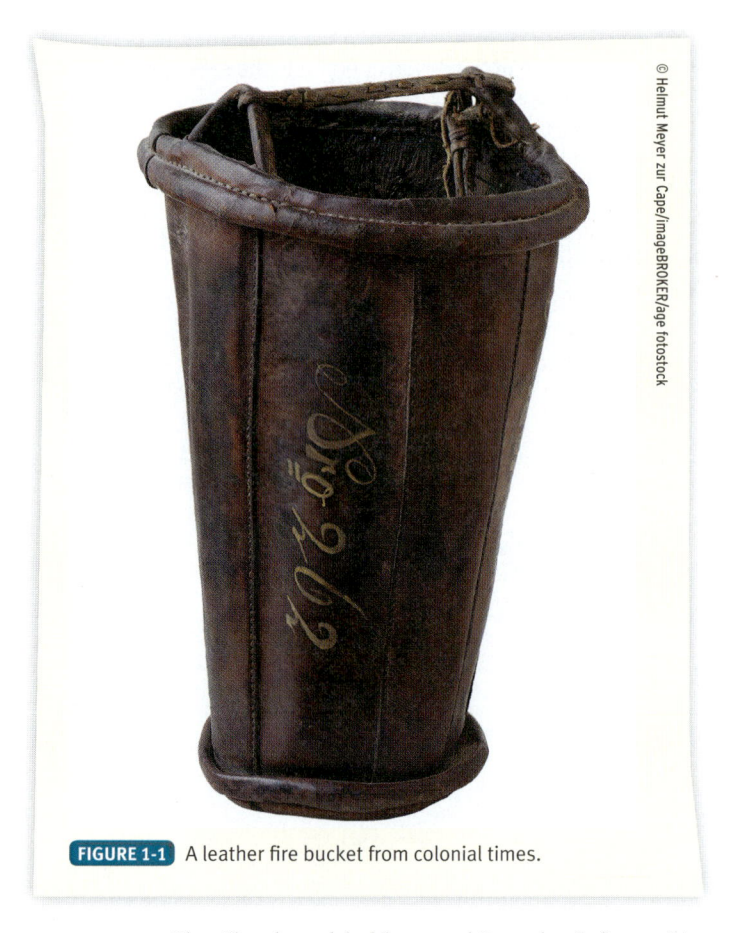

FIGURE 1-1 A leather fire bucket from colonial times.

structures. The "hook-and-ladder truck" evolved from this early equipment.

DRIVER/OPERATOR Tip

Buckets made of leather could not hold water for any length of time, so in some parts of the country, fire buckets were filled with sand. After the sand was thrown on the fire, the bucket would be refilled with water and used in a bucket brigade.

Fire Protection in Early Cities

In the early years, many cities employed watchmen to walk the streets at night looking for fires. If a fire was spotted, the watchman would run through the streets with a rattle device alerting residents to turn out and help fight the fire—thus the term "rattle watch." In some cities, a drum was used to notify fire companies of a fire. In Cincinnati, Ohio, the beating of the drum was a duty of the night watchman.

Eventually, fire companies were formed in early American towns, and small storage buildings were erected to store one or more ladders specifically for firefighting. The first organized companies would have one or two straight ladders, a few leather buckets, a selection of axes, and a small selection of hand tools.

Hand Pumps and Hose Carts

The evolution of firefighting tools was heavily influenced by fire suppression teams in Europe, which had developed hand-operated pumping devices. The first equipment to replace the bucket brigade was the hand pump. In 1720, Richard Newsham developed the first such pumper in London. Several strong men powered the pump, making it possible to propel a steady stream of water from a safe distance.

In the early 1800s, the city of Philadelphia developed a municipal water supply using wooden water mains that could be tapped for firefighting. To get the water from the fire plugs (early hydrants), fire fighters used hose made from strips of leather held together with rivets. To access water, the fire fighters would drill into the main water pipes, access the water spilling out of the leak, and then plug the leak in the pipe when the fire was suppressed. The leather hose was stored on hose carts that had a large reel. Often these hose cart wheels were ornately decorated to reflect the name of the fire company **FIGURE 1-2**.

The couplings for the fire plugs were made by local blacksmiths. Each community had its own coupling threads based on the capabilities of the local blacksmith. The Great Baltimore Fire in 1904 resulted in the development of standardizing coupling threads after mutual aid forces supplied by Philadelphia, New York City, and other locales were stymied when their equipment could not hook up to the local Baltimore hydrants.

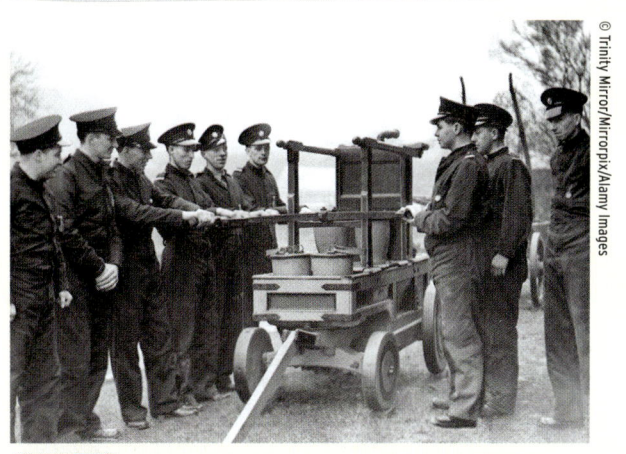

FIGURE 1-3 Larger-capacity hand pumps required more personnel to operate them.

DRIVER/OPERATOR Tip

Many communities today maintain a unique thread size for their fire hydrants. As the driver/operator, you should be familiar with any adapters that will allow you to connect to hydrants outside your normal response area.

Hand pumps were a type of piston-driven, positive-displacement pump that was pushed up and down by fire fighters manning poles at the side of the pump. Over time, these hand pumps became larger to accommodate the new, more plentiful water supplies available in municipal areas; thus they were placed on wagon wheels to allow them to be more easily transported to the fireground. The larger-capacity hand pumps also required more personnel to operate **FIGURE 1-3**; in fact, some required six to eight fire fighters to operate the pump. Many of these units maintained a fixed straight-stream nozzle, while others used a leather hose with a long pipe nozzle that was held by a crew of fire fighters.

Fire Apparatus Evolution

With the advent of the steam-powered pumps called steamers in the mid-1800s, horses replaced fire fighters in moving equipment to the fireground **FIGURE 1-4**. The first mechanized fire pumps were generally fueled by coal. A coal fire in the fire box of the steamer would be ignited, thereby creating the steam used to power the pump. Drivers of the horses, called teamsters, were hired with their horses to stay at the firehouse and transport the steamer to the fireground. While en route to the scene, a fire fighter stoked the fire in the fire box, leading to production of the needed steam pressure. One steam pumper could deliver the same volume of water as six or more hand pumpers with eight or more fire fighters working each pump handle in 15- to 20-minute shifts. The term "engineer" was used to identify the fire fighter charged with operating the steam engine. This task required knowledge of hydraulics, pressure regulators, and use of a unique source of energy to propel a pump.

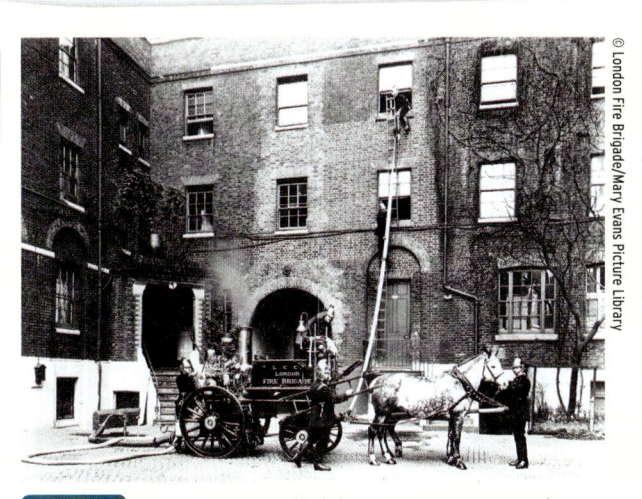

FIGURE 1-2 Horses once supplied the energy to transport the crew to the scene.

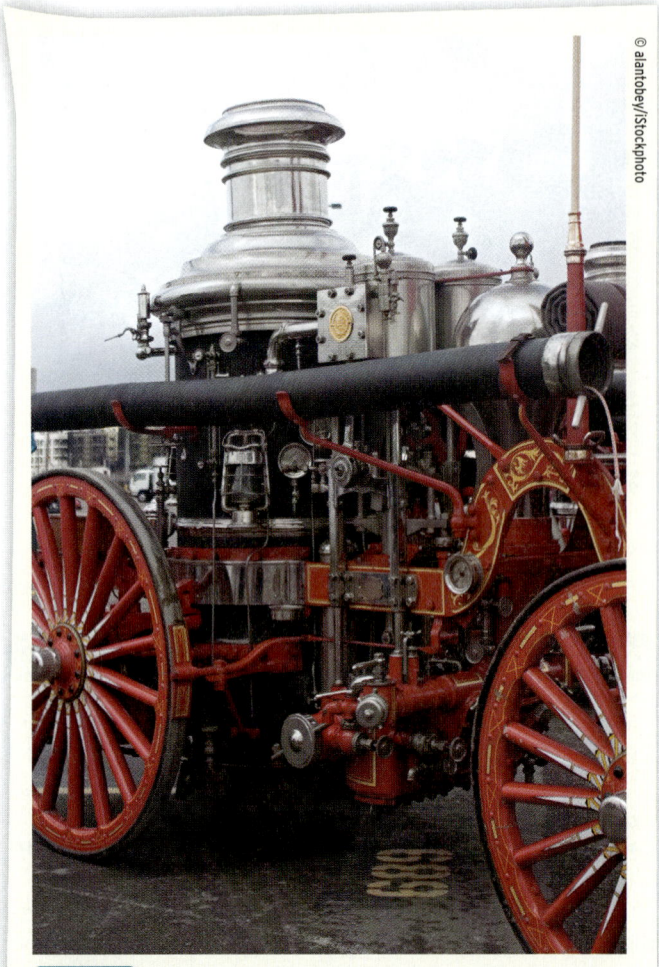

FIGURE 1-4 With the advent of the steam-powered pumps (called steamers) in the mid-1800s, horses replaced fire fighters in moving equipment to the fireground.

DRIVER/OPERATOR Tip

In early firefighting companies, a lot of excitement was generated in the streets by the sights and sounds of the horses racing through the streets, bells clanging, smoke from the steamer stack, and teamsters snapping whips. The Dalmatian dog became a friend of the teamster and fixture of the fire station. The Dalmatian had a good temperament around horses, was a good companion, and was effective in racing ahead of the belching and noisy steamer, thereby helping to clear the streets of errant animals—and people—blocking the path of the fire wagon.

■ Ladder Wagons Pulled by Horses

Wagons loaded with ladders and fire hooks were once drawn by horses and driven by teamsters **FIGURE 1-5**. Ladders were constructed with strong materials. As extension ladders were developed, wooden aerial ladders were built to serve fire fighters. These ladders were operated by hand and carried to the scene by horse-drawn cart. The wooden aerial ladder used cranks to rotate the ladder on a turntable and had a large wheel to raise, extend, or retract the wooden aerial ladder. Improvements to the wooden aerial ladder included heavy springs that caused the ladder to spring from its resting position **FIGURE 1-6**. Fire fighters would be positioned at the raising wheels when the release was pulled and used the momentum created by the compressed springs to raise the wooden aerial ladder. When the ladder was lowered, fire fighters would compress the springs so that the aerial portion of the ladder was locked in place. As the lengths of the ladders increased even further, a steering wheel was placed on the rear axle so that a tiller person could help maneuver the long ladders through the streets.

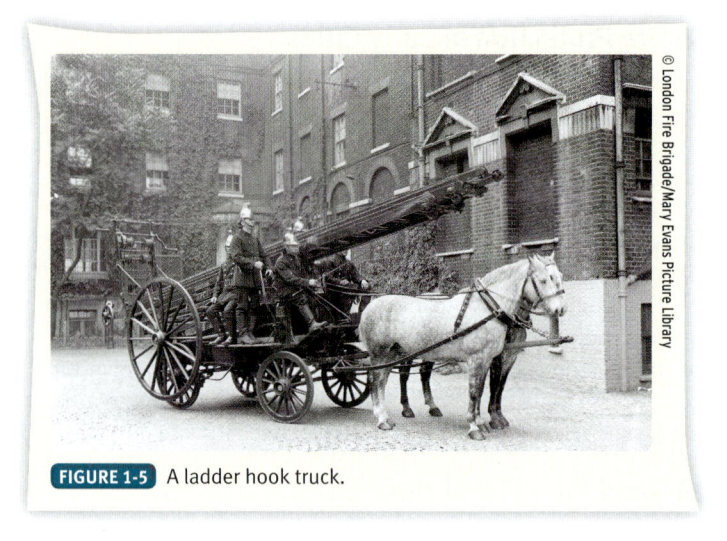

FIGURE 1-5 A ladder hook truck.

■ Elevated Streams

The first elevated streams were water towers mounted on wagons and pulled by horses. When raised, these elevated streams could raise 30 ft (9 m) in the air. Devices evolved when pipes were attached to ladders to provide elevated water streams.

■ Gasoline-Powered Fire Apparatus

The first gasoline-powered fire apparatus emerged around 1900 **FIGURE 1-7**. These units were initially small cars used by

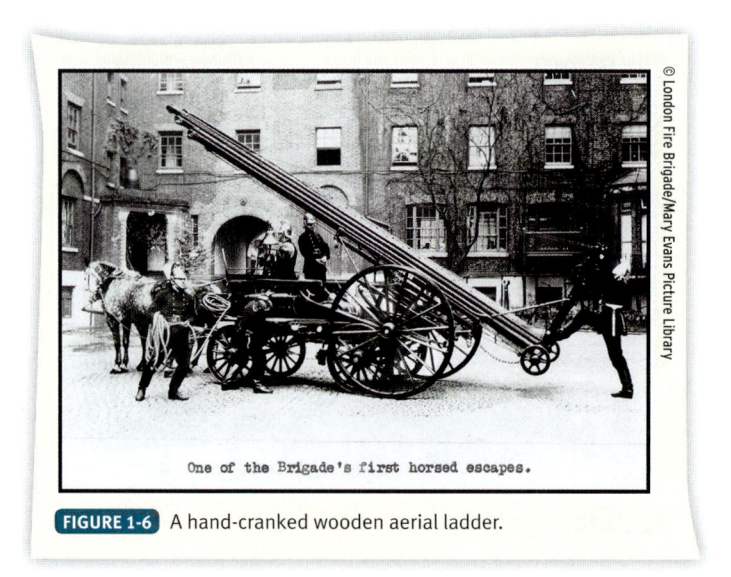

FIGURE 1-6 A hand-cranked wooden aerial ladder.

Courtesy of the National Library of Medicine

FIGURE 1-7 The first gasoline-powered fire apparatus emerged around 1900.

Courtesy of Phillip S. "Sean" Barrett

FIGURE 1-8 A booster pump.

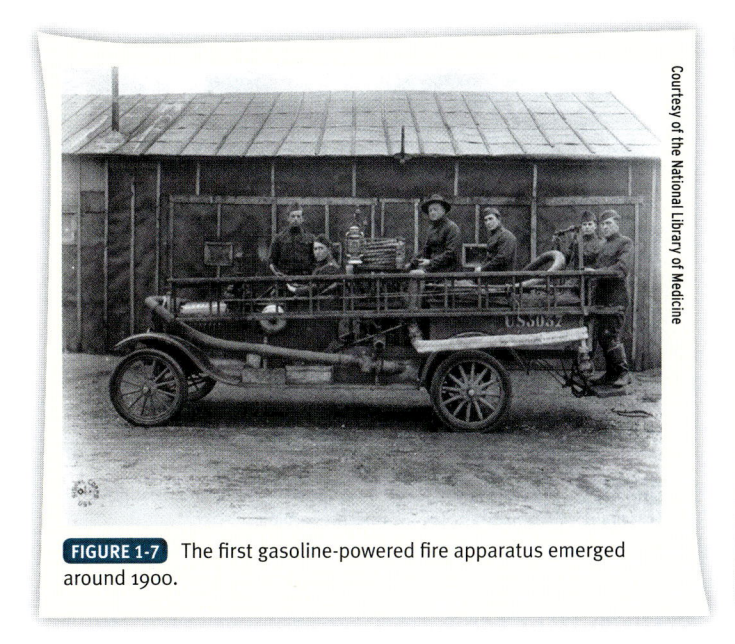

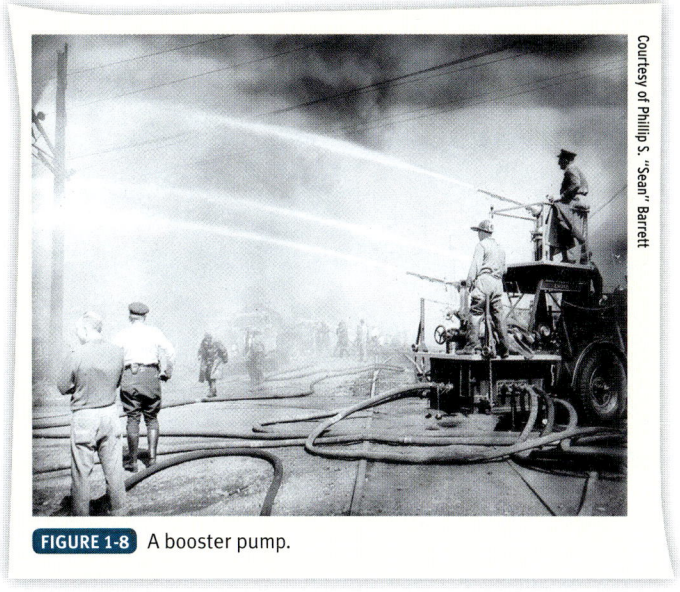

chief officers to drive to the fireground. The next gasoline-powered unit to evolve within the fire service was the ladder wagon, in which the front axle and horses were replaced by a single-axle tractor used to propel and steer the fire apparatus.

The first gasoline-powered fire apparatus to discharge water was a unit called a **chemical wagon**. This small truck carried a large soda acid extinguisher and 50 ft (15 m) or more of small hose (booster line size). It also carried a supply of double-jacked cotton hose, a short ladder, and a running board on which the fire fighters would ride. Small fires were extinguished with the soda acid device, while larger fires used the hose connected directly to the hydrant.

© London Fire Brigade/Mary Evans Picture Library/Age Fotostock

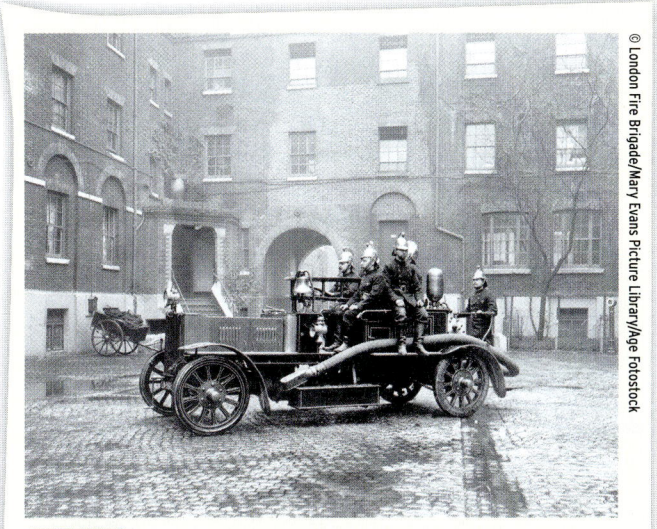

FIGURE 1-9 A major breakthrough for today's modern fire apparatus came in the early 1900s when the triple-combination pumper was introduced.

DRIVER/OPERATOR Tip

In 1911, the Savannah, Georgia, fire department became one of the first fully motorized departments.

Adding a Pump

As trucks became larger and stronger, a small pump, called a **booster pump**, was added; a small hoseline, called a **booster line**, was attached to this pump FIGURE 1-8. Many of these booster pumps were rotary gear pumps and could generate as much as 200 gallons (800 L) of water per minute. Because they could not deliver as much water as a fire hydrant, they were used mainly for small fires and to supply the booster line with water.

Triple-Combination Pumper

The real breakthrough for today's modern fire apparatus came in 1906, when the **triple-combination pumper** was introduced FIGURE 1-9. This truck carried water in a tank generally used for the booster line and commonly called the booster tank. The triple-combination pumper also had a pump capacity of 250 gallons per minute (gpm) (1000 L/min) or greater. Additionally 2½-inch (65-mm) hose was carried for water supply purposes, as well as firefighting hose, commonly 1½ inches (38 mm) in diameter. A driver/operator and a fire officer rode in the cab, and others members of the company rode on the tailboard.

Improvements in Aerial Devices

With the gasoline-powered engine, a power supply was now available to turn a hydraulic pump. Hydraulic pressure could be used to perform the tasks of lifting, rotating, and extending the aerial device. This development allowed the aerial ladders to be made of steel, reach farther, and carry greater loads—and today's modern ladder truck was born FIGURE 1-10. In the new devices, ladder fly and bed pipes were added to improve elevated streams. With the stronger metal ladders, larger-caliber nozzles could be used to flow more water onto the fire.

FIGURE 1-10 An example of a modern aerial device in action.

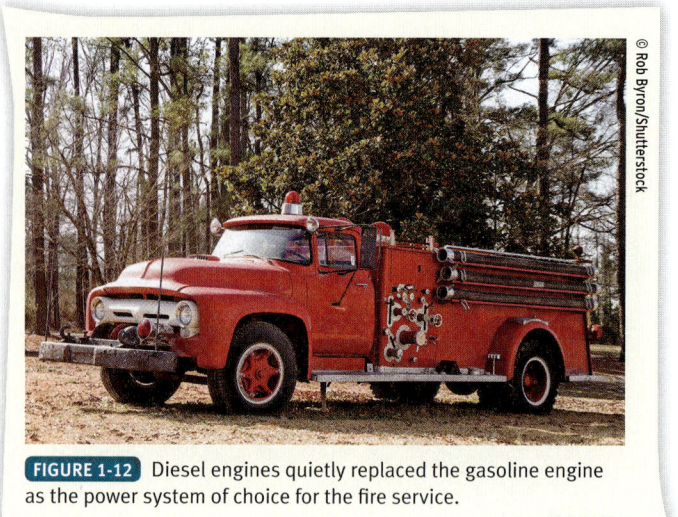

FIGURE 1-12 Diesel engines quietly replaced the gasoline engine as the power system of choice for the fire service.

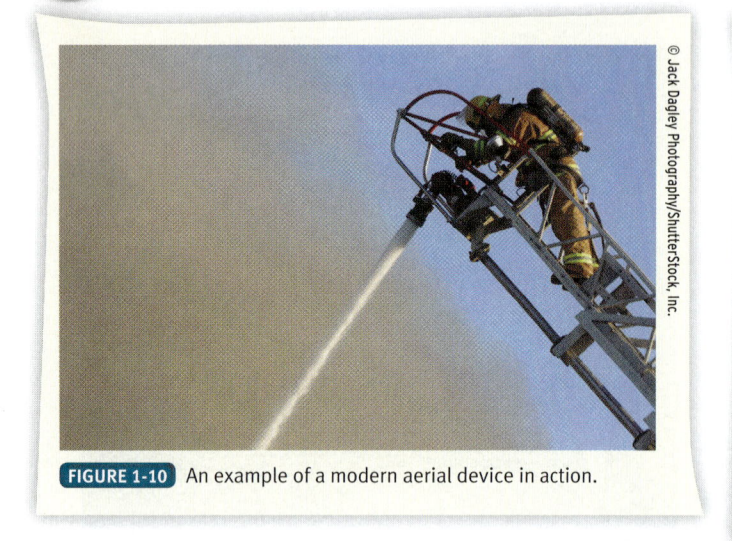

Later additional aerial devices were developed that included articulated booms and ladder towers **FIGURE 1-11**. The articulated booms provided greater flexibility in operating in areas filled with electrical wires and other obstructions. The ladder tower provided a solid platform at the end of a boom. It gave fire fighters a platform to work from, a device to use for rescue that eliminated the need for the victims to navigate down a ladder, and a platform to provide water tower equipment.

■ Other Uses for Motorized Apparatus

The gasoline engine eventually became the sole power source used to drive fire apparatus. At the same time, additional uses for apparatus emerged. A wide variety of specialty units were developed, such as salvage companies; heavy rescue squads began to use large enclosed vehicles to carry their tools and personnel hose tenders, which had the capacity to carry more hose than a standard apparatus. Air supply units carrying cascade units and compressors became available at the fireground as well.

■ Diesel-Powered Fire Apparatus

With the development of larger-capacity pumps that required greater horsepower and torque, larger vehicles carrying more equipment, and greater loads to carry, the diesel engine started to replace the gasoline engine. At the same time that greater horsepower was needed, gasoline engines were being equipped with emissions-reduction equipment that reduced their horsepower and torque. Diesel engines were more reliable, burned fuel more efficiently, and provided the desired horsepower and torque. Over time, diesel engines quietly replaced the gasoline engine as the power system of choice for the fire service **FIGURE 1-12**.

Today's Fire Apparatus

The fire apparatus being used by many fire departments today is larger, heavier, taller (with a higher center of gravity), and generally more difficult to maneuver through traffic than the devices used by earlier-era fire fighters. Growing concerns for fire fighter safety during the progression of fire apparatus resulted in the adoption of standard National Fire Protection Association (NFPA) 1500, *Standard on Fire Department Occupational Safety and Health Program* and NFPA 1901, *Standards for Automotive Fire Apparatus*. NFPA 1500 required that new fire apparatus be designed so that all members riding on the fire apparatus would be provided a seated area inside an enclosed cab. Adoption of this standard has resulted in the near elimination of rear steps on fire apparatus. Now apparatus includes large enclosed cabs, which ensure that each fire fighter can be

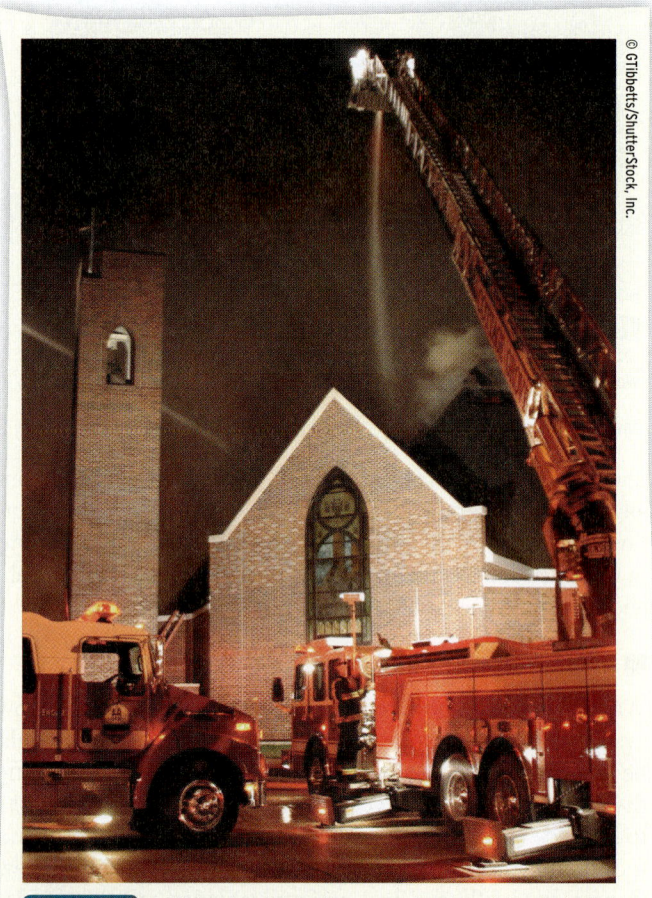

FIGURE 1-11 Additional aerial devices were developed that included articulated booms and ladder towers.

VOICES
OF EXPERIENCE

The word "SAFETY" is consistently reinforced in every fire department throughout our nation. From the East Coast to the West, whether departments are career, combination, or volunteer, it's the tie that binds us together. As a fire service instructor and company officer with more than 26 years of experience, I have encountered numerous situations where safety was only verbalized. Accomplishing an objective doesn't necessarily account for safe operations. It is important that all fire fighters understand this concept.

Three general components to safety can be instituted at any incident and must be known to accomplish specific tasks in a safe manner.

1. Take your physical fitness seriously. The number one cause of death in the fire service is stress. Being fit will assist you in performing the tasks of your job safely. Your life and the safety of those around you depend on your physical fitness.
2. Learn, know, and understand your job. Your actions throughout your career will depend on you acquiring and maintaining a working knowledge of the job. Your safety and the safety of your crew depend upon your skill set.
3. Always maintain situational awareness. In stressful situations, it is common to acquire tunnel vision. Be aware of your situation and the actions of those around you—it could save your life.

Every driver/operator is responsible for his or her own safety first. Utilizing the three components of "SAFETY" has enhanced not only my own safety, but also the safety of my crews and my students. Understanding how to operate safely is the key to your success and longevity as a driver/operator. Remember these components to "SAFETY" during your journey.

Dave Winkler
El Camino Fire Academy
Inglewood, California

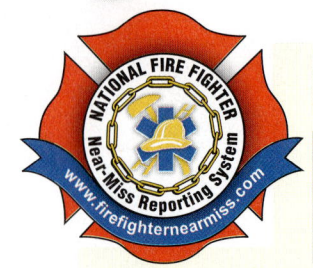

Near-Miss REPORT

Report Number: 06-0000486

Synopsis: Fire fighter falls from open cab at 50 mph (80 km/h).

Event Description: I fell from the rear cab area of a moving pumper. We were responding from a standby detail to a vehicle collision. The staffing included a driver, chief officer, and me; the only one in the open cab area. It was on a hot July Sunday morning. I was wearing only my leather helmet (unfastened), and three-quarter length boots, rolled down. I did not have my running coat on. Attempting to free a jammed restraining bar, I leaned out of the open area just as the vehicle entered into a curve. I then lost my balance and fell onto the curb side of the street. The pumper was traveling at approximately 50 mph (80 km/h). I struck the ground head-first, then slid face-down for 30 ft (9 m), stopped only by a steel post. I sustained a basal skull fracture and various facial fractures resulting in a partial hearing loss and neurological damage.

Lessons Learned: I learned to be seated and belted in a moving apparatus at all times. Full gear on a moving vehicle is a must, regardless of the weather. If I have problems with the equipment on the apparatus, I must inform the driver immediately. An SOP for use of protective gear while riding on vehicles is essential. So is an attitude adjustment among all personnel when on a call—be alert at all times!

---

seated and wear a seat belt. NFPA 1901 required that fire apparatus manufacturers install seat belt warning devices that verify that a fire fighter is seated and belted.

Additionally, fire apparatus specifications have been developed to provide a safe riding area in case of a fire apparatus rollover. The following apparatus features assist in making the apparatus safer while driving:

- **Auxiliary brakes.** The increased weight of modern fire apparatus makes it more difficult to safely and efficiently stop the vehicle. Auxiliary braking systems have been incorporated into apparatus design to supplement the service brakes. Engine brakes, also known as compression brakes, open valves in the cylinders of diesel engines to divert compression from the cylinders to create drag that slows the vehicle. Transmission retarders divert transmission fluid through a retarder chamber, which causes resistance to be applied to the driveline with the energy dissipated through heat transfer to the vehicle's cooling system. Exhaust brakes restrict exhaust flow from the engine; the compression held in the engine limits the movement of the piston and, in turn, the crankshaft, thereby slowing the vehicle. The excess compression is forced through the exhaust brake, which absorbs the energy. Driveline retarders essentially use an electrical current to create a magnetic force that slows the rotation of a driveshaft or axle. Regardless of which system is used, it is imperative that the driver/operator understands the correct operation and limitations of the system.
- **Anti-lock braking systems (ABS).** ABS uses sensors mounted on each wheel to control brake application in the event of a sudden or emergency stop. The brake application applies the correct amount of brake to each wheel to prevent the wheels from locking up and placing the vehicle in a skid, which would take steering control away from the driver/operator.
- **Automatic traction control (ATC).** ATC operates in conjunction with the vehicle's ABS system using the same wheel speed sensors and brake application devices. The ATC system detects situations in which the vehicle may enter into a skid and applies precise amounts of braking to help the vehicle maintain traction in slippery road conditions, thereby allowing the driver/operator to maintain steering control of the vehicle.
- **Cab design and crashworthiness testing.** Many manufacturers have taken steps to develop safer cab designs to protect fire fighters in the event of rollover collisions. Most fire apparatus manufacturers utilize crash testing to ensure the crashworthiness of their designs. It should be noted that while commercial and custom cabs are both subjected to rollover crash testing, only custom cabs are subjected to frontal impact testing.
- **Supplemental restraint systems.** Many custom fire apparatus manufacturers offer cabs outfitted with supplemental restraint systems for some or all riding positions, including front air bags, side air bags, and curtains. This equipment is usually combined with seat belt pretension devices and suspension seat pull-down devices. Such protective devices can reduce injury during a rollover as long as the occupants are seated and belted.

- **Lateral acceleration alert device.** Both mechanical and electronic devices are available to measure the lateral acceleration of a vehicle. Although these devices will not prevent a rollover, they can be used effectively as a driver training tool to indicate when the vehicle is approaching the rollover threshold and as a reminder to the driver that excessive lateral acceleration can lead to a rollover event.
- **Electronic stability control (ESC).** These systems are designed to assist the driver/operator with the safe operation of the apparatus by maintaining the straight orientation of the vehicle in an effort to prevent rollover collisions. Steering wheel positioning sensors, lateral positioning sensors, and accelerometers work in conjunction with the ABS system to determine when the vehicle is approaching a rollover threshold and then take action by depowering the engine and apply the appropriate amount of braking.
- <u>**Vehicle data recorders (VDRs).**</u> NFPA 1901 now requires manufacturers to equip apparatus with recording systems that monitor all aspects of the performance and operation of the apparatus. These systems are helpful in reconstructing the events of apparatus collisions and may be extremely helpful in proving that the driver/operator was operating the apparatus safely in the event of a collision. VDRs record information such as vehicle speed, acceleration and deceleration data, engine speed, throttle position, transmission status, braking system status, seats occupied and seat belt status, the use of audible and visual warning devices, as well as time and date **TABLE 1-1**. VDR data is controlled data, and the driver/operator and crew do not typically have access.

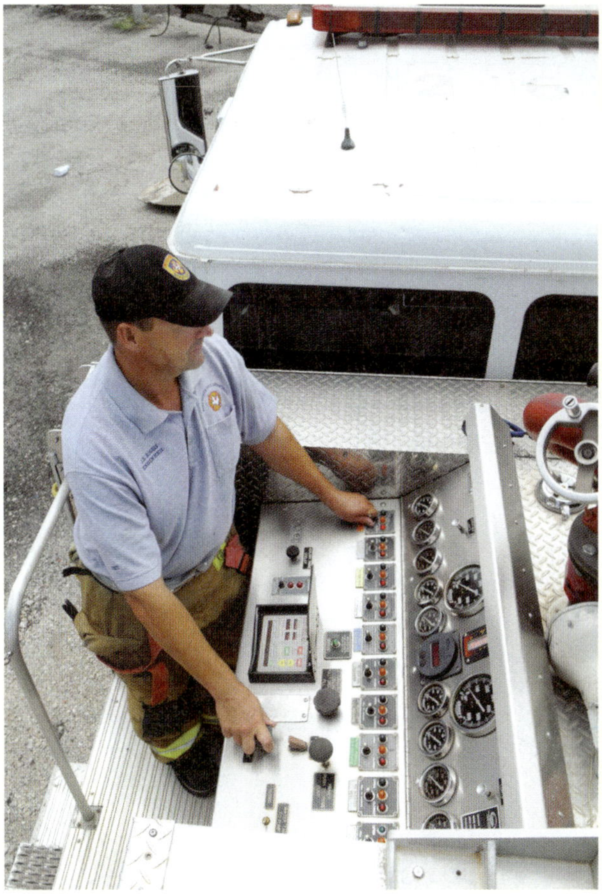

FIGURE 1-13 Top-mounted panels provide a better vantage point for viewing the entire scene.

Protecting the Driver/Operator at the Scene

Because the driver/operator of the fire apparatus is likely to be operating in the vicinity of moving traffic, efforts must be taken to guard against collisions and other traffic-related incidents. Driver/operators must wear all appropriate personal protective clothing, including the use of reflective safety vests at all times while operating on roadways. Apparatus should be positioned to provide a safe work area that shelters the crews from traffic. Additionally, cones and warning signs should be placed, not only to warn drivers of the incident, but to create traffic control zones. Care should be taken to make certain that apparatus emergency lighting is used correctly. Driver/operators should refer to the U.S. Department of Transportation, Federal Highway Administration's *Manual on Uniform Traffic Control Devices (MUTCD)* for more information.

Some fire apparatus have been designed with top-mounted pump panels that provide a better vantage point for viewing the entire scene **FIGURE 1-13**. These panels also remove fire fighters from the street. Fire apparatus have also been built with pump panels on the fire officer's side (curb side) or at the rear of the fire apparatus.

Additionally, if the fire pump is to be used, the apparatus should be positioned to protect the pump panel and driver/operator from oncoming traffic. Additional apparatus may be required to position in such a manner that creates a safe work zone in the event that the initial apparatus must be positioned to protect the pump panel. Many of today's firefighting vehicles are equipped with traffic directional arrows. Many apparatus warning light packages include rear-facing amber lights that are intended to capture the attention of drivers at a distance,

TABLE 1-1	Vehicle Data Recorder Data
Data	**Unit of Measure**
Vehicle speed	mph (km/h)
Acceleration (from speedometer)	mph (km/h)/sec
Deceleration (from speedometer)	mph (km/h)/sec
Engine speed	rpm
Engine throttle position	% of full throttle
Antilock braking system event	On/off
Seat occupied status	Occupied: yes/no by position
Seat belt status	Buckled: yes/no by position
Master optical warning device switch	On/off
Time	24-hour clock
Date	Year/month/day

FIGURE 1-14 Spotters assist in the backing up of fire apparatus.

FIGURE 1-15 The second leading cause of fire fighter fatalities is injuries sustained while responding or returning from a call.

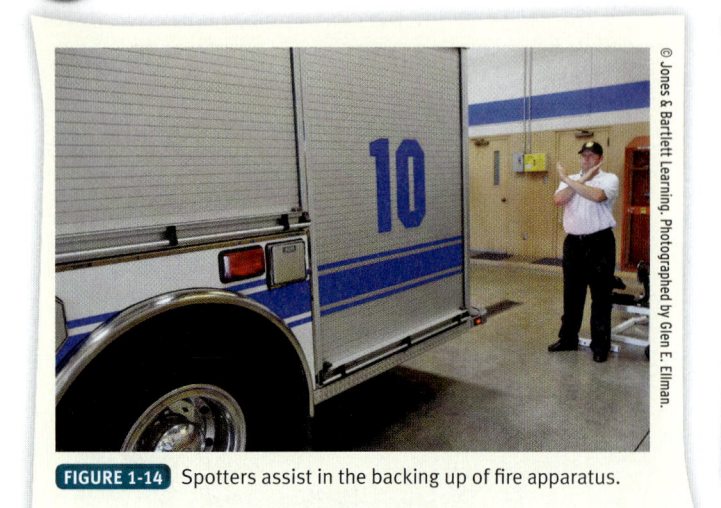

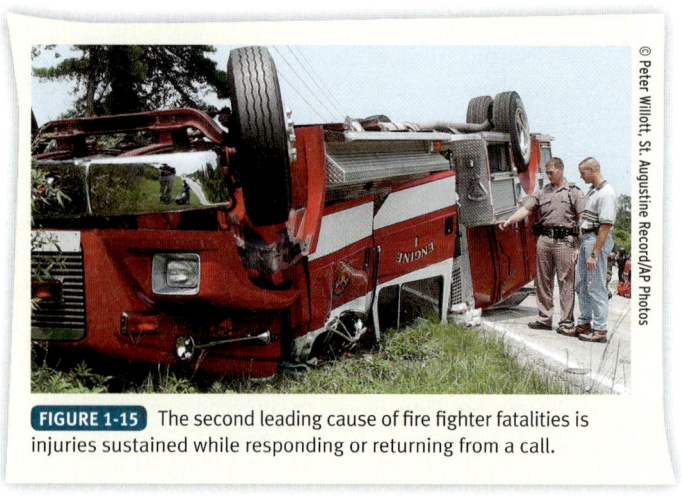

and there is an increased use of rear-facing blue lights for similar reasons. NFPA 1901 requires warning light systems to include two modes: (1) a mode that makes the apparatus visible to other drivers in order for them to yield the right-of-way to the responding apparatus, and (2) a mode for use on the emergency scene that makes the apparatus visible while on scene, especially while blocking at roadway incidents. The blocking mode shuts off all forward-facing white lights and may shed additional warning lights on the sides and rear of the apparatus once the vehicle's parking brake is set.

■ Visibility for the Driver/Operator

Fire apparatus are designed with larger windshields to provide greater visibility and with heated mirrors to prevent icing or frosting. Many are also equipped with cameras mounted on the rear of the fire apparatus so that you can view the back of the fire apparatus and reverse it more safely.

Unfortunately, fire fighter injuries and fatalities have occurred during the reversal of fire apparatus—both at fire stations and on the fireground. For this reason, many fire departments have established policies of using spotters before the fire apparatus backs up **FIGURE 1-14**. Fire apparatus are also equipped with alarms to warn persons behind the fire apparatus that the vehicle is in reverse and may be backing up. Even when such an alarm is present, the driver/operator must be cautious when backing up: Some people, such as small children, may not recognize the sound or heed the warning.

■ The Driver/Operator's Role in Safety

The second leading cause of fire fighter fatalities is injuries sustained while responding or returning from a call **FIGURE 1-15**. According to the U.S. Fire Administration (USFA), 17 fire fighters died while responding to or returning from a call in 2012.

As the driver of the fire apparatus, you are a critical factor in ensuring a safe response. You are responsible for operating the vehicle in a safe manner and driving in a defensive manner to ensure both a safe arrival at the scene and a safe return to the fire station. A critical component of this effort is the proper maintenance of the fire apparatus, which will be discussed later in this text.

While the design and features of the vehicle are important to safe driving, the most important aspect of crash prevention is the skill and experience of the driver/operator. The driver/operator's attitude, training, experience, and qualifications, and the application of those qualities, are the most important elements in crash prevention. The driver/operator must ensure that the physical limits of the vehicle are not exceeded. Driver skill is developed only through training and practice. Every fire department should develop, train members on, and enforce standard operating procedures (SOP) regarding how the fire apparatus should be driven and operated. Such SOPs should include how to follow at traffic control devices (traffic lights and stop signs), how fast the vehicle should be operated, and other safe operational procedures. Of particular importance is the process of proceeding safely through traffic control devices—such locations are where a significant number of accidents occur.

As the operator of the fire apparatus, you play a critical role in ensuring the safety of the fire fighters operating at the incident scene. Fire fighters advancing a hoseline depend on the constant flow of water at an adequate pressure not only to control the fire, but also to provide a safe retreat if needed. The sudden loss of water or pressure could result in serious injury or even death. The incorrect positioning of an aerial device adjacent to electrical power lines could result in fire fighters being electrocuted. A ladder placed at an improper angle could result in structural failure and collapse.

Modern Fire Apparatus

As noted earlier, the fire apparatus being used by many fire departments today has increased in size and weight and is generally more difficult to maneuver through traffic than the devices used by earlier-era fire fighters. Additionally, traffic continues to increase, cars are better insulated and often have stereos blaring, and drivers are generally less patient and often distracted by devices such as cell phones. Collectively, these trends present an ever-increasing challenge for the driver/operator who seeks to maneuver the fire apparatus safely through traffic.

In addition, the capacities of fire apparatus continue to increase. Fire pumps are capable of higher discharge rates, and on-board water tank capacities have also increased in many suburban and rural areas. This increased water capacity, along with enclosed cabs and other vehicle features, makes the fire apparatus heavier, larger, and more challenging to drive.

Finally, the computer age has made its way into the fire apparatus. Today's fire apparatus have computer systems to prevent the vehicle from skidding (antilock brake systems), electrical load management systems to make sure the electrical demand does not exceed the ability of the fire apparatus to produce electricity, and computer systems that monitor the engine's performance. In addition, some vehicles are able to provide monitoring information on the fire apparatus' speed and engine performance (rpm) to the fire officer's monitor.

Wrap-Up

Chief Concepts

- Early fire suppression efforts relied on buckets filled with water thrown at the fire. With buildings constructed of wood and roofs of thatch, fire was a constant threat in the colonial era.
- Formal fire protection efforts began with the adoption of response equipment such as a hand-operated pumper, a reel of hose, and a ladder.
- Fire protection has continued to improve and enhance its level of sophistication based on the improvement of fire apparatus and equipment. The key to its success is the person who will drive the fire apparatus and operate the fire apparatus at the fire incident scene.

Hot Terms

articulated booms An aerial device consisting of two or more folding boom sections whose extension and retraction modes are accomplished by adjusting the angle of the knuckle joints.

booster line A rigid hose that is ¾ inches (20 mm) or 1 inches (25 mm) in diameter. Such a hose delivers water at a rate of only 30 to 60 gpm (115 to 225 L), but can do so at high pressures.

booster pump A water pump mounted on the fire apparatus in addition to a fire pump and used for firefighting either in conjunction with or independent of the fire pump.

bucket brigade An early effort at fire protection that used leather buckets filled with water to combat fires. In many communities, residents were required to place a bucket filled with water, typically on their front steps, at night in case of a fire in the community.

chemical wagon A small truck constructed with a large soda acid extinguisher and 50 ft (15 m) or more of small hose (booster line size).

driver/operator A person having satisfactorily completed the requirements of driver/operator as specified in NFPA 1002, *Standard for Fire Apparatus Driver/Operator Professional Qualifications*.

fire hook A tool used to pull down burning structures.

fire plug A valve installed to control water accessed from wooden pipes.

fire pump A water pump with a rated capacity of 250 gpm (1000 L/min) or greater at 150 psi (1050 kPa) net pump pressure that is mounted on a fire apparatus and used for firefighting.

hand pump A piston-driven, positive-displacement pump that is pushed up and down by fire fighters manning poles at the side of the pump.

ladder tower An aerial ladder with a work platform permanently attached to the end of the ladder.

triple-combination pumper A truck that carries water in a tank generally used for the booster line and commonly called the booster tank.

vehicle data recorder (VDR) An apparatus-mounted recording system that notes what the fire apparatus was actually doing prior to a collision.

References

National Fire Protection Association (NFPA) 1002, *Standard for Fire Apparatus Driver/Operator Professional Qualifications*. 2014. http://www.nfpa.org/codes-and-standards/document-information-pages?mode=code&code=1002. Accessed March 27, 2014.

National Fire Protection Association (NFPA) 1500, *Standard on Fire Department Occupational Safety and Health Program*. 2013. http://www.nfpa.org/catalog/product.asp?pid=150013. Accessed March 27, 2014.

National Fire Protection Association (NFPA) 1901, *Standards for Automotive Fire Apparatus*. 2009. http://www.nfpa.org/codes-and-standards/document-information-pages?mode=code&code=1901. Accessed March 27, 2014.

U.S. Department of Transportation, Federal Highway Administration. *Manual on Uniform Traffic Control Devices (MUTCD)*. 2009 Edition with revision numbers 1 and 2 incorporated, May 2012. http://mutcd.fhwa.dot.gov/pdfs/2009r1r2/mutcd2009r1r2edition.pdf. Accessed February 12, 2015

U.S. Fire Administration. *Firefighter Fatalities in the United States in 2012*. FEMA, August 2013.

DRIVER/OPERATOR
in action

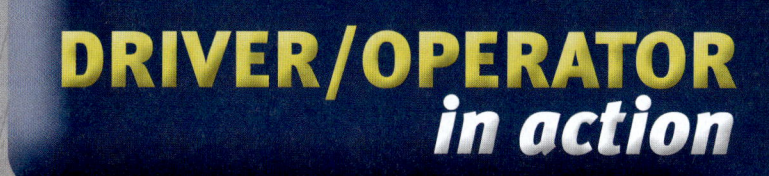

While reviewing this chapter, you have compiled a list of questions that you will ask the members of your station to test their knowledge on the evolution of fire apparatus and driver safety. Here are some of the questions that you compiled:

1. In the mid-1800s, _____ replaced fire fighters in moving equipment to the fireground.
   A. Diesel apparatus
   B. Horses
   C. Gasoline apparatus
   D. Electric vehicles

2. What was the name of the first gasoline-powered fire apparatus used to discharge water?
   A. Chemical wagon
   B. Steamer
   C. Chemical truck
   D. Steam wagon

3. NFPA _____ requires that new fire apparatus be designed with an enclosed cab so that all fire fighters can safely ride inside.
   A. 1901
   B. 1500
   C. 1002
   D. Both A and B

4. A vehicle data recorder (VDR) can store all of the following information except
   A. Vehicle speed.
   B. Seat belt status.
   C. Location of the vehicle.
   D. Engine speed.

5. What are the most important elements of the driver in preventing crashes?
   A. Attitude
   B. Training
   C. Experience
   D. All of the above

Driver Training and Selection

CHAPTER 2

Knowledge Objectives

After studying this chapter, you will be able to:

- Describe the role that the driver/operator is involved in when promoting safety, educating crew members, and promoting team building. (p 18–21)
- Describe the driver/operator's responsibility in maintaining a safe work environment. (p 21–24)
- Describe the functions and limitations of the fire apparatus and its equipment. (p 24–26)
- Identify the general requirements of a driver/operator as stated in NFPA 1002. (NFPA 1002, 4.1, 5.1 ; p 26–28)
- Identify the medical and physical requirements of a driver/operator as stated in NFPA 1500. (p 28)
- Describe the driver training requirements as stated in NFPA 1451. (p 28–29)
- Describe the testing and selection process for a driver/operator. (p 29–30)

Skills Objectives

There are no skill objectives for driver/operator candidates. NFPA 1002 contains no driver/operator Job Performance Requirements for this chapter.

Additional NFPA Standards

- NFPA 1001, *Standard for Fire Fighter Professional Qualifications*
- NFPA 1451, *Standard for a Fire and Emergency Service Vehicle Operations Training Program*
- NFPA 1500, *Standard on Fire Department Occupational Safety and Health Program*
- NFPA 1582, *Standard on Comprehensive Occupational Medical Program for Fire Departments*

You Are the Driver/Operator

Now that you have worked as a fire fighter for several years, you have decided to seek a promotion to the next higher rank—driver. After completing the required driver training that your department offers to its members, you are now eligible for promotion to the driver rank. Your department has a testing process and you must score well to be placed on the list of eligible candidates. As you prepare for the promotional exam, you think about the following questions:

1. What is the driver/operator responsible for?
2. Which training is required to operate different fire apparatus in the department?
3. What are the qualities that the department is looking for in a driver/operator?

Introduction

As a **driver/operator**, you have obligations to yourself, to your crew, and to the community that you serve. Internal and external expectations hinge on your ability to perform and complete your initial response assignments, as well as to fulfill any extra duties that arise at the scene. You know the ones—those little problems that occur at almost every call. You hear about them time after time: the generator that is difficult to get running or the power unit that will not start. You are charged with the responsibility to prevent, manage, or rectify those little requests that can make or break the ongoing operations at the scene.

To be successful in your new role, you must first understand and accept the responsibilities that come with the job. You may have moved from the attack crew to the driver/operator position, but that transition does not remove you from any frontline responsibilities. As a driver/operator, you are now involved in a greater role in the efficiency and success of your crew. Preventive maintenance, regular inspections of apparatus and equipment, and adherence to jurisdictional operating guidelines will support your and your crew's success and offer some relief from the pressures created by your new challenges.

New driver/operators may not always realize the responsibilities that this position entails. Fire fighters are injured or killed every year as a result of accidents that occur while responding and returning from emergency and nonemergency incidents. You must first acknowledge the hazards associated with driving and operating apparatus, and then you must accept the responsibility to prevent these hazards. The position itself is not hazardous——it is the risks associated with driving and operations that are hazardous. You have a responsibility to fulfill this role through the "lead by example" process.

When you complete regularly scheduled fire apparatus and equipment inspections, you instill confidence in the other crew members that the fire apparatus and equipment will function when needed. Suppression, rescue, hazardous materials, and emergency medical crews have enough to deal with during the normal course of an emergency. If they have confidence in your ability and the reliability of the fire apparatus and equipment, the fireground situation becomes much easier to manage.

Despite your best inspection and preventive maintenance efforts, situations may still arise in which the equipment fails. If you have a solid foundation of knowledge, experience, and skill, however, a variety of backup plans and alternative methods for accomplishing specific assignments will be readily available to you. Simply stated, more knowledge offers more options, and more options lead to better outcomes.

The Many Roles of the Driver/Operator

A driver/operator is a vital crew member and a safety advocate. You may be expected to fix components that are broken, offer alternative methods, maintain a state of constant readiness, and support every function that your apparatus can provide. In addition, you have a duty to educate other crew members on their roles and responsibilities to support you, much in the same way that you support their efforts on an emergency scene. For example, if you drive a ladder apparatus, you should ensure that all of the fire fighters in your company understand how to assist in the setup and deployment of the aerial device.

Crew members may not always understand the problems created by their small and seemingly insignificant actions during the response and return phases of an assignment. Consider what happens when fire fighters remove a tool from the fire apparatus and do not inform you. If you do not know the tool has been taken away, you may not account for it when the fire apparatus leaves the scene—and then you have a missing tool. It is your job to bring these problems to light so that success is shared by all.

To build crew confidence and efficiency, you must demonstrate your commitment to the department, the crew, your officer, and the community. To accomplish this goal, you must follow operating guidelines and applicable laws and regulations; create and maintain a safe work environment; and follow sound risk management principles. Team synergy begins with confidence and trust. These attributes initially begin with your words, and are later demonstrated through your actions.

> **DRIVER/OPERATOR Tip**
>
> You and your fire officer are a team. By working together and being on the same page, you set an example of teamwork and leadership for the entire department.

■ Promoting Safety

There are several key roles that an effective driver/operator must play. As with all of the positions within the fire service, safety is always your first priority. Your safety and the safety of your crew and the community is an important motivating factor for the manner in which you conduct yourself.

Getting to the incident is important to the operation, but you should also consider the events that occurred prior to your response. Were the required preventive maintenance actions taken? Is the fire apparatus in a proper state of readiness? These are all good questions—but what are the real answers?

Driver/operators play an important role in the safety and efficiency of fire service operations. As such, there are many steps you can take to support a safer work environment. You begin by recognizing the associated hazards and then taking measures to reduce or eliminate these hazards.

Many fire departments utilize standard operating procedures/standard operating guidelines (SOPs/SOGs) to maintain work-safe environments. In most cases, SOPs were developed to prevent injuries, establish uniformity, and serve as a basic foundation for effective operations at an incident. As a driver/operator, you have an obligation to acknowledge the importance of these SOPs/SOGs. Additionally, acceptance and demonstration of these procedures are critical to the overall safety of the crew and the community.

Seat belts are one safety device that is all too often underutilized by many crew members. According to chapter 4 of National Fire Protection (NFPA) 1002, *Standard for Fire Apparatus Driver/Operator Professional Qualifications*, it is the driver/operator's responsibility to ensure that passenger restraints are used. You can demonstrate the importance of wearing a seat belt by being the first one to buckle up and by insisting that your crew members follow suit. A variety of excuses may be cited for not using these safety devices; however, if you educate crew members on the consequences of ignoring this safety measure, compliance is usually achieved and safety is maintained **FIGURE 2-1**. Safety is an attitude, and changing attitudes may not come easy. Your job is to demonstrate the importance of utilizing vehicle safety systems by being the first to comply with them. Driver/operators should also emphasize the importance of passive safety systems such as seat belt monitoring systems.

Another area of concern is the equipment carried on the fire apparatus to support its function. This equipment, including heavy tools, is often stored in elevated areas that may present a significant risk to fire fighters when they are retrieving or restoring this equipment by themselves during preventive maintenance

FIGURE 2-1 Seat belts have saved many fire fighter lives; you can promote safety by being the first crew member to buckle up.

> **Safety Tip**
>
> Many older apparatus built on both commercial and custom chassis did not include seats (to include regular seats as well as those designed to hold self-contained breathing apparatus [SCBA]) and seat belts that would accommodate the extra bulk of fire fighter personal protective equipment (PPE) and clothing. Restraint systems should be evaluated with fire fighters wearing full PPE seated in the seat. Older apparatus may need to be retrofitted with longer-than-normal seat belts; however steps should be taken to make certain that any conversions are approved by the chassis and/or seat manufacturer.

activities, training activities, and emergency response activities **FIGURE 2-2**. You should demonstrate to crew members the safest technique to accomplish this task with proper use of the fire apparatus' mounted steps, ladders, and rails.

Heavy equipment, regardless of the location in which it is stored, can present a significant safety problem for fire fighters. To minimize their risk of injury, you can educate crew members on the proper removal and lifting techniques for specific

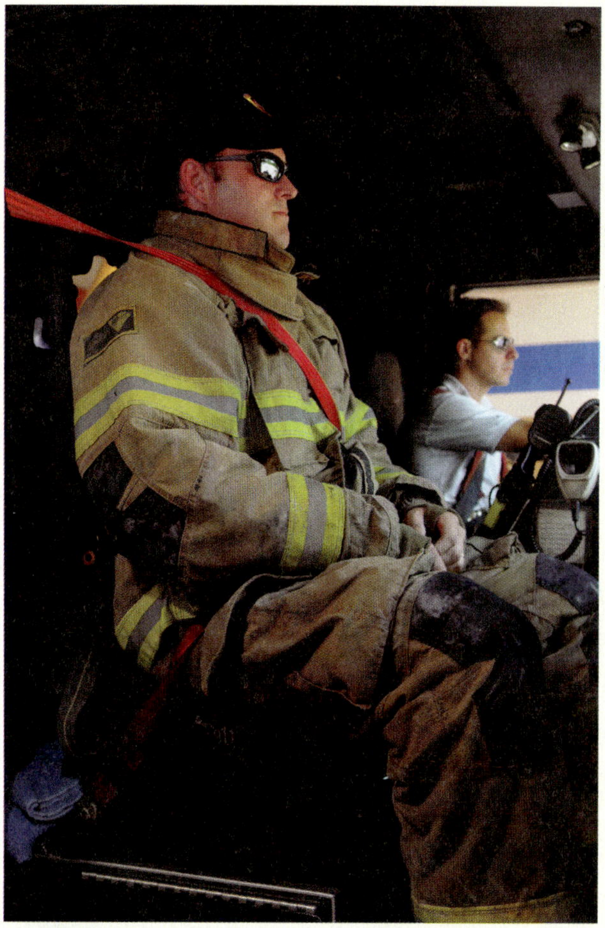

FIGURE 2-2 Equipment and heavy tools are often stored in areas that present a significant risk to fire fighters.

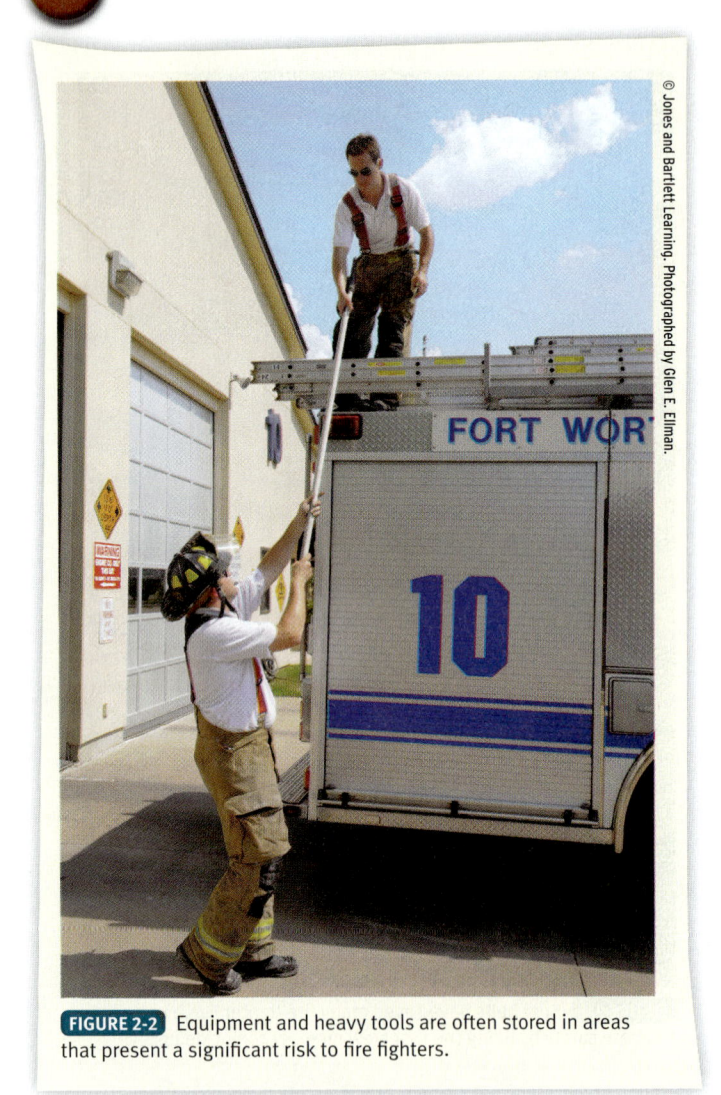

pieces of equipment. Mounting devices such as racks, brackets, or trays are not standardized; consequently, each device may have a specific process for tool and equipment removal. It is your role to explain and demonstrate the proper techniques for removing and restoring equipment to its proper location.

As a safety advocate, you can play an important role in influencing future fire apparatus and equipment purchases as well as modifications to existing equipment. Explaining and demonstrating the potential hazards to management is a proactive approach toward maintaining a safe work environment. For example, you might demonstrate what can be accomplished by installing the proper rails and steps on the fire apparatus so that fire fighters can safely retrieve equipment. By considering fire apparatus design needs, your department will save in the long term on injury and lost-time compensation costs.

■ Educating Crew Members

You must educate your crew members on the many potential hazards associated with the fire apparatus and its equipment. All too often, fire fighters have been injured while working around fire apparatus-mounted equipment, such as pike poles and ground ladders that stick out on the fire apparatus.

Here is one simple philosophy to follow: Knowing the "why" makes the "how" come easy. In other words, determining why hazards or dangerous conditions exist makes it easier to reduce or prevent these conditions. As a driver/operator, you can offer many safety tips to your crew members; knowing which information to present is the key to ensuring an effective and safe response. For example, when you are positioning the fire apparatus at an emergency scene, you are observing the traffic conditions while approaching the scene. In contrast, the rest of the crew members do not have the luxury of viewing mirrors and facing forward all of the time. The crew may be unaware of hazards as they exit the fire apparatus—and it is up to you to make sure they are properly informed of any dangers before they leave the cab.

You must address rider positioning to the crew members. Crew members may inadvertently create a hazard during the response or return phase simply by blocking your view. For example, if a crew member attempts to don SCBA in the front cab area while en route to a call, his or her actions may obstruct your view of the side-view mirror. By placing an arm out the open window while sitting in the front passenger position, a fire fighter may obstruct your view of a spot mirror during critical apparatus positioning maneuvers. Explaining or demonstrating the hazards created makes other crew members aware of such dangerous conditions so that these situations are not repeated in the future.

Riding assignments are used by many fire departments, where each seat or riding position represents a specific task or function. For example, most fire departments designate the front passenger seat to the fire apparatus fire officer in charge (OIC). Other assigned positions may include the fire fighter on the nozzle, backup line, ventilation, or forcible entry (irons). Assigned riding positions are a proactive means to ensure that critical functions are assigned to team members prior to arrival. You can extend the responsibilities of these riding positions by explaining to the crew members the response and return hazards associated with driving the fire apparatus. Fire fighters positioned in the other seats can communicate when they see vehicles attempting to pass the fire apparatus or vehicles hanging back in one of the fire apparatus' many **blind spots**. Taking advantage of the existing riding positions is an effective safety measure to make the response safer.

Sometimes communicating on the fireground or en route to the scene can be difficult. You can educate crew members on the various distractions that hinder effective communications, such as sirens, engine noise, equipment noise, and other radio traffic. Collectively, this barrage of noise can make effective communications almost impossible; it may also contribute to long-term hearing loss. Having prior knowledge of these possible conditions allows the crew members to develop a backup plan to reduce possible delays in critical communications during emergency situations. Some apparatus are equipped with a **vehicle intercom system**. A vehicle intercom system provides a headset and microphone for each rider on the fire apparatus. It enables the fire fighters on the fire apparatus to communicate clearly, without interference from outside noise. This intercom system may also be connected to the fire department's communication system, allowing these personnel to listen to and transmit information over a radio channel. Some intercom systems are hard-wired while others are wireless, which enhance the ability for the driver and spotters to communicate while backing up or positioning the apparatus at emergency scenes.

You must be familiar with SOPs regarding emergency communications such as Mayday, emergency traffic, urgent communications, or emergency evacuation signals. In many cases, fire departments rely on air horns from the fire apparatus to signal an emergency evacuation of the structure. If you are not familiar with this process or if you are not fully focused on the events of the incident, the outcome could be catastrophic. Paying strict attention to the **tactical benchmarks** of the incident will keep you ready to initiate life-preserving actions.

■ Trust and Team Building

The more the crew knows about the driver/operator's roles and responsibilities, the stronger the crew synergy becomes. The best way to impart this knowledge and ensure cohesiveness is to educate the other members of the crew on what you do. Show them how you operate the aerial device, the fire pump, and other features of the fire apparatus. The crew members may not be responsible for the actual operation of the equipment at a fire scene, but they will have more of an appreciation of what you and the rest of the team are trying to accomplish.

Staying focused on the tasks at hand makes for a more effective effort. Team building begins with confidence and finishes with trust. Trusting someone means that you believe in that person's abilities. In the fire service, crew members must believe in your ability as a driver/operator. They must believe that you have prepared the fire apparatus, the equipment, and yourself to the best of your abilities. They must believe that your decisions are calculated and that your actions are precise. This all sounds good, but how do you make it a reality? Trust is built through your communications and your actions. Consistency is the foundation needed to gain someone's trust. The more consistent you become with your decisions and your actions, the more trust you will gain.

Building a solid team takes time and patience. It is important to have support when you need it most. A working team makes successful outcomes look easy, even though that is not always the case. Consider this scenario: Do you and your crew perceive packing hose as a meaningless task, or do you perceive it as an action of readiness to meet the demands of the next alarm, thereby making your job easier at the next call? If you have ever pulled a "spaghetti mess" hose load, you can relate to the importance of team building—effective teams do not demonstrate such carelessness.

How does this issue relate to the roles and responsibilities of a driver/operator? All members of the crew must be able to perform their assignments without reservation or hesitation. As the nozzle person at a fire scene, have you ever stood at the front door of a burning building waiting for the driver to charge the hoseline? When you are in this position and ready to make an attack on the fire, it is frustrating to not have the line immediately charged with water. Crews want a driver they can trust to get them a sustained water supply quickly and efficiently. As the driver/operator, you are obligated to your crew members to provide them with the best possible on-scene support that you can muster up. Members of sports teams rely on one another to win championships; fire fighters rely on one another to survive.

> **Safety Tip**
>
> No nonessential conversation should be allowed while responding to an emergency call. All communication should be limited to mission-critical information, and crew members should be instructed to listen for essential radio messages.

Maintaining a Safe Work Environment

Maintaining a safe work environment is a tough job. Keeping fire apparatus and equipment service-ready can be a challenge to the newly appointed driver/operator. To make the process flow seamlessly, experienced driver/operators should start training future candidates for this position early in their careers.

Educating crew members is a major responsibility for any driver/operator. You must teach them how to recognize operational errors or equipment malfunctions that occur at emergency and nonemergency events. In addition, you should help them understand the **stressors** that challenge the driver/operator on a regular basis and emphasize that everyone plays a role in maintaining a safe work environment. Buy-in is what you wish to achieve; have the entire crew onboard with your work-safe philosophy. In time, you will create a work-safe ethic that will accommodate future changes in emergency and nonemergency operations.

Safety is embedded in all aspects of firefighting. As a driver/operator, you are charged with performing apparatus and equipment inspections and undertaking basic preventive maintenance operations. When the hydraulic rescue system will not start, things can become very stressful, very quickly. Regularly scheduled inspections, operational service checks, and scheduled preventive maintenance actions make major contributions to ensuring the reliability of the fire apparatus and equipment carried onboard. Routine inspections must be taken seriously. Fire apparatus and equipment operational checks must not only be performed, but also documented by the driver/operator—after all, it's your job.

What should you be doing in the course of a day? First, you should actively promote the work-safe philosophy by completing daily inspections of equipment and fire apparatus systems such as tank, tank water, and fuel levels; hydraulic rescue systems; electrical power plants and cables; pneumatic equipment and supply hoses; portable and mobile radios; fire pump operation; gas detection meters; ladder main or boom operation; thermal imagers; SCBA; hand lights; apparatus braking systems; tires and wheels; and audible and visual warning devices. The key to completing a thorough inspection is to develop a routine that allows the driver/operator to conduct the inspection the same way every time. **Job aids**, such as check lists or inspection sheets, are critical to ensuring the accuracy of inspections. If supported by an inspection process, these inspection sheets or checklists will quickly become routine parts of the job. Their ongoing use will provide the consistency that you desire for ensuring fire apparatus and equipment reliability. Cutting corners has no place in the fire service. An upfront commitment to completing your assigned responsibilities is paramount.

Other informational sources that should be used during routine inspection and preventive maintenance processes include operating and general service manuals. These manuals are required to be provided by the manufacturer with the purchase of its fire apparatus or equipment. Operating manuals are key tools for any preventive maintenance and general service program. The purchasing of fire apparatus and equipment is a competitive market for manufacturers; the continuing stream of apparatus system upgrades, equipment functionality revisions, product design changes, and newly introduced safety features makes it imperative for you to stay on top of the ongoing process of upgrading and redesigning equipment and fire apparatus. Unfortunately, not all fire pumps, rescue and suppression equipment, and apparatus systems are created equal. Different manufacturers require specific procedures, service and maintenance schedules, and lubricants to comply with their warranty obligations and life-cycle expectations. The task of keeping fire apparatus and equipment in good working order becomes much easier when you remember to refer to the manufacturer's recommendations—in other words, always check the manual.

After completing your inspections, your day is not done. Training and education continue at the fire station. There, you should educate crew members on the importance of using the safety equipment. Demonstrate how to preset, start, and operate specialized equipment. This task can be accomplished during the daily inspection and maintenance process. Get everyone involved—after all, their involvement supports their own personal safety. Teach company members how to troubleshoot problems in the field and how to correct problems as they occur through the use of a process or routine.

Consider the gasoline-powered equipment carried on the apparatus. "I started it this morning but it wouldn't start at the rescue scene"—does that complaint sound familiar? Give crew members something to work with, something to remember. In basic training, you were taught the PASS mnemonic as a tool to help you execute the procedure for operating a fire extinguisher: Pull the pin, Aim the nozzle, Squeeze the handle, and Sweep the base of the fire. Even to this day, you remember that memory aid. If this technique works for fire extinguishers, it should also work for starting power units. Try something like FCSP (fire fighters can save people) to help crew members remember the right sequence: Fuel, Choke, Switch, and Pull. This acronym may help fire fighters remember to first check the fuel level and fuel shut-off valve, then set the choke, then turn the start/engine cutoff switch to "start" or "run," and finally pull the cord or engage the start/ignition switch. To reinforce this sequence, you might write the acronym on the top of the engine cover.

Tools such as phrases and acronyms are used often in the fire service to help fire fighters remember important information. Commercial driving instructors use ABCDE to emphasize key points to be covered in fire apparatus tire inspections: Abrasions, Bulging, Cuts, Dry rot, and Even-wear inspection. Remember the "everything under pressure is worse" philosophy? That statement holds true for fire fighters whether they are attempting to do 10 things at once while people are screaming for help or whether they are performing their routine preventive maintenance procedures. Your role is to relieve some of the stress on the job by educating the crew on the basic mechanics of how equipment operates and functions.

> **DRIVER/OPERATOR Tip**
>
> You can make a difference by educating your crew, maintaining your knowledge and skill levels, and following the rules that are in place for your safety.

With experience, you may discover other roles and responsibilities that are charged to the driver/operator position. For example, while operating at the scene of a motor vehicle accident, you may not only position the fire apparatus so as to protect the scene, but also act as a lookout for the crew in heavy traffic conditions. If you anticipate and prepare for these additions and changes in your role, you will maintain your consistency and reliability while completing your assignments. Know your fire apparatus, your equipment, and your community; how you perform will reflect your knowledge of these three areas. In time, you will gain confidence and experience. Your reliability will be acknowledged and your consistency will be steadfast.

■ Lead by Example

As a driver/operator, you must lead by example. Follow the rules yourself. SOPs are for everyone—so lead by adhering to them. Follow and promote compliance with all SOPs. For example, by completing and documenting your fire apparatus inspections as part of your normal routine, you demonstrate to the crew your commitment to everyone's success. This will give you credibility with the other crew members and keep you safe at the same time. SOPs cover many fire department service areas, such as responding to and departing from incidents, required personal protective equipment for highway incidents, fire apparatus positioning, and general company assignments. Examples of such procedures include having the first-due engine company lay a supply line and connect to the fire department connection (FDC) and having the first-due ladder company go to the address side of the structure.

> **Safety Tip**
>
> Always follow the rules of your fire department to the best of your ability. Whether you are driving, pumping, or operating a specialized piece of equipment, your actions invariably fall under a law, regulation, local ordinance, or SOP. Do the right thing; exercise **due regard** on and off the street. You should always advocate safety and compliance with SOPs to others.

There are many critical life-preserving guidelines that you must know. Evacuation signals, Mayday or urgent communications, and water supply hand signals are a few examples. Remember, each fire department operates in a manner intended to best meet the needs of its community and the situation at hand. You must fully understand the strategies and tactics used by your department's fire officers. For example, some fire departments may have their driver/operators perform horizontal ventilation of a structure fire by breaking a window while the attack team calls for ventilation.

VOICES
OF EXPERIENCE

I remember the first pump operations class I attended as a fire fighter. The instructor was a veteran engineer/operator and took enormous pride in his skill. He informed me and my fellow fire fighters that anyone can be a driver/operator, but only a few select individuals truly earn the title of Engineer. I remember feeling overwhelmed by all the gauges, levels, and lights. I never thought that I would truly be able to earn the title of Engineer. After a few years however, I was promoted to Engineer and was determined to truly earn the title. I made it my mission to learn my way around a pump panel, not just the physical skill set; but, also the science and hydraulics of being an Engineer.

A number of years later I was the Engineer on the first due Truck Company to a large (36,000 sq. ft. [3345 m²]) commercial occupancy fire. The building was located in a part of our district that just had fire hydrants installed by the local taxing district. Prior to the installation of the hydrant system, our pre-fire plans had us establish a water shuttle along with drafting from a large community pool.

Upon our arrival there was heavy smoke showing. We initiated an aggressive interior attack. I set up the aerial device in preparation; in the event the incident commander decided he wanted it. Fortunately the incident commander remembered the new fire hydrants and had the second-in company lay a supply to me. The interior was not successful due to a large fire load inside the building and we had to go defensive. Two more Truck Companies were requested and set up in opposite locations to us and we began extinguishing the fire. Although we had the one fire hydrant, it was not enough and additional supply lines had to be laid from nearby hydrants along with water being shuttled to the scene.

The fire taught us the value of understanding hydraulics. If we had been better prepared in regards to understanding our potential water supply, we would have known that additional supply lines could have been attached to the hydrant providing more water in the terms of volume. From that point forward, as a department, we began attaching a shutoff valve to the 2½-inch (64-mm) outlet of the hydrant when connecting large-diameter hose (LDH) to a hydrant in preparation for additional water if the need arose.

We eventually extinguished the fire. The contents were a complete lost due to either fire and or smoke damage, but the Fire Marshal's Office felt that the building was salvageable.

Captain Robert Barron
Prairie View Fire Department
Prairie View, Texas

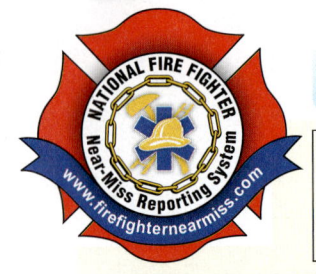

Near-Miss REPORT

Report Number: 07-0000943

Synopsis: Near-miss accident returning to station.

Event Description: I was driving the engine while returning to the station after being cancelled from a motor vehicle accident. We had responded to the far north part of our response district from our main station. On the way back, we were heading down a moderate hill at driving speed when a vehicle pulled out in front of the engine. The vehicle stopped to wait for oncoming traffic, to pass, and to make a left hand turn south of the intersection where the vehicle was. I applied the brakes firmly and the engine was slowing, but not fast enough since the vehicle that pulled out in front of me stopped to make a left turn. I had about 250 ft (76 m) to make a choice that could result in nothing happening or possibly death.

If the vehicle in front of me would have started to make the turn, I had planned to move slightly to the right towards the shoulder, which would have resulted in a partial rear-end collision to the passenger vehicle and pose the least danger to my crew. The other thought going through my head was to not continue on my path, which could have resulted in a T-bone type accident that most likely would have killed the driver of the passenger car. Under God's grace, the oncoming traffic could tell that something was not right and that the engine was not going to be able to stop and moved over to their shoulder. The car that had pulled out in front of me and then stopped to make the turn must have also noticed that something wasn't right and remained stopped. I chose to gracefully challenge traffic and pass the stopped car without incident, stopping approximately 150 ft (46 m) beyond the intersection where the passenger car had stopped.

It is still unknown if vehicle maintenance was a factor in the incident. I truly learned the limitations of such large vehicles that day. It served as a reminder that at driving speeds, it's all physics once something bad happens. I'm also glad that I remained calm during the incident. Had I panicked and made a sudden move, I could have very easily harmed my crew or a civilian.

Weather was not a factor. Being more aware and anticipating a similar situation at that location is something to be learned.

Lessons Learned: I learned to be more aware of the situation ahead of me while driving. I truly learned the full limitations of braking systems on large vehicles. The engine involved does not have an auxiliary braking system on it. Adding a secondary braking system and decreasing speed will help avoid similar situations. Pay attention and anticipate the unthinkable. Had the car that pulled out in front of me kept driving and not stopped I wouldn't be writing this.

If you put a concerted effort into learning the fire apparatus and equipment systems and acknowledge and comply with SOPs, you will be recognized as a leader and a valued crew member. Your colleagues will respond to your successes and actions by following your example. Over the long haul, equipment may begin to run a little better or the tactical operations may be executed a little more smoothly.

DRIVER/OPERATOR Tip

Personal protective equipment requirements for driver/operators always seem to be a point of discussion; however, this debate can be easily resolved by following your department's SOPs. Get involved in the process of developing these SOPs. Demonstrate safety concerns as they relate to the process of evaluating the effectiveness of each SOP.

Fire Apparatus and Equipment: Functions and Limitations

Successful driver/operators understand the primary function of each fire apparatus they are expected to operate, as well as recognize the limitations of the apparatus and the specialized equipment that it carries. For example, the primary mission for a pumper is to supply water to attack lines or other units. Water tenders haul large volumes of water, whereas brush units are primarily used to suppress vegetation fires. Regardless of the fire apparatus' function, you must know the expectations of the crew and the fire officers. Missing an assignment or not completing an assignment properly is not an option in the firefighting business. You must communicate immediately if a problem arises that cannot be quickly managed in the field. The only way to accomplish this is to fully understand the functions and limitations of the fire apparatus.

Consider the different water supplies that may be available at incident: onboard supplies, municipal water supplies, and static water supplies. How many hoselines or gallons per minute (liters per minute) can be deployed until the demand for water surpasses your available water supply? Will your process for supplying water change with different types of water supplies? The fireground is not the place to seek out the answers to these questions. Although the answers are in reach, it takes the proper training to identify them. Before these questions arise on the fireground, take the fire apparatus out and flow some water with the equipment that you have on it. Try out different scenarios that you and your crew might face, such as a broken hydrant or a burst hoseline. The complexity of knowledge and skills needed to become proficient in the driver/operator position is high, but great driver/operators should be able to troubleshoot a problem and find a way to resolve it.

Have you ever seen a fire fighter use a tool for something other than the purpose for which it was intended? For example, a pike pole with a fiberglass handle would be a poor choice of equipment for trying to pry open a door or window. This application would be using the wrong tool for the job and would create a safety hazard. Because safety is critical to a successful operation, you must know the functions and limitations of the equipment and the onboard systems. What can each rescue tool cut and what can it not cut? What are the stabilization limitations and restrictions on the operation of the aerial device? You need to know the answers to these questions or, at the very least, know where to find them quickly. Operating manuals are the best sources for retrieving the answers to specific operational questions. Educate your crew members on the limitations of the equipment established by the manufacturers. Over the long term, this kind of education and training will save your fire department money by keeping the equipment in proper working condition. It will also reduce the risk that personnel will be exposed to avoidable hazards because they have used the equipment for unintended assignments.

Not all restrictions are associated with the fire apparatus' equipment and systems, however; the fire apparatus itself presents some challenges. What happens when you cross a bridge with a 6-ton (5.4-metric-ton) weight limit while driving a 15-ton (13.6-metric-ton) truck? Knowing the height and weight restrictions for each fire apparatus is always helpful. This is easily accomplished by displaying the height and weight in the cab so that it is visible to the driver/operator and the fire officer in charge of the unit. **Vehicle dynamics** are also critical to the safe operation of the fire apparatus. Weight added or subtracted will change the handling characteristics of the fire apparatus as well as the vehicle dynamics. Simply stated, a fire apparatus may not handle in the same way with a full tank of water as it does when it carries a quarter tank of water. Prior knowledge of these conditions will provide for a much safer return.

Keeping all of these details in your head sounds like a tall order; however, it makes perfect sense. You should know the capabilities and limitations of the fire apparatus that you drive and operate, as well as the equipment that it carries and the systems that support operations. The driver/operator is the crew's "go-to person." When you fill this position, you always need to be on your game—to have the correct answers or the perfect backup plan. Education, training, and repetition will support your ability and enable you to develop alternative options during critical situations.

DRIVER/OPERATOR Tip

You should know your response area well, so that there are no weight limitation or vertical clearance surprises. Also, be aware of hills or dips where the fire apparatus could potentially "bottom out" from a low chassis clearance.

Fire Apparatus and Equipment Inspections

All onboard systems and all carried equipment should be subject to routine inspections. If equipment is not used on a regular basis, it may be forgotten. As a consequence, it may not always be in service-ready condition.

The best place to start is with a complete inventory of the fire apparatus. This exercise will provide you with a working document; at the same time, it will ensure that you and your crew learn where the equipment is kept and how to perform operational checks for each device. Although this inventory process sounds basic, it really is not. You may be surprised by the knowledge and skill levels of your crew members when it comes to the equipment carried on the rig; it is not always at the level you might expect.

Cleaning equipment is another method of inspection. Teach crew members to inspect the equipment as they clean it **FIGURE 2-3**. This "double duty" saves time and offers another level of protection from personal injury.

As a driver/operator, you are responsible for routine inspections and basic preventive maintenance procedures pertaining to the fire apparatus and the equipment it carries. To assist in this effort, you should identify resources from which to retrieve accurate information, proper specifications, and timelines for periodic inspections or maintenance schedules. For instance, when should you bring the fire apparatus in to have the transmission fluid changed? When does the pump need to be tested? At what point does tire wear become a major concern? Other areas of fire apparatus safety include coolant systems, steering components, batteries and charging systems, engine lubrication,

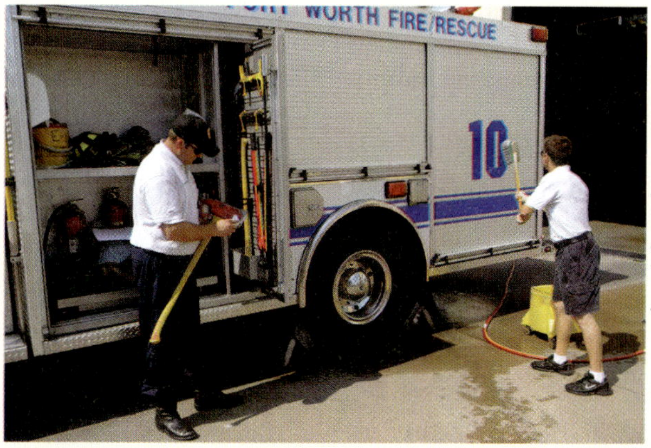

FIGURE 2-3 Encourage fire fighters to inspect equipment as they clean it. This "double duty" saves time and offers another level of protection from personal injury.

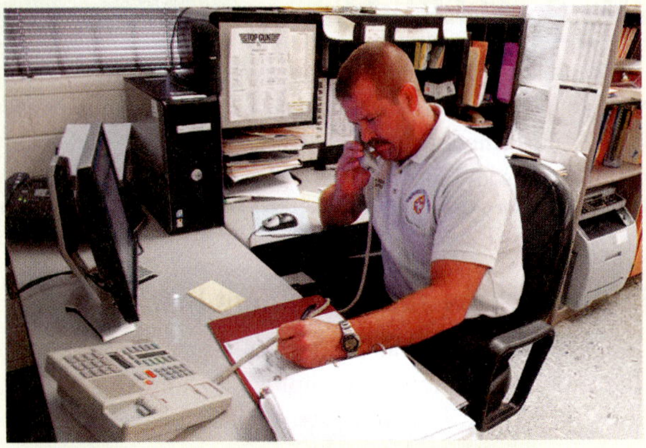

FIGURE 2-4 Specific information on maintenance schedules and indications of component wear can be obtained from a certified emergency vehicle technician.

and fuel systems. Driver/operators should always consult the manufacturer's operator's manuals as well as service and maintenance manuals. Certified emergency vehicle technicians are also a good source of information and advice **FIGURE 2-4**.

The driver/operator must also ensure that tools and equipment are in good repair. Making sure handles are secure to the tool head, tools are sharp and rust free, nozzles operate correctly, battery packs are charged, and air cylinders are full are just a few areas that require attention.

Safety Across the Board

Many different types of fire apparatus are used in the fire service. Some fire apparatus, such as the vehicles used by engine companies, are equipped with the water and hoselines necessary to extinguish a fire. Ladder companies' apparatus are equipped to help crew members gain access to structures and effect support functions at a fire scene. A heavy rescue company will be equipped for technical rescue and special operations.

No matter what the fire apparatus is used for or which type of emergency scene it may respond to, all fire apparatus are operated in two basic ways:

1. **Driving operations.** This includes all operations when the apparatus is traveling. It may include both emergency and nonemergency responses.
2. **On-scene operations.** This includes the operation of the apparatus and any of the apparatus equipment at the incident.

Both operations are critical components of fire services and will dramatically affect the outcome of the incident.

As the driver/operator, you set the tone for the rest of the team members with your response to the incident. If you drive the fire apparatus in a calm, defensive, and safe manner, your behavior will have an effect on the other members of your crew. The fire officer will be able to focus on the communications and scene size-up instead of worrying about your driving abilities. The fire fighters in the back of the apparatus will be less likely to get too excited and lose focus on the upcoming tasks. Conversely, if you drive in an erratic, out-of-control manner and allow your emotions to get the best of you, the entire crew may be in jeopardy. If the crew does not get to the call safely, they won't be able to help anyone. When responding to an emergency, remember this mantra: It's not my emergency. Always respond in a safe manner no matter what the situation is.

Once at the scene, you will have to effectively operate the equipment found on the fire apparatus. You must be capable of operating alone. While the other members of the crew may be tasked with various duties at the scene, your job is to support the crew. If you are part of an engine company, you may need to establish a water supply and charge the attack lines for the crew. Members of a ladder company may rely on you to set up the aerial device so that the ladder company can perform vertical ventilation. Whatever the circumstance, your job is not done once you reach the scene. You must be well trained and use your equipment effectively to support the crew.

NFPA 1002 Requirements

According to National Fire Protection Association (NFPA) 1002, *Standard for Fire Apparatus Driver/Operator Professional Qualifications*, the driver/operator is responsible for getting the fire apparatus to the scene safely, setting up, and operating the pump or aerial device. In the fire service, a driver/operator may also be referred to as an engineer, chauffeur, or technician **FIGURE 2-5**. This function is a permanently assigned role in some fire departments; in other fire departments, it is rotated among the fire fighters.

The operation of fire apparatus and equipment is a critical life-safety issue for all fire fighters. Too many lives are lost every year as a result of fire apparatus accidents. In fact, driving to and from the scene can be as dangerous as operating on the fireground itself. In addition, if the equipment fails on the fireground, the consequences can be disastrous. An unexpected loss of water could jeopardize the safety of an attack line crew, an overextended aerial device could suddenly fail with fire fighters on the device, or difficulty in troubleshooting a mechanical problem could result in the inability to prime a pump. For all these reasons, the driver/operator has a tremendous responsibility for the success and safety of the entire company.

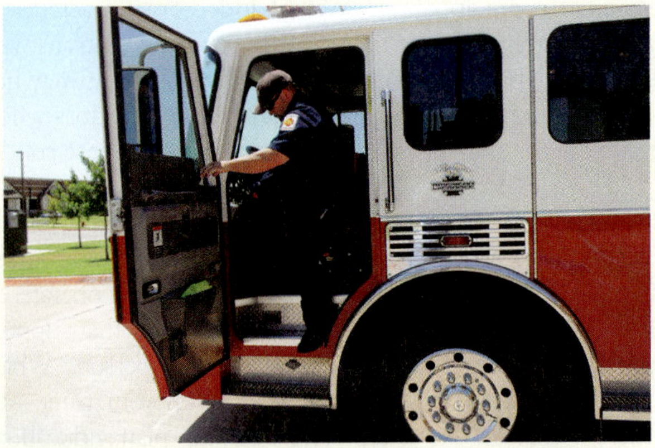

FIGURE 2-5 A driver/operator in action at the scene of fire.

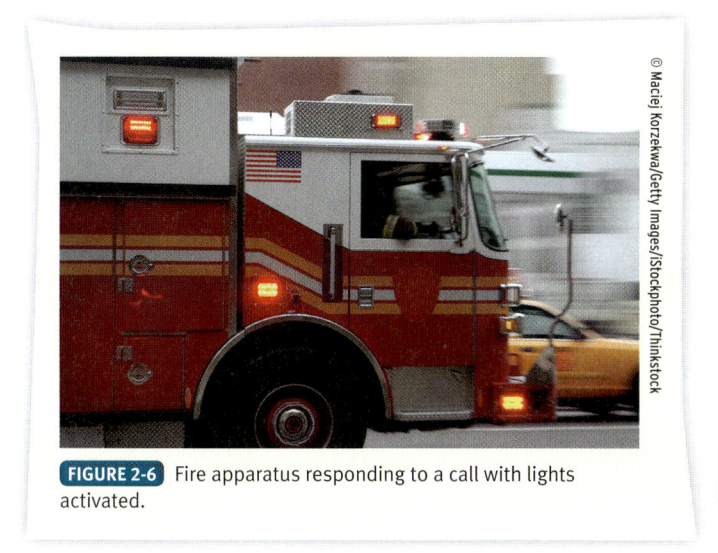

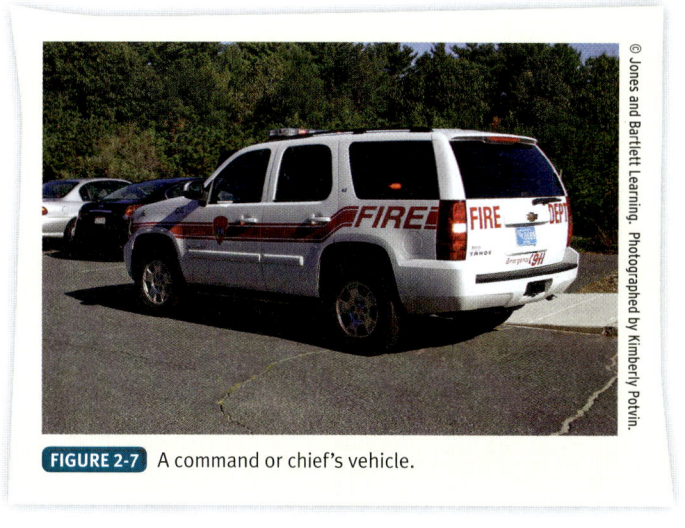

FIGURE 2-6 Fire apparatus responding to a call with lights activated.

FIGURE 2-7 A command or chief's vehicle.

As the driver/operator, you will be responsible for all aspects of the call, including the following issues:
- Preparation of the fire apparatus and equipment for a safe response
- Driving the fire apparatus in an emergency response mode to a call **FIGURE 2-6**
- Placing the fire apparatus at the scene to ensure fire fighter safety and the maximum effectiveness of the equipment
- Safely and properly operating the equipment to support all operations on the fireground
- Securing the equipment and safely returning the fire apparatus and members of the company to the fire station

■ NFPA 1002: General Requirements of a Driver/Operator

All drivers must meet the general requirements of NFPA 1002 before they are allowed to operate a **fire department vehicle**, which includes all apparatus and vehicles operated by the fire department. NFPA 1002 also outlines the minimum job performance requirements (JPRs) for personnel who will drive and operate specific types of fire apparatus. The purpose of the standard is to ensure that each member meets these minimum requirements before he or she is allowed to operate a specific fire apparatus. The following NFPA 1002 chapters identify requirements to operate specific fire apparatus:
- **Chapter 4**: General Requirements (all members who operate fire department vehicles must meet these requirements)
- **Chapter 5**: Apparatus Equipped with a Fire Pump
- **Chapter 6**: Apparatus Equipped with an Aerial Device
- **Chapter 7**: Apparatus Equipped with a Tiller
- **Chapter 8**: Wildland Fire Apparatus (not included in this text)
- **Chapter 9**: Aircraft Rescue and Fire-Fighting Apparatus (not included in this text)
- **Chapter 10**: Mobile Water Supply Apparatus

For example, if a department has only one fire department pumper and no other apparatus, the drivers would require training from Chapters 4 and 5 of NFPA 1002. Each department should ensure that its members are properly trained and authorized before they operate the apparatus.

Personnel must meet those provisions that pertain to the types of apparatus they will be expected to drive and operate, and the authority having jurisdiction (AHJ) may add additional requirements. Driver/operators of vehicles not specifically identified are expected to meet the general requirements of the standard—Chapter 4 of NFPA 1002. These vehicles may include staff or command vehicles and rescues or utility vehicles **FIGURE 2-7**. This text covers the general requirements of NFPA 1002, apparatus equipped with a fire pump, apparatus equipped with an aerial device or a tiller, and mobile water supply apparatus.

To meet the general requirements of NFPA 1002, the fire department vehicle driver/operator must be licensed to drive the vehicle that he or she expected to operate. Some states may require driver/operators to have a **commercial driver's license (CDL)**; others may exempt their drivers from certain licensing requirements altogether. A CDL ensures the driver has met the requirements to operate certain types of commercial vehicles depending on the weight of the vehicle, the number of passengers, and the presence (or not) of any hazardous materials. The U.S. Department of Transportation (DOT)/Ministry of Transportation (MOT) has established requirements for licensing drivers. However, each state or provincial/territorial government usually dictates these licensing requirements to meet its own requirements. Each fire department is responsible for ensuring that its members are properly licensed at the appropriate level for the jurisdiction. All fire fighters should be familiar with their department's requirements. For example, some departments require their driver/operators to hold a commercial driver's license (CDL), even though they are not mandated by state law.

NFPA 1002 also requires that driver/operators meet the requirements of NFPA 1001, *Standard for Fire Fighter Professional Qualifications*, for Fire Fighter I, if they will be responsible for operating a fire pump or aerial device on the fire apparatus. Any fire fighter who has been qualified as a Fire Fighter I

FIGURE 2-8 Apparatus on a fire department training ground completing a cone course or driver course.

FIGURE 2-9 A fire fighter being evaluated by a doctor.

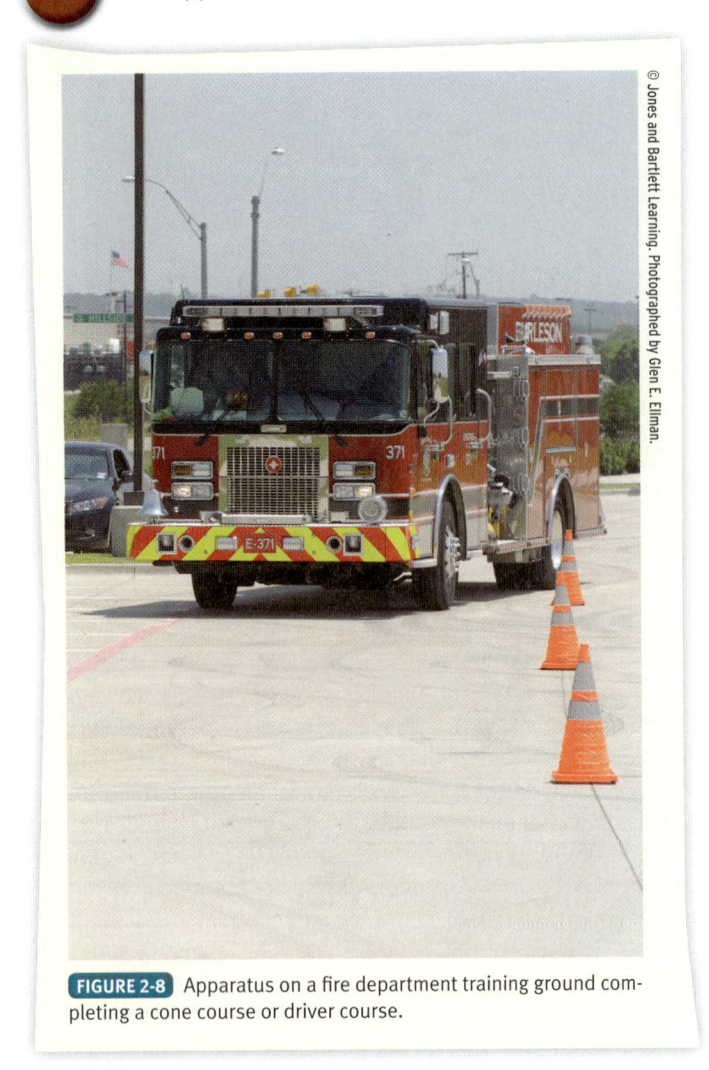

should review the requirements related to fire hose, nozzles, appliances, fire streams, water supplies, and sprinklers, as they may be tested on this information to confirm that they meet the requirements of NFPA 1002. All of the requirements in this standard should be evaluated using a vehicle that is similar in weight, wheelbase, and function as those expected to be operated in the performance of the driver/operator's normal duties **FIGURE 2-8**.

■ NFPA 1002: Medical and Physical Requirements of a Driver/Operator

According to NFPA 1002, the driver is subject to a medical evaluation, as required by NFPA 1500, *Standard on Fire Department Occupational Safety and Health Program*, to determine that the driver/operator is medically fit to perform the duties required. Just as fire fighters need to be in good physical condition to perform their job, so the driver needs to be physically ready to meet the challenges of this position. NFPA 1500 states that the driver shall be medically evaluated and qualified for duty by a physician. Such a medical evaluation shall take into account the risks and the functions associated with the individual's duties and responsibilities **FIGURE 2-9**. All drivers who will engage in fire suppression should meet the medical requirements specified in chapter 8 of NFPA 1582, *Standard on Comprehensive Occupational Medical Program for Fire Departments*. These medical requirements include, but are not limited to, a medical history review, physical examination, and several laboratory tests.

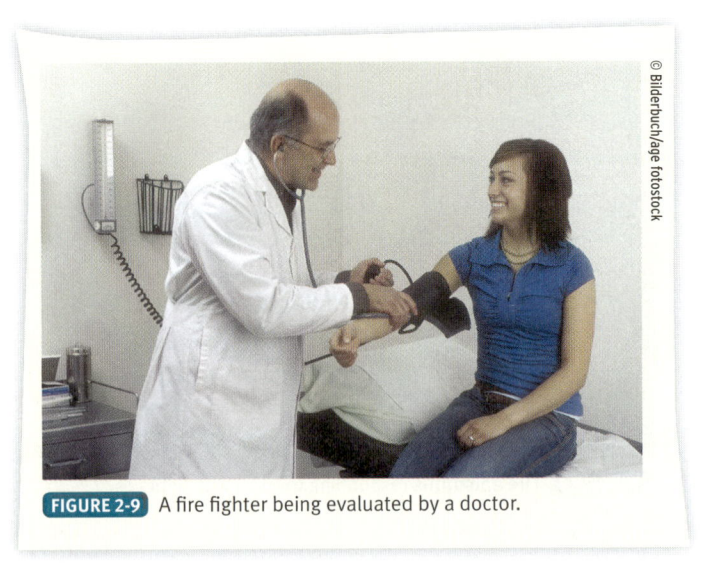

Driver/Operator Training

Training drivers to operate their apparatus safely and efficiently is critical to the success of any fire department. NFPA 1451, *Standard for a Fire and Emergency Service Vehicle Operations Training Program*, contains the minimum requirements for such program. This standard includes development of a driver/operator training program, including the organizational procedures for training drivers, maintaining vehicles, and identifying equipment deficiencies.

According to NFPA 1451, each fire department should:

- Establish and maintain a driver training program with the goal of preventing vehicle crashes, deaths, and injuries to its members and the public.
- Institute a program of post-crash drug and alcohol testing for any driver involved in a crash involving an injury or fatality **FIGURE 2-10**.
- Adopt a risk management plan, which includes risk reduction, risk evaluation, risk control techniques, and risk management monitoring.
- Evaluate the effectiveness of the vehicle training program once every 3 years.
- Establish written SOPs for safe driving of, riding within, and operating vehicles during emergency and nonemergency responses.
- Ensure all members are trained to operate specific vehicles before being authorized to drive the vehicle.
- Ensure all members are reauthorized annually for all vehicles they are expected to operate.
- Provide driver training for all members as often as necessary, but no less than twice each year, with at least one training session to include actual hands-on exercises with the vehicle the member is expected to drive.
- Ensure all members receive training when new or unfamiliar vehicles are placed into service.

CHAPTER 2 Driver Training and Selection

FIGURE 2-10 A fire apparatus and civilian vehicle crash scene.

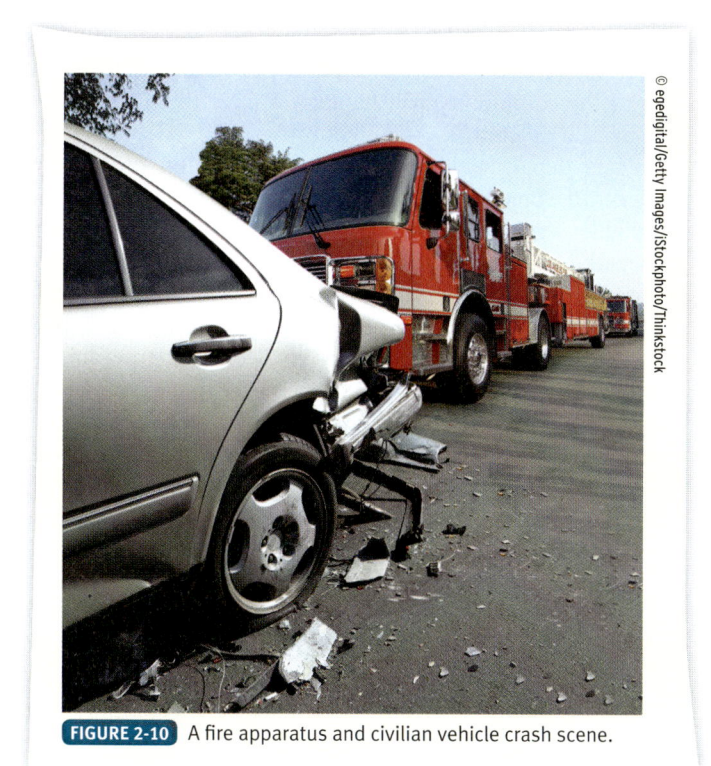

Driver/Operator Selection

What makes a good driver/operator candidate? Knowledge, skill, and attitude are some key attributes. Driver/operators must be knowledgeable in the services provided by their fire departments. They must understand how consistent delivery of excellent services provides for a safe and successful outcome. Driver/operators must be educated and trained in operating at emergency scenes. They must possess the required skills to complete critical life-preserving actions, and these skills must be developed through a continuing process of performance and repetition. Reviewing the JPRs identified in NFPA 1002 will give potential candidates a better understanding of their fire department's expectations regarding their performance.

DRIVER/OPERATOR Tip

To gain and maintain proficiency in the role of the driver/operator, you should take every opportunity to engage in skill exercises or training sessions requiring the use of the onboard systems and equipment. The more familiar you are with the related processes, the more effective you will be in solving the problems that may arise during emergency responses.

Always attempt to train as if you were on an assignment, using the same crew sizes, same fire apparatus, and same equipment resources as you would on a real call. During these training sessions, you may discover better methods that will make you and your crew more efficient. Be sure to pass on the lessons that you learn to other driver/operators and other crew members.

Remember—do not just train for the large-scale or unusual. It is usually the basic skills needed at the bread-and-butter responses that cause the most problems.

An effective driver/operator is a good problem solver. When fire apparatus or equipment malfunctions arise, he or she must be able to quickly evaluate all possible solutions to rectify the problem and seamlessly implement a backup plan. To attain this level of efficiency, driver/operators must understand the basic and complex systems of the fire apparatus and the equipment that it carries. Just as driver/operators need a working knowledge of fireground hydraulics to achieve positive results during fire suppression efforts, so they must also know all of the onboard devices and systems carried on the fire apparatus. Today, fire apparatus provides many functions to support fire department services to the community. The modern fire apparatus is a multitasking unit, and many of the functions it performs require a variety of support and power systems. Hydraulic, electrical, and pneumatic energy sources are present on many modern fire apparatus. Driver/operators, therefore, must be proficient in correcting the problems that are related to all of these onboard systems. One of the best sources for understanding these systems is the manufacturer's operating manual, many of which are available in an electronic format **FIGURE 2-11**.

Selecting a driver/operator candidate can be difficult, so the selection process is based on a candidate's knowledge, ability, and willingness to pursue the challenge. To start this selection process, fire officers may consider a few basic qualities: excellent written and verbal communication skills, physical and mental fitness, basic mechanical ability, and attitude. Driver/operators must be thorough when completing reporting forms, inspections forms, and documentation of deficiencies or corrective actions. Reporting is a major job function of the driver/operator. Do you remember being told sometime in your career, "If it's not documented, it didn't happen"? This holds true for the driver/operator. Undocumented events, conditions, or actions may lead to disaster. Crews cannot be expected to perform their assignments without the required equipment, in proper working condition. Driver/operators must explain the importance of reporting to their respective crews. Educating the other crew members will make your job easier and begin to shift the paradigm away from the notion

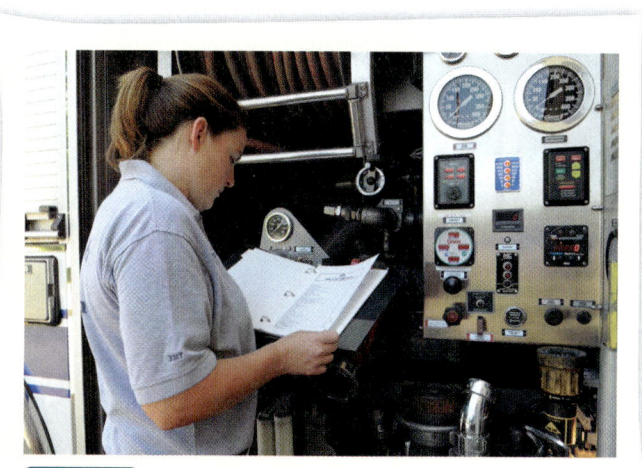

FIGURE 2-11 One of the best methods for understanding apparatus systems is to reference the manufacturer's operating manual.

that "reporting is complaining." Explain to your crew that reporting is preventing a problem or dangerous situation.

Another desirable quality is for the driver/operator to be physically capable of performing the assigned tasks. Good vision, hearing, and physical ability are all characteristics that a driver/operator will need to be safe and successful. Fire apparatus and equipment can be very unforgiving; you will be challenged both mentally and physically by the malfunctions and errors that occur on scene. Your patience will be tested and your reactions watched. Remaining focused on your assignment and being acutely aware of the ongoing operation will better position you to handle the various stressors headed your way.

Next on this list of preferred driver/operator qualities is mechanical ability. Driver/operators should have a basic understanding of mechanics. Familiarity with basic preventive maintenance processes such as lubricating components, adding fluids, and inspecting equipment and onboard systems for proper operation forms an essential skill set for driver/operators **FIGURE 2-12**. Driver/operators are charged with handling minor system repairs and preventive maintenance servicing only; qualified emergency vehicle technicians should perform major repairs or adjustments.

Finally, attitude is a key consideration for the driver/operator. The right attitude demonstrated by the driver/operator is critical for building a successful team, instilling confidence in crew members, and supporting positive response outcomes. Driver/operators must take their roles and responsibilities seriously. Many variables hinge on the ready availability of a well-maintained apparatus and service-ready equipment. Having a positive attitude toward the job will breed additional support and confidence from your crew members. You will inevitably experience operational setbacks; these come with the job.

However, a driver/operator who is committed to the mission of the fire department and dedicated to providing excellent service to the community will be able to meet these challenges and make a difference when it counts.

Each department is unique in its selection process for drivers. In some departments, the driver may be a senior fire fighter assigned to the apparatus or a promoted position within the department, while other departments may rotate all fire fighters' driving duties. If the driver position is considered a promotion, a testing process for this position is usually required. The testing process may involve a written examination and sometimes an **assessment center**, which is a series of simulation exercises **FIGURE 2-13**. Such written examinations usually include information from the department's policies, procedures, and guidelines concerning driving and positioning apparatus, hydraulic calculations, emergency vehicle driving, vehicle maintenance and operation, and material pertaining to the position of apparatus driver. The assessment center may include several practical skill exercises that determine how well a candidate can perform the essential skills required for the position. These tasks may include driving and positioning the apparatus, performing maintenance checks, pumping water from the apparatus, or operating aerial devices. Once the testing process is completed, candidates are usually placed on a promotional eligibility list, which ranks them according to how well they scored. The department then promotes members of the list as positions become available. Such a testing process can be very expensive to administer, so many departments offer such tests only once every few years. If your department has a testing process for the rank of driver, you should make sure that you know how the process works and what is required to be eligible for the testing process.

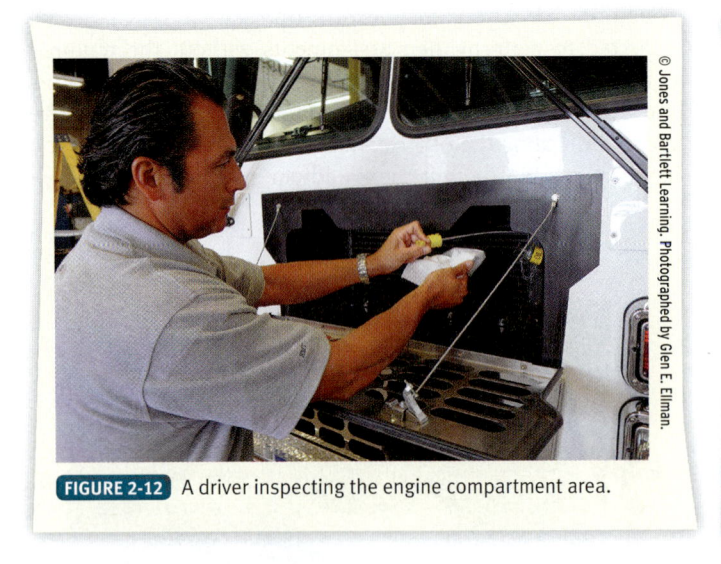

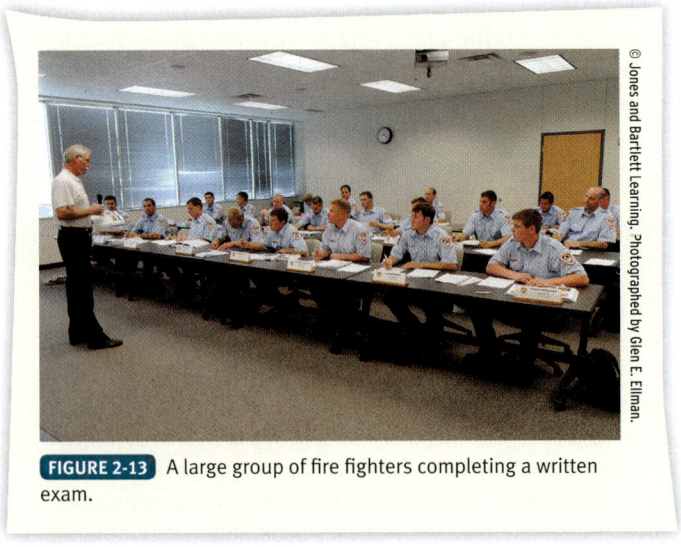

FIGURE 2-12 A driver inspecting the engine compartment area.

FIGURE 2-13 A large group of fire fighters completing a written exam.

Wrap-Up

Chief Concepts

- To be successful in your role as a driver/operator, you must fully understand and accept the responsibilities that come with the job.
- As a driver/operator, you have many obligations to your crew and to the community. Internal and external expectations hinge on your ability to perform your initial response assignments.
- You have a duty to educate other crew members on their roles and responsibilities to support your function.
- As a driver/operator, you are a teacher, a mentor, a vital crew member, and a safety advocate. You must lead by example—so remember that you are a safety advocate.
- Compliance with standard operating procedures or guidelines is essential. Always follow these procedures, and promote compliance among your crew members.
- All fire apparatus are operated in two basic ways: driving operations and on-scene operations.
- The driver is responsible for the safe and efficient operation of the vehicle.
- NFPA 1002 identifies the minimum requirements for a driver/operator.
- NFPA 1451 identifies the requirements for a fire departments driver training program.

Wrap-Up, continued

Hot Terms

assessment center A series of simulation exercises for a promotional examination.

blind spots Areas around the fire apparatus that are not visible to the driver/operator.

commercial driver's license A government-issued license that ensures the driver has met the requirements to operate certain types of commercial vehicles depending on the weight of the vehicle, the number of passengers, and the presence (or not) of any hazardous materials.

driver/operator A person who has satisfactorily completed the requirements of driver/operator as specified in NFPA 1002, *Standard for Fire Apparatus Driver/Operator Professional Qualifications*.

due regard The care exercised by a reasonably prudent person under the same circumstances.

fire department vehicle Any vehicle, including fire apparatus, operated by a fire department.

job aids A tool, device, or system used to assist a person with executing specific tasks.

stressors Conditions that create excessive physical and mental pressures on a person's body; any type of stimulus that causes stress.

tactical benchmarks Objectives that are required to be completed during the operational phase of an incident.

vehicle dynamics Vehicle construction and mechanical design characteristics that directly affect the handling, stability, maneuverability, functionality, and safeness of a vehicle.

vehicle intercom system A communication system that is permanently mounted inside the cab of the fire apparatus to allow fire fighters to communicate more effectively.

References

National Fire Protection Association (NFPA) 1001, *Standard for Fire Fighter Professional Qualifications*. 2013. http://www.nfpa.org/codes-and-standards/document-information-pages?mode=code&code=1001. Accessed March 27, 2014.

National Fire Protection Association (NFPA) 1002, *Standard for Fire Apparatus Driver/Operator Professional Qualifications*. 2014. http://www.nfpa.org/codes-and-standards/document-information-pages?mode=code&code=1002. Accessed March 27, 2014.

National Fire Protection Association (NFPA) 1451, *Standard for a Fire and Emergency Service Vehicle Operations Training Program*. 2013. http://www.nfpa.org/codes-and-standards/document-information-pages?mode=code&code=1451. Accessed March 27, 2014.

National Fire Protection Association (NFPA) 1500, *Standard on Fire Department Occupational Safety and Health Program*. 2013. http://www.nfpa.org/catalog/product.asp?pid=150013. Accessed March 27, 2014.

National Fire Protection Association (NFPA) 1582, *Standard on Comprehensive Occupational Medical Program for Fire Departments*. 2013. http://www.nfpa.org/codes-and-standards/document-information-pages?mode=code&code=1582. Accessed March 27, 2014.

DRIVER/OPERATOR in action

While studying for the promotional exam, you and several other candidates form a study group. The group decides that each fire fighter should make up several questions and bring the questions to the next study group session. All of the questions will then be compiled, and each of you will have a practice test to take before the promotional examination. Here are some of the questions that your study group created:

1. Which NFPA standard identifies the requirements of a driver/operator?
   A. NFPA 1001
   B. NFPA 1002
   C. NFPA 1003
   D. NFPA 1004

2. A driver/operator must be certified to the level of Fire Fighter I if he or she operate an apparatus equipped with a fire pump and/or
   A. Dump tank.
   B. Lights and sirens.
   C. A hydraulic system.
   D. An aerial device.

3. NFPA 1451 requires that fire departments evaluate the effectiveness of the vehicle-training program once every _____ year(s).
   A. 1
   B. 3
   C. 5
   D. 10

4. What is the acronym to remember the correct sequence to start power units?
   A. FCSP (fuel, choke, switch, pull)
   B. FSPC (fuel, switch, pull, choke)
   C. SCFP (switch, choke, fuel, pull)
   D. CFSP (choke, fuel, switch, pull)

5. At the fire scene, the driver is usually responsible for all of the following except
   A. Safely operating equipment to support operations.
   B. Placement of the apparatus at the scene.
   C. Securing equipment before leaving the scene.
   D. Repairing the apparatus if it is broken.

Types of Fire Apparatus

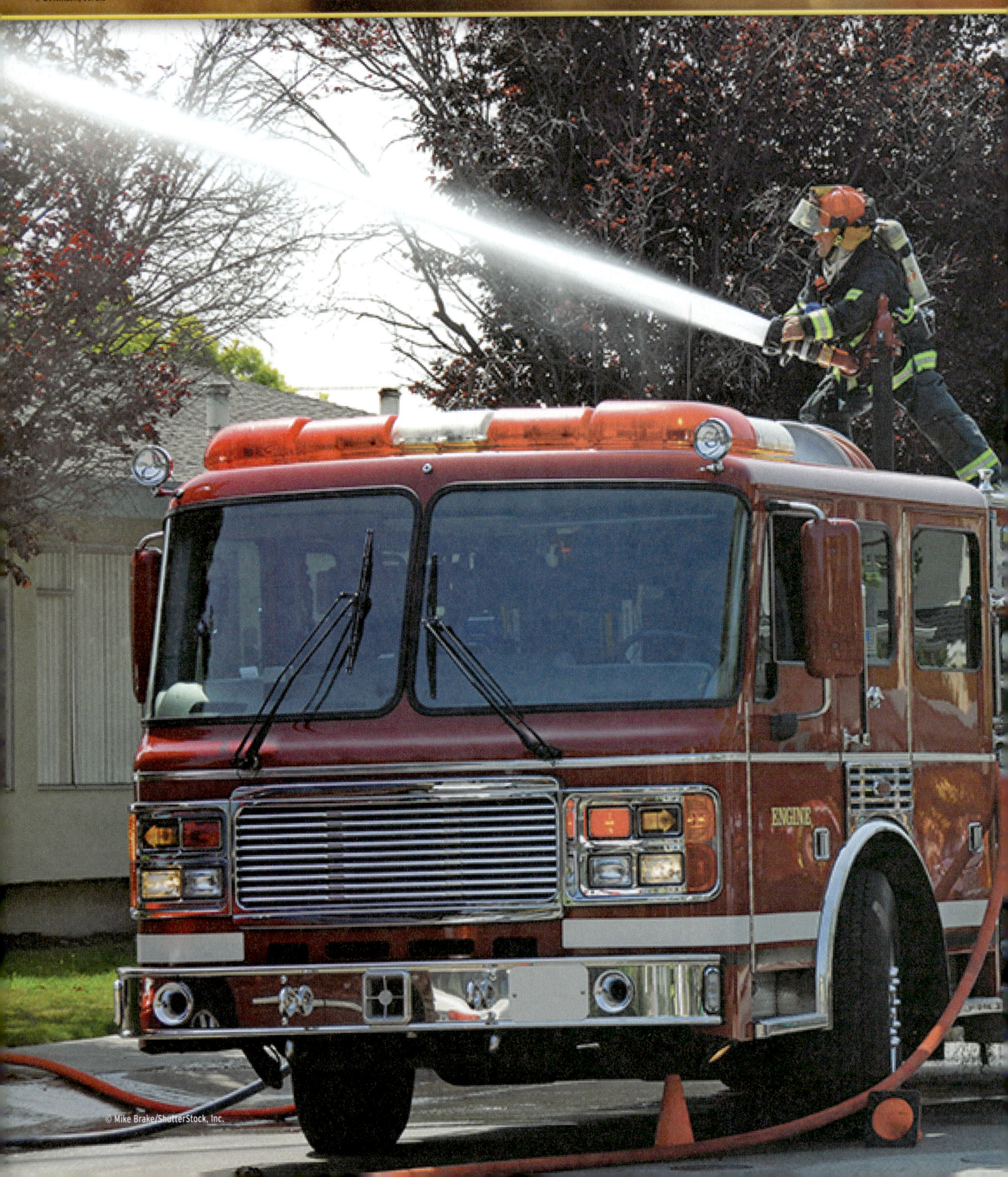

CHAPTER 3

Knowledge Objectives

After studying this chapter, you will be able to:

- Describe the general components required for a fire apparatus. (NFPA 1002, 4.1, 4.2.1(A) ; p 36–37)
- Describe which components are needed to classify a piece of fire apparatus as a pumper. (NFPA 1002, 5.1, 5.1.1(A) ; p 37–38)
- Describe the function of a pumper in the fire service. (p 37–38)
- Describe which components are needed to classify a piece of fire apparatus as an initial attack fire apparatus. (p 38–41)
- Describe the function of an initial attack fire apparatus in the fire service. (p 38–41)
- Describe which components are needed to classify a piece of fire apparatus as a mobile water supply. (NFPA 1002, 10.1.1 ; p 41–42)
- Describe the function of a mobile water supply apparatus in the fire service. (NFPA 1002, 10.1, 10.1.1(A) ; p 41–42)
- Describe which components are needed to classify a piece of fire apparatus as an aerial apparatus. (NFPA 1002, 6.1 ; p 42–44)
- Describe the function of aerial apparatus in the fire service. (NFPA 1002, 6.1, 6.2.1(A) ; p 42–44)
- Describe which components are needed to classify an apparatus as a tiller. (NFPA 1002, 7.1 ; p 42–44)
- Describe the function of tiller apparatus in the fire service. (NFPA 1002, 7.1, 7.2.1(A) ; p 42–44)
- Describe which components are needed to classify a piece of fire apparatus as a quint. (p 44–45)
- Describe the function of a quint in the fire service. (p 44–45)
- Describe which components are needed to classify a piece of fire apparatus as a special service fire apparatus. (p 44–45)
- Describe the function of a special service fire apparatus in the fire service. (p 44–45)
- Describe which components are needed to classify a piece of fire apparatus as a mobile foam apparatus. (NFPA 1002, 10.1.1(4); p 46–47)
- Describe the function of a mobile foam apparatus in the fire service. (NFPA 1002, 10.1.1(4), 10.1.1(A) ; p 46–47)

Additional NFPA Standards

- NFPA 1901, *Standard for Automotive Fire Apparatus*
- NFPA 1931, *Standard for Manufacturer's Design of Fire Department Ground Ladders*
- NFPA 1981, *Standard on Open-Circuit Self-Contained Breathing Apparatus for Fire and Emergency Services*
- NFPA 1983, *Standard on Life Safety Rope and Equipment for Emergency Services*

Skills Objectives

There are no skill objectives for driver/operator candidates. NFPA 1002 contains no driver/operator Job Performance Requirements for this chapter.

You Are the Driver/Operator

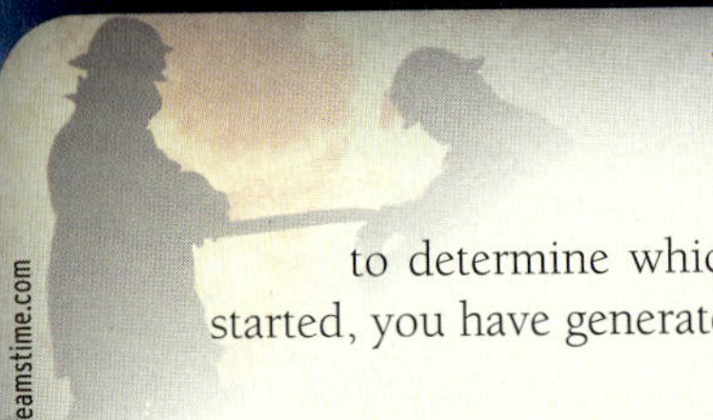

You are a new driver and have just been selected to join your fire department's apparatus specifications committee. The committee will work with a manufacturer to design a fire apparatus that will meet the needs of your community. The committee members will need to determine which type of apparatus is needed and what its capabilities should be. Before the committee gets started, you have generated a few questions:

1. What are the different types of fire apparatus that are available?
2. Is there a minimum amount of water that the fire department pumper has to carry?
3. How different is an initial attack apparatus from a mobile water supply apparatus?

Introduction

The nature of the calls to which today's fire fighters respond vary from day to day. The need to respond solely to wood-structure building fires is a thing of the past. Instead, the modern-day fire service's duties include responding to high-rise building fires, hazardous chemicals spills, brush fires, confined-space rescues, and many other emergency incidents, all of which may occur in large cities, small towns, and rural areas.

Given these many variables, no single **fire apparatus** is adequate for responding to all calls. Rather, specialized equipment has been developed for particular situations. These types of fire apparatus are distinguished based on their function and their capabilities at the emergency scene. You should know what each piece of fire apparatus in your department is capable of doing and which equipment each brings to the emergency scene. For example, you should know the difference between an aerial apparatus and a quint; although these fire apparatus may look similar, they are not identical. Put simply, you should understand that all fire apparatus are not created equal.

In this chapter, you will learn about various fire apparatus and what they are designed to do. Pump sizes, tank sizes, ladders, storage, and more are discussed, in addition to the equipment that must be on a fire apparatus to meet the criteria specified by the National Fire Protection Association (NFPA) 1901, *Standard for Automotive Fire Apparatus*.

Fire Apparatus Requirements

Working with a Manufacturer

With so many types of fire apparatus available for performing a wide variety of jobs, the fire apparatus used by different departments will inevitably vary. Nevertheless, many general requirements apply to all fire apparatus. With any fire apparatus, the jurisdiction purchasing the fire apparatus must convey the following specifications to the manufacturer:

- The specific performance requirements
- The maximum number of fire fighters who will ride on the fire apparatus
- The specific electrical loads required
- Any hoselines, ground ladders, or equipment to be carried by the apparatus that exceed the minimum requirements

The jurisdiction must also inform the manufacturer of any additional equipment that will be on the fire apparatus above and beyond what is required **FIGURE 3-1**. For example, if the jurisdiction needs room on the fire apparatus for swiftwater rescue equipment that may be purchased in the future, the department should inform the manufacturer. This way the fire apparatus can be designed to accommodate this type of equipment and space will be provided to store it. Waiting until the fire apparatus is complete and then attempting to cram additional equipment into it may not work.

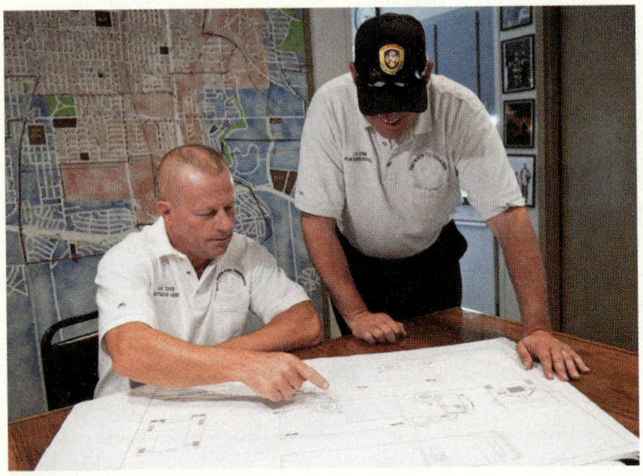

FIGURE 3-1 The jurisdiction must inform the manufacturer of any additional equipment that will be on the fire apparatus above and beyond what is required.

It is the responsibility of the jurisdiction purchasing the fire apparatus to conduct ongoing training to ensure its personnel's proficiency with regard to the safe and proper use of the fire apparatus and its equipment. If a fire department has never had an aerial apparatus, then it should ensure that all of the fire fighters operating it receive proper training. Many times, the manufacturer is available to provide this initial operational training for the department members.

The manufacturer must also describe the fire apparatus, including the estimated weight, wheelbase, turning radius, principal dimensions, transmission, axle ratios, and capacity of the aerial platform, if applicable. While designing a new fire apparatus, it is easy to keep adding features and equipment to the vehicle without realizing what problems may occur with their inclusion. Too many added features may make the vehicle grossly overweight; also, some of the equipment may not be designed to work together. The manufacturer should ensure that all of the components will interact correctly and that the vehicle does not exceed the required weight limits.

The jurisdiction and the manufacturer must work together cohesively to construct the fire apparatus. When a city or town purchases a piece of firefighting equipment whose price could exceed $500,000, it is incumbent upon the two entities to produce an excellent piece of equipment that will do the job. Once the fire apparatus is delivered to the purchasing jurisdiction, the manufacturer will typically supply a qualified representative to demonstrate the fire apparatus and provide training. This training should include all aspects of the apparatus' operation, maintenance, and equipment.

DRIVER/OPERATOR Tip

Before investing in a new fire apparatus, it is well worth the time and effort to seek out the feedback of other fire departments. You should make every effort to speak with representatives from fire departments that have purchased fire apparatus from any manufacturer that you are considering working with. Do not just take the salesperson's recommendations at face value: What are the experts in the field saying about this vehicle? The negative experience of another fire department could save your department hundreds of thousands of dollars and untold hours of frustration! Also consider using apparatus design and consulting services.

NFPA 1901 defines all of the documents and components that should be incorporated for a piece of equipment to be considered an NFPA-compliant fire apparatus. For example, all fire service apparatus must, when loaded to its estimated in-service weight, be capable of the following performance while on dry, paved roads that are in good condition:

- From a standing start, the apparatus must be able to attain a speed of 35 mph (55 km/h) within 25 seconds on a level road.
- The apparatus must be able to attain a minimum top speed of 50 mph (80 km/h) on a level road.
- The apparatus must be able to maintain a speed of at least 20 mph (32 km/h) on any grade up to and including 6 percent.
- The maximum top speed of fire apparatus with a gross vehicle weight rating (GVWR) of more than 26,000 lb (11,800 kg) must not exceed either 68 mph (109 km/h) or the manufacturer's maximum fire service speed rating for the tires installed on the apparatus, whichever is lower.

DRIVER/OPERATOR Tip

Bear in mind that your new fire apparatus will probably be sitting at the fire station for a good month or so while training on the new vehicle and its features occurs. During this month, your old fire apparatus will continue to be used to respond to incidents.

Fire Department Pumper

The **pumper fire apparatus** is the bread-and-butter of the fire service **FIGURE 3-2**. The most common type of fire apparatus, it is a part of almost every fire department. This equipment is used to respond to small incidents such as dumpster fires, vehicle fires, and brush fires in urban settings. It is also the main source of fire attack for larger fires that involve residential and commercial structures. The pumper is the piece of fire apparatus that is critical for the initial extinguishment of the fire because it brings the initial water supply as well as tools to the fire scene. The term pumper and engine are used interchangeably in this textbook.

Per NFPA 1901, a pumper must be equipped with a permanently mounted pump with a minimum rating of 750 gpm (2840 L/min) and an on-board water tank holding a minimum of 300 gallons (1135 liters). Many engines have tank sizes of at least 500 gallons (1900 liters), although 750- to 1000-gallon (2840- to 3785-liter) tanks are also very common. Each fire department should determine which types of fires the fire apparatus will respond to and, therefore, what the appropriate pump capacity is. Because the pumper is usually the first

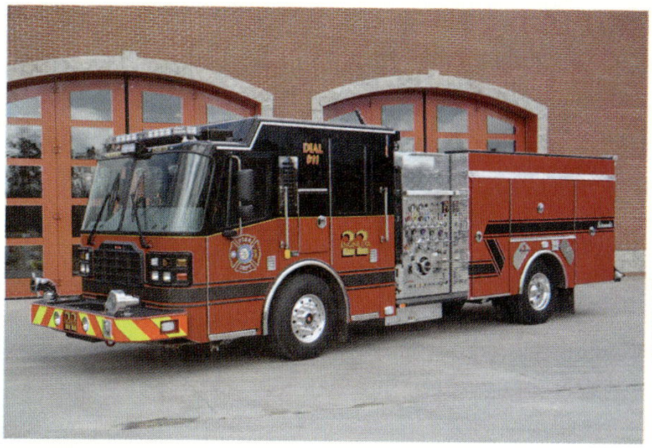

FIGURE 3-2 The pumper secures the water source and extinguishes the fire.

TABLE 3-1	Miscellaneous Equipment on a Pumper
Amount	Equipment
1	6-lb (2.7-kg) or greater flathead axe mounted in a bracket fastened to the pumper
1	6-lb (2.7-kg) pickhead axe mounted in a bracket fastened to the pumper
1	6-ft (2-m) pike pole or plaster hook mounted in a bracket fastened to the pumper
1	8-ft (2.4-m) or longer pike pole mounted in a bracket fastened to the pumper
2	Portable hand lights mounted in a bracket fastened to the pumper
1	Approved dry chemical portable fire extinguisher with a minimum 80-B:C rating mounted in a bracket fastened to the pumper
1	2 1/2-gal (9.5-L) or larger water extinguisher mounted in a bracket fastened to the pumper
1	Self-contained breathing apparatus (SCBA) complying with NFPA 1981, *Standard on Open-Circuit Self-Contained Breathing Apparatus for Emergency Services*, for each assigned seating position, but not fewer than 4 units, mounted in a bracket fastened to the apparatus or containers supplied by the SCBA manufacturer
1	Spare cylinder for each SCBA unit carried, mounted in a bracket fastened to the fire pumper or stored in a specially designed storage space
1	First-aid kit
4	Combination spanner wrenches mounted in a bracket fastened to the pumper
2	Hydrant wrenches mounted in a bracket fastened to the fire pumper
1	Double female 2 1/2-inch (65-mm) adapter with National Hose threads, mounted in a bracket fastened to the pumper
1	Double male 2 1/2-inch (65-mm) adapter with National Hose threads, mounted in a bracket fastened to the pumper
1	Rubber mallet, suitable for use on suction hose connections, mounted in a bracket fastened to the pumper
2	Salvage covers, each a minimum size of 12 × 14 ft (3.7 × 4.3 m)
2	Wheel chocks, mounted in readily accessible locations, each designed to hold the pumper, when loaded to its maximum in-service weight, on a 10 percent grade with the transmission in neutral and the parking brake released

piece of fire department equipment on scene, it needs its own water supply to sustain operation. Each fire department should determine the water supply needs of its jurisdiction and adjust the tank size accordingly.

The pumper does more than just haul water; it also carries a multitude of tools and equipment. At a minimum, this fire apparatus must carry one straight ladder with roof hooks, one extension ladder, and one attic ladder. It must carry several types of hoses as well. At a minimum, it must have 15 ft (4.5 m) of supply hose equipped with hydrant connection threads on one end and pump intake connection threads on the other, or 20 ft (6 m) of hard suction hose with a strainer. The fire department specifies to the manufacturer whether supply hose or hard suction hose is needed. The following types of fire hose and nozzles are required by NFPA 1901:

- 800 ft (240 m) of 2½-inch (65-mm) or larger supply/attack hose
- 400 ft (120 m) of 1½-inch (38-mm), 1¾-inch (45-mm), or 2-inch (50-mm) attack hose
- One combination spray nozzle capable of delivering 200 gpm (750 L/min) at a minimum
- Two combination spray nozzles capable of delivering 95 gpm (360 L/min) at a minimum
- One playpipe, with shut-off and 1-inch (25-mm), 1 1/8-inch (29-mm), and 1 1/4-inch (32-mm) tips

Each pumper must be designed with a minimum of 40 ft³ (1.1 m³) of enclosed weather-resistant compartments to store miscellaneous equipment. As stated in NFPA 1901, the **miscellaneous equipment** listed in TABLE 3-1 is the minimum carried on the fire apparatus. Most fire departments exceed this list and will add the equipment that best suits the needs of their jurisdiction.

Initial Attack Fire Apparatus

The **initial attack fire apparatus** is used much like the pumper, but its specifications are much different FIGURE 3-3. This type of fire apparatus is not as commonly encountered as the pumper, but is nevertheless used by many fire departments. The initial

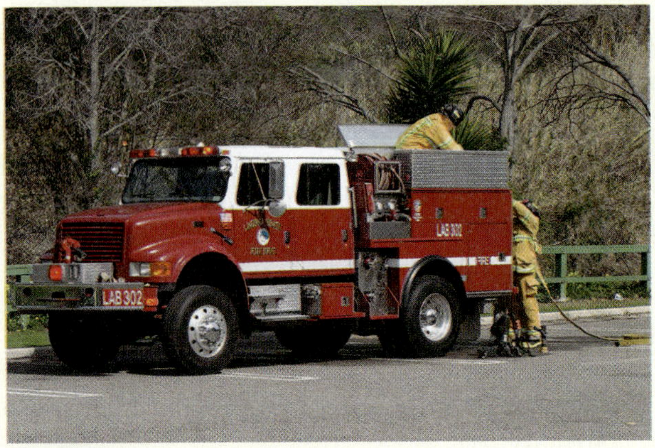

FIGURE 3-3 An initial attack fire apparatus.

attack fire apparatus is a smaller version of the pumper that is designed to be more maneuverable than the pumper, especially in off-road terrain. This apparatus is usually equipped with four-wheel drive and used to fight fires in urban and rural settings. For example, a fire department may have an area in its jurisdiction that is difficult for larger pumpers to access. Because of narrow roads and small bridges, a pumper may not be capable of accessing the buildings in this area. In such circumstances, the initial attack fire apparatus provides a scaled-down version of a pumper for responding to hard-to-reach areas.

Many initial attack fire apparatus are built on a commercial **chassis** with a custom-built body. Fire fighters should be aware of the potential for overloading the chassis with too much weight, thereby creating a safety hazard. The manufacturer's allowance for equipment and hose is often limited on initial attack apparatus due to the gross vehicle weight (GVW) rating of the chassis.

NFPA 1901 states that if a fire apparatus is to be used as an initial attack fire apparatus, then it *shall* conform to these guidelines. The initial attack fire apparatus is equipped with a fire pump as defined in NFPA 1901. The fire pump must have the minimum rated capacity of 250 gpm (1000 L/min). The apparatus' water tank must have, at a minimum, a certified capacity of 200 gal (750 L).

Hose bed areas, compartments, and reels must meet the specifications in NFPA 1901. A minimum of 15 ft (4.5 m) of supply hose equipped with hydrant connection threads on one end and pump intake connection threads on the other, or 20 ft (6 m) of hard suction hose with a strainer must be carried. The purchaser of the initial attack fire apparatus specifies whether hard or soft suction is needed. The following fire hose and nozzles are required by NFPA 1901:

- 300 ft (90 m) of 2½-inch (65-mm) or larger fire supply hose
- 400 ft (120 m) of 1½-inch (38-mm), 1¾-inch (45-mm), or 2-inch (50-mm) attack fire hose
- Two combination spray nozzles with a minimum capacity of 95 gpm (360 L/min)

Like the pumper, the initial attack fire apparatus needs storage compartments. NFPA 1901 mandates a minimum of 22 ft^3 (0.62 m^3) of enclosed weather-resistant compartments, which are to be used for storage of equipment. The compartment space is usually a custom body that is added to a commercial cab and chassis.

The initial attack fire apparatus is also used to bring equipment to the scene of the fire. Most of these tools are the same ones found on the larger pumper. Remember—the initial attack fire apparatus responds to basically the same types of fires as the larger pumpers, but is capable of accessing hard-to-reach areas.

A 12 ft (3.7 m) or longer combination or extension-type ground ladder is carried on the initial attack fire apparatus. All ground ladders must conform to the requirements in NFPA 1931, *Standard for Manufacturer's Design of Fire Department Ground Ladders*. Hand tools and other miscellaneous equipment must also be carried on the initial fire attack apparatus.

As stated in NFPA 1901, the initial attack fire apparatus must carry the miscellaneous equipment listed in **TABLE 3-2**. This equipment is the minimum that is required by NFPA

TABLE 3-2	Miscellaneous Equipment on an Initial Attack Fire Apparatus
Amount	Equipment
1	6-lb (2.7-kg) pickhead axe mounted in a bracket fastened to the initial attack fire apparatus
1	6-ft (2-m) pike pole or plaster hook mounted in a bracket fastened to the initial attack fire apparatus
2	Portable hand lights mounted in a bracket fastened to the initial attack fire apparatus
1	Approved dry chemical portable fire extinguisher with a minimum 80-B:C rating mounted in a bracket fastened to the initial attack fire apparatus
1	2½-gal (9.5-L) or larger water extinguisher mounted in a bracket fastened to the initial attack fire apparatus
1	SCBA complying with NFPA 1981, for each assigned seating position, but no fewer than two units, mounted in a bracket fastened to the apparatus or stored in containers supplied by the SCBA manufacturer
1	Spare SCBA cylinder for each SCBA unit carried, each mounted in a bracket fastened to the initial attack fire apparatus or in a specially designed storage space(s)
1	First-aid kit
2	Combination spanner wrenches mounted in a bracket fastened to the initial attack fire apparatus
1	Hydrant wrench mounted in a bracket fastened to the initial attack fire apparatus
1	Double female adapter, sized to fit 2½-inch (65-mm) or larger fire hose, mounted in a bracket fastened to the initial attack fire apparatus
1	Double male adapter, sized to fit 2½-inch (65-mm) or larger fire hose, mounted in a bracket fastened to the initial attack fire apparatus
1	Rubber mallet, for use on suction hose connections, mounted in a bracket fastened to the initial attack fire apparatus
2	Wheel chocks, mounted in readily accessible locations, each designed to hold the initial attack fire apparatus, when loaded to its maximum in-service weight, on a 10 percent grade with the transmission in neutral and the parking brake released

VOICES OF EXPERIENCE

A number of years ago, I was the chief of a fire department in rural Vermont. One February evening, the air temperature was 20°F (–7°C) and falling. The call came in for a fire in a large two-story wood-frame hardware store. The hardware store was approximately 40 × 30 ft (12 × 9 m) above the ground, with inventory in both the basement and the attic. The hardware store abutted the owner's residence of the same size and construction type. The building was built in the 1940s.

The first-arriving company found fire on the first floor of the hardware store and proceeded with search and rescue operations. Multiple additional companies were immediately requested. The initial water supply consisted of a 1000 gpm (3800 L/min) pump drafting from a large local river. This drafting pump supplied three tankers, all carrying 1200 gallons (4500 L) of water. Due to the short travel distance between the fill site and the fire scene, the tankers were able to initially support the attack engines and four handlines.

Because of the building construction type and the fuels within the structure, the operation was declared defensive. All companies were evacuated from the hardware store and the adjoining residence. Master stream devices were required to suppress the fire and protect the one wooden 80 × 40 ft (24 × 12 m) exposure to the east of the store and a 20 × 30 ft (6 × 9 m) wooden storage shed on the north side. Additional companies laid a large-diameter hose (LDH) line from the initial fill site to the fire scene. A second water supply site was set up to support an additional elevated master stream device. Large flows from the LDH lines enabled constant, uninterrupted water for the defensive operation.

The investigation after the fire found two origins for the fire: one in the hardware store and one in the residence. In the end, the fire was confined to the building(s) of origin, with no loss in the exposed structures. Thanks to the water supply, this fire was suppressed safely.

Todd Poole
Tunbridge Volunteer Fire Department
Tunbridge, Vermont

CHAPTER 3 Types of Fire Apparatus 41

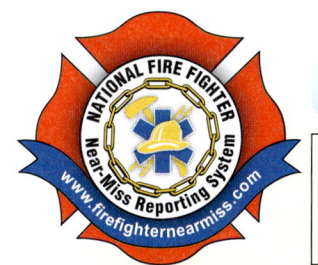

Near-Miss REPORT

Report Number: 08-0000394

Synopsis: Tanker slides off driveway and rolls over.

Event Description: We were responding to a working confirmed barn fire. As we were traveling down the snow covered dirt lane, our 2500-gallon (9464-L) tanker-pumper started to slide off of the actual driveway and onto the farmer's field, about a 2-ft (610-mm) drop. Once the tanker hit flat ground, it rolled over on its passenger side, landing in a 3-ft (1-m) snow drift. Speed was not a factor; neither was driver error. What contributed were the snow-covered narrow driveway and the weight of the tanker. Once it came to rest, the driver and crew, including myself, crawled out of the apparatus. The one fire fighter who was riding in the jump seat was thrown clear of the tanker and landed head first into the snow drift. The only damage that occurred was the right rear compartment door sustained a dent when it hit a big rock under the snow. No one was hurt, and we all stood there in shock, not really believing what had just happened.

Lessons Learned: Be aware of weather conditions and the condition of the road or driveway surface you are traveling on at all times. Also know the restrictiveness of your apparatus (height, weight, and maneuverability).

1901. Most fire departments exceed this list and add equipment that best suits the needs of their jurisdiction.

Mobile Water Supply Apparatus

Many rural communities do not have hydrants or readily accessible water for use at the fire scene. For this reason, fire fighters need fire apparatus with large-capacity water tanks at their disposal. These mobile water supply fire apparatus are commonly referred to as tenders and can provide enough onboard water to extinguish most fires that are held to only one or two bedrooms of a home. When fires are larger and more water is needed, a water shuttle operation may be used by these types of fire apparatus to establish a sustained water supply for fire attack.

Mobile water supply apparatus are defined in NFPA 1901 **FIGURE 3-4**. Such an apparatus may be designed with or without a fire pump. If the mobile water supply apparatus has a fire pump, then that fire pump must meet the criteria stated in NFPA 1901, chapter 16. This type of fire apparatus is designed to carry a large capacity of water to the fire scene. It is equipped with one or more water tanks that meet the requirements of NFPA 1901 and have a minimum certified capacity of 1000 gal (4000 L).

If the mobile water supply apparatus is equipped with a fire pump, then a minimum of 15 ft (4.5 m) of supply hose equipped with hydrant connection threads on one end and pump intake connection threads on the other, or 20 ft (6 m) of hard suction hose with a strainer is carried. Fire hose and nozzles are needed as well. At least 200 ft (60 m) of 2½-inch (65-mm) or larger supply hose must be available on the mobile water supply apparatus. If the mobile water supply apparatus is equipped with a fire pump, 400 ft (120 m) of 1½-inch (45-mm) or 2-inch (52-mm) attack hose and two combination spray nozzles with a minimum capacity of 95 gpm (360 L/min) are required.

Equipment storage is very important. A minimum of 20 ft³ (0.57 m³) of enclosed weather-resistant compartment space must be provided for the storage of equipment. Minor equipment should be organized and mounted in brackets or compartments. At a minimum, to comply with NFPA 1901 the mobile water supply fire apparatus must carry the equipment listed in **TABLE 3-3**. Most fire departments exceed this list and will add equipment that best suits the needs for their jurisdiction.

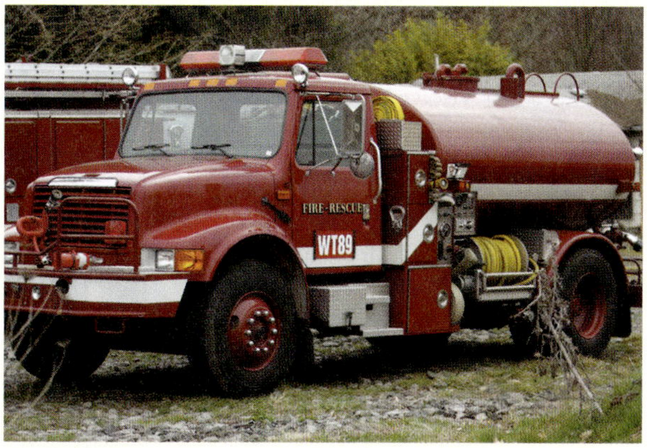

FIGURE 3-4 Mobile water supply apparatus are commonly referred to as tenders, and in the eastern U.S., they are referred to as tankers.

TABLE 3-3	Miscellaneous Equipment on Mobile Water Supply Apparatus
Amount	Equipment
1	6-lb (2.7-kg) pickhead axe mounted in a bracket fastened to the mobile water supply apparatus
1	6-ft (2-m) pike pole or plaster hook mounted in a bracket fastened to the mobile water supply apparatus
2	Portable hand lights mounted in a bracket fastened to the mobile water supply apparatus
1	Approved dry chemical portable fire extinguisher with a minimum 80-B:C rating mounted in a bracket fastened to the mobile water supply apparatus
1	2 1/2-gal (9.5-L) or larger water extinguisher mounted in a bracket fastened to the mobile water supply apparatus
1	SCBA complying with NFPA 1981 for each assigned seating position, but no fewer than 2 units, mounted in a bracket fastened to the mobile water supply apparatus or stored in containers supplied by the SCBA manufacturer
1	Spare SCBA cylinder for each SCBA unit carried, each mounted in a bracket fastened to the mobile water supply apparatus or in a specially designed storage space(s)
1	First-aid kit
2	Combination spanner wrenches mounted in a bracket fastened to the mobile water supply apparatus
1	Hydrant wrench mounted in a bracket fastened to the mobile water supply apparatus
1	Double female adapter, sized to fit 2 1/2-inch (65-mm) or larger fire hose, mounted in a bracket fastened to the mobile water supply apparatus
1	Double male adapter, sized to fit 2 1/2-inch (65-mm) or larger fire hose, mounted in a bracket fastened to the mobile water supply apparatus
1	Rubber mallet, for use on suction hose connections, mounted in a bracket fastened to the mobile water supply apparatus
2	Wheel chocks, mounted in readily accessible locations, each designed to hold the mobile water supply apparatus, when loaded to its maximum in-service weight, on a 10 percent grade with the transmission in neutral and the parking brake released

Aerial Fire Apparatus

With so many multistory buildings in their jurisdictions, what would fire fighters do without ladders? With the growth of city populations, the need for multilevel dwellings increased. Fire fighters relied on ladders to enter the upper levels to fight fires and rescue people. In 1830, Abraham Wivell, an English fire fighter, created the first fly ladder. Wivell's ladder could reach the second story with the main ladder, with the next two flies then being extended to the upper floors. Known as "escapes" in Europe, these ladders became a necessity. All too soon, however, cities began outgrowing this ladder's reach.

In the late 19th century, companies such as Scott-Uda began to design height extension ladders. The Scott-Uda design used eight extensions countered by weights and balances. These aerials were short-lived, as many people died due to their collapse. In 1868, Daniel Hayes successfully patterned an 85-ft (26-m) hand-cranked aerial ladder. As mechanics, pneumatics, and hydraulics became more popular, the race for the perfect aerial ladder began. In 1916, American LaFrance used pneumatics to raise the ladders.

Aerial fire apparatus are defined in NFPA 1901 **FIGURE 3-5**, and may be classified as on aerial ladder, an elevating platform, or a water tower **FIGURE 3-6**. Aerial apparatus may or may not be equipped with a fire pump and/or an on-board water tank. If the aerial fire apparatus is designed with any of these configurations, it is subject to the requirements outlined in specific chapters of NFPA 1901. This chapter discusses the basic fire apparatus without specialties.

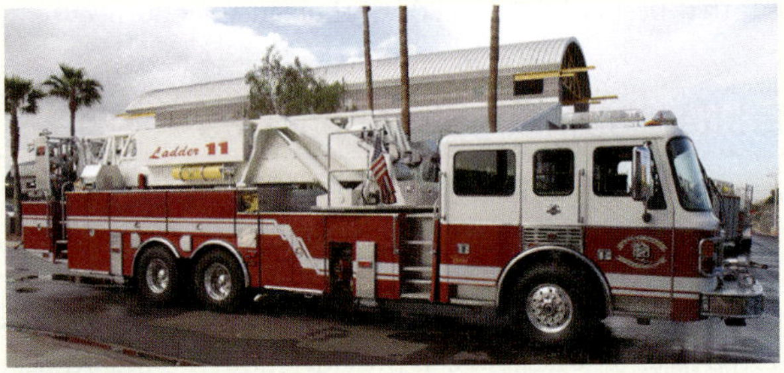

FIGURE 3-5 An aerial apparatus can be configured in many different ways.

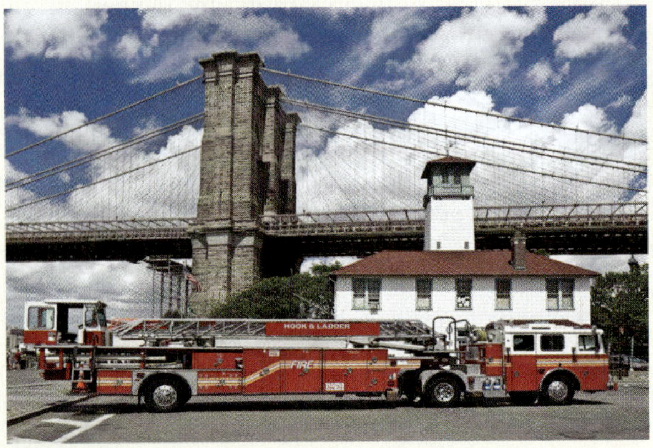

FIGURE 3-6 A tiller is a type of aerial apparatus that is also known as a hook and ladder truck.

To be considered an aerial fire apparatus as defined by NFPA 1901, the apparatus must include, at a minimum, a 115 ft (35 m) total complement of ground ladders that are supplied and installed by the manufacturer. NFPA 1901 states that, at a minimum, the following ladders shall be provided:

- One attic ladder
- Two straight ladders (with folding roof hooks)
- Two extension ladders

All ground ladders shall be mounted with brackets provided by the manufacturer and shall meet all requirements stated in NFPA 1931. In addition, NFPA 1901 states that the apparatus must include a minimum of 40 ft³ (1.1 m³) of enclosed weather-resistant compartment space for equipment storage. These vehicles are designed to assist fire fighters more with support functions than with extinguishment functions while on the fireground. Aerial fire apparatus are designed for search and rescue, forcible entry, and ventilation—all of which are support functions.

The items listed in **TABLE 3-4** are found on the aerial fire apparatus. The equipment listed in the table is the minimum that is required by NFPA 1901. Most fire departments exceed this list and will add equipment that best suits the needs of their jurisdiction. If the fire apparatus is equipped with a fire pump, the equipment in **TABLE 3-5** must be provided to be compliant with NFPA 1901.

TABLE 3-4 Equipment on an Aerial Fire Apparatus

Amount	Equipment
2	6-lb (2.7-kg) or larger flathead axes mounted in brackets fastened to the aerial fire apparatus
3	6-lb (2.7-kg) pickhead axes mounted in brackets fastened to the aerial fire apparatus
4	Pike poles mounted in brackets fastened to the aerial fire apparatus
2	3-ft to 4-ft (1-m to 1.2-m) plaster hooks with D handles mounted in brackets fastened to the aerial fire apparatus
2	Crowbars mounted in brackets fastened to the aerial fire apparatus
2	Claw tools mounted in brackets fastened to the aerial fire apparatus
2	12-lb (5-kg) sledgehammers mounted in brackets fastened to the aerial fire apparatus
4	Portable hand lights mounted in brackets fastened to the aerial fire apparatus
1	Approved dry chemical portable fire extinguisher with a minimum 80-B:C rating mounted in brackets fastened to the aerial fire apparatus
1	2½-gal (9.5-L) or larger water extinguisher mounted in brackets fastened to the aerial fire apparatus
1	SCBA complying with NFPA 1981, for each assigned seating position, but not fewer than 4 units, mounted in brackets fastened to the aerial fire apparatus or stored in containers supplied by the SCBA manufacturer
1	Spare SCBA cylinder for each unit carried, each mounted in brackets fastened to the aerial fire apparatus or stored in a specially designed storage space(s)
1	First-aid kit
6	Salvage covers, each a minimum size of 12 ft × 18 ft (3.6 m × 5.5 m)
4	Combined spanner wrenches mounted in brackets fastened to the aerial fire apparatus
2	Scoop shovels mounted in brackets fastened to the aerial fire apparatus
1	Pair of bolt cutters, 24 inches (0.6 m) at a minimum, mounted in brackets fastened to the aerial fire apparatus
4	Ladder belts meeting the requirements of NFPA 1983, *Standard on Life Safety Rope and Equipment for Emergency Services*
1	150-ft (45-m) light-use life safety rope meeting the requirements of NFPA 1983
1	150-ft (45-m) general-use life safety rope meeting the requirements of NFPA 1983
2	150-ft (45-m) utility ropes having a breaking strength of at least 5000 lb (2300 kg)
1	Box of tools including the following: • One hacksaw with three blades • One keyhole saw • One 12-inch (0.3-m) pipe wrench • One 24-inch (0.6-m) pipe wrench • One ballpeen hammer • One pair of tin snips • One pair of pliers • One pair of lineman's pliers Assorted types and sizes of screwdrivers Assorted adjustable wrenches Assorted combination wrenches
2	Wheel chocks, mounted in readily accessible locations, each designed to hold the aerial fire apparatus, when loaded to its maximum in-service weight, on a 10 percent grade with the transmission in neutral and the parking brake released

TABLE 3-5	Additional Equipment for the Aerial Fire Apparatus
Amount	Equipment
1	Double female 2 1/2-inch (65-mm) adapter with National Hose threads, mounted in a bracket fastened to the aerial fire apparatus
1	Double male 2 1/2-inch (65-mm) adapter with National Hose threads, mounted in a bracket fastened to the aerial fire apparatus
1	Rubber mallet, for use on suction hose connections, mounted in a bracket fastened to the aerial fire apparatus
2	Hydrant wrenches mounted in a bracket fastened to the aerial fire apparatus
Note:	If the supply hose carried does not use sexless couplings, an additional double female adapter and double male adapter, size 2 1/2-inch (65-mm) or larger fire hose, mounted in a bracket fastened to the aerial fire apparatus

Quint Fire Apparatus

What is a quint? Is it a pumper or is it an aerial fire apparatus? Or is it both? This debate began in 1912, when Metz of Germany patented the first quint. In the United States, American LaFrance built its first quint in 1935; Seagrave followed with its own model in 1940. "Quint" is short for "quintuple," meaning five. A quint has five functions associated with it: pump, water tank, fire hose storage, aerial, and ground ladders.

NFPA 1901 defines what an apparatus needs to be defined as a **quint** FIGURE 3-7. As previously discussed, the quint is equipped with a fire pump. This standard states that the fire pump shall meet the fire pump requirements and shall have a rated capacity of 1000 gpm (4000 L/min). NFPA 1901 also states that the quint shall be equipped with an aerial ladder or elevating platform with a permanently installed waterway, as well as a water tank that has a minimum certified capacity of 300 gal (1100 L). The quint shall carry a minimum total complement of 85 ft (26 m) of ground ladders, to include at least one extension ladder, one straight ladder equipped with roof hooks, and one attic ladder; all of these ladders must satisfy the requirements in NFPA 1931.

Because the quint has a fire pump, hose is a necessity, consisting of a minimum of 15 ft (4.5 m) of supply hose equipped with hydrant connection threads on one end and pump intake connection threads on the other with compatible couplings, or 20 ft (6 m) of hard suction hose with strainer. It is up to the purchaser to specify whether hard or soft suction will be provided. TABLE 3-6 lists the fire hose and nozzles that must be carried on a quint.

Like the pumper, the quint must have a minimum of 40 ft^3 (1.1 m^3) of enclosed weather-resistant compartment space for storage of equipment. This fire apparatus will need some of the same equipment required for a pumper and an aerial apparatus. NFPA 1901 specifies that the miscellaneous equipment listed in TABLE 3-7 shall be carried on a quint. This equipment is the minimum that is required by NFPA 1901; most fire departments exceed this list and will add equipment that best suits the needs for their jurisdiction.

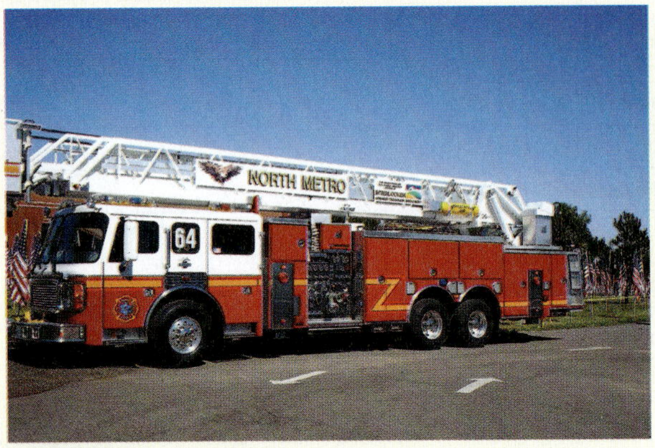

TABLE 3-6	Fire Hose and Nozzles for the Quint
Amount	Hose
	800 ft (240 m) of 2 1/2-inch (65-mm) or larger supply hose, in any combination 400 ft (120 m) of 1 1/2-inch (38-mm), 1 1/2-inch (45-mm), or 2-inch (50-mm) attack hose, in any combination
1	Combination spray nozzle, 200 gpm (750 L/min) minimum
2	Combination spray nozzles, 95 gpm (360 L/min) minimum
1	Playpipe with shut-off and 1-inch (25-mm), 1 1/8-inch (29-mm), and 1 1/2-inch (32-mm) tips

FIGURE 3-7 A quint has five functions associated with it: pump, water tank, fire hose storage, aerial, and ground ladders.

Special Service Fire Apparatus

The special service fire apparatus is designed for a particular purpose and does not quite fit into the other categories FIGURE 3-8. For example, a hazardous materials apparatus or a heavy technical rescue apparatus would fall into this category. The majority of the special service fire apparatus is devoted to providing compartment space for the unique equipment that it carries. However, if the fire apparatus is to be equipped with a fire pump, then the fire pump shall meet all of the requirements listed in NFPA 1901, chapter 16. If the special service fire apparatus is equipped with ground ladders, it shall meet all of the requirements listed in NFPA 1931.

TABLE 3-7 Miscellaneous Equipment on the Quint

Amount	Equipment
1	6-lb (2.7-kg) flathead axe mounted in a bracket fastened to the quint
1	6-lb (2.7-kg) pickhead axe mounted in a bracket fastened to the quint
1	6-ft (2-m) pike pole or plaster hook mounted in a bracket fastened to the quint
1	8-ft (2.4-m) or longer pike pole or plaster hook mounted in a bracket fastened to the quint
2	Portable hand lights mounted in a bracket fastened to the quint
1	Approved dry chemical portable fire extinguisher with a minimum 80-B:C rating mounted in a bracket fastened to the quint
1	2½-gal (9.5-L) or larger water extinguisher mounted in a bracket fastened to the quint
1	SCBA complying with NFPA 1981, for each assigned seating position, but not fewer than 4 units, mounted in brackets fastened to the quint or stored in containers supplied by the SCBA manufacturer
1	Spare SCBA cylinder for each unit carried, each mounted in brackets fastened to the quint or stored in a specially designed storage space(s)
1	Spare SCBA cylinder for each SCBA unit carried
1	First-aid kit
4	Combination wrench mounted in a bracket fastened to the quint
2	Hydrant wrenches mounted in a bracket fastened to the quint
2	Double female 2½-inch (65-mm) adapter with National Hose threads, mounted in a bracket fastened to the quint
1	Double male 2½-inch (65-mm) adapter with National Hose threads, mounted in a bracket fastened to the quint
1	Rubber mallet, for use on suction hose connections, mounted in a bracket fastened to the quint
4	Salvage covers, each a minimum size of 12 ft × 14 ft (3.7 m × 4.3 m)
4	Ladder belts meeting the requirements of NFPA 1983
1	150-ft (45-m) light-use safety rope meeting the requirements of NFPA 1983
1	150-ft (45-m) general-use safety rope meeting the requirements of NFPA 1983
2	Wheel chocks, mounted in readily accessible locations, each designed to hold the quint, when loaded to its maximum in-service weight, on a 10 percent grade with the transmission in neutral and the parking brake released

Because the primary function of this fire apparatus is to supply a certain type of equipment for the incident, it is required to have more compartment space than the other types of fire service apparatus. NFPA 1901 states it must have a minimum of 120 ft³ (3.4 m³) of enclosed, weather-resistant compartment space for storage of equipment. According to NFPA 1901, the minimum equipment that must be carried comprises the items listed in **TABLE 3-8**. Most fire departments exceed this list and will add equipment that best suits the needs of their jurisdiction.

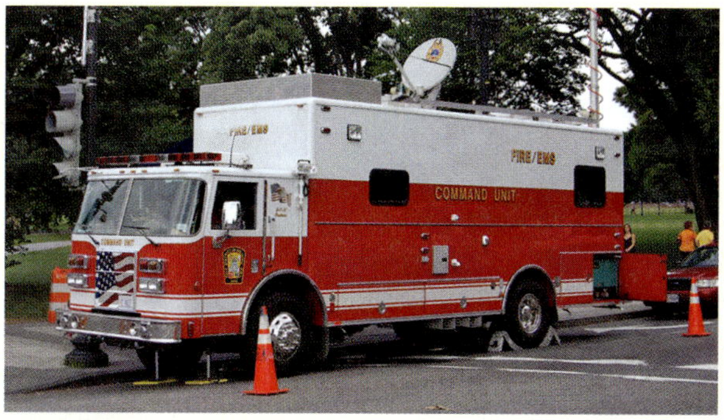

FIGURE 3-8 The special service fire apparatus is designed for a particular purpose and does not quite fit into the other categories.

TABLE 3-8 Minimum Equipment on a Special Service Fire Apparatus

Amount	Equipment
2	Portable hand lights mounted in a bracket fastened to the special service fire apparatus
1	Approved dry chemical portable fire extinguisher with a minimum 80-B:C rating mounted in a bracket fastened to the special service fire apparatus
1	2½-gal (9.5-L) or larger water extinguisher mounted in a bracket fastened to the special service fire apparatus
1	SCBA complying with NFPA 1981, for each assigned seating position, but not fewer than 4 units, mounted in brackets fastened to the special service fire apparatus or stored in containers supplied by the SCBA manufacturer
1	Spare SCBA cylinder for each unit carried, each mounted in brackets fastened to the special service fire apparatus or stored in a specially designed storage space(s)
1	First-aid kit
2	Wheel chocks, mounted in readily accessible locations, each designed to hold the special service fire apparatus, when loaded to its maximum in-service weight, on a 10 percent grade with the transmission in neutral and the parking brake released

Mobile Foam Fire Apparatus

The mobile foam fire apparatus is a fire apparatus with a permanently mounted fire pump, foam proportioning system, and foam concentrate tank(s) whose primary purpose is use in the control and extinguishment of flammable and combustible liquid fires in storage tanks and other flammable liquid spills **FIGURE 3-9**. The mobile foam fire apparatus can be configured with or without an aerial device. Its job is to deliver foam immediately at the scene without requiring fire fighters to attach special containers or change nozzles. This task may be accomplished through use of a turret attached to the top of the mobile foam fire apparatus or an aerial device that extends to reach the fire; both can be operated from inside the cab of the fire apparatus. This type of apparatus is also commonly referred to as an aircraft rescue and firefighting (ARFF) vehicle.

The mobile foam fire apparatus, as defined in NFPA 1901, shall be equipped with a fire pump that has a minimum rated capacity of 750 gpm (3000 L/min), or an industrial supply pump that meets the requirements of NFPA 1901. Because the mobile foam fire apparatus is designed to produce foam, a foam proportioning system is needed. The mobile foam fire apparatus shall be equipped with one or more foam concentrate tanks that meet the NFPA requirements and have a minimum capacity (combined if applicable) of 500 gal (2000 L).

A minimum of 15 ft (4.5 m) of supply hose equipped with hydrant connection threads on one end and pump intake connection threads on the other with compatible couplings, or 20 ft (6 m) of hard suction hose with strainer shall be carried on the mobile foam fire apparatus. NFPA 1901 identifies the fire hose and nozzles to be carried on the mobile foam fire apparatus, which are also listed in **TABLE 3-9**.

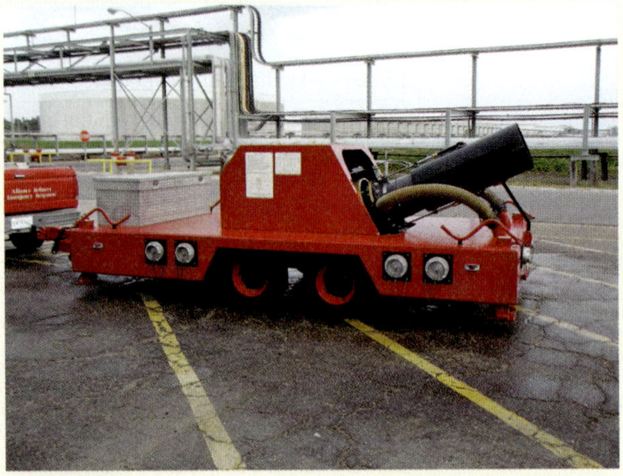

Equipment storage on a mobile foam fire apparatus must include a minimum of 40 ft³ (1.13 m³) of enclosed weather-resistant compartment space. According to NFPA 1901, the minimum equipment that must be carried comprises the items listed in **TABLE 3-10**. Most fire departments exceed this list and will add equipment that best suits the needs of their jurisdiction.

FIGURE 3-9 The mobile foam fire apparatus is a fire apparatus with a permanently mounted fire pump, foam proportioning system, and foam concentrate tank(s).

TABLE 3-9	Equipment on Mobile Foam Fire Apparatus
Amount	**Equipment**
	800 ft (240 m) of 2½-inch (65-mm) or larger supply hose, in any combination 400 ft (120 m) of 1½-inch (38-mm), 1¾-inch (45-mm), or 2-inch (50-mm) attack hose, in any combination
4	Foam or spray nozzles, 200 gpm (750 L/min)
2	Foam or spray nozzles, 95 gpm (360 L/min)
1	Preconnected monitor, rated to discharge a minimum of 1000 gpm (4000 L/min), mounted on top of the fire apparatus with a spray or foam nozzle rated at a minimum of 1000 gpm (4000 L/min)

TABLE 3-10	Minimum Equipment on Mobile Foam Fire Apparatus
Amount	Equipment
1	6-lb (2.7-kg) pickhead axe mounted in a bracket fastened to the mobile foam fire apparatus
1	6-ft (2-m) pike pole or plaster hook mounted in a bracket fastened to the mobile foam fire apparatus
2	Portable hand lights mounted in a bracket fastened to the mobile foam fire apparatus
1	Approved dry chemical portable fire extinguisher with a minimum 80-B:C rating mounted in a bracket fastened to the mobile foam fire apparatus
1	SCBA complying with NFPA 1981, for each assigned seating position, but not fewer than 4 units, mounted in a bracket fastened to the mobile foam fire apparatus
1	Spare SCBA cylinder for each SCBA unit carried, each mounted in a bracket fastened to the mobile foam fire apparatus or stored in a specially designed storage space
1	First-aid kit
4	Combination wrench mounted in a bracket fastened to the mobile foam fire apparatus
2	Hydrant wrenches mounted in a bracket fastened to the mobile foam fire apparatus
1	Double female 2½-inch (65-mm) adapter with National Hose threads, mounted in a bracket fastened to the mobile foam fire apparatus
1	Double male 2½-inch (65-mm) adapter with National Hose threads, mounted in a bracket fastened to the mobile foam fire apparatus
1	Rubber mallet, for use on suction hose connections, mounted in a bracket fastened to the mobile foam fire apparatus
2	Wheel chocks, mounted in readily accessible locations, each designed to hold the mobile foam fire apparatus, when loaded to its maximum in-service weight, on a 10 percent grade with the transmission in neutral and the parking brake released

Wrap-Up

Chief Concepts

- To obtain a fire apparatus that meets the needs of your fire department, you must work closely with the apparatus manufacturer.
- The fire pump is the key component in getting water from the fire apparatus, through the hose, and onto the fire.
- The pumper is the most common fire apparatus and is a part of almost every fire department.
  - The pumper is used on small fires such as dumpster fires, vehicle fires, and brush fires in urban settings.
  - It is also the main source of fire attack for larger fires that involve structures.
- The initial attack fire apparatus is utilized much like the pumper, but its specifications are much different. This type of apparatus is designed to be more maneuverable than the pumper, especially in off-road terrain.
- Mobile water supply fire apparatus (commonly referred to as tenders) provide enough onboard water to extinguish most fires that are held to only one or two bedrooms of a home.
- An aerial fire apparatus is a vehicle equipped with an aerial ladder, elevating platform, or water tower that is designed and equipped to support firefighting and rescue operations by positioning personnel, handling materials, providing continuous egress, or discharging water at positions elevated from the ground.
- A quint has five functions associated with it: pump, water tank, fire hose storage, aerial, and ground ladders.
- The special service fire apparatus is designed for a particular purpose and does not quite fit into the other categories. For example, a hazardous materials apparatus or a heavy technical rescue apparatus would fall into this category.
- The mobile foam fire apparatus is a fire apparatus with a permanently mounted fire pump, foam proportioning system, and foam concentrate tank(s), whose primary purpose is for use in the control and extinguishment of flammable and combustible liquid fires in storage tanks and other flammable liquid spills.

Hot Terms

aerial fire apparatus A vehicle equipped with an aerial ladder, elevating platform, or water tower that is designed and equipped to support firefighting and rescue operations by positioning personnel, handling materials, providing continuous egress, or discharging water at positions elevated from the ground.

aerial ladder A self-supporting, turntable-mounted, power-operated ladder of two or more sections permanently attached to a self-propelled automotive fire apparatus and designed to provide a continuous egress route from an elevated position to the ground.

aircraft rescue and firefighting (ARFF) vehicle A vehicle intended to carry rescue and firefighting equipment for rescuing occupants and combating fires in aircraft at, or in the vicinity of, an airport.

chassis The basic operating motor vehicle, including the engine, frame, and other essential structural and mechanical parts, but exclusive of the body and all appurtenances for the accommodation of driver, property, passengers, appliances, or equipment related to other than control. Common usage might, but need not, include a cab (or cowl).

fire apparatus A fire department emergency vehicle used for rescue, fire suppression, or other specialized functions.

initial attack fire apparatus Fire apparatus with a fire pump of at least 250 gpm (1000 L/min) capacity, water tank, and hose body, whose primary purpose is to initiate a fire suppression attack on structural, vehicular, or vegetation fires, and to support associated fire department operations.

miscellaneous equipment Portable tools and equipment carried on a fire apparatus, not including suction hose, fire hose, ground ladders, fixed power sources, hose reels, cord reels, breathing air systems, or other major equipment or components specified by the purchaser to be permanently mounted on the apparatus as received from the apparatus manufacturer.

mobile foam fire apparatus Fire apparatus with a permanently mounted fire pump, foam proportioning system, and foam concentrate tank(s), whose primary purpose is use in the control and extinguishment of flammable and combustible liquid fires in storage tanks and other flammable liquid spills.

mobile water supply apparatus A vehicle designed primarily for transporting (pickup, transporting, and delivering) water to fire emergency scenes to be applied by other vehicles or pumping equipment. Also known as a tanker or tender.

pumper fire apparatus Fire apparatus with a permanently mounted fire pump of at least 750 gpm (3000 L/min) capacity, water tank, and hose body, whose primary purpose is to combat structural and associated fires.

quint Fire apparatus with a permanently mounted fire pump, a water tank, a hose storage area, an aerial ladder or elevating platform with a permanently mounted waterway, and a complement of ground ladders.

References

National Fire Protection Association (NFPA) 1002, *Standard for Fire Apparatus Driver/Operator Professional Qualifications*. 2014. http://www.nfpa.org/codes-and-standards/document-information-pages?mode=code&code=1002. Accessed March 27, 2014.

National Fire Protection Association (NFPA) 1901, *Standards for Automotive Fire Apparatus*. 2009. http://www.nfpa.org/codes-and-standards/document-information-pages?mode=code&code=1901. Accessed March 27, 2014.

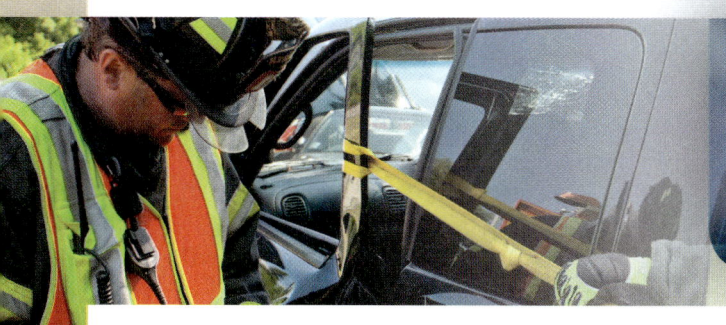

National Fire Protection Association (NFPA)1931, *Standard for Manufacturer's Design of Fire Department Ground Ladders*. 2010. http://www.nfpa.org/catalog/product.asp?pid=193110. Accessed March 27, 2014.

National Fire Protection Association (NFPA) 1981, *Standard on Open-Circuit Self-Contained Breathing Apparatus for Fire and Emergency Services*. 2013. http://www.nfpa.org/catalog/product.asp?pid=198113. Accessed March 27, 2014.

National Fire Protection Association (NFPA) 1983, *Standard on Life Safety Rope and Equipment for Emergency Services*. 2012. http://www.nfpa.org/codes-and-standards/document-information-pages?mode=code&code=1983. Accessed March 27, 2014.

DRIVER/OPERATOR in action

The committee has worked hard over the last few weeks to design a fire apparatus that will meet the needs of your community. During the last formal committee meeting, you discuss some of the detailed information that you have learned with the other committee members:

1. Which of the following is not one of the specifications that the jurisdiction must specify to the manufacturer?
   - **A.** Additional equipment requested that exceeds the minimum requirements
   - **B.** The specific performance requirements
   - **C.** Electrical load specifications
   - **D.** The number of fire fighters who will ride on the exterior of the apparatus

2. All NFPA 1901-compliant fire apparatus must be capable of attaining a minimum top speed of ___mph (km/h).
   - **A.** 35 (56)
   - **B.** 40 (64)
   - **C.** 50 (80)
   - **D.** 68 (109)

3. What is the minimum amount of tank water a pumper should hold?
   - **A.** 200 gal (800 L)
   - **B.** 1000 gal (4000 L)
   - **C.** 500 gal (2000 L)
   - **D.** 300 gal (1200 L)

4. A quint and an aerial fire apparatus carry the same total complement of ground ladders.
   - **A.** True
   - **B.** False

5. Which NFPA standard covers automotive fire apparatus?
   - **A.** NFPA 1002
   - **B.** NFPA 1021
   - **C.** NFPA 1901
   - **D.** NFPA 1931

Water

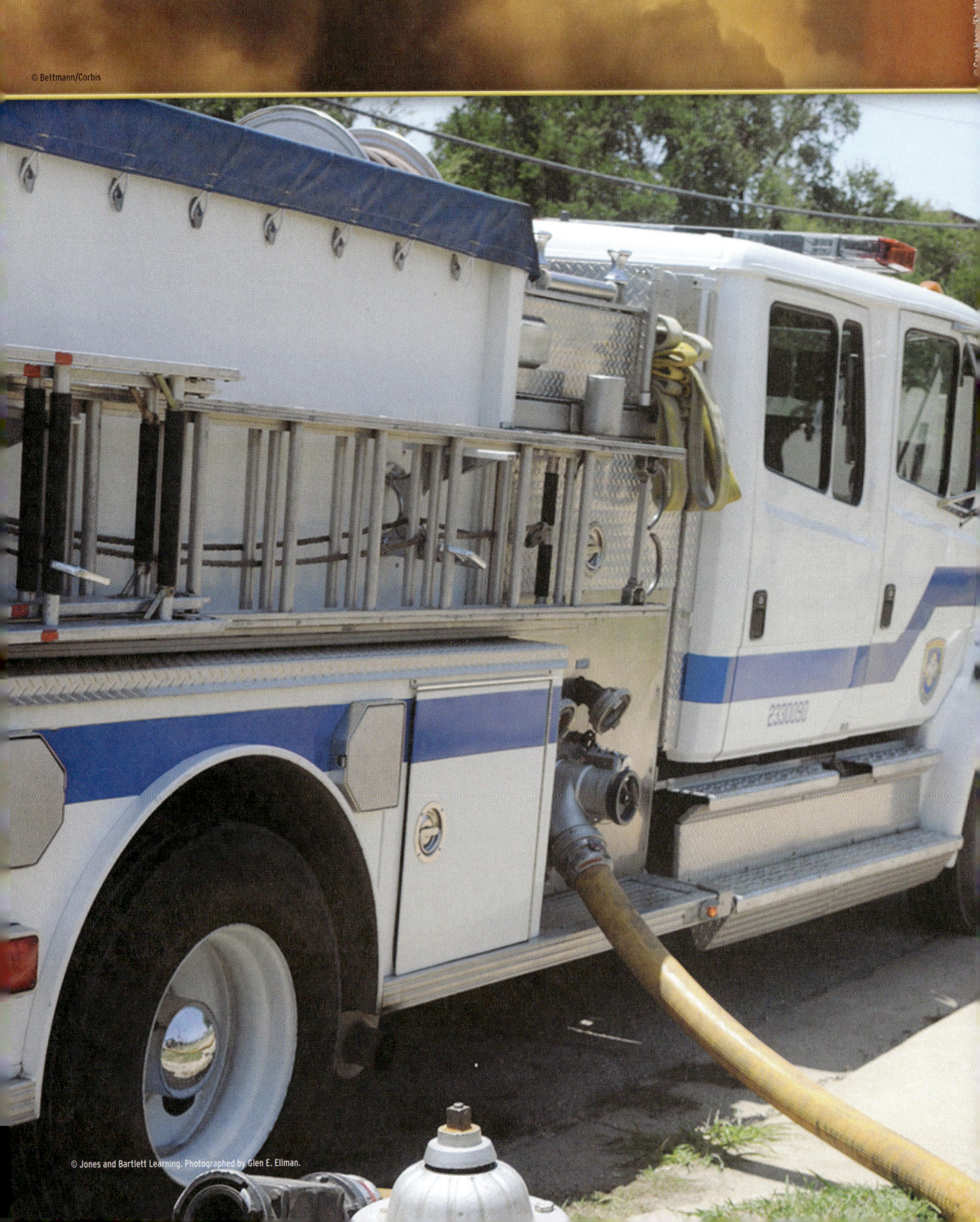

CHAPTER 4

Knowledge Objectives

After studying this chapter, you will be able to:

- Describe the properties of water. (p 53–54)
- Describe water's role in extinguishing a fire. (p 52–53)
- Describe the major features of a municipal water supply system. (p 54–56)
- Discuss the six principles of fluid pressure. (p 56–58)
- Discuss static pressure, residual pressure, flow pressure, and normal operating pressure. (p 58–59)
- Describe dry-barrel fire hydrants and wet-barrel hydrants. (p 59–61)
- Discuss maintaining and testing a fire hydrant. (p 62, 64–68)

Skills Objectives

After studying this chapter, you will be able to:

- Operate a hydrant. (p 61–63)
- Shut down a hydrant. (p 62, 64)
- Demonstrate how to obtain the static pressure. (p 66–68)
- Demonstrate the correct use of a Pitot gauge. (p 66, 68–69)

Additional NFPA Standards

- NFPA 291, *Recommended Practice for Fire Flow Testing and Marking of Hydrants*

You Are the Driver/Operator

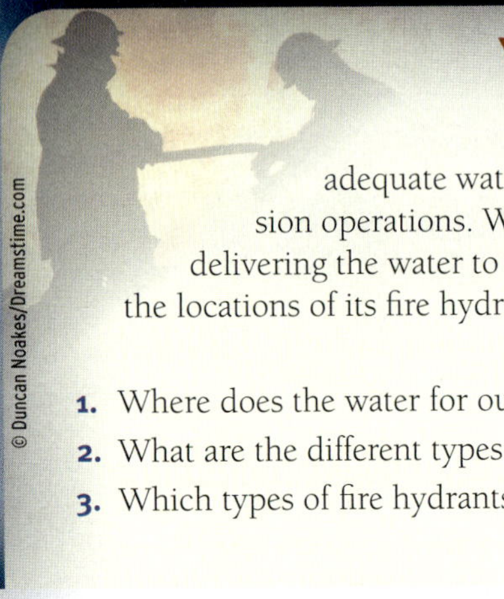

You are the driver in an engine company assigned to a district on the edge of town. Companies from the stations in the surrounding areas will have to travel a long distance to respond to your district. As the first-arriving engine company, it is essential that you establish an adequate water supply as soon as possible. You know that an adequate water supply is critical for fire suppression operations. Without water, the fire fighters cannot extinguish the fire. As the driver/operator, your job is safely delivering the water to the fire fighters from the pump on your apparatus. While reviewing the map of your district and the locations of its fire hydrants, several questions start to pop into your head.

1. Where does the water for our fire suppression activities come from?
2. What are the different types of fluid pressures that I will encounter?
3. Which types of fire hydrants will I encounter in my response district?

Introduction

The importance of a dependable and adequate **water supply** for fire suppression operations is self-evident. The hoseline is not just the primary weapon for fighting a fire; it is also the fire fighter's primary defense against being burned or driven out of a burning building. The basic plan for fighting most fires depends on having an adequate supply of water to confine, control, and extinguish the fire. If the water supply is interrupted while crews are working inside a building, fire fighters could be trapped, injured, or killed. Fire fighters entering a burning building need to be confident that their water supply is both reliable and adequate to operate hoselines for their protection and to extinguish the fire.

Ensuring a dependable water supply is a critical fireground operation that must be accomplished as soon as possible. A water supply should be established at the same time as the other initial fireground operations take place. At many fire scenes, the processes of size-up, forcible entry, raising ladders, search and rescue, ventilation, and establishing a water supply all occur concurrently.

At any scene, you will obtain water from one of two means: pressurized systems and **static water sources**. Pressurized sources may be either **municipal water systems** or **private water systems**, which furnish water under pressure through fire hydrants FIGURE 4-1. Static water supplies are sources such as lakes, ponds, rivers, and streams. These resources serve as drafting sites for fire department apparatus to obtain and deliver water to the fire scene. Often, the water carried in the tanks of the first-arriving vehicles is used in the initial attack. Although many fires are successfully controlled using tank water, this tactic does not ensure the ongoing adequacy and reliability of the water supply throughout the incident. The establishment of an adequate, continuous water supply then becomes the primary objective to support the fire attack FIGURE 4-2. The operational

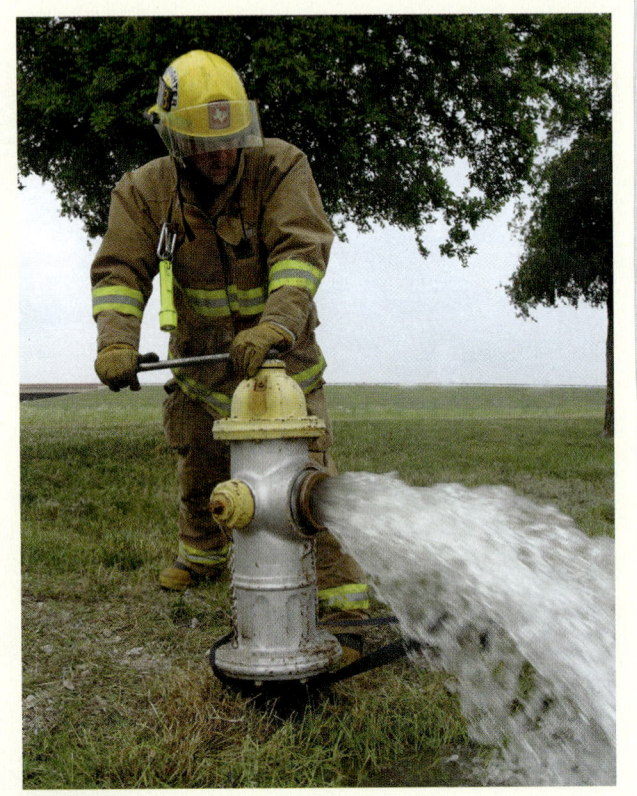

FIGURE 4-1 The water that comes from a hydrant is provided by a municipal or private water system.

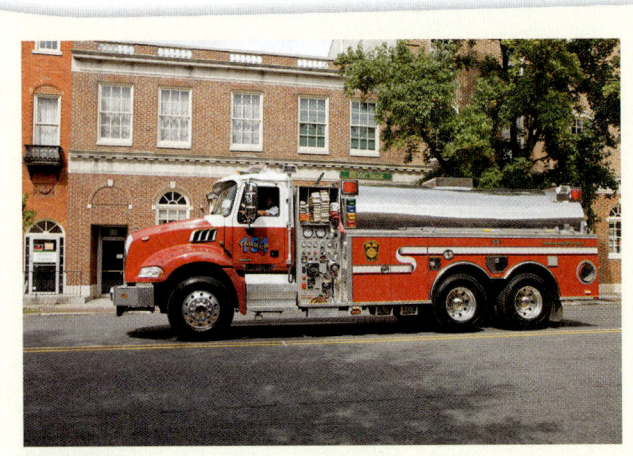

FIGURE 4-2 Mobile water supply fire apparatus can deliver large quantities of water to the scene of the fire.

plan must ensure that an adequate and reliable water supply is available before the tank is empty.

Chemical Properties of Water

Approximately 70 to 75 percent of the earth's surface is covered by water. Water is so abundant that it is often easy to take for granted. According to the U.S. Geological Survey, the U.S. population consumes 408 billion gallons of water per day.

Water is a virtually colorless, odorless, and tasteless liquid. It has many hidden qualities contained in its chemical description: H_2O. That is, in water, one atom of oxygen is bound to two atoms of hydrogen attached on the same side. This arrangement gives the water molecule a positive charge at the hydrogen side and a negative charge on the oxygen side **FIGURE 4-3**. Opposite electrical charges attract each other (hydrogen bonding), making water molecules stick to one another. As a result of this attraction, the bond between the molecules becomes stronger and forms a surface film that makes it more difficult to move an object through the surface than to move it when it is completely submersed. This **surface tension** allows water to flow, puddle, and remain together even after leaving a nozzle. It is not until gravity acts upon the water stream that it starts to break up into smaller droplets. Likewise, as water is heated, the surface tension decreases. The lower surface tension allows the water to soak into an object with which it comes into contact, rather than just skating over its outer surface.

The bond between hydrogen and oxygen in water is so strong that water dissolves more substances than any other liquid. As water passes through or moves by a substance, the positive and negative charges of the molecule take the various chemicals, minerals, and solvents along with it, thus earning water the title of **universal solvent**. For example, pour a teaspoon of salt into a glass of water and note the result: The salt dissolves into the water. The mixing of the water molecules with the sodium chloride causes the sodium and chloride molecules to separate from each other and be carried away in the solution. Whether a substance dissolves into water is determined by whether the substance's components can break the hydrogen bond of water. If they cannot, the substance's molecules pass among the water molecules but do not dissolve (i.e., interact with the water molecules). Substances dissolved in water are referred to as **aqueous**. For example, Class A foam dissolves in water, which reduces the water's surface tension and allows it to saturate the fuel.

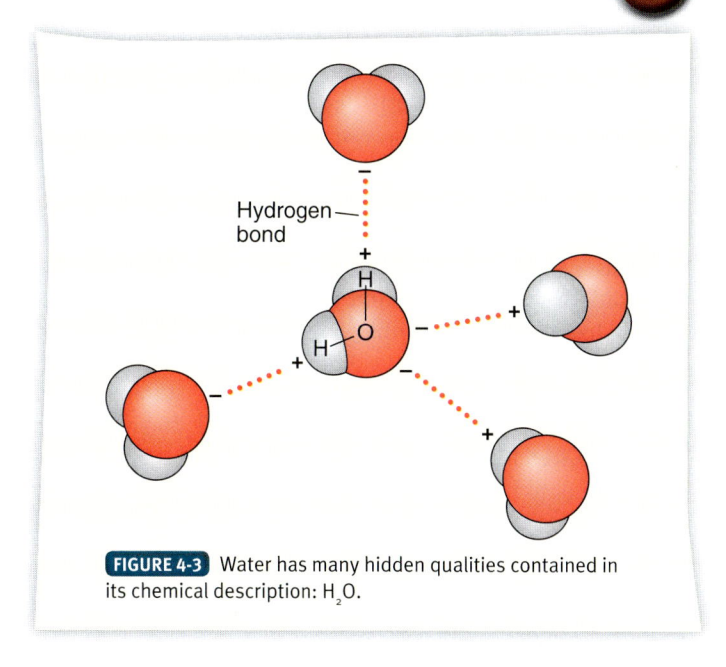

FIGURE 4-3 Water has many hidden qualities contained in its chemical description: H_2O.

Water has been used as the primary extinguishing agent in the fire service from the earliest days, mostly because of its widespread availability. Water, however, possesses other properties that make it ideal for extinguishing fires. For example, water is able to absorb heat because of its hydrogen-bonding characteristics. The amount of heat energy required to increase the temperature of a substance is known as its **specific heat index**. Water has one of the highest specific heat indexes of any known chemical compound. For example, sodium bicarbonate—a chemical once used in fire extinguishers—has a specific heat index of 0.22; water's specific heat index is 1. Thus it would take almost five times as much heat to raise the temperature of water as it does to raise the temperature of an equal amount of sodium bicarbonate. Simply stated, water absorbs almost five times more heat than sodium bicarbonate.

■ Physical Properties of Water

Water exists in all three property states on earth: liquid (oceans, rivers), gas (clouds), and solid (ice) **FIGURE 4-4**. All three property states affect the use of water in firefighting operations. Water in its liquid form weighs 8.33 pounds (3.79 kg) per gallon, adding 6248 pounds [3.124 tons (2839 kg)] of weight to the chassis of an engine with a 750-gallon (2840-L) tank—1 L of water weighs 1 kg, and 1000 kg = 1 metric ton (or tonne).

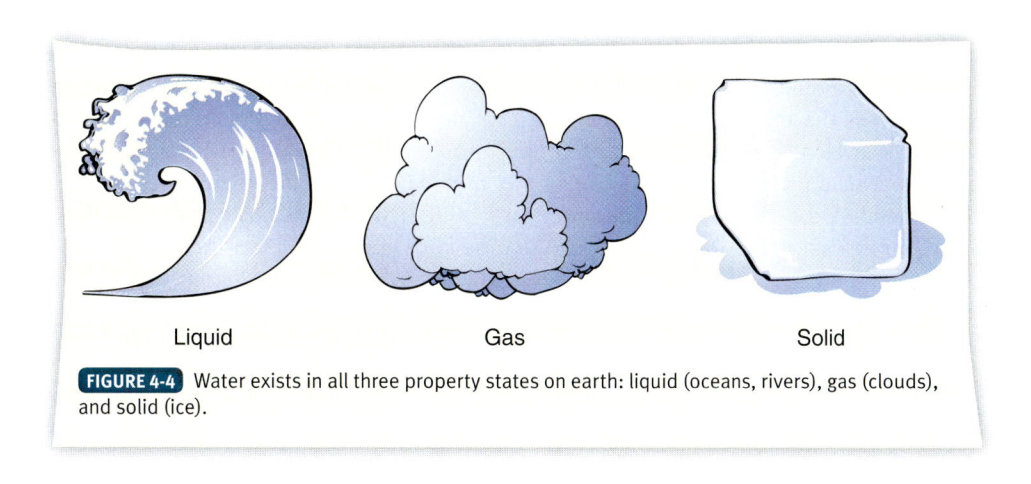

Liquid Gas Solid

FIGURE 4-4 Water exists in all three property states on earth: liquid (oceans, rivers), gas (clouds), and solid (ice).

Temperature has a significant effect on the weight of water. Water at 32°F (0°C) is almost one-half pound per cubic foot heavier than water at 100°F (38°C). Water freezes at 32°F (0°C). When in its solid form, it has a unique characteristic: Water is less dense as a solid than it is as a liquid. The molecular geometry of water when frozen causes ice to float—a very unique property. With a few exceptions, most other substances are denser when in solid form compared to their liquid form. In addition, water freezes from the top down as it gradually cools. Open lakes, for example, freeze from the top down and the ice thickens over time.

On the other end of the heat spectrum, water boils at 212°F (100°C) at sea level (184.4°F [84°C] at an altitude of 14,000 feet [4300 m]). Whereas its high heat absorption allows water to have notable cooling effects, water may also be converted to a gas (steam) through the application of heat, an effect attributable to its high **heat of vaporization**.

In summary, water is the primary substance used to extinguish a fire for the following reasons:

- Water turns to a vapor (steam) when it comes in contact with a fire. The volume of water vapor is 1700 times greater than that of an equal amount of liquid water; as a consequence, water displaces oxygen and effectively smothers the fire.
- Water absorbs heat and cools the smoke, air, and room and its contents, thereby reducing the ignition temperature and decreasing the amount of fuel available for continued combustion.
- The water molecules in steam vapor carry the elements of smoke with them as the steam is ventilated from the area.

■ Harmful Characteristics of Water

A common misconception is that water is a good conductor of electricity. Technically, pure H_2O has a relatively low ability to conduct electricity. Thus the ability of water to conduct electrical current actually depends on the amount of dissolved solids in the water. Salt water, for example, is highly conductive.

The amount of particulate matter suspended in water is known as **turbidity**. The color of the water is directly related to the level of turbidity present. Limestone turns water turquoise, whereas iron compounds turn water reddish-brown, copper compounds create an intense blue color, and algae commonly color the water green. Turbidity also affects the care and maintenance of the fire pump. As the particulates settle in the pump housing and water tank, they start to cause a breakdown of valves, gaskets, seals, and piping, which can lead to leaks and operational deficiencies.

Another effect that water has on pump maintenance derives from its **hardness**. The amount of dissolved calcium and magnesium, which increases the mineral content within water, determines the water's level of hardness. The surface tension of "hard water" is lower than that of pure water, which in turn allows for more minerals to be present. The presence of these minerals may ultimately affect the operation of fire pumps, valves, and piping. As the calcium collects in equipment over time, it starts breaking down the seals; when not regularly exercised, the valves begin to stick.

Water will also allow galvanic corrosion to take place. Galvanic corrosion takes place when two dissimilar metals are immersed in water. An example is the stainless steel piping and the cast pump casing. This essentially creates an electrical charge, and an electrical current will flow between the two metals. Sacrificial anodes prevent or limit the flow between the two metals, thus limiting the erosion or pitting of the metals.

Municipal Water Systems

Municipal water systems make clean water available to people in populated areas and provide water for fire protection. As the name suggests, most municipal water systems are owned and operated by a local government agency, such as a city, county, or special water district. Some municipal water systems are privately owned; however, the basic design and operation of both private and government systems are very similar.

Municipal water supplies domestic water to homes, commercial establishments, and industries. These systems typically make the same water supply available for fire department use through hydrants and may also supply building fire protection systems, such as automatic sprinkler systems and standpipes. In some instances, municipal water systems may exist solely to provide water for fire protection and may not have domestic water function. A municipal water system consists of three components: the water source, the treatment plant, and the distribution system.

DRIVER/OPERATOR Tip

Driver/operators are responsible for modern fire apparatus, which are complex and costly pieces of equipment. Water quality plays a large role in the wear and tear placed on a fire pump; the design of the apparatus, preventative maintenance, and your role in caring for the vehicle can significantly reduce wear and tear. The corrosion process that takes place in municipal water systems may introduce scale and sediment into the pump, while water from static sources may introduce debris. Designing the apparatus with protective features like pump anodes (sacrificial metal pieces intended to prevent corrosion of the pump components and piping), flushing the pump after using static sources, and conducting regular preventative maintenance based on the pump manufacturer's recommendations will go a long way towards ensuring the safety and reliability of your apparatus.

■ Water Sources

Municipal water systems can draw water from wells, rivers, streams, lakes, or human-made storage facilities called **reservoirs**. The source will depend on the geographic and hydrologic features of the area. Many municipal water systems draw water from several sources to ensure a sufficient supply. Underground pipelines or open canals supply some cities with water from sources that are many miles away.

The water source for a municipal water system needs to be large enough to meet the total demands of the service area. Most municipal water systems include large storage facilities, which are intended to ensure they will be able to meet the community's water supply demands if access to the primary water source is interrupted. The backup supply for some systems can provide water for several months or years; in other systems, this supply may last for only a few days.

FIGURE 4-5 Impurities are removed at the water treatment facility.

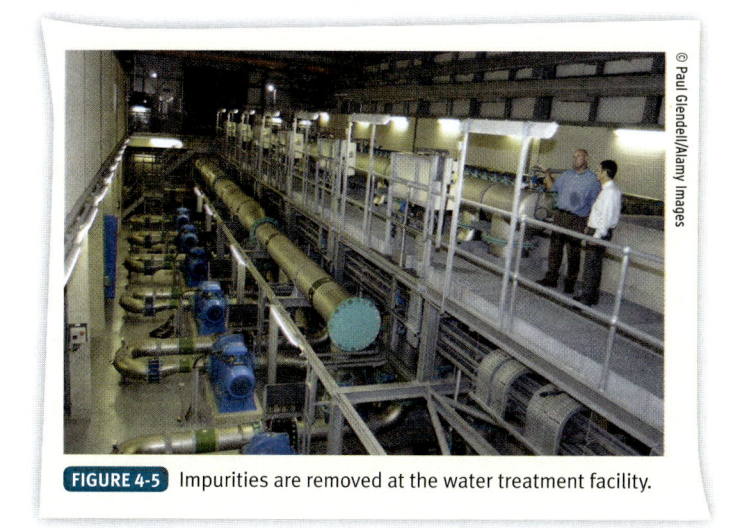

FIGURE 4-6 A gravity-feed system can deliver water to a low-lying community without the need for pumps.

■ Water Treatment Facilities

Municipal water systems also include a water treatment facility, where impurities from the water are removed **FIGURE 4-5**. The nature of the water treatment system depends on the quality of the untreated source water. Water that is clean and clear from the source requires little treatment. By comparison, other systems must use extensive filtration to remove impurities and foreign substances. Some treatment facilities use chemicals to remove impurities and improve the water's taste. In the end, all of the water in the system must be suitable for drinking. Chemicals also are used to kill bacteria and harmful organisms and to keep the water pure as it moves through the distribution system to individual homes or businesses. After the water has been treated, it enters the distribution system.

■ Water Distribution System

The distribution system delivers water from the treatment facility to the end users and fire hydrants through a complex network of underground pipes, known as **water mains**. In most cases, the distribution center also includes pumps, storage tanks, reservoirs, and other necessary components to ensure that the required volume of water can be delivered where and when it is needed, at the required pressure.

Water pressure requirements differ, depending on how the water will be used. Generally, the water pressure ranges from 20 pounds per square inch (psi) (140 kPa) to 80 psi (560 kPa) at the delivery point. Driver/operators must understand their water distribution systems and typical operating pressures; however it is recommended that hydrants have a minimum operating pressure of 20 psi (140 kPa).

Most water distribution systems rely on an arrangement of pumps to provide the required pressure, either directly or indirectly. Some water distribution systems use pumps to supply direct pressure. If the pumps stop operating, the pressure is lost, and the system will be unable to deliver the adequate water to the end users or to hydrants. Most municipal systems have multiple pumps and backup power supplies to reduce the risk of a service interruption due to a pump failure. The extra pumps can sometimes be used to boost the flow for a major fire or a high-demand period.

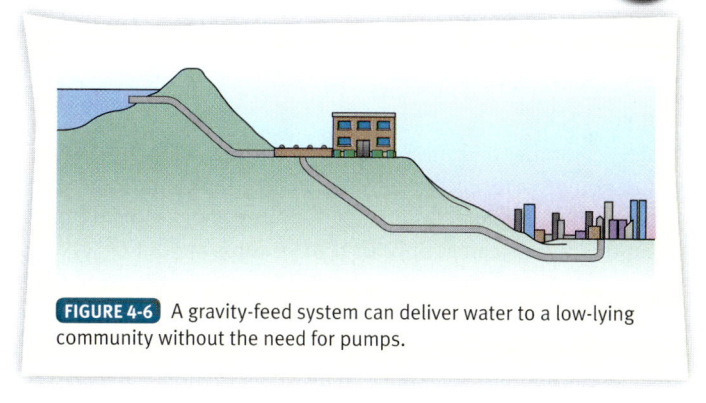

In a **gravity-feed system**, the water source, treatment plant, and storage facilities are located on high ground while the end users live in lower-lying areas, such as a community in a valley **FIGURE 4-6**. This type of system may not require any pumps, because gravity, through the elevation differentials, provides the pressure necessary to deliver the water. In some systems, the elevation pressure is so high that pressure-control devices are needed to keep from over-pressurizing parts of the system.

Most municipal water supply systems use a combination of pumps and gravity to deliver water. Pumps may be used to deliver the water from the treatment plant to **elevated water storage towers** or to reservoirs located on hills or high ground areas. The elevated storage facilities maintain the desired water pressure in the distribution system, so that water can be delivered under pressure, even if the pumps are not operating **FIGURE 4-7**. When the elevated storage facilities need

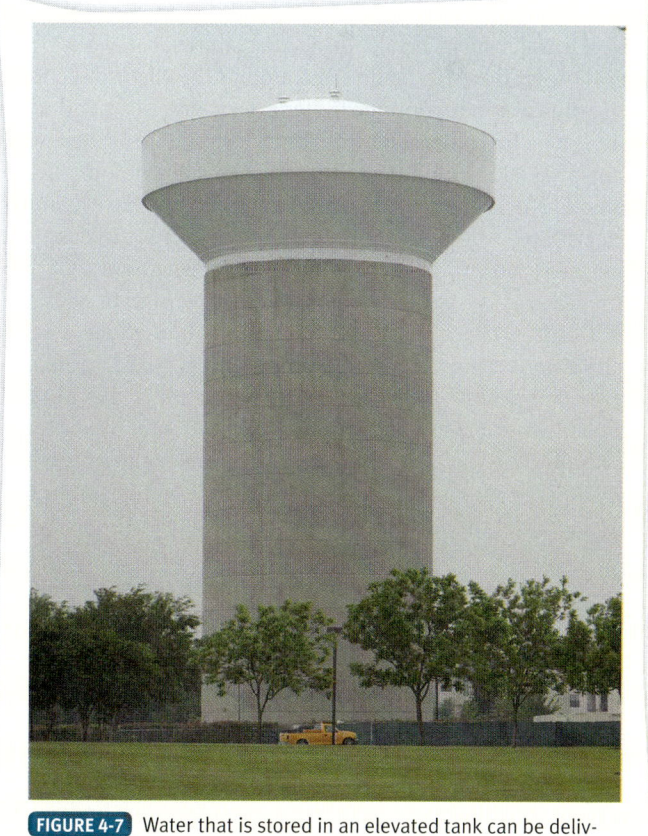

FIGURE 4-7 Water that is stored in an elevated tank can be delivered to the end users under pressure.

refilling, large supply pumps are used. Additional pumps may be installed to increase the pressure in particular areas, such as a booster pump that provides extra pressure to deliver water to a hilltop neighborhood.

A combination pump-and-gravity-feed system must maintain enough water in the elevated storage tanks and reservoirs to meet the anticipated demands. If more water is being used than the pumps can supply, or if the pumps are out of service, some systems will be able to operate for several days using only their elevated storage reserves, whereas others will be able to function for only a few hours.

The underground water mains that deliver water to the end users come in several different sizes. Large mains, known as <u>primary feeders</u>, carry large quantities of water to a section of the town or city. Smaller mains, called <u>secondary feeders</u>, distribute the water to a smaller area. The smallest pipes, called <u>distributors</u>, carry water to the users and hydrants along individual streets.

The size of the water mains required depends on the amount of water needed both for normal consumption and for fire protection in that location. Most jurisdictions specify the minimum-size main that can be installed in a new municipal water system to ensure an adequate flow. Other municipal water systems, however, may have undersized water mains in older areas of the community. You must know the arrangement and capacity of the water systems in your department's response areas.

Water mains in a well-designed system will follow a grid pattern. A grid arrangement provides water flow to a fire hydrant from two or more directions and establishes multiple paths from the source to each area. This helps to ensure an adequate flow of water for firefighting. In addition, the grid design helps to minimize downtime for the other portions of the system if a water main breaks or needs maintenance work. With a grid, water flow can be diverted around the affected section.

Some water distribution systems may have dead-end water mains, which supply water from only one direction. Such water mains may also be found in the outer reaches of a municipal system. Hydrants on a dead-end water main will have a limited water supply. If two or more hydrants on the same dead-end main are used to fight a fire, the upstream hydrant will have more water and water pressure than the downstream hydrants.

Control valves installed at intervals throughout a water distribution system allow different sections to be turned off or isolated. These valves are used when a water main breaks or when work must be performed on a section of the system.

<u>Shut-off valves</u> are located at the connection points where the underground mains meet the distributor pipes. Shut-off valves control the flow of water to individual customers or to individual fire hydrants **FIGURE 4-8**. If the water system in a building or to a fire hydrant is damaged, fire fighters can close the shut-off valves to prevent further water flow.

The fire department should notify the water department when fire operations will require prolonged use of large quantities of water. The water department may be able to increase the normal volume and/or pressure by starting additional pumps. In some systems, the water department can open valves to increase the flow to a certain area in response to fire department operations at major fires.

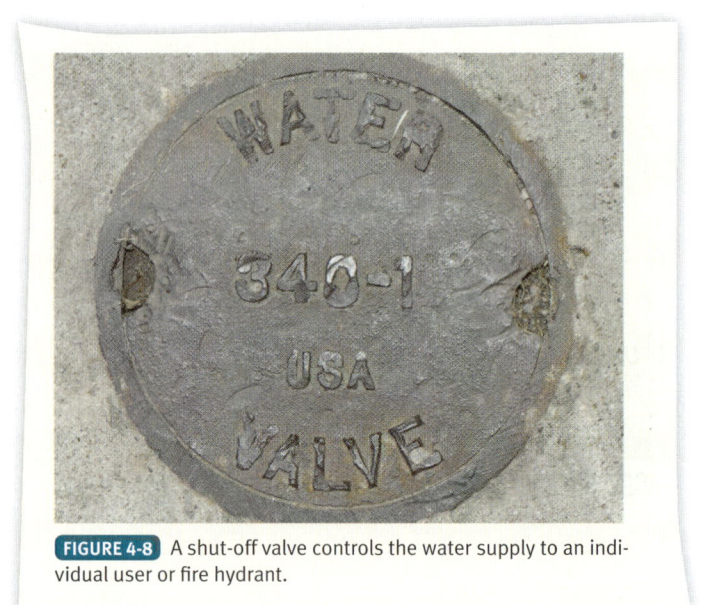

FIGURE 4-8 A shut-off valve controls the water supply to an individual user or fire hydrant.

Fluid Dynamics

<u>Water pressure</u> refers to the force per unit area, and is measured in psi (or kilopascals [kPa]). The <u>water flow</u> or quantity of water moving through a pipe, hose, or fittings is measured by its <u>volume</u>, usually in terms of gallons (or liters) per minute. Pressure and flow are two different but mathematically related measurements. As a driver, you need to understand how pressure and flow relate to one another.

Water that is not moving has potential energy. When the water is moving, it has a combination of <u>potential energy</u> and <u>kinetic energy</u>. The following six principles of fluid pressure will help you to better understand the affect pressure has on fluids.

- **Principle 1: Fluid pressure is exerted perpendicular to any surface on which it acts.** This means that the pressure of the water acts at right angles on its container. For example, if you had a container of water with flat sides, the water will exert pressure at right angles to the sides **FIGURE 4-9**. If it did not, the water would simply flow out of the container or bunch up in the center.

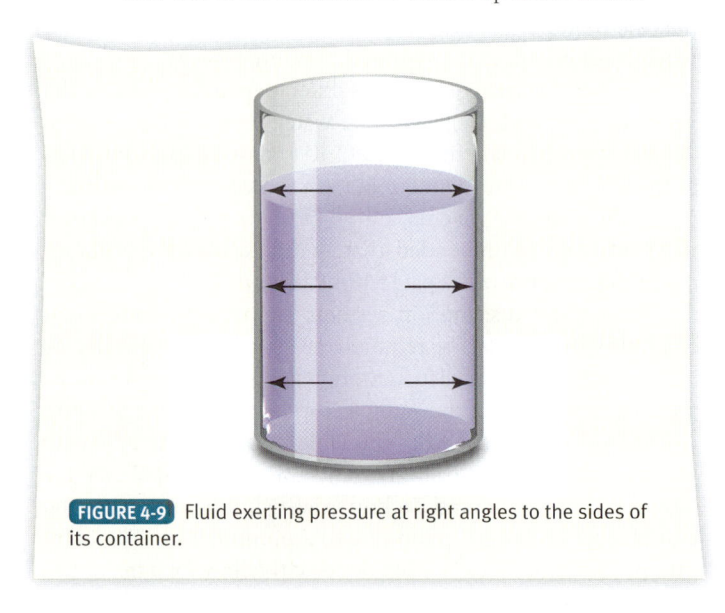

FIGURE 4-9 Fluid exerting pressure at right angles to the sides of its container.

CHAPTER 4 Water   57

FIGURE 4-10 Water pressure is exerted in all directions equally, which gives the fire hose its shape.

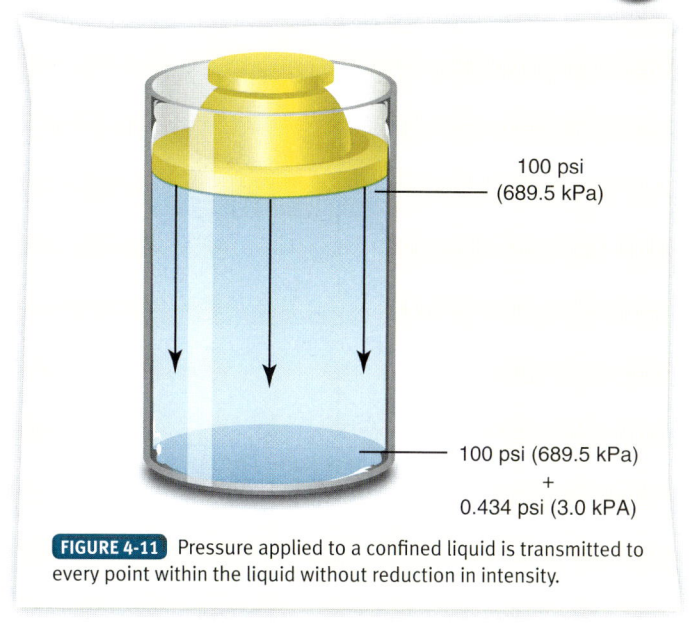

FIGURE 4-11 Pressure applied to a confined liquid is transmitted to every point within the liquid without reduction in intensity.

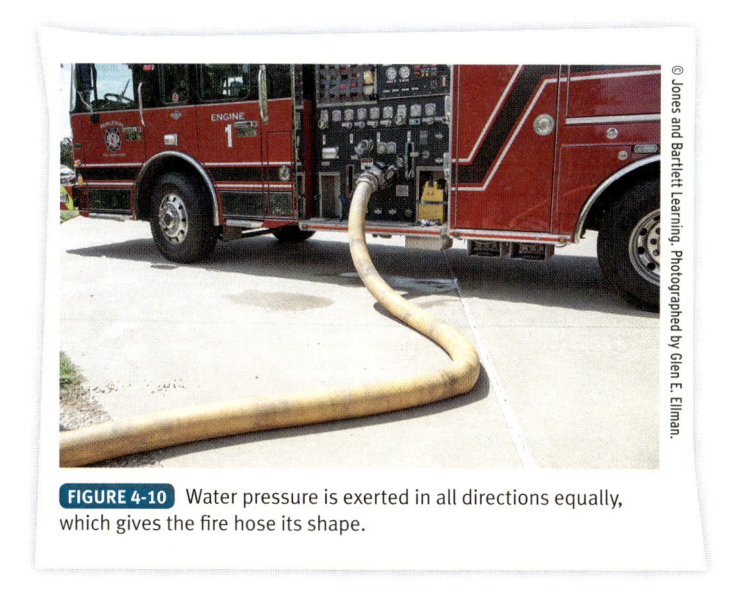

- **Principle 2: Pressure in a fluid acts equally in all directions.** For example, when filling a fire hose with water, the pressure inside is equal in all directions and fills the hose to the shape of the container—that is, the cylindrical hose **FIGURE 1-10**.
- **Principle 3: Pressure applied to a confined fluid from without is transmitted equally in all directions.** If, for example, a 1-ft (0.3-m)-tall cylinder of water is filled and no pressure is applied from the top, the water at the top of the cylinder would be at 0 psi (0 kPa) and the water at the bottom would have a pressure of 0.434 psi (3.0 kPa), because the weight of a 1-square-inch (645-mm^2) column of water exerts a pressure at the bottom of 0.434 psi (3.0 kPa). If the top of the cylinder was now closed and 100 psi (689.5 kPa) of pressure was applied from the top, the water at the top would also have 100 psi (689.5 kPa), and the water at the very bottom would have a pressure of 100.434 psi (692.5 kPa). If pressure is applied to a confined liquid, that pressure is transmitted to every point within the liquid without reduction in intensity **FIGURE 4-11**.
- **Principle 4: The pressure of a liquid in an open vessel is proportional to the depth of the liquid.** This means that if you have a cylinder filled with water that is 1 ft (0.3 m) tall, the pressure at the bottom of the cylinder would be 0.434 psi (3.0 kPa). If you had another cylinder filled with water that was 2 ft (0.6 m) tall, the water pressure at the bottom would be 0.868 psi (6.0 kPa). If you had a third container that was 3 ft (0.9 m) tall and filled with water, the pressure at the bottom would be 1.302 psi (9.0 kPa) **FIGURE 4-12**.

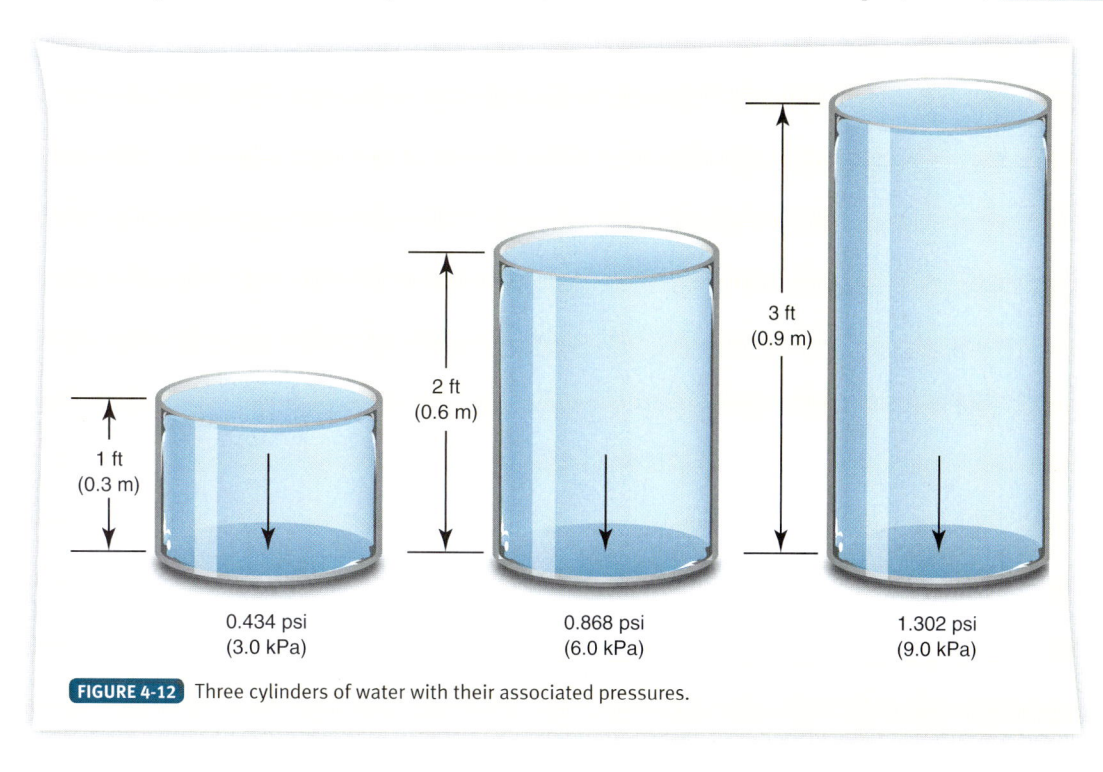

FIGURE 4-12 Three cylinders of water with their associated pressures.

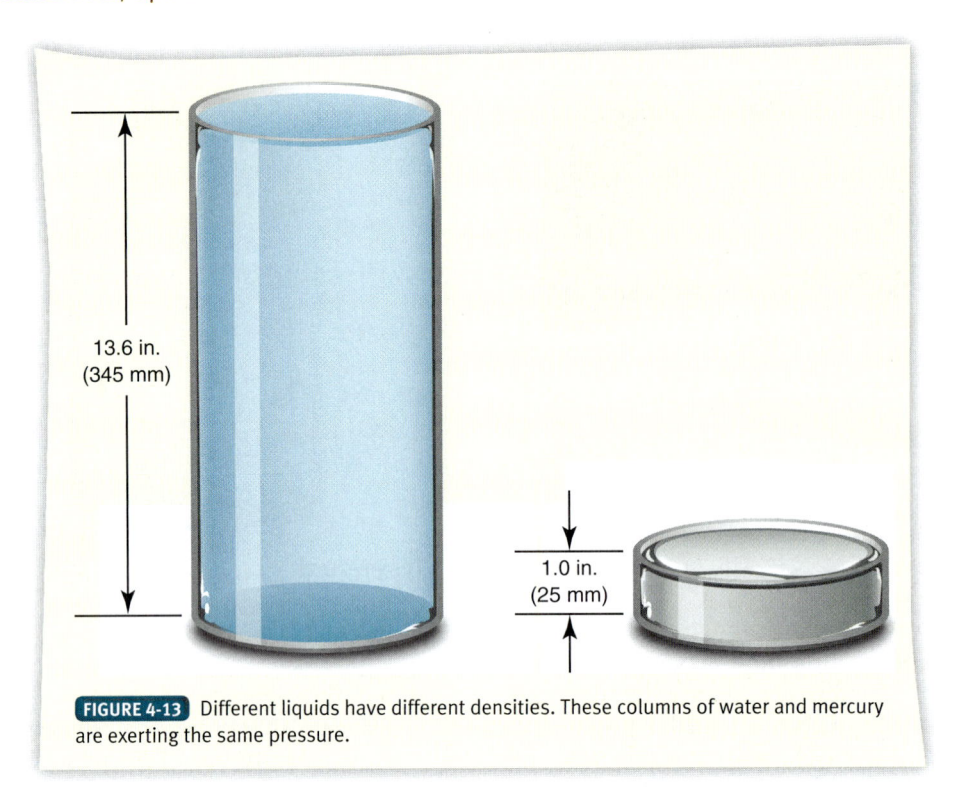

FIGURE 4-13 Different liquids have different densities. These columns of water and mercury are exerting the same pressure.

- **Principle 5: The pressure of a liquid in an open container is proportional to the density of the liquid.** Different liquids have different densities, so the pressure they exert at the same elevation also differs. For example, mercury is much denser than water. It would take a column of water 13.6 inches (345 mm) tall to exert the same pressure as a column of mercury only 1 inch (25 mm) tall **FIGURE 4-13**.
- **Principle 6: Liquid pressure on the bottom of a container is unaffected by the size and shape of the container.** Only the distance between the top and the bottom of the liquid—not the shape or size of the container—has any effect on the pressure. Along the horizontal plane of the container, the pressure is always the same **FIGURE 4-14**.

<u>Static pressure</u> is the pressure in a system when the water is not moving. Static pressure is potential energy, because it would cause the water to move if there were some place the water could go. This type of pressure causes the water to flow out of an opened fire hydrant. If there was no static pressure, nothing would happen when the hydrant was opened.

Static pressure is generally created by <u>elevation pressure</u> and/or pump pressure. An elevated storage tank, for example,

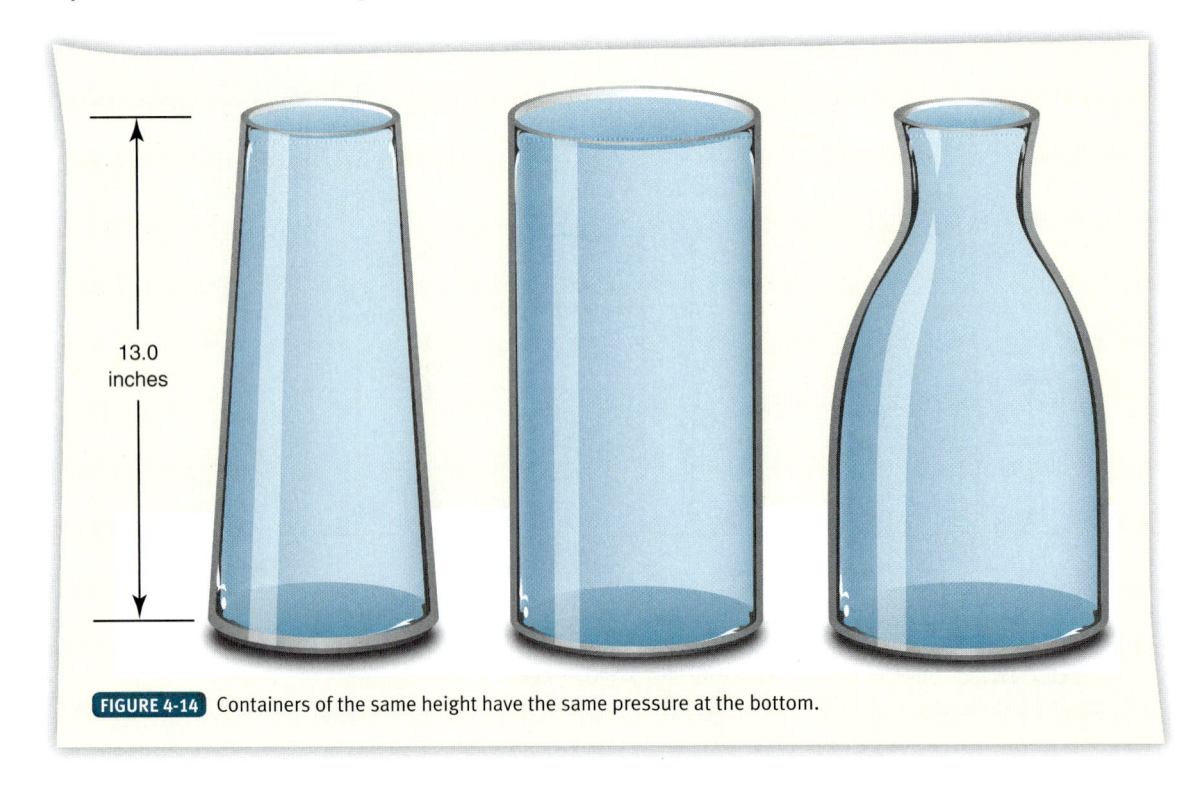

FIGURE 4-14 Containers of the same height have the same pressure at the bottom.

creates elevation pressure in the water mains. Gravity continues to exert its effects on flowing water based on the stream's elevation and altitude. For the driver/operator, elevation refers to the position of the pump (above or below) as it relates to the nozzle. Pressure will increase when the nozzle is below the location of the pump and decrease when the nozzle is above the location of the pump. Atmospheric pressure changes depending on the location of the pump as compared to sea level. Atmospheric pressure drops as altitude increases, and this drop in pressure causes pumps to work harder to generate the same pressures at lower altitudes. Atmospheric pressure decreases approximately 0.5 psi (3.4 kPa) for every 1000 ft (305 m) that the geographic location rises above sea level. Gravity also creates elevation pressure in the water system as the water flows from a hilltop reservoir to the water mains in the valley below. Pumps create pressure by bringing the energy from an external source into the system.

Placing a pressure gauge on a hydrant port and opening the hydrant valve can measure static pressure in a water distribution system. No water can be flowing out of the hydrant when the static pressure is measured; static pressure measured in this way assumes that there is no flow in the system. Because municipal water systems deliver water to hundreds or thousands of users, there is almost always water flowing within the system. Thus, in most cases, a static pressure reading is actually measuring the normal operating pressure of the system.

Normal operating pressure refers to the amount of pressure in the water distribution system during a period of normal consumption. In a residential neighborhood, for example, people are constantly using water to care for lawns, wash clothes, bathe, and do other normal household activities. In an industrial or commercial area, normal consumption occurs during a normal business day as water is used for various purposes. The system uses some of the static pressure to deliver this water to residents and businesses. A pressure gauge connected to a hydrant during a period of normal consumption will indicate the normal operating pressure of the system.

As a fire fighter, you need to know how much pressure will be in the system when a fire occurs. Because the regular users of the system will be drawing off a normal amount of water even during firefighting operations, the normal operating pressure is sufficient for measuring available water.

Residual pressure is the amount of pressure that remains in the system when the water is flowing. For example, when you open a hydrant and start to draw large quantities of water out of the system, some of the potential energy of still water is converted into the kinetic energy of moving water. However, not all of the potential energy turns into kinetic energy; some of it is used to overcome friction in the pipes. The pressure remaining after this loss is subtracted while the water is flowing is the residual pressure.

Residual pressure is an important measurement because it provides the best indication of how much more water is available in the system. The more water that is flowing, the less residual pressure there is. In theory, when the maximum amount of water is flowing, the residual pressure is zero, and there is no more potential energy to push more water through the system. In the fire service, 20 psi (140 kPa) is considered the minimum usable residual pressure, as this level reduces the risk of damage to underground water mains or pumps.

Flow pressure is the forward pressure measured at a discharge opening while water is moving. When a stream of water flows out through an opening (known as an orifice), all of the pressure is converted to kinetic energy. When a fire hydrant is opened and water flows freely into the street, the flow pressure can be measured to determine the actual volume of water flowing. To calculate the volume of water flowing, use a Pitot gauge to measure the pressure at the center of the water stream as it passes through the opening and then factor in the size and flow characteristics of the orifice. Pressure acts in all directions equally. If you know the static pressure, the flow in gallons (liters) per minute, and the residual pressure, you can calculate the amount of water that can be obtained from a hydrant or a group of hydrants on the same water main (this subject is discussed further in the chapter *Fireground Operations*).

When water is flowing through hoses, pipes, and fittings, the water is slowed by the contact it has with the walls of the hose or pipe, which results in **friction loss**. This loss is further defined as the drop in pressure while the water maintains its speed (velocity). The result of the interaction between the hose or pipe and the flowing water is a reduction in pressure at the point of discharge. The farther the water must flow through the hose or pipe, the greater the friction loss will be.

Water hammer is a pressure surge or wave caused by the kinetic energy of a fluid in motion when it is forced to stop or change direction suddenly. Quickly closing valves, nozzles, or hydrants can create damaging pressure spikes, leading to blown diaphragms, seals, and gaskets and destroyed hoses, piping, and gauges. Liquids, for the most part, are not compressible; any energy that is applied to a liquid is instantly transmitted back through it. This energy becomes dynamic in nature when a force created by, for example, quickly closing a valve or a nozzle applies velocity to the fluid. This is why nozzles and valves must be closed slowly and all large-diameter discharge gates are required to be slow-open and -close types of valves.

> **Safety Tip**
>
> Water hammer is a serious condition that can cause injuries on the fireground. Improperly closing valves at the pump panel can result in hoselines bursting. Many driver/operators work right next to the hoselines that discharge from the pump. A burst line may injure the driver/operator as well as endanger crews operating in the fireground area. Opening and closing all valves slowly will prevent water hammer.

Fire Hydrants

Fire hydrants provide water for firefighting purposes. Public hydrants are part of the municipal water distribution system and draw water directly from the public water mains. Hydrants also can be installed on private water systems supplied by the municipal water system or from a separate source. The water source as well as the adequacy and reliability of the supply to private hydrants must be identified to ensure that they will be sufficient in fighting fires.

Most fire hydrants consist of an upright steel casing (barrel) attached to the underground water distribution

VOICES OF EXPERIENCE

During the 1990s, I participated in one of the most rewarding experiences of my fire service career; assisting in building the fire service for the Riviera Mia region of Mexico. This included Playa Del Carmen, Cozumel, Tulum, and other Quintana Roo communities on the Yucatan peninsula.

The volunteer effort was led by Captain Bill Salmon of Poudre Fire Authority in Ft. Collins, Colorado, who coordinated a team of trainers, mechanics, and equipment delivery for a 2-week fire academy held every year. My contributions focused on water delivery. Attempting to replace a 5-gallon (19-L) bucket brigade approach with sustained effective fire streams was a daunting task.

The Colorado Fire Mechanic volunteers did an amazing job getting the trucks, pumps, and equipment into serviceable condition. Basic hose and nozzle handling was taught, as well as basic hydraulics, drafting, and water supply. This is when a significant problem was identified. There are no fire hydrants in these communities. Domestic water is delivered to community residents in Peepas, or 1000-gallon (3785-L) water trucks that fill cisterns at a maximum rate of 50 gpm (190 L/min). While most buildings have cisterns and many of the resorts have swimming pools, few were accessible to draft from. The majority of the cities' larger buildings were built within a quarter mile of the ocean; however 100 ft (30 m) of sandy beach made this water inaccessible as well. Clearly, a solution to adequately supply the two pumpers after the booster tank water was gone was needed.

The answer was found in a newly released appliance by Turbo Draft. By redesigning an old forest fire and shipboard firefighting eductor, designers created a tool that would provide 600 to 800 gpm (2271 to 3028 L/min) from a water source up to 150 ft (46 m) away. This was the key to solve our problem. The first engine went to the fire and initiated fire attack, while the second engine went to the closest swimming pool or beach access point. A pickup truck loaded with 2000 ft (610 m) of 3-inch (76-mm) hose laid a supply line between the two. What was a limited 50 gpm (190 L/min) supply was increased 10-fold to an effective 500 gpm (1893 L/min) supply. Problem solved!

Ron Lindroth
Central Valley Fire District
Belgrade, Montana

system. The two main types of hydrants are the dry-barrel hydrant and the wet-barrel hydrant. All hydrants are equipped with one or more valves to control the flow of water through the hydrant. One or more outlets are provided to connect fire department hoses to the hydrant. The outlets may be of various sizes depending upon the local jurisdiction, although two 2½-inch (65-mm) connections and one larger connection (4½-, 5-, or 6-inch [114-, 127-, or 154-mm]) are common.

■ Dry-Barrel Hydrants

Dry-barrel hydrants are used in climates where temperatures can be expected to fall below the freezing level. The valve that controls the flow of water into the barrel of this type of hydrant is located at the base, below the frost line, to keep the hydrant from freezing. The length of the barrel depends on the climate and the depth of the valve. Water enters the barrel of the hydrant only when it will be used. Turning the nut on the top of the hydrant rotates the operating stem, which opens the valve so that the water flows up into the barrel of the hydrant.

Whenever this kind of hydrant is not in use, the barrel must remain dry. If the barrel contains standing water, it will freeze in cold weather and render the hydrant inoperable. After each use, the water drains out through an opening at the bottom of the barrel. The drain is fully open when the hydrant valve is fully shut. When the hydrant valve is fully opened, the drain closes, which prevents water from being forced out of the drain when the hydrant is under pressure.

A partially opened valve means that the drain is also partially open, so pressurized water can flow out. This kind of drainage can erode (undermine) the soil around the base of the hydrant and may damage the hydrant. For this reason, a dry-barrel hydrant should always be either fully opened or fully closed. A fully opened hydrant also makes maximum flow available to fight a fire.

Most dry-barrel hydrants have only one large valve controlling the flow of water **FIGURE 4-15**. Each outlet must be connected to a hose or an outlet valve, or have a hydrant cap firmly in place before the valve is turned on. Many fire departments place valves on all hydrant outlets so that additional connections can be made after the hydrant is charged and water is flowing through the hose attached to the first outlet. Some departments use special hydrant-assist valves such that connections can be made to a fire department pumper in order to boost low hydrant supply pressure.

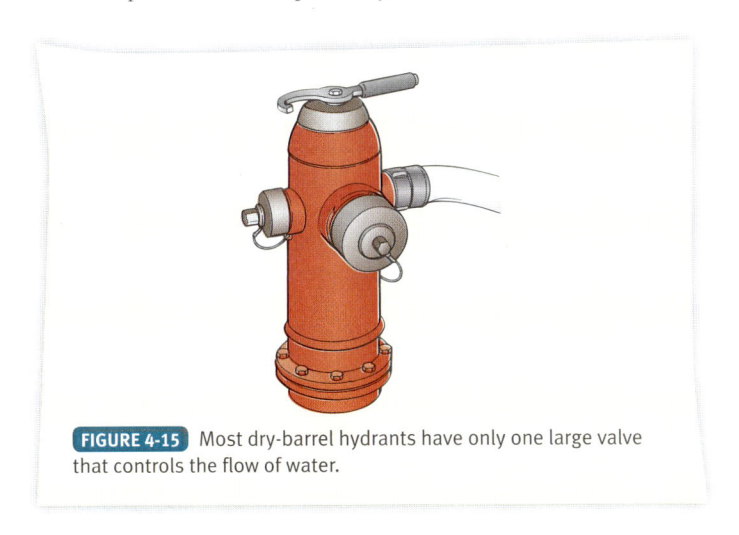

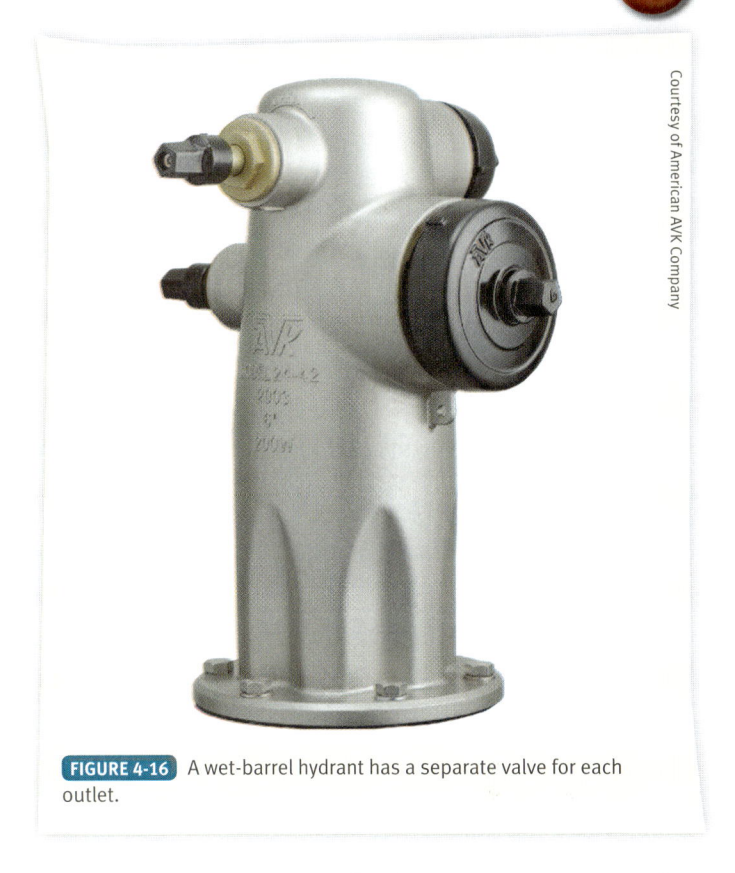

Fire fighters should always ensure that a hydrant is operational before use. Debris in the water distribution system may be forced into the barrel of a hydrant, a leaking ground valve may allow water to enter the hydrant barrel and freeze during inclement weather, and vandals may remove caps and place trash or foreign objects into the hydrant. In all instances, these problems must be identified before any hose is deployed, and this can easily be accomplished by flushing the hydrant before each use. The fire fighter making the connection opens a large outlet cap and then releases the valve just enough to ensure that water flows into the hydrant and flushes out any foreign matter. This step should take just a few seconds. The fire fighter then closes the valve, connects the hose, and reopens the valve all the way. Fire departments or water departments should also perform regular inspections and tests to keep hydrants operating smoothly.

■ Wet-Barrel Hydrants

Wet-barrel hydrants are used in locations where the temperatures do not drop below the freezing mark. These hydrants always have water in the barrel and do not have to be drained after each use. Wet-barrel hydrants usually have separate valves that control the flow to each individual outlet **FIGURE 4-16**. You can hook up one hoseline and begin flowing water, and later attach a second hoseline and open the valve for that outlet, without shutting down the hydrant.

Operation of Fire Hydrants

As a driver/operator, you must be proficient in operating a fire hydrant. **SKILL DRILL 4-1** outlines the steps in obtaining

FIGURE 4-16 A wet-barrel hydrant has a separate valve for each outlet.

FIGURE 4-15 Most dry-barrel hydrants have only one large valve that controls the flow of water.

water from a dry-barrel hydrant efficiently and safely. These same steps, with the modifications noted, apply to wet-barrel hydrants as well.

1. Remove the cap from the outlet you will be using. (**STEP 1**)
2. Quickly look inside the hydrant opening for any objects that may have been thrown into the hydrant. (**STEP 2**) (Omit this step for a wet-barrel hydrant.)
3. Check to ensure that the remaining hydrant caps are snugly attached. (**STEP 3**) (Omit this step for a wet-barrel hydrant.)
4. Place the hydrant wrench on the stem nut. Check the top of the hydrant for the arrow indicating which direction to turn the nut to open the hydrant valve. (**STEP 4**)
5. Open the hydrant just enough to determine that a good flow of water is available and to flush out any objects that may have been put into the hydrant. (**STEP 5**) (Omit this step for a wet-barrel hydrant.)
6. Shut off the flow of water. (**STEP 6**) (Omit this step for a wet-barrel hydrant.)
7. Attach the hose or valve to the hydrant outlet. (**STEP 7**)
8. When instructed, start the flow of water. Turn the hydrant wrench to fully open the valve. The average hydrant takes 12 to 14 turns to open; however some may take considerably more turns before they are fully opened. (**STEP 8**)
9. Open the hydrant slowly to avoid a pressure surge. Once the flow of water has begun, you can open the hydrant valve more quickly. Make sure that you open the hydrant valve completely. If the valve is not fully opened, the drain hole will remain open. (**STEP 9**)

Note: This skill drill applies to a dry-barrel hydrant. For a wet-barrel hydrant, omit steps 2, 3, 5, and 6, and simply open the valve for the particular outlet that will be used.

Individual fire departments may vary the procedures they specify for opening a hydrant. For example, some fire departments specify that the wrench be left on the hydrant. Other fire departments require that the wrench be removed and returned to the fire apparatus so that an unauthorized person cannot interfere with the operation. Always follow the standard operating procedures (SOP) for your fire department.

Shutting Down a Hydrant

Shutting a hydrant down properly is just as important as opening a hydrant properly. If the hydrant is damaged during shutdown, it cannot be used until it has been repaired. Following the steps shown in **SKILL DRILL 4-2** will enable you to shut down a hydrant efficiently and safely.

1. Turn the hydrant wrench slowly until the valve is closed. (**STEP 1**)
2. Allow the hose to drain by opening a drain valve or disconnecting a hose connection downstream. Slowly disconnect the hose from the hydrant outlet, allowing any remaining pressure to escape. (**STEP 2**)
3. On dry-barrel hydrants, leave one outlet open until the water drains from the hydrant. (**STEP 3**)
4. Replace the hydrant cap. (**STEP 4**)

Note: Do not leave or replace the caps on a dry-barrel hydrant until you are sure that the water has completely drained from the barrel. If you feel suction on your hand when you place it over the opening, the hydrant is still draining. In very cold weather, you may have to use a hydrant pump to remove all the water and prevent the hydrant from freezing.

DRIVER/OPERATOR Tip

Establishing an uninterruptible water supply is a critical fire-ground factor needed to ensure the safety of the fire company operating in a fire building. This can most efficiently be accomplished through teamwork within the fire company. A fire fighter dropped off at a hydrant with the proper tools can begin the process of establishing the water supply while the other crew members are deploying handlines and you complete the connection to the engine.

Locations of Fire Hydrants

Fire hydrants are located according to local standards and nationally recommended practices. Fire hydrants may be placed a certain distance apart, about every 500 ft (150 m) in residential areas and every 300 ft (90 m) in high-value commercial and industrial areas. In many communities, fire hydrants are located at every street intersection, with mid-block fire hydrants being established if the distance between intersections exceeds a specified limit.

In some cases, the requirements for locating fire hydrants are based on occupancy, construction, and size of a building. A builder may be required to install additional fire hydrants when a new building is constructed so that no part of the building will be more than a specified distance from the closest fire hydrant.

Knowing the plan for installing fire hydrants makes them easier to find in emergency situations. Fire companies that perform fire inspections or develop preincident plans should identify the locations of nearby fire hydrants for each building or group of buildings as part of their survey.

Inspecting and Maintaining Fire Hydrants

Because fire hydrants are essential to fire suppression efforts, you must understand how to inspect and maintain them. Fire hydrants should be checked on a regular basis—no less than once a year—to ensure that they are in proper operating condition. During inspections, you may encounter some common problems and should know how to correct them.

The first factors to check when inspecting fire hydrants are visibility and accessibility. Fire hydrants should always be visible from every direction, so they can be easily spotted. A fire hydrant should not be hidden by tall grass, brush, fences, debris, dumpsters, or any other obstructions **FIGURE 4-17**. In

CHAPTER 4 Water 63

SKILL DRILL 4-1 Operating a Fire Hydrant

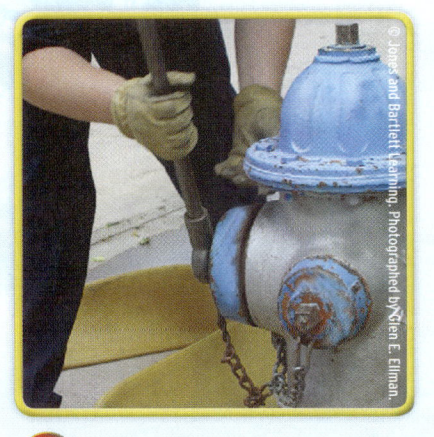

1. Remove the cap from the outlet you will be using.

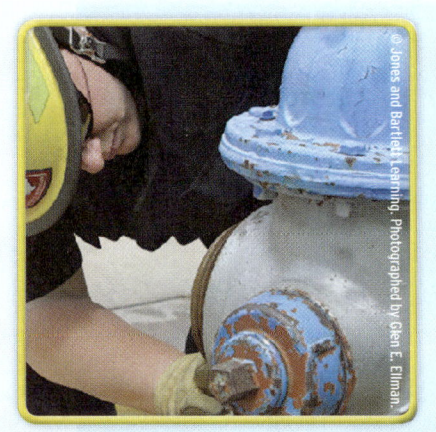

2. Quickly look inside the hydrant opening for foreign objects (dry-barrel hydrant only).

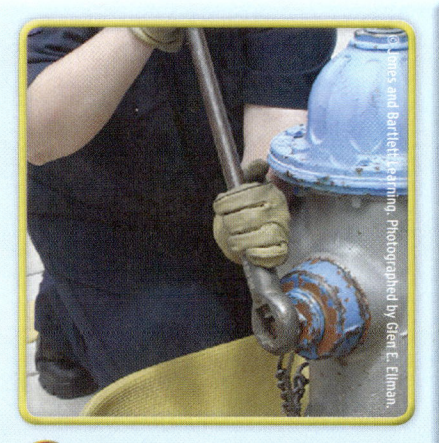

3. Check that the remaining caps are snugly attached (dry-barrel hydrant only).

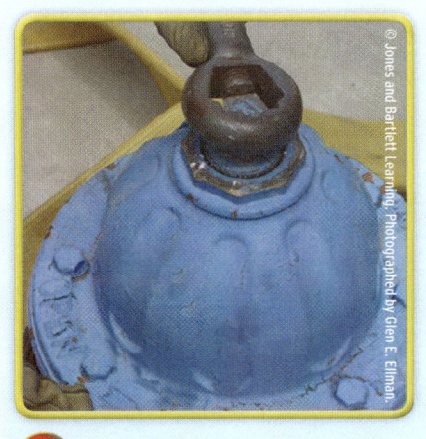

4. Attach the hydrant wrench on the stem nut. Check for an arrow indicating the direction to turn to open.

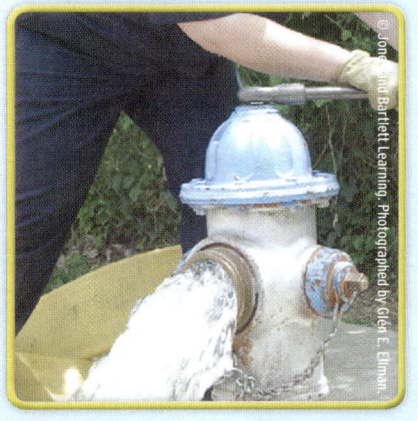

5. Open the hydrant enough to verify the flow and flush the hydrant (dry-barrel hydrant only).

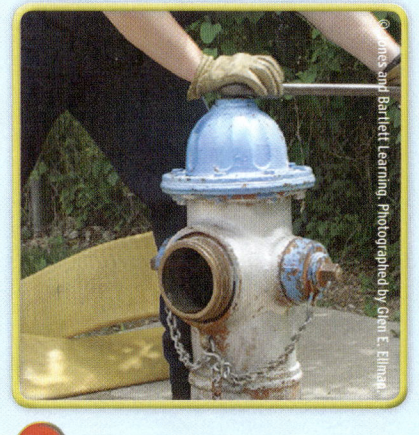

6. Shut off the flow of water (dry-barrel hydrant only).

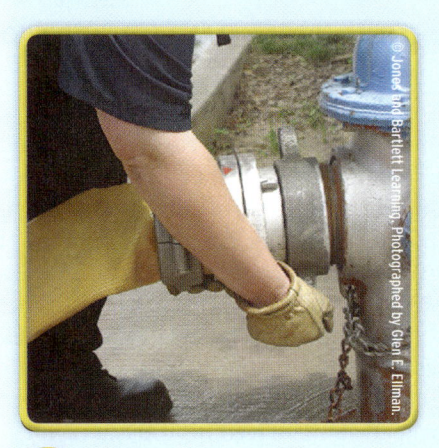

7. Attach the hose or valve to the hydrant outlet.

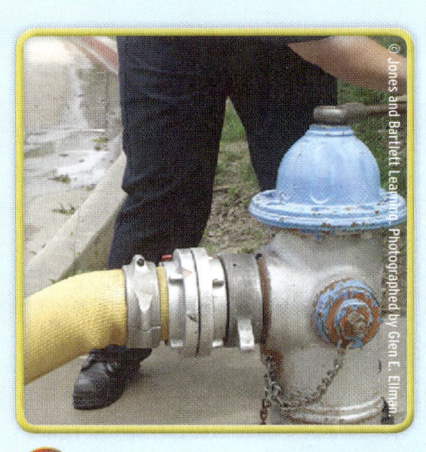

8. When instructed, turn the hydrant wrench to fully open the valve.

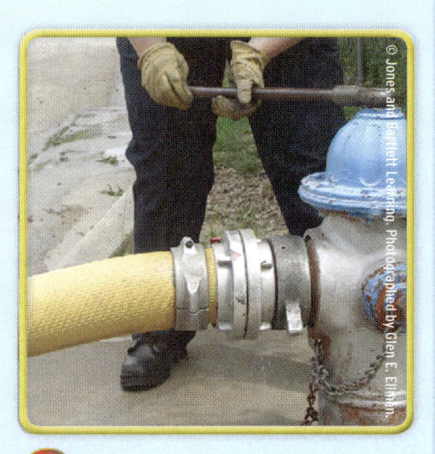

9. Open the hydrant slowly to avoid a pressure surge.

© LiquidLibrary

SKILL DRILL 4-2   Shutting Down a Hydrant

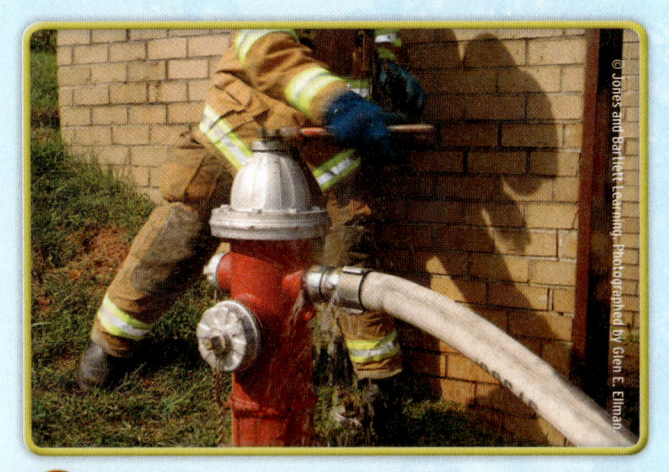

1. Turn the hydrant wrench slowly until the hydrant valve is shut.

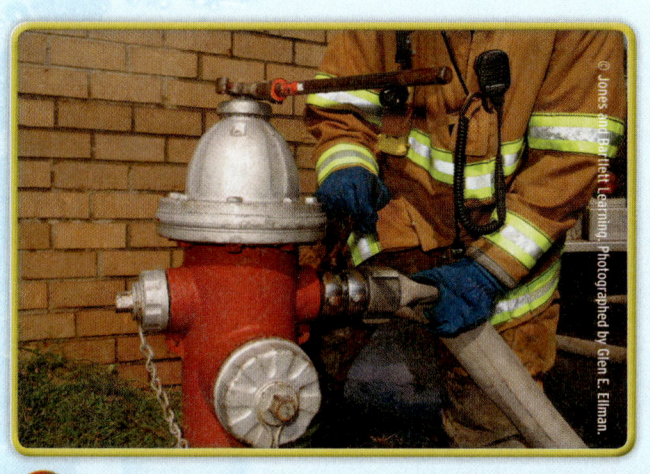

2. Drain the hoseline. Slowly disconnect the hose from the hydrant outlet.

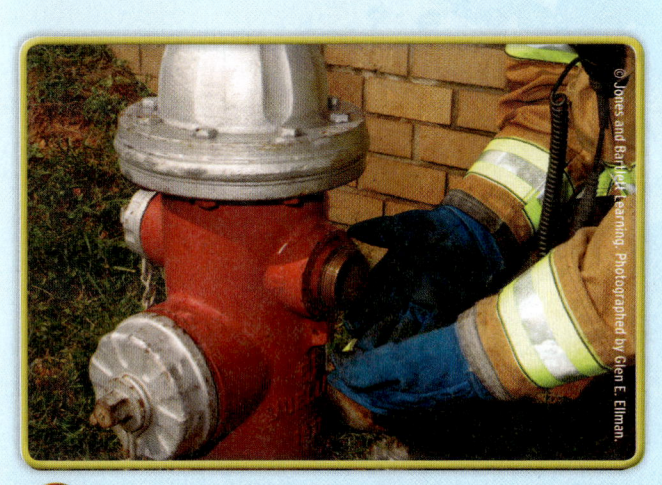

3. Leave one hydrant outlet open until the hydrant is fully drained (dry-barrel hydrant only).

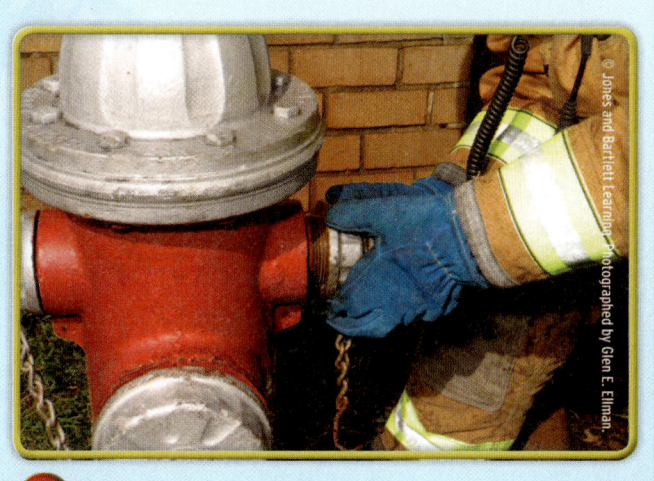

4. Replace the hydrant cap.

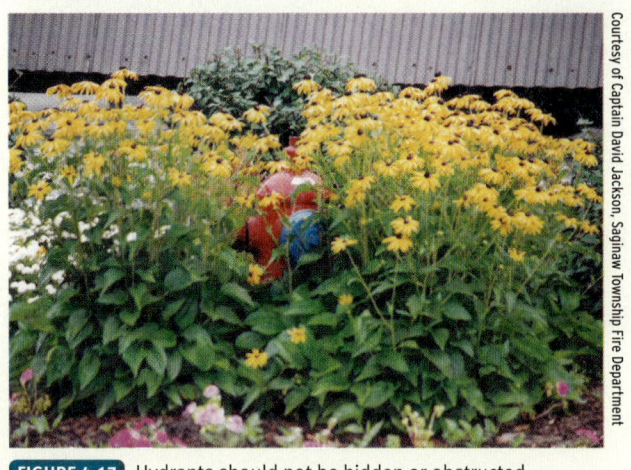

FIGURE 4-17 Hydrants should not be hidden or obstructed.

winter, fire hydrants must be clear of snow. No vehicles should be allowed to park in front of a fire hydrant.

In many communities, fire hydrants are painted in bright reflective colors for increased visibility. The bonnet (the top of the fire hydrant) may also be color-coded to indicate the available flow rate of a fire hydrant **TABLE 4-1**. While some jurisdictions use their own color coding system, it is recommended that NFPA 291 be followed. Colored reflectors are sometimes mounted next to the fire hydrants or placed in the pavement in front of them to make them more readily visible at night.

Fire hydrants should be installed at an appropriate height above the ground. The outlets should not be so high or so low that the fire companies have difficulty connecting hoselines to them. NFPA 291 requires a minimum of 8 inches (0.2 m) from the center of a hose outlet to the finish grade. Areas

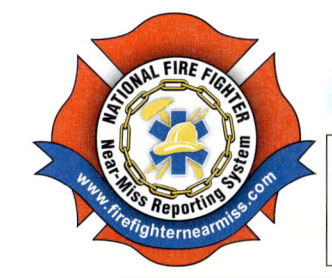

Near-Miss REPORT

Report Number: 09-0001045

Synopsis: Water hammer causes coupling to shear.

Event Description: During a pump training class, the tanker was being filled by a "hot" hydrant. I, along with the other fire fighters, was at the rear of the tanker as it was being filled. As the tanker started to overflow, it was communicated to shut off the direct-fill ball valve. One fire fighter ran to shut off the valve and slammed it shut. This caused a water hammer from the heavy flow hydrant, resulting in the male quick-connect coupling shearing apart. The jagged, pot-metal connector, still attached to the fill hose, whipped by our faces and snaked wildly on the apron. The burst connector missed our faces by inches (millimeters).

Lessons Learned: If the fire fighter had slowed down and not rushed his actions, the water hammer would not have occurred. Additionally, if the hydrant had been shut off at the same time, the flow would not have been so forceful when the coupling broke loose. The coupling should have also been inspected before being put to use, as it could have been cracked or had signs of a defect or failure. It's always important to think about what you are about to do. Do not rush your actions and always stay aware of the situation you are in. Training is where our skills are fine-tuned.

TABLE 4-1 Fire Hydrant Colors

National Fire Protection Association (NFPA) 291, *Recommended Practice for Fire Flow Testing and Marking of Hydrants*, recommends that fire hydrants be color-coded to indicate the water flow available from each hydrant at 20 psi (140 kPa). It is recommended that the top bonnet and the fire hydrant caps be painted according to the following system, which provides an idea of how much water can be obtained from a fire hydrant during a fire.

Class	Flow Available at 20 psi (140 kPa)	Color
Class C	Less than 500 gpm/1893 L	Red
Class B	500 to 999 gpm/1893 to 3782 L	Orange
Class A	1000 to 1499 gpm/3785 to 5674 L	Green
Class AA	1500 gpm/5678 L and higher	Light blue

that experience snow accumulations may require placement of hydrants further above the finish grade. Fire hydrants should be positioned so that the connections—and especially the large steamer connection—face the street.

During a fire hydrant inspection, check the exterior of the hydrant for signs of damage. Open the steamer port of each dry-barrel hydrant to ensure that the barrel is dry and free of debris. Make sure that all caps are present and that the outlet hose threads are in good working order **FIGURE 4-18**.

The second part of the inspection ensures that the hydrant is working properly. Open the hydrant valve just enough to confirm that water flows out and flushes any debris out of the barrel. After flushing, shut down the hydrant. A properly draining hydrant will create suction against a hand placed over the outlet opening **FIGURE 4-19**. When the hydrant is fully drained, replace the cap on a wet-barrel hydrant; leave the cap off a dry-barrel hydrant to ensure that it drains properly.

If the threads on the discharge ports need cleaning, use a steel brush and a small triangular file to remove any burrs in

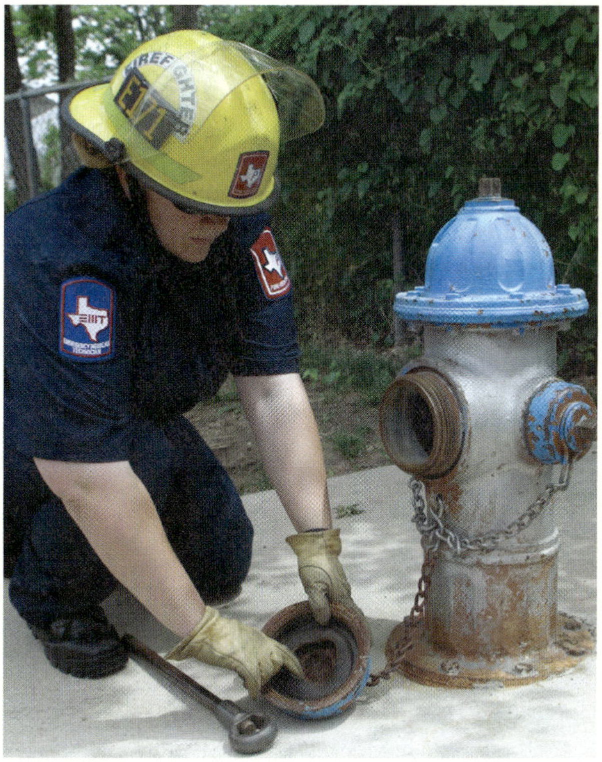

FIGURE 4-18 All fire hydrants should be checked at least annually.

the threads. Also check the gaskets in the caps to make sure they are not cracked, broken, or missing. Replace worn gaskets with new ones, which should be carried with each apparatus. Always follow the manufacturer's recommendations for any parts that require lubrication.

FIGURE 4-19 Feel suction to indicate the fire hydrant is draining.

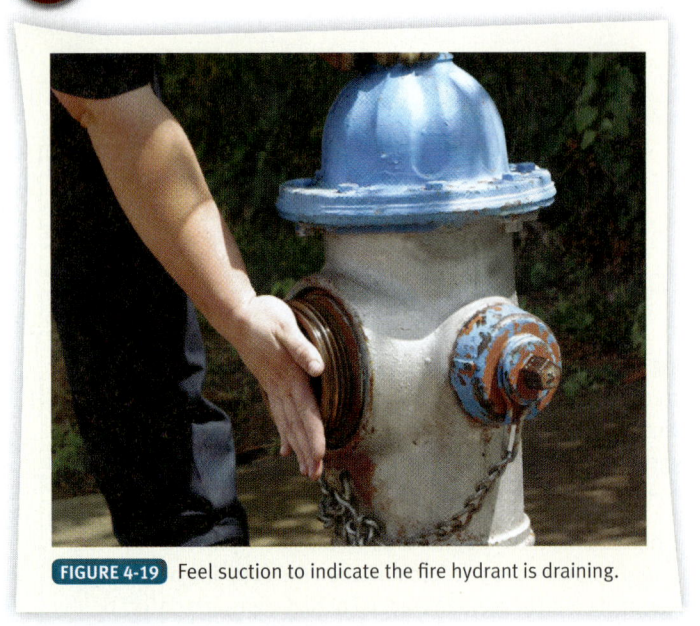

Testing Fire Hydrants

The amount of water available to fight a fire at a given location is a crucial factor in planning an attack. Will the fire hydrants deliver enough water at the needed pressure to enable fire fighters to control a fire? If not, what can be done to improve the water supply? How can you obtain additional water if a fire does occur?

Fire-suppression companies are often assigned to test the flow from fire hydrants in their districts. The procedures for testing fire hydrants are relatively simple, but a basic understanding of the concepts of hydraulics and careful attention to detail are required. This section explains some of the basic theory and terminology of hydraulics and describes how the tests are conducted and the results are recorded.

■ Fire Hydrant Testing Procedure

The procedure for testing fire hydrant flows requires two adjacent hydrants, a Pitot gauge, and an outlet cap with a pressure gauge. A **Pitot gauge** is used to measure flow pressure in psi (or kilopascals) and to calculate the flow in gallons (liters) per minute. As part of testing, fire fighters measure static pressure and residual pressure at one hydrant, and open the other hydrant to let water flow out. The two hydrants should be connected to the same water main and preferably at about the same elevation **FIGURE 4-20**.

The cap gauge is placed on one of the outlets of the first hydrant. The hydrant valve is then opened to allow water to fill the hydrant barrel. The initial pressure reading on this gauge is recorded as the static pressure. To obtain the static pressure, follow the steps in **SKILL DRILL 4-3**:

1. Remove the cap from the hydrant port, open the hydrant, and allow water to flow until it runs clear. Do your best to avoid property damage with the flowing water. (**STEP 1**)
2. Close the hydrant valve. (**STEP 2**)
3. Install a cap gauge on the port. (**STEP 3**)
4. Open the hydrant valve fully to fill the barrel. No water should be flowing. (**STEP 4**)
5. Note the pressure reading on the gauge; this is the static pressure of the system. (**STEP 5**)
6. Close the hydrant fully.
7. Bleed down the pressure.
8. Remove the cap gauge and replace it with the hydrant cap. (**STEP 6**)

At the second hydrant, fire fighters remove one of the discharge caps and open the hydrant. They put the Pitot gauge into the middle of the stream and take a reading. This value is recorded as the Pitot pressure. At the same time, fire fighters at the first hydrant record the residual reading.

Using the size of the discharge opening (usually 2½ inches [65 mm]) and the Pitot pressure, fire fighters can calculate the flow in gallons per minute or look it up in a table; such a table usually incorporates factors to adjust for the shape of the discharge opening. Fire fighters can use special graph paper or computer software to plot the static pressure and the residual

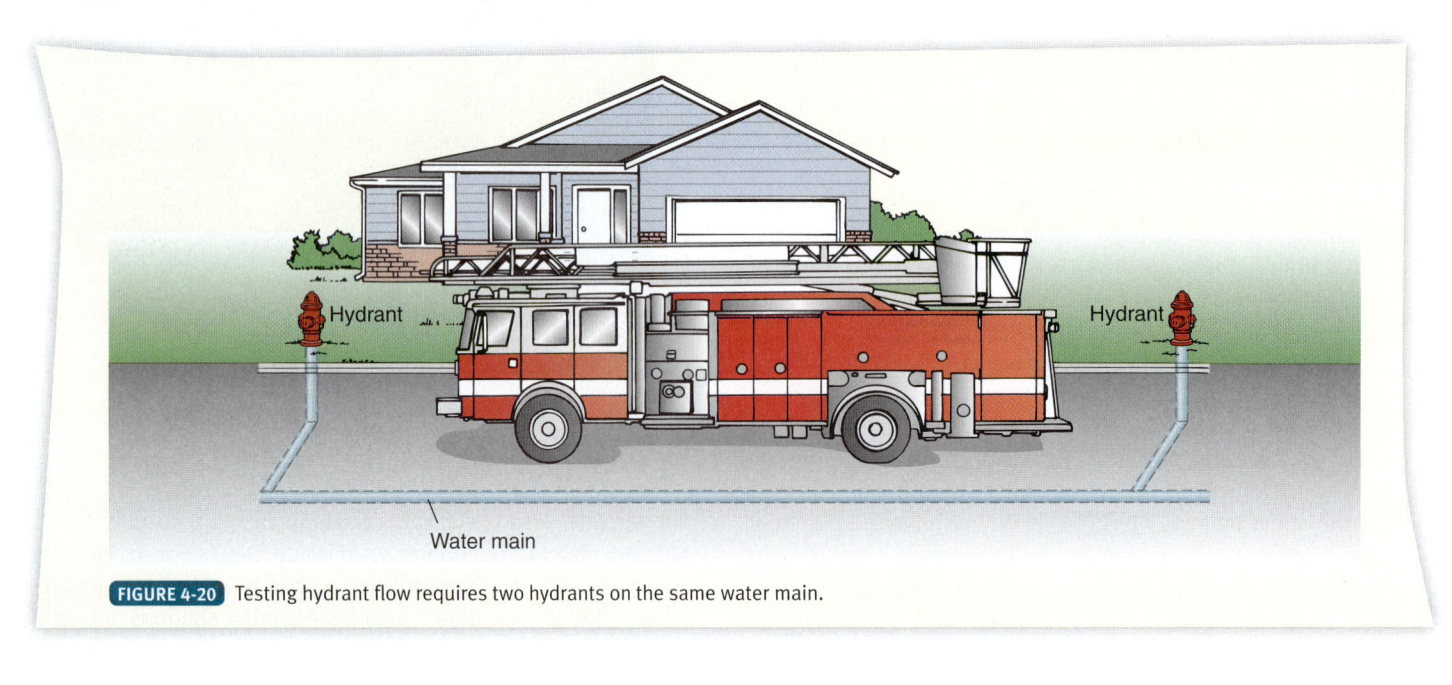

FIGURE 4-20 Testing hydrant flow requires two hydrants on the same water main.

CHAPTER 4 Water 67

SKILL DRILL 4-3 Obtaining the Static Pressure

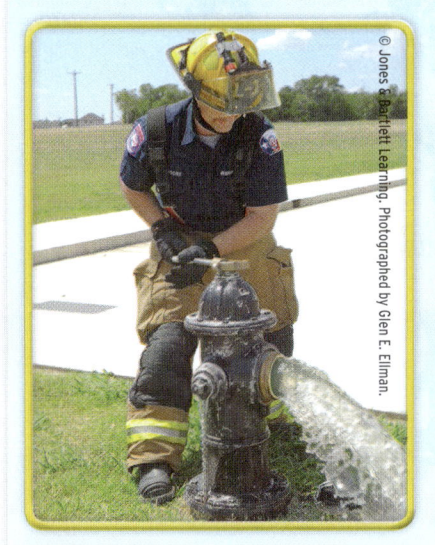

1 Remove the cap from the hydrant port, open the hydrant, and allow water to flow until it runs clear.

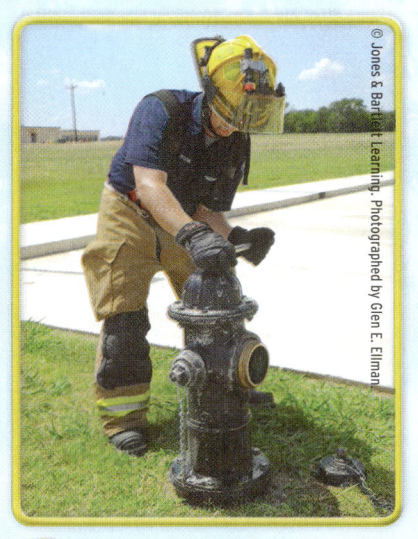

2 Close the hydrant valve.

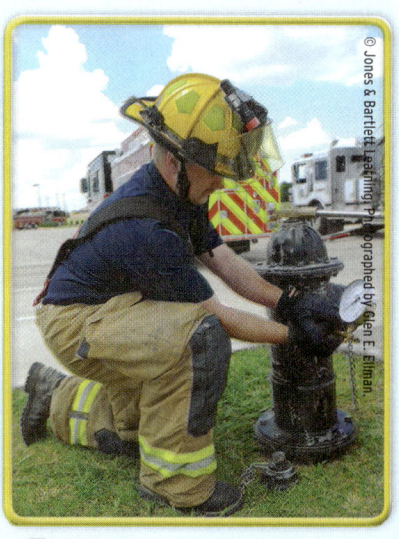

3 Install a cap gauge on the port.

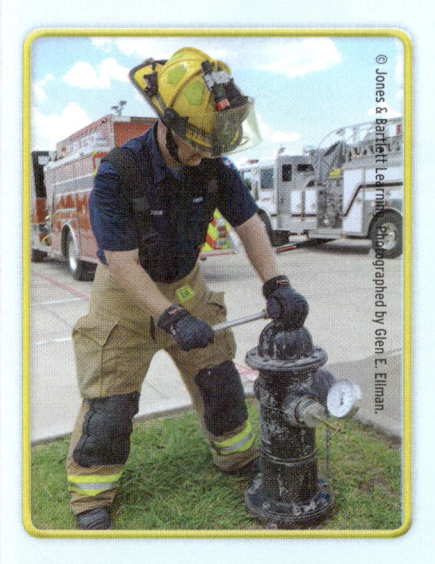

4 Open the hydrant valve fully to fill the barrel. No water should be flowing.

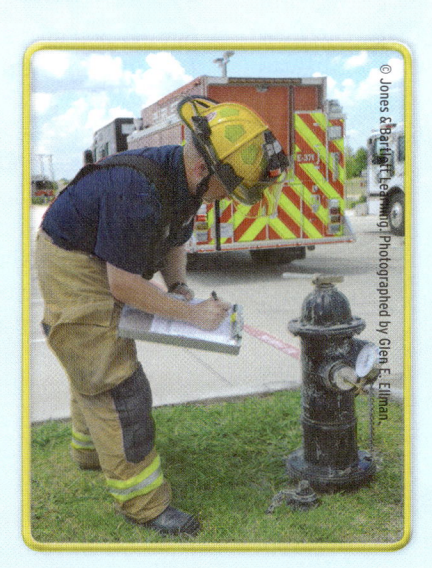

5 Note the pressure reading on the gauge; this is the static pressure of the system.

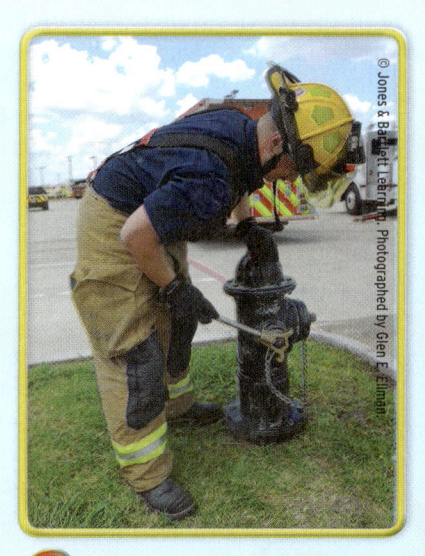

6 Close the hydrant fully, bleed down the pressure, remove the cap gauge, and replace it with the hydrant cap.

© LiquidLibrary

FIGURE 4-21 The Pitot gauge.

FIGURE 4-22 Any accessible body of water can be used as a static source.

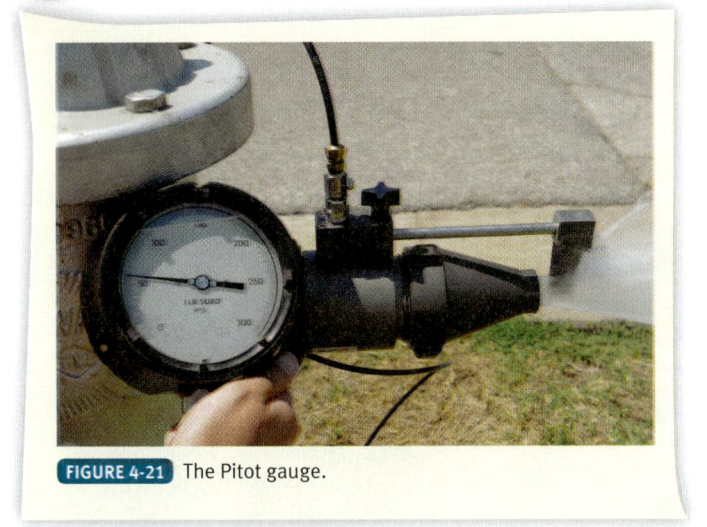

pressure at the test flow rate. The line defined by these two points shows the number of gallons (liters) per minute that is available at any residual pressure. The flow available for fire suppression is usually defined as the number of gallons (liters) per minute available at 20 psi (140 kPa) residual pressure.

Several special devices are available to simplify the process of taking accurate Pitot readings. Some outlet attachments have smooth tips and brackets that hold the Pitot gauge in the exact required position **FIGURE 4-21**. The flow can also be measured with an electronic flow meter instead of a Pitot gauge.

To operate a Pitot gauge, follow the steps in **SKILL DRILL 4-4**:

1. Remove the cap from a hydrant port, preferably the 2½-inch (65-mm) discharge port. (**STEP 1**)
2. Measure the inside diameter of the discharge port, and record the size. (**STEP 2**)
3. Fully open the hydrant and allow water to flow. (**STEP 3**)
4. Hold the Pitot gauge into the center of the flow and place it parallel to the discharge opening at a distance one-half of the inside diameter of the discharge port. (**STEP 4**)
5. Record the pressure reading. (**STEP 5**)
6. Close the hydrant valve fully and replace the cap. (**STEP 6**)

Hydrant flow testing should be conducted during the water distribution system's peak flow times. For instance, if the greatest demand on the system is between 6:00 A.M. and 8:00 A.M., the flow testing should be conducted during that time period.

Rural Water Supplies

Many fire departments protect areas that are not serviced by municipal water systems. In these areas, residents usually depend on individual wells or cisterns to supply the water needed for domestic uses. Because there are no fire hydrants in these areas, fire fighters must depend on water from other sources. In rural areas, you must know how to get water from the sources that are available.

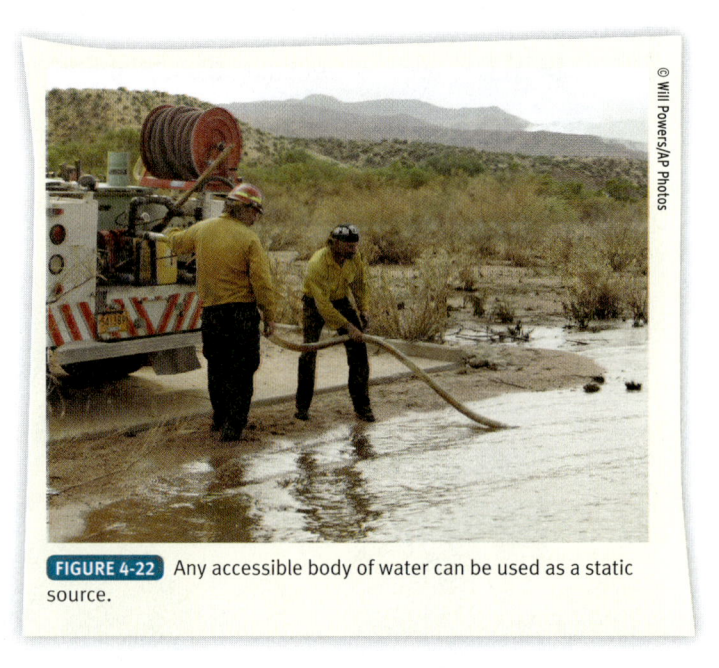

Static Sources of Water

Several potential static water sources can be used for fighting fires in rural areas. Both natural and human-made bodies of water such as rivers, streams, lakes, ponds, oceans, reservoirs, swimming pools, and cisterns can be used to supply water for fire suppression **FIGURE 4-22**. Some areas have many different static sources, whereas others have few or none at all. Water from a static source can be used to fight a fire directly, if it is close enough to the fire scene. Otherwise, water must be transported to the fire using long hoselines, engine relays, or mobile water supply tankers.

Static water sources must be accessible to a fire engine or portable pump. Rural fire departments should identify these areas and practice establishing drafting operations at all of these locations. Some fire departments construct special access points so engines can approach the water source.

Dry hydrants also provide quick and reliable access to static water sources. A dry hydrant is a pipe with a strainer on one end and a connection for a hard suction hose on the other end. The strainer end should be placed below the water's surface and away from any silt or potential obstructions. The other end of the pipe should be accessible to fire apparatus, with the connection at a convenient height for an engine hook-up **FIGURE 4-23**. When a hard suction hose is connected to the dry hydrant, the engine can draft water from the static source.

Dry hydrants are often installed in lakes and rivers and close to clusters of buildings where there is a recognized need for fire protection. They may also be installed in farm cisterns or connected to swimming pools on private property to make water available for the local fire department. In some areas, dry

SKILL DRILL 4-4 Operating a Pitot Gauge

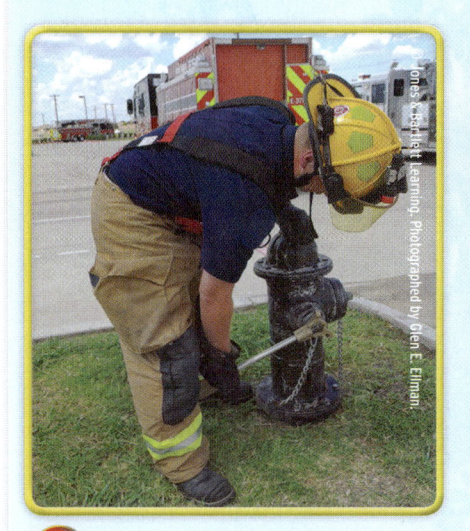

1 Remove the cap from a hydrant port, preferably the 2½-inch (65-mm) discharge port.

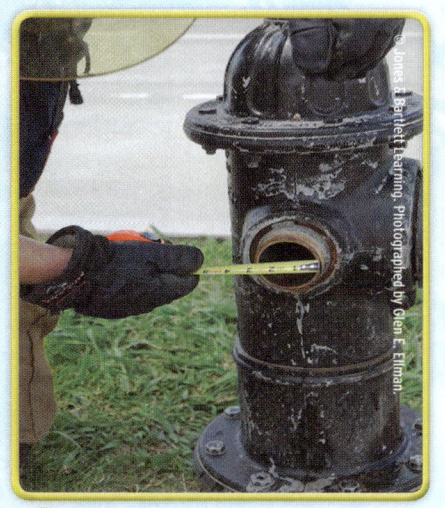

2 Measure the inside diameter of the discharge port and record the size.

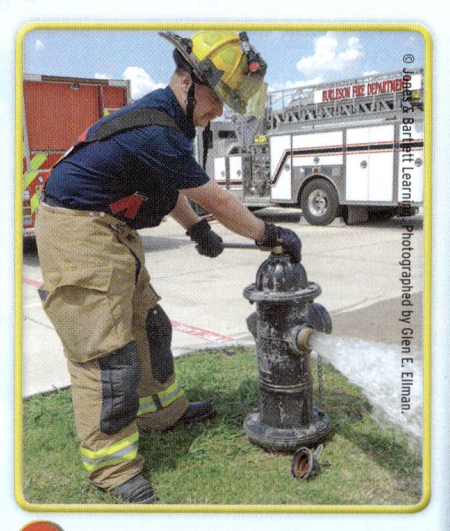

3 Fully open the hydrant and allow water to flow.

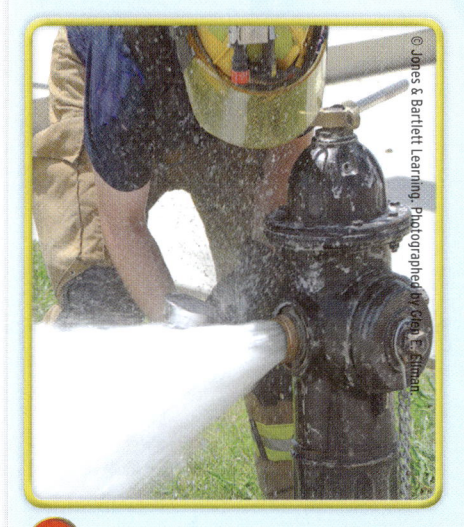

4 Hold the Pitot gauge into the center of the flow and place it parallel to the discharge opening at a distance one-half of the inside diameter of the discharge port.

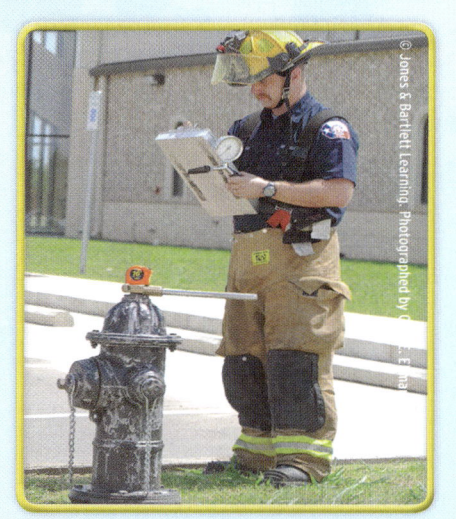

5 Record the pressure reading.

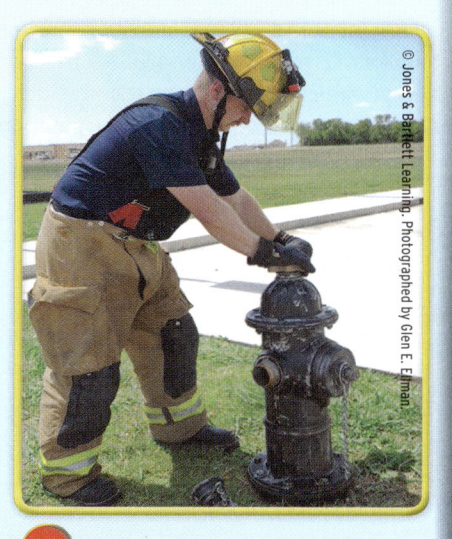

6 Close the hydrant valve fully and replace the cap.

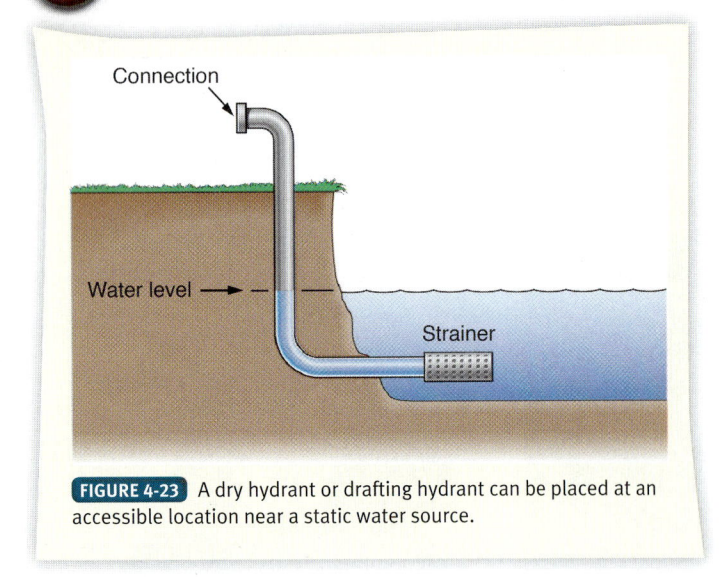

FIGURE 4-23 A dry hydrant or drafting hydrant can be placed at an accessible location near a static water source.

hydrants are used to enable fire fighters to reach water under the frozen surface of a lake or river. Dry hydrants should be flow-tested at least on an annual basis and should be back-flushed prior to use.

The portable pump is an alternative means of obtaining water in areas that are inaccessible to fire apparatus **FIGURE 4-24**. The portable pump can be hand-carried or transported by an off-road vehicle to the water source. Such pumps can deliver up to 500 gallons (1893 liters) of water per minute.

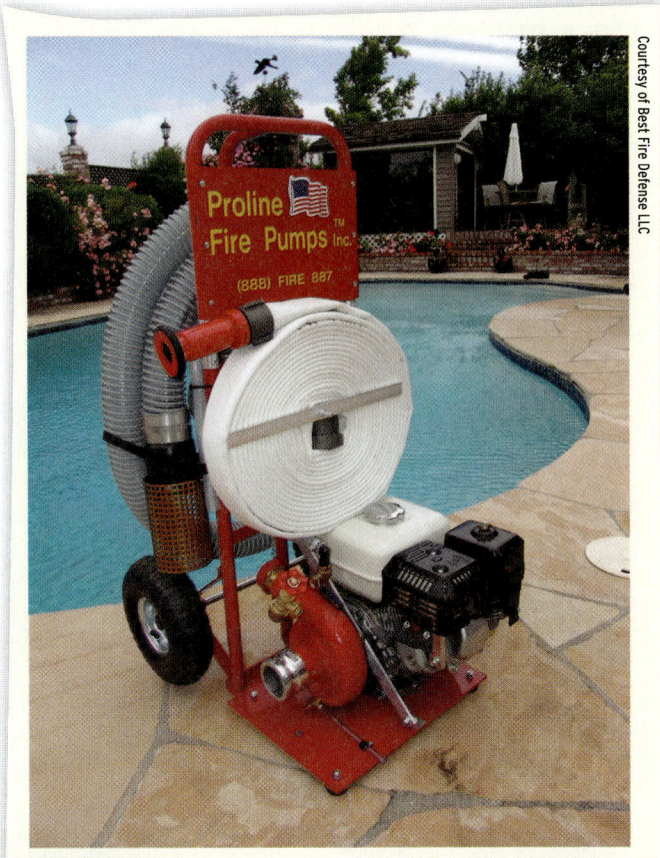

FIGURE 4-24 A portable pump can be used if the water source is inaccessible to a fire department engine.

Wrap-Up

Chief Concepts

- The basic plan for fighting most fires depends on having an adequate supply of water to confine, control, and extinguish the fire.
- Understanding fluid dynamics is an important aspect of the driver/operator's job.
- Three types of fire hydrants are available: wet-barrel, dry-barrel, and dry hydrants.
- Fire hydrants are located according to local standards and nationally recommended practices.
- Fire fighters must be proficient in operating a fire hydrant, including being able to turn on and shut down a fire hydrant.

Hot Terms

aqueous Pertaining to, related to, similar to, or dissolved in water.

distributors Relatively small-diameter underground pipes that deliver water to local users within a neighborhood.

dry-barrel hydrant The most common type of hydrant; it has a control valve below the frost line between the footpiece and the barrel. A drain is located at the bottom of the barrel above the control valve seat for proper drainage after operation.

dry hydrant An arrangement of pipes that is permanently connected to a water source other than a piped, pressurized water supply system; it provides a ready means of water supply for firefighting purposes, and takes advantage of the drafting (suction) capability of fire department pumpers.

elevated water storage tower An above-ground water storage tank that is designed to maintain pressure on a water distribution system.

elevation pressure The amount of pressure created by gravity.

flow pressure Forward pressure at a discharge opening while water is flowing.

friction loss The result of the interaction between the hose or pipe and the flowing water, which leads to a reduction in flow pressure at the point of discharge.

gravity-feed system A water distribution system that depends on gravity to provide the required pressure. The system storage is usually located at a higher elevation than the end users of the water.

hardness The mineral content of the water; it usually consists of calcium and magnesium, but can also include iron, aluminum, and manganese.

heat of vaporization The energy required to transform a given quantity of a substance into a gas.

kinetic energy The energy possessed by an object as a result of its motion.

municipal water system A government-owned and -operated water distribution system that is designed to deliver potable water to end users for domestic, industrial, and fire protection purposes.

normal operating pressure The observed static pressure in a water distribution system during a period of normal demand.

Pitot gauge A type of gauge that is used to measure the velocity pressure of water that is being discharged from an opening. It is used to determine the flow of water from a hydrant.

potential energy The energy that an object has stored up as a result of its position or condition. A raised weight and a coiled spring have potential energy.

primary feeder The largest-diameter pipe in a water distribution system, which carries the largest amount of water.

private water system A privately owned water system that operates separately from the municipal water system.

reservoir A water storage facility.

residual pressure The pressure that exists in the distribution system, measured at the residual hydrant at the time the flow readings are taken at the flow hydrant.

secondary feeder A smaller-diameter pipe that connects the primary feeder to the distributors.

shut-off valve Any valve that can be used to shut down water flow to a water user or system.

specific heat index The amount of heat energy required to raise the temperature of a substance. These values are determined experimentally and then made available in tabular form.

static pressure The pressure in a water pipe when there is no water flowing.

static water source A water source such as a pond, river, stream, or other body of water that is not under pressure.

surface tension The elastic-like force at the surface of a liquid, which tends to minimize the surface area, causing water drops to form.

turbidity The amount of particulate matter suspended in water.

universal solvent A liquid substance capable of dissolving other substances, which does not result in the first substance changing its state when forming the solution.

volume The quantity of water flowing; usually measured in gallons (liters) per minute.

water flow The amount of water flowing through pipes, hoses, and fittings, usually expressed in gallons (liters) per minute (gpm or L/min).

Wrap-Up, continued

water hammer The surge of pressure caused when a high-velocity flow of water is abruptly shut off. The pressure exerted by the flowing water against the closed system can be seven or more times that of the static pressure.

water main A generic term for any underground water pipe.

water pressure The application of force by one object against another. When water is forced through the distribution system, it creates water pressure.

water supply A source of water that provides the flows (L/min) and pressures (kPa) required by a water-based fire protection system.

wet-barrel hydrant A hydrant used in areas that are not susceptible to freezing. The barrel of this type of hydrant is normally filled with water.

References

National Fire Protection Association (NFPA) 291, *Recommended Practice for Fire Flow Testing and Marking of Hydrants*. 2013. http://www.nfpa.org/catalog/product.asp?pid=29113&cookie%5Ftest=1. Accessed March 27, 2014.

National Fire Protection Association (NFPA) 1002, *Standard for Fire Apparatus Driver/Operator Professional Qualifications*. 2014. http://www.nfpa.org/codes-and-standards/document-information-pages?mode=code&code=1002. Accessed March 27, 2014.

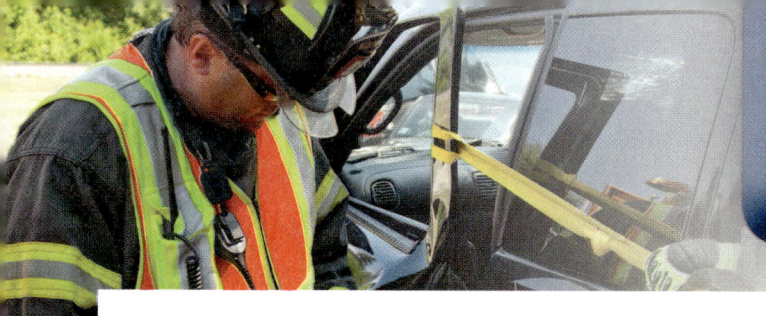

DRIVER/OPERATOR
in action

While your company is performing hydrant tests in your response district, the new fire fighter starts to ask you questions about the water system and the different types of fire hydrants. While you are working, you explain to him how the water distribution system is set up, how the system is pressurized, and which types of pressures are found in the system. After returning to the station, you will quiz the fire fighter on what he has learned by asking him to answer the following questions:

1. What allows water to flow, puddle, and remain together even after leaving the nozzle?
   A. Heat of vaporization
   B. Surface tension
   C. Specific gravity
   D. The drain works before using it.

2. There are _____ principles of fluid pressure.
   A. 4
   B. 5
   C. 6
   D. 7

3. What is the pressure that remains in the system when water is flowing?
   A. Residual pressure
   B. Flow pressure
   C. Static pressure
   D. Normal operating pressure

4. Fire hydrants are located according to local standards and nationally recommended practices.
   A. True
   B. False

5. NFPA 291, *Recommended Practice for Fire Flow Testing and Marking of Hydrants*, recommends that fire hydrants be color-coded to indicate the water flow available from each hydrant at __ psi (kPa).
   A. 10 (70)
   B. 20 (140)
   C. 30 (210)
   D. 40 (280)

The Fire Pump

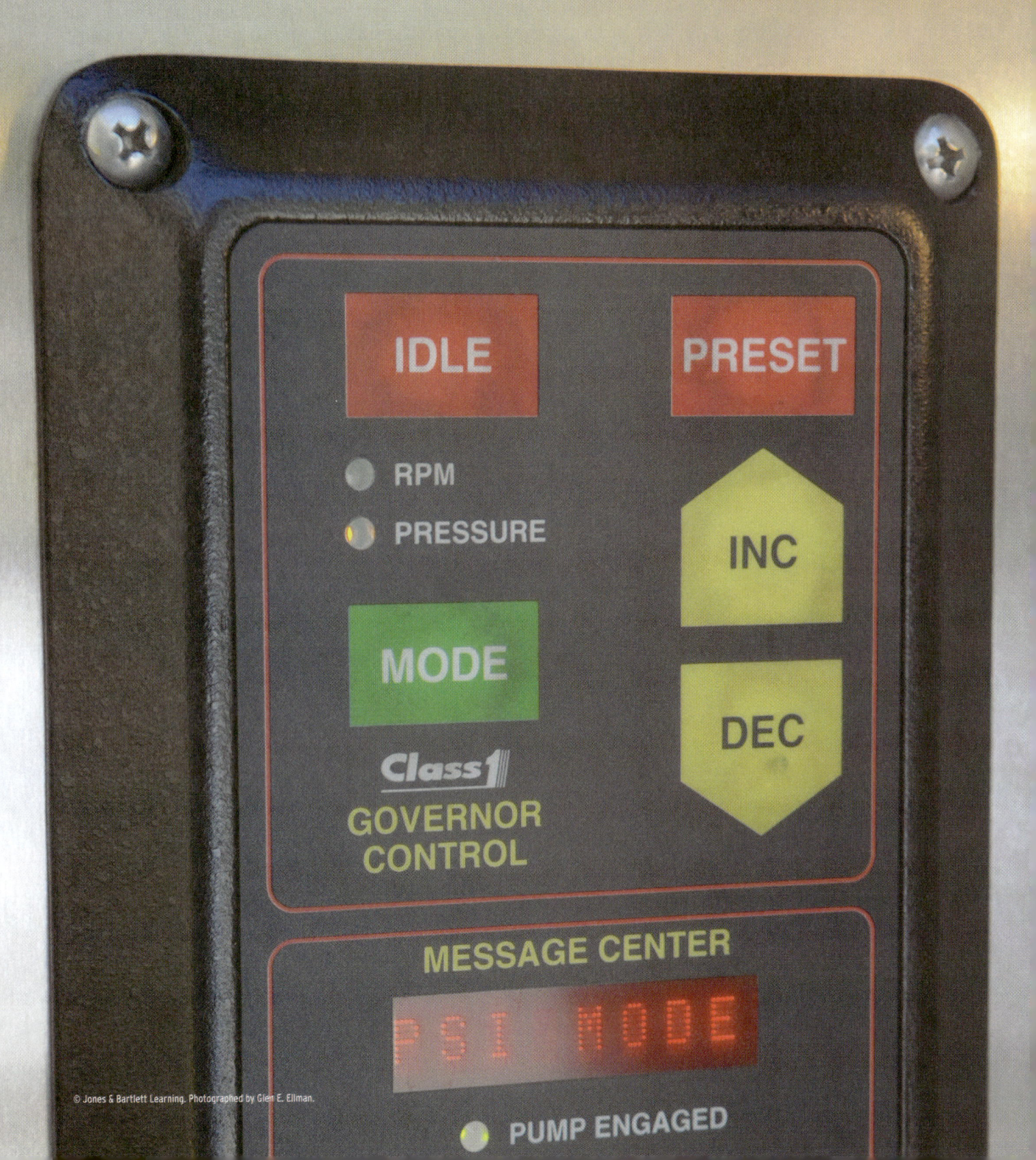

CHAPTER 5

Knowledge Objectives

After studying this chapter you will be able to:
- Explain the importance of understanding the fire pump and its systems. (p 76)
- Describe the exterior and interior features of a pumper. (p 76–77)
- Define the term *pump*. (p 77–79)
- Explain the basic operations of positive-displacement pumps and centrifugal pumps. (p 79–86)
- Explain the different types of positive-displacement pumps. (p 79–81)
- Explain the different types of centrifugal pumps. (p 81, 83–86)
- Describe a single-stage pump and a two-stage pump. (p 83–86)
- Describe the intake side of the fire pump. (p 86–87)
- Describe the discharge sides of a pump. (p 87–88)
- Describe the pump valves and drains. (p 86–88)
- Describe the components of the pump panel. (p 88–94)

Skills Objectives

There are no skill objectives for Driver/Operator candidates. NFPA 1002 contains no Driver/Operator Job Performance Requirements for this chapter.

Additional NFPA Standards

- NFPA 20, *Standard for the Installation of Stationary Pumps for Fire Protection*
- NFPA 1901, *Standard for Automotive Fire Apparatus*

You Are the Driver/Operator

As the driver/operator, one of your responsibilities is to teach the other members of the crew about your job. The new fire fighter in the station has asked that you teach him about the fire apparatus pump, including how it works. Before you can make your way from the kitchen to the apparatus bay, the new fire fighter starts to pepper you with questions about the pump:

1. What are the different types of pumps that are used in the fire service?
2. What powers the pump on the engine apparatus?
3. What are the different gauges, valves, and controls on the pump panel for?

Introduction

This chapter discusses the basic principles underlying the use of pumps in the fire service. Pumps are vital to the operations of firefighting. Without them, fire fighters would be unable to discharge water under pressure to extinguish fire **FIGURE 5-1**. As the driver/operator of the fire department pumper, you must understand how pumps operate so that you will be able to fix any problems that you may encounter on the fireground.

The fire service has an old saying, "Don't just be a knob puller—know what you are doing." That means you should not just memorize a specific sequence of tasks to operate the fire pump, but instead should make sure that you have a thorough understanding of how each pump operates. For example, if you understand that a **centrifugal pump** is capable of pumping only fluids (and not air), then you will know that you have to **prime the pump** before it can operate.

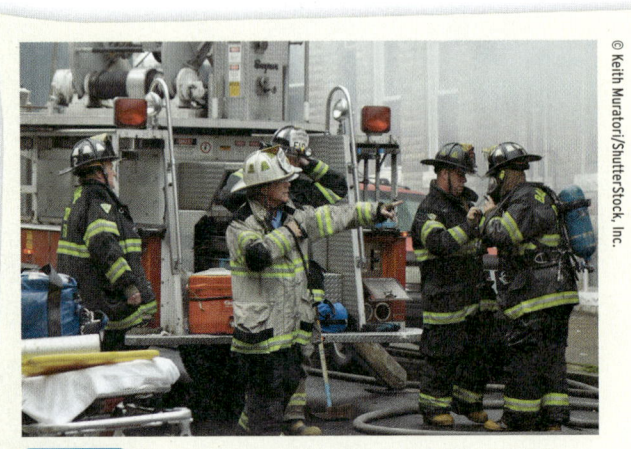

FIGURE 5-1 Pumps are essential to a successful fire attack.

Exterior of the Fire Department Pumper

The fire department pumper, whose crew is known as an engine company, is, essentially, a large fire pump with hose and tools to extinguish fires. The pumper is the most common fire apparatus, being found in almost every fire department's fleet. The cab of the fire apparatus, where the fire fighters ride to the emergency, sits on a steel frame. Attached to this frame are the storage compartments and the fire pump. The compartments on the fire apparatus hold all of the various tools and equipment needed for firefighting operations. Ground ladders may be mounted on the side of the apparatus on a side-mounted ladder rack (stowed position is on top of the apparatus), in a special compartment in the hose bed, adjacent to the hose bed, or in a through-the-tank compartment.

Supply hose and attack lines are stored in the hose bed, which may be either left uncovered or covered with a tarp to protect it from the elements. Some fire apparatus may provide a metal cover to further protect the hose. Most pumpers carry preconnected attack lines for quick deployment of such lines; these hoselines are usually located above or on the side of the pump panel.

The pump panel is the most notable device on the fire apparatus **FIGURE 5-2**. It is usually covered in stainless steel and has multiple levers and gauges mounted on it. Although this panel might seem intimidating to the new driver/operator, once you have a thorough understanding of the pump behind it and the functioning of this system, you will be capable of confidently operating the fire pump.

Interior of the Fire Department Pumper: The Cab

Inside the cab of the pumper, you will find all of the necessary controls to operate the fire apparatus **FIGURE 5-3**. When you are sitting in the driver's seat, many of the controls and features will seem similar to those found in any other large vehicle.

CHAPTER 5 The Fire Pump 77

FIGURE 5-3 The interior vehicle controls on an engine apparatus are very similar to those found on many other large vehicles, with a few exceptions.

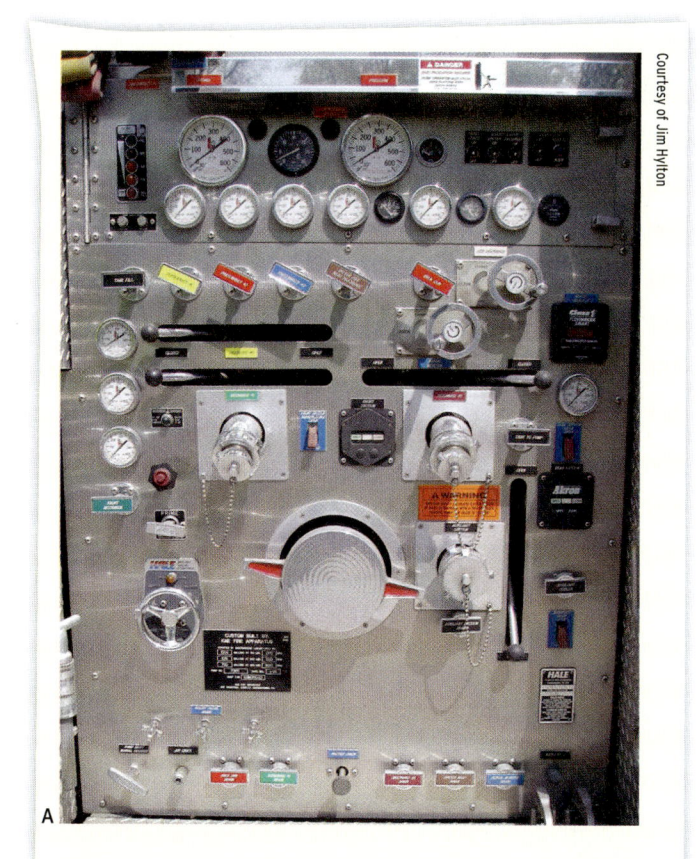

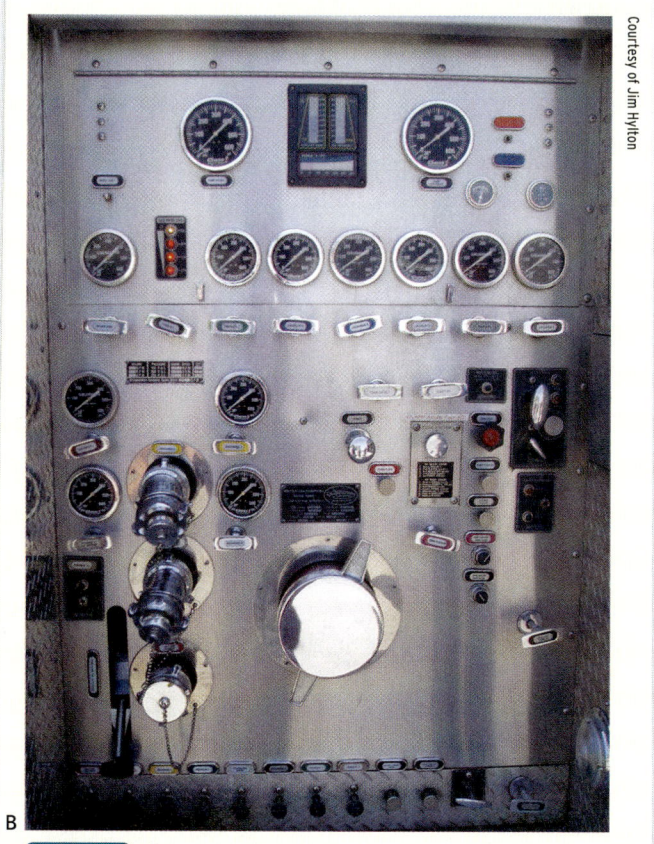

FIGURE 5-2 The pump panel may seem very confusing. Once you learn the basics of pump operations, you will become more comfortable with its components. **A.** A 1998 KME Quint 1500 gpm single-stage pump with no pressure governor. **B.** A 1500 gpm waterous two-stage pump.

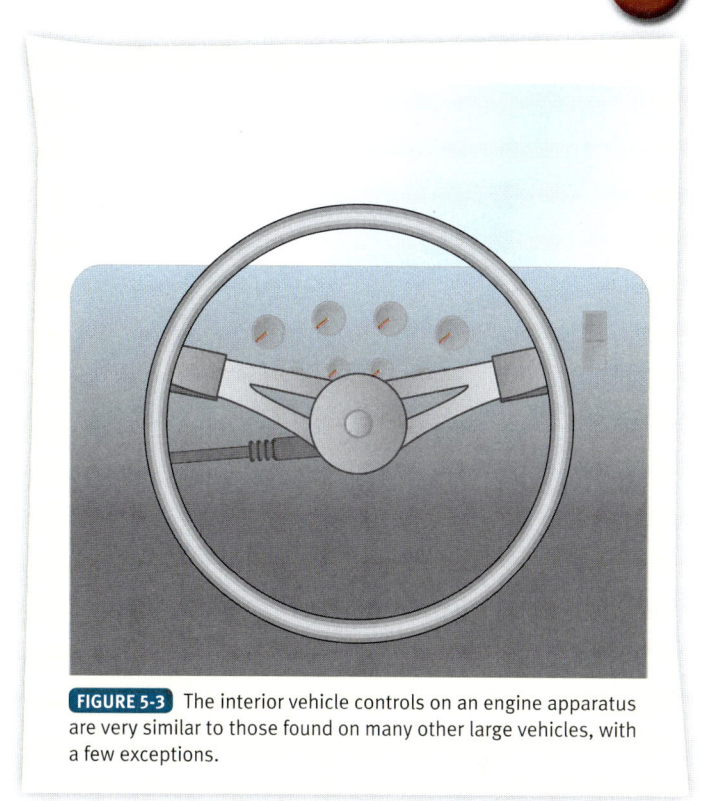

There are switches to operate the seats, mirrors, headlights, and windshield wipers, just as in any other vehicle. Some of the controls, however, are very different. For example, the controls to engage the fire pump or operate the emergency lights will not be found in other types of vehicles. It is important for the new driver/operator to understand that the fire apparatus is not like any other vehicle—and, therefore, should not be operated like other vehicles.

Fire Pumps

A major component of fire attack is water. To get the water on the fire, or "put the wet stuff on the red stuff," you must first pressurize it. To do so, you need a fire pump. National Fire Protection Association (NFPA) 1901, *Standard for Automotive Fire Apparatus*, defines a fire pump as a water pump that is mounted on the fire apparatus and used for firefighting. The fire pump must be capable of delivering a minimum capacity of 250–3000 gallons per minute (gpm) (1000–12,000 L/min) at 150 pounds per square inch (psi) (1000 kilopascals [kPa]) net pump pressure or over 3000 gpm (12,000 L/min) at 100 psi (700 kPa) net pump pressure. When the fire apparatus is designed for pump-and-roll operations, the fire apparatus engine and drive train must be arranged so that the unit can pump at least 20 gpm (80 L/min) at a gauge pressure of 80 psi (560 kPa) while the fire apparatus is moving at a speed of 2 mph (3.2 km/h) or less **FIGURE 5-4**.

Some fire apparatus are designed for responding to small vegetation fires and have relatively small capacities because they do not carry large amounts of water. These devices are usually mounted on the fire apparatus and have a separate engine to power them, other than the one that drives the fire

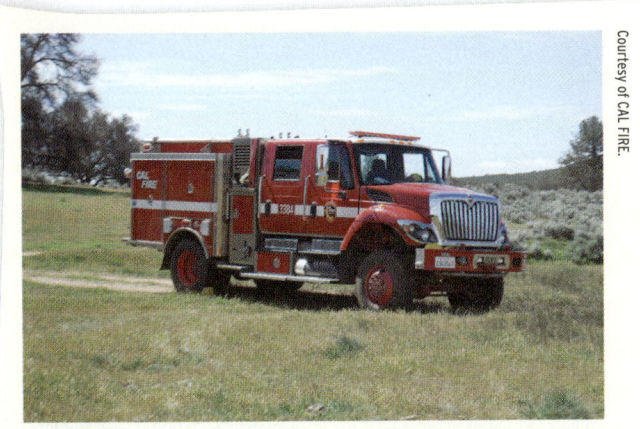

FIGURE 5-4 A fire apparatus designed for pump and roll operations.

FIGURE 5-5 A fire apparatus with a water tank.

apparatus. Other fire pumps are operated in a stationary position; they tend to be much larger and have a greater capacity. These fire pumps, which are typically used to combat fires that involve structures such as homes and commercial buildings, are powered through the transmission in the fire apparatus' engine. Still other fire pumps may be equipped with pump-and-roll capabilities.

No matter what size the fire pump, it must meet certain requirements. For example, NFPA 1901 states that if the pumping system is rated at 3000 gpm (12,000 L/min) or less, it shall be able to deliver water at the following rates:

- 100 percent of rate capacity at 150 psi (1000 kPa) net pump pressure
- 70 percent of rated capacity at 200 psi (1350 kPa) net pressure
- 50 percent of rated capacity at 250 psi (1700 kPa) net pressure

These requirements indicate that the maximum amount of water (gpm) the fire pump can deliver is at 150 psi (1000 kPa) net pump pressure. As the fire pump's psi rate increases, the amount of water that can be delivered decreases. After the fire pump reaches capacity, the only thing to gain by increasing the revolutions per minute (rpm) rate is an increase in pressure. Caution must be exercised to avoid cavitation when increasing pressure output and not increasing the amount of water being delivered. Cavitation occurs when you attempt to flow water faster than it is being supplied to the pump. This information may be useful if you are supplying attack lines for a high-rise fire and need the added pressure but not the entire capacity of the fire pump.

While drafting, if the fire pump is rated at less than 1500 gpm (6000 L/min), it is capable of taking suction through 20 ft (6 m) of suction hose and can discharge water in less than 30 seconds. If the fire pump is rated at greater than 1500 gpm, it is capable of taking suction through 20 ft (6 m) of suction hose and can discharge water in less than 45 seconds. Larger fire pumps are allowed more time to operate from a draft because they have more space inside that must be exhausted of air before water can enter the pump.

The fire apparatus manufacturer shall certify that the fire pump has the capability to pump water at 100 percent of the rated capacity at 150 psi (1000 kPa) with a net pump pressure from draft through 20 ft (6 m) of suction hose with a strainer at an atmosphere of 1000 ft (300 m) above sea level, an atmospheric pressure of 759 mm Hg (101 kPa), and a water temperature of 60°F (15.6°C). The size and number of suction lines required vary according to the size of the fire pump. All fire pumps are rated from a draft, meaning that no added water pressure from an external source is used to offset the capacity of the fire pump. The pump test is usually conducted at the manufacturer by a third party—for example, to determine Underwriters Laboratories (UL) certification.

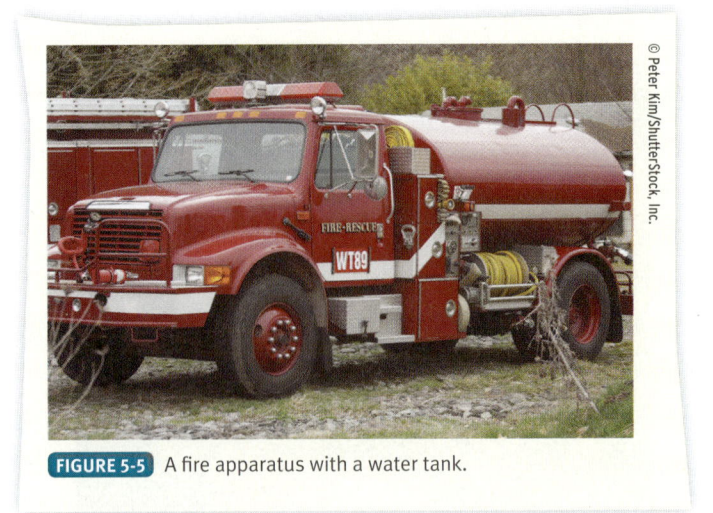

Once you engage the fire pump, you need to have a mechanism to ensure that it is running. When a separate engine is used to drive the fire pump, an indicator light in the driving compartment is illuminated when the fire pump is running. This indicator light is marked with a label such as "Pump Engine Running." If a fire apparatus is equipped with an automatic **chassis** transmission, the fire pump is driven by the transmission. This type of fire pump is used for stationary pumping only. A "Pump Engaged" indicator in the driver/operator's compartment signals when the pump shift process is complete, and an "OK to Pump" indicator in the driver/operator's compartment identifies when the fire pump is engaged. A separate "Throttle Ready" indicator is provided at the pump panel to signal when all necessary steps have been taken to ensure proper safe pumping. Other indicators of pump engagement include that the speedometer in the cab is operating and that the pressure is indicated on the master discharge gauge of the pump panel.

What good would a fire pump be without water? NFPA 1901 defines the requirements of fire apparatus equipped with water tanks **FIGURE 5-5**. Depending on the type of fire apparatus, the water tank may hold several hundred or several thousand gallons of water. Each fire department should carefully evaluate its water supply needs and the available water delivery systems when considering the size of water tank on the fire apparatus. Regardless of the tank's size, NFPA 1901 states that all water tanks shall be constructed with noncorrosive materials or other materials that are treated against corrosion and deterioration. In addition, all water tanks should be equipped with a baffling system with a minimum of two transverse or longitudinal vertical baffles that cover at least 75 percent of the area of the plane that contains the baffle. Each tank should include one or more cleanout sumps with 3-inch (77-mm) or larger removable pipe plugs. These plugs are often used to clean out the silt and debris that may become trapped in the water tank over time. NFPA 1901 covers many other aspects of water tanks, including water-level indicators, tank-to-pump intakes, filling, and venting, as well as external filling issues.

Fires are extinguished when the proper amount of water (or gallons per minute [gpm] or liters per minute [L/min] rate) is applied to the fire. This volume of water is directed through a nozzle at the required pressure to give the fire stream enough reach so that it can penetrate to the seat of the fire. A pump pressurizes the water used to attack the fire. According to the 2013 edition of NFPA 20, *Standard for the Installation of Stationary Pumps for Fire Protection*, a **fire pump** is defined as a provider of liquid flow and pressure dedicated to fire protection. It is a mechanical device used to move fluids. This concept is very important for fire fighters because they want the pump to move the water from the source, such as the onboard water tank, to the fire through the attack lines. To do so successfully, you must understand how each type of pump works.

Pumps displace the fluid, which causes this fluid to move or flow; resistance to this flow, in turn, creates pressure. With higher pressures, you will have less volume or flow; with higher flows, you will have less pressure. Pumps cannot provide both high pressure and high volume of water at the same time.

Types of Fire Pumps

The fire service primarily uses two types of pumps: positive-displacement pumps and centrifugal pumps. Each type relies on very different operating principles and offers a very different set of features.

■ Positive-Displacement Pumps

According to NFPA 20, a **positive-displacement pump** produces a flow by capturing a specific volume of fluid per pump revolution and reducing the fluid void by a mechanical means to displace the pumping fluid. It traps a fixed amount of fluid and forces that amount into the discharge stream during every revolution of the pumping element. The pump displaces the liquid by creating a space between the pumping elements and trapping the liquid in the space. As the pumping element moves, it reduces the size of this space, which in turn forces the fluid out of the pump.

Positive-displacement pumps rely on tightly fitting parts to function properly. Although these models are self-priming, they still require proper conditions, such as no excessive air leaks, to function properly. They can move air or water during every revolution because the parts fit together so closely. This makes the positive-displacement pump an ideal choice for use as a priming pump for centrifugal pumps.

As a priming pump, the positive-displacement pump is connected to the top of the centrifugal pump. When the positive-displacement pump is operated, it draws air and water from the top of the centrifugal pump until a constant flow of water is achieved, thereby ensuring that only water is inside the centrifugal pump casing.

Positive-displacement pumps may also be used as high-pressure auxiliary pumps or portable pumps. Because their efficiency depends on their close-fitting moving parts, the performance of these pumps will begin to deteriorate as they wear down over time and with excessive use. The presence of sand and other debris can cause the moving parts to wear out prematurely, further diminishing their performance.

The two broad classifications of positive-displacement pumps for firefighting purposes are the piston pump and the rotary pump. Rotary pumps exhibit a circular motion, whereas piston pumps have an up-and-down action.

Piston Pumps

Piston pumps use a cylinder to contain the fluid; a piston then moves back and forth inside the unit to move the liquid out of the cylinder. As the piston moves, water is drawn in from the intake side of the pump and expelled out the discharge side of the pump. This output of fluid is directly related to the cycles per minute of the piston: As the piston moves faster, the liquid will be discharged faster.

Piston pumps have three moving parts: the piston, the intake valve, and the discharge valve. Inside the cylinder is the piston, which creates a seal in the cylinder to separate the intake side and the discharge side of the pump. The intake and discharge valves create or block their respective openings so as to direct the water toward the target.

Two types of piston pumps are available: single-acting piston pumps and double-acting piston pumps.

Single-Acting Piston Pump

The operation of a **single-acting piston pump** is very simple. This type of pump has one intake side and one discharge side, both of which are located at the same ends of the cylinder. As the piston moves upward, away from the intake side, a vacuum is created in the cylinder. This vacuum causes the intake valve to open and fill the cylinder with water. Water continues to fill the cylinder until the piston stops. At the same time, at the discharge side of the pump, the discharge valve remains in the closed position. Once the piston moves in the opposite direction, the intake valve closes and the discharge valve opens to expel the water.

The single-acting piston pump is similar to a squirt gun. As you depress the trigger, water inside a cylinder is compressed and discharged out the tip **FIGURE 5-6**. When you release the trigger, the cylinder refills with water and waits to be discharged again **FIGURE 5-7**.

DRIVER/OPERATOR Tip

The first hand pump used in the first fire brigades consisted of a single-acting piston pump.

With every pump on the lever, a definite amount of fluid is discharged from the single-acting piston pump. Water is discharged only on the downward movement of the piston, which creates a pulsating effect because water flow is not constant. As a consequence, single-acting piston pumps are not suitable for use on an attack line. The fire stream from this type of pump

FIGURE 5-6 As you depress the trigger, water inside a cylinder is compressed and discharged out the tip.
Adapted from Hale Products, Inc.

FIGURE 5-7 When the trigger is released, the cylinder refills with water and waits to be discharged again.
Adapted from Hale Products, Inc.

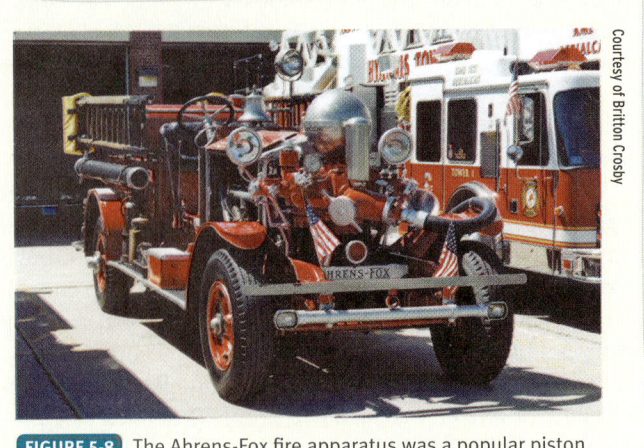

FIGURE 5-8 The Ahrens-Fox fire apparatus was a popular piston pump fire apparatus for years.

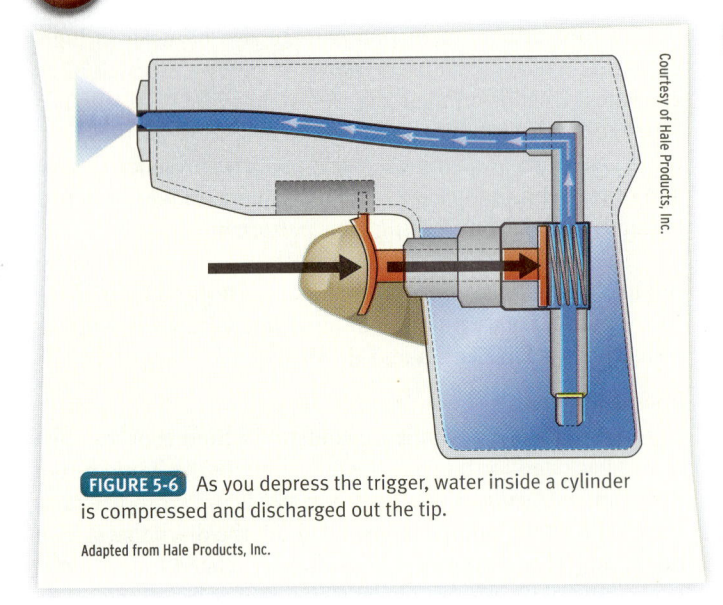

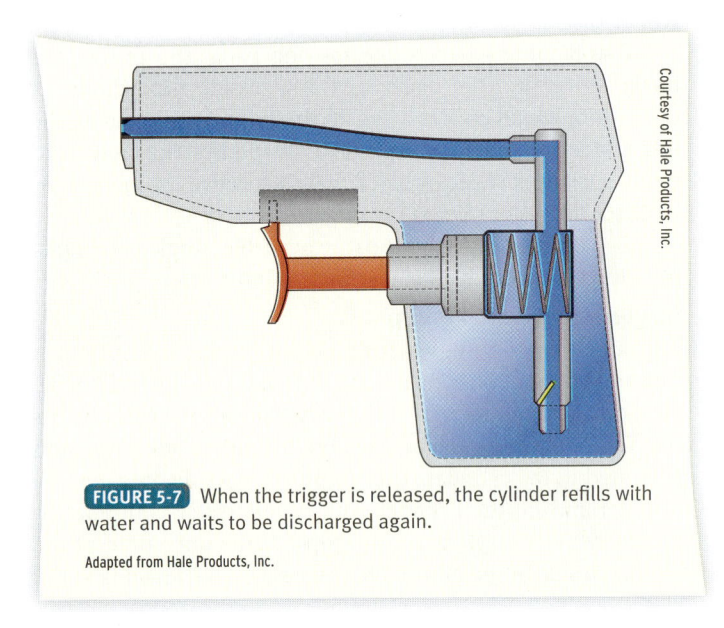

would be inconsistent and have moments without any water discharged. An additional piston can be added to increase the water flow and provide a more constant flow. With this setup, the two pistons would operate in opposite directions to maintain the water flow. While one piston is filling with water, the other would be discharging the water.

Double-Acting Piston Pump

A <u>double-acting piston pump</u> allows water to flow more continuously than a single-acting piston pump while using only one piston. This double-acting piston pump still has periods of limited flow—specifically, when the pistons are at the top of their stroke before changing direction. Instead of having only one intake valve and discharge valve at one end of the cylinder, however, this pump has both valves at each end. As a consequence, the cylinder fills with water on both the up and down strokes of the piston. When the piston is pulled upward, the water flows into the cylinder through the intake valve; at the same time, water flows through the discharge valve on the other side of the piston.

DRIVER/OPERATOR Tip

Steam-powered pumps used the same pump design as piston pumps to move water. Some of the first motorized fire apparatus used piston pumps that were able to deliver a flow volume of as much as 500 gpm (2000 liters per minute [L/min]). The Ahrens-Fox fire apparatus was a popular piston pump fire apparatus for many years **FIGURE 5-8**.

Rotary Pumps

<u>Rotary pumps</u> are typically used as the priming pump for a centrifugal pump. These pumps operate in a circular motion and discharge a constant flow of water with each revolution. To accomplish this task, some <u>pumping element</u>, such as a gear or vane encased in the pump casing, rotates, expanding the volume inside to allow water to enter the pump. As the pumping elements rotate, the area in which the fluid is contained is reduced, which in turn forces the water out of the pump. This results in a smooth continuous flow of water discharged from the pump. The internal components fit together tightly and allow for very little water to slip back from the discharge side to the intake side of the pump during operation.

Rotary Gear Pumps

One type of positive-displacement pump commonly encountered in the fire service is the <u>rotary gear pump</u>, which is typically used as a priming pump **FIGURE 5-9**. The rotary gear pump uses two gears, most often driven by a 12-volt electric motor. Inside the pump casing, two gears rotate in opposite directions. These gears are positioned closely to each other and to the inside of the pump casing, forming a watertight seal. As the two gears mesh together, they trap water and move it to the discharge side of the pump. Usually, a motor powers one gear, which then powers the second gear. Oil may be fed into the pump to maintain as watertight a seal as possible. The oil will fill any open spaces to make the pump work more efficiently.

Rotary Vane Pumps

A <u>rotary vane pump</u> uses small movable elements called <u>vanes</u>, which freely move in and out of the slots of the <u>rotor</u>

CHAPTER 5 The Fire Pump 81

move independently, as the surface of the vane itself wears down over time, it will continue to maintain a watertight fit: It can automatically adjust itself to compensate for the wear and tear in the unit. Centrifugal force keeps the vane tightly pressed against the pump casing, thereby ensuring a tight seal. This makes the pump operate very efficiently.

FIGURE 5-9 Rotary gear pump.

DRIVER/OPERATOR Tip

Operating the priming valve on the pump panel opens a valve from the priming pump to the centrifugal pump and engages the electric motor of a rotary pump. With every revolution of the rotary pump, the pump moves air or water. As a priming pump, it is designed to pump the air from the centrifugal pump, thereby ensuring that only water is available inside the centrifugal pump.

DRIVER/OPERATOR Tip

Other devices that do not use a pump may also be used to prime the main pump. For example, an intake manifold priming device uses the vacuum of the truck's engine on the intake manifold to prime the pump. The two chambers of this device prevent water from entering the engine—an arrangement commonly known as an **exhaust primer**. The engine's exhaust is directed through a device that causes a **Venturi effect**, which creates a vacuum. This vacuum is connected to the main fire pump, drawing air out of it. While some fire apparatus use this type of priming device, it is most often found on portable pumps.

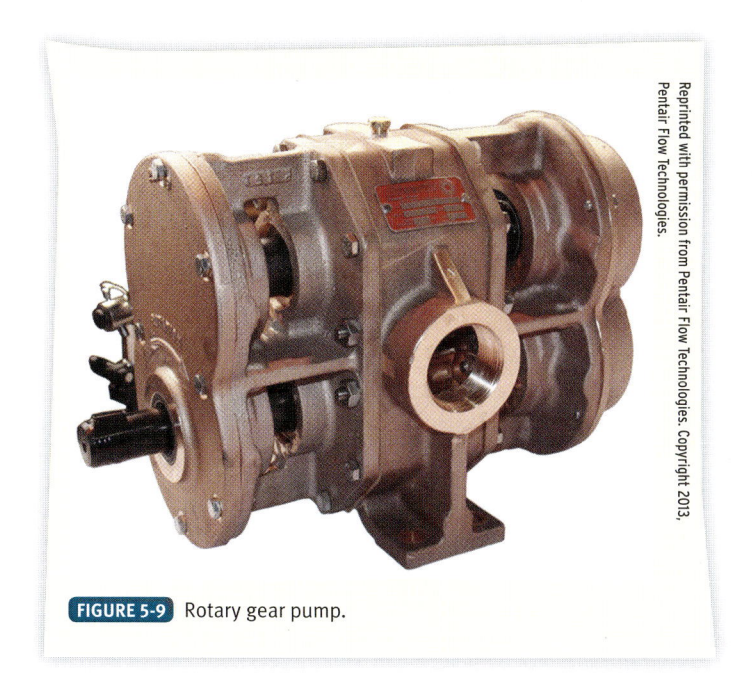

to maintain a tight seal against the pump casing **FIGURE 5-10**. The vanes are positioned off-center inside the pump casing and automatically maneuver in and out to compensate for changes in the pump casing. As the vanes approach the intake side of the pump, the void space increases and the vanes slide farther out of their slots. Water then flows in between these vanes, becoming trapped there. When the vanes approach the discharge side of the pump, the void space decreases and the vanes slide farther back into their slots. Water that is trapped in between the vanes is then discharged from the pump. Because the vanes in the rotor

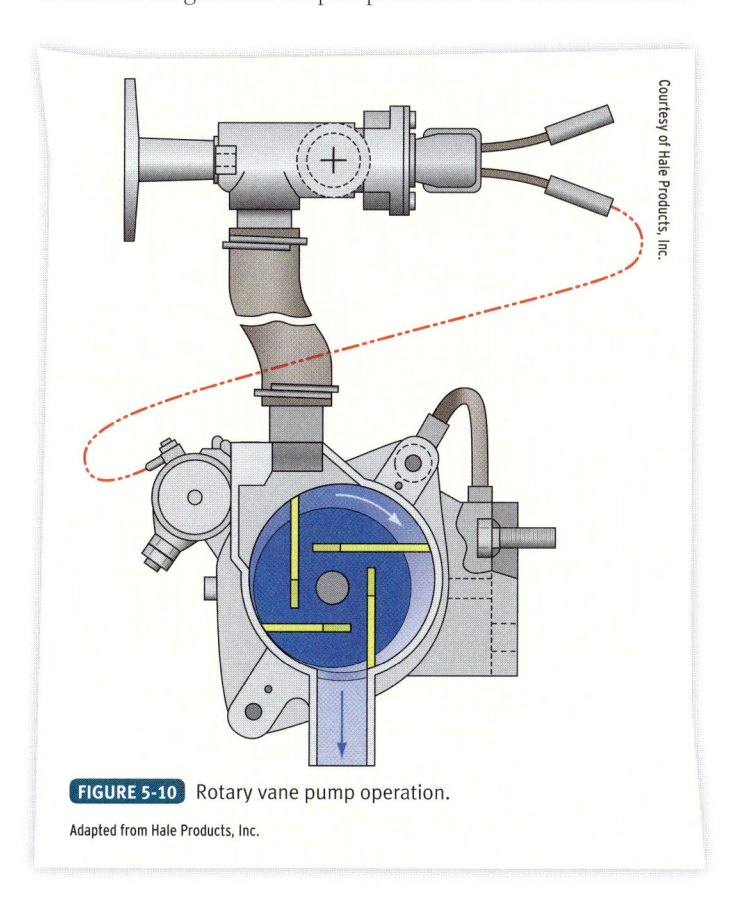

■ Centrifugal Pump

The most common fire pump in use today is the centrifugal pump **FIGURE 5-11**. This type of pump has largely replaced positive-displacement pumps on modern fire apparatus. Centrifugal pumps do not flow a definite amount of water with each revolution; instead, the flow or amount of water discharged is based on the pressures at the discharge side of the pump. At higher discharge pressures (psi), the pump will flow lower volumes of water. Consequently, as the pump spins more slowly, it will flow higher volumes (gpm) of water at lower pressure on the discharge side. This flexibility makes the centrifugal pump a very versatile piece of equipment on the fireground. As the driver/operator, you need to understand how this pump works to maximize its potential as part of firefighting operations.

This pump operates on the basic principle of **centrifugal force**—that is, the outward force from the center of rotation. The centrifugal pump receives water into the center or eye of an **impeller** **FIGURE 5-12** that is mounted (as an offset) inside the pump casing. The pump impeller forms the heart of the pumping device: This metal rotating component transfers energy from the vehicle's motor to discharge the incoming water. Inside the impeller are **impeller vanes**, which divide the impeller. As the impeller spins, it accelerates the movement

FIGURE 5-10 Rotary vane pump operation.
Adapted from Hale Products, Inc.

VOICES OF EXPERIENCE

One of the most valuable skills I have learned is being calm while under extreme duress. When a driver/operator becomes traumatized and panics, that behavior has a detrimental effect on his or her performance, endangers the lives of team members, and can endanger everyone involved in the incident. Driver/operators must be able to function within the team, which is part of the reason why the camaraderie is so strong among fire fighters. Literally, you must be willing to trust your life to your fellow fire fighters. You must train extensively to develop a sense of calm so that you can function effectively when everyone and everything around you appear to be in a chaotic state. Driver/operators routinely operate in environments that endanger life and property. The old adage, "Fire fighters run in, when everyone else is running away," still holds true.

The best driver/operators are always seeking knowledge to enhance their ability to perform. This knowledge should be obtained from a variety of sources:

- College-based instruction and formal education
- Local, regional, state, and national fire schools and academies
- Institutional knowledge such as thorough knowledge of the department and local mutual aid resources available
- Experiential learning by hands-on practical application of techniques
- Community knowledge: pertinent information about community demographics, water mains, water sources, utilities, building design and construction, potential community hazards, traffic routes, evacuation routes, and location of fire protection systems

The importance of each driver/operator's contribution to the overall mission of public safety and the department's role must be extolled. Fire fighters are called when people do not know what to do; an incident may involve a seemingly insignificant operation such as water in the basement, but it may also involve a devastating fire with multiple fatalities. The only way a driver/operator can effectively respond to this task is by being calm and constantly learning.

Charles Garrity
Berkshire Community College
Pittsfield, Massachusetts

FIGURE 5-11 Centrifugal pump operation.
Adapted from Hale Products, Inc.
Courtesy of Hale Products, Inc.

FIGURE 5-12 A centrifugal pump impeller.

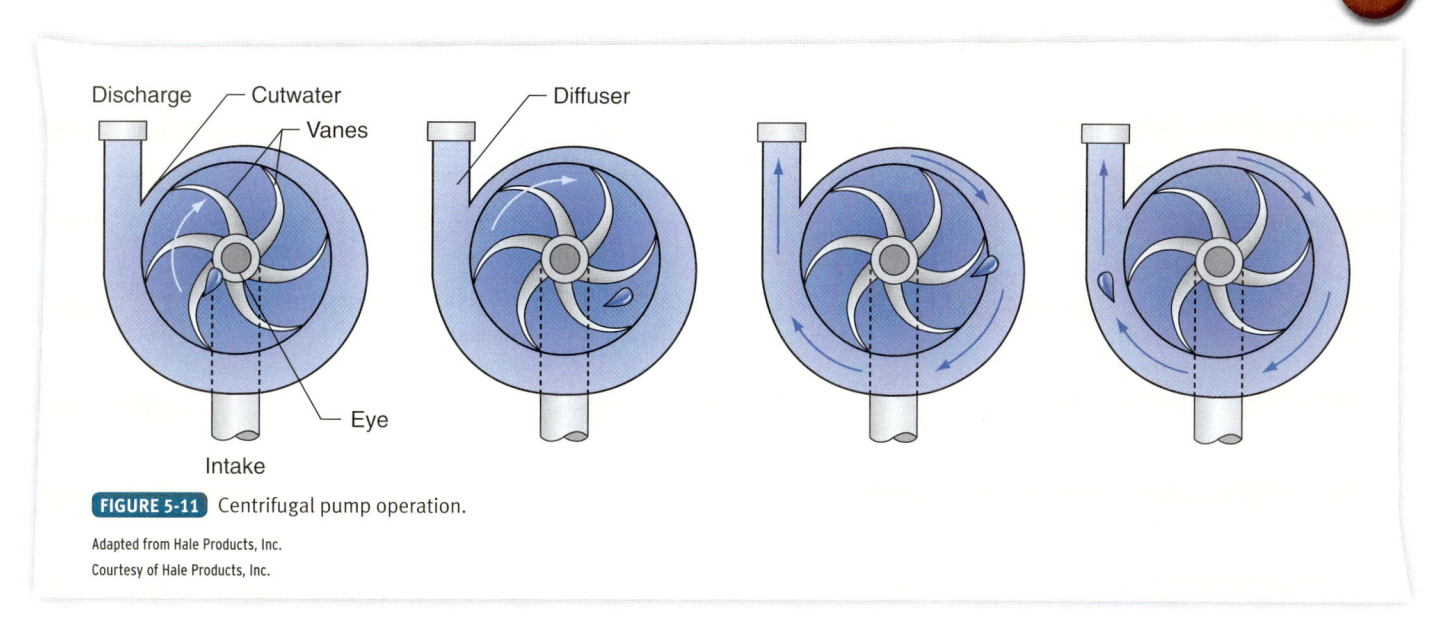

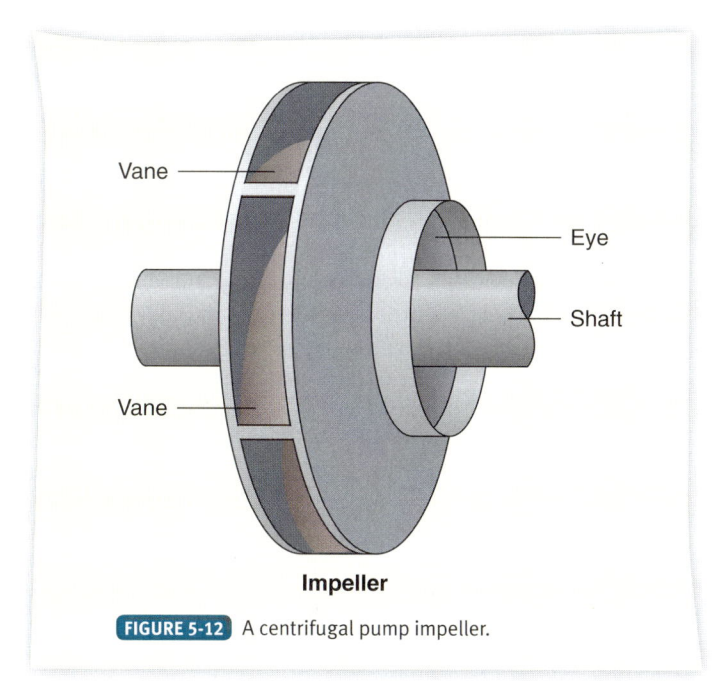

of water between the vanes and discharges the fluid radially outward into a collection area called a **volute**. The volute gradually increases in area, causing the water pressure to increase; it then directs the water into the **discharge header**, where piping is attached and valves are arranged to deliver water to the intended hoselines or devices.

DRIVER/OPERATOR Tip

The eye of the impeller is where the water enters the centrifugal pump. Some pumps have water enter from only one side of the impeller. Other models, called double-intake impellers, have the water enter from each side.

A centrifugal pump can pump only water or other liquids. This kind of pump is completely devoid of any valves from the intake to the discharge side. Water is free to move between either side of the impeller when it is not spinning. When the impeller is spinning, the water is taken from the intake side and flows out the discharge side. If the discharge valves are all closed, the water inside the pump simply churns around inside. The centrifugal pump relies on the movement of water from the intake side to the discharge side to operate effectively. Unlike a positive-displacement pump, this device is not self-priming; therefore the centrifugal cannot pump air—only liquids (typically water).

Also unlike positive-displacement pumps, centrifugal pumps are able to take advantage of any incoming pressure on the intake side of the pump. This additional intake pressure will simply increase the discharge pressure of the pump. For example, if the pump is receiving water at a pressure of 60 psi (420 kPa) from a hydrant at the intake side of the pump, and you need to supply the attack line at 100 psi (700 kPa), the pump will have to create only an additional 40 psi (280 kPa) to achieve the desired pressure.

Single-Stage and Multistage Pumps

Centrifugal pumps can be single-stage models (one impeller) or multistage units (two or more impellers within one pump housing turning on the same shaft).

Single-Stage Pump

A **single-stage pump** has one impeller, which both takes the water in and discharges it out of the pump. This single impeller is responsible for supplying 100 percent of the total amount of water for the pump. Such a design makes the pump easier to operate because the pump can operate in only one mode **FIGURE 5-13**.

Two-Stage Pump

The most common type of multistage pump is the two-stage pump. A two-stage pump has two impellers, which are enclosed in their own pump casings but are part of a common housing. Each impeller is identical in size and capacity, and each is mounted on the same drive shaft and, therefore, spins at the same speed. At the discharge side of the first impeller, a

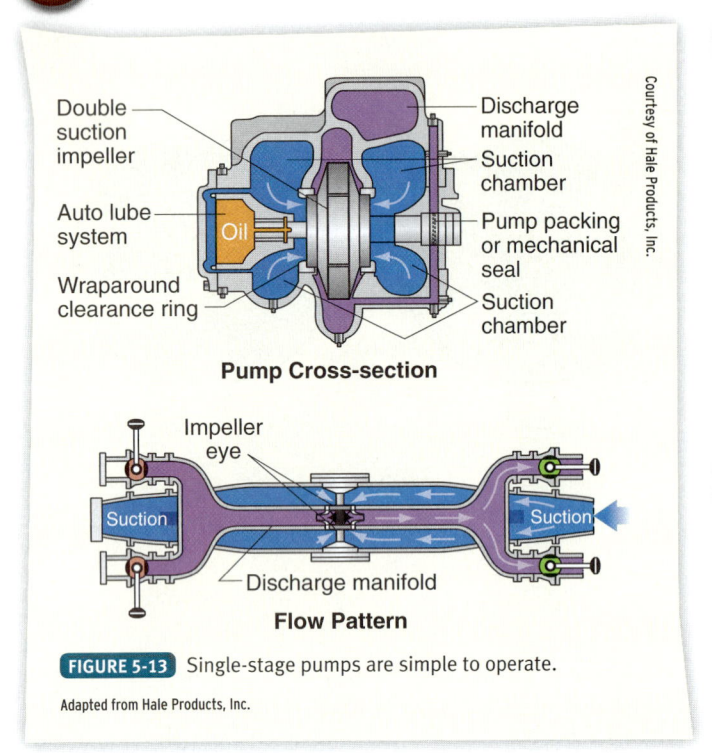

FIGURE 5-13 Single-stage pumps are simple to operate.
Adapted from Hale Products, Inc.

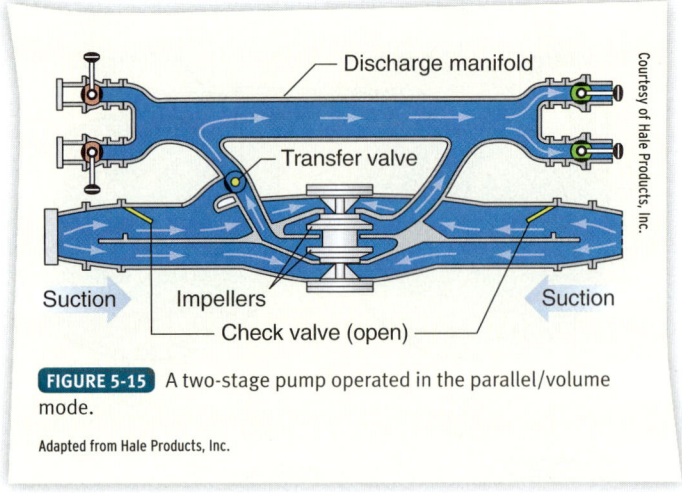

FIGURE 5-15 A two-stage pump operated in the parallel/volume mode.
Adapted from Hale Products, Inc.

transfer valve directs the water to either the pump's discharge header or the intake side of the second impeller **FIGURE 5-14**. A transfer valve determines whether the pump will be operated in series/pressure mode or parallel/volume mode. Both positions have their own strengths and weaknesses.

Parallel/Volume Mode

When water is directed in the **parallel/volume mode**, it enters each impeller from a common intake side and is discharged into a common discharge header **FIGURE 5-15**. This results in the pump's maximum volume of water being discharged. In this mode, each of the two impellers pumps 50 percent of the pump's total capacity. For example, if the pump is rated as a 2000 gpm (8000 L/min) pump, then each impeller would discharge a flow of 1000 gpm (4000 L/min). When more than 50 percent of the pump's rated capacity is needed on the fireground, the pump should be operated in parallel/volume mode to ensure that the desired flow can be achieved.

Series/Pressure Mode

When water is discharged in **series/pressure mode**, it travels through one impeller at a time or in series **FIGURE 5-16**. Water enters the first-stage pump impeller's intake side, gains pressure, and is discharged to the second-stage impeller's intake side. The second impeller then pumps the water out of the discharge header. The water will have more pressure as it enters the second-stage impeller than when it entered the first impeller, and it will gain additional pressure after being discharged from the second impeller. Series/pressure mode is the position in which two-stage pumps are most commonly operated. Most fire responses do not require the pump to deliver more than 50 percent of the pump's rated capacity. Therefore, the pump is left in series/pressure mode so that the desired pressure is achieved by operating at a lower rate (rpm).

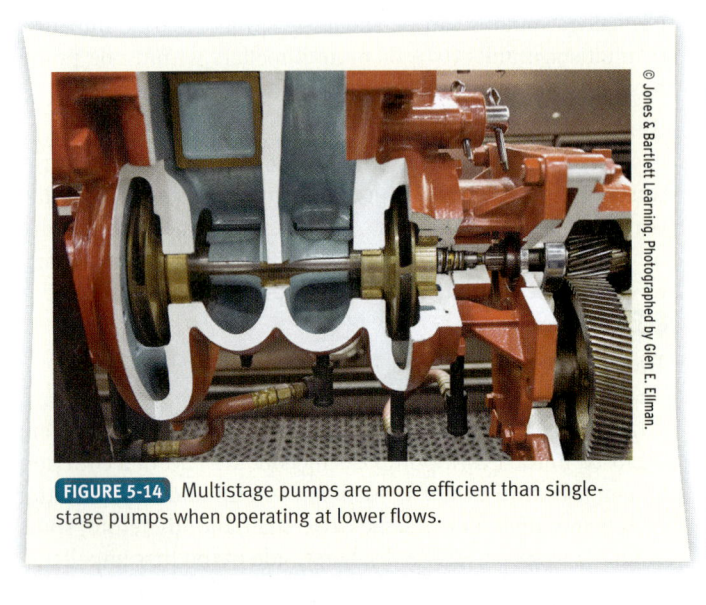

FIGURE 5-14 Multistage pumps are more efficient than single-stage pumps when operating at lower flows.

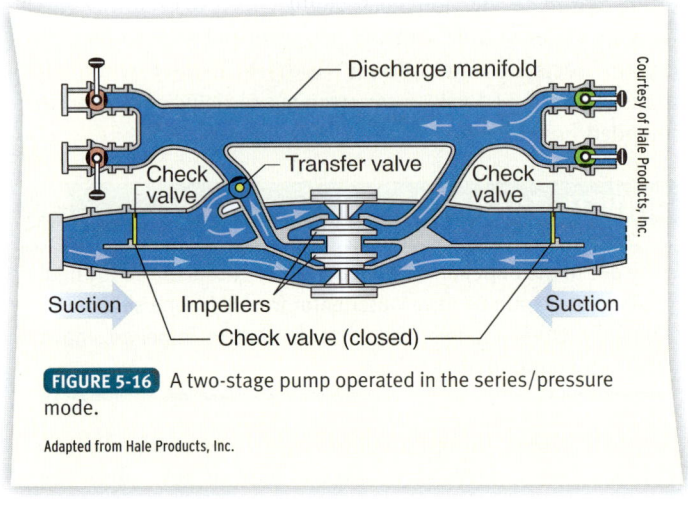

FIGURE 5-16 A two-stage pump operated in the series/pressure mode.
Adapted from Hale Products, Inc.

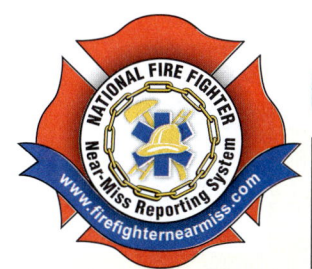

Near-Miss REPORT

Report Number: 10-0000559

Synopsis: Missed step in pump operation causes pump failure.

Event Description: We responded to a reported dumpster fire up against a building. We had a box assignment dedicated to the call (three pumps, one ladder, and one rescue). Deputy, on arrival, reported a dumpster fully involved. I was on the second pump, so our responsibility was to secure a hydrant if needed. The first pump on scene started stretching a line with no result—no water pressure. It turned out that the pump operator had failed to engage the maxi-brake, which prevented the pump from engaging. The operator attempted to correct the issue but wasn't able to successfully troubleshoot.

Lessons Learned: I believe this problem could have been corrected on-scene in time to extinguish the fire. There was a lot of standing around and leaving the fire fighter to attempt to rectify the problem himself. A lot of confusion on-scene and several fire fighters assumed that the problem was mechanical in nature. The lessons learned include reinforcing teamwork and accountability. The pump operator didn't acknowledge an issue.

A fire pump is rated by and tested to UL specifications. To satisfy the UL standards, it must produce 100 percent of its rated capability at 150 psi (1000 kPa) for 20 minutes, 70 percent of its rated capability at 200 psi (1350 kPa) for 10 minutes, and 50 percent of its rated capability at 250 psi (1700 kPa) for 10 minutes. No additional rating is provided for pressures greater than 250 psi (1700 kPa); such pressures can be generated by using one pump impeller or multiple pump impellers inside the pump. Alternatively, the pump can be configured to provide pressures significantly greater than 250 psi (1700 kPa) by directing the water from the first impeller directly to the second impeller and then to the discharge, thereby doubling the pressure. With this configuration, 50 percent of the flow rate of the pump is lost because the first impeller does not send its water to the discharge side, but rather sends it to the second impeller (second stage).

As a driver/operator, you will find a control valve on the pump panel of a multistage pump indicating whether the impellers are being operated in parallel/volume mode or series/pressure mode. If the pump operation requires a large volume of water, then the pump should be operated in parallel/volume mode. In most pumping operations, you will supply one or two handlines with a total flow of 300–400 gpm (1200–1600 L/min) of water. A 1000-gal (4000-L) two-stage pump can easily supply this amount while operating in series/pressure mode. The advantage of this configuration is not attributable to any need for excessive pressure; rather, this setting allows the pumper engine and power supply to produce the water at lower engine speed (rpm), which is more efficient.

Think of a two-stage pump as similar to working from a hydrant water supply and pumper. When you start operating from the onboard water tank and pump water at a pressure of 100 psi (700 kPa), the total pressure available on the discharge is 100 psi (700 kPa). When a hydrant line is opened, it provides 100 psi (700 kPa) to the intake side of the pump, which is combined with the 100 psi (700 kPa) flow that the pump is already supplying. Therefore the pressure will be increased at the discharge to 200 psi (1400 kPa). The same concept applies when water is directed from the first impeller to the second impeller instead of being allowed to flow out of the discharge. The pressure is doubled in the pump, but the total flow capability depends on the capability of the first impeller because the second impeller now receives its water from the first impeller.

Special multistage pumps have been built to produce extraordinarily high pressures for special pumping requirements. In addition, some fire departments want to preserve the ability to use high-pressure booster lines while still having volume pumping capabilities of 500 gpm (2000 L/min) or more. One method of achieving this goal is to place both a piston pump and a volume pump on the same fire apparatus. Another approach is to use a three-stage pump; the first two stages operate as a two-stage pump as previously described, while a small amount of water is directed to a third stage that produces higher pressures, typically supplying one or two booster hoselines.

Pump capacity over the years has increased significantly as larger pumps with larger impellers have been developed. In the 1950s, pumps typically delivered flows at 500 or 750 gpm (2000 or 3000 L/min). By comparison, today's fire pumps can flow water at 2000 gpm (8000 L/min) or larger. The other element driving the increases in pump capacity is the increase in diesel engines' horsepower, which has doubled from 250 horsepower to more than 500 horsepower since the 1950s. To turn a pump fast enough to produce a flow of 2000 gpm (8000 L/min) at 150 psi (1000 kPa) from draft requires a significant power supply, which is readily achieved with modern fire apparatus.

DRIVER/OPERATOR Tip

When pumping requirements exceed 50 percent of the rated capacity of a two-stage pump, then you should operate the pump in parallel/volume mode. This will allow for the rated capacity of the pump to be used based on the availability of water on the intake side of the pump. A 1500 gpm (6000 L/min) two-stage pump would provide this capacity at 150 psi (1000 kPa) when operating from draft. When operating from a residual source, such as a hydrant, it will produce additional flow (gpm) and pressure. There is a point at which only so much water can be pushed through an opening, however—so do not expect the pump to deliver heroic amounts of water or water at an unusually high pressure simply because you are connected to a hydrant with a good flow rate and pressure.

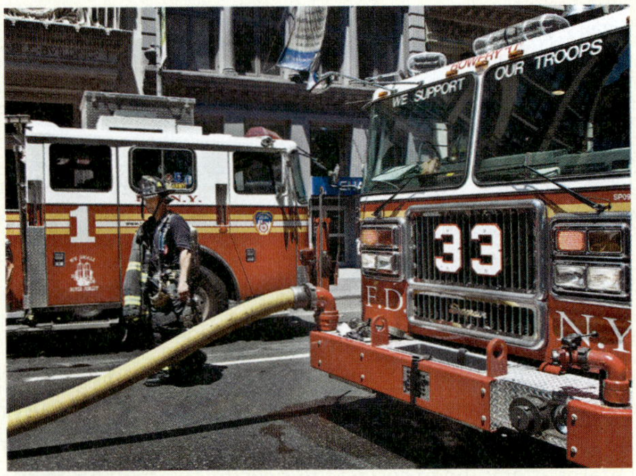

FIGURE 5-17 A front intake connection on engine apparatus.

Fire Pump Anatomy

The two main sides of all pumps are the intake and discharge sides. The <u>intake side</u> of the pump is where the water enters the pump. It is also referred to as the supply side of the pump because it is where water is supplied to the pump. On most pumps, the pipes and connections for the intake are set lower than the discharge piping and connections. The location where the water exits the pump is called the <u>discharge side</u>. Valves may be located on either side of the pump. They are necessary to control the flow of water both to and from the pump. Drains allow operators to empty the pump for repairs and to ensure that the water in the pump does not freeze in cold weather situations. NFPA 1901 further describes these components of fire service pumps: pump intake connections and pump discharge outlet connections.

■ Pump Intake Connections

Water enters the pump from either the on-board water tank or an intake connection pipe. The pipe that leads from the apparatus water tank to the fire pump is commonly referred to as the <u>tank-to-pump</u>. This pipe can be of various sizes but must meet certain performance requirements. If the water tank has a certified capacity of less than 500 gallons (2000 liters), the piping and valve arrangement must be capable of delivering water to the pump at a minimum rate of 250 gpm (1000 L/min). If the water tank has a certified capacity of greater than 500 gallons (2000 liters), the piping and valve arrangement must be capable of delivering water to the pump at a minimum rate of 500 gpm (2000 L/min). The tank-to-pump piping also contains a check valve, which allows water to flow only from the tank into the pump and not back inside the tank. This helps to prevent damage to the tank in situations where excessive intake pressure is encountered—such as relay pumping (this topic is covered further in the chapter *Relay Pump Operations*).

When the internal water tank is not used to supply the fire pump, an external water supply is needed to fulfill this purpose. This water enters the pump directly through the intake side via an intake connection pipe. The pump should have a sufficient number and size of intake connections to perform the pump certification test successfully. Most common intake connections are National Standard Thread (NST) or sexless type connections, such as a Storz connector. These intake connection pipes are usually located on both sides of the pump; if intake piping were located at the front or the rear of the apparatus, that arrangement might not allow for drafting at the pump's rated capacity due to the length of the piping **FIGURE 5-17**.

Most pumps also include one or more valves connected to the intake connection piping to control the water flow at the intake to the pump. At least one valve should be a minimum of 2½ inches (65 mm) nominal size. Most fire service pumps rated up to 2000 gpm (8000 L/min) have a large-diameter hose (LDH) intake that is 4–6 inches (100–150 mm) in diameter on both sides of the pump. Several LDH intake valve designs may be used, including a ball valve, a butterfly valve, or a piston intake valve, which is connected to the threaded intake piping **FIGURE 5-18**.

Each intake valve that has a connection larger than 3 inches (77 mm) must be equipped with an adjustable <u>automatic intake pressure relief device</u> installed on the supply (intake) of the valve to bleed off excess pressure coming into the valve **FIGURE 5-19**. The excess pressure is required to discharge away from the pump operator, and the valve should be adjustable from 90 psi (630 kPa) to at least 185 psi (1295 kPa). If the pump is equipped with one or more intakes larger than 3 inches (76 mm) that are not valved, an adjustable automatic intake pressure relief device must be installed on the pump system to bleed off excess pressure from hose connected to the intake side of the pump. This automatic intake pressure relief device must be adjustable from 90 psi (630 kPa) to at least 185 psi (1295 kPa) and discharge to the atmosphere and away from the pump operator.

Each intake valve must also be equipped with a bleeder valve to remove any air trapped in the hose before it enters the centrifugal fire pump **FIGURE 5-20**. All intake piping must also have a removable or accessible strainer to prevent debris from entering the impeller of the pump and causing damage to the pump. All intakes must be provided with caps or plugs and

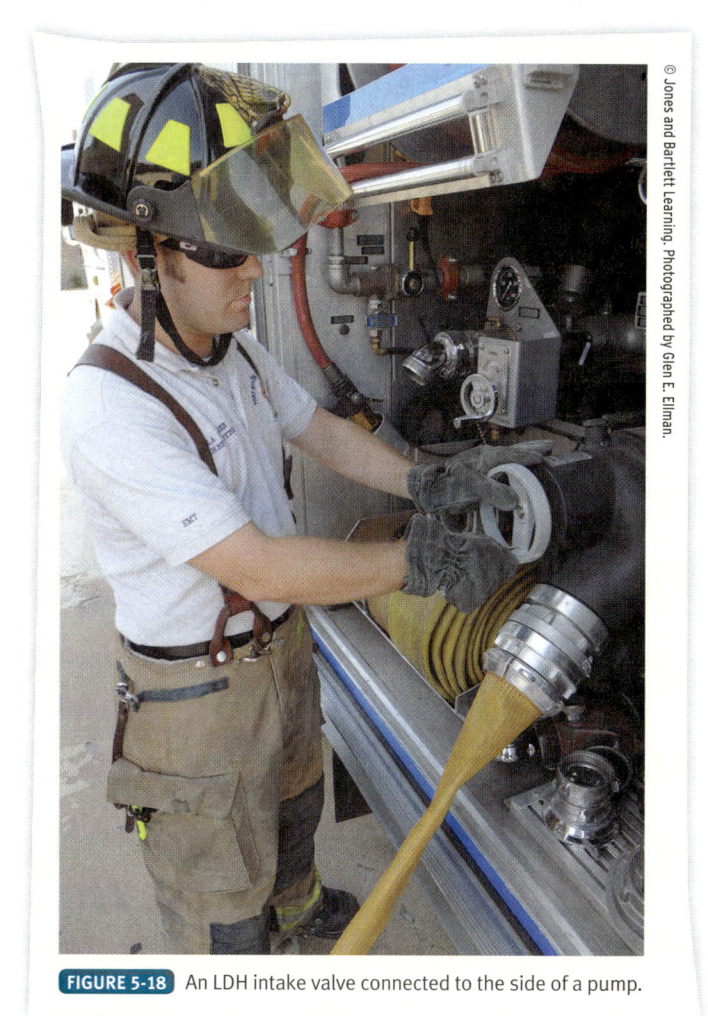

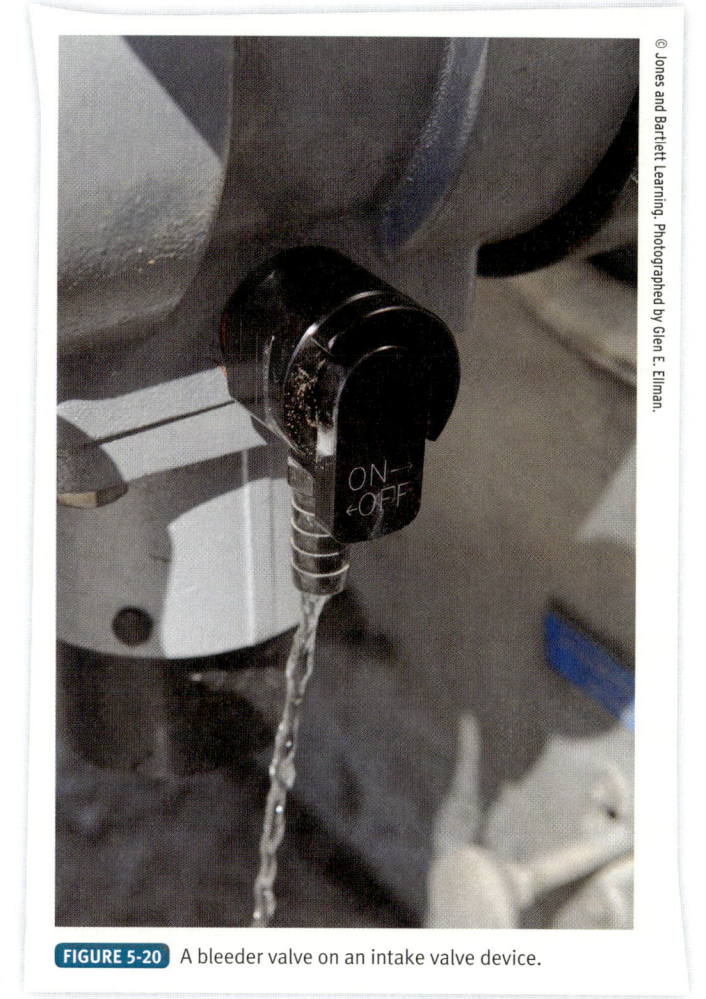

FIGURE 5-18 An LDH intake valve connected to the side of a pump.

FIGURE 5-20 A bleeder valve on an intake valve device.

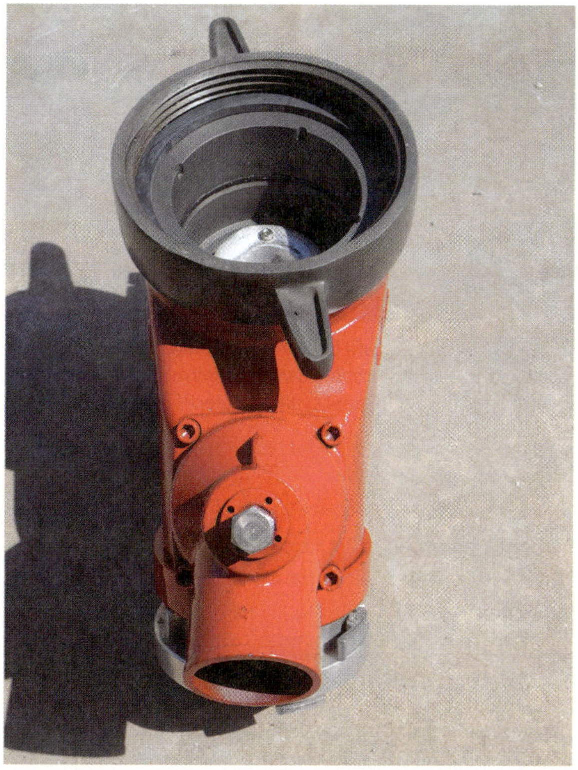

FIGURE 5-19 An automatic intake pressure relief valve.

should remain secured to the apparatus when removed; this ensures that they will not be lost.

Pump Discharge Outlet Connections

The discharge side of the pump is where the pressurized water is expelled from the pump and distributed to discharge outlets. One of the outlets from the discharge side of the pump goes to the apparatus-mounted water tank and is used to fill the tank and circulate water. These outlets have piping that is usually 1 to 2 inches (25 to 50 mm), depending on the size of the water tank. A valve to operate this discharge, called the <u>tank fill</u> valve, is located on the pump panel **FIGURE 5-21**. Another outlet from the discharge is a pump cooling/recirculation line, whose operation may be either automatic or manual. This, which line is smaller than the tank-fill line, is used to circulate water in the system to prevent overheating the fire pump.

Discharge outlets of 2½ inches (65 mm) or larger must be provided to discharge the rated capacity of the pump. Generally, a minimum of two 2½-inch (65-mm) outlets will be provided on any pump that is rated at 750 gpm (3000 L/min) or greater and a minimum of one 2½-inch (65-mm) outlet will be provided on any pump rated less than 750 gpm (3000 L/min). All 2½-inch (65-mm) or larger discharge outlet connections must be equipped with male National Hose threads. This

FIGURE 5-21 A tank fill valve on a pump panel.

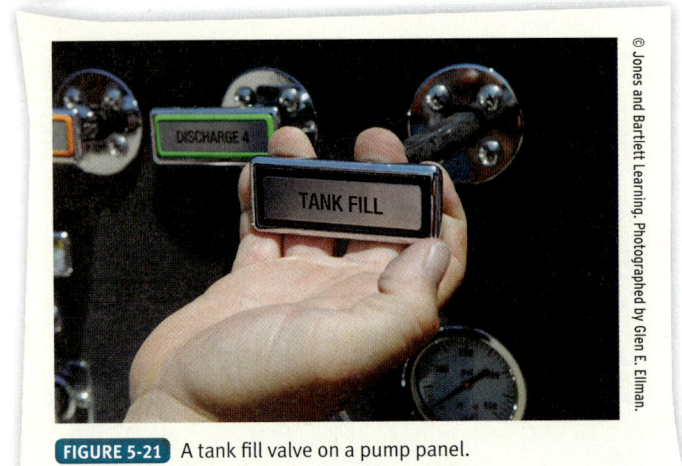

requirement is intended to ensure interoperability between fire departments at major incidents. The piping and valves supplying preconnected 1½-, 1¾-, and 2-inch (38-, 45-, and 50-mm) hoselines must be at least 2 inches (50 mm) in size.

Any discharge that is not directly connected to a preconnected hoseline must be equipped with a cap and secured to the apparatus so they are not lost **FIGURE 5-22**. Each discharge outlet must be equipped with a valve that can be opened and closed smoothly while operating at 250 psi (1750 kPa). Each discharge must have a valve that can be operated from the pump operator's position and have an indicator to show when the valve is open or closed. Control of discharges may achieved by pull-type actuators, swing valves, flexible push/pull controls, gear operated hand wheel controls, or hydraulic, air, and electric operators **FIGURE 5-23**. These controls may either be quick operating or slow operating. If the discharge valve is 3 inches (77 mm) or larger, it must be equipped with a slow-operating control mechanism. All 1½-inch (38-mm) or larger discharge outlets must be equipped with a drain or bleeder for draining off pressure from a hose connected to an outlet.

A pump drain must be provided to allow the draining of the pump and all water-carrying pipes and accessories. Fire department personnel must be able to operate this drain valve without getting under the apparatus.

FIGURE 5-22 A cap on a discharge outlet.

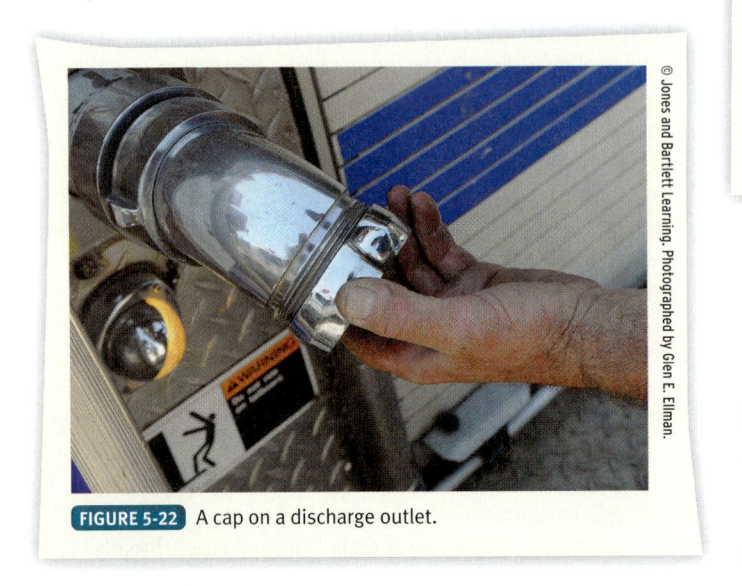

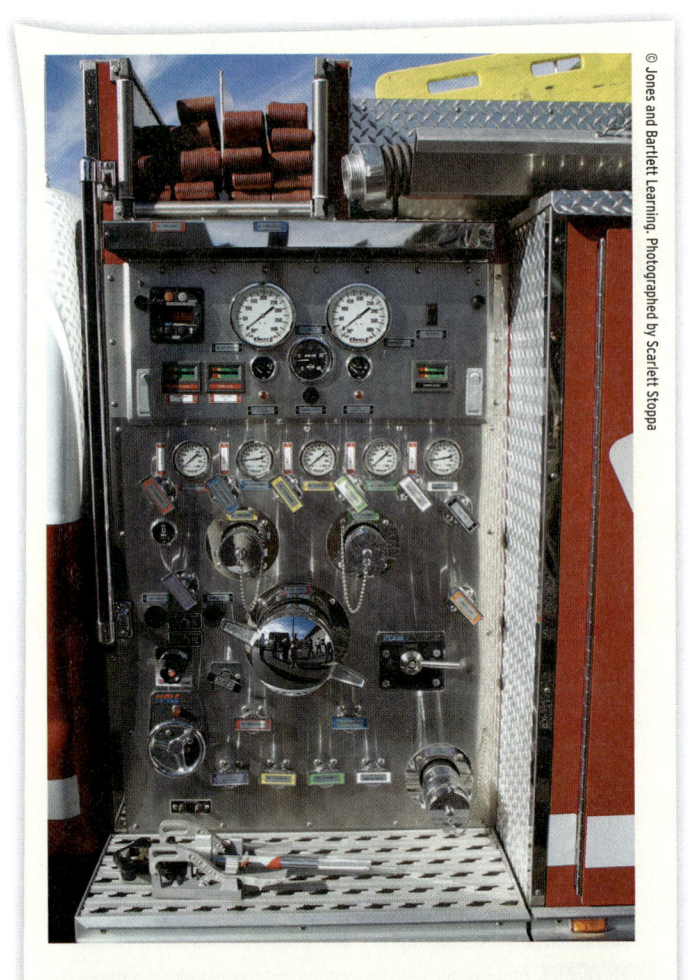

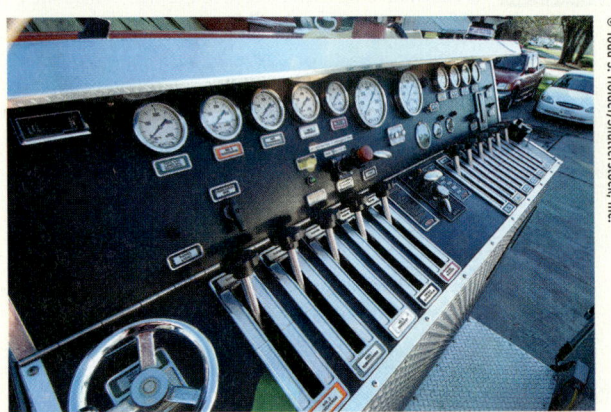

FIGURE 5-23 Discharge outlets may be controlled by pull-type actuators, swing valves, flexible push/pull controls, gear-operated hand wheel controls, or hydraulic, air, and electric operators.

The Pump Panel

The gauges, instruments, and controls necessary to operate the pump are located on a panel known as the **pump operator's panel**. Each gauge, instrument, and control must be marked

CHAPTER 5 The Fire Pump

FIGURE 5-24 An illuminated pump panel.

FIGURE 5-25 A master pump intake gauge.

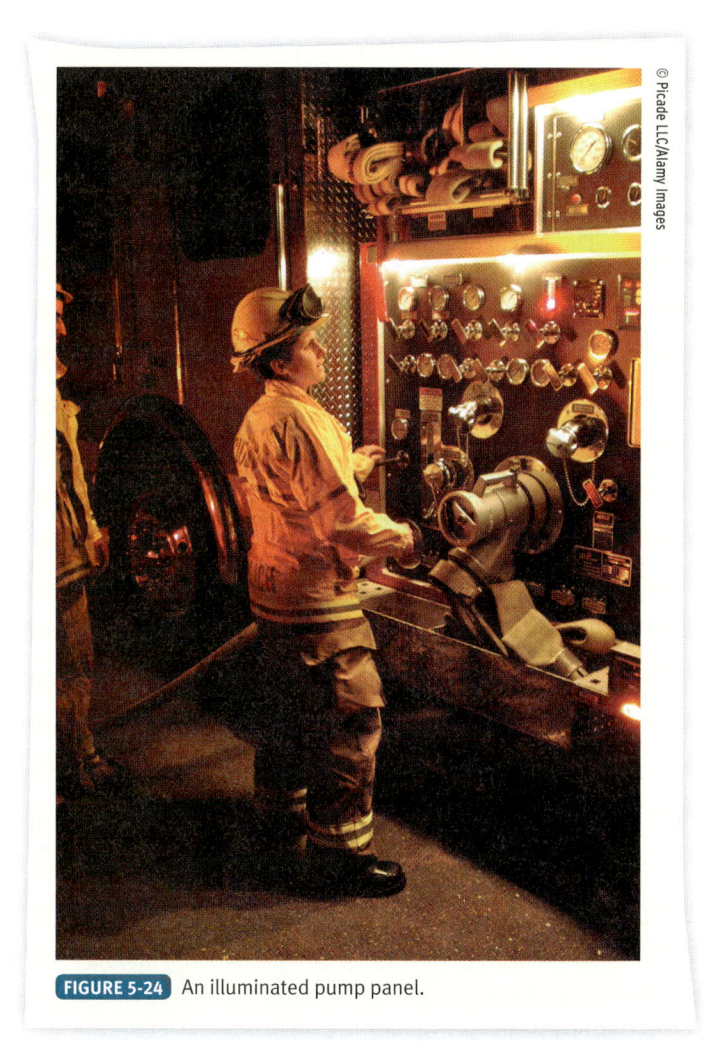

with a label as to its function and must be illuminated for the operator to see it during night operations **FIGURE 5-24**. NFPA 1901 requires the following controls and instruments be provided and installed as a group on the pump operator's panel:
- Master pump intake pressure gauge
- Master pump discharge gauge
- Pumping engine tachometer
- Pumping engine coolant temperature gauge
- Pumping engine oil pressure gauge
- Voltmeter
- Pump pressure controls
- Pumping engine throttle
- Primer control
- Water tank-to-pump valve control
- Water tank fill valve control
- Water tank level gauge
- Fuel level indicator
- Pump overheat indicator

Master Pump Intake Pressure Gauge

This gauge is connected to the intake side of the pump and measures both a positive pressure and a vacuum. It must be capable of reading 30 inches Hg (100 kPa) vacuum to at least a gauge pressure of 300 psi (2100 kPa). The gauge must be labeled as "Pump Intake" **FIGURE 5-25**.

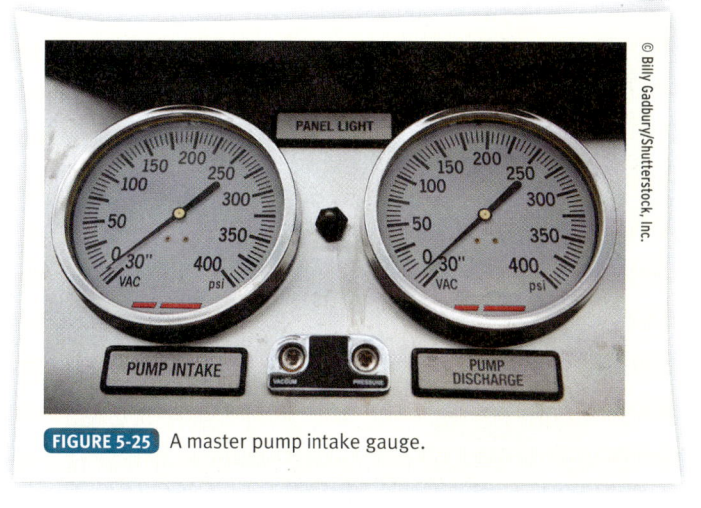

Master Pump Discharge Gauge

This gauge measures the pressure as it leaves the pump and is connected to the discharge side of the pump. It must be capable of reading from 0 to 300 psi (0 to 2100 kPa). The master pump discharge gauge must be labeled as "Pump Discharge" and located within 8 inches (200 mm) of the master pump intake gauge. This gauge must be at least 1 inch (25 mm) larger than all of the other discharge gauges **FIGURE 5-26**.

Pressure Gauges

A pressure gauge must also be provided for each discharge outlet that is 1½ inches (38 mm) or larger in size; the gauge must be marked to indicate the outlet to which it is connected. This pressure gauge must be connected to the outlet of discharge valve. Two types of gauges may be used—analog **FIGURE 5-27** and digital **FIGURE 5-28**.

Analog gauges must meet the following requirements:
- The gauge must be resistant to vibrations, pulsations, corrosion, condensation, and shock.
- The master intake and discharge gauges' numerals must be a minimum of 0.25 inch (6 mm) high.
- Numerals must be a minimum of 5/32 inch (4 mm) high for all other discharge gauges.

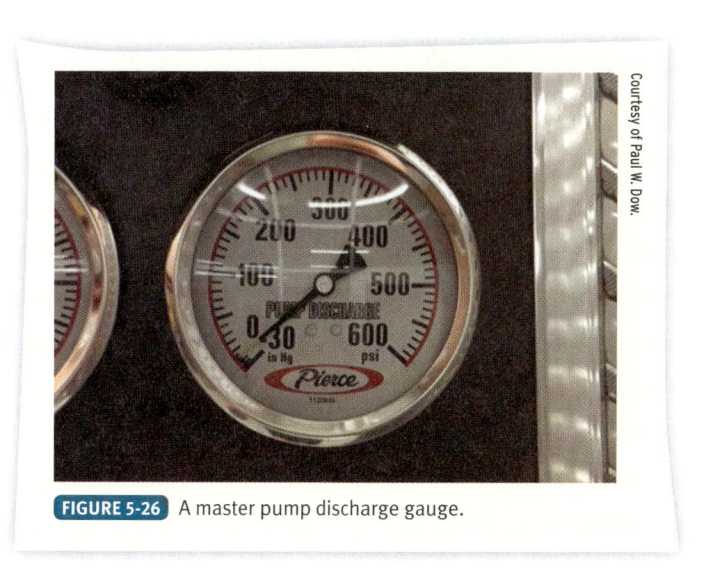

FIGURE 5-26 A master pump discharge gauge.

- The gauge must have internal mechanisms that are factory lubricated for the life of the gauge.

Digital gauges must meet the following requirements:
- Digital master pressure gauges must have an accuracy of ±3 percent over the full scale.
- All digits must be at least 0.5 inch (13 mm) in height.
- The gauge must display pressure in increments of not more than 10 psi (70 kPa).

Flow Meters

The <u>flow meter</u> is a device on a straight section of pipe, that measures volumetric flow rates, is threaded on each end, and is placed between two sections of hose **FIGURE 5-29**. A sensing device on top of the meter is designed to measure the flow (gpm) through the hose. In the fire service, these sensors are generally of spring probe or paddlewheel design. The paddlewheel version has the paddlewheel on top of the pipe, thereby ensuring that sediment cannot settle on the paddlewheel; the speed of the wheel indicates the flow. The spring probe flow meter injects a stainless steel spring probe into the stream to measure resistance and read the amount of flow (in either gpm or L/min), with measurements being read in increments of 10 gpm (40 L/min) or less.

Flow meters give an indication of the actual volume of water being discharged through each line. This flow is sent as a signal to the gauge. The indicator gauge may be either digital or analog.

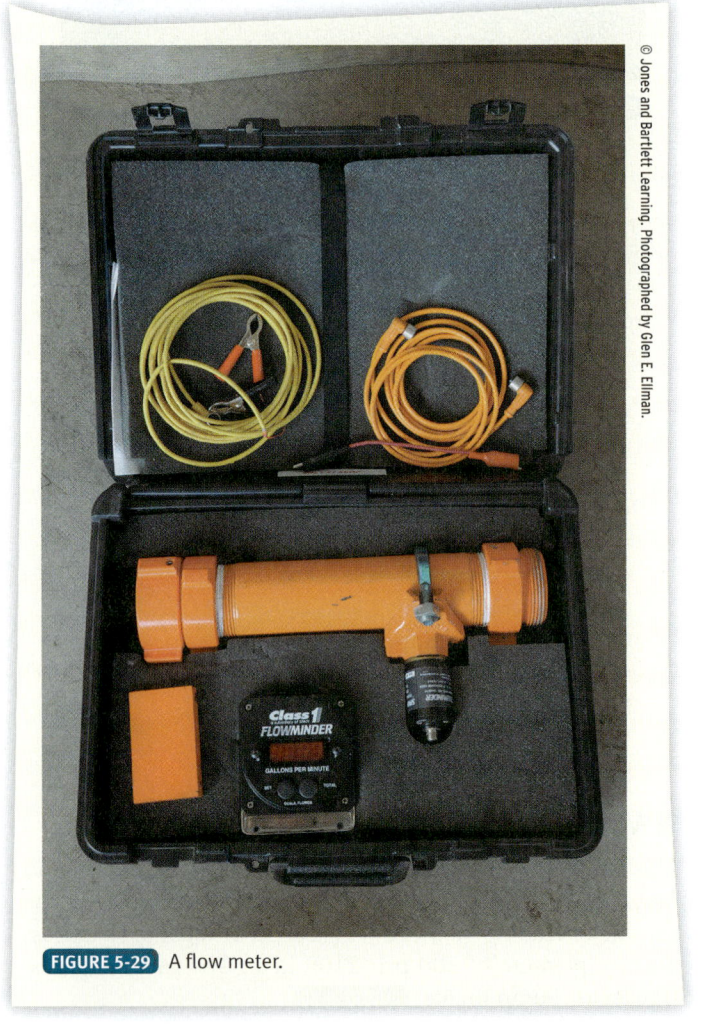

FIGURE 5-27 An analog gauge.

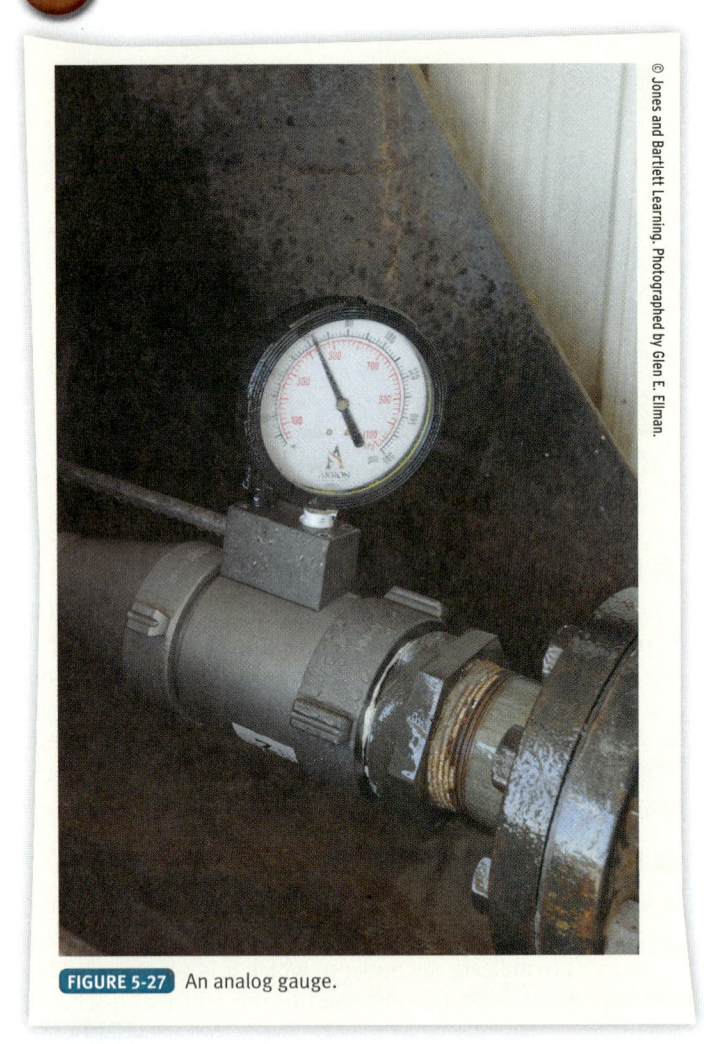

- The gauge must have graduation lines showing at least every 10 psi (70 kPa), with major and intermediate graduation lines emphasized and figures at least every 100 psi (700 kPa).

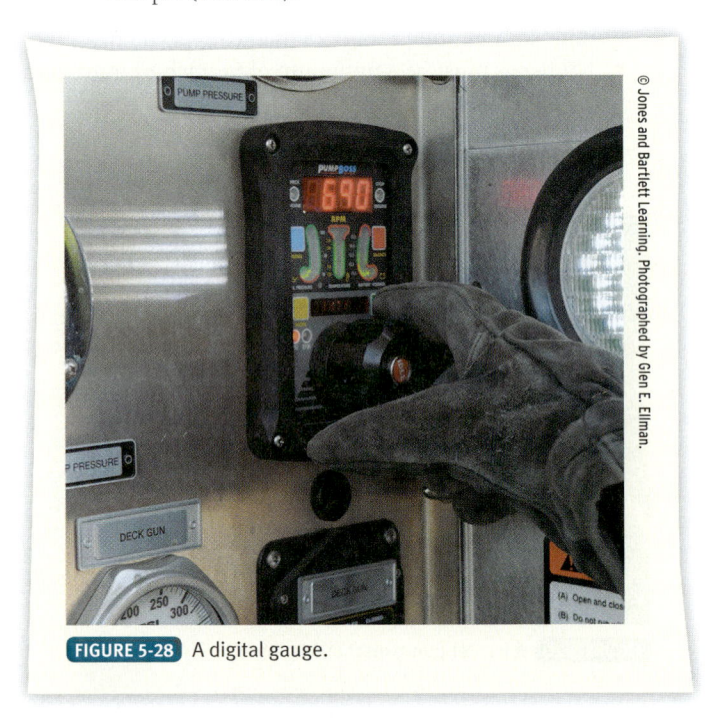

FIGURE 5-28 A digital gauge.

FIGURE 5-29 A flow meter.

The use of a flow meter can lessen the amount of calculations required to determine pump discharge pressure (PDP). With this approach, the driver/operator communicates with the attack team and, by reading the flow meter, increases or decreases the pressure to achieve the desired flow as directed.

Many types of flow meters are available, from a variety of manufacturers. NFPA 1901 allows flow meters on discharges from 1½ inches (38 mm) to 3 inches (77 mm) in diameter. All discharge outlets equipped with a flow meter must also use a pressure gauge as well. Combination models offer both flow and pressure gauges. Some indicate the flow of only one discharge, whereas others provide a total flow button that displays the total amount flowing from the pump. Flow meters generally boast accuracy within 1 to 3 percent, but require periodic calibration to maintain this accuracy.

One important characteristic of the flow meter is that it reports the discharge port flow without the engine operator having to calculate it. As a consequence, use of flow meters is associated with several advantages:

- Flow meters are very useful in multistory buildings, as hose length, friction loss, and elevation vary in incidents involving these structures and may be undetermined.
- The flow from master stream appliances with automatic nozzles may look good but may be actually smaller than required. Flow meters eliminate this problem.
- Flow meters eliminate the math needed to carry out a relay operation because the flow meter is automatically set to the desired flow.

Engine Tachometer

The tachometer is an instrument used for measuring rotational speed, defined as revolutions per minute (rpm) of the apparatus engine **FIGURE 5-30**. The pump operator may reference the tachometer when troubleshooting any issue with the pump. Each pump will identify on a nomenclature plate the rpm required to pump a specific number of gpm at a certain psi. If the psi does not match the rpm of the engine, the operator may recognize a problem with the pump and have to stop its operation.

Engine Coolant Temperature Gauge and Engine Cooling Devices

This gauge indicates the temperature of the coolant inside the engine of the apparatus. If the temperature is too high, it can cause severe damage to the engine and possibly cause it to shut down. If the temperature is too low, the engine may not operate as efficiently. An engine-cooling device may be installed to assist with maintaining the temperature of the engine coolant for optimal performance **FIGURE 5-31**. Such a device uses the water from the fire pump (when the pump is operating) and directs water to cool the pipes that carry the coolant around the engine through an exchanger. This lowers the temperature of the engine coolant, thereby lowering the temperature of the engine. However, it may also raise the temperature of the water that is circulating inside the fire pump if no external water source is being used.

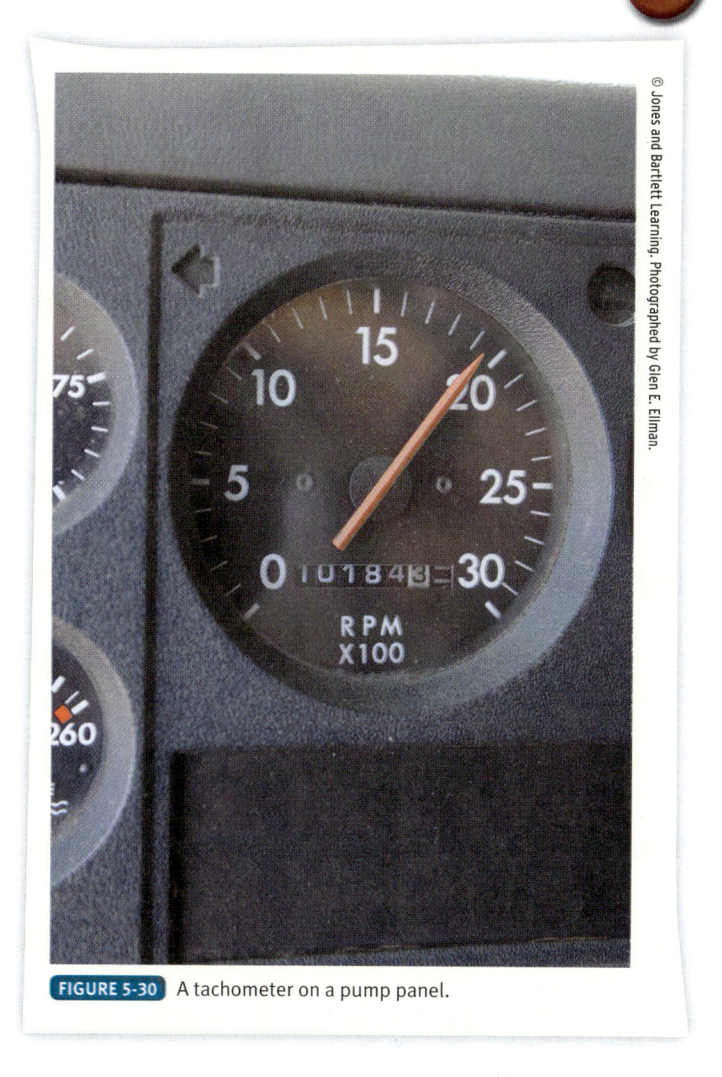

FIGURE 5-30 A tachometer on a pump panel.

Engine Oil Pressure Gauge

This gauge indicates whether an adequate supply of oil is being distributed to all of the necessary areas of the engine **FIGURE 5-32**. If the engine is not properly lubricated with oil, it can overheat and seize. Different engines operate at different oil pressures, so the operator must be familiar with the normal operating range for the oil pressure in each apparatus they operate.

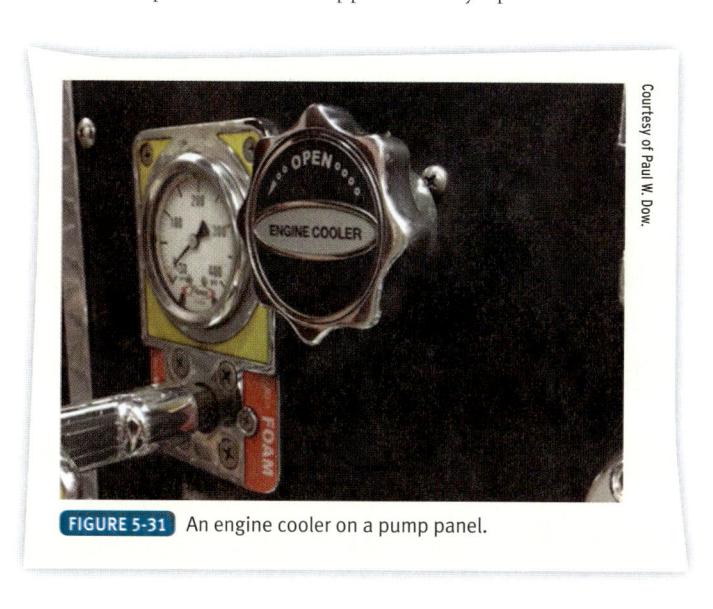

FIGURE 5-31 An engine cooler on a pump panel.

© Andrew Macdonald/Alamy Images

FIGURE 5-32 An oil pressure gauge on a pump panel.

© Jones and Bartlett Learning. Photographed by Glen E. Ellman.

FIGURE 5-34 A water tank level indicator.

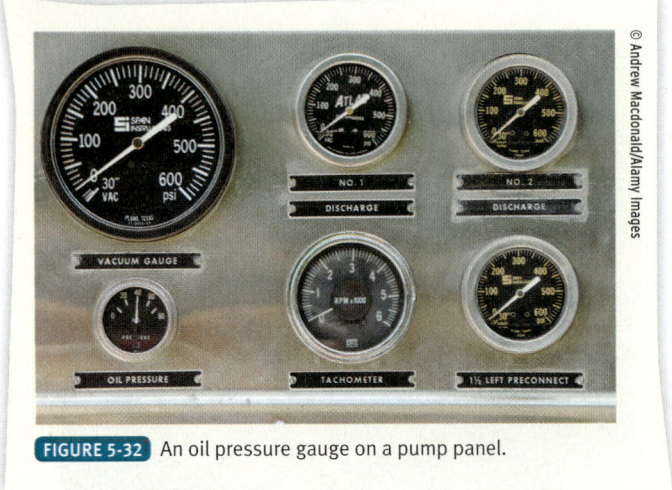

Voltmeter

The voltmeter measures the voltage across the battery terminals and gives an indication of the electrical condition of the battery FIGURE 5-33. Operating voltage while the alternator is charging may vary between vehicles depending on the regulator setting. Always refer to the manufacturer's operation manual to determine these parameters.

Water Tank Level Indicator

The pump operator must be capable of determining the amount of water that is inside the on-board water tank of the apparatus. This information must be visible on the pump panel, which usually indicates the water level in one-quarter increments FIGURE 5-34. Some apparatus manufacturers may install large lights on the side of the apparatus so that the water level inside the water tank can be seen from a greater distance.

Fuel Level Indicator

The pump operator needs to be aware of the fuel level of the apparatus. A fuel level indicator or red warning light indicating when the fuel level falls below one-quarter of the capacity of the tank must be provided on the pump operator's panel.

Courtesy of Paul W. Dow.

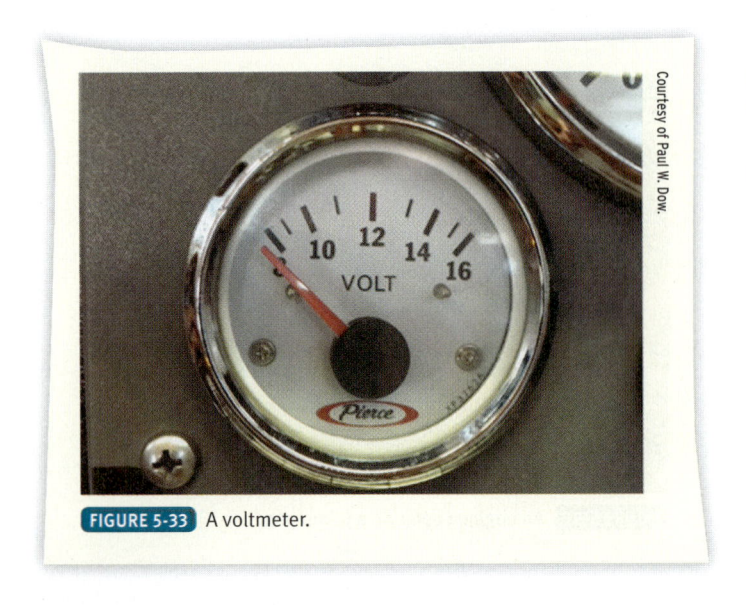

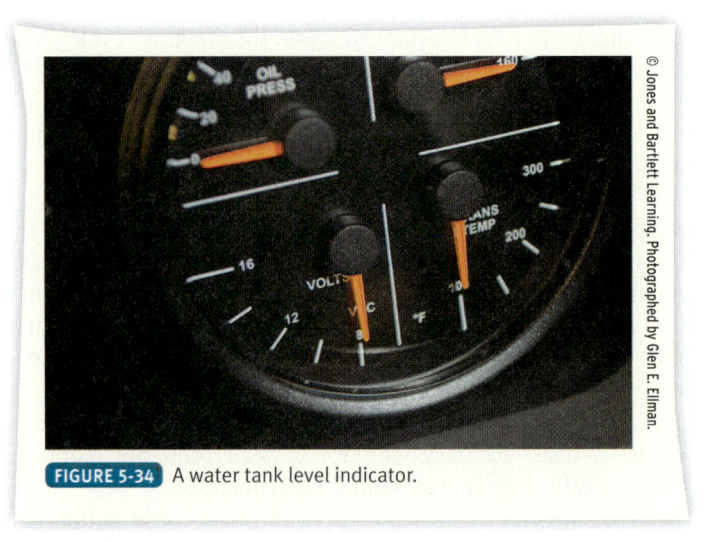

FIGURE 5-33 A voltmeter.

Primer Control

The pump operator must be capable of operating the pump's priming system from the pump panel. This primer control is used to expel any air that may be trapped inside the pump and during drafting operations (this topic is discussed further in the chapter *Drafting and Water shuttle Operations*). The priming system must be capable of operating with no lubricant or with a biodegradable nontoxic lubricant.

Pump Pressure Control Systems

The purpose of a pressure control system is to control the discharge pressures and thereby protect fire fighters who are operating hose streams as well as to protect the discharge hose from damage in the event attack hose streams are shut off or other valves are closed, reducing flow rates. When multiple attack lines are flowing, they may be operating at different pressures. As one attack line is shut down, the excess pressure may be transferred to the other attack lines—causing the fire fighters on the nozzle to lose control of the line. By using the pressure control system on the discharge side of the pump, the driver can ensure that the fire fighters on the nozzle do not receive an excessive amount of pressure as hoselines are opened and closed.

Two systems may be used to control the discharge pressure of the pump: a discharge pressure relief valve or a pressure governor. The **discharge pressure relief valve** controls pressure by passing water from the discharge side of the pump back into the intake side of the pump FIGURE 5-35. The **pressure governor** controls the engine speed, which relates directly to the net pump pressure; if the speed is raised, the pressure goes up, and if the speed is lowered, the pressure goes down FIGURE 5-36.

Regardless of the system used, NFPA 1901 requires the following:

- The system must be equipped with a means to indicate when the system is in control of the pressure. For the discharge relief valve, an indicator light on the pump panel usually accomplishes this. With a discharge relief valve, the light will illuminate when the valve is operating and dim when it is closed. For the pressure governor, a light or digital screen will show when the system is turned on and whether it is controlling the engine speed or the pump pressure.

CHAPTER 5 The Fire Pump

- The system must automatically control the pump pressure to a maximum of 30 psi (207 kPa) pressure rise no faster than 3 seconds and no slower than 10 seconds from the time the pressure surge is detected.
- The system must operate over a range of pressure from 70 to 300 psi (490 to 2100 kPa) discharge pressure and flows greater than 150 gpm (600 L/min) up to the rated capacity of the fire pump.

Pressure control systems will relieve excess pressure when valves are closed in a normal manner, but some water hammer conditions could occur due to valves being closed so quickly that the system cannot respond fast enough to eliminate damage to equipment. Proper fireground procedures are still required.

FIGURE 5-35 A discharge pressure relief valve on a pump panel.

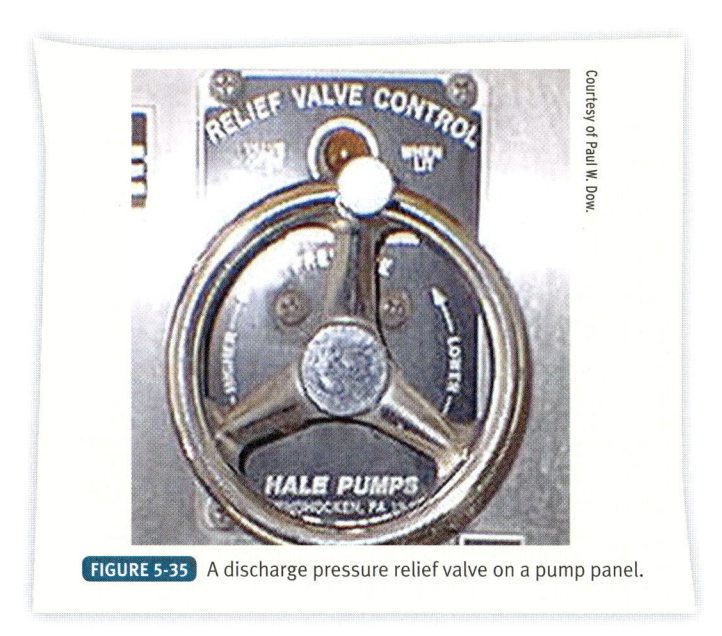

- One person at the pump panel position must control either system.
- If the system discharges water to the atmosphere, the discharge must not expose the operator to high-pressure water streams.

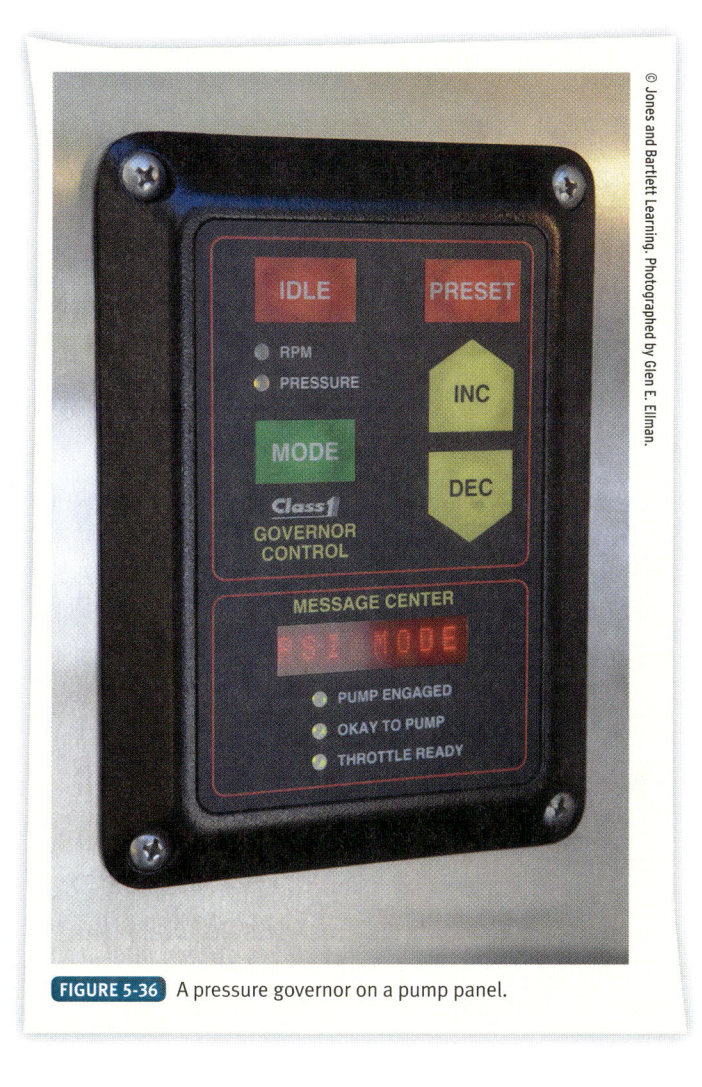

Pumping Engine Throttle

The apparatus engine powers the fire pump; in turn, the operator must have a way of increasing or decreasing the engine speed from the pump panel. The pump panel must be equipped with a throttle control that holds its set position to control the engine speed. Many older apparatus have a **manual throttle control**, whereas newer apparatus may be equipped with an electric throttle control or an **electronic pump controller**.

Electronic Pump Controllers

In recent years, technology has reduced the amount of calculations that the driver/operator must perform. In addition, technology is constantly changing the electronic systems found on fire trucks and has influenced the way the pump panel operates. **Multiplexing** is a term used in electrical engineering to refer to the process of combining information from several different sources. In the fire service, this means that different sensors and controls on a pumper are brought to one control board or indicating panel **FIGURE 5-37**. The trend in modern fire apparatus is to use electronic control and monitoring equipment. Many new pumping apparatus, for example, include electronic throttle and pressure controls.

Electronic components are often designed by an independent contractor and integrated into the manufacturer's apparatus. Two examples are the Electronic Fire Commander (EFC)

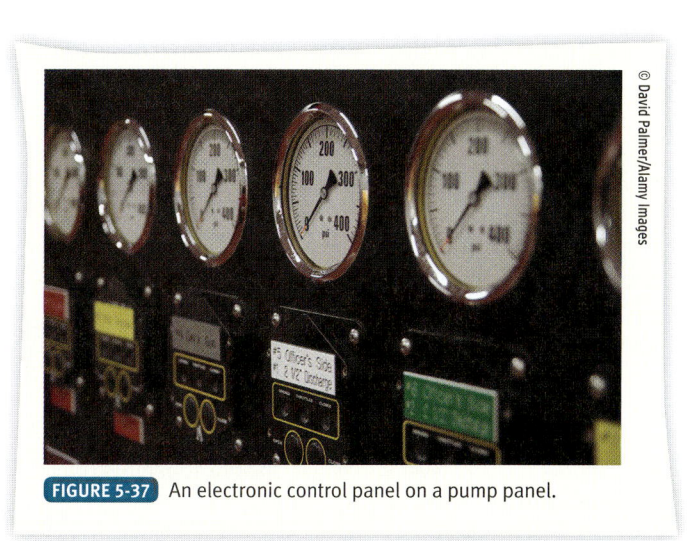

FIGURE 5-36 A pressure governor on a pump panel.

FIGURE 5-37 An electronic control panel on a pump panel.

offered by Class 1 and the Incontrol mechanism developed by Fire Research Group. These companies provide a small computer panel (keypad and display) for controlling the pump. Placed on the pump panel, these panels contain both a pressure governor and an engine speed governor, and include a preset function that eliminates the need for a separate throttle or pressure relief valve. They also feature an LED information center that displays engine-related data such as temperature, oil pressure, speed (rpm), and voltage. A one-touch button advances the pressure to the preprogrammed pressure, and another button returns the engine speed to the idle level. If the preprogrammed pressure is not needed, the pressure may be increased or decreased by pushing an increase pressure button or a decrease pressure button, respectively.

While this technological innovation assists the driver/operator, the concern that arises with its use is the possibility of an electrical failure disabling the fire apparatus. The threat of an electrical malfunction is increased with such technology because of the frequent absence of manual overrides on fire apparatus with these features. This fact further highlights the necessity of the driver/operator having a thorough understanding of the fire apparatus and pumping procedures should problems occur.

Power Supplies for Pumps

As the driver/operator, you must be familiar with how the various types of pumps receive their power. Given that much of this equipment is located out of sight, you should study the fire apparatus schematics and manuals and examine the underside of the fire apparatus to observe how the power train is designed.

The simplest form of power supply is available with the portable pump FIGURE 5-38. This pump is typically carried by two or more fire fighters to a water source and used to pump water from that source. It has a small engine attached directly to the pump and provides power on a one-to-one basis: For every revolution of the engine, there is one revolution of the pump. With this type of unit, there is typically no gear box, clutch, shifting level, or other devices to operate. You simply start the engine and the pump starts. This same concept is often used for aircraft crash rescue apparatus so they can have a pump-and-roll capability—that is, the ability to discharge water as the apparatus is moving.

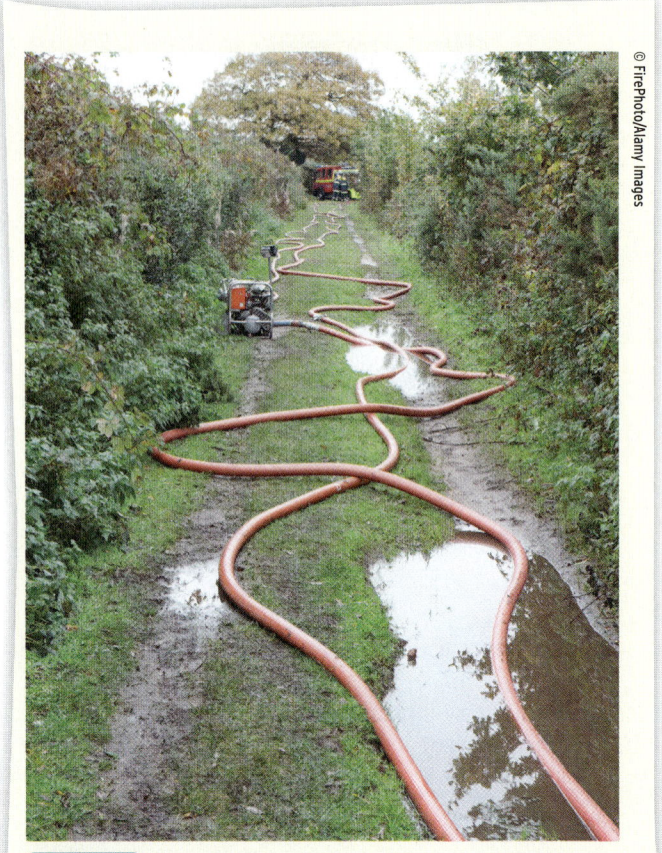

FIGURE 5-38 A portable pump is designed for use in remote areas.

Some fire apparatus may have a pump mounted on the front bumper, known as a front mount FIGURE 5-39. The power for this pump is taken from the crankshaft on the front of the engine. It is transferred via a drive shaft to the pump transmission that operates the pump. This same concept is often used to power large snowplow trucks, cement mixers, and other heavy equipment.

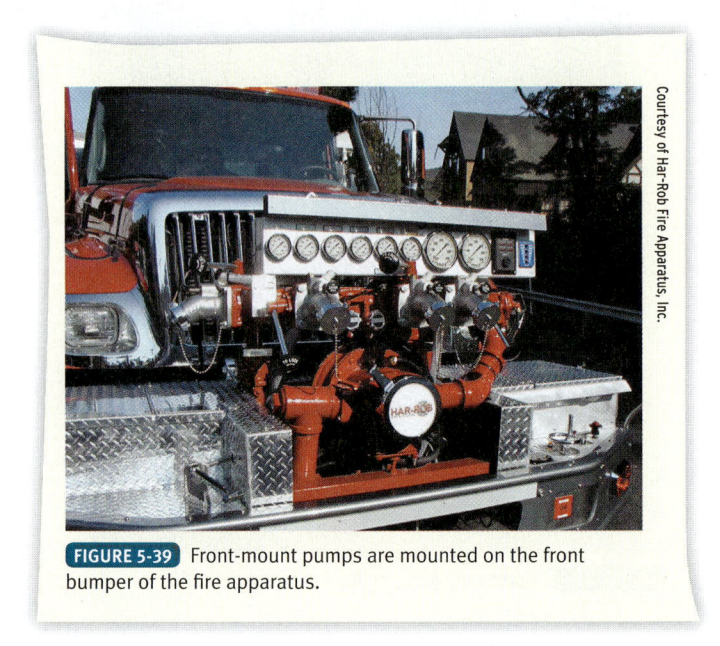

FIGURE 5-39 Front-mount pumps are mounted on the front bumper of the fire apparatus.

Driver/Operator Safety

With both the front-mount pump and the pump that uses a power take-off supply, it is absolutely critical that the fire apparatus be secured when it is parked and the pump is being operated. The brakes need to be set and locked, the wheels chocked, and the gear shift locked into neutral, especially with automatic transmissions. Imagine what might happen if a front-mount pump is operating at 2000 rpm when someone accidentally knocks the shift lever into drive—the fire apparatus could become a lethal weapon.

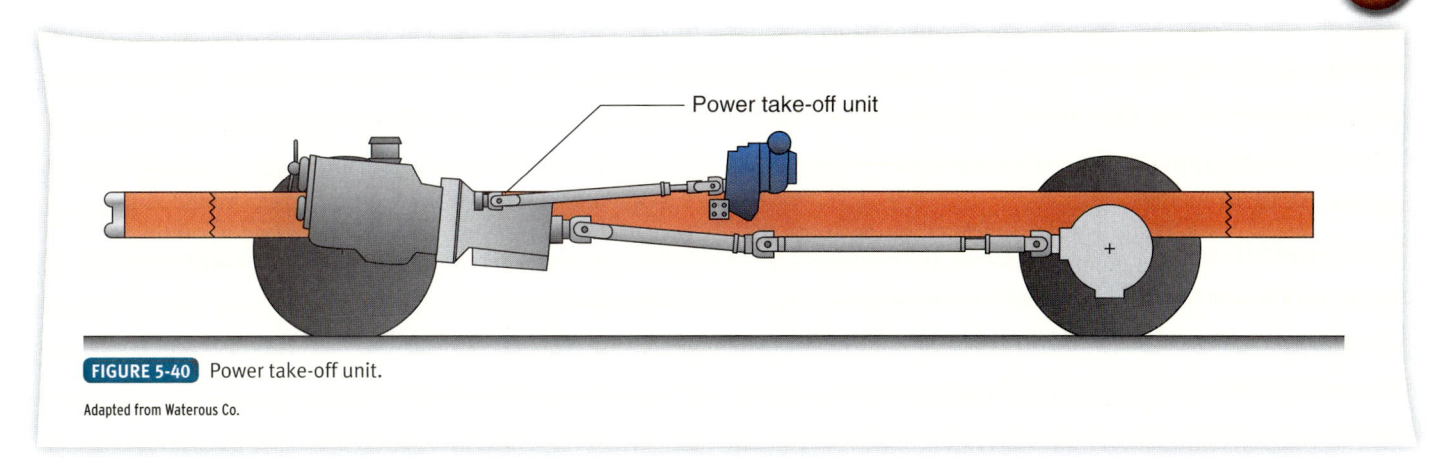

FIGURE 5-40 Power take-off unit.
Adapted from Waterous Co.

Power take-off (PTO) units **FIGURE 5-40** are commonly used for small pumps such as those found on tankers or tenders. A power take-off unit is mounted to the side of the transmission and through a shaft directed to the gear case on the pump. It provides a less expensive method of developing power for the pump, especially when the pump has only limited capacity. This approach also provides a pump-and-roll capability for apparatus such as wildland firefighting trucks.

The most common power system found in pumps is the **transfer case** **FIGURE 5-41**. This gear box is mounted to the fire apparatus frame between the transmission and the rear axle. A drive shaft connects the fire apparatus' transmission to the

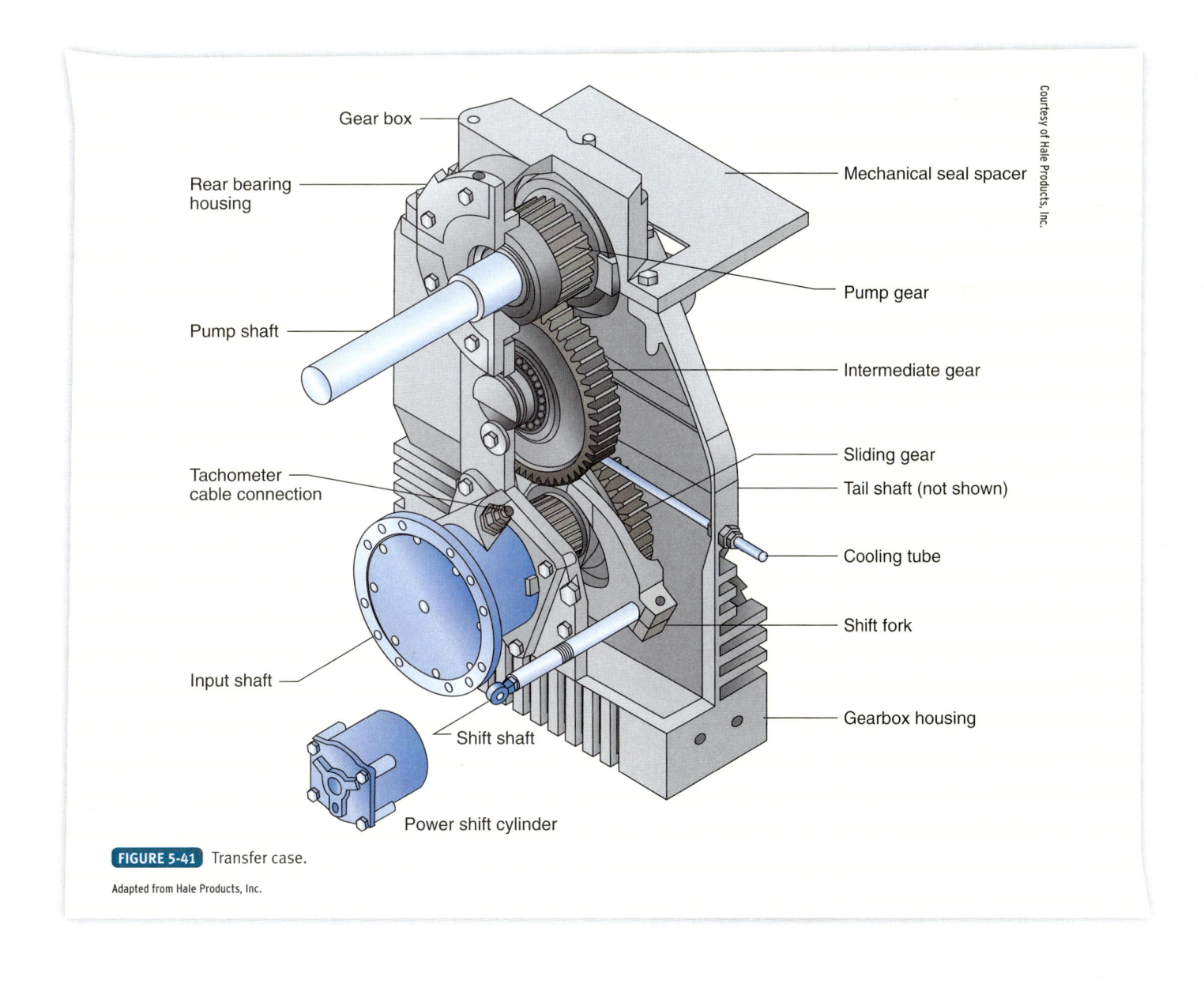

FIGURE 5-41 Transfer case.
Adapted from Hale Products, Inc.

transfer case, so that the transfer case has the ability to direct the power to the rear axle or to the pump. When you place the pump into pump gear in the cab, you are transferring the power from the rear axle to the pump. The gear ratio is typically 1:1. The purpose of this configuration is simply to divert the power from one usage to another.

The speed of the pump is directly related to the speed of the transmission. A transmission placed in first gear will propel the pump at a slow pace; by comparison, a transmission placed in fifth gear will turn it at a much faster rate. The fire apparatus manufacturer determines the most effective gear to use for the engine and the optimal transmission arrangement for each fire apparatus. The manufacturer must also consider how much power is required for the pump application.

Automatic transmissions are specifically made for pumping operations that will lock into the gear intended for pump operations once the fire apparatus is placed in pumping mode. This setup prevents the transmission from shifting gears and ensures that the pump operates only in the selected gear (typically the highest gear).

Wrap-Up

Chief Concepts

- As the driver/operator of the pump apparatus, you must understand how pumps operate so that you are able to fix any problems that you may encounter on the fireground.
- The pump panel is the most notable device on the fire apparatus. It is usually covered in stainless steel and has multiple levers and gauges mounted on it. Once you have a thorough understanding of the pump behind it and the way in which the pump functions, you will be capable of confidently operating the fire pump.
- It is important for the new driver/operator to understand that the fire apparatus is not like any other vehicle—and, therefore, should not be operated like other vehicles.
- According to the NFPA, a pump is defined as a provider of liquid flow and pressure dedicated to fire protection. It is a mechanical device used to move fluids.
- The goal in firefighting is for the pump to move water from a source, such as the onboard water tank, to the fire through the attack lines. To do so successfully, the driver/operator must understand how each different type of pump works.
- The fire service primarily uses two types of pumps: positive-displacement pumps and centrifugal pumps. Each type relies on very different operating principles and offers a very different set of features.
- Positive-placement pumps produce a flow by capturing a specific volume of fluid per pump revolution and reducing the fluid void by mechanical means to displace the pumping fluid.
- Two broad classifications of positive-displacement pumps exist: the piston pump and the rotary pump.
- Centrifugal pumps—the most common fire pumps in use today—do not flow a definite amount of water with each revolution; instead, the flow or amount of water discharged is based on the pressures at the discharge side of the pump.
    - At higher flow rates (rpm), the pump will flow less volume but will create higher pressures.
    - As the pump spins more slowly, it will create less pressure on the discharge side but will flow a greater volume of water.
    - This flexibility makes the centrifugal pump a very versatile piece of equipment on the fireground.
- The two main sides of all pumps are the intake and discharge sides.
- Intake relief valves prevent excessive pressure from building up on the intake side of the pump.
- Discharge relief valves prevent excessive pressure from building up on the discharge side of the pump.
- The pump panel consists of several gauges, controls and valves to operate the pump.

Wrap-Up, continued

Hot Terms

automatic intake pressure relief device A device installed on the supply side of a valve to bleed off excessive pressure coming into the valve.

centrifugal force The outward force that is exerted away from the center of rotation or the tendency for objects to be pulled outward when rotating around a center.

centrifugal pump A pump in which the pressure is developed principally by the action of centrifugal force.

chassis The basic operating motor vehicle, including the engine, frame, and other essential structural and mechanical parts, but exclusive of the body and all appurtenances for the accommodation of driver, property, passengers, appliances, or equipment related to other than control. Common usage might, but need not, include a cab (or cowl).

discharge header The piping and valves on the discharge side of the pump.

discharge pressure relief valve A device to control pressure by passing water from the discharge side of the pump back into the intake side of the pump.

discharge side The side of a pump where water is discharged from the pump.

double-acting piston pump A positive-displacement pump that discharges water on both the upward and downward strokes of the piston.

electronic pump controller A device to control the engine and pump speed by means of a digital panel.

exhaust primer A means of priming a centrifugal pump by using the fire apparatus' exhaust to create a vacuum and draw air and water from the pump.

fire pump (fire apparatus) A device that provides for liquid flow and pressure and that is dedicated to fire protection.

flow meter A device for measuring volumetric flow rates of gases and liquids.

front mount An apparatus pump that is permanently mounted to the front bumper of the apparatus and is directly connected to the motor.

impeller A metal rotating component that transfers energy from the fire apparatus' motor to discharge the incoming water from a pump.

impeller vanes Sections that divide the impeller.

intake side The side of a pump where water enters the pump.

manual throttle control A device to control the engine speed and pump speed.

multiplexing Combining several different sensors or controls into one panel.

parallel/volume mode Positioning of a two-stage pump in which each impeller takes water in from the same intake area and discharges it to the same discharge area. This mode is used when pumping water at the rated capacity of the pump.

piston pump A positive-displacement pump that operates in an up-and-down action.

portable pump A type of pump that is typically carried by hand by two or more fire fighters to a water source and used to pump water from that source.

positive-displacement pump A pump that is characterized by a method of producing flow by capturing a specific volume of fluid per pump revolution and reducing the fluid void by a mechanical means to displace the pumping fluid.

power take-off (PTO) unit A direct means of powering a pump with the fire apparatus' transmission and through a shaft directed to the gear case on the pump.

pressure governor A device that controls the engine speed, which relates directly to the net pump pressure.

prime the pump To expel all air from a pump.

pump operator's panel The gauges, instruments, and controls necessary to operate the pump.

pumping element A rotating device such as a gear or vane encased in the pump casing of a rotary pump.

rotary gear pump A positive-displacement pump that uses two gears encased inside a pump casing to move water under pressure.

rotary pump A positive-displacement pump that operates in a circular motion.

rotary vane pump A positive-displacement pump characterized by the use of a single rotor with vanes that move with pump rotation to create a void and displace liquid.

rotor A metal device that houses the vanes in a rotary vane pump.

series/pressure mode Positioning of a two-stage pump in which the first impeller sends water into the second impeller's intake side and water is then discharged out the pump's discharge header, thereby creating more pressure with less flow.

single-acting piston pump A positive-displacement pump that discharges water only on the downward stroke of the piston.

single-stage pump A pump that has one impeller that takes the water in and discharges it out using only one impeller.

tank fill A discharge directly into the on-board water tank.

tank-to-pump A pipe that leads from the apparatus water tank to the fire pump.

transfer case A gear box that transfers power, thereby enabling a fire apparatus' motor to operate a pump.

transfer valve An internal valve in a multistage pump that enables the user to change the mode of operation to either series/pressure or parallel/volume.

vane A small, movable, self-adjusting element inside a rotary vane pump.

Venturi effect The creation of a low-pressure area in a chamber so as to allow air and water to be drawn in.

volute The part of the pump casing that gradually decreases in area, thereby creating pressure on the discharge side of a pump.

References

National Fire Protection Association (NFPA) 20, *Standard for the Installation of Stationary Pumps for Fire Protection*. 2013. http://www.nfpa.org/codes-and-standards/document-information-pages?mode=code&code=20. Accessed March 27, 2014.

National Fire Protection Association (NFPA) 1002, *Standard for Fire Apparatus Driver/Operator Professional Qualifications*. 2014. http://www.nfpa.org/codes-and-standards/document-information-pages?mode=code&code=1002. Accessed March 27, 2014.

National Fire Protection Association (NFPA) 1901, *Standard for Automotive Fire Apparatus*. 2009. http://www.nfpa.org/codes-and-standards/document-information-pages?mode=code&code=1901. Accessed March 27, 2014.

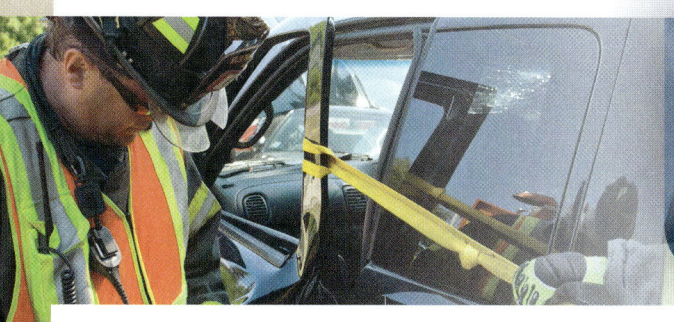

DRIVER/OPERATOR in action

The new fire fighter is a great listener and grasps the material very quickly. As you cover the different types of pumps, the ways in which they work, pump anatomy, and the controls of the pump panel, other members of the station start to come out into the apparatus bay for a quick lesson. The officer adds in his experience and knowledge as well as the more senior driver/operator. Afterward, you decide to quiz one another on some of the material you just covered. These are some of the questions that you ask of your fellow fire fighters:

1. The centrifugal pump receives water into the center or eye of a(n) _____.
   A. Volute
   B. Intake header
   C. Impeller
   D. Vane

2. To satisfy the Underwriters Laboratories (UL) specifications, the pump must produce 100 percent of its rated capacity at ___ psi (kPa).
   A. 100 (700)
   B. 150 (1000)
   C. 200 (1350)
   D. 250 (1700)

3. In the tank-to-pump piping, there is also a _____, which allows water to flow only from the tank into the pump and not back inside the tank.
   A. Check valve
   B. Intake valve
   C. Discharge valve
   D. Flow valve

4. Which instrument is used for measuring rotational speed?
   A. Rotator
   B. Speedometer
   C. Auxiliary Cooler
   D. Tachometer

5. A _____ valve determines if a two-stage pump will be operated in series/pressure or parallel/volume mode.
   A. Ball
   B. Transfer
   C. Timing
   D. Relay

Fire Hose, Appliances, and Nozzles

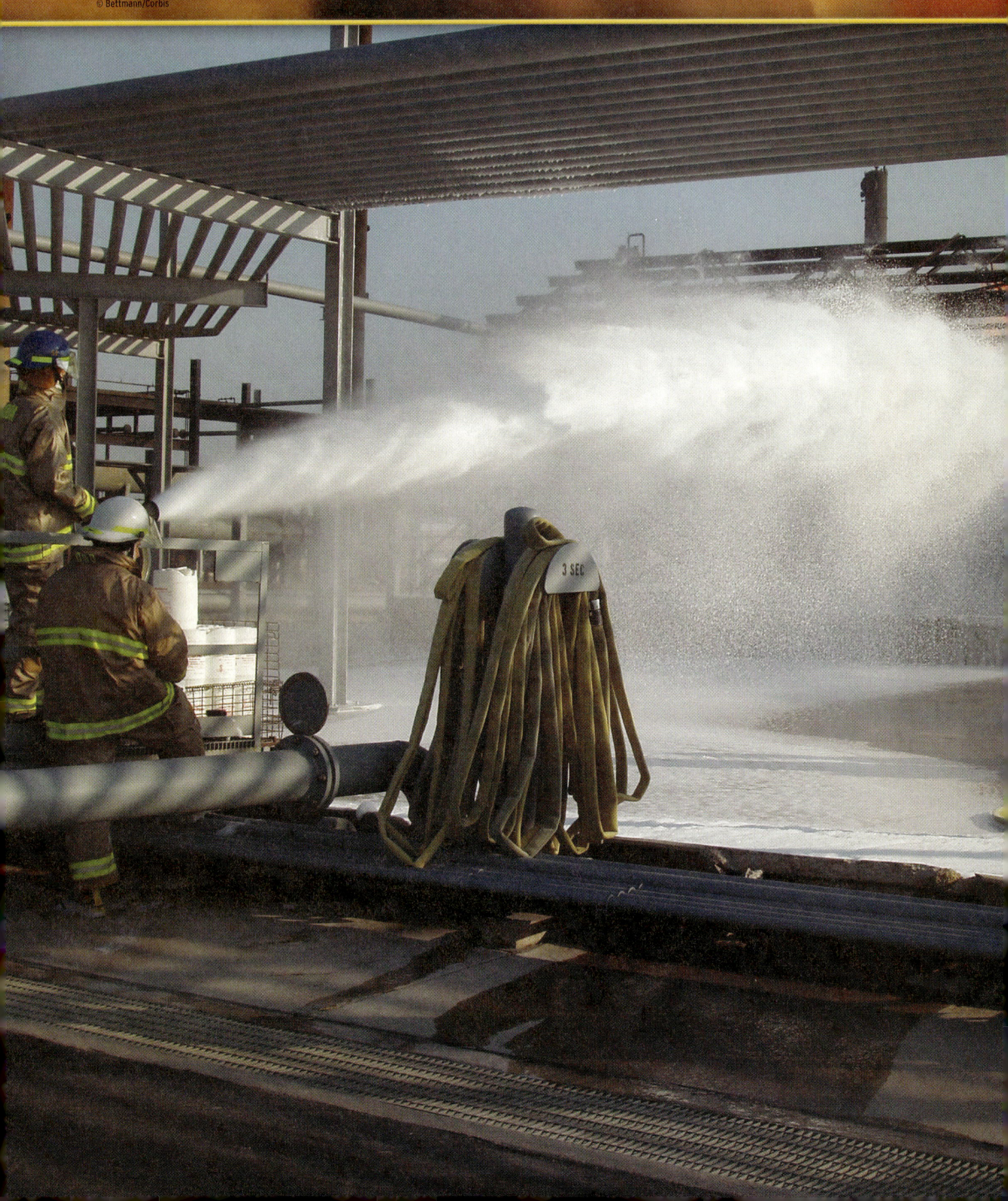

CHAPTER 6

Knowledge Objectives

After studying this chapter, you will be able to:

- Describe the types of hoses used in the fire service. (NFPA 1002, 4.3.7, 4.3.7(A) ; p 102–106)
- Describe connecting a hose to a hydrant. (NFPA 1002, 5.2.4, 5.2.4(A) ; p 105–106)
- Describe fire hose appliances. (NFPA 1002, 4.3.7(A), 5.1.1 ; p 105, 107–109)
- Describe the types and designs of nozzles. (NFPA 1002, 4.3.7(A), 5.1.1 ; p 111–114)
- Describe nozzle maintenance and inspection. (NFPA 1002, 4.3.7(A), 5.1.1 ; p 114–115)

Skills Objectives

After studying this chapter, you will be able to:

- Assemble a hoseline from a hydrant to a pump. (NFPA 1002, 4.3.7, 4.3.7(B), 5.2.4, 5.2.4(B) ; p 105–106)
- Inspect a solid-stream nozzle. (p 112–113)
- Inspect a fog nozzle. (p 114–115)

Additional NFPA Standards

- NFPA 1961, *Standard on Fire Hose*
- NFPA 1962, *Standard for the Inspection, Care, and Use of Fire Hose, Couplings, and Nozzles, and the Service Testing of Fire Hose*
- NFPA 1963, *Standard for Fire Hose Connections*
- NFPA 1964, *Standard for Spray Nozzles*
- NFPA 1965, *Standard for Fire Hose Appliances*

You Are the Driver/Operator

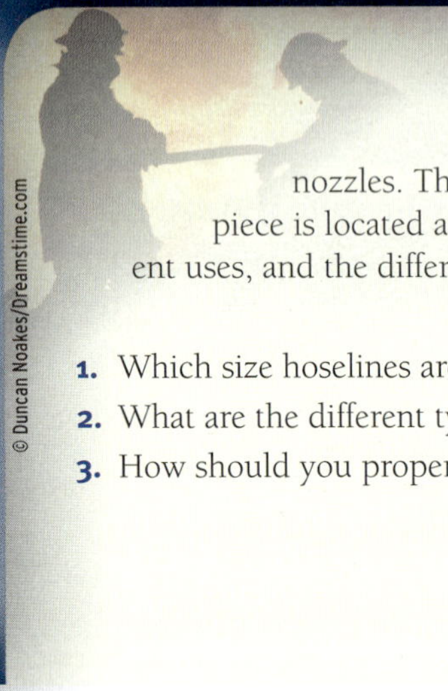

© Duncan Noakes/Dreamstime.com

It is 8 a.m. and your shift has just begun. You are the driver/operator on Engine 5 and have just started to inspect its equipment. This is your apparatus for the remainder of the shift, and you take great pride in the inspection of its equipment—especially the hoselines, appliances, and nozzles. This equipment is essential to the function of an engine company, and you enjoy knowing where every piece is located and what its capabilities are. Each nozzle has a unique application, each appliance is capable of different uses, and the different-size hoselines can flow dramatically different amounts of water.

1. Which size hoselines are carried on your apparatus?
2. What are the different types of appliances that you carry and how are they used?
3. How should you properly care for the nozzles that are assigned to your apparatus?

Fire Hose, Appliances, and Nozzles Overview

Functions of Fire Hose

Fire hose is used for two main purposes: as supply hose and as attack hose. **Supply hose** (also known as **supply lines**) FIGURE 6-1 is used to deliver water from a static source or from a fire hydrant to an attack pumper. The water can come directly from a hydrant, or it can come from another engine that is being used to provide a water supply for the attack pumper. Supply line sizes include 3½-inch (90-mm), 4-inch (100-mm), 5-inch (125-mm), and 6-inch (150-mm) hoses. Supply hose is designed to carry larger volumes of water at lower pressures compared to attack lines.

Attack hose (also known as **attack lines**) FIGURE 6-2 is used to discharge water from an attack pumper onto the fire. Attack lines usually operate at higher pressures than do supply lines. These lines can also be attached to the outlet of a standpipe system inside a building.

© Jones and Bartlett Learning. Photographed by Glen E. Ellman.

FIGURE 6-2 Attack hose is used to discharge water from the pump to the fire.

© Jones and Bartlett Learning. Photographed by Glen E. Ellman.

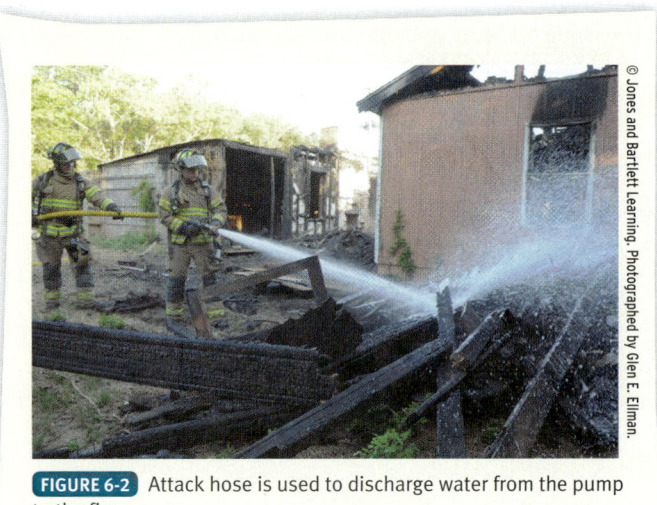

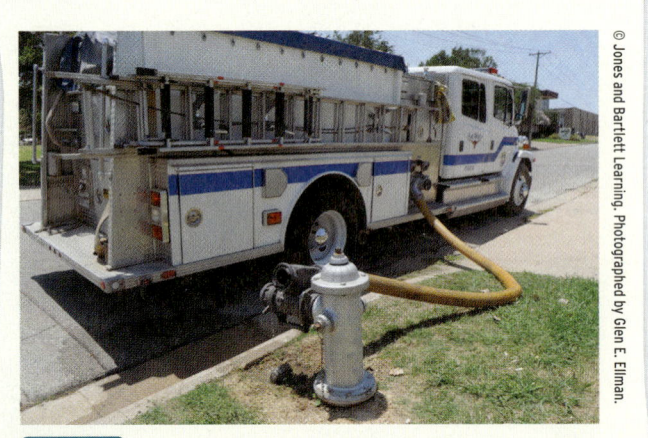

FIGURE 6-1 Supply hose brings the water from a water source to the pump.

Sizes of Hose

Fire hose ranges in size from 1 inch (25 mm) to 6 inches (150 mm) in diameter FIGURE 6-3. The nominal hose size refers to the inside diameter of the hose when it is filled with water. Smaller-diameter hose is used as attack lines; larger-diameter hose is almost always used as supply lines. Medium-diameter hose can be used as either attack lines or supply lines.

Small-diameter hose (SDH) ranges in size from 1 inch (25 mm) to 2 inches (50 mm) in diameter FIGURE 6-4. Many fire department vehicles are also equipped with a reel of ¾-inch (19-mm) or 1-inch (25-mm) hard rubber hose called a **booster hose** (or **booster line**), which is used for extinguishing small outdoor fires.

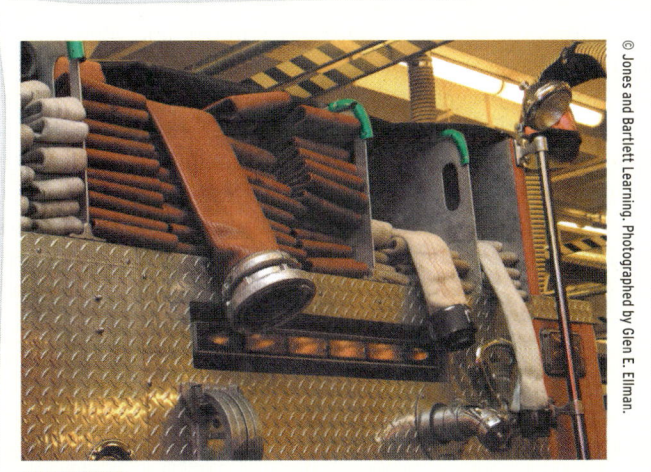

FIGURE 6-3 Fire hose comes in a wide range of sizes for different uses and situations.

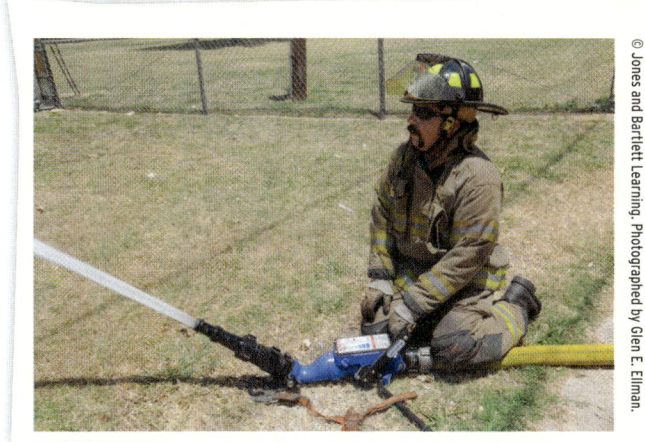

FIGURE 6-5 Medium-diameter hose has multiple uses, including serving as attack lines for commercial buildings, supplying master stream devices, and in some cases serving as supply hose for small fires.

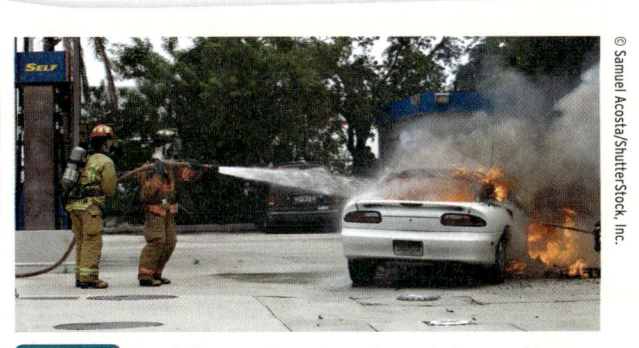

FIGURE 6-4 Small-diameter hose is used mostly for attacking vehicle fires and dumpster fires.

The hose that is most commonly used to attack interior residential structure fires is either 1½ inches (38 mm) or 1¾ inches (45 mm) in diameter. These lines are usually preconnected directly to a discharge so that they are ready for quick deployment. Some fire departments also use 2-inch (50-mm) attack lines. Each length of attack hose is usually 50 ft (15 m), although 100-ft (30-m) sections are available.

Medium-diameter hose (MDH) has a diameter of 2½ inches (65 mm) or 3 inches (77 mm) **FIGURE 6-5**. Hose in this size range can be used as either supply lines or attack lines. Large handline nozzles are often used with 2½-inch (65-mm) hose to attack larger fires. When used as an attack line, the 3 inch (77 mm) size is more often used to deliver water to a master stream device or a fire department connection. These hose sizes are typically available in 50-ft (15-m) and 100-ft (30-m) lengths.

Large-diameter hose (LDH) has a diameter of 3½ inches (90 mm) or more. Standard LDH sizes include 4-inch (100-mm) and 5-inch (125-mm) diameters; these hoselines are used as supply lines by many fire departments. The largest LDH size is 6 inches (150 mm) in diameter. Standard lengths of 50 ft (15 m) and 10 ft (3 m) are available for LDH.

Fire hose is typically designed to be used as either attack hose or supply hose, although some hose may serve both purposes. Attack hose must withstand higher pressures and is designed to be used in a fire environment where it can be subjected to high temperatures, sharp surfaces, abrasion, and other potentially damaging conditions. LDH supply hose is constructed to operate at lower pressures than attack hose and in less severe operating conditions; however, it must still be durable and resistant to external damage. Attack hose can be used as supply hose, but LDH supply hose must never be used as attack hose unless that usage is recommended by its manufacturer.

Attack hose must be tested annually at a pressure of at least 300 psi (2100 kPa) and is intended to be used at pressures up to 275 psi (1900 kPa). Supply hose must be tested annually at a pressure of at least 200 psi (1400 kPa) and is intended to be used at pressures up to 185 psi (1300 kPa). Most LDH is constructed for use as supply lines; however, some fire departments use special LDH that can withstand higher pressures. This hose may be used in water supply operations in case of high-rise fires or large industrial fires.

■ Attack Hose

Attack hose is designed to be used for fire suppression. During this activity, it may be exposed to heat and flames, hot embers, broken glass, sharp objects, and many other potentially damaging conditions. For this reason, attack hose must be tough, yet flexible and light in weight.

Most fire departments use two sizes of hose as attack lines for fire suppression. The smaller size is usually either 1½ inches (38 mm) or 1¾ inches (45 mm) in diameter. Medium-diameter (2½-inch [65-mm]) hose is most often used for heavy interior attack lines and for certain types of exterior attacks. These lines can be either double-jacket or rubber-covered construction.

1½-Inch (38-mm) and 1¾-Inch (45-mm) Attack Hose

Most fire departments use either 1½-inch (38-mm) or 1¾-inch (45-mm) hose as the primary attack line for most fires. Both sizes of hose use the same 1½-inch (38-mm) couplings. Handlines of this size can usually be operated by one fire fighter, although having a second person on the line makes it much easier to advance and control the hose. This hose is often stored on fire apparatus as preconnected attack lines in lengths ranging from 150 ft (45 m) to 250 ft (75 m), ready for immediate use.

The primary difference between 1½-inch (38-mm) and 1¾-inch (45-mm) hose is the amount of water that can flow though the hose. Depending on the pressure in the hose and the type of nozzle used, a 1½-inch (38-mm) hose can generally flow water at a rate between 60 gpm (225 L/min) and 125 gpm (475 L/min). An equivalent 1¾-inch (45-mm) hose can flow water at a rate between 120 gpm (455 L/min) and 200 gpm (757 L/min). This difference is important, because the fire-extinguishing capability is directly related to the amount of water that is applied to the fire. A 1¾-inch (45-mm) hose can deliver much more water and is only slightly heavier and more difficult to advance than a 1½-inch (38-mm) hoseline. As a consequence, the 1¾-inch (45-mm) hose is one of the most widely used primary attack lines in the fire service.

2½-Inch (65-mm) Attack Hose

A 2½-inch (65-mm) hose is used as an attack line for fires that are too large to be controlled by a 1½-inch (38-mm) or 1¾-inch (45-mm) hoseline. A 2½-inch (65-mm) handline is generally considered to deliver a flow of approximately 250 gpm (945 L/min). It takes at least two fire fighters to safely control this size of handline owing to the combined weight of the hose and the water and the nozzle reaction force. A 50-ft (15-m) length of dry 2½-inch (65-mm) hose weighs approximately 30 lb (14 kg). When the hose is charged and filled with water, however, it may weigh as much as 200 lb (90 kg) per 100 ft (30 m) of length.

Higher flows—up to approximately 350 gpm (1325 L/min)—can be achieved with higher pressures and larger nozzles. It is difficult to operate a handline at these high flow rates, however. For this reason, such flows are more likely to be used to supply a master stream device.

Booster Hose

A booster hose is usually carried on a hose reel that holds 150 ft (45 m) or 200 ft (60 m) of rubber hose. Booster hose contains a steel wire that gives it a rigid shape. This rigid shape allows the hose to flow water without pulling all of the hose off the reel. Booster hose is light in weight and can be advanced quickly by one person.

The disadvantage of booster hose is its limited flow. The normal flow from a 1-inch (25-mm) booster hose is in the range of 40 gpm (150 L/min) to 50 gpm (190 L/min), which is not an adequate flow for extinguishing structure fires. As a consequence, the use of booster hose is typically limited to small outdoor fires and trash dumpsters. This type of hose should not be used for structural firefighting.

■ Supply Hose

Supply hose is used to deliver water to an attack pumper from a pressurized source, which could be a hydrant or another engine working in a relay operation. Supply lines range from 3½ inches (90 mm) to 6 inches (150 mm) in diameter. The choice of diameter is based on the preferences and operating requirements of each fire department. It also depends on the amount of water needed to supply the attack pumper, the distance from the source to the attack pumper, and the pressure that is available at the source.

Fire department engines are normally loaded with at least one bed of hose that can be laid out as a supply line. When **threaded hose couplings** are used, this hose can be laid out from the hydrant to the fire (known as a forward lay) or from the fire to the hydrant (known as a reverse lay). Sometimes engines are loaded with two beds of hose so they can easily drop a supply line in either direction. If Storz-type sexless couplings are used or the necessary adapters are provided, hose from the same bed can be laid in either direction.

When 2½-inch (65-mm) hose is used as a supply line, it typically comprises the same type of hose that is used for attack lines. This size of hose has a limited flow capacity, but it can be effective at low to moderate flow rates and over short distances. Sometimes two parallel lines of 2½-inch (65-mm) hose are used to provide a more effective water supply.

Large-diameter supply lines are much more efficient than 2½-inch (65-mm) hose for moving larger volumes of water over longer distances. Given this fact, many fire departments use 4-inch (100-mm) or 5-inch (125-mm) hose as their standard supply line. A single 5-inch (125-mm) supply line can deliver flows exceeding 1500 gpm (5678 L/min) under some conditions. LDH is heavy and difficult to move after it has been charged with water, however. This hose comes in 50-ft (15-m) and 100-ft (30-m) lengths. A typical fire engine may carry anywhere from 600 ft (180 m) to 1250 ft (380 m) of supply hose.

Soft Sleeve Hose

A **soft sleeve hose** is a short section of LDH that is used to connect a fire department pumper directly to the large streamer outlet on a hydrant **FIGURE 6-6**. Use of this type of hose allows as much water as possible to flow from the hydrant to the pump through a single hose. A soft sleeve hose may have Storz or similar connections on both ends or a female connection on each end. If it has two Storz connections, an adapter is required to connect the large-diameter inlet to the engine and the hydrant. Many Storz connections have locks to prevent the couplings from coming loose. New ones will have locks, but older couplings may not. As the driver/operator,

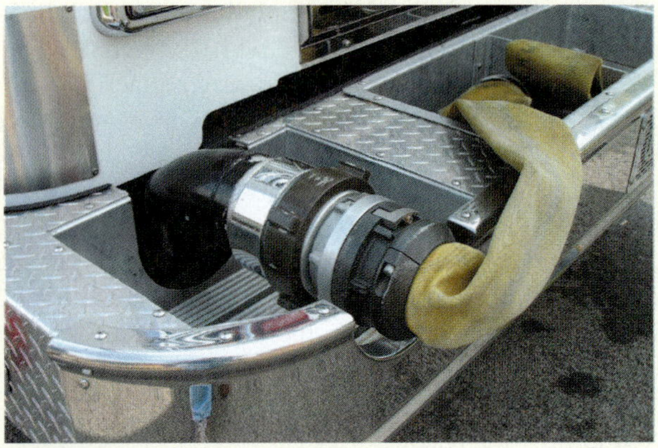

FIGURE 6-6 Soft sleeve hose.

you should always make sure the coupling is locked before charging the line. Hydrant valves are becoming used more often in areas with low water pressure. The use of a hydrant valve allows a second pumper to increase the water pressure in most cases. If the hose uses two female threaded connections, one end should match the local hydrant threads and the other end should match the threads on a large-diameter inlet to the engine. The couplings may have large handles to allow for quick tightening by hand. The hose can range from 4 inches (100 mm) to 6 inches (150 mm) in diameter and is usually between 10 ft (3 m) and 25 ft (7.5 m) in length.

Hard Suction Hose

A hard suction hose is a special type of supply hose that is used to draft water from a static source such as a river, lake, or portable drafting basin **FIGURE 6-7**. The water is drawn through this hose into the pump on a fire department engine or into a portable pump. This type of line is called a hard suction hose because it is designed to remain rigid and will not collapse when a vacuum is created in the hose to draft the water into the pump.

Hard suction hose normally comes in 10-ft (3-m) or 20-ft (6-m) sections. The diameter of this type of hose is based on the capacity of the pump and can be as large as 6 inches (150 mm). Hard suction hose can be made from either rubber or plastic; the newer plastic versions are much lighter and more flexible than the older rubber hoses.

Long handles are provided on the female couplings of hard suction hose to assist in tightening the hose. To draft water, it is essential to have an airtight connection at each coupling. Sometimes it may be necessary to gently tap these handles with a rubber mallet to tighten the hose or to disconnect it. Tapping these handles with anything metal, however, could cause damage to the handles or the coupling—so always use the right tool for the job.

How to Connect from a Hydrant to a Pump

Follow the steps in **SKILL DRILL 6-1** to connect a coupling for a soft sleeve hose from a hydrant to a pump:

1. Using a hydrant wrench, remove the large-diameter discharge cap on the hydrant. (**STEP 1**)
2. Open the hydrant and flush the hydrant until any debris is cleared. (**STEP 2**)
3. Unroll the 15-ft (4.5-m) to 25-ft (7.5-m) length of soft sleeve hose. (**STEP 3**)
4. Connect the matching threaded side of the hydrant adapter to the hydrant. (**STEP 4**)
5. Connect the hose's coupling to the end of the hydrant adapter. (**STEP 5**)
6. Connect the coupling at the other end of the hose to the large-diameter inlet on the pump, using another adapter if necessary. (**STEP 6**)

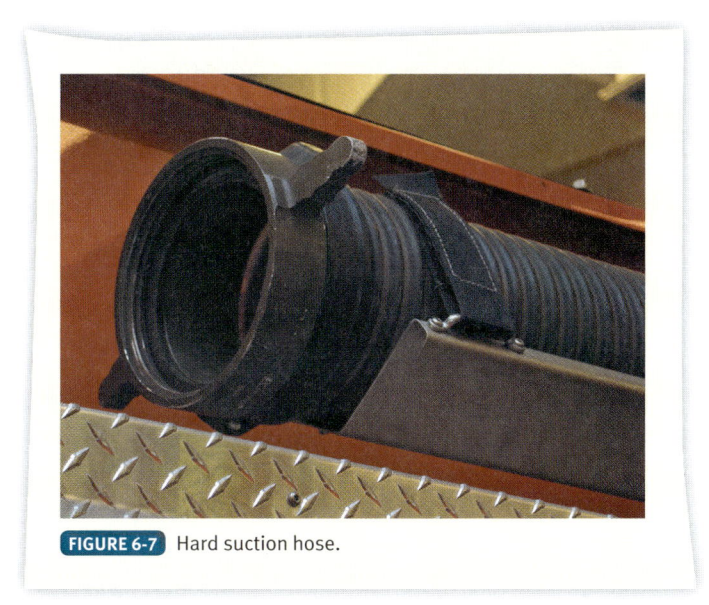

■ Fire Hose Appliances

A fire hose appliance is any device used in conjunction with a fire hose for the purpose of delivering water. As a driver/operator, you should be familiar with wyes, water thiefs, Siamese connections, double-male and double-female adapters, reducers, hose clamps, hose jackets, and hose rollers. It is important for you to learn how to use the various hose appliances and tools required by your fire department; that is, you should understand the purpose of each device and be able to use each appliance correctly. Some hose appliances are used primarily with supply lines, whereas others are most often used with attack lines. Many hose appliances can be employed with both supply lines and attack lines.

Wyes

A wye is a device that splits one hose stream into two hose streams. The word "wye" refers to a Y-shaped part or object. When threaded couplings are used, a wye has one female connection and two male connections. Unless the wye is preassembled to the hoseline, you should use the foot-tilt method to connect the wye to the hoseline. This method helps to prevent cross-threading the two couplings.

The wye that is most commonly used in the fire service has one 2½-inch (65-mm) inlet and splits into two 1½-inch (38-mm) outlets. It is used primarily for 1¾-inch (45-mm) attack lines that stretch for long distances from the fire apparatus. A gated wye is equipped with two quarter-turn ball valves so that the flow of water to each of the split lines can be controlled independently **FIGURE 6-8**. A gated wye enables fire fighters to

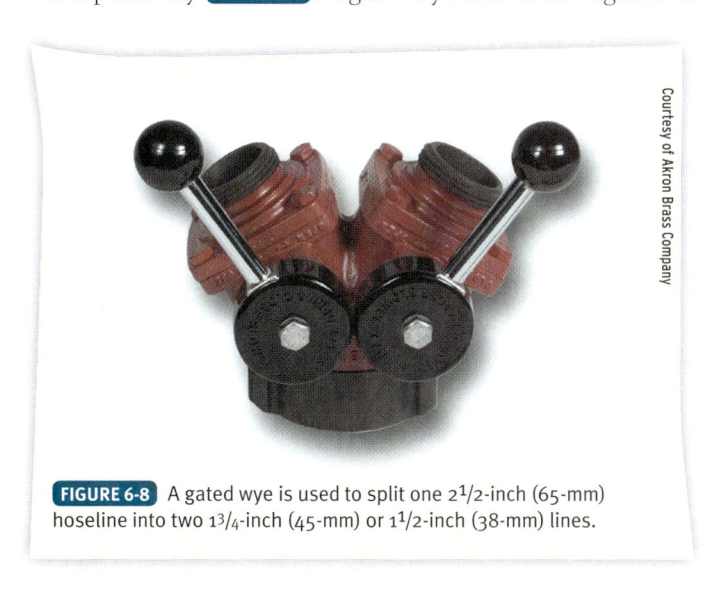

FIGURE 6-7 Hard suction hose.

FIGURE 6-8 A gated wye is used to split one 2½-inch (65-mm) hoseline into two 1¾-inch (45-mm) or 1½-inch (38-mm) lines.

Courtesy of Akron Brass Company

SKILL DRILL 6-1

Connecting a Coupling for a Soft Sleeve Hose from a Hydrant to a Pump
(NFPA 1002, 5.2.4(A), 5.2.4(B))

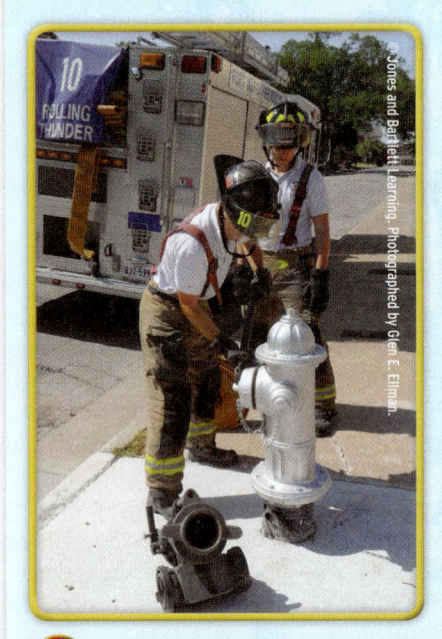

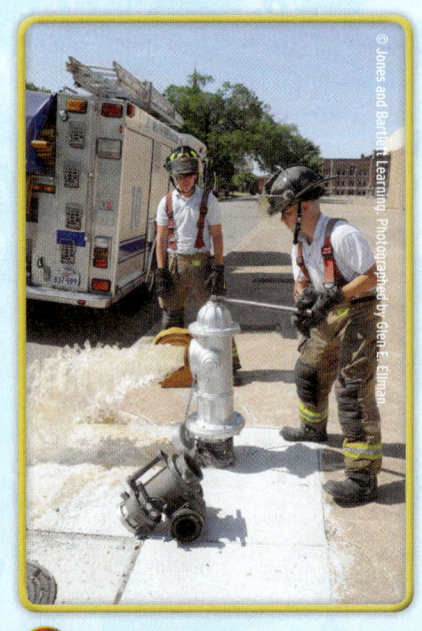

1 Remove the large-diameter cap on the hydrant.

2 Flush the hydrant.

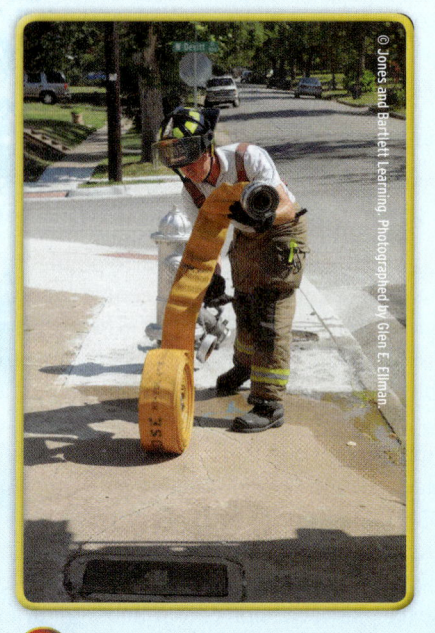

3 Unroll the hose.

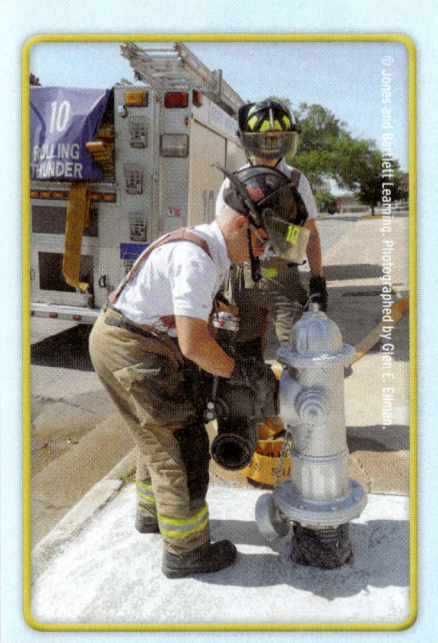

4 Connect the hydrant adapter to the hydrant.

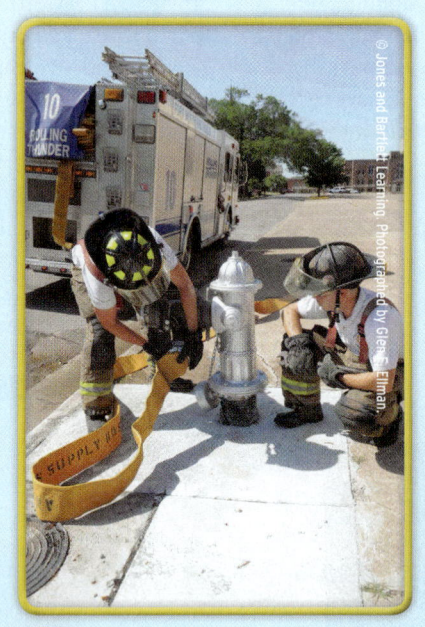

5 Connect the hose to the hydrant adapter.

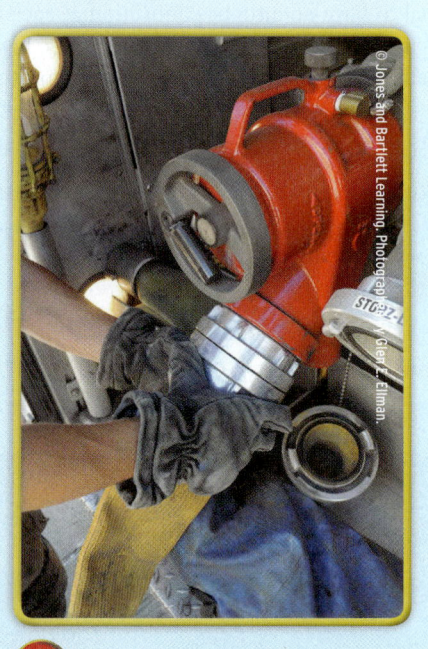

6 Connect the hose to the large-diameter inlet on the pump.

FIGURE 6-9 A water thief.

FIGURE 6-10 A typical Siamese connection has two female inlets and a single outlet.

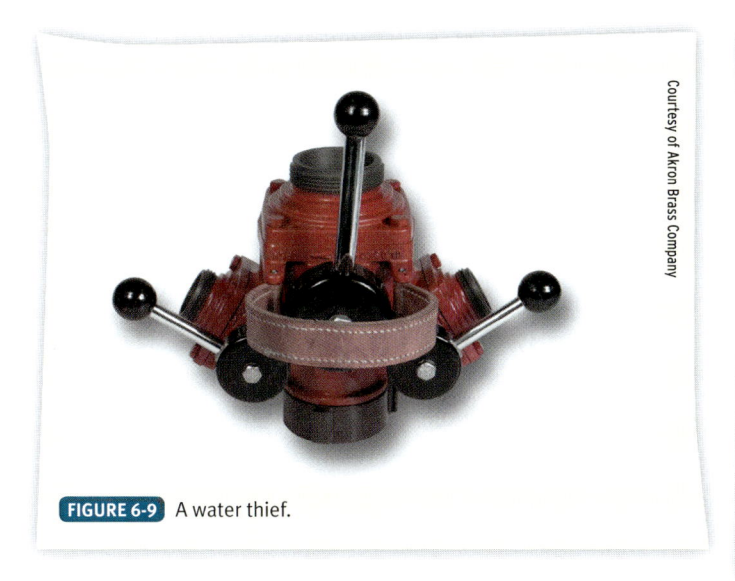

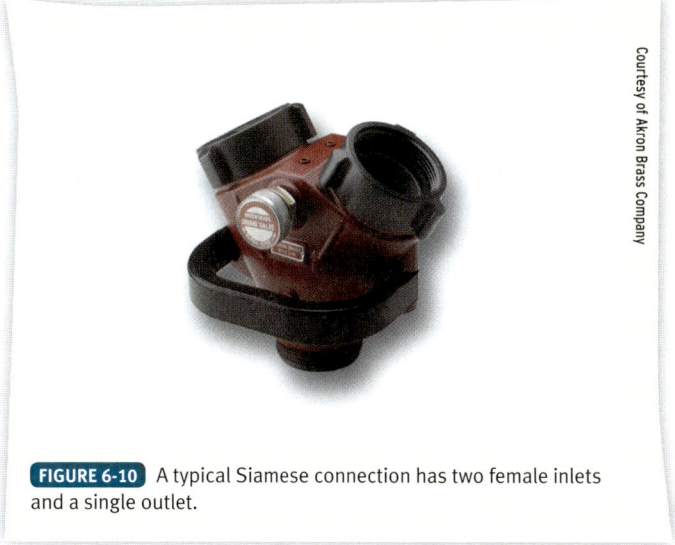

initially attach and operate one hoseline, and then to add a second hose later if necessary. The use of a gated wye avoids the need to shut down the hoseline supplying the wye while attaching this second line. To use this appliance correctly, you must know where it is positioned relative to the hoseline. As the driver/operator, you are responsible for providing the correct water flow to the nozzles. Using this appliance may change the required pressure for the attack line.

Water Thief
A water thief is similar to a gated wye, but includes an additional 2½-inch (65-mm) outlet **FIGURE 6-9**. It is used primarily on attack lines. With this appliance, the water that comes from a single 2½-inch (65-mm) inlet can be directed to two 1½-inch (38-mm) outlets and one 2½-inch (65-mm) outlet. Under most conditions, it will not be possible to supply all three outlets at the same time because the capacity of the supply hose is limited. You should attach the water thief to the 2½-inch (65-mm) hoseline and then connect the other lines to the appliance as needed. When using different-size hoses that require different operating pressures, you may adjust the pressure by opening or closing the valves.

A water thief can be placed near the entrance to a building to provide the water for interior attack lines. One or two 1½-inch (38-mm) attack lines can be used in such cases. If necessary, they can then be shut down and a 2½-inch (65-mm) line substituted for them. Sometimes the 2½-inch (65-mm) line is used to knock down a fire, while the two 1½-inch (38-mm) lines are used during overhaul.

Siamese Connection
A Siamese connection is a hose appliance that combines two hoselines into one. The most commonly encountered type of Siamese connection combines two 2½-inch (65-mm) hoselines into a single 2½-inch (65-mm) hoseline **FIGURE 6-10**. This scheme increases the flow of water on the outlet side of the Siamese connection. A Siamese connection that is used with threaded couplings has two female connections on the inlets and one male connection on the outlet. It can be used with supply lines and with some attack lines. For example, you may connect a Siamese appliance to the 2½-inch (65-mm) inlet on the engine's pump, which allows for more water to be delivered from the pump. When making this type of connection, hold the Siamese connection level with the inlet and make sure you do not cross-thread the couplings. Once the Siamese connection is attached to the pump, connect first one hoseline and then the other. Most Siamese appliances contain a built-in clapper valve to allow for one hoseline to be charged before the other one is connected.

A Siamese connection is sometimes used on an engine inlet to allow water to be received from two different supply lines. This type of connection is also used to supply master stream devices and ladder pipes. Siamese connections are commonly installed on the fire department connections that are used to supply water to standpipe and sprinkler systems in buildings. Fire fighters should be familiar with their department's policies on the correct procedures for supplying fire department Siamese connections.

Adapters
Adapters are used for connecting hose couplings that have the same diameter but dissimilar threads. Dissimilar threads might be encountered when different fire departments are working together or in industrial settings where the hose threads of the building's equipment do not match the threads of the municipal fire department. Adapters are also used to connect threaded couplings to Storz-type couplings. They are useful for both supply lines and attack lines.

Adapters can also be used when it is necessary to connect two female couplings or two male couplings. A double-female adapter is used to join two male hose couplings. A double-male adapter is used to join two female hose couplings. Such double-male and double-female adapters are often used when performing a reverse hose lay **FIGURE 6-11**. With the reverse lay, the fire apparatus stops at the incident site and deploys hose; it then drives to the water source. If the engine company has its hose set up for a forward hose lay (water source to the fire scene), the first coupling to come off will be female. The fire fighters may then connect a double-male adapter to the hose,

FIGURE 6-11 Double-male and double-female adapters are used to join two couplings of the same sex.

FIGURE 6-13 A hose jacket is used to repair a leaking hoseline.

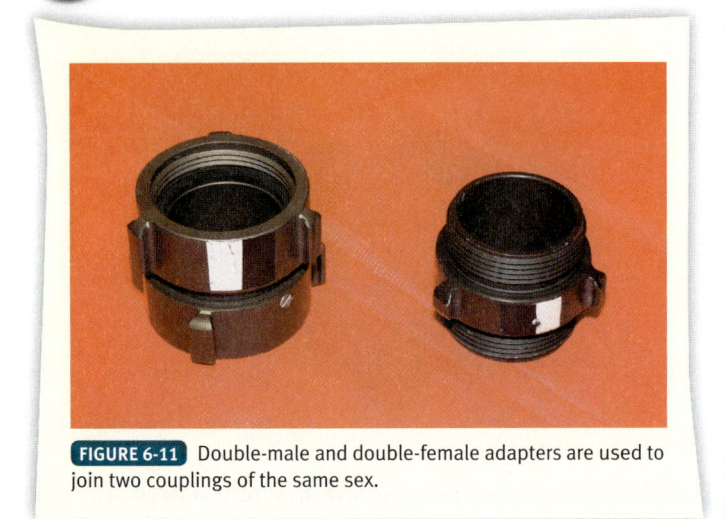

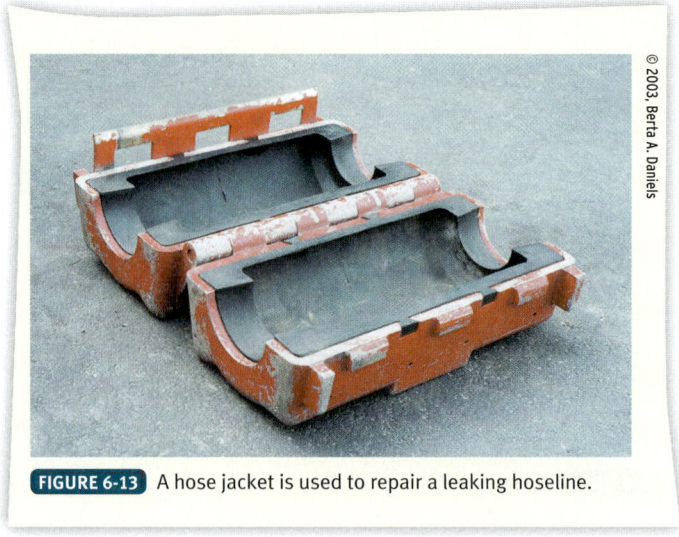

followed by connection of a nozzle to the double-male adapter. After the engine company is positioned at the water source and a sufficient amount of hose is pulled, you would first connect a double-female adapter to the end of the hose and then connect it to a discharge on the pump.

Reducers

A <u>reducer</u> is used to attach a smaller-diameter hose to a larger-diameter hose **FIGURE 6-12**. Usually the larger end has a female connection and the smaller end has a male connection. One type of reducer is used to attach 2½-inch (65-mm) couplings to 1½-inch (38-mm) couplings. Many 2½-inch (65-mm) nozzles are constructed with a built-in reducer, so that a 1½-inch (38-mm) line can be attached for overhaul. For example, after the main fire is knocked down, fire fighters operating a 2½-inch (65-mm) attack line would shut off the water flow at the nozzle's bale (the handle that controls the quarter-turn valve) and remove the tips on the nozzle, exposing the 1½-inch (38-mm) male threads. The driver/operator would then bring a smaller-diameter hoseline with 1½-inch (38-mm) couplings to the end of the hoseline and attach the smaller hose with a smaller nozzle to continue fire suppression activities. Use of a smaller hose allows the crew to move around more easily and requires fewer personnel to operate the attack line. Reducers may also be used to attach a 2½-inch (65-mm) supply line to a larger suction inlet on a fire pumper.

Hose Jacket

A <u>hose jacket</u> (also called a burst hose jacket) is a device that is placed over a section of hose to stop a leak **FIGURE 6-13**. Of course, the best way to handle a leak in a section of hose is to replace the defective section of hose. A hose jacket, however, can provide a temporary fix until the section of hose can be replaced. This device should be used only in cases where it is not possible to quickly replace the leaking section of hose. It can be applied to both supply lines and attack lines.

As the driver/operator, you will often be in the best position to deploy a hose jacket if necessary. The hose jacket consists of a split metal cylinder that fits tightly over the outside of a hoseline. This cylinder is hinged on one side to allow it to be positioned over the leak. A fastener is then used to clamp the cylinder tightly around the hose. Two thick rubber gaskets at each end are provided to trap the water inside the appliance. To deploy the hose jacket, you place the section of hose with the leak between the two rubber gaskets and securely lock the device in position.

Hose Clamp

A <u>hose clamp</u> **FIGURE 6-14** is used to temporarily stop the flow of water in a hoseline. Hose clamps are often applied to supply lines so as to allow a hydrant to be opened before the line is hooked up to the intake of the attack pumper. In such a case, the fire fighter at the hydrant does not have to wait for the pump operator to connect the supply line to the pump intake before opening the hydrant. At the fire scene, one of the fire fighters or the driver/operator should immediately place the hose clamp on the dry supply line. It is important to place the clamp past the coupling, in case the clamp slides when the line is charged. This will prevent the clamp getting knocked open on the coupling. Once you pull enough supply hose from the hose bed and connect it to the intake, the clamp can be released. Ensure that the

FIGURE 6-12 A reducer is used to connect a smaller-diameter hoseline to the end of a larger-diameter line.

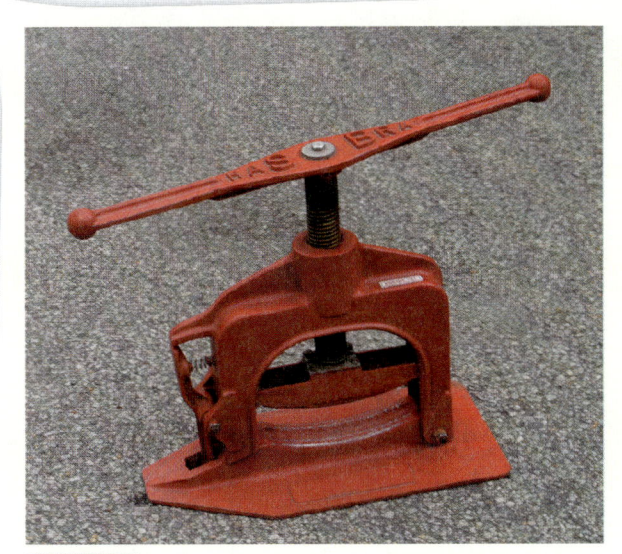

FIGURE 6-14 A hose clamp is used to temporarily interrupt the flow of water in a hoseline.

clamp is opened slowly so it does not injure you or cause water hammer. A hose clamp can also be used to stop the flow in a line if a hose ruptures or if an attack line needs to be connected to a different appliance.

Valves

Valves are used to control the flow of water in a pipe or hoseline. Several types of valves are used on fire hydrants, fire apparatus, standpipe and sprinkler systems, and attack hoselines. The important thing to remember when opening and closing any valve or nozzle is to do it s-l-o-w-l-y so as to prevent water hammer.

The following types of valves are commonly encountered on the fireground FIGURE 6-15:

- Ball valves: Ball valves are used on nozzles, gated wyes, and engine discharge gates. These valves consist of a ball with a hole in the middle. When the hole is lined up with the inlet and the outlet, water flows through it. As the ball is rotated, the flow of water is gradually reduced until it is shut off completely. Ball valves are the most common discharge valves found on fire pumps.
- Gate valves: Gate valves are found on hydrants and on sprinkler systems. With this type of valve, rotating a spindle causes a gate to move slowly across the opening for the water flow. The spindle is rotated by turning it with a wrench or a wheel-type handle.
- Butterfly valves: Butterfly valves are often found on the large pump intake connections where a hard suction hose or soft sleeve hose is connected. They are opened or closed by rotating a handle for one-quarter turn.
- Relay or hydrant valves: This appliance, which is attached to a fire hydrant, is used in conjunction with a pumper to increase water pressure in relaying operations.

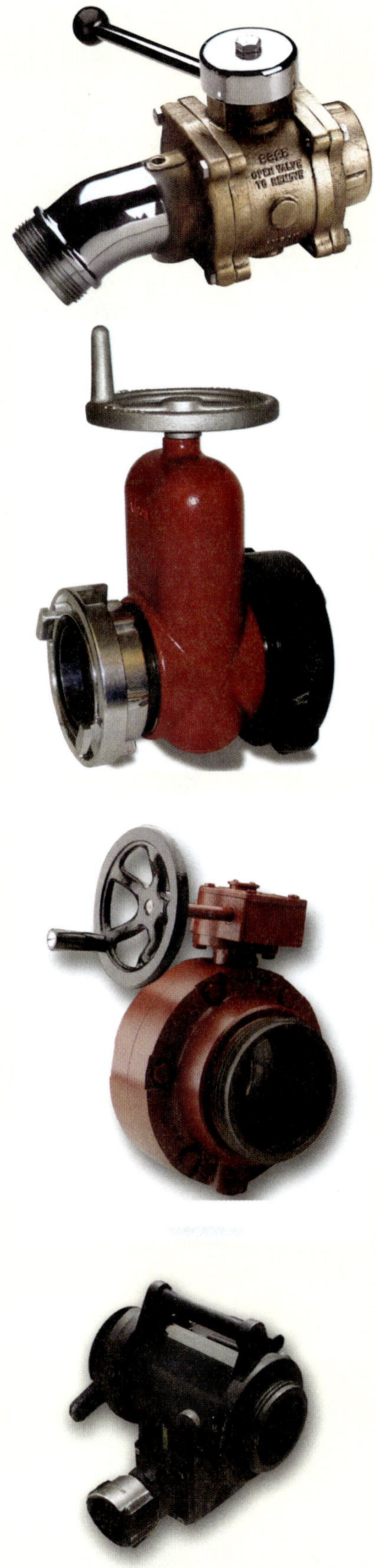

A

Courtesy of Akron Brass Company

B

Courtesy of Akron Brass Company

C

Courtesy of Akron Brass Company

D

Courtesy of Jim Hylton

FIGURE 6-15 Types of valves. **A.** Ball valve. **B.** Gate valve. **C.** Butterfly valve. **D.** Hydrant valve.

VOICES OF EXPERIENCE

A driver/operator must know the capabilities and limitations of their equipment and themselves. This will separate an average driver/operator from an exceptional one. The operator must know how to deal with problems as they arise in a timely manner. Our department SOPs have the first Engine go directly to the fire, while the second lays in from a hydrant. Occasionally the second due does not arrive in a timely manner, and the driver/operator is then faced with a problem.

As the driver/operator, do you know where the closest hydrant is? Can you pull a supply to it, using a standard 5-inch (127-mm) or 3-inch (76-mm) supply line? If you have practiced this scenario, you will know how far you can pull a 5-inch (127-mm) vs. a 3-inch (76-mm) line. It is true that the 5-inch (127-mm) line delivers more water with less friction loss, but does that volume make up for the speed that will be required to achieve a continuous supply? When should the driver/operator decide to take the hydrant: ¾ of a tank, ½ of a tank, or ¼ of a tank? How long would it take to accomplish this task on your own?

While you consider the above questions, you must keep in mind the most important priority of any operation—the safety of the fire fighters at the end of the attack line. The water you keep coming out of the attack line is the difference between life and death. Before you make any decision, you must ensure the safety of the fire fighters. Can you communicate with them? All interior fire fighters are required to have a radio—do they have it on the right channel and can they hear your radio traffic that you are running out of water? What is your secondary plan to communicate with them? If you come to a situation where you cannot make a continuous supply to support the attack line before running out of water, then the only priority is to get the fire fighters to pull back out of harm's way and then deal with the supply issue.

A new driver/operator will be taught the standard pumping techniques, and after that must challenge themselves to deal with the possible problems that can arise. There are no shortage of possible problems that can happen: rocks in the pump, a hose bursting, a faulty hydrant, poor positioning, a lack of communication, conflicting orders, and the list goes on and on. The driver/operator that anticipates and practices for when problems arise will always be successful because they know their capabilities and limitations. My mentor had a saying, "I am not afraid of what I know can go wrong, I am afraid of what I don't know can go wrong."

Captain Mario Minoia
San Jose Fire Department
San Jose, California

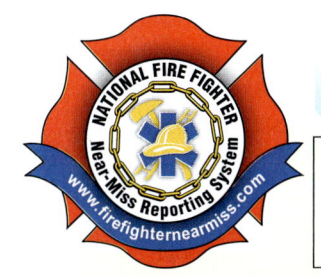

Near-Miss REPORT

Report Number: 10-0001084

Synopsis: Unattended hose appliance strikes fire fighter.

Event Description: During a training evolution on an exterior third floor stairwell, a 2½-inch (65-mm) hose was being used with a gated wye to a high rise pack. There were four fire fighters at the entry door awaiting water on the 2½-inch (65-mm) hose. Once the hose was deployed, water was called for 2½-inch (65-mm) hoseline. Another fire fighter and I were preparing for entry by donning our masks and checking equipment as the water was coming up to the wye. As the 2½-inch (65-mm) hoseline was charged, the pressure lifted the gated wye off the landing, and it first hit my helmet and then hit my breathing apparatus bottle. After that happened, the wye was controlled by a member of the rapid intervention crew (RIC).

Lessons Learned: The gated wye needs to be controlled at all times. With the fire attack crew getting ready for entry, a member of the RIC might be a good candidate to handle the gated wye, but whoever is controlling the wye needs to communicate that information. There is a lot going on at the entry point but situational awareness must be maintained and fire fighters should not be so focused on one area that they fail to see other issues.

■ Nozzles

Nozzles are attached to the discharge end of attack lines to give fire streams shape and direction. Without a nozzle, the water discharged from the end of a hose would reach only a short distance. Nozzles are used on all sizes of handlines as well as on master stream devices.

Nozzles can be classified into three groups:

1. **Low-volume nozzles** flow 40 gpm (150 L/min) or less. They are primarily used on booster hoses; their application is limited to small outside fires.
2. **Handline nozzles** are used on hoselines ranging from 1½ inches (38 mm) to 2½ inches (65 mm) in diameter. Handline streams usually flow water at a rate between 60 gpm (225 L/min) and 350 gpm (1325 L/min).
3. **Master stream nozzles** are used on deck guns, portable monitors, and ladder pipes that flow more than 350 gpm (1325 L/min).

Low-volume and handline nozzles incorporate a shut-off valve that is used to control the flow of water. In contrast, the control valve for a master stream is usually separate from the nozzle itself. All nozzles have some type of device or mechanism to direct the water stream into a certain shape. Some nozzles also incorporate a mechanism that can automatically adjust the flow based on the water's volume and pressure.

Nozzle Shut-Offs

The **nozzle shut-off** enables the fire fighter at the nozzle to start or stop the flow of water. The most commonly encountered nozzle shut-off mechanism is a ball valve or quarter-turn valve. The handle that controls this valve is called a bale. Some nozzles incorporate a rotary control valve that is operated by rotating the nozzle in one direction to open it and in the opposite direction to shut off the flow of water.

Two types of nozzles are manufactured for the fire service: **smooth-bore nozzles** and **fog-stream nozzles** (also called combination or fog nozzles). Smooth-bore nozzles produce a solid column of water, whereas fog-stream nozzles separate the water into droplets. With a fog nozzle, the fire fighter can change the size of the water droplets and the discharge pattern by adjusting the nozzle setting. Nozzles must have an adequate volume of water and an adequate pressure to produce a good fire stream. These volume and pressure requirements vary according to the type and size of nozzle.

Smooth-Bore Nozzles

The simplest smooth-bore nozzle consists of a shut-off valve and a **smooth-bore tip** that gradually decreases the diameter of the stream to a size smaller than the hose diameter **FIGURE 6-16**. Smooth-bore nozzles are manufactured to fit both handlines and master stream devices. Those used for master streams and ladder pipes often consist of a set of stacked tips, where each successive tip in the stack has an increasingly smaller-diameter opening. Tips can be quickly added or removed to provide the desired stream size, which allows different sizes of streams to be produced under different conditions.

A smooth-bore nozzle has several advantages over a fog-stream nozzle. For example, this type of nozzle has a longer reach than a combination fog nozzle operating at a straight stream setting. In addition, a smooth-bore nozzle is capable of deeper penetration into burning materials, resulting in quicker fire knockdown and extinguishment. Smooth-bore nozzles also operate at lower pressures than many adjustable-stream nozzles: Most smooth-bore nozzles are designed to operate at 50 psi (350 kPa), whereas many adjustable-stream nozzles generally require pressures of 75 psi (525 kPa) to 100 psi (700 kPa). Lower nozzle pressures result in less nozzle reaction, which makes it easier for a fire fighter to handle the nozzle.

FIGURE 6-16 A smooth-bore nozzle.

Fog-Stream Nozzles

Fog-stream nozzles produce fine droplets of water **FIGURE 6-17**. The advantage of creating these droplets of water is that they absorb heat much more quickly and efficiently than does a solid column of water. This characteristic is important when immediate reduction of room temperature is needed to avoid a flashover. Discharging 1 gallon (3.8 L) of water in 100 ft^3 (2.8 m^3) of involved interior space may produce enough steam to extinguish a fire in 30 seconds. Fog nozzles can produce a variety of stream patterns, ranging from a straight stream, to a narrow fog cone of less than 45 degrees, to a wide-angle fog pattern that is close to 90 degrees.

The straight streams produced by fog nozzles have openings in the center; in other words, a fog nozzle cannot produce a solid stream. The straight stream from a fog-stream nozzle will break up more quickly and will not have the reach of a solid stream delivered by a smooth-bore nozzle. In addition, this straight stream will be affected more dramatically by wind than will a solid stream.

The use of fog-stream nozzles offers several advantages over the use of smooth-bore nozzles, however. First, fog nozzles can be used to produce a variety of stream patterns by rotating the tip of the nozzle. In addition, fog streams are

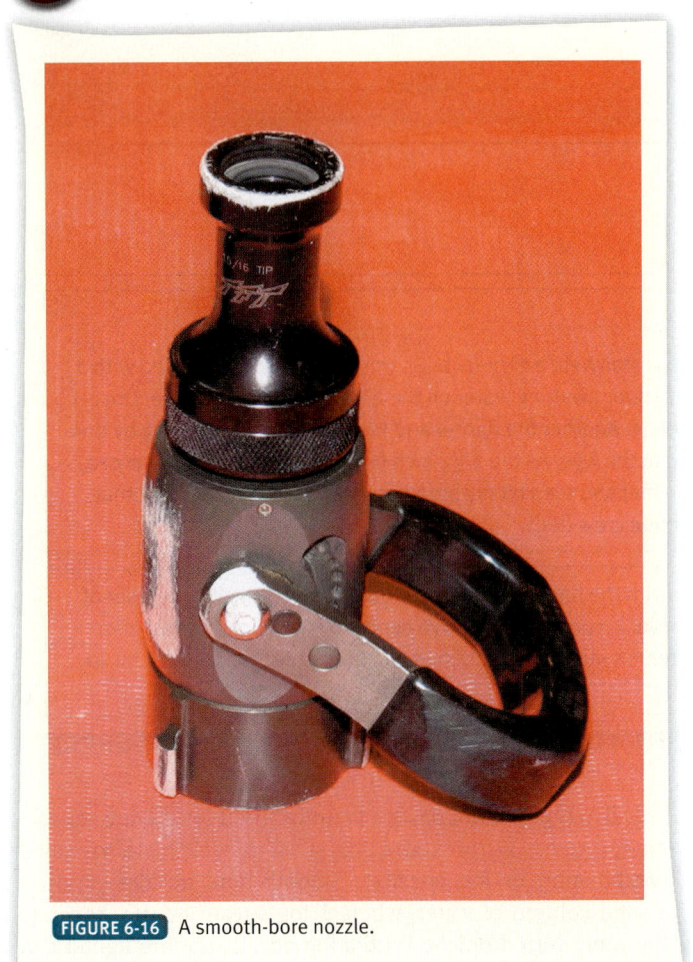

A solid stream extinguishes a fire with less air movement and less disturbance of the thermal layering than does a fog stream; this, in turn, renders the heat conditions less intense for fire fighters during an interior attack. It is also easier for the hose operator to see the pathway of a solid stream than a fog stream.

There are also some disadvantages associated with smooth-bore nozzles. Specifically, the streams from these nozzles do not absorb heat as readily as fog streams and are not as effective for hydraulic ventilation. A fire fighter cannot change the setting of a smooth-bore nozzle to produce a fog pattern; in contrast, a fog nozzle can be set to produce a straight stream.

To inspect a solid-stream nozzle, follow the steps in **SKILL DRILL 6-2**:

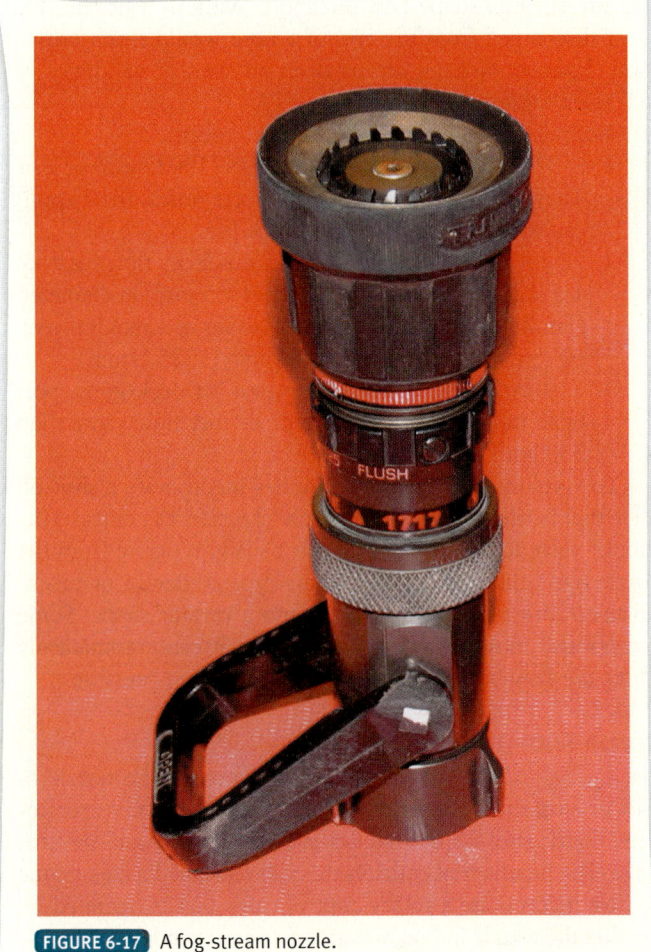

1. Inspect the nozzle for any damage. Remove the nozzle from the hose, and look at the exterior as well as the inside for any dents, broken parts, or missing pieces. (**STEP 1**)
2. Ensure that the gasket located in the female swivel is in place and in good condition. (**STEP 2**)
3. Ensure that the nozzle tips are properly labeled with their size and are attached. (**STEP 3**)
4. Operate the shut-off valve from the closed position to the open position. The valve should not stick or be difficult to operate. (**STEP 4**)

FIGURE 6-17 A fog-stream nozzle.

CHAPTER 6 Fire Hose, Appliances, and Nozzles

SKILL DRILL 6-2 Inspecting a Solid-Stream Nozzle

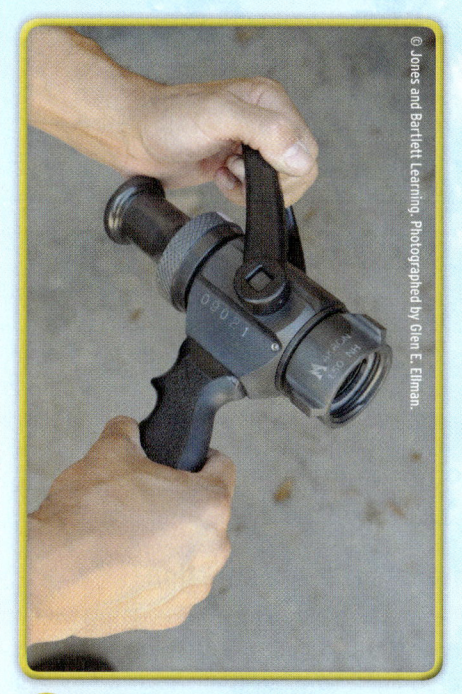

1 Inspect the nozzle for damage.

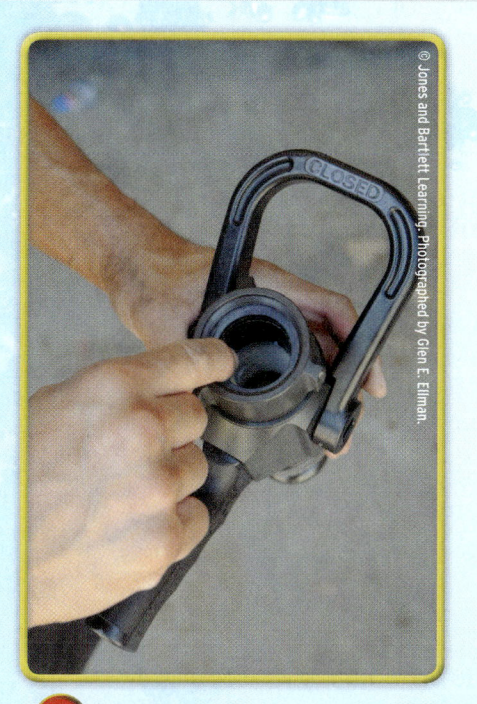

2 Check the gasket.

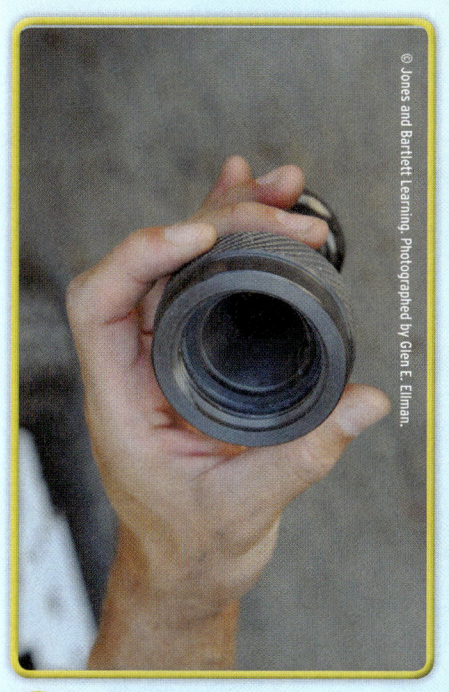

3 Inspect the nozzle tips.

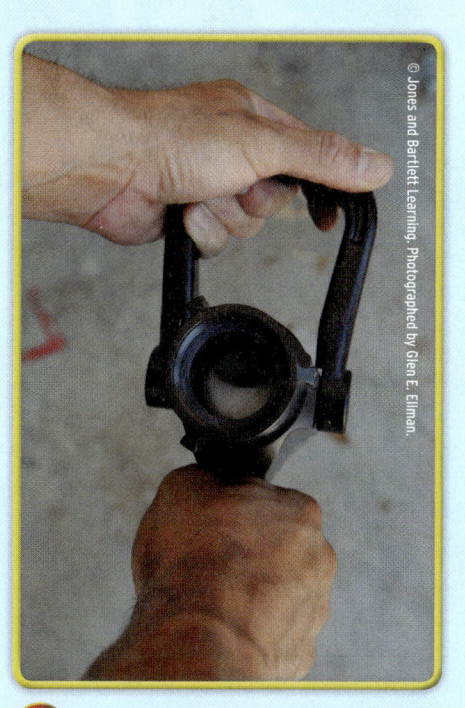

4 Operate the shut-off valve.

effective at absorbing heat and can be used to create a water curtain to protect fire fighters from extreme heat.

Fog nozzles move large volumes of air along with the water, which can be an advantage or a disadvantage, depending on the situation. For example, a fog stream can be used to exhaust smoke and gases through hydraulic ventilation. Unfortunately, this air movement can also result in sudden heat inversion in a room, which then pushes hot steam and gases down onto the fire fighters.

To produce an effective stream, nozzles must be operated at the pressure recommended by the manufacturer. For many years, the standard operating pressure for fog-stream nozzles was 100 psi (700 kPa). In recent years, some manufacturers have produced low-pressure nozzles that are designed to operate at 50 psi (350 kPa) or 75 psi (525 kPa). The advantage of low-pressure nozzles is that they produce less reaction force, which makes them easier to control and advance. Lower nozzle pressure also decreases the risk that the nozzle will get out of control.

Three types of fog-stream nozzles are available, with the differences among the types being related to the water delivery capability:

- A fixed-gallonage fog nozzle delivers a preset flow at the rated discharge pressure. The nozzle could be designed to flow 30, 60, or 100 gpm (115, 225, or 375 L/min).
- An adjustable-gallonage fog nozzle allows the operator to select a desired flow from several settings by rotating a selector bezel to adjust the size of the opening. For example, a nozzle could have the options of flowing 60, 95, or 125 gpm (225, 360, or 475 L/min). Once a setting is chosen, the nozzle will deliver the rated flow only as long as the rated pressure is provided at the nozzle.
- An automatic-adjusting fog nozzle can deliver a wide range of flows. As the pressure at the nozzle increases or decreases, its internal spring-loaded piston moves in or out to adjust the size of the opening. The amount of water flowing through the nozzle is adjusted to maintain the rated pressure and produce a good stream. A typical automatic nozzle could have an operating range of 90 to 225 gpm (340 to 850 L/min) while maintaining a discharge pressure of 100 psi (700 kPa).

To inspect a fog-stream nozzle, follow the steps in **SKILL DRILL 6-3**:

1. Inspect the nozzle for any damage. Remove the nozzle from the hose, and look at the exterior as well as the inside for any dents, broken parts, or missing pieces. (STEP 1)
2. Ensure that the gasket located in the female swivel is in place and in good condition. (STEP 2)
3. Ensure that the nozzle tip is operating properly. Rotate the nozzle tip through all positions several times; it should not bind or stick. (STEP 3)
4. Operate the shut-off valve from the closed position to the open position. The valve should not stick or be difficult to operate. (STEP 4)

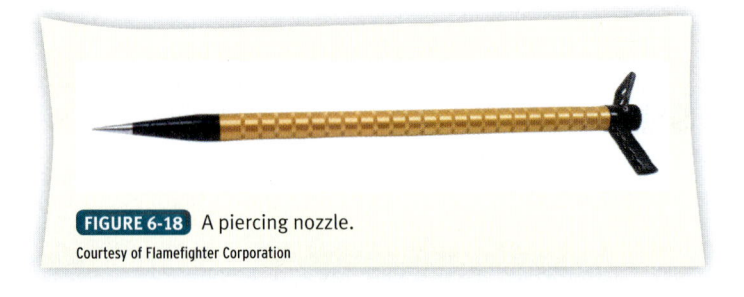

FIGURE 6-18 A piercing nozzle.
Courtesy of Flamefighter Corporation

Other Types of Nozzles

Several other types of nozzles are used for special purposes. Piercing nozzles, for example, are used to make holes in automobile sheet metal, aircraft, or building walls or ceilings, so as to extinguish fires behind these surfaces **FIGURE 6-18**.

Cellar nozzles and Bresnan distributor nozzles are used to fight fires in cellars and other inaccessible places such as attics and cocklofts **FIGURE 6-19**. These nozzles discharge water in a wide circular pattern as the nozzle is lowered vertically through a hole into the cellar. They work much like a large sprinkler head.

If your fire department has other types of specialty nozzles, you need to become proficient in their use and operation.

Nozzle Maintenance and Inspection

Nozzles should be inspected on a regular basis, along with all of the equipment on every fire department vehicle. In particular, nozzles should be checked after each use at an incident before they are placed back on the apparatus. They should be kept clean and clear of debris. Debris inside the nozzle will affect the performance of the nozzle, including possibly reducing flow. Dirt and grit can also interfere with the valve operation and prevent the nozzle from opening and closing fully. Applying a light grease to the valve ball will keep it operating smoothly.

On fog nozzles, inspect the teeth on the face of the nozzle. Make sure all teeth are present and that the finger ring can spin freely. Any missing teeth or failure of the ring to spin will dramatically affect the fog pattern. Any problems noted should be referred to a competent technician for repair.

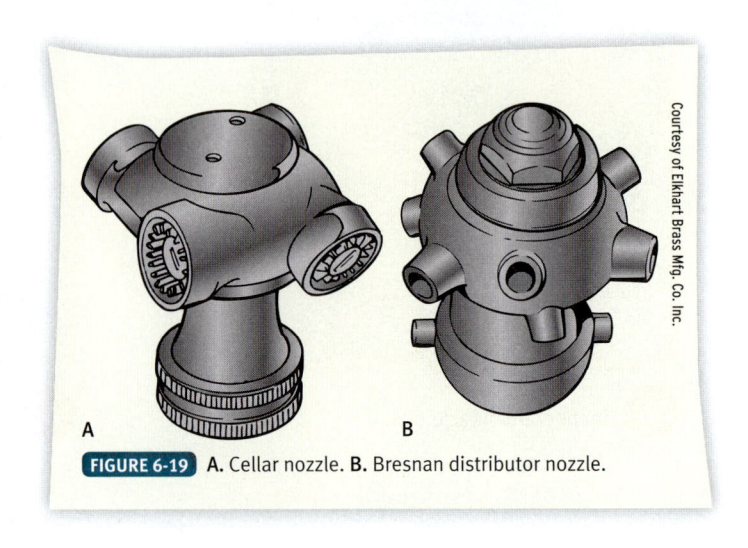

FIGURE 6-19 A. Cellar nozzle. B. Bresnan distributor nozzle.
Courtesy of Elkhart Brass Mfg. Co. Inc.

CHAPTER 6 Fire Hose, Appliances, and Nozzles

SKILL DRILL 6-3 Inspecting a Fog-Stream Nozzle

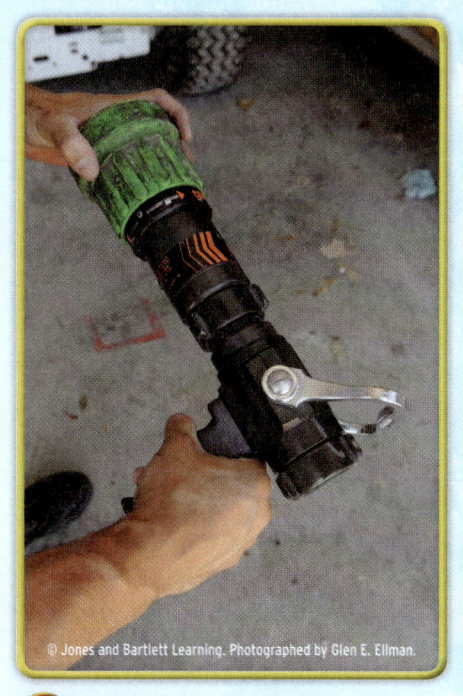

1 Inspect the nozzle for damage.

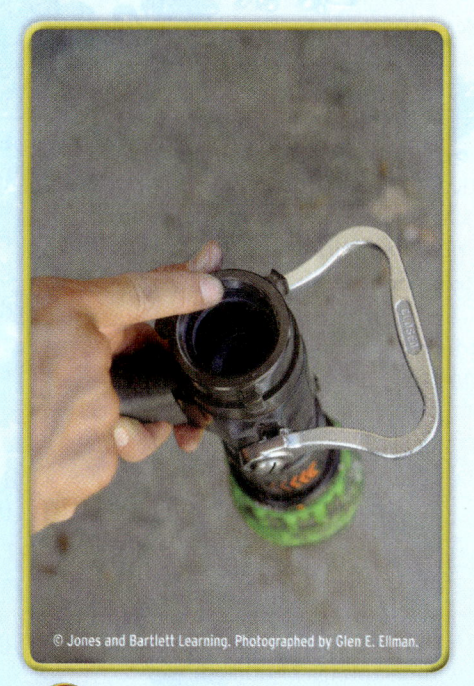

2 Check the gasket.

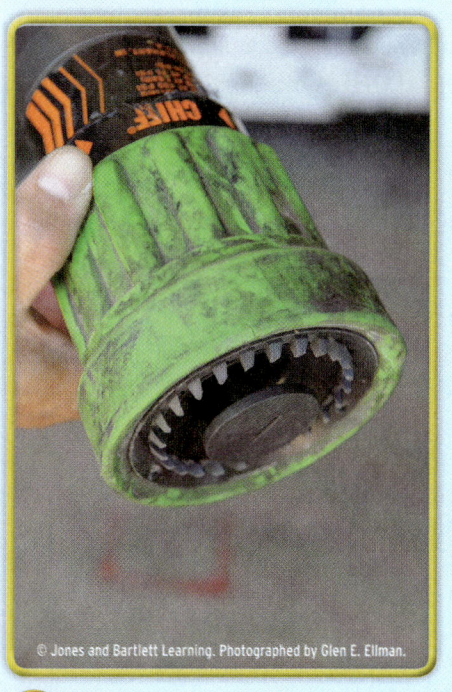

3 Inspect the nozzle tip.

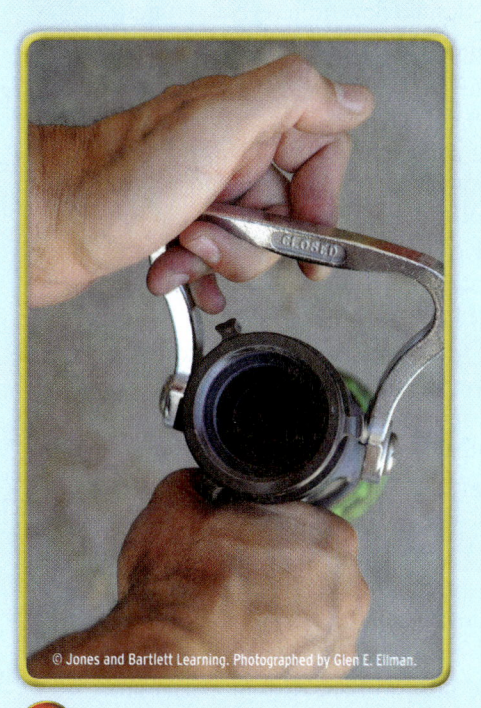

4 Operate the shut-off valve.

© LiquidLibrary

Wrap-Up

Chief Concepts

- Fire hoses are used for two main purposes: as supply hoses and as attack hoses.
- Small-diameter hoses are used as attack lines, large-diameter hoses are almost always used as supply hoses, and medium-diameter hoses can be used for both purposes.
- Supply hose can be classified into two categories: soft sleeve hose and hard suction hose.
- A fire hose appliance is any device used in conjunction with a fire hose for the purpose of delivering water.
- Nozzles can be classified as low-volume, handline, or master stream devices.
- Both smooth-bore and fog-stream nozzles have distinct advantages and disadvantages.
- Three types of fog-stream nozzles are available: fixed gallonage, adjustable gallonage, and automatic adjusting.
- Nozzle maintenance and inspection are critical to their performance.

Hot Terms

adapter Any device that allows fire hose couplings to be safely interconnected with couplings of different sizes, threads, or mating surfaces, or that allows fire hose couplings to be safely connected to other appliances.

adjustable-gallonage fog nozzle A nozzle that allows the operator to select a desired flow from several settings.

attack hose (attack line) Hose designed to be used by trained fire fighters and fire brigade members to combat fires beyond the incipient stage.

automatic-adjusting fog nozzle A nozzle that can deliver a wide range of water stream flows. It operates by means of an internal spring-loaded piston.

ball valve A type of valve used on nozzles, gated wyes, and engine discharge gates. It consists of a ball with a hole in the middle of the ball.

booster hose (booster line) A noncollapsible hose that is used under positive pressure and that consists of an elastomeric or thermoplastic tube, a braided or spiraled reinforcement, and an outer protective cover.

Bresnan distributor nozzle A nozzle that can be placed in confined spaces. The nozzle spins, spreading water over a large area.

butterfly valve A valve found on the large pump intake valve where the hard suction or soft sleeve hose connects to it.

cellar nozzle A nozzle used to fight fires in cellars and other inaccessible places.

double-female adapter A hose adapter that is used to join two male hose couplings.

double-male adapter A hose adapter that is used to join two female hose couplings.

fire hose appliance A piece of hardware (excluding nozzles) generally intended for connection to fire hose to control or convey water.

fixed-gallonage fog nozzle A nozzle that delivers a set number of gallons per minute as per the nozzle's design, no matter what pressure is applied to the nozzle.

fog-stream nozzle A nozzle that is placed at the end of a fire hose and separates water into fine droplets to aid in heat absorption.

gated wye A valved device that splits a single hose into two separate hoses, allowing each hose to be turned on and off independently.

gate valve A type of valve found on hydrants and sprinkler systems.

handline nozzle A nozzle with a rated discharge of less than 350 gpm (1325 L/min).

hard suction hose A hose used for drafting water from static supplies (e.g., lakes, rivers, wells). It can also be used for supplying pumpers from a hydrant if designed for that purpose. The hose contains a semi-rigid or rigid reinforcement designed to prevent collapse of the hose under vacuum.

hose clamp A device used to compress a fire hose so as to stop water flow.

hose jacket A device used to stop a leak in a fire hose or to join hoses that have damaged couplings.

large-diameter hose (LDH) A hose of 3½ inches (90 mm) size or larger.

low-volume nozzle A nozzle that flows 40 gpm (150 L/min) or less.

master stream device A large-capacity nozzle supplied by two or more hoselines of fixed piping that can flow 300 gpm (1135 L/min). These devices include deck guns and portable ground monitors.

master stream nozzle A nozzle with a rated discharge of 350 gpm (1325 L/min) or greater.

medium-diameter hose (MDH) Hose with a diameter of 2½ inches (65 mm) or 3 inches (77 mm).

nozzle A constricting appliance attached to the end of a fire hose or monitor to increase the water velocity and form a stream.

nozzle shut-off A device that enables the fire fighter at the nozzle to start or stop the flow of water.

piercing nozzle A nozzle that can be driven through sheet metal or other material to deliver a water stream to that area.

Wrap-Up, continued

reducer A device that connects two hoses with different couplings or threads together.

relay or hydrant valve A specialized type of valve that can be placed on a hydrant and is used in conjunction with a pumper to increase water pressure in relaying operations.

Siamese connection A device that allows two hoses to be connected together and flow into a single hose.

small-diameter hose (SDH) Hose with a diameter ranging from 1 inch (25 mm) to 2 inches (50 mm).

smooth-bore nozzle A nozzle that produces a straight stream that consists of a solid column of water.

smooth-bore tip A nozzle device that is a smooth tube and is used to deliver a solid column of water.

soft sleeve hose A large-diameter hose that is designed to be connected to the large port on a hydrant (steamer connection) and into the engine.

supply hose (supply line) Hose designed for the purpose of moving water between a pressurized water source and a pump that is supplying attack lines.

threaded hose coupling A type of coupling that requires a male fitting and a female fitting to be screwed together.

water thief A device that has a 2½-inch (65-mm) inlet and a 2½-inch (65-mm) outlet in addition to two 1½-inch (38-mm) outlets. It is used to supply many hoses from one source.

wye A device used to split a single hose into two separate lines.

References

National Fire Protection Association (NFPA) 1002, *Standard for Fire Apparatus Driver/Operator Professional Qualifications.* 2014. http://www.nfpa.org/codes-and-standards/document-information-pages?mode=code&code=1002. Accessed March 27, 2014.

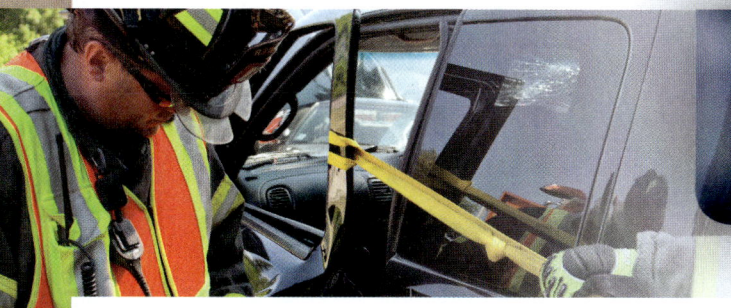

DRIVER/OPERATOR in action

While completing your inventory of equipment on the apparatus, you test your knowledge of the equipment by having another driver/operator quiz you. He tests your expertise by asking you questions about the hose, appliances, and nozzles to make sure that you are competent:

1. Large-diameter hose (LDH) has a diameter of ___ or more.
   A. 3½ inches/90 mm
   B. 5 inches/125 mm
   C. 6 inches/150 mm
   D. 7 inches/175 mm

2. Which appliance combines two hoselines into one?
   A. Water thief
   B. Siamese connection
   C. Adapter
   D. Wye

3. Which of the following is not one of the three groups that nozzles are classified into?
   A. Low-volume nozzles
   B. Handline nozzles
   C. Master stream nozzles
   D. Foam nozzles

4. Which of the following nozzles allows the operator to select a desired flow from several settings by rotating a selector bezel to adjust the size of the opening?
   A. Piercing nozzle
   B. Adjustable-gallonage nozzle
   C. Fixed-gallonage nozzle
   D. Automatic-adjusting nozzle

5. Most smooth-bore nozzles are designed to operate at ___ psi (kPa).
   A. 25 (175)
   B. 35 (245)
   C. 50 (350)
   D. 85 (595)

Mathematics for the Driver/Operator

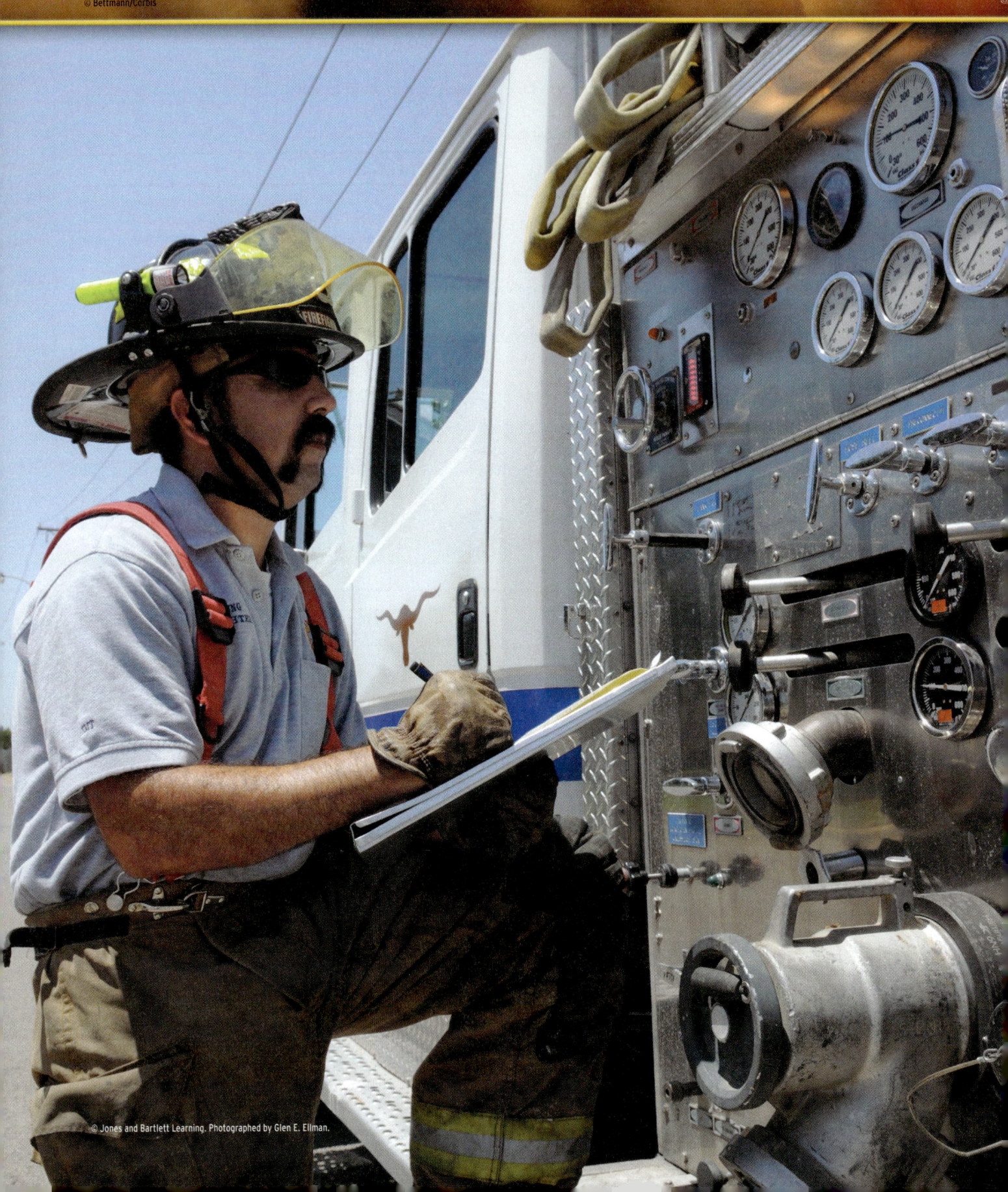

CHAPTER 7

Knowledge Objectives

After studying this chapter, you will be able to:

- Describe pump discharge pressure. (NFPA 1002, 5.2.1, 5.2.1(A) ; p 121–122)
- Describe nozzle pressure. (NFPA 1002, 5.2.1, 5.2.1(A) ; p 122–124)
- Describe nozzle reaction. (NFPA 1002, 5.2.1, 5.2.1(A) ; p 124)
- Describe the four principles of friction loss. (NFPA 1002, 5.2.1, 5.2.1(A) ; p 127)
- List the elements needed to calculate pump discharge pressure. (NFPA 1002, 5.2.1, 5.2.1(1), 5.2.1(2), 5.2.1(3), 5.2.1(4), 5.2.1(A) ; p 121–127)
- Describe the concepts underlying theoretical hydraulic calculations. (NFPA 1002, 5.2.1, 5.2.1(1), 5.2.1(2), 5.2.1(3), 5.2.1(4), 5.2.1(A) ; p 121, 156–158)
- Describe the concepts underlying fireground hydraulic calculations. (NFPA 1002, 5.2.1, 5.2.1(1), 5.2.1(2), 5.2.1(3), 5.2.1(4), 5.2.1(A) ; p 156–157)
- Describe how to utilize fireground hydraulic calculations during an incident. (NFPA 1002, 5.2.1, 5.2.1(1), 5.2.1(2), 5.2.1(3), 5.2.1(4), 5.2.1(A) ; p 156–161)
- Describe how to calculate additional water available from a hydrant. (NFPA 1002, 5.2.1, 5.2.1(1), 5.2.1(2), 5.2.1(3), 5.2.1(4), 5.2.1(A) ; p 161–162)

Skills Objectives

After studying this chapter, you will be able to perform the following skills:

- Calculate nozzle reaction. (NFPA 1002, 5.2.1, 5.2.1(B) ; p 124)
- Calculate the smooth-bore nozzle flow rate. (NFPA 1002, 5.2.1, 5.2.1(B) ; p 125–127)
- Calculate the friction loss in single hoselines. (NFPA 1002, 5.2.1, 5.2.1(B) ; p 127–131)
- Calculate the friction loss in multiple hoselines. (NFPA 1002, 5.2.1, 5.2.1(B) ; p 128–129, 132–133)
- Calculate the elevation pressure loss and gain. (NFPA 1002, 5.2.1, 5.2.1(B) ; p 129–130, 134)
- Calculate the friction loss in an appliance. (NFPA 1002, 5.2.1, 5.2.1(B) ; p 131, 135–139)
- Use a Pitot gauge to test the friction loss in a portable master stream appliance through 3-inch (77-mm) hose. (NFPA 1002, 5.2.1, 5.2.1(B) ; p 136, 138)
- Use in-line gauges to test the friction loss in a specific hose. (NFPA 1002, 5.2.1, 5.2.1(B) ; p 138–139)
- Determine the pump discharge pressure in a wye scenario with equal lines. (NFPA 1002, 5.2.1, 5.2.1(B) ; p 140–141)
- Determine the pump discharge pressure in a wye scenario with unequal lines. (NFPA 1002, 5.2.1, 5.2.1(B) ; p 140–143)
- Determine the pump pressure for a Siamese connection line by the split flow method. (NFPA 1002, 5.2.1, 5.2.1(B) ; p 143–144)
- Calculate the friction loss in Siamese connection lines by coefficient. (NFPA 1002, 5.2.1, 5.2.1(B) ; p 144–145)
- Calculate the friction loss in Siamese connection lines by percentage. (NFPA 1002, 5.2.1, 5.2.1(B) ; p 145–147)
- Calculate the pump discharge pressure for a prepiped elevated master stream device. (NFPA 1002, 5.2.1, 5.2.1(B) ; p 145–147, 150–151)
- Calculate the pump discharge pressure for an elevated master stream. (NFPA 1002, 5.2.1, 5.2.1(B) ; p 145–147, 152–153)
- Calculate the pump discharge pressure for a standpipe during preplanning. (NFPA 1002, 5.2.4, 5.2.4(A), 5.2.4(B) ; p 147, 149–150, 152–153)
- Calculate the pump discharge pressure for a standpipe. (NFPA 1002, 5.2.4, 5.2.4(A), 5.2.4(B) ; p 150–151, 154–155)
- Calculate the flow rate (gpm) for a given hose size and nozzle pressure using a slide rule calculator. (NFPA 1002, 5.2.1, 5.2.1(B) ; p 158)
- Calculate the friction loss for a given hose size and nozzle pressure using a slide rule calculator. (NFPA 1002, 5.2.1, 5.2.1(B) ; p 158)
- Perform calculations by hand. (NFPA 1002, 5.2.1, 5.2.1(B) ; p 158–160)
- Perform the hand method of calculation for 2½-inch (65-mm) hose. (NFPA 1002, 5.2.1, 5.2.1(B) ; p 158–159)
- Perform the hand method of calculation for 1¾-inch (45-mm) hose. (NFPA 1002, 5.2.1, 5.2.1(B) ; p 159–160)
- Perform the subtract 10 method of calculation. (NFPA 1002, 5.2.1, 5.2.1(B) ; p 160)
- Perform the condensed Q method of calculation. (NFPA 1002, 5.2.1, 5.2.1(B) ; p 160–161)
- Perform a calculation to determine the additional water available from a hydrant. (NFPA 1002, 5.2.1, 5.2.1(B) ; p 161–162)

Additional NFPA Standards

- NFPA 13, *Standard for the Installation of Sprinkler Systems*
- NFPA 14, *Standard for the Installation of Standpipe and Hose Systems*
- NFPA 25, *Standard for the Inspection, Testing, and Maintenance of Water-Based Fire Protection Systems*
- NFPA 99, *Standard for Health Care Facilities*
- NFPA 600, *Standard on Industrial Fire Brigades*
- NFPA 921, *Guide for Fire and Explosion Investigations*
- NFPA 1500, *Standard on Fire Department Occupational Safety and Health Program*
- NFPA 1620, *Recommended Practice for Preincident Planning*
- NFPA 1901, *Standard for Automotive Fire Apparatus*

You Are the Driver/Operator

Your engine company has been assigned to career day at the local high school. The school has asked that the fire department share some information about being a fire fighter and answer questions from the audience. The company officer informs the group of teens about the department schedule, benefits, and application process, while you and the other members of the crew stand in front of the audience. One of the students raises his hand and asks, "Do I have to be good at math to be a fire fighter?" The company officer smiles, then turns and looks at you. "Do you want to handle this one?" he asks. Immediately you recall your last fire, where you had multiple lines flowing of various sizes and lengths. You begin to explain to the audience the importance of mathematics as it relates to the driver/operator position and the effects that it can have on the fireground operations.

1. How do you start to calculate the pump discharge pressure?
2. What are the different formulas that you need to know?
3. How do you determine friction loss?

Introduction

Fire service hydraulic calculations are used to determine the required **pump discharge pressure (PDP)** for fireground operations. As the driver/operator, you have a great deal of responsibility at each incident. You must maneuver the fire apparatus through traffic and weather and arrive safely at the correct address. You must secure an adequate water supply and position the fire apparatus to strategic advantage. With the strategy and tactics selected, you must apply the appropriate hoselines or combination of hoselines and/or master stream devices to provide enough water to overcome the heat produced by the fire. The hoselines must be charged quickly and at the correct pump discharge pressure (PDP).

Clearly, the driver/operator is critical to the success of the firefighting attack. When you take on this position, your actions are also critical to ensuring the safety of the attack team, any occupants within the fire-involved structure, the personnel on the scene, and any exposures. The driver/operator fills a very serious role whose decisions are often a matter of life and death.

The fundamentals of theoretical hydraulic calculations are a necessary building block in the professional fire fighter's education. Although many concepts, formulas, and constants are used in hydraulic calculations, hydraulics can be described as an art rather than a science because of the large number of variables that influence the ultimate decisions made. Calculations are influenced by specific factors such as the apparatus manufacturer's design specifications; the characteristics of the fire apparatus, hose, nozzles, appliances, adapters, and couplings; and the relevant departmental policies. The way in which these influences interact is specific to each fire department; as a consequence, no standard set of rules will apply. You must know the requirements of the equipment on your fire apparatus to make the appropriate calculations correctly. This chapter covers the most common calculations that you will need to know as a driver/operator.

Fire service **hydraulics** is the study of the characteristics and movement of water as they pertain to calculations for fire streams and fireground operations. These calculations are generally categorized as theoretical hydraulics and fireground hydraulics. The scientific or more exact calculations are commonly referred to as **theoretical hydraulics**. The concepts underlying this field are fundamental to the understanding of fire streams; they enable you to correctly calculate pump discharge pressures for fire streams and increase your ability to troubleshoot problems and perform professionally on the fireground. Fireground operations are very dynamic, however, so situations can change very quickly. **Fireground hydraulics** is the term for the less exact—but certainly more user-friendly and forgiving—calculation methods used on the fireground.

While much of hydraulics is scientific, much is inexact. Achieving the right balance is an art. The major variables affecting hydraulics are the many numerical values influencing calculations.

Manufacturers offer a wide variety of nozzles, appliances, and hose, each with individual specifications that may vary from those identified on traditional charts. Different brands of hose will flow slightly more or less water than other brands, and different nozzles will vary in their performance. To be as accurate as possible when performing hydraulics calculations, you should use the manufacturer's recommended nozzle pressure specific to the actual nozzle used on your hose or appliance, with your fire apparatus and under the guidelines of your fire department. Flow tests with your equipment will confirm the most precise pressures to use.

As the driver/operator, you must combine your knowledge of the specific equipment on your fire apparatus with the methodology underlying hydraulic theory. There is an art to figuring out this relationship, however, and you must be prepared to adjust it based on the variables in the scenario at hand. Practice and experience with hydraulics calculations are imperative so that you can perform as a skilled driver/operator.

DRIVER/OPERATOR Tip

The driver/operator may work alone on the fireground while operating the pump or other apparatus, but should work as a team on the outside of the fire building to facilitate apparatus operations. A new driver/operator may arrive first on the fireground. If the second-arriving engine has a more experienced driver/operator who does not have a more pressing assignment, it is often a good idea for the experienced driver/operator to assist the less experienced operator. This practice can be an unwritten policy or may be determined by the company officer.

DRIVER/OPERATOR Tip

When two or more fire pumpers are in use, a water supply officer may be assigned to verify adequate supply and support operations.

Pump Discharge Pressure

Fighting fire with water is a matter of water flow rate (gallons per minute [gpm] or liters per minute [L/min]) versus heat generation (British thermal units [Btu], joules [J], or kilocalories [kcal]). To extinguish a fire, sufficient flow must be applied to overcome the heat generated by the fire—a rate referred to as the critical rate of flow. For this reason, one of the most important attack decisions after securing the water supply is which hose and nozzle will produce adequate flow to extinguish the fire. The selected line or lines then must be placed strategically, using the correct tactics, so as to protect lives and confine and extinguish the fire.

The real goal of the driver/operator is to deliver the correct flow (adequate gpms [L/min]) to the nozzle. This may be accomplished by providing the correct PDP, but the goal is always gpms (L/min). Too great a pressure will cause the stream to break up and lessen its effectiveness. It will also create a greater nozzle reaction, which will hinder the attack team's ability to advance the hoseline and cause the team members to become fatigued more quickly. Conversely, inadequate pressure will produce insufficient flow to overcome the fire, possibly endangering the safety of the attack team. It may also contribute to more kinks in the hoseline, further restricting the water flow. Each hose and nozzle combination has an optimal delivery pressure. As the driver/operator, you must make the necessary calculations to determine the correct PDP for the scenario to be supplied.

The PDP is the total pressure needed to overcome all friction, appliance, and elevation loss while maintaining adequate nozzle pressure to deliver effective fire streams. Several factors must be addressed to achieve this goal, including nozzle pressure, friction loss in the hoseline, elevation gain or loss, and friction loss in the appliances. Calculations become more complicated as the complexity of the fire attack operation increases, but all must start with the basic PDP formula:

$$PDP = NP + FL$$

where:

PDP = pump discharge pressure
NP = nozzle pressure
FL = friction loss

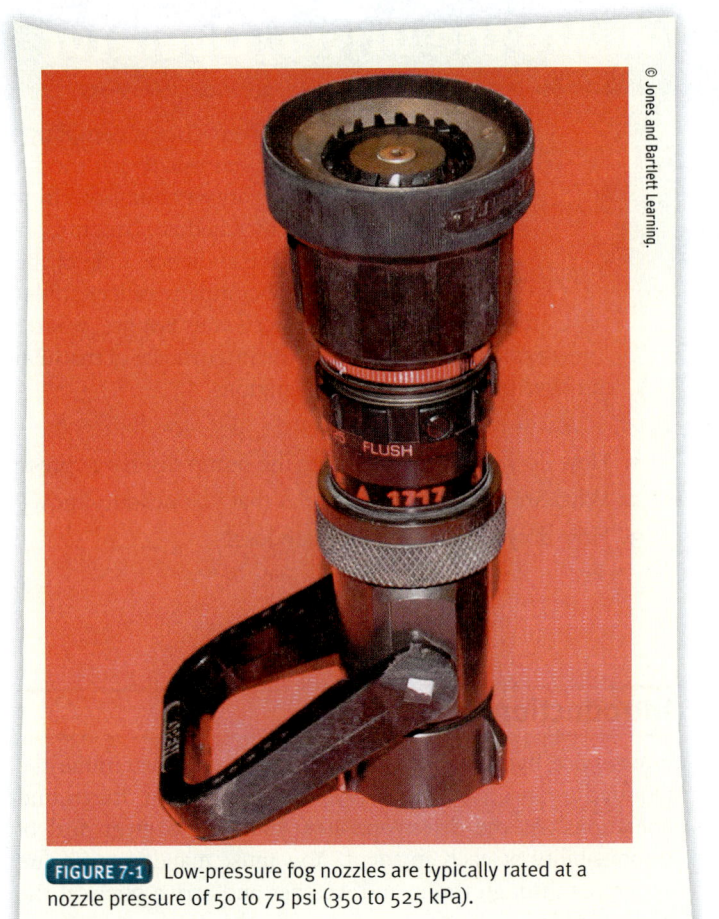

FIGURE 7-1 Low-pressure fog nozzles are typically rated at a nozzle pressure of 50 to 75 psi (350 to 525 kPa).

Nozzle Pressures

To determine the PDP, you use the formula PDP = NP + FL. Next you must establish the appropriate nozzle pressure (NP) given the scenario to inject into the formula. Nozzle pressure is the pressure required at the nozzle to deliver the fire stream and flow rate for which the nozzle was designed. This pressure is defined by the manufacturer of the nozzle and is determined through testing to deliver an efficient amount of water while maintaining an NP at or below safe thresholds.

Combination nozzles (fog nozzles) traditionally have a NP of 100 pounds per square inch (psi) (700 kilopascal [kPa]), but come with different features that have varied NP levels. Low-pressure fog nozzles have a NP that varies from 50 to 75 psi (350 to 525 kPa) **FIGURE 7-1**. Smooth-bore nozzles, also referred to as solid-stream or solid-tip nozzles, have a NP of 50 psi (350 kPa) for handlines and 80 psi (560 kPa) for master streams **FIGURE 7-2**. Smooth-bore nozzles on a handline are normally flowed at a NP of 50 psi (350 kPa). Some master stream smooth-bore nozzles are rated at less than 80 psi (560 kPa), however **FIGURE 7-3**. The actual maximum flow from a master stream nozzle may decrease when the nozzle is detached from the fire apparatus and used from the portable base **FIGURE 7-4**.

The manufacturer's specifications for maximum water flow from an aerial device are listed along with the nozzle specifications. If the nozzle is rated at a higher flow than the aerial device can handle, then fire fighters should limit the nozzle pressure based on the capability of the aerial; usually, this scenario arises

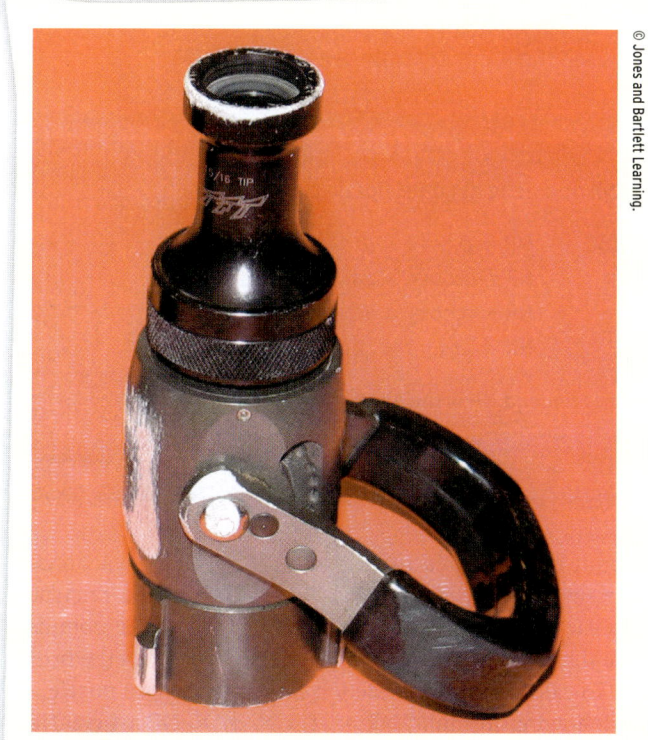

FIGURE 7-2 Smooth-bore handline nozzles are commonly rated at a nozzle pressure of 50 psi (350 kPa).

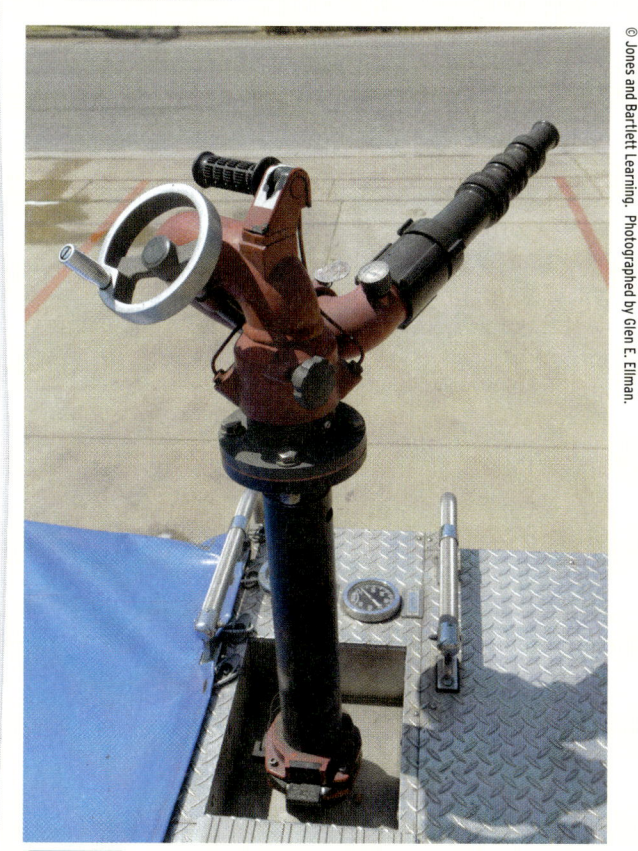

FIGURE 7-3 Smooth-bore nozzles on prepiped elevated master streams are commonly rated at a nozzle pressure of 80 psi (560 kPa).

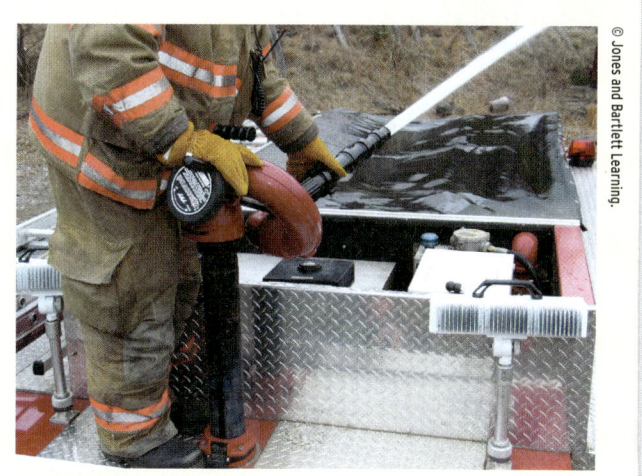

FIGURE 7-4 Master stream devices that are attached to a deck gun are commonly rated at a higher flow (gpm [L/min]) than devices that are attached to the portable base because the truck provides added stability to counteract nozzle reaction.

only with older aerial devices. Unless manufacturer's instructions vary, limit the nozzle pressure for smooth-bore nozzles on elevated master streams to a maximum of 80 psi (560 kPa).

Nozzles are available in both fog and smooth-bore varieties. Fog nozzles are generally rated at 100 psi (700 kPa) and smooth-bore nozzles at 50 psi (350 kPa) **FIGURE 7-5**. Distributor nozzles constantly spin and present centrifugal forces that are symmetrical. Because these forces occur perpendicular to the hose, they do not produce a corresponding nozzle reaction.

Given the many types of products on the market, it is not possible to provide instructions for all of them here. Therefore this text focuses on the most common specifications while addressing the fundamental concepts of hydraulic calculations. Once you understand the fundamentals, you will be able to master the variables you encounter on the actual fireground.

Three standard nozzle pressures (SNPs), all of which are dictated by the type and use of the nozzle, are generally

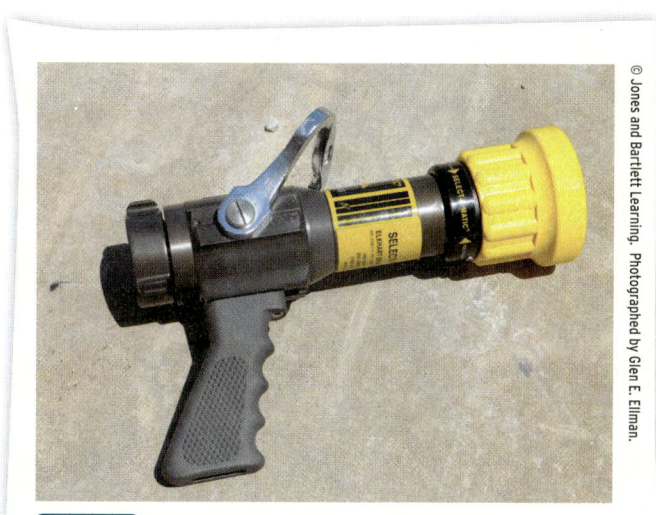

FIGURE 7-5 Combination variable fog and straight stream nozzle.

SKILL DRILL 7-1: Calculating the Nozzle Reaction from a Smooth-Bore Nozzle

Example 1: Calculate the nozzle reaction for a 1-inch tip operating at 50-psi nozzle pressure.

Standard:
$NR = 1.5 \times d^2 \times NP$
$NR = 1.5 \times 1^2 \times 50$
$NR = 1.5 \times 1 \times 50$
$NR = 75$ pounds

Metric:
$NR = 0.0015 \times d^2 \times NP$
$NR = 0.0015 \times 29^2 \times 350$
$NR = 0.0015 \times 841 \times 350$
$NR = 441.53$ or 442 N

where NR is nozzle reaction, d is the diameter of the nozzle, and NP is the nozzle pressure.

© LiquidLibrary

---

sufficient for most fireground operations. For the purpose of this text, we will use these three SNPs:

- 70 psi (480 kPa) NP for all fog nozzles
- 50 psi (350 kPa) NP for smooth-bore handline nozzles
- 80 psi (560 kPa) NP for smooth-bore master stream nozzles

■ Nozzle Reaction

Newton's third law of motion states: "When one body exerts a force on a second body, the second body simultaneously exerts a force equal in magnitude and opposite in direction to that of the first body." Nozzle reaction is the opposing reaction that occurs as water is expelled from the nozzle or the force that pushes back on the fire fighter when he or she flows water. It is a factor of both the amount of the water as it leaves the nozzle and the velocity at which the water travels. If you make a change to both or one of the factors it will change the nozzle reaction.

For practical purposes, it is only necessary to understand how the nozzle reaction will change as the amount of water and the nozzle pressure change. Calculating nozzle reaction should not be attempted at the fire scene but rather determined during training sessions. It is important for the driver/operator to know the nozzle reaction for the preconnected attack lines on the apparatus and to recognize what constitutes a realistic amount of nozzle reaction for the crew. Nozzle reactions for both smooth-bore nozzle and fog nozzles can be calculated, with each reaction being expressed in terms of the pounds of force that the fire fighter must overcome to control the nozzle.

To calculate nozzle reaction in a smooth-bore nozzle, use the following formula: $NR = 1.5 \times d^2 \times NP$, where NR is nozzle reaction, d is the diameter of the nozzle in inches, and NP is the nozzle pressure in psi. Thus, to calculate the nozzle reaction, you need to know the nozzle pressure and the diameter of the smooth-bore nozzle. Use the formula presented in **SKILL DRILL 7-1** to determine the nozzle reaction for smooth-bore nozzles.

To calculate nozzle reaction in a fog nozzle, use the following formula: $NR = 0.0504 \times gpm \times \sqrt{NP}$ (Metric: $NR = 0.0156 \times L/min \times \sqrt{NP}$), where NR is nozzle reaction and $\sqrt{NP}$ is the square root of the nozzle pressure. This calculation works for fog nozzles that are operating in a straight stream pattern only. As the nozzles pattern widens, the nozzle reaction will lessen slightly. For our purposes, we will determine the nozzle reaction for fog nozzles only as they operate in a straight stream pattern. To calculate the nozzle reaction, we need to know the nozzle pressure and the flow from the nozzle. Use the formula presented in **SKILL DRILL 7-2** to determine the nozzle reaction for fog nozzles.

SKILL DRILL 7-2: Calculating the Nozzle Reaction from a Fog Nozzle

Example 1: Calculate the nozzle reaction for a fog nozzle flowing 200 gpm operating at 100-psi nozzle pressure.

Standard:
$NR = 0.0504 \times gpm \times \sqrt{NP}$
$NR = 0.0504 \times 200 \times \sqrt{100}$
$NR = 0.0504 \times 200 \times 10$
$NR = 100.8$ pounds

Metric:
$NR = 0.0156 \times L/min \times \sqrt{NP}$
$NR = 0.0156 \times 750 \times \sqrt{700}$
$NR = 0.0156 \times 750 \times 26.46$
$NR = 309.58$ or 310 N

where NR is nozzle reaction and $\sqrt{NP}$ is the square root of the nozzle pressure.

© LiquidLibrary

Standard TABLE 7-1 — Smooth-Bore Nozzle Flows

Common Smooth-Bore Nozzle Pressures by Application and Their Square Root

Application	Nozzle Pressure	Square Root
Handline	50	7.07
Master stream	80	8.94

Smooth-Bore Nozzle Flows

Tip Size (inch)	At 50 psi	At 65 psi	At 80 psi	Round to
¾	118	135		
⅞	162	183		
15/16	185	210		
1	210	239		
1⅛	266	303		
1¼	328		414	400
1⅜			502	500
1½			597	600
1¾			813	800
2			1062	1000

Smooth-bore nozzle tips for a 2½-inch handline may be rounded off as follows:
1 inch = 210 gpm; round to 200 gpm
1⅛ inch = 266 gpm; round to 250 gpm
1¼ inch = 328 gpm; round to 300 gpm

Metric TABLE 7-1 — Smooth-Bore Nozzle Flows

Common Smooth-Bore Nozzle Pressures by Application and Their Square Root

Application	Nozzle Pressure (kPa)	Square Root
Handline	350	18.71
Master stream	560	23.66

Smooth-Bore Nozzle Flows

Tip Size (mm)	At 350 kPa	At 450 kPa	At 560 kPa	Round to
19	446	505		
22	598	678		
24	711	806		
25	772	875		
29	1038	1177		
32	1264		1599	1600
35			1913	1900
38			2255	2250
45			3163	3150
50			3905	3900

Smooth-bore nozzle tips for a 65-mm handline may be rounded off as follows:
25 mm = 772 L/min; round to 750 L/min
29 mm = 1038 L/min; round to 1050 L/min
32 mm = 1264 mm; round to 1250 L/min

■ Determining Nozzle Flow

Flow rate is the volume of water moving through the nozzle during a specific time period; it is measured in units of gpm or L/min. Fog nozzles are designed with predetermined flow rates based on a set NP. For example, the specification for a fog nozzle might state that it will flow 175 gpm (660 L/min) at a NP of 100 psi (700 kPa). The flow and pressure will differ by design and purchaser's selection (i.e., the flow will be more or less at a greater or lesser pressure, respectively). A label describing the performance ratio of flow to pressure can be found on the face of the nozzle.

To determine the flow rate of a smooth-bore nozzle, you need to employ your mathematical skills. **TABLE 7-1** lists

SKILL DRILL 7-3

Calculating the Flow of a 1¼-Inch Smooth-Bore Nozzle on a 2½-Inch Handline
NFPA 1002, 5.2.1 (standard)

Example 1: Calculate the flow rate for a 1¼-inch tip used on a 2½-inch handline.

$$\text{gpm} = 29.7 \times d^2 \times \sqrt{NP}$$
$$\text{gpm} = 29.7 \times (1¼)^2 \times \sqrt{50}$$
$$\text{gpm} = 29.7 \times (1.25)^2 \times \sqrt{50}$$
$$\text{gpm} = 29.7 \times 1.56 \times 7.07$$
$$\text{gpm} = 327.567 \text{ (round to 300 gpm)}$$

Example 2: Calculate the flow rate for a 1½-inch smooth-bore master stream nozzle.

$$\text{gpm} = 29.7 \times d^2 \times \sqrt{NP}$$
$$\text{gpm} = 29.7 \times (1.5)^2 \times \sqrt{80}$$
$$\text{gpm} = 29.7 \times 2.25 \times 8.94$$
$$\text{gpm} = 597.415 \text{ (round to 600 gpm)}$$

© LiquidLibrary

SKILL DRILL 7-3

Calculating the Flow of a 32-mm Smooth-Bore Nozzle on a 65-mm Handline
NFPA 1002, 5.2.1 (metric)

Example 1: Calculate the flow rate for a 32-mm tip used on a 65-mm handline.

$$\text{L/min} = 0.067 \times d^2 \times \sqrt{NP}$$
$$\text{L/min} = 0.067 \times (32)^2 \times \sqrt{350}$$
$$\text{L/min} = 0.067 \times 1024 \times 18.71$$
$$\text{L/min} = 1283.656 \text{ (round to 1300 L/min)}$$

Example 2: Calculate the flow rate for a 38-mm smooth-bore master stream nozzle.

$$\text{L/min} = 0.067 \times d^2 \times \sqrt{NP}$$
$$\text{L/min} = 0.067 \times (38)^2 \times \sqrt{560}$$
$$\text{L/min} = 0.067 \times 1444 \times 23.66$$
$$\text{L/min} = 2289.058 \text{ (round to 2300 L/min)}$$

© LiquidLibrary

commonly used smooth-bore nozzle flows. To calculate the flow (gpm or L/min) from smooth-bore nozzles, use the formula presented in **SKILL DRILL 7-3**:

1. Determine the diameter of the nozzle tip (it is usually stamped into the side of the nozzle). Convert the diameter fraction to a decimal and square it. For example:

$$(1¼ \text{ inch})^2 = (1.25)^2$$

2. Find the square root of the desired nozzle pressure ($\sqrt{NP}$).
3. Multiply the diameter squared (d^2) by the square root of the nozzle pressure ($\sqrt{NP}$), and then multiply the result by the constant 29.7 to find the gpm flow rate of the nozzle.

To calculate the flow rate from smooth-bore nozzles using metric measurements, follow these steps **FIGURE 7-6**:

FIGURE 7-6 Smooth-bore nozzles are commonly rated at a nozzle pressure of 50 psi (350 kPa).

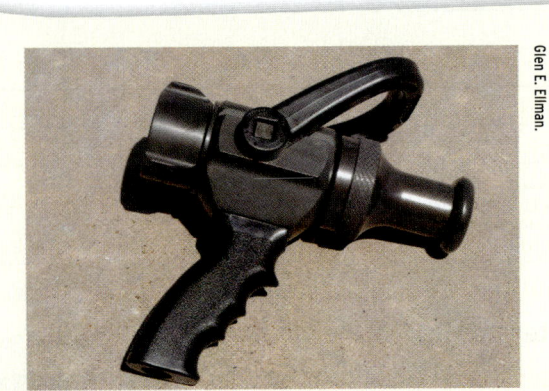

© Jones and Bartlett Learning. Photographed by Glen E. Ellman.

1. Determine the diameter of the nozzle tip (it is usually stamped into the side of the nozzle) and square it. For example:

$$(32)^2$$

2. Find the square root of the desired nozzle pressure ($\sqrt{NP}$). Note that $\sqrt{350}$ kPa = 18.71 and $\sqrt{560}$ kPa = 23.66 for future reference.
3. Multiply the diameter squared (d^2) by the square root of the nozzle pressure ($\sqrt{NP}$), and then multiply the result by the constant 0.067 to find the L/min flow of the nozzle.

DRIVER/OPERATOR Tip

A secured water supply is essential, but it is wise to think about an escalated situation that may require a secondary or supplemental water supply. Develop a habit of thinking ahead.

Friction Loss

After determining the correct NP, you must next determine the friction loss. **Friction loss (FL)** is the pressure lost from turbulence as water passes through pipes, hoses, fittings, adapters, and appliances. It is measured in units of either psi or kPa.

Four laws govern how friction loss behaves. If you understand these laws, you will better understand friction loss in general. These laws will always apply to hose evolutions but may also be practical in other hydraulic situations.

1. **Friction Loss Law 1: Provided all conditions are equal, friction loss will vary in direct proportion to the length of the hose.** Therefore, as the length of the hose increases, the friction loss will also increase. This change in friction is directly related to the change in the hose's length. For example, if the hose length is doubled and the flow remains the same, the friction loss will double.
2. **Friction Loss Law 2: In the same size hose, friction loss varies approximately as the square of the velocity.** As the speed of the water is increased, the water becomes more turbulent. Friction loss will develop much faster than the change in velocity. Therefore, if you double the speed of the water, the friction loss increases four times. For example, if you are flowing 100 gpm in a hoseline in which the friction loss per 100 ft is 10 psi, and then the flow is doubled to 200 gpm, the friction loss will quadruple to 40 psi.
3. **Friction Loss Law 3: For the same discharge, provided all conditions are equal, friction loss will vary according to the diameter of the hose.** Basically, as the diameter of the hose increases, the friction loss decreases. For example, the friction loss for a 100-ft-long, 2½-inch hose flowing 200 gpm is 16 psi, and the friction loss for the same length of 5-inch hose is less than 1 psi.
4. **Friction Loss Law 4: For a given velocity, the friction loss in the hose is approximately the same no matter what the pressure may be.** As pressure changes, it is possible for friction loss to also change. For example, when the pressure in the hose increases, the diameter of the hose will actually increase slightly. This allows more room for water to flow and decreases the friction loss. However, as the pressure increases, it may also elongate he hose slightly, thus increasing the length of the hose and increasing the friction loss.

It is important to know that theoretical FL calculations know no bounds. You can continue calculating with no end in sight, although reality suggests there are limitations to FL. For example, you might calculate a FL for a flow of 500 gpm (1900 L/min) through 1¾-inch (45-mm) hose; you will get an answer, but it is evident that this is not a realistic expectation, because 1¾-inch (45-mm) hose cannot actually flow that amount of water. If you exceed 50 psi (350 kPa) of FL per 100 ft (30 m) of hose, then the flow may begin to decrease either from the increasing turbulence in the hose or from a reduction in the pump capacity owing to the excessive PDP.

Over the years, many equations and other means of calculating FL have been suggested, most of which were designed for specific hoses and equipment. As fire service equipment has improved, hydraulic calculations have reflected these changes and evolved into the modern FL equation: **FL = C Q² L**. This equation first appeared in the National Fire Protection Association's (NFPA's) *NFPA Fire Protection Handbook*, Fifteenth Edition, in 1981; it is now widely accepted as the fire service standard. The success of this equation is due to its ability to adapt to changes in hose diameter, water flow, and length of hose.

Calculating Friction Loss

The friction loss formula in its simplest form is expressed as

$$FL = C Q^2 L$$

where:

$$FL = \text{friction loss}$$

C = the **coefficient (C)**, a numerical measure that is a constant for each specific hose diameter **TABLE 7-2**

Q = the *quantity* of water flowing (gpm or L/min) divided by 100

L = the *length* of hose in feet divided by 100, or in meters divided by 100

The FL formula may also be expressed as FL = C × (Q/100)² × L/100. Given that driver/operators use the formula so frequently, they typically divide Q by 100 and L by 100 mentally to simplify and shorten the written form of the formula to **FL = C Q² L**.

Table 7-2 lists the FL coefficients used in the FL formula. Although this list of coefficients is both typical and reliable, you must be aware of ongoing improvements in hose technology and use the manufacturer's recommendations for these values when purchasing new hose and equipment.

Standard TABLE 7-2 — Friction Loss Coefficients

Friction Loss Coefficients

Hose Diameter (inch)	Coefficient
¾	1100
1	150
1½	24
1¾	15.5
2	8
2½	2
3 with 2½-inch couplings	0.8
3 with 3-inch couplings	0.67
3½	0.34
4	0.2
4½	0.1
5	0.08
6	0.05
Siamese 2½-Inch Hose	
Two	0.5
Three	0.22
Four	0.12
Siamese 3-Inch Hose With 2½-Inch Couplings	
Two	0.2
Three	0.09

Metric TABLE 7-2 — Friction Loss Coefficients

Metric Friction Loss Coefficients

Hose Diameter (mm)	Coefficient
20	1741
25	238
32	127
38	38
45	24.6
50	12.7
65	3.17
77 mm with 65-mm couplings	1.27
77 mm with 77-mm couplings	1.06
90	0.53
100	0.305
115	0.167
125	0.138
150	0.083
Siamese 65-mm Hose	
Two	0.789
Three	0.347
Four	0.189
Siamese 77-mm Hose With 65-mm Couplings	
Two	0.316
Three	0.142

The coefficients in Table 7-2 were derived from the standard measures using the following formula:
$C_m = C_s \times (6.894757)/[(3.785412)^2 \times 0.3048]$
$ = C_s \times 1.57862$
where:
C_m = coefficient (metric)
C_s = coefficient (standard)
Given that:
1 psi = 6.894757 kPa
1 gpm = 3.785412 L/min
1 ft = 0.3048 m

To determine the FL in a hose lay, follow the steps in **SKILL DRILL 7-4**:

1. Write the FL formula: $FL = C Q^2 L$.
2. Select the coefficient (C) from Table 7-2 that matches the hose in the given scenario.
3. The coefficient for 2½-inch hose is 2. Therefore C = 2.
4. Determine the flow rate (quantity) of water through the hoseline and divide the amount by 100 to find Q. Next, square Q.
5. The flow is determined by knowing the flow of each nozzle. We know that a 1¼-inch handline nozzle tip will flow 328 gpm. On paper you may use 328, but on the fireground you may round this value off to 300 gpm. If you are flowing 300 gpm, then 300/100 = 3.
6. Because Q = 3, $Q^2 = 3^2 = 9$.
7. Determine the length of the hose you are calculating and then divide by 100 to find L. How long is the hoseline? If it is 200 ft long, then 200/100 = 2. Therefore L = 2.
8. Multiply the results from steps 1, 2, and 3 to determine FL:

$$FL = C \times Q^2 \times L$$
$$FL = 2 \times 9 \times 2$$
$$FL = 36$$

Multiple Hoselines of Different Sizes and Lengths

On the fireground, you will undoubtedly encounter a scenario where multiple water pressures are needed from one fire pumper on the fire scene. This might not sound like a problem until you understand that only one pressure—the highest pressure—can be created by the fire pumper. Knowing this fact, you need to know how to control the water pressures on those discharges requiring less pressure. When flowing two identical lines that have the same nozzle pressure and flow and that are of equal size, length, and elevation, both lines require the same pressure. Operating lines of unequal size and length with different nozzles and flows can be challenging.

Under normal conditions, you always fully open a valve to prevent excess turbulence and FL through the valve; however, partially closing a valve is sometimes necessary to prevent excessive pressure from being delivered. For those discharges requiring a lesser pressure, you must open the valve just enough to deliver the desired pressure, a practice referred to as gating a valve.

For example, suppose you are flowing water from three different discharges. The first requires 160 psi (1100 kPa), the second requires 130 psi (900 kPa), and the third requires 200 psi (1400 kPa). First, you open discharge number 3 to establish a pressure of 200 psi (1400 kPa)—the highest pressure—on the master discharge gauge. This will adequately supply all three discharge valves but will over-pressurize the first and second discharge valves. Next, you slowly open discharge number 1 while the handline from discharge number 1 is flowing. Keep an eye on the pressure to discharge number 3, as it may drop and you may need to throttle up to maintain 200 psi (1400 kPa) on this line. Repeat this process of opening discharge number 1 slowly and adjusting the throttle to maintain discharge number 3 at 200 psi (1400 kPa) until you achieve 160 psi (1100 kPa) at discharge number 1 and are maintaining discharge number 3 at 200 psi (1400 kPa). Next, open discharge number 2 slowly, once again making sure to throttle up to keep discharge number 3 at 200 psi (1400 kPa) and discharge number 1 at 160 psi (1100 kPa). Continue until discharge number 2 reaches 130 psi (900 kPa), discharge number 3 maintains 200 psi (1400 kPa), and discharge number 1 maintains 160 psi (1100 kPa). **Note:** All discharges must be flowing water to set the pressures correctly.

To calculate the FL for multiple hoselines of different size and length, follow the steps in **SKILL DRILL 7-5**:

1. Determine the correct PDP for each line in the scenario.
2. Use the pump discharge formula: PDP = NP + FL (nozzle pressure + friction loss). Also use the FL formula: FL = C Q² L, where C = coefficient for the line diameter, Q² = quantity of flow (gpm or L/min) divided by 100 and squared, and L = length divided by 100.
3. Determine which line requires the highest pressure. This pressure is the correct answer for a written problem.
4. On the fireground, pump to the highest pressure and gate back any lines requiring lower discharge pressures.

To calculate FL in multiple hoselines of different sizes and lengths using the metric system, follow these steps:

1. Determine the correct PDP for each line in the scenario.
2. Use the pump discharge formula: PDP = NP + FL (nozzle pressure + friction loss). Also use the FL formula: FL = C Q² L, where C = coefficient for the line diameter, Q² = quantity of flow (L/min) divided by 100 and squared, and L = length in meters divided by 100.
3. Determine which line requires the highest pressure. This pressure is the correct answer for a written problem.
4. On the fireground, pump to the highest pressure and gate back any lines requiring lower discharge pressures.

Elevation Pressure

Calculations must be adjusted for the distance the nozzle is above or below the pump, which is referred to as elevation pressure (EP). The pressure lost when the nozzle is above the pump is known as elevation loss; it requires pressure to be added to the discharge pressure to compensate for the loss. The pressure gained when the nozzle is below the pump is known as elevation gain; it requires pressure to be subtracted from the discharge pressure. After you calculate the EP, this value must be added to or subtracted from the PDP. Remember, EP could be zero if the nozzle and the pump are at the same elevation.

Elevation is relative to grade; altitude is relative to sea level. You will regularly encounter situations where water will have to be discharged at an elevation higher or lower than the position of the fire pumper—for example, down a hill to supply a fire apparatus or up to the upper floor of a home or office building for fire suppression. The change in elevation affects the PDP because water has weight, and this weight must be compensated for in the calculations. Thus EP may be either a gain or a loss.

Water exerts a pressure of 0.434 psi per 1 ft (9.817 kPa/m) of water column. This pressure can be either a positive or a negative factor in calculating PDP. If water is discharging below the center line of the pump, then subtract 0.434 psi per 1 ft (9.817 kPa/m) of elevation loss; conversely, add 0.434 psi per 1 ft (9.817 kPa/m) of elevation gain if water is discharging above the pump. To simplify the multiplication, multiply by 0.5 rather than 0.434 (or 10 rather than 9.817 in the metric system).

To further speed up the calculation process, simply determine the elevation change in 10-ft (3-m) increments and multiply your findings by 5 psi (5 psi per 10 ft) [30 kPa (10 kPa per 3 m)]. A common application for this rule would be 5 psi (30 kPa) per gain or loss for each floor of elevation change in a residential structure where floor spacing is commonly 10 ft (3 m) **FIGURE 7-7**. Be aware, however, that not all buildings have floors spaced every 10 ft (3 m). High-rise buildings are spaced in 12- to 14-ft (3.5- to 4.25-m) increments **FIGURE 7-8**. Just remember that using an increment of ±5 psi (±30 kPa) per floor may lead you to underestimate the EP due to alternative floor spacing in different types of structures; therefore for metric, use 35 kPa per floor.

For the purposes of this text, we will use a variance of ±5 psi (±35 kPa) per floor when calculating the elevation gain/loss. For multistory buildings, you can use the following formula: EP = 5

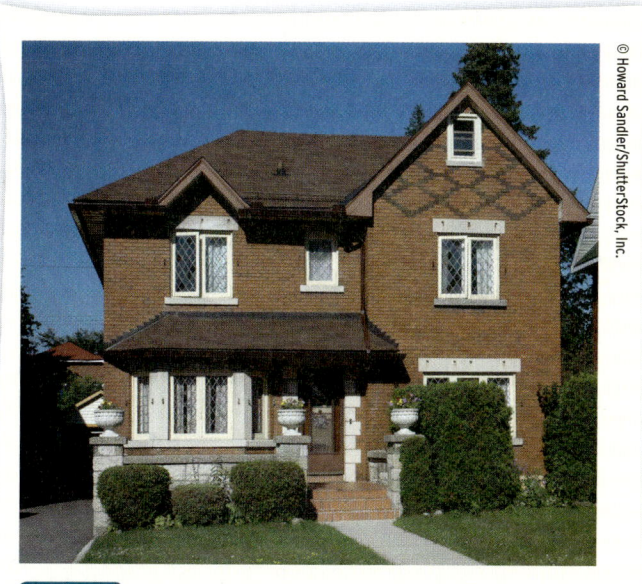

FIGURE 7-7 Floors in residential structures are typically spaced 10 ft (3 m) apart.

SKILL DRILL 7-4: Calculating Friction Loss in a Single Hoseline
NFPA 1002, 5.2.1 (standard)

Example 1: What is the PDP for 300 ft of $2^{1}/_{2}$-inch hose with a $1^{1}/_{8}$-inch smooth-bore nozzle?

In this problem, we see a smooth-bore nozzle on a handline, so we know to assign it a NP of 50 psi:

$$PDP = NP + FL$$
$$PDP = 50 + FL$$

Now we must calculate FL:
- For a $2^{1}/_{2}$-inch hose, the coefficient is 2 (C = 2).
- The nozzle has a $1^{1}/_{8}$-inch tip, which we know will flow 250 gpm (rounded).
- We know the nozzle flow from Table 7-1; alternatively, using the formula, gpm = 29.7 d^2 $\sqrt{NP}$.
- The flow is 250 gpm, so 250/100 = 2.5 and Q = 2.5.

Insert these values into the formulas:

$$FL = C\,Q^2\,L$$
$$FL = 2 \times (2.5)^2 \times 300/100$$
$$FL = 2 \times 6.25 \times 3$$
$$FL = 37.5\ \text{psi}$$

Now we return to our PDP formula and insert the FL:

$$PDP = NP + FL$$
$$PDP = 50 + 37.5$$
$$PDP = 87.5\ \text{psi}$$

Example 2: Calculate the FL in 200 ft of $1^{3}/_{4}$-inch hose with a $7/_{8}$-inch smooth-bore nozzle.

A smooth-bore handline has a NP of 50 psi, so NP = 50. A $7/_{8}$-inch tip flows 161 gpm, so Q = 1.6.

PDP = NP + FL	FL = C Q^2 L
PDP = 50 + FL	FL = 15.5 × (1.6)² × 2
PDP = 50 + 80	FL = 15.5 × 2.56 × 2
PDP = 130 psi	FL = 79.36 psi (round to 80 psi)

Calculating PDP requires the operator to determine FL so as to arrive at the PDP.

© LiquidLibrary

---

psi × (number of stories – 1) [or 35 kPa × (number of stories – 1)]. Do not count the first story of a multistory building. To calculate EP for a grade, use the following formula: EP = 0.5 H, where 0.5 is a constant and H = height in feet (or EP = 10 H, where 10 is a constant and H = height in meters).

To calculate the EP loss or gain, follow the steps in **SKILL DRILL 7-6**:

1. Determine the EP when operating in a multistory building.
2. Use the formula: EP = 5 psi × (number of stories – 1).
3. Count the number of stories to the nozzle.
4. Multiply 5 psi times the number of stories minus 1.

To calculate the EP using the metric system, follow these steps:

1. Determine the EP when operating in a multistory building.
2. Use the formula: EP = 35 kPa × (number of stories – 1).
3. Count the number of stories to the nozzle.
4. Multiply 35 kPa times the number of stories minus 1.

DRIVER/OPERATOR Tip

Mark the preconnected attack hoselines with a predetermined pressure for a predetermined flow rate. Preconnected lines are the most commonly used attack lines, so you should be able to quickly establish the needed pressures with only minimal calculations. These pressures should be determined before a fire occurs. This is a good time to do the math, especially if you are an inexperienced driver/operator.

The best way to determine correct pressures is to flow your hoselines with the nozzles on your fire apparatus. This is the only way to be sure of the exact performance of your equipment. Take your fire apparatus out onto the parking lot or drill ground. Pull the preconnected lines and flow them. Establish the pressure for each single hoseline and mark it on the individual pressure gauge with a red pen stripe on automotive tape. Now it will be effortless to pump a preconnected handline. This exercise is a great practice tool while you are mastering the calculations needed for pumping.

SKILL DRILL 7-4 Calculating Friction Loss in a Single Hoseline
NFPA 1002, 5.2.1 (metric)

Example 1: What is the PDP for 90 m of 65-mm hose with a 29-mm smooth-bore nozzle?
In this problem, we see a smooth-bore nozzle on a handline, so we know to assign it a NP of 350 kPa:

$$PDP = NP + FL$$
$$PDP = 350 + FL$$

Now we must calculate FL:
- For a 65-mm hose, the coefficient is 3.17 (C = 3.17).
- The nozzle has a 29-mm tip, which we know will flow 1050 L/min (rounded).
- We know the nozzle flow from Table 7-1; alternatively, using the formula, L/min = $0.067 \times d^2 \times \sqrt{NP}$.
- The flow is 1054 L/min, so 1054/100 = 10.54 and Q = 10.54.

Insert these values into the formulas:

$$FL = C Q^2 L$$
$$FL = 3.17 \times (10.54)^2 \times 90/100$$
$$FL = 3.17 \times 111.09 \times 0.9$$
$$FL = 316.94 \text{ (round to 300 kPa)}$$

Now we return to our PDP formula and insert the FL:

$$PDP = NP + FL$$
$$PDP = 350 + 300$$
$$PDP = 650 \text{ kPa}$$

Example 2: Calculate the FL in 60 m of 45-mm hose with a 22-mm smooth-bore nozzle.
A smooth-bore handline has a NP of 350 kPa; therefore NP = 350. A 22-mm tip flows 598 L/min; therefore Q = 5.98 (round to Q = 6).

PDP = NP + FL	FL = $C Q^2 L$
PDP = 350 + FL	FL = $24.5 \times (6)^2 \times 0.6$
PDP = 350 + 530	FL = $24.5 \times 36 \times 0.6$
PDP = 880 kPa	FL = 529.2 kPa (round to 530 kPa)

© LiquidLibrary

Appliance Loss

Appliances are devices that are used to connect and adapt hoses, and to direct and control water flow in various hose layouts. Appliances consist of, but are not limited to, adapters, reducers, gated wyes, Siamese connections, water thieves, monitors, manifolds, and elevated master stream devices **FIGURE 7-9**. Like any other water supply device, appliances may add to FL. Also, as in fire hose, the FL in an appliance is directly proportional to the volume (gpm) of water flowing through the system. Generally, the appliance FL is considered insignificant and may be recorded as zero when water flows are less than 350 gpm (1400 L/min). However, it is recommended that you test your department's appliances for FL at reasonable flows to determine how you will account for the FL associated with them.

For the purposes of this text, we will follow these guidelines:
- Allow 10 psi (70 kPa) FL in appliances when the flow rate is 350 gpm (1400 L/min) or greater.
- Friction loss in appliances will be zero when flows are less than 350 gpm (1400 L/min).
- Allow 25 psi (175 kPa) FL for all master stream appliances. The 25 psi (175 kPa) flow allows for FL in the intake and the internal piping. The loss in internal piping is specific to the apparatus, however, and may actually be quite large. One discharge may consist of a straight pipe with almost no FL, whereas the piping of another discharge on the same pump may create 10 to 30 psi (70 to 210 kPa) of FL depending on the number of turns the pipe makes and the flow rate.
- Written tests or quizzes for this text cannot account for specific piping FL, so they will use the guidelines given here.

Fire streams of less than 350 gpm (1400 L/min) are generally considered handlines, whereas fire streams of 350 gpm (1400 L/min) or greater are considered **master streams**. In your calculations, you should assume 25 psi (175 kPa) of appliance

SKILL DRILL 7-5: Calculating Friction Loss in Multiple Hoselines of Different Sizes and Lengths
NFPA 1002, 5.2.1 (standard)

Example 1: A pumper is supplying two attack lines. The first consists of 150 ft of 1¾-inch hose flowing 150 gpm with a fog nozzle. The second line consists of 200 ft of 2½-inch hose flowing 250 gpm with a smooth-bore nozzle. What is the PDP?

In this scenario, the operator will calculate the pressure for each line, then set the pump to the highest pressure and gate the other discharge back to its required pressure. The answer to the written problem is the highest pressure.

The PDP for the first line is

$$FL = C Q^2 L$$
$$FL = 15.5 \, (1.5)^2 \, 1.5$$
$$FL = 15.5 \times 2.25 \times 1.5 = 52.3$$

Insert the FL into the PDP formula:

$$PDP = 100 \, NP + 52.3 \, FL = 152.3 \text{ psi}$$

The PDP for the second line is

$$FL = C Q^2 L = 2 \, (2.5)^2 \, 2$$
$$FL = 2 \times 6.25 \times 2 = 25$$

Insert the FL into the PDP formula:

$$PDP = 50 \, NP + 25 \, FL = 75 \text{ psi}$$

The answer for this scenario is the highest pressure, which is 152.3 psi (round to 152 psi). In this example, the operator will set the pump to 152 psi and then gate down the discharge for the 2½-inch hoseline until it reads 75 psi, while the line is flowing water at a flow rate of 250 gpm.

Now that you are acquainted with the PDP formula, begin writing it with just the values for NP and FL, such as PDP = 50 + 25, so PDP = 75 psi.

Example 2: A pumper is supplying three hoselines. The first attack line is 300 ft of 2½-inch hose flowing 300 gpm with a smooth-bore nozzle. The second line is 200 ft of 1¾-inch hose flowing 150 gpm with a fog nozzle. The third line is 200 ft of 1¾-inch hose flowing 161 gpm with a ⅞-inch smooth-bore tip. What is the PDP?

In this scenario, the operator will calculate the pressure for each line, then set the pump to the highest pressure and gate the other discharges back to their required pressures. The answer to the written problem is the highest pressure.

The PDP for the first line is

$$FL = C Q^2 L$$
$$FL = 2 \, (3)^2 \, 3 = 54$$

Insert the FL into the PDP formula:

$$PDP = 50 + 54 = 104 \text{ psi}$$

The PDP for the second line is

$$FL = C Q^2 L$$
$$FL = 15.5 \, (1.5)^2 \, 2$$
$$FL = 15.5 \times 2.25 \times 2 = 69.75$$

Insert the FL into the PDP formula:

$$PDP = 100 + 69.5 = 169.75 \text{ psi}$$

The PDP for the third line is

$$FL = C Q^2 L$$
$$FL = 15.5 \, (1.61)^2 \, 2$$
$$FL = 15.5 \times 2.59 \times 2 = 80$$

Insert the FL into the PDP formula:

$$PDP = 50 + 80 = 130 \text{ psi}$$

The answer for this scenario is the highest pressure, which is 169.75 psi (round to 170 psi).

© LiquidLibrary

SKILL DRILL 7-5

Calculating Friction Loss in Multiple Hoselines of Different Sizes and Lengths
NFPA 1002, 5.2.1 (metric)

Example 1: A pumper is supplying two attack lines. The first consists of 45 m of 45-mm hose flowing 550 L/min with a fog nozzle. The second line consists of 60 m of 65-mm hose flowing 950 L/min with a smooth-bore nozzle. What is the PDP?

With this scenario, the operator will calculate the pressure for each line, then set the pump to the highest pressure and gate the other discharge back to its required pressure. The answer to the written problem is the highest pressure.

The PDP for the first line is

$$FL = C Q^2 L \quad FL = 24.5 \times (5.5)^2 \times 0.45$$
$$FL = 24.5 \times 30.25 \times 0.45 = 333.5 \text{ (round to 334)}$$

Insert the FL into the PDP formula:

$$PDP = 700 \text{ NP} + 334 \text{ FL} = 1034 \text{ kPa}$$

The PDP for the second line is

$$FL = C Q^2 L = 3.16 \times (9.5)^2 \times 0.6 \quad FL = 3.16 \times 90.25 \times 0.6 = 171$$

Insert the FL into the PDP formula:

$$PDP = 350 \text{ NP} + 171 \text{ FL} = 521 \text{ kPa}$$

The answer for this scenario is the highest pressure, which is 1034 kPa (round to 1050 psi).

Now that you are acquainted with the PDP formula, begin writing it with just the values for NP and FL, such as PDP = 350 + 171, so PDP = 521 kPa.

Example 2: A pumper is supplying three hoselines. The first attack line is 90 m of 65-mm hose flowing 1100 L/min with a smooth-bore nozzle. The second line is 60 m of 45-mm hose flowing 550 L/min with a fog nozzle. The third line is 60 m of 45-mm hose flowing 600 L/min with a 22-mm smooth-bore tip. What is the PDP?

In this scenario, the operator will calculate the pressure for each line, then set the pump to the highest pressure and gate the other discharges back to their required pressures. The answer to the written problem is the highest pressure.

The PDP for the first line is

$$FL = C Q^2 L$$
$$FL = 3.16 \times (11)^2 \times 0.9 = 344$$

Insert the FL into the PDP formula:

$$PDP = 350 + 344 = 694 \text{ kPa}$$

The PDP for the second line is

$$FL = C Q^2 L$$
$$FL = 24.5 \times (5.5)^2 \times 0.6$$
$$FL = 24.5 \times 30.25 \times 0.6 = 445$$

Insert the FL into the PDP formula:

$$PDP = 700 + 445 = 1145 \text{ kPa}$$

The PDP for the third line is

$$FL = C Q^2 L$$
$$FL = 24.5 \times (6)^2 \times 0.6$$
$$FL = 254.5 \times 36 \times 0.6 = 529$$

Insert the FL into the PDP formula:

$$PDP = 350 + 529 = 879 \text{ kPa}$$

The answer for this scenario is the highest pressure, which is 1145 kPa (round to 1150 kPa).

© LiquidLibrary

SKILL DRILL 7-6
Calculating the Elevation Pressure (Loss and Gain)
NFPA 1002, 5.2.1 (standard)

Example 1: Determine EP when the nozzle is on the 11th floor of a building.

$$EP = (11 - 1) \times 5 \text{ psi}$$
$$EP = 10 \times 5 \text{ psi}$$
$$EP = 50 \text{ psi}$$

You can also determine the EP for a grade using the formula EP = 0.5 H, where 0.5 is a constant and H = height:

1. Estimate the elevation gain or loss. When the nozzle is higher than the pump, the EP is a positive number and you will compensate for this loss in pressure by increasing pressure output from the pump. When the nozzle is below the pump, the elevation is a negative number and you will compensate for this gain by decreasing pressure output from the pump.
2. Multiply 0.5 × height, where the height will be a positive or negative number.

Example 2: Determine the EP when the nozzle is 30 ft below the pump.

$$EP = -30 \times 0.5 \quad EP = -15$$

Example 3: Determine the EP when the nozzle is 50 ft above the pump.

$$EP = 50 \times 0.5 \quad EP = 25$$

© LiquidLibrary

SKILL DRILL 7-6
Calculating the Elevation Pressure (Loss and Gain)
NFPA 1002, 5.2.1 (metric)

Example 1: Determine the EP when the nozzle is on the 11th floor of a building.

$$EP = (11 - 1) \times 35 \text{ kPa}$$
$$EP = 10 \times 35 \text{ kPa}$$
$$EP = 350 \text{ kPa}$$

You can also determine the EP for a grade using the formula EP = 10 H, where 10 is a constant and H = height in meters:

1. Estimate the elevation gain or loss. When the nozzle is higher than the pump, the EP is a positive number (compensate for the loss by increasing pressure). When the nozzle is below the pump, the elevation is a negative number (compensate for the gain by decreasing pressure).
2. Multiply 10 × height, where the height will be a positive or negative number.

Example 2: Determine the EP when the nozzle is 9 m below the pump.

$$EP = -9 \times 10 \quad EP = -90 \text{ kPa}$$

Example 3: Determine the EP when the nozzle is 15 m above the pump.

$$EP = 15 \times 10 \quad EP = 150 \text{ kPa}$$

© LiquidLibrary

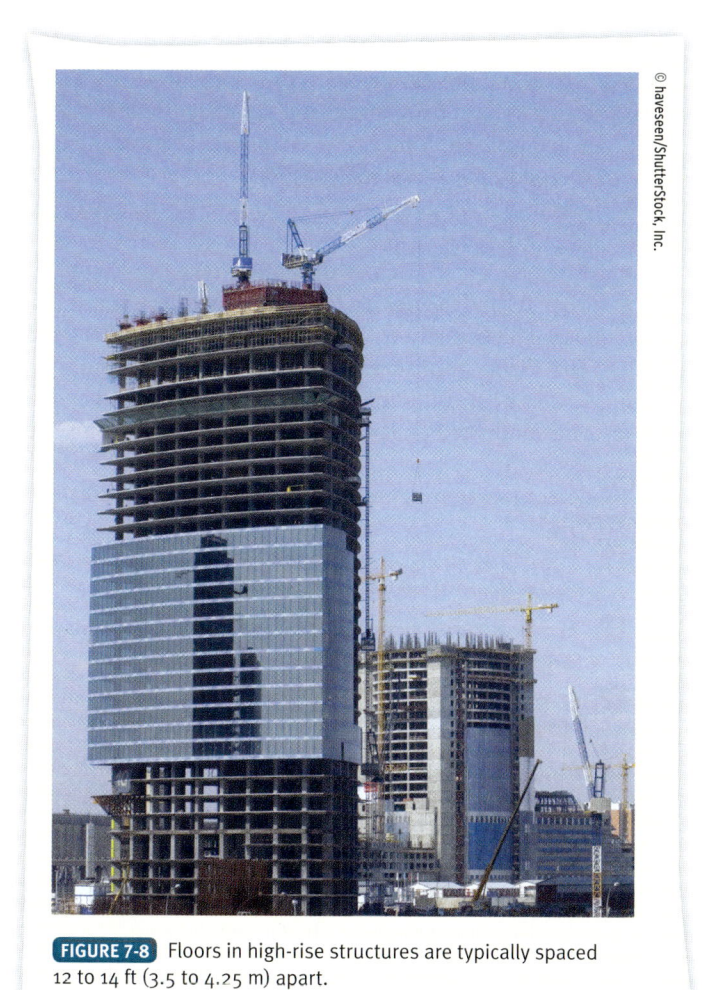

FIGURE 7-8 Floors in high-rise structures are typically spaced 12 to 14 ft (3.5 to 4.25 m) apart.

Standard TABLE 7-3	Appliance Losses for High-Flow Devices
Device	Appliance Loss (psi)
Wye, Siamese connection, FDC, manifold (if the flow rate is greater than 350 gpm)	10
Elevated master stream and ground monitor	25

Metric TABLE 7-3	Appliance Losses for High-Flow Devices
Device	Appliance Loss (kPa)
Wye, Siamese connection, manifold (if the flow rate is greater than 1400 L/min)	70
Elevated master stream and monitor	175
Standpipe	175

loss (AL) for master streams, and 10 psi (70 kPa) of AL for handlines with a flow of 350 gpm (1400 L/min) or greater.

TABLE 7-3 lists ALs for some commonly encountered devices. It is highly recommended that you conduct FL testing of your appliances and determine how they will be used on the fireground.

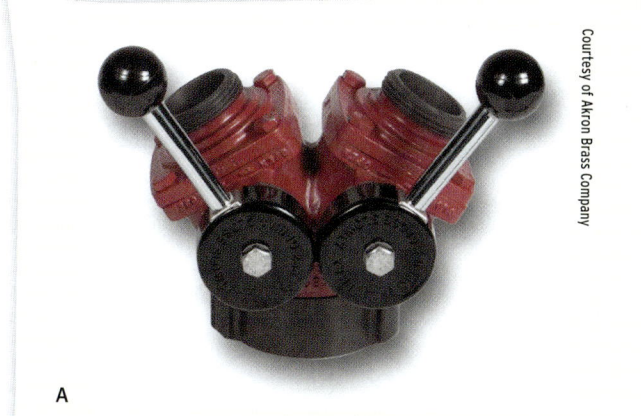

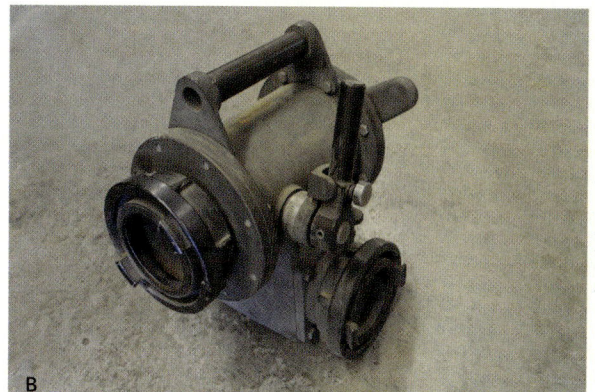

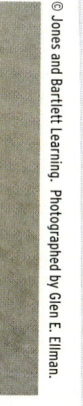

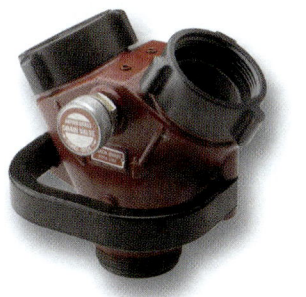

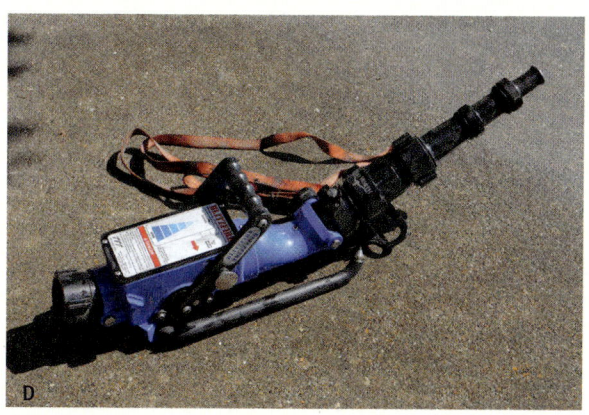

FIGURE 7-9 Appliances include adapters, reducers, gated wyes, Siamese connections, water thieves, monitors, manifolds, and elevated master stream devices, among other items. **A.** A typical gated wye device. **B.** A relay valve. **C.** A typical Siamese connection device. **D.** A typical monitor.

- The hose or appliance to be tested.
- Two in-line pressure gauges for testing hose. If you are testing a master stream device, you may use one or two in-line gauges, or they may be replaced by a manual or threaded Pitot gauge **FIGURE 7-10**.
- Nozzle of an appropriate size for the hose to control the water discharged.
- Hose necessary to make all connections.
- Adapters and fittings necessary to make all connections.

Choose which method you will use and document the results. The FL in appliances is minimal until the pump is flowing 350 gpm (1400 L/min) or greater. It is recommended that tests be conducted on level ground and that you complete the process at various flows to see how the FL changes.

To determine the FL in appliances, follow the steps in **SKILL DRILL 7-7**:

1. Attach 100 ft (30 m) of 2-inch (65-mm) or larger hose to the selected discharge. (**STEP 1**)
2. Attach one in-line pressure gauge to the hose in Step 1. (**STEP 2**)
3. Attach the appliance to be tested to the in-line gauge. (**STEP 3**)
4. Attach the second in-line gauge to the discharge side of the appliance or Pitot gauge if testing a smooth-bore nozzle on a master stream device.
5. If not testing a nozzle, connect additional hose and a nozzle to the second in-line gauge, enough to direct the discharged water to the desired location.
6. Engage the pump, flow water, and increase the throttle until the desired amount of pressure is achieved on the second in-line gauge or the Pitot gauge.
7. Record the pressure reading from both gauges.
8. Subtract the pressure on the second gauge from the pressure on the first gauge; this is the appliance FL for the specific flow rate used during the test. (**STEP 4**)

To use a Pitot gauge to test the FL in a portable master stream appliance through 3-inch (76-mm) hose, follow the steps in **SKILL DRILL 7-8**:

1. Connect 100 ft (30 m) of 3-inch (77-mm) hose to the pump. (**STEP 1**)
2. Place and safely secure a smooth-bore 1¼-inch (32-mm) tip on the end of the hose. (**STEP 2**)
3. Charge the line. Using a Pitot gauge, increase the pressure until it reads 80 psi (560 kPa). Record the PDP. (**STEP 3**)
4. Remove the nozzle and place the portable master stream appliance on the end of the hose; attach the same tip to the discharge. (**STEP 4**)
5. Use a Pitot gauge and increase the pressure until the gauge reads 80 psi (560 kPa). Record the PDP.
6. Compare the PDP before the appliance was added to the PDP after the appliance was added. This pressure difference represents the FL within the appliance. With a 1¼-inch (32-mm) tip, the PDP before the appliance was added was 93 psi (640 kPa), and

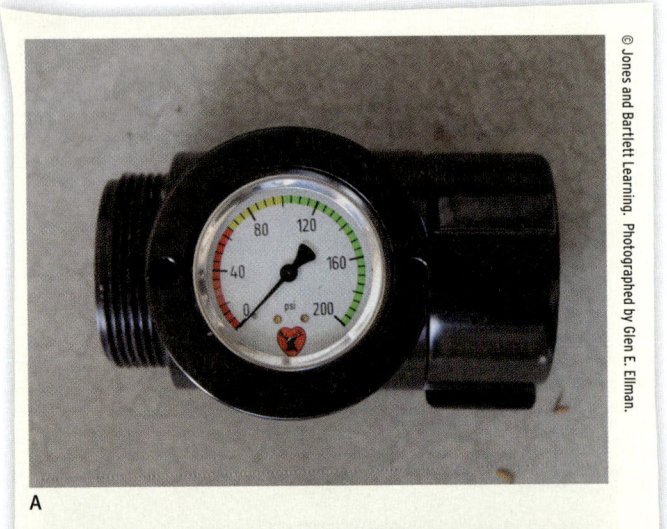

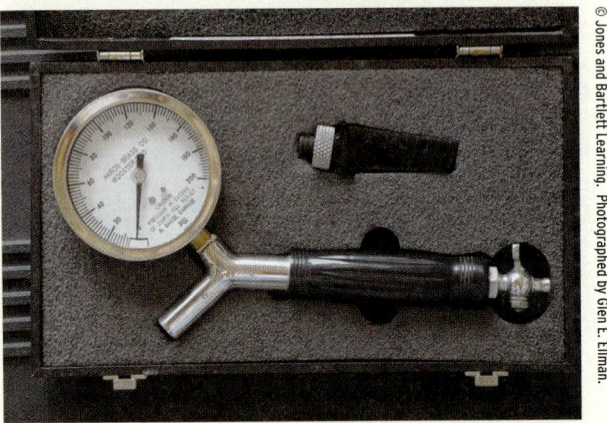

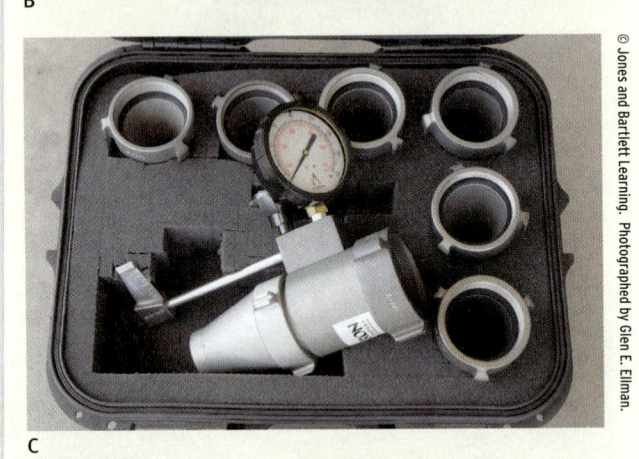

FIGURE 7-10 Two in-line pressure gauges are needed for testing hose. If you are testing a master stream device, you may use one or two in-line gauges or, alternatively, a manual or threaded Pitot gauge. **A.** In-line pressure gauge. **B.** Manual Pitot gauge. **C.** Threaded Pitot gauge.

Determining Friction Loss in Appliances

It is recommended that you check the appliances in your department for FL at the water flows that are most likely to be encountered on the fireground. The process to check for FL is very simple. You will need the following equipment:

CHAPTER 7 Mathematics for the Driver/Operator

SKILL DRILL 7-7
Determining the Friction Loss in Appliances
NFPA 1002, 5.2.1

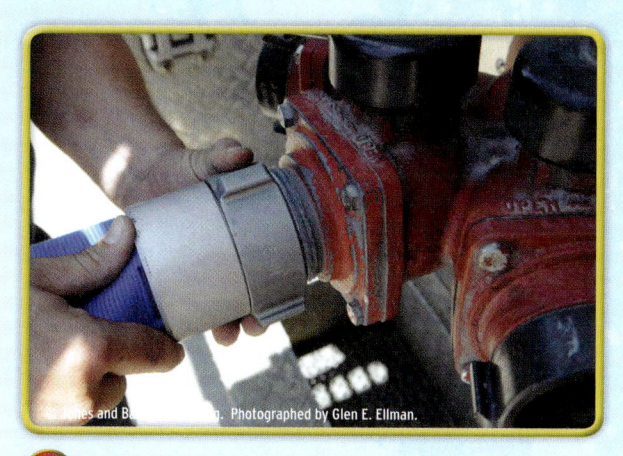

1 Attach 100 ft (30 m) of 2½-inch (65-mm) or larger hose to the selected discharge.

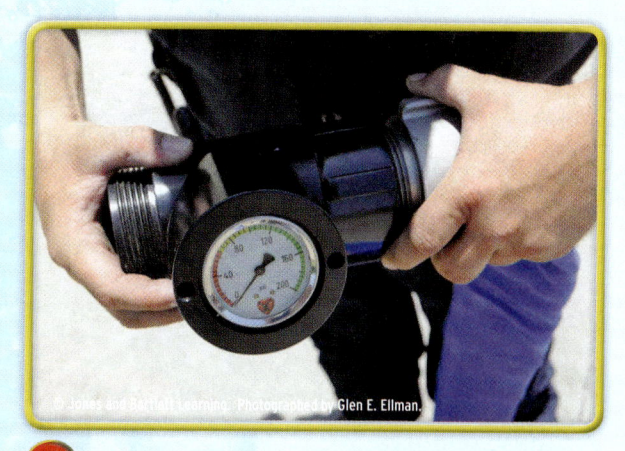

2 Attach one in-line pressure gauge to the hose.

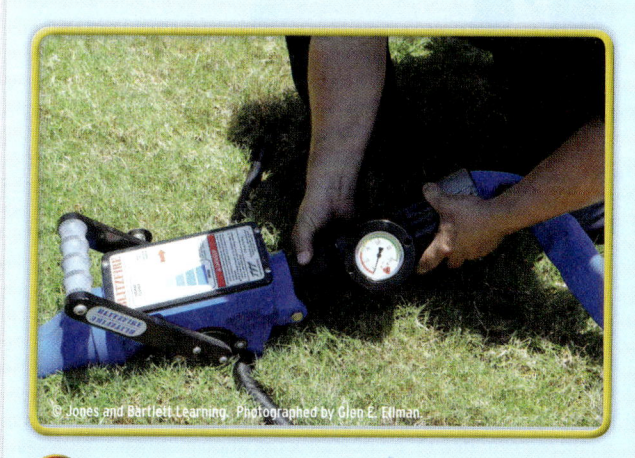

3 Attach the appliance to be tested to the in-line gauge.

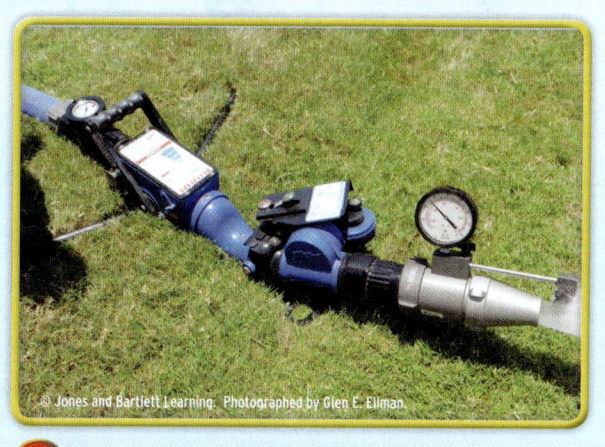

4 Attach the second in-line gauge to the discharge side of the appliance or Pitot gauge if testing a smooth-bore nozzle on a master stream device. If not testing a nozzle, connect additional hose and a smooth-bore nozzle to the second in-line gauge, enough to direct the discharged water to the desired location. Engage the pump, flow water, and increase the throttle until the desired amount of pressure is achieved on the second in-line gauge or the Pitot gauge. Record the pressure reading from both gauges. Subtract the pressure on the second gauge from the pressure on the first gauge; this is the appliance FL.

SKILL DRILL 7-8
Using a Pitot Gauge
NFPA 1002, 5.2.1

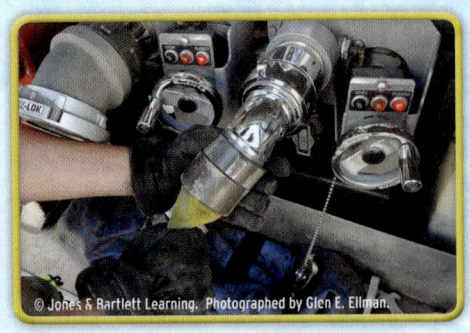

1. Connect 100 ft (30 m) of 3-inch (776-mm) hose to the pump.

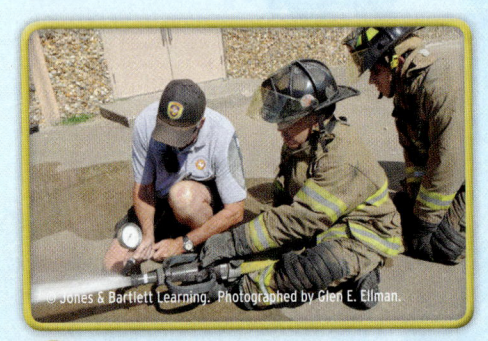

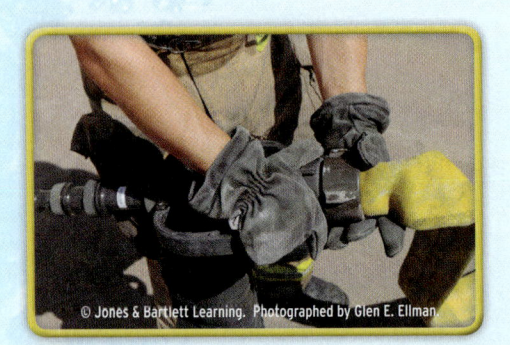

2. Place and safely secure a smooth-bore 1¼-inch (32-mm) tip on the end of the hose.

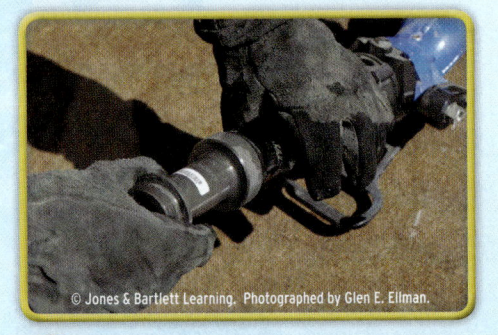

3. Charge the line. Using a Pitot gauge, increase the pressure until it reads 80 psi (560 kPa). Record the pump discharge pressure.

4. Remove the nozzle and place the portable master stream appliance on the end of the hose; attach the same tip to the discharge.

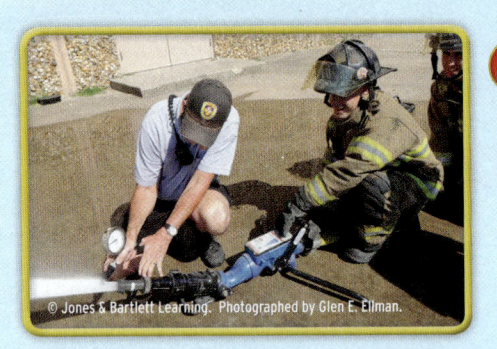

5. Use a Pitot gauge and increase the pressure until it reads 80 psi (560 kPa). Record the PDP. Compare the PDP before the appliance was added to the PDP after the appliance was added. This pressure difference represents the FL within the appliance. With a 1¼-inch (32-mm) tip, the PDP before the appliance was added was 93 psi (640 kPa) and the PDP after the appliance was added was 113 psi (780 kPa). This represents 20 psi (140 kPa) FL in the appliance at a flow rate of 400 gpm (1514 L/min).

---

the PDP after the appliance was added was 113 psi (780 kPa). This represents 20 psi (140 kPa) FL in the appliance. (**STEP 5**)

To use in-line gauges to test the FL in a specific hose, follow the steps in **SKILL DRILL 7-9**:

1. Connect 50 ft (15 m) of hose to the pump discharge with an in-line gauge on the end. (**STEP 1**)
2. Connect 200 ft (60 m) of hose to the in-line gauge. (**STEP 2**)
3. Attach a second in-line gauge to the end of the 200-ft (60-m) hose. (**STEP 3**)
4. Add 50 ft (15 m) to 100 ft (30 m) of hose with a smooth-bore nozzle on the end. (**STEP 4**)
5. Flow a specific amount of water and compare gauges.
6. Using the gauge reading, compare the pressure from the first gauge to the pressure from the second gauge. This pressure loss will illustrate the FL in the amount of hose between the gauges for this specific hose. (**STEP 5**)

CHAPTER 7 Mathematics for the Driver/Operator 139

SKILL DRILL 7-9
Using In-Line Gauges to Test Friction Loss
NFPA 1002, 5.2.1

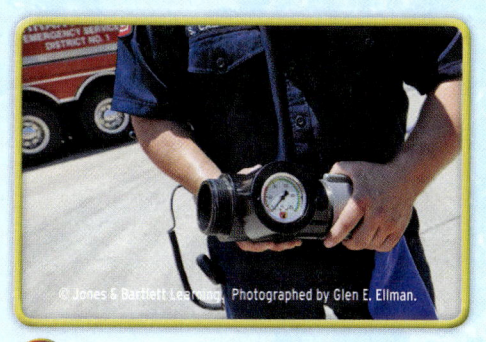

1 Connect 50 ft (15 m) of hose to the pump discharge with an in-line gauge on the end.

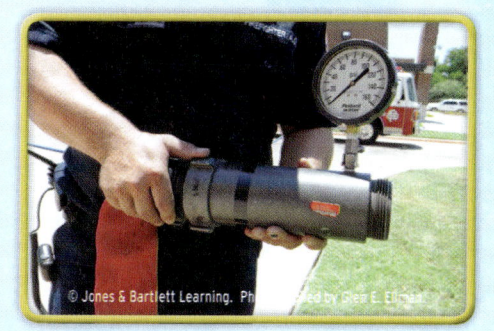

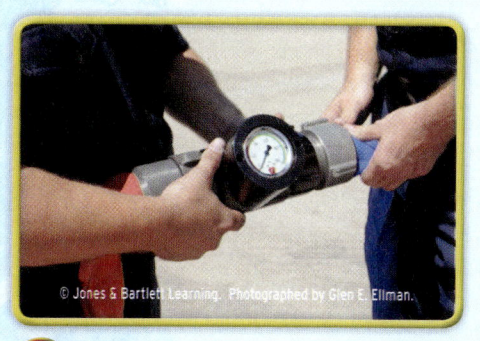

2 Connect 200 ft (60 m) of hose to the in-line gauge.

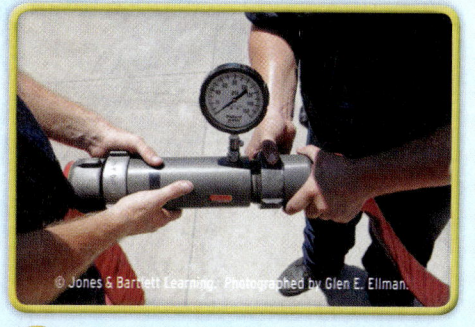

3 Attach a second in-line gauge to the end of the 200-ft (60-m) hose.

4 Add 50 ft (15 m) to 100 ft (30 m) of hose with a smooth-bore nozzle on the end.

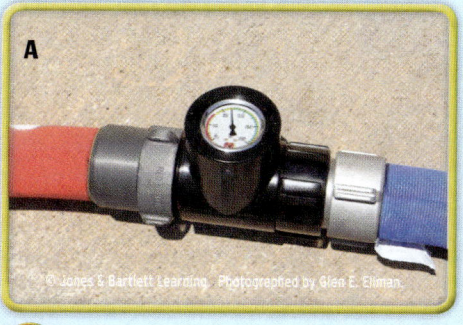

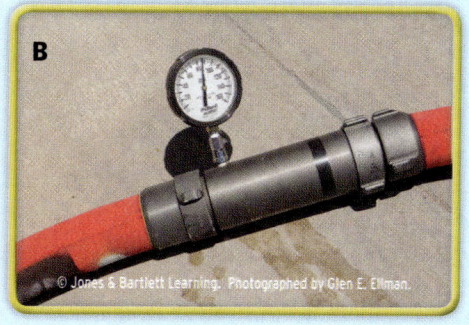

5 Flow a specific amount of water and compare the gauges.

DRIVER/OPERATOR Tip

When calculations are more complex and extend beyond a simple single line, it is often helpful to break the problem into sections. In the classroom, it is helpful to sketch the scenario, put parentheses around each section of the problem, and work from one end to the other. This way you are less likely to miss a calculation. Many driver/operators find it helpful and efficient to do this type of "chunking" mentally on the fireground as well.

■ Total Pressure Loss

In any pumping scenario, if appliances are used or elevation gain or loss is present, you must insert AL and EP into the FL formula. First start with the equation PDP = NP + FL and determine the NP. Next determine the **total pressure loss (TPL)**. The FL formula in expanded form becomes **FL = (C × Q² × L) + AL + EP**. This expanded formula reflects the TPL, so it may be expressed as follows: **TPL = (C × Q² × L) + AL + EP**. The TPL equation does not include a value for the NP.

SKILL DRILL 7-10 — Determining the Pump Discharge Pressure in a Wye Scenario with Equal Lines
NFPA 1002, 5.2.4 (standard)

Example 1: A pumper is supplying 100 ft of 2½-inch hose to a wye that has two 1¾-inch lines 200 ft long flowing 150 gpm each through fog nozzles. What is the PDP?

$$PDP = NP + FL$$
$$FL = C Q^2 L$$
$$FL \text{ for the } 2\tfrac{1}{2} \text{ inch} = 2\,(3)^2\,1 = 18 \text{ psi}$$

FL for a 1-inch line:

$$FL = C Q^2 L = 15.5\,(1.5)^2\,2$$
$$FL = 15.5 \times 2.25 \times 2 = 69.75 \text{ (round to 70 psi)}$$

It takes 70 psi to flow the first 1-inch line; the second 1-inch line is identical. Thus both lines experience the same FL and have the same NP. Insert the values in the formula:

$$PDP = NP + FL$$
$$PDP = 100 \text{ (NP)} + 18 \text{ (for the } 2\tfrac{1}{2}\text{-inch line)} + 70$$
$$\text{(for the } 1\tfrac{1}{2}\text{-inch lines)}$$
$$PDP = 100 + 18 + 70 = 188 \text{ psi}$$

As the flow did not exceed 350 gpm, do not add 10 psi AL for the wye.

Example 2: A pumper is supplying 100 ft of 3-inch (with 2½-inch couplings) to a wye with two equal lines of 2½-inch hose, each 200 ft flowing 250 gpm through smooth-bore nozzles. What is the PDP?

$$PDP = NP + FL$$

FL for the 3-inch line:

$$FL = C Q^2 L = 0.8\,(5)^2\,1$$
$$FL = 0.8 \times 25 = 20$$

FL for the 2-inch lines:

$$FL = C Q^2 L = 2\,(2.5)^2\,2$$
$$FL = 2 \times 6.25 \times 2 = 25$$
$$PDP = 50 \text{ NP} + (20 \text{ for the 3-inch line}) + 25 \text{ (for the } 2\tfrac{1}{2}\text{-inch lines)} + 10 \text{ (AP)}$$
$$PDP = 50 + 20 + 25 + 10 = 105 \text{ psi}$$

© LiquidLibrary

After calculating the TPL, apply it to the PDP formula, which can now be expressed as **PDP = NP + TPL**. You may use either form of the formula as long as you include all contributing factors in the calculation.

Wyed Hoselines

A wye is used to split a single line into two lines. Use of this appliance requires a series of calculations to find the final FL. For a wyed hose lay where all discharge lines are of equal size and length, follow the steps in SKILL DRILL 7-10 to determine the PDP:

1. Add the flow rate for all discharges from the wye together to obtain the quantity (Q) for the supply line to the wye device.
2. Calculate the FL for the supply line to the wye device using the Q value determined in Step 1.
3. Calculate the FL for one of the discharge lines from the wye device and add the nozzle pressure.
4. If the scenario is flowing 350 gpm (1400 L/min) or greater, add 10 psi (70 kPa) friction loss for the wye device.
5. Add the results of Steps 2 through 4 to determine the PDP.

For a wyed hose lay where each discharge line from the device is different (unequal), follow the steps in SKILL DRILL 7-11 to determine the PDP:

1. Add the flow rate for all discharges from the wye together to obtain the quantity (Q) for the supply line to the wye device.
2. Calculate the FL for the supply line to the wye device using the Q value determined in Step 1.

SKILL DRILL 7-10 — Determining the Pump Discharge Pressure in a Wye Scenario with Equal Lines
NFPA 1002, 5.2.4 (metric)

Example 1: A pumper is supplying 30 m of 65-mm hose to a wye that has two 45-mm lines 60 m long flowing 550 L/min each through fog nozzles. What is the PDP?

$$PDP = NP + FL$$
$$FL = C Q^2 L$$

FL for the 65-mm line = $3.16 (11)^2 \, 0.3 = 115$ kPa

$$FL \text{ for a 45-mm line} = C Q^2 L = 24.5 (5.5)^2 \, 0.6$$
$$FL = 24.5 \times 30.25 \times 0.6 = 444.6 \text{ (round to 445 kPa)}$$

It takes 445 kPa to flow the first 45-mm line; the second 45-mm line is identical. Thus both lines experience the same FL and have the same NP. Insert the values in the formula:

$$PDP = NP + FL$$
$$PDP = 700 \text{ (NP)} + 115 \text{ (for the 65-mm line)} + 445 \text{ (for the 45-mm lines)}$$
$$PDP = 700 + 115 + 445 = 1260 \text{ kPa}$$

As the flow did not exceed 1400 L/min, do not add 70 kPa AL for the wye.

Example 2: A pumper is supplying 30 m of 77-mm hose (with 65-mm couplings) to a wye with two equal lines of 65-mm hose, with each 60 m flowing 950 L/min through smooth-bore nozzles. What is the PDP?

$$PDP = NP + FL$$

FL for the 77-mm line:

$$FL = C Q^2 L = 1.26 (19)^2 \, 0.3$$
$$FL = 1.26 \times 361 \times 0.3 = 136.4 \text{ (round to 136)}$$

FL for the 65-mm lines:

$$FL = C Q^2 L = 3.16 (9.5)^2 \, 0.6$$
$$FL = 3.16 \times 90.25 \times 0.6 = 171.1 \text{ (round to 171)}$$
$$PDP = 350 \text{ NP} + (136 \text{ for the 77-mm line}) + 171 \text{ (for the 65-mm lines)} + 70 \text{ (AL)}$$
$$PDP = 350 + 136 + 171 + 70 = 727 \text{ kPa}$$

If the lines are the same diameter and length, have nozzles with the same flow and NP, and are at the same elevation, they require the same PDP. The pressure from the pump will be the same in both lines.

© LiquidLibrary

Total Pressure Loss

Example 1 (Standard): Determine the PDP of 250 ft of 2½-inch hose flowing 300 gpm where the hand-held smooth-bore nozzle is 40 ft below the pump.

$$PDP = NP + FL \qquad FL = C Q^2 L + EP$$
$$PDP = 50 + FL \qquad FL = [2 \times (3)^2 \times 2.5] - 20$$
$$PDP = 50 + 25 \qquad FL = (45) - 20$$
$$PDP = 75 \text{ psi} \qquad FL = 25$$

Example 1 (Metric): Determine the PDP of 75 m of 65-mm hose flowing 1100 L/min where the hand-held smooth-bore nozzle is 12 m below the pump.

$$PDP = NP + FL \qquad FL = C Q^2 L + EP$$
$$PDP = 350 + FL \qquad FL = [3.16 \times (11)^2 \times 0.75] - 120$$
$$PDP = 350 + 167 \qquad FL = (287) - 120$$
$$PDP = 517 \text{ kPa} \qquad FL = 167$$

SKILL DRILL 7-11: Determining the Pump Discharge Pressure in a Wye Scenario with Unequal Lines
NFPA 1002, 5.2.4 (standard)

Example 1: A pumper is supplying 100 ft of 3-inch hose (with $2\frac{1}{2}$-inch couplings) to a wye. The first attack line from the wye is 200 ft of $2\frac{1}{2}$-inch hose with a $1\frac{1}{4}$-inch smooth-bore nozzle flowing 300 gpm. The second attack line is 150 ft of $2\frac{1}{2}$-inch hose with a 1-inch smooth-bore nozzle flowing 200 gpm. What is the PDP? (Remember that when the flow is 350 gpm or greater in a wye, you must add 10 psi AL.)

FL for 3-inch hose (with $2\frac{1}{2}$-inch couplings) = C Q² L
$$= 0.8\ (5)^2\ 1$$
$$= 0.8 \times 25 \times 1$$
$$= 20\ \text{psi}$$

FL for first $2\frac{1}{2}$-inch hose = C Q² L = 2 (3)² 2 = 36 psi

PDP = 50 (NP) + 20 (FL in 3-inch hose) + 36 (FL in first $2\frac{1}{2}$-inch hose) + 10 (AL) = 116 psi

FL for second $2\frac{1}{2}$-inch hose = C Q² L = 2 (2)² 1.5 = 12 psi
PDP = 50 (NP) + 20 (FL in 3-inch hose) + 12 (FL in second $2\frac{1}{2}$-inch hose) + 10 (AL) = 92 psi

The second attack line requires less pressure; gate this line back to 92 psi. This will need to be done at the actual gated wye and not at the pump panel. The gated wye may not have a pressure gauge; therefore, you will need to estimate the amount to gate the valve on the gated wye. As the first attack line has a greater FL, pump to its pressure of 116 psi:

$$PDP = 116\ \text{psi}$$

Example 2: A pumper is supplying 100 ft of 3-inch hose to a wye. From the wye, the first attack line is 200 ft of $1\frac{3}{4}$-inch hose flowing 150 gpm through a fog nozzle. The second attack line is 200 ft of $2\frac{1}{2}$-inch hose flowing 300 gpm through a fog nozzle. What is the PDP?

FL for the 3-inch hose = C Q² L
$$= 0.67\ (4.5)^2\ 1$$
$$= 0.67 \times 20 \times 1$$
$$= 13.5\ (\text{round to } 14)$$

FL for first $1\frac{3}{4}$-inch attack line: FL = C Q² L
$$= 15.5\ (1.5)^2\ 2$$
$$= 15.5 \times 2.25 \times 2$$
$$= 69.75\ (\text{round to 70 psi})$$

PDP = 100 (NP) + 14 (FL in 3-inch hose) + 70 (FL in $1\frac{3}{4}$-inch hose) + 10 (AL) = 194 psi

FL for second attack line ($2\frac{1}{2}$-inch hose): FL = C Q² L
$$= 2\ (3)^2\ 2$$
$$= 2 \times 9 \times 2$$
$$= 36\ \text{psi}$$

PDP = 100 (NP) + 14 (FL in 3-inch hose) + 36 (FL in $2\frac{1}{2}$-inch hose) + 10 (AL) = 160 psi

The PDP for the $1\frac{3}{4}$-inch line is greater, so pump at 194 psi and gate the $2\frac{1}{2}$-inch valve down to 160 psi:

$$PDP = 194\ \text{psi}$$

© LiquidLibrary

CHAPTER 7 Mathematics for the Driver/Operator

SKILL DRILL 7-11 Determining the Pump Discharge Pressure in a Wye Scenario with Unequal Lines
NFPA 1002, 5.2.4 (metric)

Example 1: A pumper is supplying 30 m of 77-mm hose (with 65-mm couplings) to a wye. The first attack line from the wye is 60 m of 65-mm hose with a 32-mm smooth-bore nozzle flowing 1150 L/min. The second attack line is 45 m of 65-mm hose with a 25-mm smooth-bore nozzle flowing 750 L/min. What is the PDP? (Remember that when the flow is 1400 L/min or greater in a wye, you must add 70 kPa AL.)

$$\text{FL for 77-mm hose} = C Q^2 L$$
$$= 1.26 \,(19)^2 \, 0.3$$
$$= 1.26 \times 361 \times 0.3$$
$$= 136.4 \text{ kPa (round to 136 kPa)}$$

FL for first 65-mm hose = $C Q^2 L$ = 3.16 $(11.5)^2$ 0.6

$$= 250.7 \text{ kPa (round to 251 kPa)}$$

PDP = 350 (NP) + 136 (FL in 77-mm hose) + 251 (FL in first 65-mm hose) + 70 (AL) = 807 kPa

FL for second 65-mm hose = $C Q^2 L$

$$= 3.16 \,(7.5)^2 \, 0.45 = 79.9 \text{ kPa (round to 80 kPa)}$$

PDP = 350 (NP) + 136 (FL in 77-mm hose) + 80 (FL in second 65-mm hose) + 70 (AL) = 636 kPa

The second attack line requires less pressure; gate this line back to approximately 636 kPa. As the first attack line has a greater FL, pump to its pressure of 807 kPa:

$$\text{PDP} = 807 \text{ kPa}$$

Example 2: A pumper is supplying 30 m of 77-mm hose to a wye. From the wye, the first attack line is 60 m of 45-mm hose flowing 570 L/min through a fog nozzle. The second attack line is 60 m of 65-mm hose flowing 1150 L/min through a fog nozzle. What is the PDP?

FL for the 77-mm hose = $C Q^2 L$ = 10.7 $(17.2)^2$ 0.3 = 10.7 × 296 × 0.3 = 95 kPa
FL for first 45-mm attack line: FL = $C Q^2 L$

$$= 24.5 \,(5.7)^2 \, 0.6$$
$$= 24.5 \times 32.5 \times 0.6$$
$$= 477.75 \text{ (round to 478 kPa)}$$

PDP = 700 (NP) + 95 (FL in 77-mm hose) + 478 (FL in 45-mm hose) + 70 (AL) = 1343 kPa
FL for second attack line (65-mm hose): FL = $C Q^2 L$

$$= 3.16 \,(11.5)^2 \, 0.6$$
$$= 3.16 \times 132.25 \times 0.6$$
$$= 250.7 \text{ (round to 251 kPa)}$$

PDP = 700 (NP) + 95 (FL in 77-mm hose) + 251 (FL in 65-mm hose) + 70 (AL) = 1116 kPa
The PDP for the 45-mm line is greater, so pump at 1343 psi and gate the 65-mm line down to 1116 kPa:

$$\text{PDP} = 1343 \text{ kPa}$$

© LiquidLibrary

3 Calculate the FL and NP for each of the discharge lines from the wye device. Add the NP to the FL for the hoseline requiring the greatest pressure.

4 If the scenario is flowing 350 gpm (1400 L/min) or greater, add 10 psi (70 kPa) FL for the wye device.

5 Add the results of Steps 2 through 4 to determine the PDP.

■ Siamese Hoselines

A Siamese connection is a device that allows multiple hoselines to converge into one hoseline. Such a device is often used on the intake side of the pump, thereby allowing multiple lines to supply the fire pumper. A Siamese connection is used by fire departments that do not have large-diameter hose (LDH) and need to supply large amounts of water at a reasonable amount of pump

SKILL DRILL 7-12 Determining the Pump Pressure for a Siamese Line by the Split Flow Method
NFPA 1002, 5.2.4 (standard)

Example: A pumper is supplying 1200 gpm through three 2½-inch lines that are 300 ft long to a Siamese connection. What is the FL to the Siamese connection as calculated using the split flow method?

1200 gpm/3 hoselines = 400 gpm each

$FL = CQ^2L$

$C = 2$

$Q = 400/100 = 4$

$L = 300 \text{ ft}/100 = 3$

$FL = 2 \times 4^2 \times 3$

$FL = 96 \text{ psi}$

© LiquidLibrary

SKILL DRILL 7-12 Determining the Pump Pressure for a Siamese Line by the Split Flow Method
NFPA 1002, 5.2.4 (metric)

Example: A pumper is supplying 4500 L/min through three 65-mm lines that are 90 m long to a Siamese connection. What is the FL to the Siamese connection as calculated using the split flow method?

4500 L/min/3 hoselines = 1500 L/min each

$FL = CQ^2L$

$C = 3.16$

$Q = 1500/100 = 15$

$L = 90 \text{ m}/100 = 0.9$

$FL = 3.16 \times 15^2 \times 0.9$

$FL = 640 \text{ kPa}$

© LiquidLibrary

---

pressure. On the discharge side of the pump, this device may be used to bring two or three lines into one attack line, thereby reducing the FL in a long reach. **Portable master stream devices** (such as a removable deck gun) and the inlet of aerial waterways on squirts, quints, and ladder trucks may be supplied by a single LDH supply or a Siamese connection. The **fire department connection (FDC)** on buildings with standpipe sprinkler systems will have a Siamese connection consisting of two 2½-inch (65-mm) connections or one LDH connection.

The three methods used to calculate the FL in the lines to the Siamese connection when the lines are of equal size and length are the split flow method, the coefficient method, and the percentage method:

- In the split flow method, you divide the flow among the lines equally and calculate the pressure to supply that one line because that pressure will support all the supply lines.
- The coefficient method utilizes the FL equation with the appropriate coefficient for the lines entering the Siamese connection.
- In the percentage method, you calculate the total flow through one line. The FL in two hoselines will be 25 percent of the total flow through one hoseline, and the FL in three hoselines will be approximately 10 percent of the total flow through one hoseline.

To use the split flow method, follow the steps in **SKILL DRILL 7-12**:

1. Divide the total amount of flow desired by the number of lines in the Siamese connection.
2. Use the resulting flow amount as the quantity (Q).
3. Complete the modern FL equation with the calculated Q value.

To calculate the FL in Siamese lines by use of the coefficient method, follow the steps in **SKILL DRILL 7-13**:

1. Determine the diameter and number of hoselines going to the Siamese connection.
2. Find the corresponding arrangement on the Siamese coefficient table to assign the correct Siamese coefficient.

CHAPTER 7 Mathematics for the Driver/Operator

SKILL DRILL 7-13
Calculating Friction Loss in Siamese Lines by the Coefficient Method
NFPA 1002, 5.2.1 (standard)

Example: A fire pumper is supplying 1200 gpm through three 2½-inch lines that are 300 ft long to a Siamese line. What is the FL to the Siamese connection as calculated using the Siamese coefficient?

$$FL = C\,Q^2\,L$$
$$C = 0.22$$
$$Q = 1200/100 = 12$$
$$L = 300\text{ ft}/100 = 3$$
$$FL = 0.22 \times 12^2 \times 3$$
$$FL = 95\text{ psi}$$

© LiquidLibrary

SKILL DRILL 7-13
Calculating Friction Loss in Siamese Lines by the Coefficient Method
NFPA 1002, 5.2.1 (metric)

Example: A fire pumper is supplying 4500 L/min through three 65-mm lines that are 90 m long to a Siamese line. What is the FL to the Siamese connection as calculated using the Siamese coefficient?

$$FL = C\,Q^2\,L$$
$$C = 0.347$$
$$Q = 4500/100 = 45$$
$$L = 90\text{ m}/100 = 0.9$$
$$FL = 0.347 \times 45^2 \times 0.9$$
$$FL = 632\text{ kPa}$$

© LiquidLibrary

3. Insert the coefficient into the FL formula ($C\,Q^2\,L$) to determine the FL in the Siamese supply part of the calculation.
4. If there is no Siamese equation for the configuration, use one of the other methods to calculate the FL.

To calculate the FL in Siamese lines by use of the percentage method, follow the steps in **SKILL DRILL 7-14**:

1. Determine the total flow of the lines supplying the Siamese connection.
2. Figure out the quantity (Q) from the total flow and calculate the FL as if the total flow were going through one line.
3. If two lines supplied the flow, divide the FL based on total flow through one line by 25 percent to find the actual FL.
4. If three lines supplied the flow, divide the FL based on total flow through one line by 10 percent to find the approximate FL.

■ Calculating Elevated Master Streams
Prepiped Elevated Master Stream

The term **prepiped elevated master stream** refers to an aerial fire apparatus (ladder truck) with a fixed waterway attached to the underside of the ladder such that a water inlet at the base supplies a master stream device at the end. The master stream device may have a locking mechanism that places the nozzle on the bed section for rescue or on the fly section for water tower operations **FIGURE 7-11**. No single FL amount can be identified that will adequately encompass all prepiped elevated master stream devices; therefore it is imperative that each aerial device be tested for its unique amount of FL.

When water comes into the intake, it will have several sharp turns through the piping before it finally reaches the fire pump. All of these turns increase FL. Unless the loss in the intake, piping, and nozzle has been established for the specific apparatus, you should assume a minimum of 25 psi (175 kPa) FL for all master stream appliances.

SKILL DRILL 7-14: Calculating Friction Loss in Siamese Lines by the Percentage Method
NFPA 1002, 5.2.1 (standard)

Example 1: A fire pumper is supplying 1200 gpm through three 2½-inch lines that are 300 ft long to a Siamese connection. What is the FL to the Siamese connection as calculated using the percentage method?

$$FL = C Q^2 L$$
$$C = 2$$
$$L = 300 \text{ ft}/100 = 3$$
$$Q^2 = (1200/100)^2 = 12^2 = 144$$
$$FL = 2 \times 144 \times 3 = 864: 10\% \text{ of } 864 = 86.4$$
$$FL = 86.4$$

Working the same problem with each method produced the following results:

- Split flow method: FL = 96 psi
- Coefficient method: FL = 95 psi
- Percentage method: FL = 86.4 psi

Example 2: A pumper is supplying 1000 gpm through two 2½-inch lines that are 200 ft long to a Siamese connection. What is the FL to the Siamese connection?

Percentage method:

$$FL = C Q^2 L$$
$$C = 2$$
$$L = 200 \text{ ft}/100 = 2$$
$$Q = 500/100 = 5^2 = 25 \text{ (Each hoseline flows 500 gpm for a total of 1000 gpm)}$$
$$FL = 2 \times 25 \times 2 = 100$$
$$FL = 100 \text{ psi}$$

Split flow method:

$$FL = 2 \times 5^2 \times 2$$
$$FL = 100 \text{ psi}$$

© LiquidLibrary

FIGURE 7-11 A typical prepiped elevated master stream device.

TABLE 7-4 Standard Coefficients for Multiple Lines

Siamese 2½-Inch Hose

Two lines	0.5
Three lines	0.22
Four lines	0.12

Siamese 3-Inch Hose With 2½-Inch Couplings

Two lines	0.2
Three lines	0.09

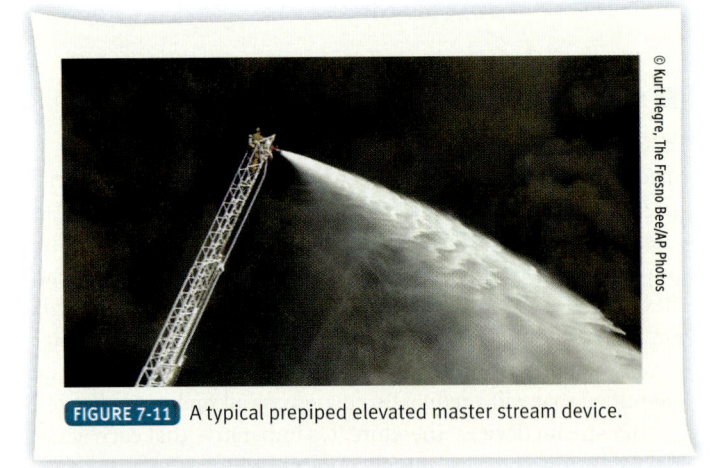

To calculate the PDP for a prepiped elevated master stream device, follow the steps in **SKILL DRILL 7-15**:

1. Determine the NP by observing which nozzle is on the tip. If it is a smooth-bore nozzle, the NP will be 80 psi (560 kPa) unless the manufacturer's specifications differ. If it is a fog nozzle, is it an automatic appliance that delivers the standard pressure of 100 psi (700 kPa) or does it meet some other specification?

2. Determine the FL in the supply line(s) from the pumper to the aerial device. Use the split flow, Siamese coefficient **TABLE 7-4**, or percentage method to find the FL in the supply line.

3. Determine the FL of the prepiped master stream. Add 25 psi (175 kPa) FL for any master stream device.

CHAPTER 7 Mathematics for the Driver/Operator

SKILL DRILL 7-14: Calculating Friction Loss in Siamese Lines by the Percentage Method
NFPA 1002, 5.2.1 (metric)

Example 1: A fire pumper is supplying 4500 L/min through three 65-mm lines that are 90 m long to a Siamese connection. What is the FL to the Siamese connection as calculated using the percentage method?

$$FL = C Q^2 L$$
$$C = 3.16$$
$$L = 90 \text{ m}/100 = 0.9$$
$$Q^2 = (4500/100)^2 = 45^2 = 2025$$
$$FL = 3.16 \times 2025 \times 0.9 = 5759: 10\% \text{ of } 5759 = 575.9 \text{ (round to 576 kPa)}$$
$$FL = 576 \text{ kPa}$$

Working the same problem with each method produced the following results:

- Split flow method: FL = 640 kPa
- Coefficient method: FL = 632 kPa
- Percentage method: FL = 576 kPa

Example 2: A pumper is supplying 3800 L/min through two 65-mm lines that are 60 m long to a Siamese connection. What is the FL to the Siamese connection?

Percentage method:

$$FL = C Q^2 L$$
$$C = 3.16$$
$$L = 60 \text{ m}/100 = 0.6$$
$$Q = 3800/100 = 38^2 = 1444$$
$$FL = 3.16 \times 1444 \times 0.6 = 2738: 25\% \text{ of } 2738 = 684$$
$$FL = 684 \text{ kPa}$$

Split flow method:

$$FL = 3.16 \times 19^2 \times 0.6$$
$$FL = 684 \text{ kPa}$$

© LiquidLibrary

Metric TABLE 7-4 Coefficients for Multiple Lines

Siamese 65-mm Hose	
Two lines	0.789
Three lines	0.347
Four lines	0.189
Siamese 77-mm Hose With 65-mm Couplings	
Two lines	0.316
Three lines	0.142

4. Calculate the EP.
5. Add the results of Steps 1 through 4 to obtain the PDP.

Calculate PDP for a Non-Prepiped Elevated Master Stream

Before the days of prepiped waterways, detachable ladder pipes were clamped onto the end of a ladder, with hose then being laid from the appliance down the ladder bed and to a Siamese connection on the ground. The only difference in calculations for this arrangement is that you must add the FL for the hose running up the ladder to the tip and allow for both appliances.

To calculate the PDP for an elevated master stream, follow the steps in **SKILL DRILL 7-16**:

1. Determine the NP.
2. Calculate the FL in the hose from the pumper to the master stream device.
3. Determine the FL in the master stream device.
4. Adjust for elevation changes between the nozzle and the pumper.
5. Add the results of Steps 1 through 4 to determine the PDP.

Standpipe Systems

Standpipe operations pose a huge firefighting and logistical challenge. Many different strategic and tactical decisions for fire attack may be made depending on the various types of standpipe-equipped buildings encountered. To make good decisions

VOICES OF EXPERIENCE

During my fire service career, I responded to and performed as a driver/operator on many of the same types of fires commonly encountered by every other fire department. Often, and especially during the initial stages of fire attack, you do not have time to think about—much less perform—complex hydraulic calculations, so I depended heavily on the preplanned pump pressures that I had determined for basic and complex fire attack scenarios.

I committed some of these simpler preplanned pressures to memory. The more complex calculations were outlined on pump charts that I could immediately consult on the fireground to save time. Without knowledge of friction loss and the steps needed to accurately calculate pump discharge pressures, I would not have been able to develop those dependable and complete pump pressures for either basic or complex fire attack scenarios.

Thorough hydraulic calculations can be very challenging when you are first learning to become a driver/operator; however, performing them correctly is well worth both your time and effort. Your knowledge of hydraulics calculations will not only make you a better pump operator, but will also ensure the safety of your fire attack crew. As a driver/operator, you must supply an adequate amount of pressure and flow to extinguish the fire and protect their lives. Hydraulic calculations will ensure the integrity of your water supply and will ensure their safety.

    Daryl Songer
    Roanoke Fire-EMS
    Roanoke, Virginia

and increase the chance of a successful operation, fire fighters must know the buildings in their jurisdiction, their occupancy, the fire load, any special hazards, and hydrant locations. They should be familiar with the FDC and standpipe locations, know whether they are equipped with pressure-regulating valves (and their types, if they are present), and know whether a fire pump is available in the building. In addition, they should have established a preincident plan for these high-hazard targets.

For these types of buildings, the water supply is critical. When the FDC has two 2½-inch (65-mm) connections, it is a good idea to advance a 2½-inch (65-mm) hoseline to the FDC and charge it before attaching the second hoseline. The goal is to get water into the **standpipe system** as soon as possible. When possible, a different pumper should supply each FDC if the building is equipped with multiple FDCs. Whenever possible, a water supply independent of the supply of the building should be available as well.

Incidents requiring use of a standpipe system can easily be one of the most demanding pumping scenarios that you as the driver/operator will encounter on the fireground. Calculating the required pressure for a standpipe system may need to be based upon several variables and the required fire flow for the given situation. Standpipe pump pressures may be calculated, identified from markings on or at the FDC, or determined by departmental standard operating procedures (SOPs). It is extremely beneficial to predetermine pump discharge pressures for high-rise structures to limit the amount of calculations needed on the fireground during the excitement of an actual incident. As a general rule, you should not exceed a PDP of 200 psi (1400 kPa) unless you know the system is designed to handle the greater pressure required.

As the driver/operator at an incident, you can control only one pressure to the standpipe, even though multiple discharge hoselines may be in use in the same structure on different floors. The one pressure that you control from the pump panel is the highest pressure needed at any one discharge (regardless of the floor it is on). As explained in the discussion of supplying lines of unequal size or length, the operator must pump to the highest pressure required. This same rule also applies to standpipes in multistory buildings: Calculate the PDP for each line being supplied, and then pump to the highest pressure. This will not necessarily be the highest point in the line's elevation.

For example, suppose a fire pumper is supplying two attack lines on the top floor of a five-story building, each consisting of 200 ft (60 m) of 2½-inch (65-mm) hose with 1⅛-inch (29-mm) smooth-bore nozzles requiring a PDP of 141 psi (987 kPa). The same fire pumper is also supplying a 1¾-inch (45-mm) hose with a fog nozzle that fire fighters are using to perform overhaul on the third floor; this line has a PDP of 181 psi (1267 kPa). The fire pumper can send only one pressure into the standpipe; it cannot pump two different pressures. Therefore the driver/operator must pump to the highest pressure, which in this case is 181 psi (1267 kPa).

The actual numbers would be rounded, but note that the hose requiring the most pressure is not on the highest floor in this example. Also note that NP is important, because a fog nozzle requires a nozzle pressure of 100 psi (700 kPa) NP, whereas a smooth-bore nozzle requires only 50 psi (350 kPa) in NP.

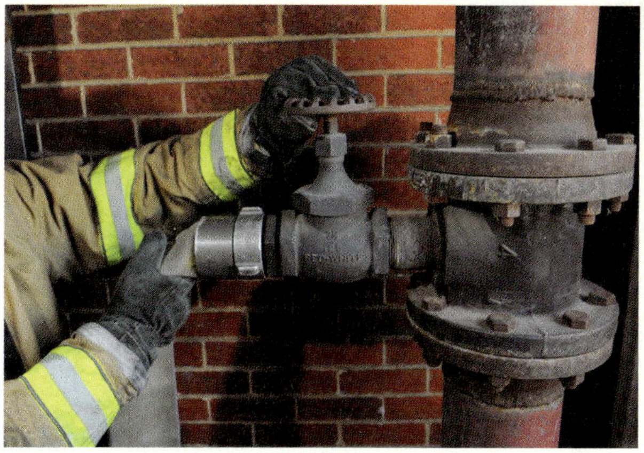

FIGURE 7-12 Lower pressures needed at subsequent discharges should be controlled by a fire fighter staged at the discharge valve of the standpipe riser used.

In commercial buildings and multistory structures, the attack hose should consist of 2½-inch (65-mm) lines with smooth-bore nozzles. In multistory buildings, the attack lines should be supplied from the floor below with an in-line gauge on the standpipe outlet. Any lower pressures needed at subsequent discharges will have to be controlled by a fire fighter staged at the discharge valve of the **standpipe riser** used **FIGURE 7-12**. A standpipe riser is the vertical portion of the system piping within a building that delivers the water supply for fire hose connections, and sprinklers on combined systems, vertically from floor to floor.

The fire fighter needs to know the required operating pressure of the attack hoselines, so he or she can adequately control the pressure from that outlet. The attack hoseline must be flowing water if the crew member is to obtain an accurate reading from the gauge. Increase the pressure until the in-line pressure gauge at the riser meets the predetermined pressure for the attack hose/nozzle combination. The use of the in-line gauge will compensate for any discrepancies if calculations are off or circumstances have changed.

Use of an in-line gauge is highly advantageous for standpipe operations. If in-line gauges are not available, you are well advised to test the flow from your high-rise hoseline and nozzle combination in a realistic simulation to set performance expectations. To calculate the discharge pressure, follow the steps in **SKILL DRILL 7-17**:

1. Determine the means by which you will connect to the standpipe, the amount of hose needed, and the desired flow rate.
2. Use the appropriate FL calculation given the size and amount of hose needed. An LDH fire department connection may require only a single line, whereas the more common 2½-inch (65-mm) FDC will require multiple hoses to be used. When using two 2½-inch (65-mm) lines, split the flow to determine the quantity value (Q) for the FL equation. For multiple 2½-inch hoselines, use the coefficient for Siamese lines.
3. Calculate the FL in the riser using the applicable coefficient for standpipe risers from **TABLE 7-5**. The height

SKILL DRILL 7-15

Calculating the Pump Discharge Pressure for a Prepiped Elevated Master Stream Device
NFPA 1002, 5.2.4 (standard)

Example 1: A pumper supplying an elevated master stream is on the hydrant. This apparatus is supplying one 5-inch line that is 200 ft long to the inlet of the ladder truck, which the ladder has extended 80 ft vertically; it is equipped with a 1½-inch smooth-bore master stream tip (600 gpm). What is the PDP?

$$PDP = NP + FL$$
$$PDP = 80 + FL$$
$$FL = (C \times Q^2 \times L) + AL + EP$$
$$FL = (0.08 \times 6^2 \times 2) + 25 + 40 = 71$$
$$FL = 6 + 25 + 40$$
$$FL = 71 \text{ psi}$$
$$PDP = 80 + 71$$
$$PDP = 151 \text{ psi}$$

Example 2: Determine the PDP for supplying a prepiped elevated master stream through 200 ft of 4-inch hose, where the aerial device is raised to 80 ft vertically and has a 2-inch tip rated at 80 psi.

$$PDP = NP + FL$$
$$PDP = 80 + FL$$
$$FL = (C \times Q^2 \times L) + AL + EP \ (FL = (0.2 \times 1062/100^2 \times 200 \text{ ft}/100) + AL + EP)$$
$$FL = (0.2 \times 10.62^2 \times 2) + AL + EP$$
$$FL = (0.2 \times 113 \times 2) + 25 + 40$$
$$FL = 45 \text{ psi} + 25 + 40$$
$$FL = 110$$
$$PDP = 80 + 110$$
$$PDP = 190 \text{ psi}$$

Standard TABLE 7-5 — Coefficients for Standpipe Risers

Friction Loss Coefficients for Standpipe Risers

Riser Diameter (inch)	Coefficient
4	0.374
5	0.126
6	0.052

Metric TABLE 7-5 — Coefficients for Standpipe Risers

Friction Loss Coefficients for Standpipe Risers

Riser Diameter (mm)	Coefficient
100	0.590
125	0.199
150	0.082

of the highest discharge used will be the value for L in the equation. Add 10 psi (70 kPa) FL for the FDC when flowing 350 gpm (1400 L/min) or greater. If the amount of water flowing is less than 350 gpm (1400 L/min), then do not add the 10 psi (70 kPa).

④ Calculate the amount of pressure lost due to the increase in elevation as described in the discussion of EP.

⑤ Calculate the friction loss in the attack hoselines, and then add the associated NP.

⑥ Add the results from Steps 1 through 5 to determine the PDP.

The PDP for standpipe operations requires that calculations be made for the supply lines to the standpipe, FL within the standpipe system, FL for the attack handlines, and pressure loss due to an increase in elevation. If no preincident plan exists and the size of the riser is unknown, then it is too late to try to measure the riser. Instead, simply add 25 psi (175 kPa) to account for the standpipe riser. When personnel are in place, the in-line gauge is on the riser outlet, and water is flowing, the person on the gauge can then radio you to increase or decrease the pressure as needed.

To calculate the PDP for standpipe operations, follow the steps in **SKILL DRILL 7-18**:

① Determine how you will connect to the standpipe and the amount of hose needed.

② Use the appropriate FL calculation given the size and amount of hose needed. An LDH fire department connection may require only a single line, whereas the

CHAPTER 7 Mathematics for the Driver/Operator

SKILL DRILL 7-15
Calculating the Pump Discharge Pressure for a Prepiped Elevated Master Stream Device
NFPA 1002, 5.2.4 (metric)

Example 1: A pumper supplying an elevated master stream is on the hydrant. This apparatus is supplying one 125-mm line that is 60 m long to the inlet of the ladder truck, which has the ladder extended 24 m vertically; it is equipped with a 38-mm smooth-bore master stream tip (2250 L/min). There is 210 kPa of FL in the fixed waterway of this particular truck. Assign 175 kPa FL for the master stream appliance. What is the PDP?

$$PDP = NP + FL$$
$$PDP = 560 + FL$$
$$FL = C \times Q^2 \times L + AL + EP$$
$$FL = 0.126 \times (22.5)^2 \times 0.6 + 175 + 240 = 453$$
$$FL = 453 + 210 \text{ specific to the waterway}$$
$$FL = 663 \text{ kPa}$$
$$PDP = 560 + 663$$
$$PDP = 1223 \text{ kPa}$$

Example 2: Determine PDP for supplying a prepiped elevated master stream through 60 m of 100-mm hose, where the aerial device is raised to 24 m and has a waterway with a 50-mm tip rated at 560 kPa, and the appliance has 175 kPa FL.

$$PDP = NP + FL$$
$$PDP = 560 + FL$$
$$FL = C \times Q^2 \times L + AL + EP \, [FL = 0.315 \times (3900/100)^2 \times 60 \text{ m}/100 + AL + EP]$$
$$FL = 0.315 \times 39^2 \times 0.6 + AL + EP$$
$$FL = 0.315 \times 1521 \times 0.6 + AL + EP$$
$$FL = 288 \text{ kPa} + AL + EP$$
$$AL = 175$$
$$EP = 24 \text{ m} \times 10$$
$$EP = 240 \text{ kPa}$$
$$PDP = NP + (FL + AL + EP)$$
$$PDP = 560 + 288 + 175 + 240$$
$$PDP = 1263 \text{ kPa}$$

© LiquidLibrary

---

more common 2½-inch (65-mm) FDC will require multiple hoses to be used. When using two 2½-inch (65-mm) lines, split the flow to determine the quantity value (Q) for the FL. For multiple 2½-inch (65-mm) hoselines, use the Siamese coefficient.

3 Calculate the FL in the riser using the applicable coefficient from **TABLE 7-5**. The height of the highest discharge used will be the value of L in the equation. Add 10 psi (70 kPa) FL for the FDC if flowing 350 gpm (1400 L/min) or greater. If the amount of water flowing is less than 350 gpm (1400 L/min), do not add the 10 psi (70 kPa). If the pump pressure has not been predetermined and the riser size and length are not known, add 25 psi (175 kPa) FL for the FDC.

4 Calculate the amount of pressure lost due to the increase in elevation as described in the discussion of elevation loss/gain.

5 Calculate the FL in the attack hoselines, and then add the associated NP.

6 Add the results of Steps 1 through 5 to determine the PDP.

■ Pressure-Regulating Valves

Pressure-regulating valves (PRV) are installed on standpipe risers where static pressures exceed 175 psi (1225 kPa) per NFPA 13, *Standard for the Installation of Sprinkler Systems*. If pressures while flowing exceed 100 psi (700 kPa), then NFPA 14, *Standard for the Installation of Standpipe and Hose Systems*, requires the installation of a device at the outlet to restrict or reduce the flow pressure to a maximum of 100 psi (700 kPa). The height of a column of water above the discharge is known as the head; the pressure in that column of water is referred to as head pressure. To determine the head pressure,

SKILL DRILL 7-16 — Calculating the Pump Discharge Pressure for an Elevated Master Stream
NFPA 1002, 5.2.4 (standard)

Example: Determine the PDP for supplying a non-prepiped elevated master stream that is raised to 60 ft and is flowing 600 gpm to a 1½-inch tip rated at 80 psi through 300 ft of 3-inch hose with 2-inch couplings. The aerial and master streams have 25 psi of FL each.

$$PDP = NP + FL$$
$$PDP = 80 + FL$$
$$FL = 0.8 \times (600/100)^2 \times 300\ ft/100\ (+ AL + EP)$$
$$FL = 0.8 \times (6)^2 \times 3 = 0.8 \times 36 \times 3$$
$$FL = 86\ psi$$
$$AL = 25\ psi$$
$$EP = 60\ ft \times 0.5$$
$$EP = 30\ psi$$
$$PDP = NP + FL + AL + EP$$
$$PDP = 80 + 86 + 25 + 30$$
$$PDP = 221\ psi$$

© LiquidLibrary

SKILL DRILL 7-17 — Calculating the Discharge Pressure for a Standpipe During Preplanning
NFPA 1002, 5.2.4, 5.2.4(A), 5.2.4(B) (standard)

Example: You have been assigned to develop a preincident plan for the use of a standpipe system for fire attack on the top floor of a 17-story building. The attack hose will consist of two lines, each of which comprises 200 ft of 2½-inch hose with a smooth-bore 1⅛-inch tip nozzle. A third 2½-inch line with a 1¼-inch tip is the backup line. The total flow is 858 gpm. The FDC is supplied with two 100-ft lengths of 2½-inch hose. The building is equipped with a 5-inch riser. (The coefficient is 0.126.) What is the PDP to operate these three lines on the seventeenth floor?

$$\text{Supply FL} = C\ Q^2\ L = 2 \times (4.29)^2\ 1 = 36.8\ (\text{round to 37 psi})$$
$$\text{FDC} = 10\ psi\ AL\ \text{when flowing 350 GPM or greater and calculating for standpipe FL}$$
$$\text{Riser FL} = C\ Q^2\ L = 0.126\ (8.58)^2\ 1.6 = 9.27 \times 1.6 = 14.84\ (\text{round to 15 psi})$$

Two attack lines with 200 ft of 2½-inch hose with 1⅛-inch smooth-bore nozzles:

$$FL = C\ Q^2\ L = 2\ (2.66)^2\ 2 = 28\ psi$$
$$PDP = 50 + 28 = 78\ psi\ \text{for these two lines (round to 80 psi)}$$

One attack line with 200 ft of 2½-inch hose with a 1¼-inch smooth-bore nozzle:

$$FL = C\ Q^2\ L = 2\ (3.26)^2\ 2 = 42.5\ psi\ (\text{round to 43 psi})$$
$$PDP = 50 + 43 = 93\ psi$$

Pump to the line requiring the highest pressure (93 psi) and add it all together:

```
  93 highest-pressure attack line
  15 for riser (14.84 psi actual)
  10 FDC
+ 37 supply to the FDC
 155 psi total PDP
```

© LiquidLibrary

SKILL DRILL 7-16 Calculating the Pump Discharge Pressure for an Elevated Master Stream
NFPA 1002, 5.2.4 (metric)

Example: Determine the PDP for supplying a non-prepiped elevated master stream that is raised to 18 m and is flowing 2250 L/min to a 38-mm tip rated at 560 kPa through 90 m of 77-mm hose with 65-mm couplings. The aerial Siamese connection has 70 kPa of friction loss and the master stream has 175 kPa of FL.

$$PDP = NP + FL$$
$$PDP = 560 + FL$$
$$FL = 1.26 \times (2250/100)^2 \times 90\ m/100\ (+ AL + EP)$$
$$FL = 1.26 \times (22.5)^2 \times 0.9 = 1.26 \times 506.25 \times 0.9$$
$$FL = 574\ kPa$$
$$AL = 70 + 175 = 245\ kPa$$
$$EP = 18\ m \times 10$$
$$EP = 180\ kPa$$
$$PDP = NP + FL + AL + EP$$
$$PDP = 560 + 574 + 245 + 180$$
$$PDP = 1559\ kPa$$

© LiquidLibrary

SKILL DRILL 7-17 Calculating the Discharge Pressure for a Standpipe During Preplanning
NFPA 1002, 5.2.4, 5.2.4(A), 5.2.4(B) (metric)

Example: You have been assigned to develop a preincident plan for the use of a standpipe system for fire attack on the top floor of a 17-story building. The attack hose will consist of two lines, each of which comprises 60 m of 65-mm hose with a smooth-bore 29-mm tip nozzle. A third 65-mm line with a 32-mm tip is the backup line. The total flow is 3350 L/min. The FDC is supplied with two 60-m lengths of 65-mm hose. The building is equipped with a 125-mm riser. (The coefficient is 0.199.) What is the PDP to operate these three lines on the seventeenth floor?

$$\text{Supply FL} = C\ Q^2\ L = 3.16 \times (16.75)^2 \times 0.6 = 532\ kPa$$
$$FDC = 70\ kPa\ AL\ \text{when flowing 1400 L/min or greater and calculating for standpipe FL}$$
$$\text{Riser FL} = C\ Q^2\ L = 0.199\ (33.5)^2\ (16 \times 3\ m/100) = 0.199 \times 1022.25 \times 0.48 = 97.6\ (\text{round to 98 kPa})$$

Two attack lines with 60 m of 65-mm hose with 29-mm smooth-bore nozzles:

$$FL = C\ Q^2\ L = 3.16\ (10.5)^2\ 0.6 = 209.1\ kPa\ (\text{round to 209 kPa})$$
$$PDP = 350 + 209 = 559\ kPa\ \text{for these two lines}$$

One attack line with 60 m of 65-mm hose with a 32-mm smooth-bore nozzle:

$$FL = C\ Q^2\ L = 3.16\ (13)^2\ 0.6 = 320.4\ kPa\ (\text{round to 320 kPa})$$
$$PDP = 350 + 320 = 670\ kPa$$

Pump to the line requiring the highest pressure (670 kPa) and add it all together:

670 highest-pressure attack line
98 for riser
70 FDC
+ 532 supply to the FDC
1370 kPa

© LiquidLibrary

SKILL DRILL 7-18: Calculating Pump Discharge Pressure for a Standpipe
NFPA 1002, 5.2.4, 5.2.4(A), 5.2.4(B) (standard)

Example: You are supplying three 200-ft attack lines consisting of 2½-inch hose with 1⅛-inch tips rated at 50 psi. The highest attack line is on the 15th floor. The other two lines are on the 14th floor. Using the split flow method for the two 2½-inch supply lines that are 200 ft long to the FDC, what is the PDP?

Friction Loss: Supply

$$\text{Total flow} = 266 \text{ gpm} \times 3 = 798 \text{ gpm (round to 800)}$$
$$800 \text{ gpm}/2 \text{ supply lines} = 400 \text{ gpm each}$$
$$\text{FL (supply)} = 2 \times (4)^2 \times 2 = 64 \text{ psi}$$

Friction Loss: Standpipe
The standpipe is made of 6-inch pipe, and the connection on the 15th floor is 180 ft in elevation (L).

$$FL = C Q^2 L$$
$$\text{FL (riser)} = 0.052 \times (798/100)^2 \times 180 \text{ ft}/100 \text{ (round 798 to 800)}$$
$$\text{FL (riser)} = 0.052 \times (8)^2 \times 1.8 \text{ (round to 2)}$$
$$\text{FL (riser)} = 6 \text{ psi}$$
$$\text{FDC} = 10 \text{ psi}$$
$$\text{AL (FDC and standpipe)} = 16 \text{ psi}$$

Elevation Pressure

$$EP = (15 - 1) \times 5 = 14 \times 5 \text{ psi}$$
$$EP = 70 \text{ psi}$$

Friction Loss: Attack Line

$$\text{FL (attack line)} = 2 \times (266/100)^2 \times 200 \text{ ft}/100$$
$$\text{FL (attack line)} = 2 \times (2.66)^2 \times 2$$
$$\text{FL (attack line)} = 2 \times 7.08 \times 2$$
$$\text{FL (attack line)} = 28 \text{ psi}$$

Nozzle Pressure

$$NP = 50 \text{ psi}$$

Pump Discharge Pressure

$$PDP = NP + \text{FL (supply)} + \text{AL (FDC and standpipe)} + EP + \text{FL (attack line)}$$
$$PDP = 50 + 64 + 16 + 70 + 28$$
$$PDP = 228 \text{ psi}$$

© LiquidLibrary

---

divide the height of the column in feet by 2.31; for calculations in the metric system, divide the column height in meters by 9.812.

In this case, the column of water is in the standpipe riser. As the height of the riser increases, the head pressure becomes so great that it could easily exceed the burst pressure of fire hose. Without the control established by restricting or regulating valves, excessive elevation pressures within the building standpipe system could burst hoselines, halting the suppression attack and possibly injuring fire fighters.

Standpipe test documentation should be on file in the building's maintenance office. The design pressure of the building's standpipe system should meet the minimum PRV pressure. You may boost the pressure to the maximum design pressure; however, if calculations require a pressure lower than the system minimum, default to the designed pressure so that the PRV can operate properly.

These valves have huge implications for fire fighters, whether installed properly or not, and can severely hinder firefighting operations. One of the most notable examples of this problem occurred during the One Meridian Plaza Fire in Philadelphia in 1991, in which three fire fighters lost their lives. Fire fighters in that incident struggled due to the lack of pressure within the standpipe system.

CHAPTER 7 Mathematics for the Driver/Operator

SKILL DRILL 7-18 Calculating Pump Discharge Pressure for a Standpipe
NFPA 1002, 5.2.4, 5.2.4(A), 5.2.4(B) (metric)

Example: You are supplying three 60-m attack lines consisting of 65-mm hose with 29-mm tips rated at 350 kPa. The highest attack line is on the 15th floor. The other two lines are on the 14th floor. Using the split flow method for the two 65-mm supply lines that are 60 m long to the FDC, what is the PDP?

Friction Loss: Supply

$$\text{Total flow} = 1050 \text{ L/min} \times 3 = 3150 \text{ L/min}$$
$$3150 \text{ L/min}/2 \text{ supply lines} = 1675 \text{ L/min each}$$
$$\text{FL (supply)} = 3.16 \times (16.75)^2 \times 0.6 = 532 \text{ kPa}$$

Friction Loss: Standpipe
The standpipe is made of 150-mm pipe, and the connection on the 15th floor is 42 m in elevation (L).

$$FL = C Q^2 L$$
$$\text{FL (riser)} = 0.082 \times (3150/100)^2 \times 42/100$$
$$\text{FL (riser)} = 0.082 \times (31.5)^2 \times 0.42$$
$$\text{FL (riser)} = 34 \text{ kPa}$$
$$FDC = 70 \text{ kPa}$$
$$\text{AL (FDC and standpipe)} = 104 \text{ kPa}$$

Elevation Pressure

$$EP = (15 - 1) \times 3 \text{ m} \times 10 \text{ kPa/m} = 42 \times 10 \text{ kPa}$$
$$EP = 420 \text{ kPa}$$

Friction Loss: Attack Line

$$\text{FL (attack line)} = 3.16 \times (1050/100)^2 \times 60/100$$
$$\text{FL (attack line)} = 3.16 \times (10.5)^2 \times 0.6$$
$$\text{FL (attack line)} = 3.16 \times 110.25 \times 0.6$$
$$\text{FL (attack line)} = 209 \text{ kPa}$$

Nozzle Pressure

$$NP = 350 \text{ kPa}$$

Pump Discharge Pressure

$$PDP = NP + \text{FL (supply)} + \text{AL (FDC and standpipe)} + EP + \text{FL (attack line)}$$
$$PDP = 350 + 532 + 104 + 420 + 209$$
$$PDP = 1618 \text{ kPa}$$

© LiquidLibrary

DRIVER/OPERATOR Tip

The PDP is set to support the line requiring the highest pressure regardless of its location.

■ Net Pump Discharge Pressure

A water supply can be either static or dynamic. Static sources such as lakes and streams require establishing a draft. Dynamic sources such as hydrants or another fire apparatus are positive-pressure sources. **Net pump discharge pressure (NPDP)** from a positive-pressure source (pps) is referred to as $NPDP_{pps}$. Net pump discharge pressure from a static source is referred to as $NPDP_{draft}$. To understand net pump pressure, remember that the pump develops pressure even at idle. If the hydrant is giving a certain pressure, and the driver/operator throttles up to achieve a given PDP, then the part of the total pressure that the pump creates is equal to the net pump pressure.

$NPDP_{pps}$, then, is the amount of pressure created by the pump after it receives water under pressure from a hydrant or another pump. For example, assume you are pumping at a PDP of 170 psi (1190 kPa) and you have 50 psi (350 kPa) of pressure coming in from a hydrant. The $NPDP_{pps}$ is the PDP minus the incoming pressure. In this case, the calculation is 170 psi

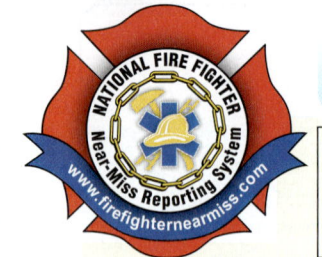

Near-Miss REPORT

Report Number: 10-0000038

Synopsis: Attack team makes entry without proper water pressure.

Event Description: The department was alerted to a report of a structure fire. The Chief arrived and reported fire evident from an end of the row unit on a single story motel. The engine arrived and stretched a 1³/₄-inch (45-mm) attack line. As the engine crew was stretching the initial line, the pump operator was hand stretching a supply line to a hydrant that was located near the engine. The pump operator did charge the initial line, and the attack crew detected low pressure in the line.

The attack crew was able to knock the bulk of the fire down and had a sufficient stream to reach the rear of the apartment. They decided to make entry into the structure to hit the hot spots and complete final extinguishment even though proper pressure had not been achieved in the attack line.

It was later discovered that the pump operator failed to open the rear intake piston valve allowing the supply to enter the pump. In addition, the attack team had kinks in the hoseline hampering the proper pressure/gpm (L/min) to reach the nozzle. The incident commander (IC) never initiated the incident command system, accountability, or a safety officer.

Lessons Learned: After discussion and review of the incident, the initial attack crew should have remained outside until proper pressure in the water line was reached, and then utilized the reach of the nozzle stream to penetrate the room and complete fire suppression. Preplanning of the structure would have informed emergency personnel of lightweight truss construction. The arriving IC needs to implement the incident command system, accountability, and a safety officer.

(1190 kPa) minus 50 psi (350 kPa), giving an $NPDP_{pps}$ of 120 psi (840 kPa).

Safety Tip

There is an old fire service saying: As the first line goes, so goes the fire! It is much better to be "over-gunned" than "under-gunned." When selecting a handline, always use a 2¹/₂-inch (65-mm) line for fires in commercial buildings or well-involved fires. Remember—small fire = small water and big fire = big water!

Fire Service Hydraulic Calculations

Fire service hydraulic calculations may generally be categorized as either theoretical hydraulics or fireground hydraulics. Theoretical hydraulic calculations are more exact, generally require more mathematical skills, and take more time to compute. Away from the fireground, they may be computed on paper, by calculator, or using a computer.

Theoretical hydraulic calculations may be used on the fireground or for preincident planning purposes, such as determining the appropriate pump pressures for high-risk or high-hazard targets as well as buildings requiring complex hose layouts and standpipe systems. On the fireground, theoretical calculations are performed mentally. As a driver/operator, you should practice these mental calculations extensively until you are competent and comfortable using the formulas.

In this role, you should be able to effortlessly calculate FL and PDP. More complex problems may require a few moments of thought and often a notepad to jot down calculations. These problems should be performed during the preincident planning stage.

Fireground hydraulic calculations employ methods intended to estimate calculations more quickly due to the urgency of the incident. These methods may also be used as a backup to mental theoretical calculations, as a system to check results, and as a means to ensure reasonable accuracy. They also reinforce the learning process as you develop the ability to perform theoretical hydraulics calculations in the field. These methods yield working approximations and are not as accurate as theoretical computations.

The two fundamental formulas for determining PDP are as follows:

$$PDP = NP + FL$$
$$FL = C Q^2 L + AL + EP$$

The acquired FL number is then added to the other components of the formula to determine the correct PDP. All of the essential components of hydraulics—those determining factors influencing PDP—must be considered when using the fireground hydraulic methods. Each provides a way to reduce the math required, although the NP, flow (gpm or L/min), size and length of hose, and FL (including AL and elevation gain/loss) must be accounted for. Common fireground hydraulic calculation methods include the following techniques:

CHAPTER 7 Mathematics for the Driver/Operator

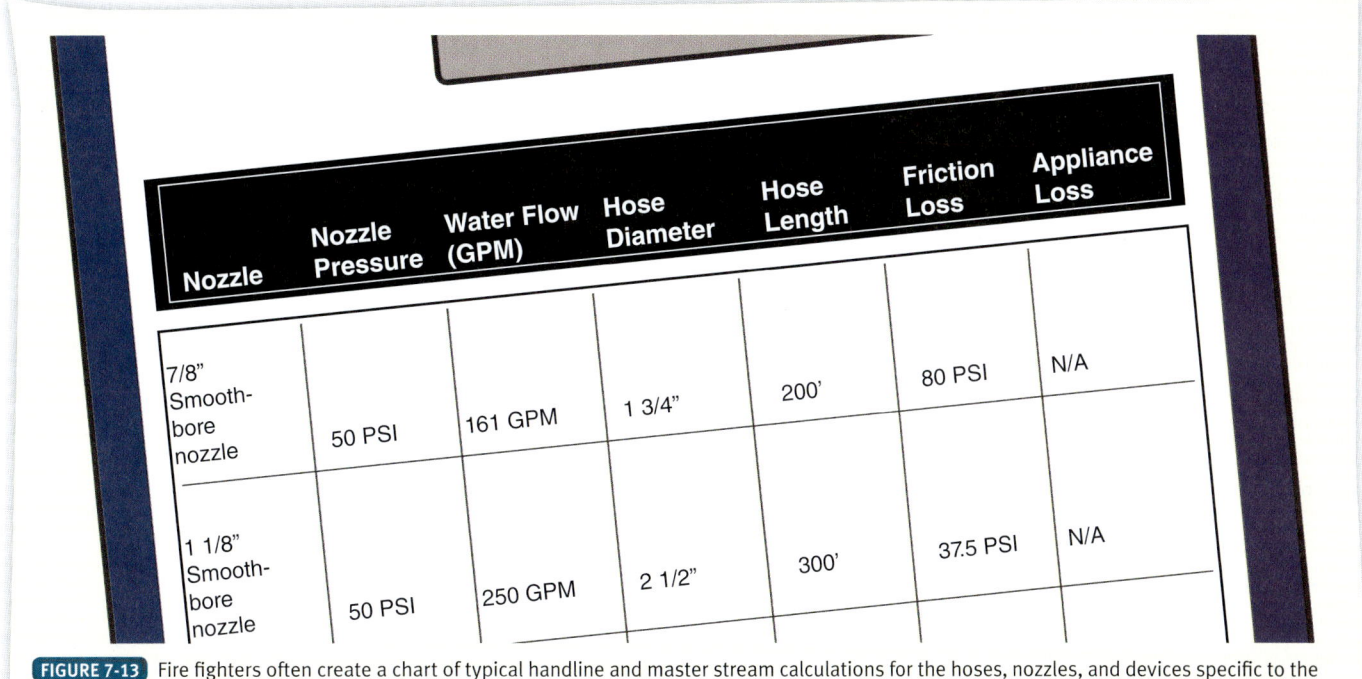

Nozzle	Nozzle Pressure	Water Flow (GPM)	Hose Diameter	Hose Length	Friction Loss	Appliance Loss
7/8" Smooth-bore nozzle	50 PSI	161 GPM	1 3/4"	200'	80 PSI	N/A
1 1/8" Smooth-bore nozzle	50 PSI	250 GPM	2 1/2"	300'	37.5 PSI	N/A

FIGURE 7-13 Fire fighters often create a chart of typical handline and master stream calculations for the hoses, nozzles, and devices specific to the fire apparatus within their fire department.

- Charts
- Hydraulic calculators
- Hand method
- "Subtract 10 method," also known as the "gpm flowing method"
- Condensed Q method
- Preincident plan data
- Additional water available from a hydrant

Charts

Fire fighters often create a **chart** of typical handline and master stream calculations for the hoses, nozzles, and devices specific to the fire apparatus within their department. These charts list the most commonly used or reasonably expected hose lays. Such charts are designed so that the driver/operator can easily find the needed discharge pressure without having to perform calculations on the fly on the fireground **FIGURE 7-13**.

The calculations chart lists the common pressures for the attack hose and nozzle combinations at different lengths as well as the pressures required for the use of master stream appliances. These represent different scenarios with different tip sizes and flows, elevations, and corresponding FL. Such charts, whether homemade or purchased from an outside source, may be pocket-size or larger. Often they consist of a laminated sheet of paper that is taped inside a compartment door, within sight of the pump panel. When creating your own pump chart, list the nozzle, NP, flow (gpm or L/min), hose diameter, hose length, FL, and AL when applicable. All elements of hydraulic calculations must be considered when compiling this kind of chart. Most importantly, the calculations must be accurate if the chart is to be reliable. When using such charts, do not allow pressures to exceed hose test pressures and be sure to stay within the pressures mandated by your fire department's SOPs.

Charts may also be prepared for complex fire problems such as multistory buildings or other high-hazard target locations. Preincident planning affords you the opportunity to establish baseline calculations before an emergency response becomes necessary. These pressures may then be placed on a chart, entered into the preincident plan book or computer, and/or labeled on the FDC.

Charts for high-rise buildings, such as the one developed by Battalion Chief David McGrail of the Denver Fire Department, suggest a pressure for a range of floors **TABLE 7-6**. As the driver/

TABLE 7-6	Friction Loss Pump Chart for High-Rise Standpipe Operations

Floors	Pump Pressure
1 to 5 stories	125 psi
6 to 10 stories	150 psi
11 to 15 stories	175 psi
15 to 20 stories	200 psi
21 to 25 stories	225 psi
26 to 30 stories	250 psi
31 to 35 stories	275 psi
36 to 40 stories	300 psi
41 to 45 stories	325 psi
45 to 50 stories	350 psi
51 to 55 stories	375 psi
56 to 60 stories	400 psi
61 to 65 stories	425 psi

Note: Friction Loss for 150 ft of 2½-inch hoseline and a 1⅛-inch smooth-bore nozzle.
Source: David McGrail of the Denver, Colorado Fire Department.

operator, you will pump to the pressure on the chart for a given floor, subsequently increasing or decreasing the pressure as instructed by personnel on that floor when they confirm the location and begin suppression operations. The members of the attack team will first flush the standpipe riser and then connect the in-line pressure gauge and gated wye. They will then connect the attack lines and advance toward the fire. As soon as water is flowing, the fire fighter assigned to the riser must read the in-line pressure gauge at the standpipe riser.

The attack team should know in advance what pressure is needed from a riser for the particular attack line and nozzle combination in the team's high-rise/standpipe bag. For example, 200 ft (60 m) of 2½-inch (65-mm) hose with a 1¼-inch (32-mm) solid tip may require a pressure of 90 psi (630 kPa) to achieve the desired flow. If you as the driver/operator increase the pressure until the in-line pressure gauge at the riser reads 90 psi (630 kPa), then the nozzle should deliver the desired flow. The fire fighter reading the gauge will advise you by radio to increase or decrease the pressure so that the target pressure is met. Be aware that this pressure is flow pressure, not static pressure; that is, water must be flowing to make this determination. Use of this fireground method simplifies a situation requiring complicated theoretical hydraulics calculations.

■ Hydraulic Calculators

Hydraulic calculators may be either manual (mechanical) or electronic. The manual hydraulic calculator may consist of a sliding card or a slide rule. These items can handle calculations involving a variety of nozzle pressures, flow rates (in gpm or L/min), and hose diameters, and indicate FL per 100 ft (30 m) of hose. Slide rule hydraulic calculators offer a fire stream calculator (gpm or L/min) on one side and a FL calculator on the other side.

To find the flow rate with a fire stream calculator, follow the steps in **SKILL DRILL 7-19**:

1. Slide the interior of the calculator until the arrow at the top points to the NP selected.
2. Choose the NP: 50 psi (350 kPa) smooth-bore nozzle, 100 psi (700-kPa) fog nozzle, or 75 psi (525 kPa) fog nozzle.
3. For a smooth-bore nozzle, find the tip size; the flow will be indicated below it.
4. For a 100 psi (700 kPa) fog nozzle, find the rating at 100 psi (700 kPa); the flow will be indicated below it.
5. For a 75 psi (525 kPa) fog nozzle, find the rating at 75 psi (525 kPa); the flow will be indicated below it.

To calculate the flow for a given hose size and nozzle pressure using a slide rule calculator and measurements in the metric system, follow these steps:

1. Slide the interior of the calculator until the arrow at the top points to the NP selected.
2. Choose the nozzle: smooth-bore nozzle, 700 kPa fog nozzle, or 525 kPa fog nozzle.
3. For a smooth-bore nozzle, find the tip size; the flow will be indicated below it.
4. For a 700 kPa fog nozzle, find the rating at 700 kPa; the flow will be indicated below it.
5. For a 525 kPa fog nozzle, find the rating at 525 kPa; the flow will be indicated below it.

To use a manual friction loss calculator, follow the steps in **SKILL DRILL 7-20**:

1. Slide the interior of the calculator to set the flow to the arrow at the top.
2. Look for the hose size (whether single or connected to a Siamese connection) and read the FL indicated.

Electronic calculators may be either mounted or hand-held devices. Mounted calculators are seldom encountered today, whereas the hand-held type is quite common. The hand-held pocket-size electronic calculator allows you to calculate engine pressure, FL, application rate, flow rate, and reaction force (RF, also known as normal reaction [NR]). All in all, the pocket calculator is a very useful tool.

■ Hand Method

The purpose of the hand method (the counting fingers method) is to quickly determine the amount of FL per 100 ft (30 m) of hose. The FL must then be multiplied by the number of 100-ft (30-m) lengths of hose. Next, add any AL, the EP, and the NP to provide the correct PDP.

To use the hand method to calculate friction, follow the steps in **SKILL DRILL 7-21**, and then complete Skill Drill 7-22:

1. Multiply the first digit of the flow by the number of 100-ft (30-m) sections used.
2. Add the other variables of AL and elevation gain or loss if applicable. This will determine the PDP for that hoseline.
3. With the FL established, add the other variables of AL and elevation gain or loss, if applicable, to the NP to determine the PDP for that hoseline.

Hand methods have been established for calculations involving almost every size of hose. The primary attack lines in the fire service today are 1¾-inch and 2½-inch hose, so naturally the methods for these two sizes are most commonly used. To perform the hand method calculation for the 2½-inch hose, follow the steps in **SKILL DRILL 7-22**:

1. Start with the left hand open and the thumb on the left.
2. Assign the flow in hundreds of gpm to the base of each finger, from left to right, in 100-gpm increments, designating the thumb as 100 gpm, then 200 gpm, 300 gpm, 400 gpm, and finally 500 gpm on the little finger.
3. Assign the spaces between fingers as the half-hundred figures (i.e., 150, 250, 350, 450). In this way, the flow designations are assigned to the hand for 2½-inch hose.
4. Assign to the fingertips the multiplier numbers of 2 for the thumb, and 4, 6, 8, and 10 across the hand to the fingertips.
5. Assign 3, 5, 7, and 9 to the spaces between the fingers.
6. The FL for 100 ft of 2½-inch hose is obtained by selecting the desired flow and multiplying the number at the tip of the finger by the first digit of the number at the base of the finger. Half-hundred flows such as 250 gpm may be translated as 2.5.

CHAPTER 7 Mathematics for the Driver/Operator

SKILL DRILL 7-21 Performing the Hand Method Calculation
NFPA 1002, 5.2.4 (standard)

Example: Calculate the PDP for 200 ft of 2½-inch hose flowing 250 gpm through a fog nozzle up a hill with an elevation of 40 ft.

The hand method calculates the FL per 100 ft of hose. When flowing 250 gpm through a 2½-inch line, we find the number on the hand that corresponds to the flow of 250 gpm. The number 5 corresponds to this flow, so we multiply 2.5 (from the flow of 250) times 5: $2.5 \times 5 = 12.5$ per 100 ft.

From the scenario we know we have 200 ft of hose, so FL = $2 \times 12.5 = 25$ psi.

Insert the values into the formula:

$$PDP = 100\ NP + 25\ FL + 20\ EP = 145\ psi$$

If there were AL, it would have been added into the calculation.

SKILL DRILL 7-22 Performing the Hand Method Calculation for 2½-Inch Hose
NFPA 1002, 5.2.4 (standard)

Example 1: When flowing 250 gpm in 100 ft of 2½-inch hose, multiply the first digit of the flow, 250 gpm = 2.5 (found at the space between the index and middle fingers), by the corresponding multiplier of 5 = 12.5 psi FL for 100 ft of 2½-inch hose.

Example 2: If flowing 300 gpm through 100 ft of 2½-inch hose, multiply the first digit of the flow, 300 gpm = 3 (found at the base of the middle finger), by the corresponding multiplier of 6 = 18 psi FL per 100 ft of 2½-inch hose.

The hand method for 2½-inch hose works so nicely because the coefficient for 2½-inch hose is 2 when using imperial units. In metric units, use the quick method for 65-mm hose. The coefficient for 65-mm hose (same as 2½-inch hose, just a different name) is 1 if you use 30-m lengths, which makes things even easier. The FL for each 30-m length of 65-mm hose can be determined by dividing the flow in L/min by 100 and squaring that number to obtain the FL in kPa. This is the same as setting both C and L equal to 1 in the FL equations.

To perform the hand method calculation for 1¾-inch hose, follow the steps in **SKILL DRILL 7-23**. Note that there is no simple metric equivalent to this method.

SKILL DRILL 7-23 Using the Hand Method Calculation for 1¾-Inch Hose
NFPA 1002, 5.2.4 (standard)

Example: When flowing 150 gpm, note that 150 gpm is the middle finger and has the number 3 at the tip and the number 12 at the base. When multiplied, $3 \times 12 = 36$ psi FL in 100 ft of 1½-inch hose. The exact FL would be 34.875 psi per 100 ft of 1¾-inch hose.

1. Start with the left hand open and the thumb on the left.
2. Assign the flow in gpm to the base of each finger, from left to right, in 25-gpm increments, designating the thumb as 100 gpm, then 125 gpm, 150 gpm, 175 gpm, and finally 200 gpm on the little finger.
3. Assign numbers to the tips of the fingers beginning with the thumb as 1, then 2, 3, 4, and 5 on the little finger.
4. Assign the multiplier number of 12 to the base of the thumb, and to the base of each of the other fingers.
5. To calculate the FL for a given flow through a 1¾-inch hose, find the gpm on the hand, and multiply the number at the tip times the number at the bottom of the finger.
6. The hand method calculates the FL per 100 ft of hose only. Multiply this value times the length and add any AL loss, elevation gain/loss, and NP to find the correct PDP.

Subtract 10 Method (gpm Flowing Method)

The subtract 10 method determines FL in 2½-inch hose only and for flows of 160 gpm or greater. It is useful for either fog or smooth-bore nozzles. The simplicity of this method is its strength; using this technique, you can determine FL in 2½-inch hose very quickly. To use this method, follow the steps in **SKILL DRILL 7-24**. Note that there is no simple metric equivalent to this method.

1. Assume a flow of 200 gpm in a 2½-inch line.
2. Subtract 10 from the first two digits of the flow to obtain the FL per 100 ft of hose: 200 gpm = 20 − 10 = 10 psi FL per 100 ft.
3. If flowing 250 gpm, subtract 10 from 25 = 15 psi FL per 100 ft.
4. If flowing 300 gpm, subtract 10 from 30 = 20 psi FL per 100 ft.
5. After obtaining the FL, multiply it times the number of 100-ft sections and add AL, EP (if any), and NP to arrive at the PDP.

Condensed Q Method

The **condensed Q method** is a quick method for calculating FL per 100 ft in 3-inch to 5-inch hoseline only. It is especially useful when the apparatus is part of a relay operation and is supplying another pumper. Note that there is no simple metric equivalent to this method. The condensed Q formulas are as follows:

$$\text{3-inch hose FL} = Q^2$$
$$\text{3½-inch hose FL} = Q^2/3$$
$$\text{4-inch hose FL} = Q^2/5$$
$$\text{5-inch hose FL} = Q^2/15$$

To use the condensed Q method, follow the steps in **SKILL DRILL 7-25**:

1. Use the appropriate formula for the size hose.
2. To calculate FL in 3-inch hose, use the formula $FL = Q^2$.
3. When flowing 300 gpm, $Q^2 = 3^2 = 9$ psi FL per 100 ft of hose.
4. To calculate FL in 3½-inch hose, use the formula $FL = Q^2/3$. For example, when flowing 300 gpm through 3½-inch hose, $Q^2/3 = 3^2/3$ or $9/3 = 3$ psi per 100 ft of 3½-inch hose.
5. To calculate FL in 4-inch hose, use the formula $FL = Q^2/5$. For example, when flowing 500 gpm, $Q^2/5 = 5^2/5 = 25/5 = 5$ psi per 100 ft of 4-inch hose.
6. To calculate FL in 5-inch hose, use the formula $Q^2/15$. For example, when flowing 700 gpm, $Q^2/15 = 7^2/15 = 49/15 = 3.2$ or 3 psi per 100 ft of 5-inch hose.

SKILL DRILL 7-24 Using the Subtract 10 Method (gpm Flowing Method)
NFPA 1002, 5.2.4 (standard)

Example 1: Calculate the PDP for 300 ft of 2½-inch hose with a 1-inch smooth-bore tip. The 1-inch tip flows 200 gpm and has a NP of 50 psi. Subtract 10 from the first two digits of the flow:

For 200 gpm: 20 − 10 = 10 psi FL per 100 ft
300 ft of hose with 10 psi loss per 10 ft = 30 psi FL
PDP = NP + FL = 50 + 30 = 80 psi

Example 2: Do the same problem using the Q formula.

$FL = C Q^2 L$ or $2 \times (2)^2 \times 3 = 24$ psi FL
PDP = 50 + 24 = 74 psi

© LiquidLibrary

DRIVER/OPERATOR Tip

As an alternative calculation on the fireground when supplying 5-inch hose, some fire fighters use a 5-inch condensed Q formula of FL = $Q^2/10$, simply because the lengths and gpm are easily divided by 10. For example, if the flow is 700 gpm, $Q^2/10 = 7^2/10$ or 49/10 = 5 psi per 100 ft of 5-inch hose. A calculation using the relationship $Q^2/10$ would result in 3.26 psi per 100 ft of hose. Approximations allow you to set up the scene quickly.

■ The Condensed Q Method in a Relay Operation

When two pumpers arrive at a fire scene at the same time or within seconds of each other, the first pumper often positions itself for attack while the other lays a line from the attack pumper to the hydrant to establish the water supply. In a rural setting, it is often essential to establish a relay operation owing to a lack of hydrants or a long distance to a hydrant.

Whenever one pumper is supplying another apparatus, the operator of the supply pumper must quickly calculate the PDP for the supply line to the attack pumper. Because most fire departments use a supply line with a diameter in the range of 3-inch to 5-inch, the condensed Q method is a quick and easy way to determine the PDP.

For example, suppose Engine 1 is on a hydrant and is supplying 600 ft of 5-inch hose to Engine 2, which is pumping 1200 gpm. What is the PDP for Engine 1? Engine 1 needs to know only the size and length of the hose and the rate at which Engine 2 is flowing water. It does not matter which hose configuration Engine 2 is using; instead, Engine 1 needs to know the total flow so Q can be determined. The driver operator for Engine 2 tells the driver/operator of Engine 1 on the radio that he is flowing 1200 gpm. The driver/operator for Engine 1 will calculate the FL for the 5-inch hose with the knowledge that Q = 12. As there is no NP, the driver/operator should allow 20 psi for the intake into Engine 2 and insert this value in place of NP.

Calculating PDP Using the Q Formula:
PDP = NP + FL
PDP = **20** + FL
FL = C Q^2 L
FL = 0.08 × $(12)^2$ × 6
FL = 0.08 × 144 × 6 = 69.12 or 70 psi
PDP = 20 + 70 = **90** psi

Alternative: Calculating PDP Using the Condensed Q–Formula:

With 5-inch FL = $Q^2/15$:
FL = $12^2/15$ = 144/15 = 9.6 per 100 ft
FL = 9.6 × 6 = 57.6
PDP = 20 + 58 = 78 psi or **80 psi**

With 5-inch FL = $Q^2/10$:
FL = $12^2/10$ = 144/10 = 14 per 100 ft
FL = 14 × 6 = 84 psi
PDP = 20 + 84 = **104 psi**

Although the numbers vary, from this example you can see that the condensed Q method will quickly present a close workable calculation.

■ Preincident Plan

When developing a suppression strategy, there is no more useful tool than knowledge of the target structure and a well-developed <u>**preincident plan**</u>. When conducted with permission from the property owner and at a convenient time, a preincident survey yields valuable information to the fire department's knowledge base. The resulting preincident plan data may be stored on paper, in a book, on the station computer, or in the onboard computer on the fire apparatus. Gathering building blueprints or diagrams and as much relevant data as possible during the survey process will enrich the plan.

The FDC on the structure, for example, may indicate whether it serves the standpipe system or the sprinkler system, or both. It may indicate the pump pressures required and the maximum pressure allowed by the system. It may also indicate which wing or part of a building the FDC serves.

Information collected as part of preincident planning and the knowledge gained by the company while conducting the preplanning process are priceless assets. This information and experience will better prepare the company and department for an emergency response.

■ Determining Additional Water from a Hydrant

It is possible to estimate the amount of water that is available from a fire hydrant and, therefore, to determine how many more additional attack lines the hydrant can supply. This kind of calculation can be very useful in situations where fire hydrants are limited and/or the fire flow required is so great that you must maximize the hydrants available. It is not intended to be exact but rather a true estimate of the available water. The driver/operator must always ensure that the pump is operating within the limits established by the department.

To calculate the available water from a hydrant, use the first-digit method. This method provides an easy calculation that can be done in the field and yields a quick estimate of the available water.

1. Determine the static pressure from the hydrant on the master intake gauge (intake pressure from the hydrant when not flowing water).
2. Flow the first attack line(s) and determine the gpm flowing.
3. Determine the residual pressure from the hydrant on the master intake gauge (intake pressure left over after the first attack lines are flowing).
4. Subtract the residual pressure from the static pressure.
5. Multiply the first digit of the static pressure by 1, 2, or 3 to determine the number of additional lines of equal flow that can be added. If the first digit of the static pressure multiplied by 1 is equal to or less than the difference between the static and residual pressures, the hydrant will supply three times the gpm

currently flowing. If the first digit of the static pressure multiplied by 2 is equal to or less than the difference between the static and residual pressures, the hydrant will supply two times the gpm currently flowing. If the first digit of the static pressure multiplied by 3 is equal to or less than the difference between the static and residual pressures, the hydrant will supply one times the gpm currently flowing.

For example, suppose the static pressure is 80 psi from the hydrant and the driver flows several attack lines with a total flow of 300 gpm. The residual pressure is now 70 psi. The hydrant would be capable of supplying two times the amount currently flowing or another 600 gpm.

1. The static pressure is 80 psi.
2. The lines are currently flowing 300 gpm.
3. The residual pressure is 70 psi.
4. Subtract the residual pressure from the static pressure (80 − 70 = 10).
5. The first digit of the static pressure (80) is **8**. When this digit is multiplied by 1 (8 × 1 = 8), the result is not more than or equal to the difference between the static and residual (10). When multiplied by 2 (8 × 2 = 16), the result is more than or equal to the difference between the static and residual pressure (10). Therefore, the hydrant can safely flow twice the amount of water it is currently flowing.

Wrap-Up

Chief Concepts

- Fire service hydraulic calculations are used to determine the required pump discharge pressure (PDP) for fireground operations.
- Fighting fire with water successfully is a matter of water flow rate versus heat release rate.
- Sufficient flow must be applied to overcome the heat generated by the fire.
- Friction loss is the pressure lost from turbulence as water passes through pipes, hoses, fittings, adapters, and appliances. It is measured in pounds per square inch (psi) or kilopascals (kPa).
- The pump discharge pressure (PDP) formula is PDP = NP (nozzle pressure) + FL (friction loss).
- Fire service hydraulic calculations may generally be categorized as either theoretical hydraulics or fireground hydraulics.
- Theoretical hydraulic calculations entail more exact calculations, generally require more mathematical skills, and take more time to compute.
- Away from the fireground, theoretical hydraulic calculations may be computed on paper, with a calculator, or on a computer.
- Fireground hydraulic calculations involve methods devised to estimate the needed data more quickly due to the urgency of the fire scene.
- Fireground hydraulic calculations may also be used as a backup to mental theoretical calculations, as a system to check results, and as a means to ensure reasonable accuracy.
- Fireground hydraulic calculations reinforce the learning process as the driver/operator develops the ability to compute theoretical hydraulics in the field.
- Fireground hydraulic calculations yield working approximations and are not as accurate as theoretical hydraulic computations.
- Determining the additional amount of water available from a hydrant can be very useful when attempting to maximize the hydrant's capabilities.

Hot Terms

British thermal unit (Btu) The quantity of heat required to raise the temperature of one pound of water by 1°F at the pressure of 1 atmosphere and a temperature of 60°F. A British thermal unit is equal to 1055 joules, 1.055 kilojoules, and 252.15 calories.

chart A document summarizing the typical handline and master stream calculations for the hoses, nozzles, and devices specific to the fire apparatus. It lists the most commonly used or reasonably expected hose lays.

coefficient (C) A numerical measure that is a constant for a specified hose diameter.

condensed Q method Fireground method used to quickly calculate friction loss in 3-inch (77-mm) to 5-inch (125-mm) hoselines.

critical rate of flow The essential flow, measured in gallons per minute, that is needed to overcome the heat generated by a fire.

elevation gain The pressure gained when the nozzle is below the pump; it requires pressure to be subtracted from the discharge pressure.

elevation loss The pressure lost when the nozzle is above the pump; it requires pressure to be added to the discharge pressure to compensate for the loss.

elevation pressure (EP) In hydraulic calculations, the distance the nozzle is above or below the pump.

fire department connection (FDC) A connection through which the fire department can pump supplemental water into the sprinkler system, standpipe, or other system, thereby furnishing water for fire extinguishment to supplement existing water supplies.

fireground hydraulics Simpler fireground methods for performing hydraulic calculations.

flow rate The volume of water moving through the nozzle measured in gallons per minute or liters per minute.

friction loss (FA) The reduction in pressure resulting from the water being in contact with the side of the hose. This contact requires force to overcome the drag that the wall of the hoses creates.

gating a valve Opening a valve just enough to deliver the desired pressure.

hydraulics The study of the characteristics and movement of water as they pertain to calculations for fire streams and fireground operations.

master stream A portable or fixed firefighting appliance supplied by either hoselines or fixed piping that has the capability of flowing in excess of 350 gpm (1400 L/min) of water or a water-based extinguishing agent.

net pump discharge pressure (NPDP) The amount of pressure created by the pump after receiving pressure from a hydrant or another pump.

nozzle pressure (NP) The pressure required at the inlet of a nozzle to produce the desired water discharge characteristics.

portable master stream device A master stream device that may be removed from a fire apparatus, typically to be placed in service on the ground.

Wrap-Up, continued

preincident plan A written document resulting from the gathering of general and detailed data to be used by responding personnel for determining the resources and actions necessary to mitigate anticipated emergencies at a specific facility.

prepiped elevated master stream An aerial ladder with a fixed waterway attached to the underside of the ladder, with a water inlet at the base supplying a master stream device at the tip.

pressure-regulating valve (PRV) The type of valve found in a multistory building, which is designed to limit the pressure at a discharge so as to prevent excessive elevation pressures under both flowing (residual) and nonflowing (static) conditions.

pump discharge pressure (PDP) The pressure measured at the pump discharge needed to overcome friction and elevation loss while maintaining the desired nozzle pressure and delivering an adequate fire stream.

standpipe The vertical portion of the system piping that delivers the water supply for hose connections, and sprinklers on combined systems, vertically from floor to floor in a multistory building. Alternatively, the horizontal portion of the system piping that delivers the water supply for two or more hose connections, and sprinklers on combined systems, on a single level of a building.

standpipe riser The vertical portion of the system piping within a building that delivers the water supply for fire hose connections, and sprinklers on combined systems, vertically from floor to floor in a multistory building.

standpipe system An arrangement of piping, valves, hose connections, and allied equipment with the hose connections located in such a manner that water can be discharged in streams or spray patterns through attached hose and nozzles, for the purpose of extinguishing a fire and so protecting designated buildings, structures, or property in addition to providing occupant protection as required.

theoretical hydraulics Scientific or more exact fireground calculations.

total pressure loss (TPL) Combination of friction loss, elevation loss, and appliance loss.

References

National Fire Protection Association. *NFPA Fire Protection Handbook, Fifteenth Edition*. Quincy, MA: National Fire Protection Association, 1981.

National Fire Protection Association (NFPA) 13, *Standard for the Installation of Sprinkler Systems*. 2013. http://www.nfpa.org/codes-and-standards/document-information-pages?mode=code&code=13. Accessed December 23, 2014.

National Fire Protection Association (NFPA) 14, *Standard for the Installation of Standpipe and Hose Systems*. 2013. http://www.nfpa.org/codes-and-standards/document-information-pages?mode=code&code=14. Accessed December 23, 2014.

National Fire Protection Association (NFPA) 1002, *Standard for fire Apparatus Driver/Operator Professional Qualification*. 2014. http://www.nfpa.org/codes-and-standards/document-information-pages?mode=code&code=1002.AccessedMarch27, 2014.

DRIVER/OPERATOR in action

After you explain the importance of mathematics in the fire service, your crew is dispatched a vehicle fire several blocks from the school. While operating at the fire scene, you recall some of the information that you shared with the students and review hydraulic calculations while the other members of the crew extinguish the vehicle fire.

1. What is the nozzle pressure for a hand-held smoothbore nozzle?
   A. 100 psi (700 kPa)
   B. 50 psi (350 kPa)
   C. 80 psi (560 kPa)
   D. Varies according to the manufacturer

2. What is the friction loss formula?
   A. FL = C Q² L
   B. FL = Q² C L
   C. FL = L² Q C
   D. FL = A/Q L

3. What is the pressure lost when the nozzle is above the pump called?
   A. Elevation gain
   B. Elevation pressure
   C. Elevation loss
   D. Friction loss

4. Generally, you will use a minimum of ___ psi (kPa) friction loss in calculations for all master stream appliances.
   A. 10 psi (70 kPa)
   B. 15 psi (105 kPa)
   C. 25 psi (175 kPa)
   D. 50 psi (350 kPa)

5. Pressure-regulating valves are installed on standpipe risers where static pressures exceed ___ psi per NFPA 13.
   A. 100 (700 kPa)
   B. 150 (1034 kPa)
   C. 175 (1225 kPa)
   D. 200 (1400 kPa)

Performing Fire Apparatus Check-Out and Maintenance

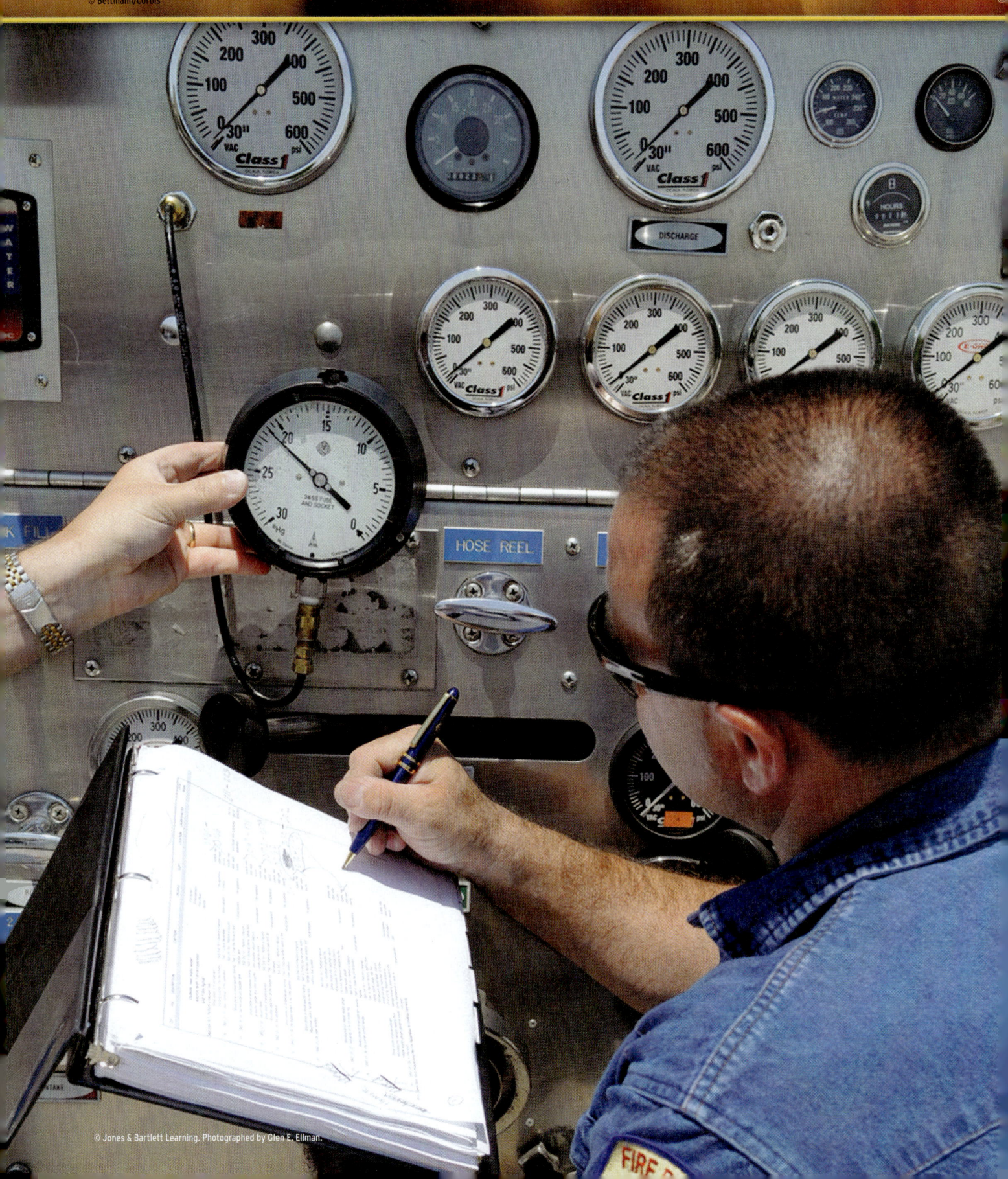

CHAPTER 8

Knowledge Objectives

After studying this chapter, you will be able to:

- Describe the inspection and maintenance procedures required by your fire department. (NFPA 1002, 4.2, 4.2.1, 4.2.1(A), 5.1.1, 5.1.1(A), 6.1.1, 6.1.1(A), 10.1.1, 10.1.1(A)); p 168–187)
- Describe the inspection and maintenance procedures recommended by the manufacturer on each of the fire apparatus that you will be required to inspect, test, or maintain. (NFPA 1002, 4.2, 4.2.1, 4.2.1(1), 4.2.1(2), 4.2.1(3), 4.2.1(4), 4.2.1(5), 4.2.1(6), 4.2.1(7), 4.2.1(8), 4.2.1(9), 4.2.1(10), 4.2.1(11), 4.2.1(A), 5.1.1, 5.1.1(1), 5.1.1(2), 5.1.1(3), 5.1.1(A), 6.1.1, 6.1.1(1), 6.1.1(2), 6.1.1(3), 6.1.1(4), 6.1.1(5), 6.1.1(6), 6.1.1(7), 6.1.1(A), 10.1.1, 10.1.1(1), 10.1.1(2), 10.1.1(3), 10.1.1(4), 10.1.1(A)); p 168–187)
- Describe the items on the written inspection and maintenance forms required to be completed by your fire department. (NFPA 1002, 4.2.2, 4.2.2(A)); p 169–172, 187)
- Describe the procedures to be followed when an inspection reveals maintenance problems beyond the scope of the driver/operator's ability to remedy. (p 187)
- Describe the type of problems found during the inspection and routine maintenance of fire apparatus that warrant taking the fire apparatus or equipment out of service. (p 187)
- Describe the equipment carried on fire apparatus that requires inspection and maintenance. (NFPA 1002, 4.2.1(1), 4.2.1(2), 4.2.1(3), 4.2.1(4), 4.2.1(5), 4.2.1(6), 4.2.1(7), 4.2.1(8), 4.2.1(9), 4.2.1(10), 4.2.1(11)); p 179–181, 184–185)
- Describe the routine maintenance procedures or adjustments to be completed by the driver/operator. (p 168–185)
- Describe the maintenance procedures and items that will be performed by specially trained personnel other than the driver/operator. (p 176, 179, 187)
- Describe the process to initiate required maintenance procedures. (p 169–172)
- Describe the schedule for routine inspection and maintenance procedures for all fire apparatus and equipment that the driver/operator will be responsible for inspecting, maintaining, or testing. (p 168–187)

Skills Objectives

After studying this chapter, you will be able to:

- Perform the daily inspection of fire apparatus and equipment in a safe and effective manner. (NFPA 1002, 4.2.1, 4.2.1(1), 4.2.1(2), 4.2.1(3), 4.2.1(4), 4.2.1(5), 4.2.1(6), 4.2.1(7), 4.2.1(8), 4.2.1(9), 4.2.1(10), 4.2.1(11), 4.2.1(B), 4.2.2, 4.2.2(B), 5.1.1, 5.1.1(1), 5.1.1(2), 5.1.1(3), 5.1.1(B), 6.1.1, 6.1.1(1), 6.1.1(2), 6.1.1(3), 6.1.1(4), 6.1.1(5), 6.1.1(6), 6.1.1(7), 6.1.1(B), 10.1.1, 10.1.1(1), 10.1.1(2), 10.1.1(3), 10.1.1(4), 10.1.1(B)); p 168–187)

Additional NFPA Standards

- NFPA 1071, *Standard for Emergency Vehicle Technician Professional Qualifications*
- NFPA 1451, *Standard for a Fire and Emergency Service Vehicle Operations Training Program*
- NFPA 1901, *Standard for Automotive Fire Apparatus*
- NFPA 1911, *Standard for the Inspection, Maintenance, Testing, and Retirement of In-Service Automotive Fire Apparatus*

You Are the Driver/Operator

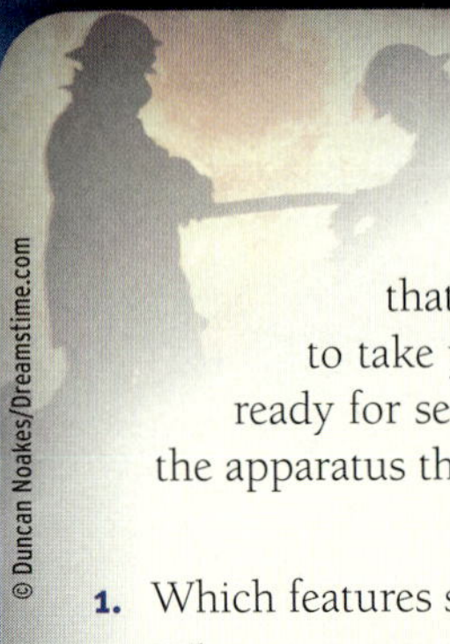

You are the driver/operator of an engine company. It is your first day on shift; your shift will last for the next 24 hours. When you talk to the driver from the preceding shift, you learn that the regular apparatus is in the maintenance shop for repairs and you have been assigned a spare apparatus for the shift. All of the spare apparatus in your department are older apparatus that have more miles on them and sometimes small issues with their operation. You know that you will have to take your time completing a very thorough apparatus inspection so that the vehicle and all of its equipment are ready for service. Before you start the inspection, you think about the differences between your original apparatus and the apparatus that you are standing in front of.

1. Which features should you inspect first?
2. What are some problems that may indicate that this fire apparatus may or may not be serviceable?
3. How are the emergency lights and sirens operated on the reserve fire apparatus?

Introduction

Being assigned as the driver/operator of a fire apparatus is a great responsibility. Duties assigned to this position include safely driving the fire apparatus and operating the equipment on the fire apparatus such as the pump or aerial device. In addition, the driver/operator is often given the responsibility to inspect and maintain the fire apparatus in as perfect condition as possible. Each fire apparatus must always be ready to respond and perform on the emergency scene in the manner for which it was designed. If the fire apparatus is equipped with a **fire pump** FIGURE 8-1, it must be capable of flowing water at the required pressures. If the fire apparatus has an **aerial device**, the driver/operator is responsible for making sure that equipment is capable of operating as required FIGURE 8-2. Maintaining the serviceability of all components of the apparatus is a key aspect of the **preventive maintenance program** that each fire department establishes for its fire apparatus. A quality preventive maintenance program ensures that the various fire apparatus in the fire department's fleet are kept in ready condition by qualified and trained personnel, the vehicles are inspected on a regular basis by the members who use the fire apparatus, and all documentation is accurate and complete.

Fire apparatus and equipment must be inspected at least weekly and within 24 hours after being used during an emergency response. Safety is the most important and obvious reason for inspecting the fire apparatus regularly. The bottom line is that the fire apparatus must be maintained in a state where it can respond to emergencies on a moment's notice FIGURE 8-3. Always be guided by your department's policies regarding apparatus inspection and maintenance.

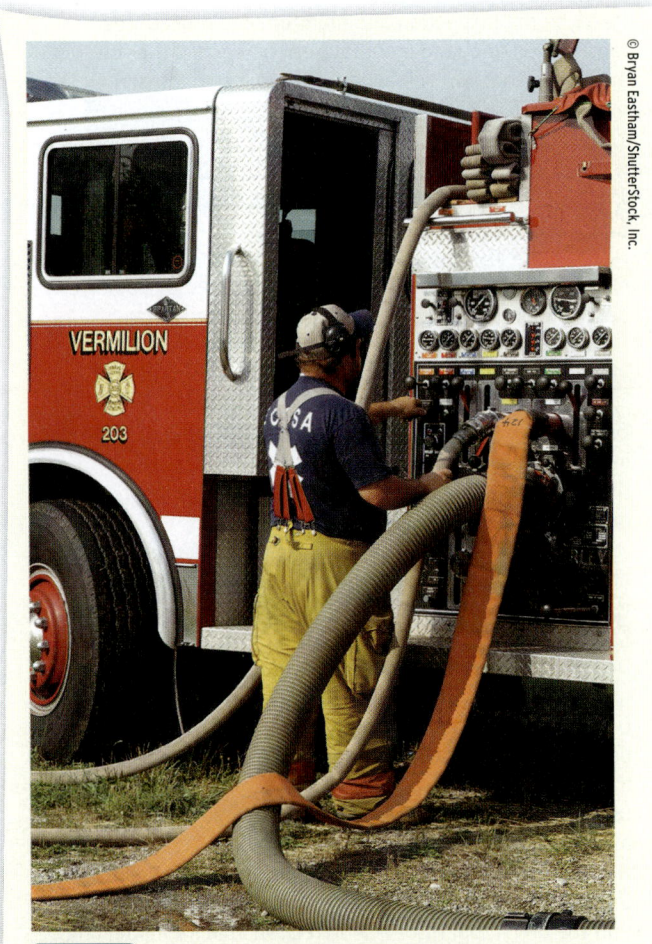

FIGURE 8-1 If the fire apparatus is equipped with a fire pump, it must be capable of flowing water at the required pressures.

FIGURE 8-2 A fire apparatus equipped with an aerial device.

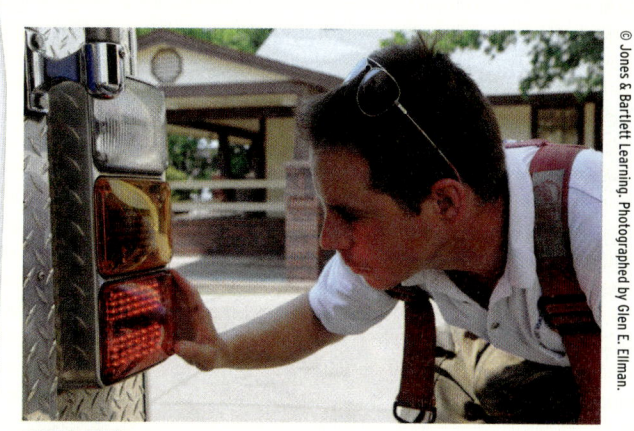

FIGURE 8-4 Some parts of the fire apparatus inspection may involve more than one crew member. Teamwork is essential to completing a thorough inspection.

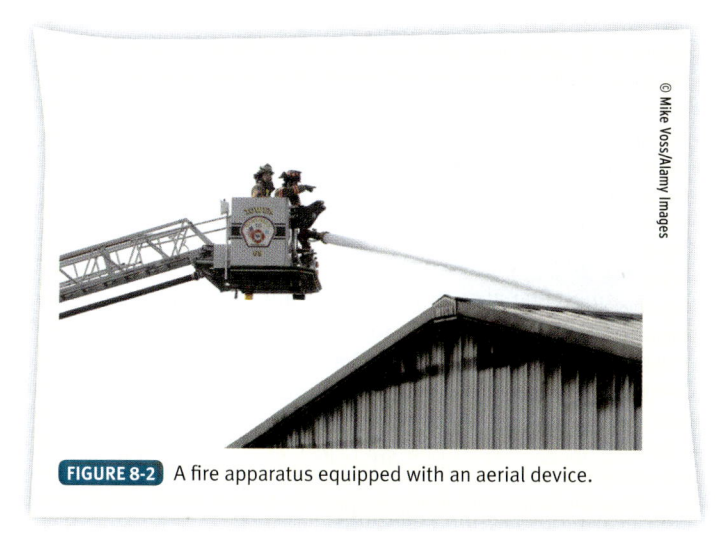

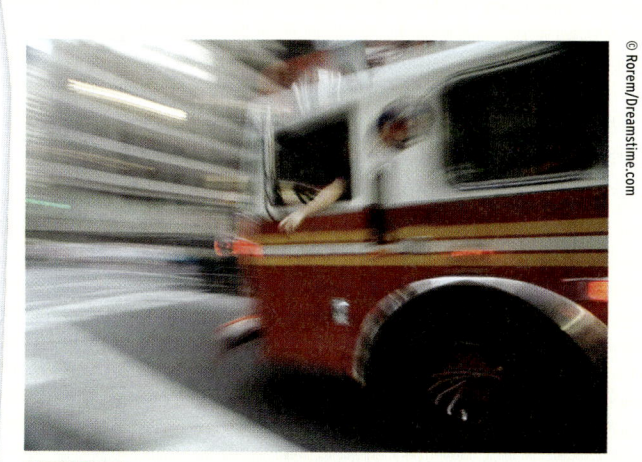

FIGURE 8-3 Fire apparatus should always be prepared to respond at a moment's notice.

Inspection

According to National Fire Protection Association (NFPA) 1451, *Standard on Fire and Emergency Service Vehicle Operations Training Program*, and NFPA 1071, *Standard for Emergency Vehicle Technician Professional Qualifications*, each department should establish and maintain a preventive maintenance program for its fleet of apparatus. A complete inspection, maintenance, and repair record for every vehicle used by the department shall be included as part of this program. These records should include the date and description of all maintenance work, repairs, and other inspections performed on the vehicle. All repairs shall be performed by a qualified person in accordance with the manufacturer's instructions.

The **fire apparatus inspection** is an evaluation of the fire apparatus and its equipment to ensure its safe operation. This inspection should be planned, methodical, and performed in an organized manner. Driver/operators typically conduct such inspections at the start of the shift, when the fire apparatus is being put back into service after repairs were made, and after a large incident during which the fire apparatus was used extensively at the scene of an emergency. This process identifies deficiencies with the fire apparatus or the equipment that might limit or incapacitate the fire apparatus from performing as required. Although most of the inspection can be performed by a single individual, thoroughly inspecting some of the features of the fire apparatus requires two crew members. For example, when inspecting the brake lights on the fire apparatus, one crew member will need to be behind the fire apparatus while the other member operates the brake pedal inside the cab **FIGURE 8-4**.

To perform the inspection, you must have some basic knowledge and skills related to vehicle maintenance. That is not to say that you should be capable of *performing* the actual maintenance of the fire apparatus; rather, you should be capable of *identifying* any potential problems before they become critical safety issues. Some fire departments prohibit their members from making any repairs on the fire apparatus, whereas other fire departments encourage fire station crews to make simple repairs to these apparatus. If the fire apparatus is under factory warranty, be aware that you may void the warranty by completing any repairs on the fire apparatus. Always refer to your fire department's inspection procedures before attempting to make any repairs to the fire apparatus.

Conducting an inspection may require using basic vehicle maintenance equipment such as tire pressure gauges, screwdrivers, wrenches, flashlights, creeper, and other small tools **FIGURE 8-5**. Every fire station should have a basic set of tools to aid the driver in performing the fire apparatus inspection. You should also have access to replacement fluids if you are required to maintain the fluid levels of the fire apparatus.

It is critical that the driver/operator performing the inspections, tests, or maintenance be familiar with the operating procedures of the fire department as well as the recommendations of the fire apparatus manufacturer. NFPA 1901, *Standard for Automotive Fire Apparatus*, requires each fire apparatus manufacturer to provide documentation of the following items for the entire fire apparatus and each major operating system of the fire apparatus:

- The manufacturer's name and address, for contact purposes
- Country of manufacture
- Source for service and technical information regarding the fire apparatus

© Jones & Bartlett Learning. Photographed by Glen E. Ellman.

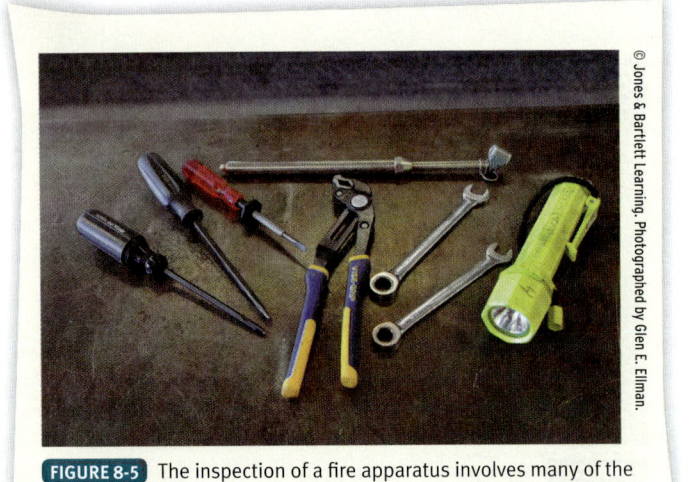

FIGURE 8-5 The inspection of a fire apparatus involves many of the same tools that you might use to maintain your personal vehicle.

- Parts replacement information
- Descriptions, specifications, and ratings of the chassis, pump (if applicable) and aerial device (if applicable)
- Wiring diagrams for low-voltage and line-voltage systems
- Lubrication charts
- Operating instructions for the chassis, any major components such as a pump or aerial device, and any auxiliary systems
- Precautions related to multiple configurations of aerial devices, if applicable
- Instructions regarding the frequency and procedure for recommended maintenance
- Overall fire apparatus operating instructions
- Safety considerations
- Limitations of use
- Inspection procedures
- Recommended service procedures
- Troubleshooting guide
- Fire apparatus body, chassis, and other component manufacturers' warranties
- Copies of required manufacturer test data or reports, manufacturer certifications, and independent third-party certifications of test results
- A material safety data sheet (MSDS) for any fluid that is specified for use on the fire apparatus

As a driver/operator, you should use the fire department's procedures and the manufacturer's recommendations as a reference to help you properly maintain the fire apparatus. For example, if the fluid level is low in a radiator cooling system, should you add water or antifreeze coolant? If the oil level is found to be low following a **dip stick** test, which type of oil should be added? Specific fluids are required to ensure proper functioning of specific systems. For instance, oil for a hydraulic system may need to be of a different type or viscosity than oil for the engine. Likewise, the transmission will likely require a different type of oil than either the engine or the hydraulic system. You must adhere to the manufacturer's specifications when adding fluids to the fire apparatus; otherwise, you risk damaging the equipment. Each department is responsible for educating members on how to properly maintain its fire apparatus.

Before you are assigned to perform the task of inspecting the fire apparatus, it is critical that the tasks are made clear and are well understood. It is also important that you consider your safety. Loosening a **radiator cap** on a hot engine, for example, may lead to a sudden release of hot liquid and steam. Working near a running engine may cause a shirt sleeve or body part to become entangled in a belt. Getting battery acid on your skin will cause burns and could damage your eyesight if this corrosive fluid gets into your eyes. Each department is responsible for training its members on how to inspect a fire apparatus both safely and thoroughly. Always wear the appropriate personal protective equipment (PPE) while performing the fire apparatus inspection, including safety glasses, work gloves, and hearing protection FIGURE 8-6.

Safety Tip

© Photos.com

When performing any maintenance functions on the fire apparatus or equipment, appropriate safety precautions must always be taken. Appropriate eye protection, hand protection, hearing protection, and inspection procedures must be utilized.

© Jones & Bartlett Learning. Photographed by Glen E. Ellman.

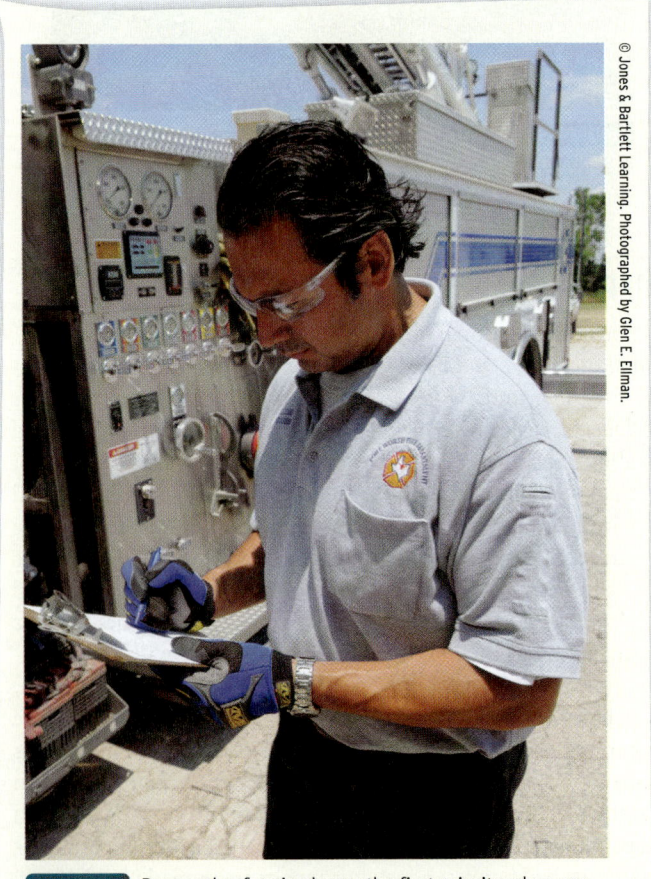

FIGURE 8-6 Personal safety is always the first priority when conducting an inspection of a fire apparatus.

CHAPTER 8 Performing Fire Apparatus Check-Out and Maintenance

DRIVER/OPERATOR Tip

If the inspection form is not organized in a logical format and process, then the inspection will not be performed properly. Make sure you take the time to organize the process you will use to complete the inspection process. As an example, similar items that will be examined in one process may be color-coded on the inspection form. Groupings such as electrical system components, drive-train components, pump-related components, and so on can all be logical methods of organizing your inspection. Being organized can help you manage your time effectively and ensure that items are not overlooked.

Inspection Process

The inspection process should begin with a review of the apparatus inspection form that was completed after the previous inspection FIGURE 8-7. This document identifies who performed the inspection and when it was performed. It also identifies any equipment that is damaged or has been repaired and points out any other preventive maintenance procedures performed on the fire apparatus. For example, the last member who inspected the fire apparatus may have documented items such as "one quart oil added to the engine," "right rear outside dual tire low and reinflated to the correct pounds per square inch (psi)/kilopascal (kPa)," and "right rear warning light located on top

DAILY ENGINE INSPECTION SHEET

Week of _____ Unit I.D. _____ Shop # _____

Date:

	Mon.	Tues.	Wed.	Thurs.	Fri.	Sat.	Sun.
Name:							
Knox box serial number							
Fuel level							
Motor oil							
Radiator							
Wipers							
Gauges							
Brakes							
Starter							
Lights/siren							
Generator							
Mirrors							
Body condition							
Water level							
Pump controls/gauges							
Press control device							
Hydrant tools							
Hose/nozzles							
Appliances							
Tools/ladders							
SCBA—PPE							
Radios							
Box-lights							
Map-books/computer							
Keys							
Accountability							
Clipboard							
Tire pressure							
Batteries							
Transmission fluid							
Bleed air tanks							
Primer fluid							
Drain valves							
Tool box							
Power toolsw							

Comments:

FIGURE 8-7 The fire apparatus inspection form is essential for maintaining an accurate record of the condition of the fire apparatus.

rail not working and bulb replaced by mechanic." If during your inspection process you note that the engine is low on oil again, this finding may indicate some type of ongoing mechanical problem or leak. If the rear right dual tire is low again, it could indicate the tire is leaking and in need of repairs.

In many fire departments, the fire apparatus inspection form is simply attached to a clipboard and stored in the station, usually in the main office. Other departments may have an electronic version of the fire apparatus inspection form and use a computer program to track the inspections of their fire apparatus. Either way, the driver/operator must review this material before beginning the inspection. If the driver/operator does not take the time to examine the previous inspection report, some information identified in the current inspection may not seem relevant. Driver/operators from different shifts should also communicate to one another about the fire apparatus and any problems they encounter. Sometimes talking to the other members of the fire department who inspect the same fire apparatus can help to locate a potential problem. Taken in conjunction with the information from the previous report, your inspection process could reveal a need for an appropriate mechanic or qualified person to inspect the vehicle for defects.

Next, you must perform the actual inspection of the fire apparatus. This investigation may take some time depending on the size and complexity of the fire apparatus and its components. Fire apparatus inspections should be performed in a systematic manner. In other words, you should perform the inspection the same way each time to reduce the likelihood that you will miss something. While you are conducting your survey, the fire apparatus should be located in a safe area—either inside the fire apparatus bay, on the fire station driveway, or on an open lot devoid of traffic. The fire apparatus should be parked on a flat, level surface if possible. Check the area around the fire apparatus to determine if it is safe to operate the various components of the fire apparatus, such as lifting the cab of the fire apparatus or lowering the ladder rack on the side of the apparatus **FIGURE 8-8**.

During the inspection process, you should thoroughly document your findings on the fire apparatus inspection report. This step will help ensure that all documentation is as accurate as possible and no items are overlooked. Most of the items are inspected visually. When performing this step, you are looking for any signs of damage, excessive wear, or defects. Some items must be operated during the inspection to ensure they function properly. For example, the emergency lights can be inspected visually by simply turning them on and walking around the fire apparatus looking for any inoperable lights.

Remember, it does not always take a mechanic to recognize a problem. By visually inspecting and operating the equipment during every shift, you will become familiar with the fire apparatus and its normal condition. You will then be able to quickly recognize when components break down or are in need of maintenance and can recommend the fire apparatus undergo repairs when necessary. Always be guided by your fire department's policies regarding fire apparatus inspections, and do not be afraid to ask for a second opinion if you are unsure about something you find in the inspection.

After the inspection is complete, review the report and make sure that no items were missed. Many fire departments require their members to complete the inspection of the fire apparatus by a certain time each day or else face disciplinary actions. The inspection of fire apparatus should be taken very seriously—because it *is* a serious matter. Failure to complete a thorough inspection may result in an unsafe fire apparatus operating on the road and the emergency scene.

DRIVER/OPERATOR Tip

Each fire department's fire apparatus inspection forms should reflect the policies of the fire department and identify which items need to be checked. Some fire departments have set up inspection procedures that include items to be inspected daily, items to be inspected weekly, items to be inspected monthly, and items to be inspected quarterly.

While you may be responsible for the daily and weekly items, fire officers may be responsible for carrying out the more comprehensive inspections, tests, or maintenance procedures to be performed. For example, the fire officer may be accountable for scheduling the annual fire hose and ground ladder tests for the fire apparatus, although it is your responsibility as the driver/operator to ensure that the equipment is prepared for this inspection. You must be familiar with all of your fire department's required inspection and maintenance procedures.

DRIVER/OPERATOR Tip

A good inspection of a fire apparatus will get you dirty. If you do not walk into the station after checking out the fire apparatus with dirt and grease from your elbows to your fingertips, then you probably did not do an adequate inspection.

Fire Apparatus Sections

Often the inspection process is broken down into sections. Dividing the inspection in this way allows you to focus on a single aspect of the fire apparatus and discourages you from jumping from one element of the inspection to another without

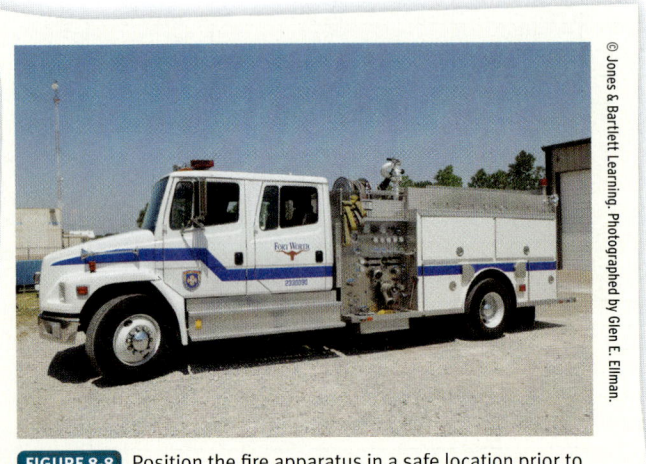

FIGURE 8-8 Position the fire apparatus in a safe location prior to starting the inspection process.

a plan. Jumping around randomly leads to the possibility that critical elements may be missed. Each driver/operator should use whatever system or sequence is recommended by his or her fire department.

The following is a suggested fire apparatus inspection procedure that has been broken down into several sections. The first five sections apply to all fire apparatus. The last two apply only to those fire apparatus that meet the criteria for that section. Not all of the items in each section will apply to every fire apparatus; it is up to the driver/operator to determine which items are applicable to his or her fire apparatus. These sections should be inspected in the following order unless otherwise stated by your fire department:

- Exterior inspection
- Engine compartment
- Cab interior
- Brake inspection
- General tools/equipment inspection
- Pump inspection
- Aerial device inspection

■ Exterior Inspection

The first section to be completed is the inspection of the fire apparatus exterior. Physically walk around and look at the fire apparatus' general condition. Is the fire apparatus clean and well maintained, or is it worn and in need of several minor repairs? Determine whether the fire apparatus is leaning to one side; this may indicate a broken suspension system or tires not inflated to the correct pressure. Visually inspect under the fire apparatus for any fresh oil, coolant, or other fluid leaks. Check for any damage to the body such as dents, scratches, and paint chips. Look for signs of stress or cracks on the body. Inspect the compartment doors, hinges, and latches for proper operation.

DRIVER/OPERATOR Tip

As part of the exterior inspection, you may need to tilt the cab or crawl under the fire apparatus to properly inspect the items.

Safety Tip

If the fire apparatus will be moved outside to the apron for engine and pump operation, first make sure it is safe to do so. Confirm that all compartment doors are closed, all personal protective equipment is secure, and all cab doors are closed. Whenever the vehicle is operated inside the station, make sure that it is connected to an **extractor exhaust system**—a system designed to draw the fire apparatus exhaust to the outside so that it does not fill the fire apparatus bay with harmful gases. When the inspection is complete, before backing the vehicle into the station, verify that no one is behind the fire apparatus and have a spotter maintain a visual observation behind the fire apparatus while it is operating in reverse.

Tires are critical to many aspects of the safe operation of the fire apparatus—namely, proper stability of the fire apparatus, stopping capability, and ability to carry loads. When inspecting the tires, use a flashlight to get a better look at their overall condition. It is very dangerous to drive with tires in bad condition. Look for problems such as cuts, cracks, or fabric showing through the tread or sidewall.

The valve stems on all tires should be accessible and devoid of cracks and cuts, with the valve caps securely fastened. The size and make of all tires should match those recommended by the manufacturer. Dual tires should not be in contact with each other or with other parts of the fire apparatus. Determine whether the tread on the tire is wearing unevenly, as this may indicate a possible problem with the suspension system, an issue related to the steering system, or inflation of the tire to an incorrect pressure. When inspecting the wear, the tire should have at least $4/32$ inch (3 mm) of tread depth in every major groove on all tires on turning axles and $2/32$ inch (2 mm) of tread depth on drive axles. U.S. coins can be substituted for a tire tread depth gauge as tires wear to the critical final few thirty-secondths of an inch of their remaining tread depth. To use this technique for measuring tread depth, place a quarter into several tread grooves across the tire. If part of George Washington's head is always covered by the tread, the tire has more than $4/32$ inch (3 mm) of tread depth remaining.

Refer to the manufacturer's recommendations to determine the appropriate tire pressures for each fire apparatus. Using a pressure gauge, check the tire pressure by removing the valve cap and applying the pressure gauge. If the tire pressure is adequate per the manufacturer's or department's specifications, then return the valve cap. If the tire pressure is low, then use an air hose to inflate the tire to the correct pressure. Check the tire again to obtain the pressure level. If necessary, add more air until the desired pressure level is obtained. Replace the valve cap and note that air was added to the tire on the inspection form.

A damaged wheel or rim can cause a tire to lose pressure or even slip off. This event can cause a motor vehicle accident if it occurs while the apparatus is operating on the roadway. Look for any sign of damage, including dents or large scratches along the edge that meets the tire. If rust is found around the wheel nuts, it may be an indication that the nuts are loose and need to be retightened. The wheel should not be missing any clamps, spacers, studs, lugs, or protective covers. Stainless wheel covers could hide a dangerous situation. If your apparatus has these, they should be removed to thoroughly check the rims.

Today's fire apparatus are equipped with a **power steering system**. This system reduces the effort required to steer the vehicle by using an external power source to assist in turning the apparatus' wheels. While inspecting the steering system, look for any bent, loose, or broken parts, such as the steering column or tie rods. With the engine compartment exposed, examine the power steering pump, hoses, and fittings for leaks. While in the cab of the fire apparatus, inspect the amount of free play in the steering wheel. If the steering wheel has more than 10 degrees of free play, a mechanic should service the fire apparatus. Ten degrees of free play is equivalent to 2 inches (51 mm) of movement at the rim of a 20-inch (51-cm) steering wheel **FIGURE 8-9**.

FIGURE 8-9 Ten degrees of play is equivalent to 2 inches (51 mm) of movement at the rim of a 20-inch (51-cm) steering wheel.

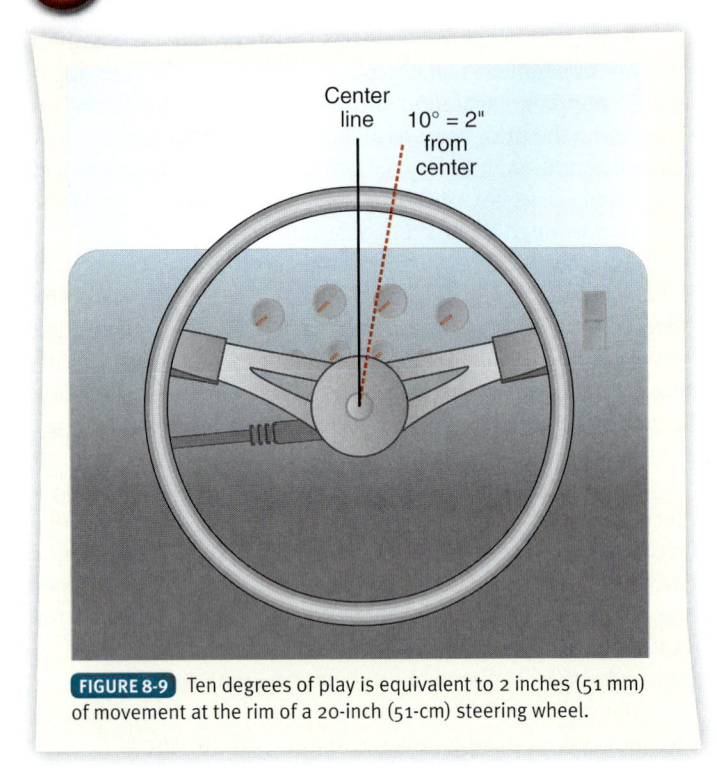

The suspension system keeps the vehicle's axles in place and holds up the fire apparatus and its load. A defect in this system may cause problems with the fire apparatus' braking or power steering system. Inspect the frame assembly to ensure that no parts are cracked, loose, broken, or missing. Look for any spring hangers or other axle positioning parts that are broken and might allow the axle to move out of position. Also, look for any broken sections or sections that have shifted out of place in the leaf springs. Identify whether the shock absorbers are leaking fluids or are bent out of shape. Torque rods and torsion bars should be free of damage. If your apparatus is equipped with air bag suspension, check that the bags are properly inflated. If your system dumps (i.e., an ambulance), check that this system is functioning properly.

Visually inspect the fire apparatus exhaust system to check for any loose, broken, or missing mounting brackets or parts. The exhaust piping should not rub against the tires or other moving parts of the fire apparatus, and no leaks should be found. A broken exhaust system may allow poisonous fumes to enter the cab, harming the crew members who are aboard the fire apparatus.

The fuel cap should be securely fastened to prevent any spillage or fumes leaking from the tank. This cap should also be labeled with the appropriate fuel. Although larger fire apparatus use diesel fuel, some vehicles may require a specific grade or biodiesel. Always consult the operator's manual provided by the manufacturer to determine which type of fuel to add to the fire apparatus. The fuel tank should be checked to make sure that no leaks are present and the mounting brackets are properly secured.

■ Engine Compartment

This section focuses on the process of inspecting the fluid levels, battery charge, cooling system, motor components such as belts, charging system, and drive train elements. NFPA 1901 requires that all fire apparatus be designed so that the manufacturer's recommended routine maintenance checks of lubricants and fluid levels can be performed through a limited-access port without lifting the cab of the fire apparatus or without the need of special tools for routine maintenance checks of lubricants and fluid levels **FIGURE 8-10**. On most fire apparatus, you will still need to raise the cab to inspect most portions of the engine,

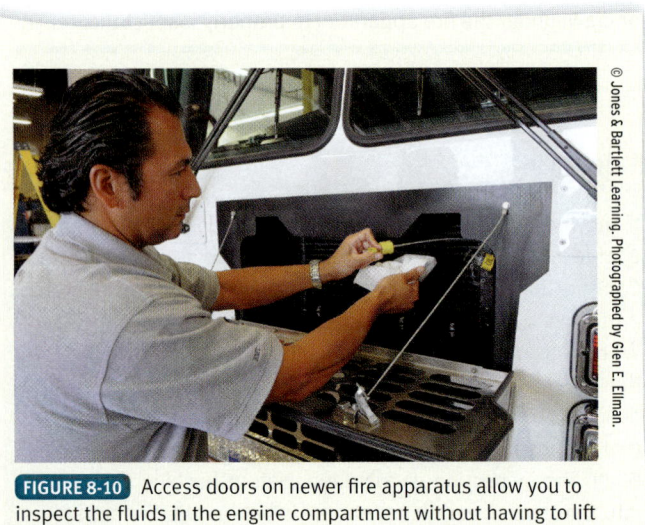

DRIVER/OPERATOR Tip

Cleanliness is a very important part of proper fire apparatus maintenance. A clean fire apparatus not only is a source of pride in the station and its crew, but also is safer than a dirty fire apparatus. Dirt and grime build-up will damage moving parts and cover defects. By keeping the fire apparatus clean, you are gaining intimate knowledge of the equipment, thereby ensuring that any defects will be identified sooner.

To clean the fire apparatus, you must first rinse it with clean water to remove any loose dirt. This action also reduces the chance of scratching the paint during the remainder of the clean-up procedure. Wash the fire apparatus with an automotive soap, as recommended by the manufacturer. The entire fire apparatus should be thoroughly washed, including the top of the cab, wheel wells, and diamond plate surfaces, among other components. Rinse the vehicle with clean water, and then dry the fire apparatus with an approved chamois or towel. All trash should be removed from the cab's interior; this compartment should then be dusted, swept, or vacuumed and dressed with the appropriate surface treatment.

Glass should be cleaned and all painted surfaces waxed as necessary after the fire apparatus is completely dry. Metal surfaces should be polished to prevent tarnish and dull surfaces. Compartments should be cleaned out and all equipment maintained as necessary. If the engine compartment is clean, it makes the inspection process easier. Never use gasoline or other unapproved solvents to clean painted surfaces, as they may cause discoloration and damage.

FIGURE 8-10 Access doors on newer fire apparatus allow you to inspect the fluids in the engine compartment without having to lift the cab.

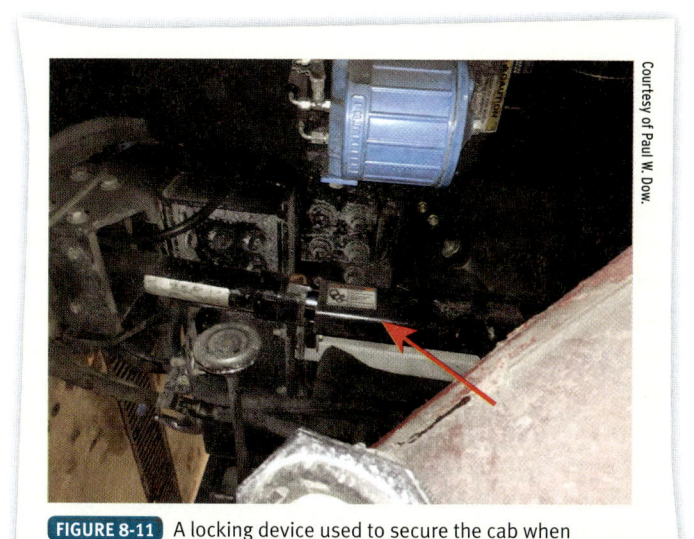

CHAPTER 8 Performing Fire Apparatus Check-Out and Maintenance 175

FIGURE 8-11 A locking device used to secure the cab when anyone is operating underneath it.

including belts, hoses, and fan blades. Older fire apparatus may not have an access door through which to check the fluids; as a consequence, the cab must be tilted to determine the fluid levels in these vehicles. If this is the case, the cab should be secured with a locking device to make that the cab cannot fall on anyone operating underneath it **FIGURE 8-11**.

While the engine is off, you can inspect the engine compartment. Examine this area for any fluid leaks; broken, cracked, or damaged hoses; and electrical wiring that shows signs of wear, chaffing, or damage from heat. Also, confirm that the cooling fan is free of any obstructions or defects. The air intake filter should be replaced as necessary and its housing should not have any cracks, loose fasteners, or broken supports.

Depending on your fire department's policy, the driver/operator may be required to maintain the appropriate fluid levels in the fire apparatus. Remember, when adding any fluids, you must record the amount on the fire apparatus inspection form. You should not rely solely on sensors and computer systems to give an accurate reading of fluid level—always physically check the fluid levels.

Be sure to consult the owner's manual or the fluid chart that was provided with the apparatus. On new apparatus, NFPA 1901 requires that a fluid chart is provided (usually in the cab or the engineer's compartment) that list types and quantities of all fluid on that particular apparatus. Most larger apparatus are using automatic transmission fluid (ATF) or motor oil-based fluids in the power steering system. The coolants in the larger apparatus have special additives that are not always found in the smaller vehicles, so just because the fluid in the apparatus is red, for example, do not assume it is the same red coolant that might be in your car.

The engine oil level is checked with a dip stick, usually after the engine has been turned off for at least 15 minutes; this delay allows the oil to settle back down and gives an accurate reading. The dip stick is pulled, wiped clean, and then replaced. It is then pulled a second time and the oil level compared to the marking on the dip stick. Generally a range is provided between "low" and "full." If the engine was operated just before the oil is checked, the dip stick level may appear low, as oil is still in the engine components and not totally drained to the crankcase. If the oil level is truly low, then the recommended amount of oil should be added via the correct port. After waiting a few minutes, check the level again to confirm that the proper level has been achieved and record the amount of oil added on the inspection form.

The coolant level should be measured, observed, or checked in the manner recommended by the manufacturer. Most systems in use today do not require the removal of the radiator cap, but rather provide an exterior coolant reservoir that is marked with the appropriate level. Some manufacturers provide a sight glass on the radiator to determine the coolant level **FIGURE 8-12**. If the coolant system is low on coolant, then you should consult your fire department's procedures to determine which coolant should be added to bring the reservoir to the proper level. Adding water will diminish the protection from freezing. Additionally, antifreeze fluid contains other materials designed to prevent rusting and act as a lubricant; it may be the only appropriate liquid to add to the cooling system. If the fire apparatus has been run recently, be aware that the coolant itself may be hot.

If you must remove the radiator cap, use caution. The coolant may be under pressure and be hot; if it boils over, it could cause an injury. For this reason, it is not recommended

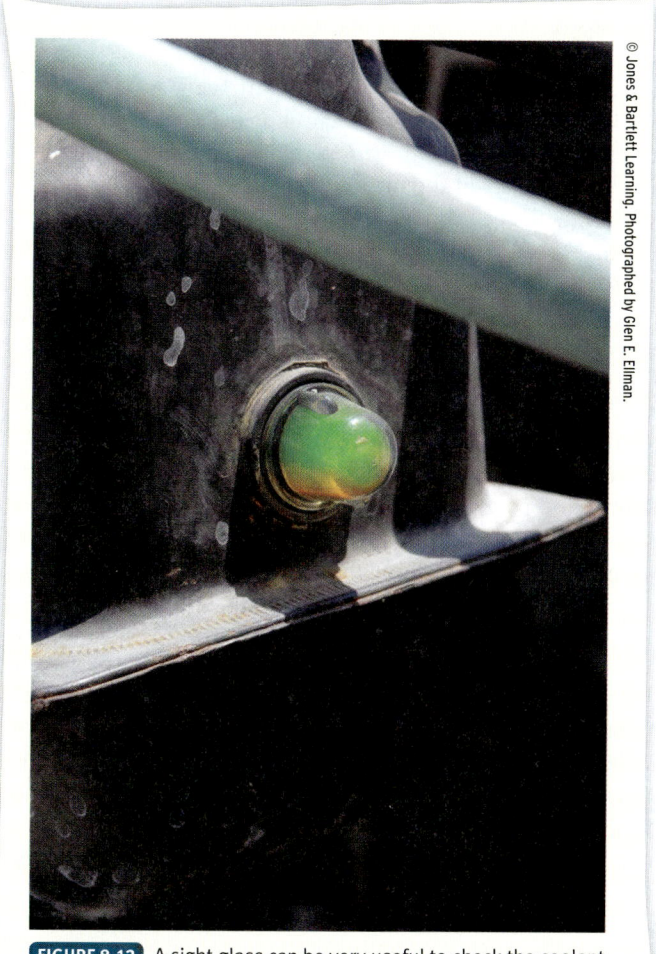

FIGURE 8-12 A sight glass can be very useful to check the coolant levels.

that you remove the cap when the fire apparatus is running or when the fire apparatus is hot.

Power steering system fluid is checked in the same way as the engine oil. A small dip stick is inserted to determine the fluid level. If it is low, add power steering fluid as required.

The transmission fluid is the only fluid that may need to be inspected while the engine is running, although some manufacturers also recommend checking power steering fluid at operating temperature. Many manufacturers recommend that the transmission be operated at the normal operating temperature (usually 170°F [77°C]) after the apparatus has run through all of its gears and that the vehicle be parked in neutral when the fluid is checked. To check the transmission fluid, use a dip stick in a similar manner as when performing an engine oil check. Most of the larger apparatus are using automatic transmissions that have the ability to check the fluid without pulling the dipstick via the keypad shift selector (consult with the owner's manual).

Other fluid levels, such as the rear differential fluid (axle), hydraulic oil, and pump gear box oil levels, are often checked by a fire department mechanic on a periodic basis. Always refer to the manufacturer's recommendations when determining the correct levels of these fluids.

Belts that drive engine components such as alternators, the power steering pump, the air compressor, and other equipment may become loose due to wear. To check the tension on a belt, push against the belt in an area where there is no pulley. Depending on the manufacturer's recommendations, the belt may be able to be pushed to some extent, but should not have any excess slack. In some fire departments, a mechanic or specially trained inspector will check items such as belts on a frequent basis; thus the driver/operator may not be required to perform this part of the inspection. Nevertheless, you should ensure that the belts do not show any signs of excessive wear or fraying. Always refer to the manufacturer's recommendations regarding belt inspections.

The fire apparatus' (one or more) batteries should be examined for signs of corrosion on the terminals where the wires connect to the battery post. When performing this part of the inspection, it is important that you protect yourself from corrosion and the liquid inside the battery. Appropriate eye, hand, and/or body protection should be provided and worn during this part of the fire apparatus inspection. Corrosion may be removed by scraping the terminal with a wire brush; always wear eye protection when performing this activity.

The physical process of removing the electrical wire connection from the terminal is normally performed by a mechanic or other person specially trained to perform this task. Given that most of today's fire apparatus have computerized systems on board, severe damage could occur if removal of the battery cables is done improperly **FIGURE 8-13**. For example, the computer system that operates the fire apparatus may have to be reset by a qualified technician if it loses power for a significant amount of time. Although older vehicle batteries may have fluid cells that can be refilled as often as needed, many newer batteries are sealed, meaning there is no way to check the fluid cells. You should refer to the manufacturer's recommendations when inspecting batteries on any fire apparatus.

Voltage levels may be checked by observing the **voltage meter** on the dashboard if the vehicle is so equipped. A voltmeter registers the voltage of the battery system. For example, the voltage of a 12-volt battery will typically be recorded as a number such as 14 volts. Batteries that are equipped with removable caps on the cells of the battery should be checked for appropriate liquid levels. Liquid should cover the cells, albeit not to overflowing. If the liquid level is low, follow the fire department's or manufacturer's recommendations regarding which liquid to use to refill the battery.

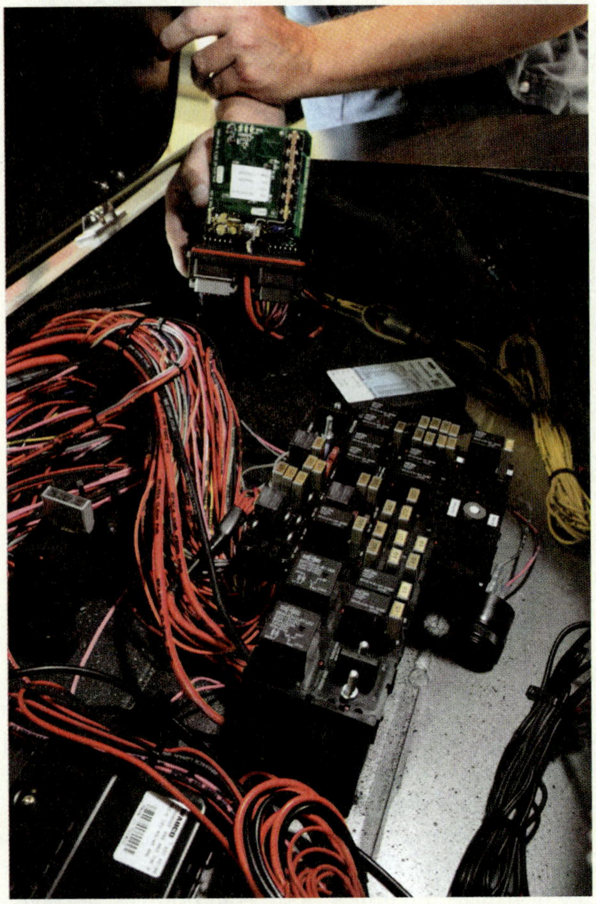

New apparatus manufactured after 2010 may have an additional tank of diesel exhaust fluid (DEF), which is 30 percent urea and 70 percent water. This fluid is used in the emission system to meet the new emission requirements. This tank will have a blue cap and will range typically from 2 to 10 gallons (8 to 38 liters) depending on the type of vehicle. The tank location will also depend on the manufacturer. Consult the owner's manual prior to refilling DEF.

■ Cab Interior

When inspecting the cab interior, first check that all cab-mounted equipment is present and accounted for, including the following items:

- Portable radios
- Self-contained breathing apparatus (SCBA)
- Maps
- Traffic vests

FIGURE 8-13 Do not disconnect the batteries on newer-model fire apparatus, as this step may cause damage to the computer system.

© Jones & Bartlett Learning. Photographed by Glen E. Ellman.

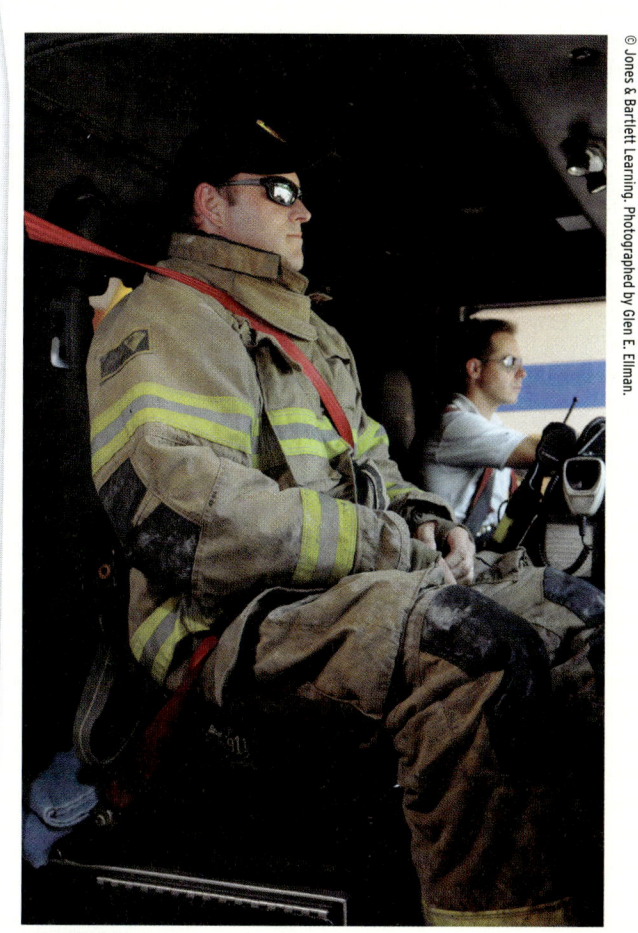

FIGURE 8-14 NFPA 1901 requires that seat belts be red or orange so that fire fighters can tell them apart from the waist belts on SCBA units.

- Hearing protection
- Medical gloves
- Box lights

Also, check for worn or torn seats, cushions, dashboards, and headliners. Ensure that all seat belts are functioning properly and are free of cuts and frays. NFPA 1901 requires that all seated positions in the modern-day fire apparatus cab be equipped with bright orange or red seat belts so they are not confused with seat-mounted SCBA belts and straps FIGURE 8-14.

The interior of the cab is where most of the controls for the fire apparatus are located. For this section of the inspection, set the parking brake and start the fire apparatus by engaging its normal starting sequence. This provides the opportunity to observe the gauges such as those measuring oil pressure, electrical system, engine temperature, and air pressure. Once you are sitting inside the cab, adjust the seat and the mirrors and familiarize yourself with the functional controls. As a driver/operator, you must be familiar with all of the controls in the cab so that you do not need to take your eyes off the road to make any adjustments while driving.

Make sure that all of the gauges indicate performance within the normal operating ranges. Each fire apparatus may have different ranges for normal operations; refer to the manufacturer's recommendations. Determine whether any indicator lights are activated and need attention. For example, if the oil light is activated and you have recently added more oil to the engine, either the sensor is faulty or another problem may exist. Check the operation of the functional control switches—that is, the controls that operate interior functions as well as those that operate exterior functions.

Interior Functional Control Switches

Interior functional control switches include the controls for items that are located inside the cab itself—for example, the heater, air conditioner, defroster, map lights, dash lights, mobile data terminal (MDT), radio, and other devices. All of these items should be inspected to ensure that they are operating correctly. Some fire departments require members to check the MDT and radio to confirm that they are transmitting information appropriately. Always refer to your department's policies when conducting this part of the fire apparatus inspection.

Exterior Functional Control Switches

Exterior functional control switches include the controls for items that are located outside of the cab but are operated from controls in the cab—for example, the emergency lights, headlights, directional lights, brake lights, side marker lights, spotlights, and taillights. All of the lights should be clean and operating correctly. To inspect the lights of the fire apparatus, you must activate the lights and walk around the fire apparatus visually inspecting their operation FIGURE 8-15. Another fire fighter should assist you in checking the brake and reverse lights.

Check the mirrors, windows, and windshield. All of the windows of the fire apparatus should be clean and free of cracks or chips. If any defects are found during the inspection, document them on the report. All of the windows should roll down properly, whether they are manually or electronically controlled. Windshield wipers and fluid level should be checked as well. The wiper blades should be soft, flexible, and clean. If the blades are too hard or cracked, then they should be replaced. The wiper fluid level should be topped off with the appropriate liquid as recommended by the manufacturer.

© Jones & Bartlett Learning. Photographed by Glen E. Ellman.

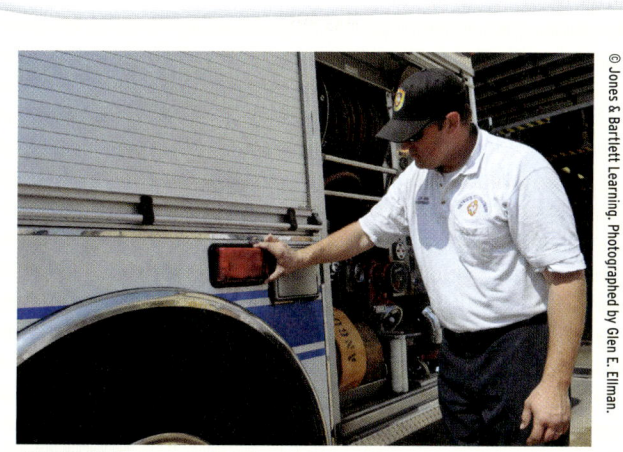

FIGURE 8-15 You will have to walk around the fire apparatus and visually inspect the operation of the lights on the fire apparatus.

DRIVER/OPERATOR Tip

The emergency warning equipment must be checked to confirm that all components are functioning appropriately. Driving lights (head, tail, marker) and warning lights should be checked for appropriate function, and audible warning devices should be tested to ensure they operate correctly. Likewise, all other electrical equipment—such as scene lighting devices and traffic directional arrows—should be tested to verify that they are functioning correctly. If the emergency lights do not operate properly, for example, the fire apparatus is not capable of operating safely during an emergency response.

■ Brake Inspection

The brakes of the fire apparatus should receive special attention during the driver/operator's inspection, as this equipment is clearly vital to the safe and efficient operation of the fire apparatus. First, you should inspect the brakes for the following conditions: cracked drums or rotors; shoes or pads contaminated with oil, grease, or brake fluid; and shoes or pads that are worn dangerously thin, missing, or broken. Next, you should test the brakes of the apparatus. Your department's policies and procedures will dictate if and when the following tests are to be completed.

DRIVER/OPERATOR Tip

The vehicle's fuel level can easily be checked by observing the fuel gauge when the electrical system is energized. Be familiar with your fire department's policies stating when the fuel tank must be replenished or topped off. Many fire departments have a policy that states the fuel level for any fire apparatus should never go below half a tank.

Parking Brake Test

NFPA 1901 requires the parking brake to hold the apparatus on a 20 percent grade. The best way to check the parking brake is to place the apparatus on a 20 percent grade and apply the parking brake. If the brakes do not hold the apparatus in place, the vehicle needs to be removed from service. Applying the parking brake while moving causes damage to the brake system.

Brake Pedal Test

National Federal Motor Carrier requires that vehicles stop at 20 mph (32 km/h) within 35 ft (10 m). The brake pedal test should be part of the vehicle inspection. When the brake pedal is pushed firmly, if the fire apparatus demonstrates excessive pulling to one side or the other, if it exhibits a delayed stopping action, or if the "feel" of the pedal is off, this may indicate a potential problem. In such a case, have the fire apparatus inspected by a qualified mechanic.

The following tests are applicable only to fire apparatus equipped with air brake systems. Your department's policies and procedures will dictate if and when the following tests are to be completed. Those vehicles without air brake systems may not be required to complete any additional brake tests. For the following tests, you should chock both sides of the front left wheel with the fire apparatus' wheel chocks **FIGURE 8-16**.

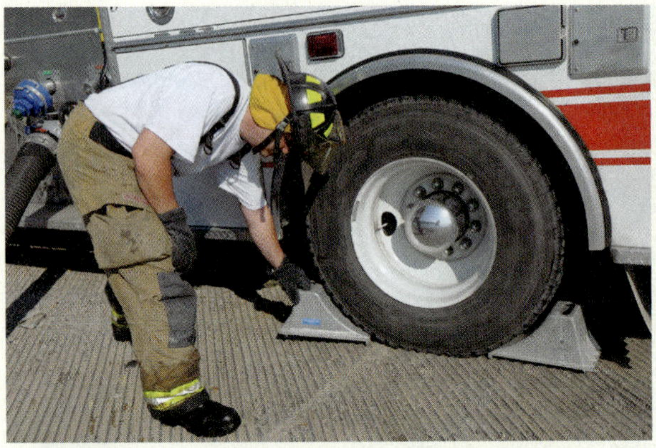

FIGURE 8-16 Chock the wheels of the fire apparatus when conducting a dual air brake system warning and buzzer test.

Air Brake System Warning Light and Buzzer Test

Many fire apparatus are operated with an air brake system. With this system, a mechanically operated parking brake is activated in the event of a service brake failure. An air brake system actually consists of two separate air brake systems, primary and secondary, that use a single set of brake controls—a setup that provides more air capacity and, therefore, a safer system. Each system has its own air tank and hoses; they are split so that one system operates the front of the fire apparatus and the other operates the rear. On the dash of the fire apparatus, the gauges for each system are labeled as "front" and "rear," respectively.

To complete the test, follow these steps. First, turn the fire apparatus on and allow time for the air compressor to build up to a minimum of 110 psi (758 kPa) in both the front and rear systems. Next, shut the engine off. Leave the battery in the "on" position, and step on and off the brake pedal to reduce air tank pressure. An audible alarm should signal before the pressure drops to less than 60 psi (414 kPa) in the air tank with the lowest air pressure. Have the fire apparatus inspected by a qualified mechanic if the audible alarm does not work properly, as such a malfunction could cause the system to lose air pressure without your knowledge. Without the proper air pressure, the brakes will become less effective, thereby increasing the stopping distance of the fire apparatus and leading to unsafe operation.

Spring Brake Test

This test ensures that the parking brake operates as it was designed. The parking brakes should engage whenever brake pressure drops below 40 psi (275 kPa) in the rear brake system. The spring brake test is performed by allowing enough air pressure to build up in the braking system to release the parking brake. Depress the parking brake knob to release it. Next, step on and off the brake pedal to reduce the pressure in the system. The parking brake knob should activate when the air pressure drops below 40 psi (275 kPa). The spring brakes will then activate and help to prevent the vehicle from moving.

CHAPTER 8 *Performing Fire Apparatus Check-Out and Maintenance* 179

FIGURE 8-17 Manual valves to drain the moisture in the brake system are found underneath the fire apparatus.

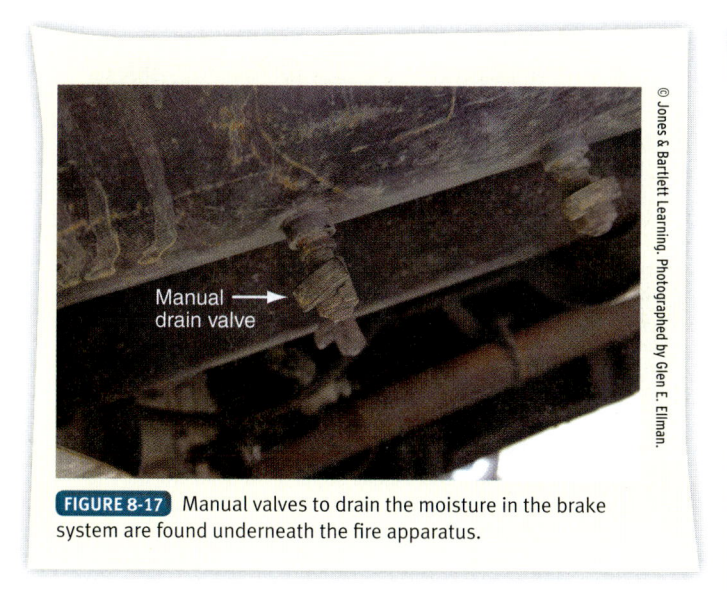

As a result of normal condensation of moisture in the air and moisture created during the compression phase, some water may enter into the air supply of the braking system. The danger from the presence of moisture in the air supply is that in cold weather it may collect and freeze, thereby preventing the braking system from operating properly. Fire apparatus equipped with air brakes may be equipped with automatic moisture exhaustion valves to overcome this problem. In addition, some fire apparatus have a manual water drain valve that must be opened to drain moisture from the air system **FIGURE 8-17**. Refer to the operator's manual to determine which procedures are recommended to maintain this system. Automatic moisture reduction systems will make a spitting noise when they are removing moisture from the system; this is normal and not a cause for alarm. As a driver/operator, you must become familiar with the air brakes and the moisture removal system with which your fire apparatus is equipped.

DRIVER/OPERATOR Tip

During major maintenance checks, emergency vehicle technicians (EVTs) will check the brake slack adjuster to make sure the proper stroke length is available for safe stopping. EVTs may employ the use of a heat gun to check brake drum temperatures to ensure that braking is applied evenly to all wheels.

■ General Tools/Equipment Inspection

All other equipment carried on the fire apparatus—such as breathing apparatus, cascade systems (including compressors), generators, fans, hydraulic rescue tools, hand tools, power tools, hose, nozzles, ground ladders, and so on—must also be inspected to make sure that it is operational **FIGURE 8-18**. The SCBA should be checked in accordance with the fire department's respiratory protection program, which may require completion of a separate inspection form. A record of this inspection process must be kept by the member in charge of the respiratory protection equipment in accordance with

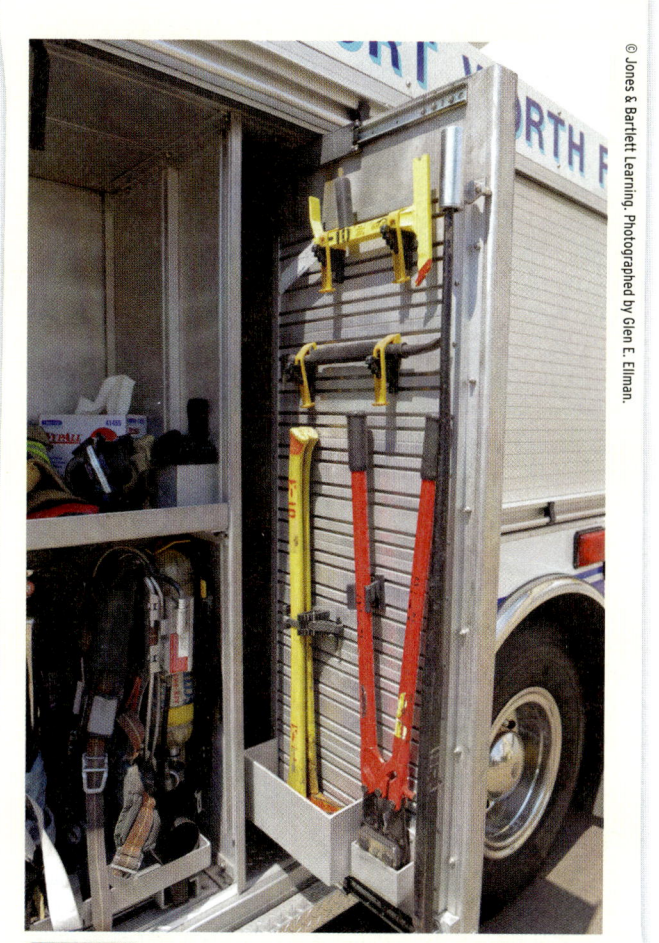

FIGURE 8-18 Equipment found in the compartments of the fire apparatus must be inspected, and the results of the investigation documented on the inspection report.

Occupational Safety and Health Administration (OSHA) 29 Code of Federal Regulations (CFR) 1910.134.

Power tools such as saws, fans, and hydraulic rescue tools should be checked for oil level (if appropriate) and fuel supply. All equipment should be started and operated. Equipment such as power saws may have two-cycle engines, in which the lubricating oil is mixed with the gasoline or another fuel; that is, they may not have a crankcase with a separate oil supply serving as the lubricant. Devices such as portable pumps will typically have four-cycle engines and an oil reservoir that must be checked. When refueling power tools, it is critical to make sure the appropriate fuel is used.

Many fire apparatus carry equipment on board that needs to be recharged as the fire apparatus sits in the station bay. This equipment may include portable radios, thermal imaging cameras, and batteries for electrical equipment **FIGURE 8-19**. If the fire apparatus is not operated for an extended duration, its batteries may be drained of power by the ongoing recharging of equipment stored on board the fire apparatus. Therefore, it is critical to keep the vehicle's batteries properly charged at all times. To do so, many fire apparatus are equipped with a charging system that connects to an electrical outlet in the fire station. This electrical line recharges the

FIGURE 8-19 Small electrical equipment may be charged while mounted on the fire apparatus.

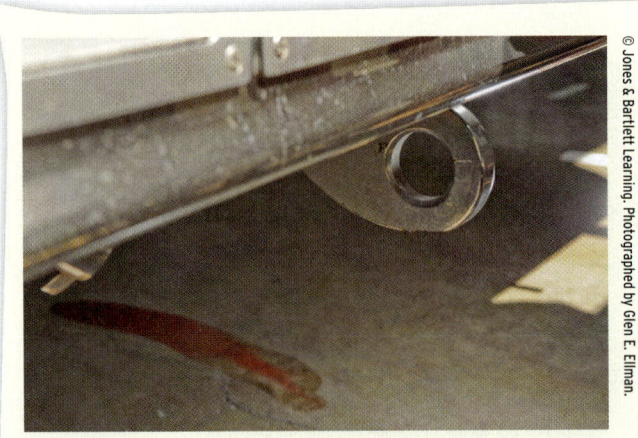

FIGURE 8-20 Water or other liquids dripping from underneath the fire apparatus should be inspected to determine whether the leak is serious.

battery(s) while the fire apparatus is not running, thereby ensuring that the fire apparatus has enough electrical power in its batteries to recharge any equipment and start the fire apparatus as required.

Safety Tip

Extreme caution should be used when adding fuel to power tools. Never fuel equipment inside the station, and never fuel equipment while it is running. If the engine is hot, allow it to cool before refueling the equipment. Use the appropriate fuel dispensing device(s).

Pump Inspection

The pump inspection process includes the following items:
- Water supply tank
- Foam supply tank
- Intakes and discharges
- Primer pump
- Centrifugal fire pump

A visual inspection of the water supply tank should be conducted, even if it has a water tank level gauge. This step will help verify that the gauge is correct. Tank gauges may not be accurate because of fluctuations caused by the materials in "hard water" and electrical malfunctions. Always visually confirm that the water tank is full.

In fire apparatus that is equipped with foam systems, the foam tank levels should be checked. This inspection is typically completed at the same time as the water tank check. As with the water tank, always visually confirm the fluid level in the foam tank.

Before opening any valve and allowing water to drain, check the floor area under the fire apparatus for the presence of water. A puddle of water or dripping water may indicate a loose pump seal or some other leak in the system **FIGURE 8-20**. A loose pump seal may not be considered a significant problem if the pump is always operated from a pressurized water supply, such as a hydrant. It is a problem, however, if the pump needs to be operated in draft mode. It may not be possible to prime the pump in such a case owing to the leaking seal. Repairing this problem requires a mechanic who is specially trained to adjust the seals. In addition, leaking water from the pump seals during operations in cold weather will cause ice to build up in and around the fire apparatus.

In areas subject to cold weather, pumps may be kept in a dry state during winter months. If this is the case, do not open the tank-to-pump valve, as this maneuver will cause the pump to fill with water. Always refer to your department's policy regarding the use of wet versus dry fire pumps.

During your inspection of the fire apparatus, while the pump is not engaged, open and close each discharge valve several times to ensure that it operates properly. Remove all of the caps on the discharges and open the drain valve for each discharge to ensure it functions properly. Confirm that all caps are easily operated and free of corrosion.

The intakes—that is, the piping that allows water to enter the fire pump—are inspected next. To do so, remove the plugs, caps, or **piston intake valve (PIV)** and visually inspect the piping. The PIV is a large appliance that connects directly to the pump's intake and controls the amount of water that flows from a pressurized water source into the pump. Hard water and corrosion can cause the plugs or caps from the intakes or at the end of the PIV to stick and make it difficult to open them. In such a case, it is better to fix the problem at the fire station during the fire apparatus inspection than to wait until it happens at the next fire scene.

Intake strainers are located at the front of all intakes directly on the pump. These small screens prevent debris such as rocks from entering the pump and causing damage. These screens should be checked at least weekly or as directed by your department. Be careful when completing this portion of the inspection, because water will be released as the pump partially drains. Check the grids of the strainers to make sure they are clear and no pieces are bent or missing **FIGURE 8-21**.

FIGURE 8-21 The intake strainers should be in good condition and should not have any missing or damaged pieces.

If the priming pump is wet, then a stream of water should be observed within a few seconds. If the pump is being carried dry, then no water should be seen. If the pump drains are open, then no negative pressure will be recorded on the compound gauge.

DRIVER/OPERATOR Tip

Newer apparatus are equipped with oil-less priming pumps due to environmental factors. These primers work in the same manner, but do not require oil to create a vacuum-tight seal. Just like the oil primers, however, they should be run daily to eliminate a scale build-up from hard water.

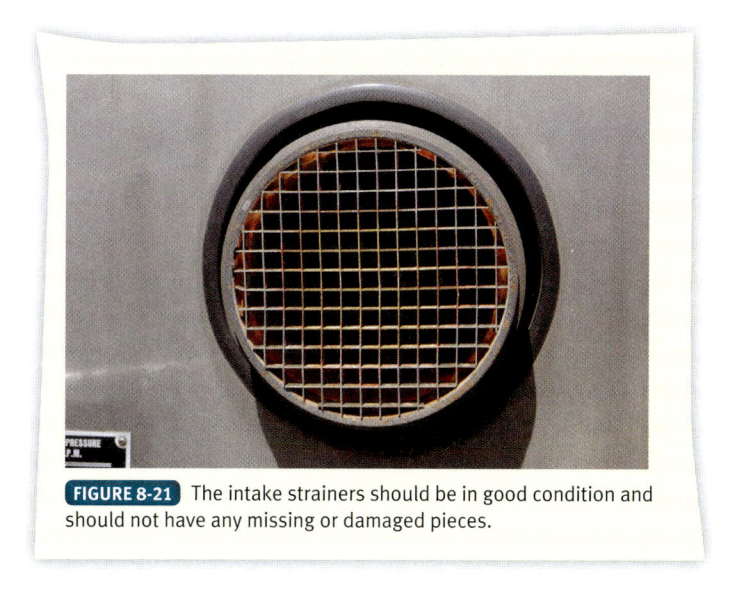

Repeat this process for each intake. After the intake strainers are checked and the caps or PIV replaced, it is critical that the fire pump be refilled with water as required.

Because the fire apparatus is equipped with a centrifugal pump, it will have a priming pump; the oil reservoir of this priming pump most likely must be checked daily **FIGURE 8-22**. The priming pump is used to draw air out of the centrifugal pump for proper operation. Some of these pumps allow a small amount of oil to enter the centrifugal pump during priming operations to help seal and lubricate the pump.

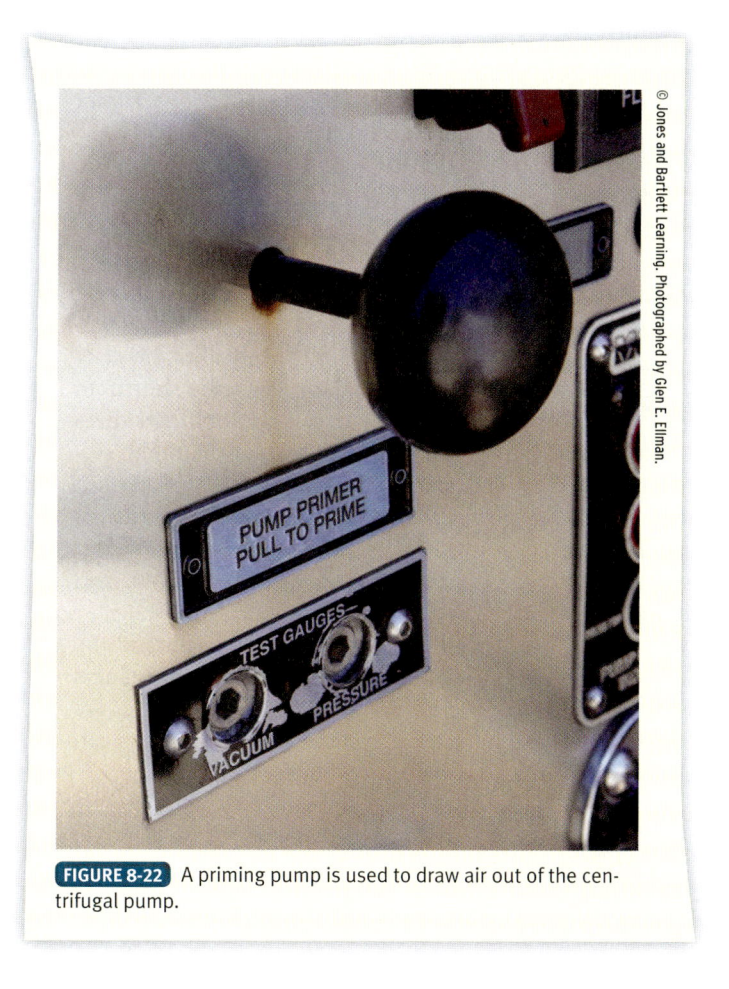

If the priming pump is being carried in a wet condition, after the pump valves and components have been operated, the fire apparatus engine should be started and the pump engaged in the appropriate gear. Before starting the engine, make sure that the parking brake is set and the wheels are chocked. Once the engine is started and the pump engaged, observe the fire apparatus' speedometer to see whether a speed is being recorded, indicating the pump is in gear. On the pump panel, observe the tachometer to observe that the pump is activated. Also on the pump panel, the pump indicator light will indicate when the engine is in pump. Ensure that all of the gauges and instruments are operating properly.

To set the pressure relief valve, open the tank-to-pump valve and the tank fill valve. Next, increase the engine speed to bring the pump pressure up to an operating pressure, such as 125 psi (875 kPa). Then set the pressure relief valve and confirm that it is functioning properly. To do so, increase the engine speed and the pressure enough to cause the relief valve to operate or open. If the relief valve is functioning properly, the pressure will not increase more than the set pressure. For engines equipped with a pressure governor, both the tank-to-pump and tank fill valves should be open and the pressure governor should be turned to the "on" position. Increase the pressure to about 125 psi (875 kPa), which will in turn set the pressure governor at this pressure. Once water flow is established and the governor set, close the tank fill valve halfway. The governor should adjust the engine speed to maintain the desired pressure. Reopen the tank fill valve all the way.

Be sure not to operate the pump for more than a few minutes without circulating water back to the tank or the other discharge line. Without the cooling provided by the circulating water, friction will cause the water to heat and boil, which may damage the pump. The larger the pump, the more heat is created. The smaller the tank, the less the tank capacity is able to dissipate the heat.

For fire apparatus with multistage pumps, the **transfer valve** should be set to change from pressure to volume operation or from series to parallel operation. The pressure should change appropriately with about half the pressure in parallel (volume) from the series (pressure) setting. This change should be made two or three times to exercise the valve.

FIGURE 8-22 A priming pump is used to draw air out of the centrifugal pump.

VOICES OF EXPERIENCE

Routine maintenance is just that: routine. Daily apparatus checks, however, are not an area where shortcuts can be taken. That expectation needs to be made clear on the first day a new driver/operator reports to the company. In addition, senior driver/operators must stay diligent in taking these checks seriously every single day of their careers.

The criteria and sequence for fire apparatus maintenance are established by detailed fire department check-off lists. However, the steps for developing a positive safety attitude toward fire apparatus maintenance within the company are not written down—that is up to the driver/operator.

Remember, the fire apparatus is both your office and your toolbox. Daily apparatus checks will ensure its safety. The following tips will help you make sure that your daily apparatus check is both thorough and effective:

- The vibration that takes place while the fire apparatus is on the road tends to loosen certain pieces of equipment. All attack lines, whether preconnected or not, have a nozzle attached and have to be physically checked. Ensure that the nozzle is firmly attached to the hose and that the tip of the nozzle is screwed down tightly at the ball-valve shut-off.
- Many departments carry their monitor tips "stacked" at the end of the deck gun. Ensure that all tips are firmly screwed onto the appliance.
- Whenever sections of hose are changed out, make sure there is a gasket inside the female swivel of the coupling.
- Confirm that your fire extinguishers are properly charged and that the gauge is "in the green."
- Check the chain on the chainsaw. In some cases, a fire fighter has unknowingly put the chain on backward on the bar.
- The apparatus floors should be swept and mopped immediately after the daily apparatus checks. Be alert to any puddles forming throughout the shift from water, oil, fuel, or other fluids. They may be your only indication that there is a slow leak in the tank, a loose pump seal, or an oil, fuel, or hydraulic system leak. Some companies have members wipe down the apparatus before shift change with a chamois. Some even go so far as to wipe down the undercarriage. Although this step may seem excessive, it gets the members under the rigs with creepers and forces them to take notice of the inside tires, belts, bolts, and mounting brackets, among other components.

Daily apparatus checks are more than checking a diesel engine for fuel and oil. Take these checks seriously; your own life and the lives of your fellow fire fighters may be put at risk by faulty fire apparatus. Your crew members and their families are depending on you to prepare that apparatus for a safe response. Taking shortcuts can make your rig unsafe on the road and unreliable on the fireground.

Raul A Angulo
Seattle Fire Department
Seattle, Washington

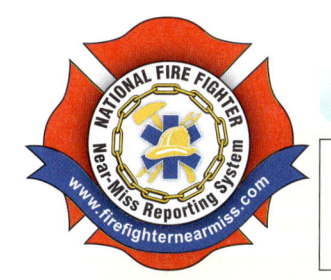

Near-Miss REPORT

Report Number: 10-0000185

Synopsis: Brakes fail on truck while driving.

Event Description: A hazardous materials truck was returning from a training exercise to its home station. The truck was driven by an acting engineer with 14 years of experience, and a fire fighter was the front seat passenger. As the hazardous materials truck was exiting the highway eastbound at a reported 45 mph (72 km/hr), the acting engineer attempted to slow the vehicle down for a red light, but the vehicle would not stop. He told the fire fighter that he did not have any brakes and noted that the brake pedal was depressed all the way down to the floor. As he approached the intersection, he did not see any traffic, but he did have a red light. He decided to proceed through the intersection hoping to clear it without hitting anything. He did not try to swerve or turn to the right, as there was a raised median and he was worried about causing a rollover if his wheels struck the curb. As he approached the intersection eastbound, he observed a passenger car proceeding south into the intersection. He swerved to the right attempting to avoid a collision. The passenger car swerved to the left, and both vehicles collided and continued eastbound through the intersection. There was minor damage to the hazardous material truck and moderate damage to the passenger car. The front seat occupant in the passenger car had a minor injury that was treated on scene. The acting engineer later reported that if the passenger car had approached a second sooner, they would have killed one or both occupants of the passenger car.

An Automotive Service Excellence (ASE) Master mechanic with Emergency Vehicle Technician (EVT) certification evaluated the vehicle on scene and found the vehicles brakes to be completely out of adjustment. The rear brakes were so far out of adjustment that they were totally ineffective. The braking system had to be adjusted manually, as automatic slack adjusters were not installed. In his opinion, at the last mechanical service, the mechanic must have turned the adjustment nut in the wrong direction. His opinion was based on the low number of miles from when the brakes were inspected and adjusted to the time of the accident. In addition, this vehicle is a manually operated stick shift transmission with a "split" rear end. The acting engineer exited the highway in "neutral" because he was unable to downshift the truck due to grinding of the gears. This was said to be normal, because the truck is old and the transmission was loose. The vehicle also had a manually activated supplemental braking system (driveline electromagnetic retarder) commonly known as a "Telma." The retarding system was in the Off position, because the acting engineer did not think it was necessary for normal vehicle operation on the highway. Fatigue did not appear to be a factor, as the acting engineer had 9 hours of continuous sleep the previous night. A review of maintenance records revealed that the vehicle had inadequate maintenance intervals by certified mechanics (commonly known as B service per NFPA) even though the vehicle had very low miles due to lack of use. The weekly checks by the fire fighters were reported to have occurred but no log or documentation was found. Due to the infrequency of driving the vehicle, it is unlikely the brake problem would have been discovered during a weekly check.

The root cause of this event was improper vehicle maintenance (out of adjustment brakes and inadequate inspection) followed by improper operation of the vehicle (failure to remain in gear and failure to use supplemental braking system). The acting engineer did not have vehicle-specific training to include the use of a manual transmission with a split shaft or manually activated retarding system. All of our other apparatus have automatic transmissions with automatic supplemental braking systems.

Lessons Learned: We learned that a combination of factors came together and almost caused a fatal collision. Vehicle maintenance performed by properly trained mechanics at the appropriate time intervals is critical. Nonstandard vehicles or equipment require additional special training to ensure their safe operation. Replace older vehicles when possible to take advantage of safer operations and better safety standards. Safety division recommendations:

1. Ensure vehicle maintenance is performed properly in accordance with fleet maintenance requirements and NFPA standard 1911 (2007 edition).
2. Ensure vehicles driven by employees are maintained and repaired by fleet services and not outside contractors.
3. Install automatic slack adjusters on all vehicles that are not currently equipped.
4. Request installation of automatic slack adjusters on all nondepartment owned vehicles that are driven by our employees.
5. Ensure daily and weekly checks are performed with specific emphasis on air brake system inspection and testing.
6. Ensure proper documentation of all daily and weekly checks on a vehicle maintenance form.
7. Provide formalized training on all vehicles that have a manual transmission and/or manually activated supplemental braking system.
8. Establish minimum certification requirements in policy for drivers and apparatus operators.
9. Establish continuing education requirements in policy for drivers and apparatus operators.
10. Replace the Hazmat-1 vehicle as soon a practically feasible with a newer vehicle that includes an automatic transmission, automatic supplemental braking system, and a lap/shoulder seatbelt system.

Aerial Device Inspection

The aerial device should be inspected according to the manufacturer's recommendations. NFPA 1911, *Standard for the Inspection, Maintenance, Testing, and Retirement of In-Service Automotive Fire Apparatus*, requires that aerial devices be tested annually. As part of this inspection, you should record the amount of time it takes to perform each of the three recommended tests: full lift, extension, and 90-degree rotation. An increase in the amount of time it takes to complete a test may indicate problems with the hydraulic system. All tests are meant to check for the proper operation and adjustment of components if necessary. Inspection that ensures the availability of a properly maintained and adjusted aerial device may prevent an accident or a catastrophic failure of the device.

Many departments require the driver/operator to not only inspect the aerial device, but also to clean and lubricate it. Follow the manufacturer's recommended maintenance schedule for the replacement of hydraulic filters, hydraulic fluid, and proper lubricants.

Always follow your department's policies for this inspection process. Many different aerial devices exist, and each has different features. Before operating the aerial device, always make sure that it is in a safe position and that no overhead obstructions are present in the immediate area.

The components most commonly found on an aerial device include the following items:

- Aerial device hydraulic system
- Stabilizing system
- Cable systems
- Slides and rollers
- Aerial device safety system
- Breathing air system
- Communications system

The main component of the aerial device is the hydraulic system that powers it. Using the hydraulic fluid and large cylinders that constitute this system, the aerial device can be maneuvered into almost any position. The hydraulic system consists of a reservoir of hydraulic fluid, a pump, pressurized lines, and hydraulic cylinders that power the stabilizers and the aerial device.

To inspect this system, with the aerial device and stabilizers in the stored position, you should first check the fluid stored in the reservoir. Depending on the manufacturer, a simple dip stick or a sight glass may be used to determine the fluid level. The hydraulic lines should also be visually inspected for any leaks or signs of chafing. In addition, engage the hydraulic system and verify that all of the functions and alarms are operating correctly.

Next, place the wheel chocks on the fire apparatus and prepare to deploy the stabilizers. The stabilizers should be checked for their full range of motion; they should also operate smoothly and evenly. Check the stabilizer arms for any leaks, cracks, broken welds, or loose parts. The stabilizers should be clean and free of rust, and all working parts should be lubricated as required **FIGURE 8-23**. All of the controls should be properly labeled.

Once the stabilizers are set, put the aerial device through its full range of operation using the main controls. The controls' response should be smooth and even with no unusual noise or vibration.

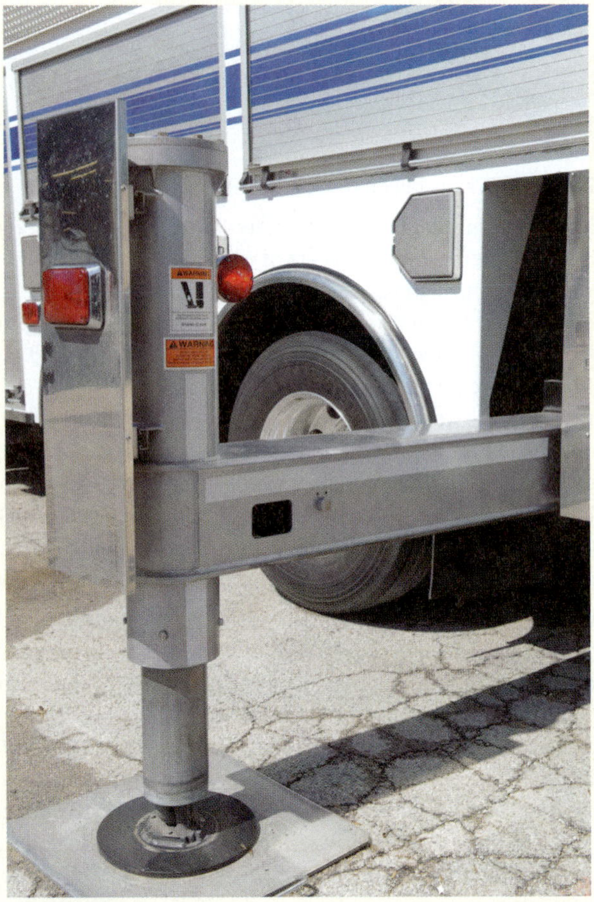

FIGURE 8-23 Clean stabilizers are easier to inspect for defects.

Inspect the aerial device for any cracks, loose parts, damage, or signs of heat stress. Check the turntable gears for any missing teeth, broken welds, leaking hydraulic lines/cylinders, or damage to the lifting cylinders. Inspect the cables for looseness, frays, broken strands, or other signs of damage. Next, inspect the slides and rollers of the aerial, which allow the different sections of the aerial device to move in and out without rubbing against each other **FIGURE 8-24**. Ensure that there is no metal-to-metal contact and that the slides and rollers are properly lubricated and functioning properly.

Many aerial devices are equipped with safety systems that will not allow the device to perform specific functions if the apparatus is not in a safe position. For example, if the stabilizers are not fully extended on one side of the fire apparatus, the aerial device will not be allowed to operate on that side. Specifically, a sensor will stop the aerial device from operating on that side so as to prevent the fire apparatus from tipping over. Each manufacturer provides different safety systems and overrides for its systems. You must be very comfortable operating the aerial device and know how and why to perform an override of any system. Remember, however, that these safety systems are designed for the protection of the fire fighter. Overriding a safety system should only be done by a trained driver/operator. Any extra personnel not part of the override process should be moved to a safe area away from the apparatus. Departments should have standard operating procedures/standard operating

CHAPTER 8 Performing Fire Apparatus Check-Out and Maintenance   185

FIGURE 8-24 The slides and rollers prevent the sections of the aerial device from contacting each other. **A.** The roller. **B.** The aerial.

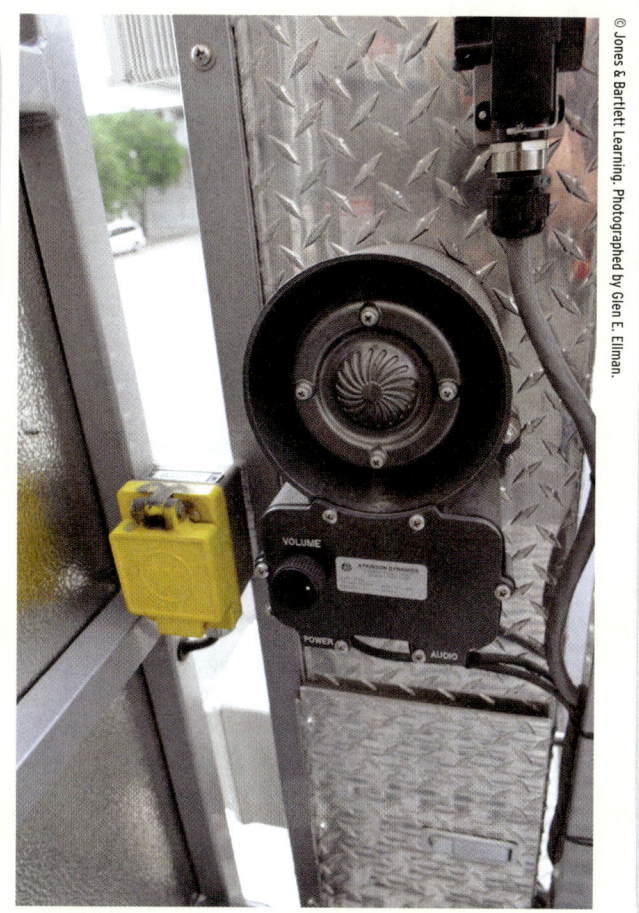

FIGURE 8-25 A communication system allows the driver/operator at the turntable to remain in contact with the crew members who are working at the tip of the aerial device.

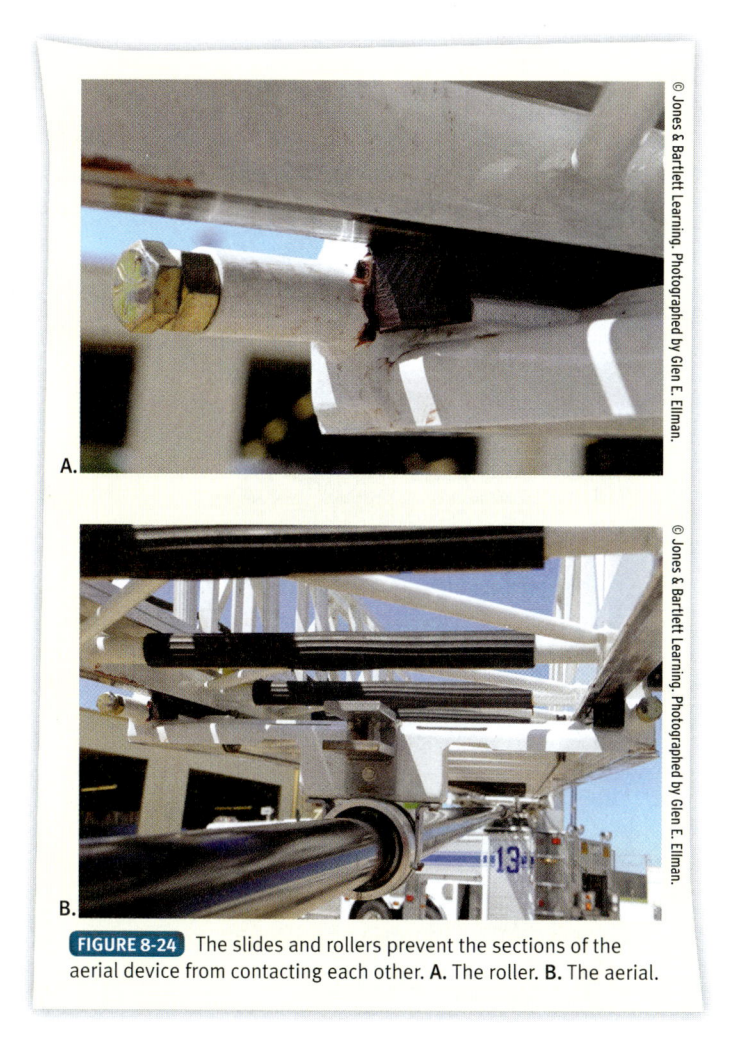

guidelines (SOPs/SOGs) in place detailing who and how the override process should happen.

Many times fire fighters will operate at the tip of the aerial device during firefighting operations. While doing so, the fire fighters may use the air supply from the fire apparatus rather than the SCBA that they carry on their backs—a strategy that allows them to work for longer periods of time than would be possible with SCBA. To check the functioning of the fire apparatus' air supply system, first make sure the air tanks are full. Many fire departments have the driver/operator document this information on the fire apparatus inspection form. Look for any cracked hoses or loose parts.

A communication system at the turntable enables the driver/operator of the fire apparatus to speak with a fire fighter working at the tip of the aerial device. This system should be checked for proper operation as part of the fire apparatus inspection **FIGURE 8-25**.

Follow the steps in **SKILL DRILL 8-1** to perform an inspection of a fire apparatus:

1. Review the previous apparatus inspection reports for information regarding the fire apparatus. (**STEP 1**)
2. Inspect the exterior of the apparatus in accordance with the department's policies and procedures. (**STEP 2**)
3. Inspect the engine compartment of the fire apparatus in accordance with the department's policies and procedures. (**STEP 3**)
4. Inspect the cab interior of the fire apparatus in accordance with the department's policies and procedures. (**STEP 4**)
5. Complete a brake inspection of the fire apparatus in accordance with the department's policies and procedures. (**STEP 5**)
6. Inspect the tools and equipment of the fire apparatus in accordance with the department's policies and procedures. (**STEP 6**)
7. Inspect the pump of the fire apparatus and all of the features associated with its function in accordance with the department's policies and procedures (if applicable). (**STEP 7**)
8. Inspect the aerial device and all of the features associated with its function in accordance with the department's policies and procedures (if applicable). (**STEP 8**)

Safety

Not only is it critical that you perform the fire apparatus inspection in a safe manner, but you must also ensure that the fire apparatus is prepared for a safe response. This includes

SKILL DRILL 8-1

Performing an Apparatus Inspection
(NFPA 1002, 4.2.1, 4.2.1(B), 5.1.1, 5.1.1(B), 6.1.1, 6.1.1(B), 10.1.1, 10.1.1(B))

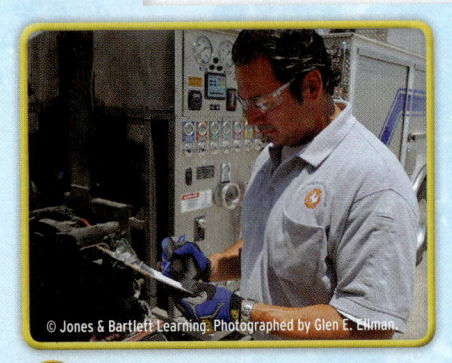

1. Review the previous fire apparatus inspection report.

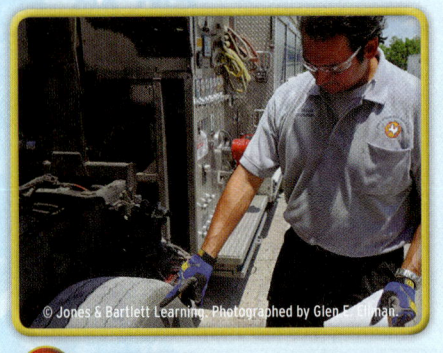

2. Inspect the exterior of the fire apparatus.

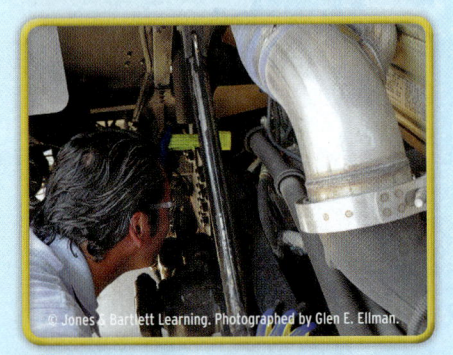

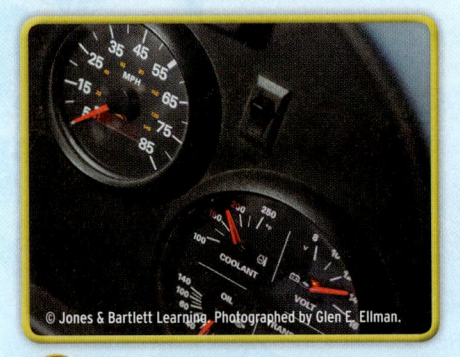

3. Inspect the engine compartment.

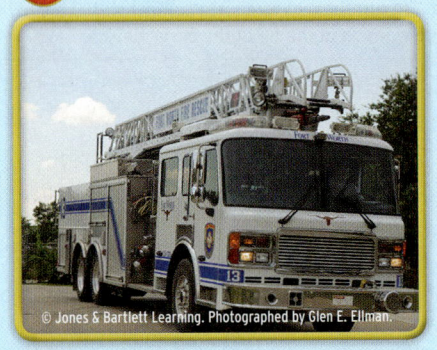

4. Inspect the cab interior.

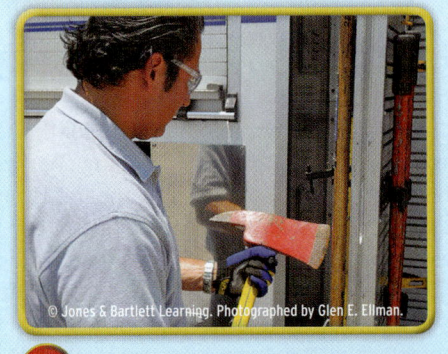

5. Inspect the fire apparatus brakes.

6. Inspect the tools and equipment carried on the fire apparatus.

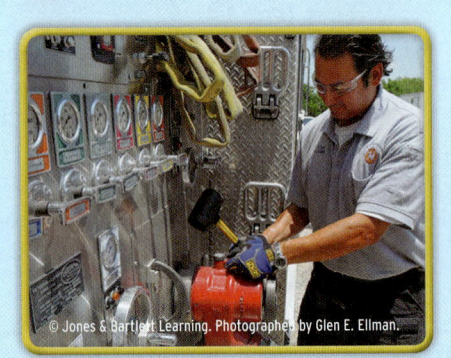

7. If applicable, inspect the pump of the fire apparatus and all the features associated with its function.

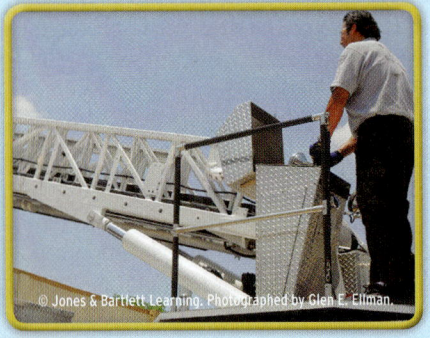

8. If applicable, inspect the aerial device and all the features associated with its function.

making sure that the fire apparatus is in proper working condition, the emergency warning equipment is operating correctly, tools and equipment are functional, and the vehicle is ready to support sustained operations.

The final portion of the safety evaluation focuses on making sure that the fire apparatus is safe to ride on and operate. As part of that safety check, all tools and equipment should be secured, breathing apparatus secured, equipment properly placed and secured on compartment shelves, and equipment carried on the outside of the apparatus properly secured. Hoselines should be loaded and ready for deployment, ground ladders securely nested, portable tanks secured on water tankers/ tenders, and other tools or equipment properly secured to the fire apparatus **FIGURE 8-26**. In case of a sudden stop or use of evasive driving techniques, all equipment in the passenger compartment must stay firmly secured. A sudden stop can cause a hammer, for example, to become a dangerous projectile.

Weekly, Monthly, or Other Periodic Inspection Items

In addition to undergoing its daily inspection, each fire apparatus will typically be subject to other inspections that are performed on a less frequent basis. For example, some elements of the inspection process—such as checking hydraulic oil levels, checking pump bearing oil reservoir levels, and so on—may be done on a weekly, monthly, or even quarterly basis. These inspections should be performed in accordance with existing NFPA testing standards, manufacturers' recommendations, local experience, and accepted good maintenance practices. The manufacturer's instructions should be considered minimum criteria for the maintenance, inspection, and repair of equipment.

■ Completing Forms

The forms recording the inspection and maintenance process are filled out as the inspection takes place. At the conclusion of the fire apparatus and equipment inspection, these forms should be completed and filed in accordance with the fire department's procedures. Any abnormalities should be reported to the officer in charge so that he or she can make a determination on the best method of corrective action. In some instances, a situation found during your inspection may require that the fire apparatus be immediately taken out of service. In other situations, appropriate maintenance and repairs may be scheduled to be performed at a later date.

■ Removing Vehicles from Service

According to NFPA 1451, each department shall establish in writing the conditions that require the vehicle to be taken out of service. These conditions may include problems or deficiencies in the brakes, emergency lights, steering mechanism, tires, fuel system, electrical system, coolant system, suspension, and other systems. Each department shall also establish a procedure to remove unsafe vehicles from service and schedule them for repair. Any department vehicle found to be unsafe shall be taken out of service immediately. No member should operate an unsafe vehicle until it has been properly repaired. Reference NFPA 1911 for more information on these requirements.

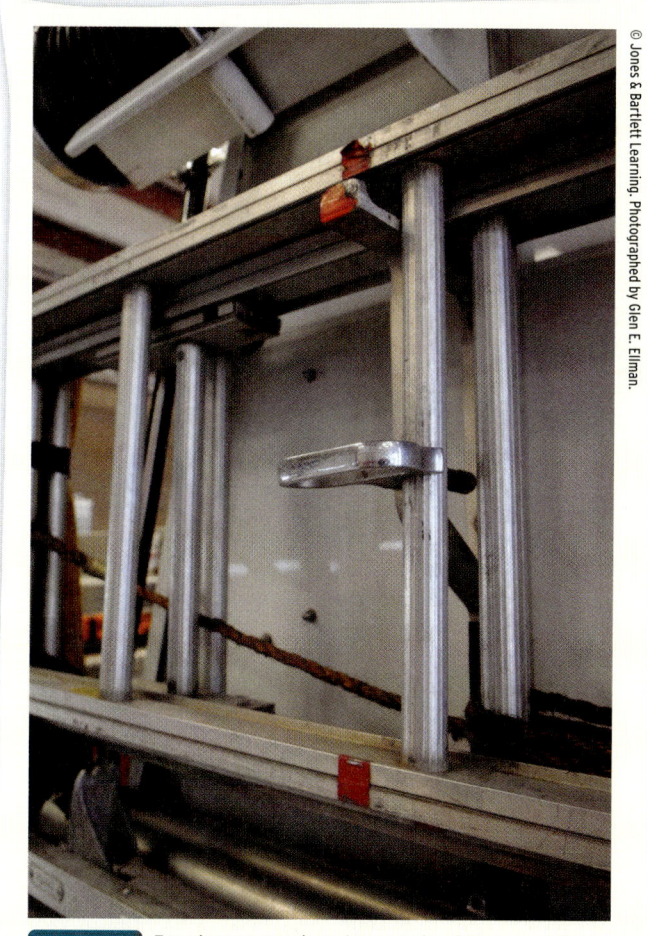

FIGURE 8-26 Exterior-mounted equipment should be properly stored before the fire apparatus moves.

Wrap-Up

Chief Concepts

- The fire apparatus inspection is an evaluation of the fire apparatus and its equipment that is intended to ensure its safe operation.
- The inspection should be planned, methodical, and performed in an organized manner.
- The inspection process should begin with a review of the apparatus inspection form that was completed after the previous inspection.
- Dividing the inspection into sections allows you to focus on a single aspect of the fire apparatus and discourages you from jumping from one element of the inspection to another without a plan; jumping during an inspection leads to the possibility that critical elements may be missed.
- Not only is it critical that you perform the inspection in a safe manner, but you must also ensure that the fire apparatus is prepared for a safe response. This includes making sure that the fire apparatus is in proper working condition, the emergency warning equipment is operating, tools and equipment are functional, and the vehicle is ready for sustained operations.

Hot Terms

aerial device An aerial ladder, elevating platform, aerial ladder platform, or water tower that is designed to position personnel, handle materials, provide continuous egress, or discharge water.

apparatus inspection form A document that identifies who performed the inspection and when the fire apparatus inspection was performed, identifies any equipment that is damaged and/or repaired, and details other preventive maintenance procedures performed on the apparatus.

dip stick A graduated instrument for measuring the depth or amount of fluid in a container, such as the level of oil in a crankcase.

extractor exhaust system A system used inside the fire apparatus bay that connects to the fire apparatus tailpipe and draws its exhaust outside the building.

fire apparatus inspection An evaluation of the fire apparatus and its equipment that is intended to ensure its safe operation.

fire pump A water pump with a rated capacity of 250 gpm (1000 L/min) or greater at 150 psi (1034 kPa) net pump pressure that is mounted on an fire apparatus and used for firefighting.

piston intake valve (PIV) A large appliance that connects directly to the pump's intake and controls the amount of water that flows from a pressurized water source into the pump.

power steering system A system for reducing the steering effort on vehicles in which an external power source assists in turning the vehicle's wheels.

preventive maintenance program A program designed to ensure that apparatus are capable of functioning as required and are maintained in working order.

radiator cap The pressure cap that is screwed onto the top of the radiator, and through which coolant is typically added.

transfer valve An internal valve in a multistage pump that enables the user to change the mode of operation to either series/pressure or parallel/volume.

voltage meter A device that registers the voltage of a battery system.

References

National Fire Protection Association (NFPA) 1002, *Standard for Fire Apparatus Driver/Operator Professional Qualifications*. 2014. http://www.nfpa.org/codes-and-standards/document-information-pages?mode=code&code=1002. Accessed March 27, 2014.

National Fire Protection Association (NFPA) 1071, *Standard for Emergency Vehicle Technician Professional Qualification*. 2016. http://www.nfpa.org/codes-and-standards/document-information-pages?mode=code&code=1071. Accessed November 17, 2014.

National Fire Protection Association (NFPA) 1451, *Standard for a Fire and Emergency Service Vehicle Operations Training Program*. 2013. http://www.nfpa.org/codes-and-standards/document-information-pages?mode=code&code=1451. Accessed April 9, 2014.

National Fire Protection Association (NFPA) 1901, *Standard for Automotive Fire Apparatus*. 2009. http://www.nfpa.org/codes-and-standards/document-information-pages?mode=code&code=1901. Accessed April 9, 2014.

National Fire Protection Association (NFPA) 1911, *Standard for the Inspection, Maintenance, Testing, and Retirement of In-Service Automotive Fire Apparatus*. 2012. http://www.nfpa.org/codes-and-standards/document-information-pages?mode=code&code=1911. Accessed April 9, 2014.

DRIVER/OPERATOR
in action

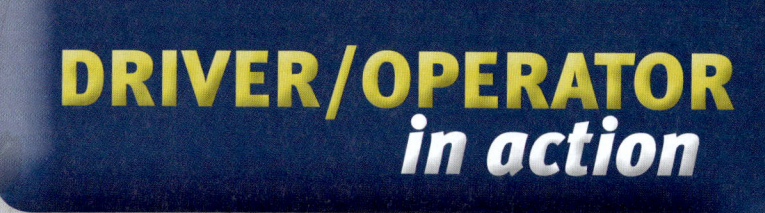

While you are inspecting the fire apparatus for any deficiencies, a fire fighter asks if he can assist you. His help would be very beneficial to you because several items on the fire apparatus are difficult—if not impossible—to inspect by yourself, such as the brake lights. In the past, you have found that it is very useful to have another set of eyes looking for any problems with the fire apparatus or the equipment on the fire apparatus. An extra set of eyes helps to ensure that nothing critical is missed and makes for a better inspection.

1. The inspection process should begin with a review of the _____.
   A. Department policy
   B. Apparatus inspection form
   C. Operator's manual
   D. Daily report

2. To ensure their readiness, the fire apparatus and equipment must be inspected at least weekly and within __ hours after being used during an emergency response.
   A. 24
   B. 12
   C. 2
   D. 48

3. An audible alarm should signal before the pressure drops to less than __ psi (kPa) in the air tank with the lowest air pressure.
   A. 40 (275)
   B. 50 (345)
   C. 60 (414)
   D. 110 (758)

4. Which of the following is not one of the standard brake tests a driver/operator should perform?
   A. Spring brake test
   B. Parking brake test
   C. Brake pedal test
   D. Speed brake test

5. Many fire departments have a policy that requires that their fire apparatus fuel tanks do not go below what level?
   A. One-fourth of a tank
   B. One-half of a tank
   C. Three-fourths of a tank
   D. None of the answers is correct

Driving Fire Apparatus

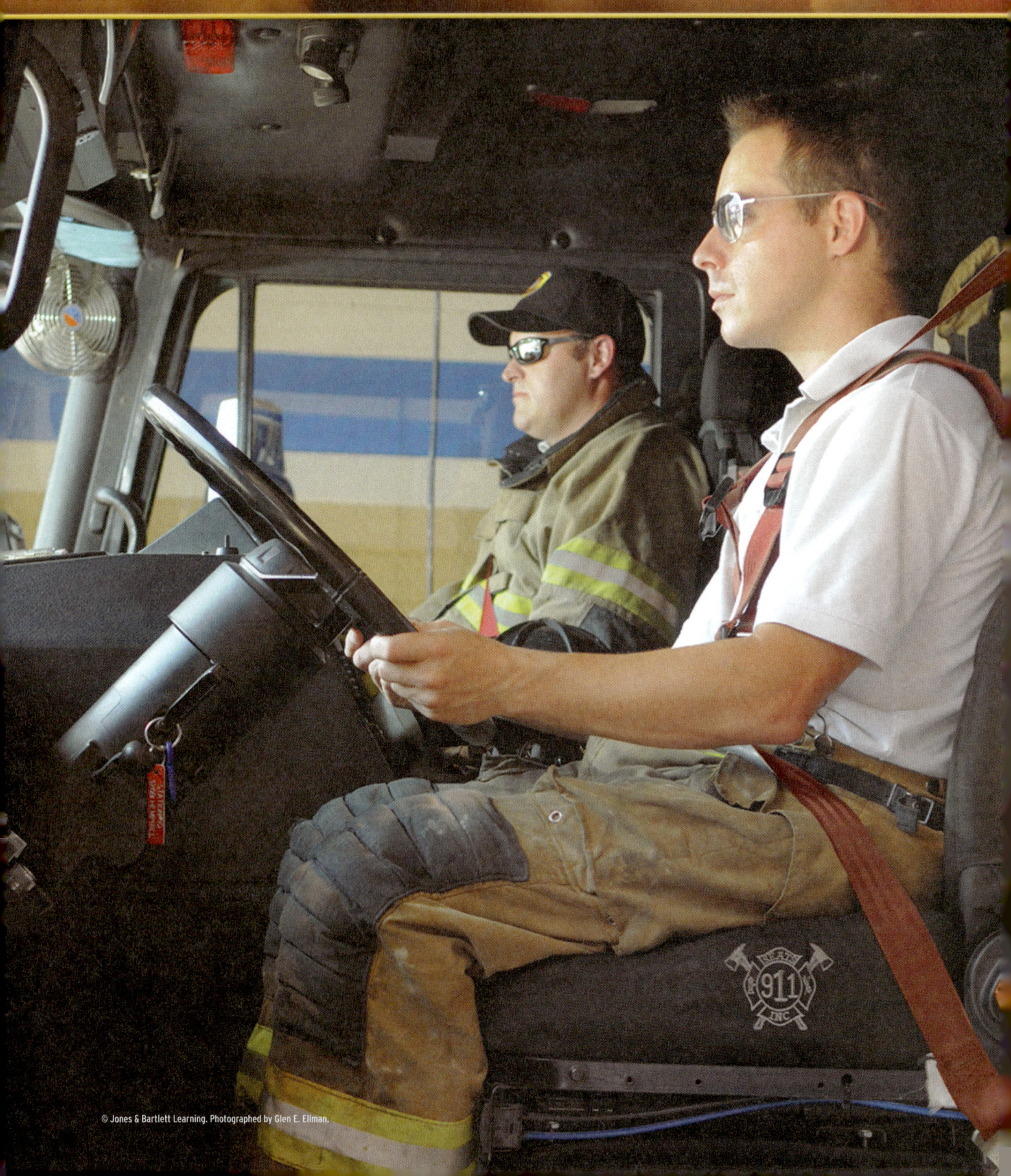

CHAPTER 9

Knowledge Objectives

After studying this chapter, you will be able to:

- Describe the 360-degree inspection. (p 192–193)
- Describe the process to start the apparatus, get it underway, and shut it down. (NFPA 1002, 4.3, 4.3.1, 4.3.1(A); p 194–199, 207, 209–210)
- Describe the seat belt requirements of NFPA 1500. (NFPA 1002, 4.3.1(A); p 196)
- Describe the various driver-training exercises required by NFPA 1002. (NFPA 1002, 4.3.1, 4.3.1(A), 4.3.2, 4.3.2(A), 4.3.3, 4.3.3(A), 4.3.4, 4.3.4(A), 4.3.5, 4.3.5(A); p 200–204)
- Describe the procedure to back up the apparatus. (NFPA 1002, 4.3.2, 4.3.2(A); p 205–208)

Skills Objectives

After studying this chapter, you will be able to:

- Perform a 360-degree inspection. (p 192–193)
- Start the fire apparatus. (NFPA 1002, 4.3.1, 4.3.1(B); p 194, 196–199)
- Perform the serpentine exercise. (NFPA 1002, 4.3.3, 4.3.3(B); p 200–201)
- Perform a confined-space turnaround. (NFPA 1002, 4.3.4, 4.3.4(B); p 201–203)
- Perform a diminishing clearance exercise. (NFPA 1002, 4.3.5, 4.3.5(B); p 203–204)
- Back a fire apparatus into a fire station bay. (NFPA 1002, 4.3.2, 4.3.2(B); p 205–208)
- Shut down and secure a fire apparatus. (NFPA 1002, 4.3.1, 4.3.1(B); p 207, 209–210)

Additional NFPA Standards

- NFPA 1901, *Standard for Automotive Fire Apparatus*
- NFPA 1500, *Standard on Fire Department Occupational Safety and Health Program*

You Are the Driver/Operator

You are the driver/operator for Engine Company 5. While your company is operating at the scene of a large commercial structure fire, your apparatus is reassigned to the rear of the building. The Incident Commander has informed you that there is a hydrant somewhere at the rear of the building, and you are to connect to it and supply an aerial device that is already positioning for a defensive attack. As you get to the rear of the large building, you see numerous parked cars, dumpsters, and obstacles blocking a clear path. You maneuver through the area and locate the hydrant at the end of a long alley. Your officer asks you to back the apparatus down the alley so you can lay the supply hoseline from the hydrant to a position closer to the aerial apparatus.

1. Have you been trained to operate the fire apparatus in narrow alley ways?
2. Do you know how to complete a confined-space turnaround?
3. What are the proper hand signals for backing the apparatus?

Introduction

The most fundamental task of a driver/operator is actually "driving" the fire apparatus to and from emergency incidents. The driver/operator must safely get the members of the crew, the fire apparatus, and the equipment that it carries to the scene of the incident. This response should not be taken lightly. Fire apparatus are not designed like many other vehicles on the road. They are usually bigger and heavier, which will change the characteristics of the vehicle—and, therefore, change how it should be driven. Do not assume that the fire apparatus can be driven like your own personal vehicle. Fire apparatus can be very dangerous machines when individuals who have not been properly trained in safe and efficient operational techniques drive them. It takes training and time to become a skilled fire apparatus driver. New driver/operators should not attempt the same maneuvers that more experienced drivers may perform until they are capable. This chapter discusses how to properly prepare to drive the apparatus, start the apparatus, perform several basic maneuvers, and shut down the fire apparatus. It also covers the use of seat belts—essential safety equipment on the fire apparatus that protects both the driver/operator and the other members of the company.

Preparing to Drive

360-Degree Inspection

Before entering the cab and starting the apparatus, you must complete a preliminary inspection of the fire apparatus, also known as a 360-degree inspection. A 360-degree inspection is a quick check of the fire apparatus and its surroundings to ensure that the apparatus is prepared for a response, either to an emergency or to a nonemergency. Failure to complete this inspection may result in damage to life and/or property. For example, an open compartment door may be sheared off by the fire station walls as the fire apparatus leaves the bay. Unsecured equipment stored on the outside of the fire apparatus may fly off and strike a civilian. The preliminary inspection must be performed every time that you move the fire apparatus, regardless of the emergency. Remember—complacency kills.

If the fire apparatus is responding from inside the fire station, the first step in a preliminary inspection is to open the fire apparatus bay door. While the door is opening, continue with the inspection—do not waste valuable time waiting for the door to open later. Walk around the fire apparatus and physically check that the cab doors are completely shut. All compartments should be checked to ensure that they are secure for travel. Ground ladders and equipment mounted to the exterior must be properly secured. Many fire apparatus have an interior warning light or buzzer to notify you that a compartment is open or not completely latched. Inspect the hose for any signs that it may come loose during a response. Remove any cups, equipment, or debris that may have been improperly placed on the running boards, front bumper, or tailboard. Visually verify that the area underneath the fire apparatus is free of debris. Your review should take only a matter of seconds. By making this inspection a habit, you will ensure that the fire apparatus is safe to respond.

To perform a 360-degree inspection, follow the steps in **SKILL DRILL 9-1**:

1. Open the fire apparatus bay door completely. (**STEP 1**)
2. Walk completely around the fire apparatus. (**STEP 2**)
3. Check that all doors are secured. (**STEP 3**)
4. Check that all compartment doors are secured. (**STEP 4**)
5. Check that all exterior-mounted equipment is properly secured. (**STEP 5**)
6. Remove any debris from the running boards, front bumper, and tailboard. (**STEP 6**)
7. Check that the area underneath the fire apparatus is clear of debris. (**STEP 7**)
8. Check that the area in front of the fire apparatus is clear and free of debris. (**STEP 8**)

CHAPTER 9 Driving Fire Apparatus 193

SKILL DRILL 9-1 Performing a 360-Degree Inspection

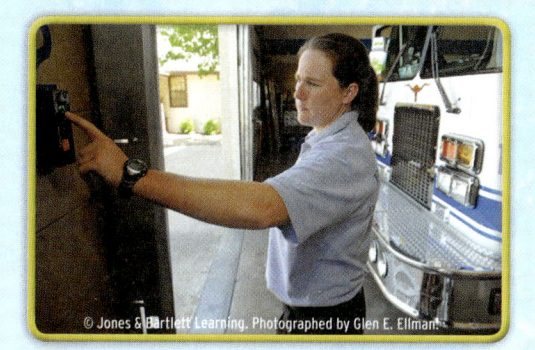

1. Open the fire apparatus bay door completely.

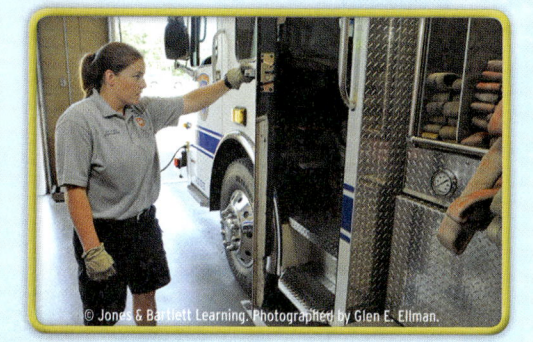

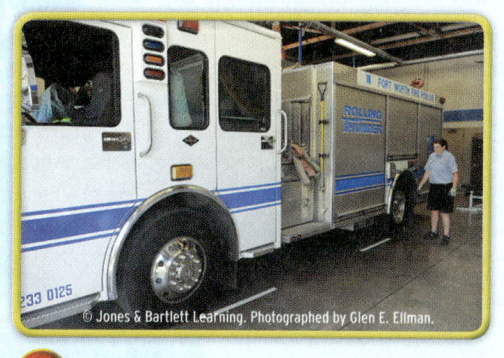

2. Walk completely around the fire apparatus.

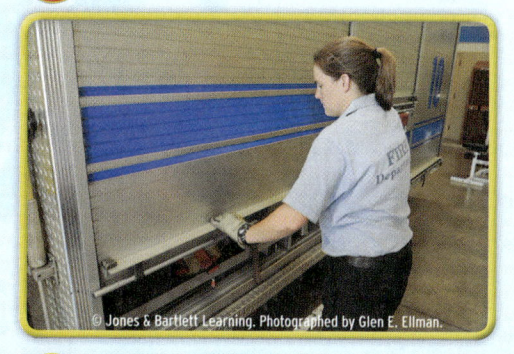

3. Check that all doors are secured.

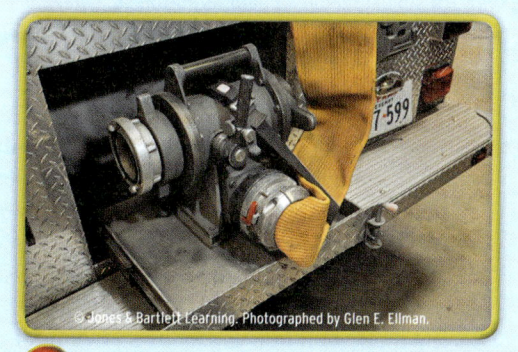

4. Check that all compartment doors are secured.

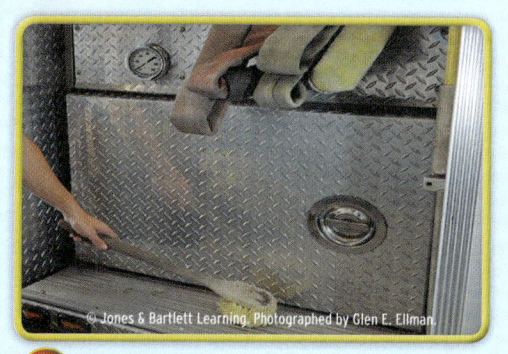

5. Check that all exterior-mounted equipment is properly secured.

6. Remove any debris from the running boards, front bumper, and tailboard.

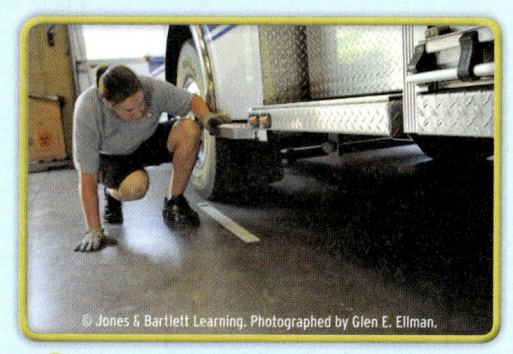

7. Check that the area underneath the fire apparatus is clear of debris.

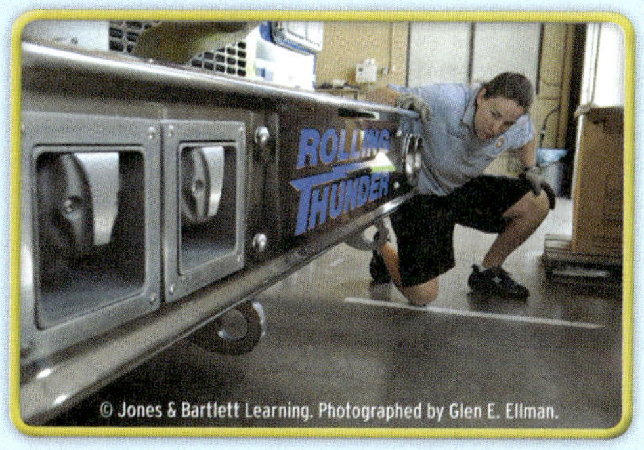

8. Check that the area in front of the fire apparatus is clear and free of debris.

© LiquidLibrary

Starting the Apparatus

After the 360-degree inspection is complete, you will enter the cab and initiate the sequence to start the fire apparatus. Modern fire apparatus are usually powered by a diesel engine. This engine requires a significant amount of current during the starting process. Before starting the fire apparatus, always ensure that unnecessary electrical loads are shut off (i.e., headlights, heater, and air conditioning). Verify that the **parking brake** is set. This brake is required by National Fire Protection Association (NFPA) 1901, *Standard for Automotive Fire Apparatus*, to hold the fire apparatus on at least a 20 percent grade. If the fire apparatus has an automatic transmission (most modern fire apparatus do), make sure it is in the neutral position.

For most fire apparatus, the battery selector switch is turned on next. The **battery selector switch** is used to disconnect all electrical power to the fire apparatus to prevent discharge while it is not in use. Once the power has been transferred to the electrical system, in some fire apparatus it will initiate the system check sequence. A **system check sequence** is a series of checks that an electrical system performs to ensure that all systems are functioning properly before the fire apparatus is started. This check usually takes just a few seconds to complete. If the fire apparatus is started without allowing the system check sequence to finish, it may cause intermittent alarms to occur. For any nonemergency response, always allow the prove-out sequence to continue until the cycle is complete. During an emergency situation, this time delay may not be practical, however.

Once the system check sequence is complete, the fire apparatus is ready to start. Some newer models are equipped with an ignition switch and one or two starter switches. The **ignition switch** delivers operational power to the chassis; engage this switch. The **starter switch** engages the starter motor for cranking. If two starter switches are available, they are provided for redundancy. Engage either or both of these switches to operate the starter motor. When the engine starts, release the starter switch. If the engine does not start within 30 seconds (or in accordance with the manufacturer's recommendations), release the starter switch and allow the starter motor to cool off for 2 minutes before attempting to start it again.

The seats and mirrors should all be adjusted during the daily fire apparatus inspection. If they are not adjusted correctly, readjust them now while the fire apparatus is not in motion. It is very dangerous to attempt to make any changes to the seating or mirror configurations while operating a moving vehicle. Many driver/operators prefer to adjust the mirrors so that the side of the fire apparatus is barely in view of the mirror; this way they can see the side of the apparatus if necessary and can observe any objects to the side of the vehicle **FIGURE 9-1**.

Before you leave for the incident, you must look over the instrument panel. The following items on the instrument panel should always be checked:

- Fuel. The **fuel gauge** indicates the amount of fuel in the apparatus tank. All fire apparatus should be in a constant state of readiness. No fire apparatus fuel tank should ever drop below the halfway level. Always monitor the fuel gauge during operations.

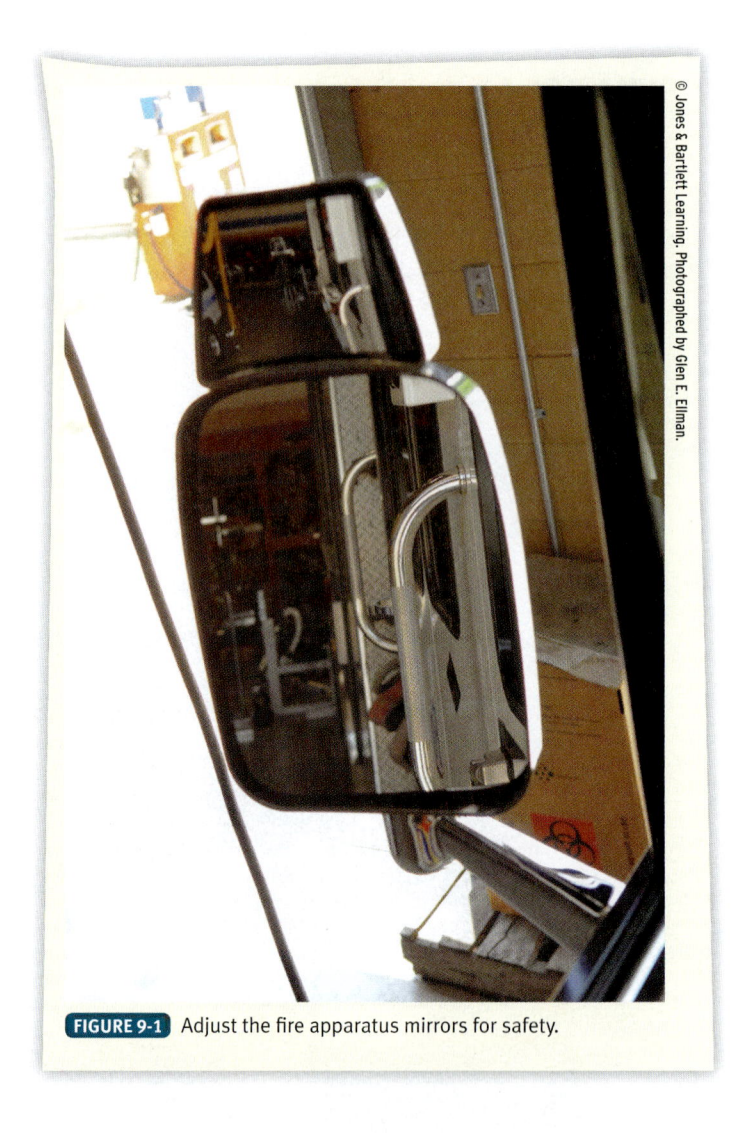

FIGURE 9-1 Adjust the fire apparatus mirrors for safety.

- **Air pressure gauges**. These gauges identify the air pressure stored in the tanks or reservoirs of apparatus equipped with an air braking system. This air pressure is used to slow down and stop the apparatus while it is responding on the roadway. NFPA 1901, *Standard for Automotive Fire Apparatus*, requires that the fire apparatus have a quick build-up capability so that if the apparatus has a completely discharged air system, it is able to move within 60 seconds of start-up. On a chassis that cannot be equipped with a quick recharge air brake system, an onboard automatic electric compressor or a fire station compressed-air shore-line hookup is permitted so as to maintain full operating air pressure while the vehicle is not running. The fire apparatus is also required to have a warning alarm to indicate a low level of air pressure in the system. This alarm is activated when the pressure falls below 60 psi (414 kPa) and remains active until adequate pressure has built up to release the parking brake. For most fire apparatus equipped with air braking systems, a pressure between 100 and 120 psi (690 and 827 kPa) is the normal operating pressure for an air braking system. Always consult the manufacturer's recommendations to determine the appropriate pressure.

VOICES OF EXPERIENCE

I began my career in the fire service and was trained as a driver/operator in an urban area with wide streets and plenty of lanes. Later in my career, my wife and I decided to relocate to the southern part of our state, which happens to be more rural. When I joined my current department, I felt confident in my abilities as a driver/operator and informed the chief that I was ready to drive as soon as he was ready to let me. Back then, our certification process was nonexistent.

During training one day, the chief decided that he was ready to let me drive and prove my abilities. I confidently assumed the driver's seat and began the work of proving to the chief that I was everything that I claimed to be behind the driver's wheel. Just as I had predicted, everything went fine and there were no problems in my driving proficiency. However, during this evaluation time, we spent all of our time on wider "in-town" roads and kept off the narrower country roads.

Finally it was time for me to drive beyond the confines of training. My sergeant told me where we were going. I was familiar with the road and knew that it was one of the narrowest in our district, but I felt confident that I could handle it. We turned onto the narrow road and at first there were no issues; however, there was no oncoming traffic yet either.

Then it happened, I met my first oncoming vehicle. Unfortunately, the vehicle did not feel like yielding to our much larger fire engine. So I moved over to the side of the road a little bit more than I should have and accidentally dropped the rear tire into a shallow ditch. I thought that my heart was going to jump out of my chest and that my sergeant was going to pass out.

Luckily, we were able to get the rear tire back up onto the road without any incident or damage, but I learned that day that there is a huge difference in driving a large fire engine in the city than in the country. I also learned to never yield too much road. If a motorist decides not to give me enough room, I stop and allow the car to pass before I proceed. It's better to get there a few seconds later than not at all.

Jesse Vacra
New Mexico Firefighters Training Academy
Socorro, New Mexico

CHAPTER 9 Driving Fire Apparatus

FIGURE 9-2 A voltmeter.

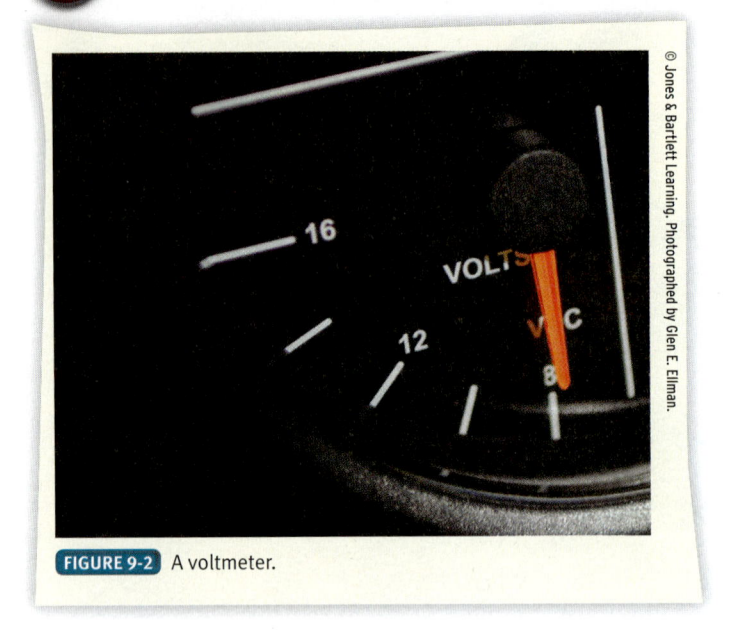

- **Voltmeter.** The voltmeter measures the voltage across the battery terminals of the apparatus and gives an indication of the electrical condition of the battery **FIGURE 9-2**. Operating voltage while the alternator is charging may vary among vehicles depending on the regulator setting. The voltmeter allows for direct observation of the system voltage. If this kind of monitoring is provided, an alarm will sound if the system voltage drops below 11.8 V for 12-V nominal systems or below 23.6 V for 24-V nominal systems for more than 120 seconds. Newer apparatus are extremely sensitive to drops in voltage; it is imperative that the correct voltage be maintained at all times. Many apparatus are equipped with on-board chargers for various pieces of auxiliary equipment, such as flashlights, thermal imaging cameras, and mobile data computers, and it is imperative that the apparatus be plugged into shoreline electrical power when parked in the apparatus bays of the firehouse.
- **Oil pressure gauge.** This gauge identifies the pressure of the lubricating oil in the engine. When the fire apparatus is started, it should provide a reading within a few seconds. If it does not, stop the engine and have a trained technician check the oil pressure.

Seat Belt Safety

Before the fire apparatus moves, you must visually check that all members are wearing a seat belt. You should never move an emergency vehicle with members unsecured. NFPA 1901 requires that all seats of fire apparatus be enclosed and provided with an approved seat belt.

Safety Tip

Newer fire apparatus have alarms to notify you if a fire fighter is not wearing a seat belt. Some fire apparatus will not move unless a weight sensor indicates that all fire fighters are properly wearing their seat belts.

Safety Tip

NFPA standards are not exclusive to just emergency vehicle responses. During funeral processions, parades, or public relations/education events, standing or riding on the tailboard, sidesteps, running board, or any other exposed position should be specifically prohibited. This action is unprofessional and needlessly jeopardizes the safety of fire fighters and the public they serve. Whenever the fire apparatus moves, everyone should be seated and belted—no exceptions!

NFPA 1500, *Standard on Fire Department Occupational Safety and Health Program*, requires the driver/operator not to move the fire apparatus until all persons on the vehicle are seated and secured with seat belts in approved riding positions. While the vehicle is in motion, fire fighters shall not release or loosen their seat belts for any purpose, including the donning of personal protective equipment (PPE) or self-contained breathing apparatus (SCBA).

Getting Underway

Once all members are secure in the cab of the fire apparatus, verify once again that all exterior compartment doors, ladder racks, telescoping scene lights, and any other fire apparatus-mounted equipment are secure **FIGURE 9-3**. Some fire apparatus are equipped with compartment-door indicator lights. These lights are activated only if the fire apparatus compartment doors are open and the parking brake is in the off position. Other fire apparatus may have a digital display that shows any open compartment doors or other equipment that may be damaged if the vehicle moves **FIGURE 9-4**. A 360-degree inspection is always required to ensure safe operation; use these apparatus-mounted systems only as a secondary resource. Double-check the sides of the fire apparatus by using the mirrors.

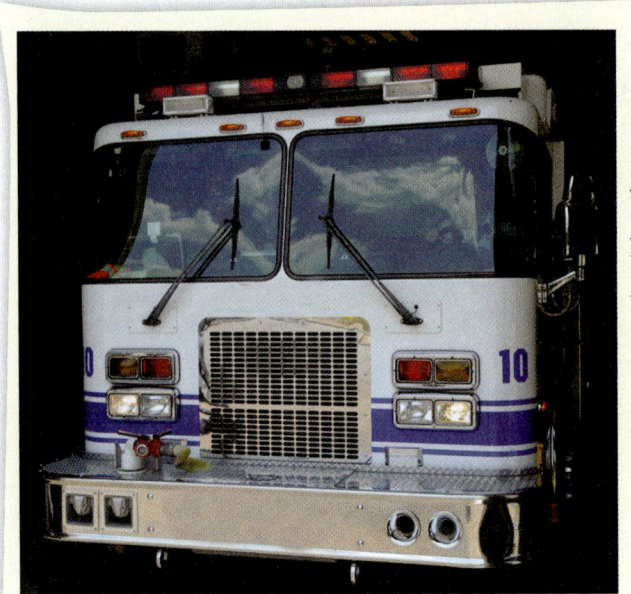

FIGURE 9-3 Before leaving the bay, the driver/operator must verify that all exterior compartment doors, ladder racks, telescoping scene lights, and any other fire apparatus mounted equipment are secure.

FIGURE 9-4 The fire apparatus may have a digital display that shows open compartment doors or other equipment that may be damaged if the vehicle moves.

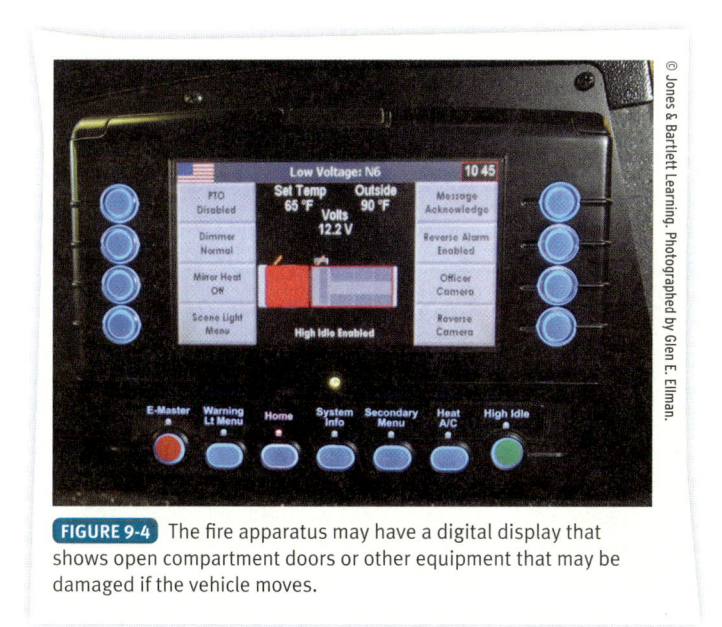

Interior compartment doors also need to be secured in the closed position while the apparatus is responding to an incident. Otherwise, the items that are stored in these compartments may fly out if the fire apparatus is involved in an accident. No fire fighter should ever be injured because someone failed to secure equipment that is stored inside the cab. In particular, equipment such as axes and Halligan tools should never be stored in the cab unless they are secured in an approved bracket. If a compartment or mounting system is provided for equipment, use it!

When applicable, the engine should be allowed to warm up before the response begins. Of course, this may not always be possible depending on the nature of the emergency. Be aware that operating a cold engine and transmission under very hard conditions (emergency response) may have a damaging effect to the engine. Whenever possible, allow the engine to warm up for 3 to 5 minutes. This will help to extend the life of the fire apparatus and may prevent future breakdowns.

The headlights should be turned on whenever the fire apparatus is moving, not just during the night. Research has shown that a vehicle is easier for other drivers and pedestrians to identify during any conditions if it has its headlights on.

Once the overhead garage door is fully open, the fire apparatus may be driven out of the station. Be aware that other fire apparatus at the station may be leaving at the same time or that the exhaust extractor system and electrical cords may not eject properly. For these reasons, you should not exceed 5 mph (8 km/h) while pulling out of the fire station.

Look to the sides of the fire apparatus and ensure that the cords and extractor are clear. Always remember to close the doors after clearing the building. If responding in an emergency mode, activate the emergency lights and audible warning devices at this time.

To start a fire apparatus and ensure that it is ready for a response, follow the steps in **SKILL DRILL 9-2**:

1. Enter the fire apparatus cab. (**STEP 1**)
2. Verify that the parking brake is set in the "on" position. (**STEP 2**)
3. Check that the transmission is in the neutral position. (**STEP 3**)
4. Verify that any unnecessary electrical loads (including the air conditioner/heater and headlights) are turned off before activating the battery. (**STEP 4**)
5. Turn on the battery selector switch. (**STEP 5**)
6. Allow the fire apparatus to complete the system check sequence.
7. Engage the ignition switch. (**STEP 6**)
8. Engage the starter switch. (**STEP 7**)
9. Adjust the seat and mirrors, if necessary. (**STEP 8**)
10. Check the gauges: fuel, air pressure, voltmeter, and oil pressure. (**STEP 9**)
11. Ensure that each crew member is wearing a seat belt before moving the fire apparatus. (**STEP 10**)
12. Check the compartment-door indicator light, if applicable, to ensure that no compartments are open. (**STEP 11**)
13. Turn on the headlights. (**STEP 12**)
14. Allow the engine to warm up before moving, if applicable.
15. Place the transmission in "drive." (**STEP 13**)
16. Release the parking brake. (**STEP 14**)
17. Activate the emergency lights and audible warning devices. (**STEP 15**)
18. Drive the fire apparatus out of the fire station at a speed less than 5 mph (8 km/h).
19. Check the sidewalk to confirm that all pedestrian traffic has stopped. (**STEP 16**)
20. Activate any signal control system to stop traffic in front of the fire station. (**STEP 17**)
21. Close the fire station doors with the remote control to ensure security. (**STEP 18**)

Safety Tip

According to a Texas State Fire Marshal's Office Fire Fighter Fatality Investigation Report, a fire fighter fell from a moving fire apparatus while responding to a structure fire. On April 23, 2005, fire fighter Brian Hunton of the Amarillo Fire Department was riding in the left-rear seat of a Ladder 1 apparatus when the door opened and he fell out. Hunton struck his head on the street and sustained severe head injuries; he died two days later. During the response, he had been donning his SCBA and not wearing his seat belt.

All fire fighters are responsible for their own safety. During an emergency response, all members should wear their seat belts. This type of accident is preventable with the proper use of seat belts. Each fire department should have a SOP in place that requires the use of seat belts, and this policy must be enforced by all members. Requiring fire fighters to wear seat belts is a simple rule that could prevent 10 to 15 fatalities every year.

Fire Apparatus Driver/Operator

SKILL DRILL 9-2 Starting a Fire Apparatus
NFPA 1002, 4.3.1, 4.3.1(B)

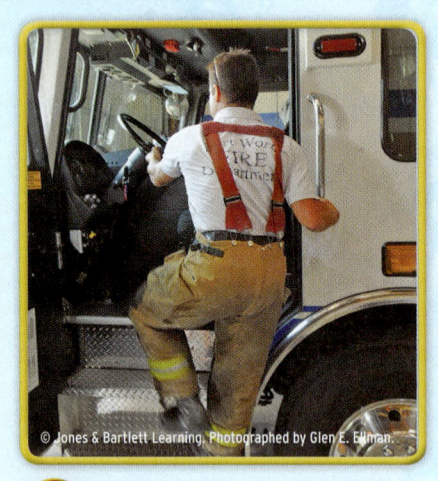

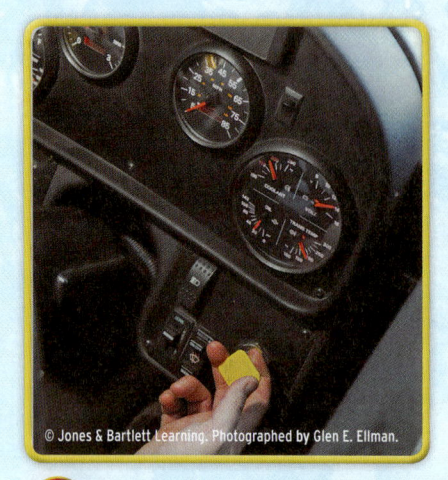

1. Enter the fire apparatus cab.

2. Verify that the parking brake is set in the "on" position.

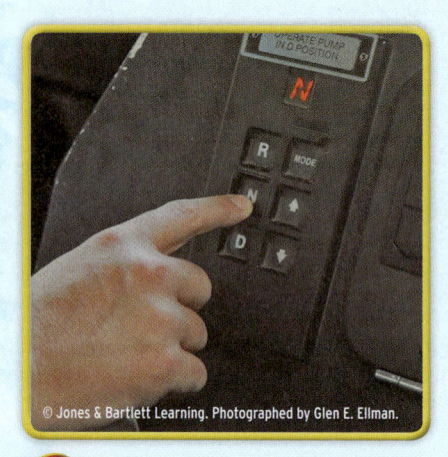

3. Check that the transmission is in the neutral position.

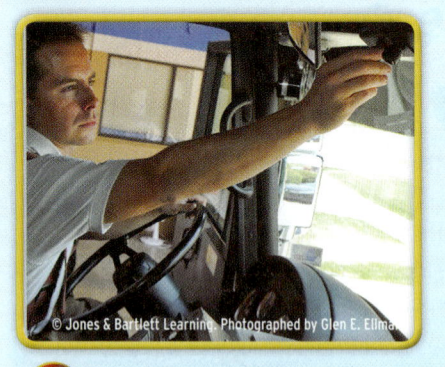

4. Verify that any unnecessary electrical loads (including the air conditioner/heater and headlights) are turned off before activating the battery.

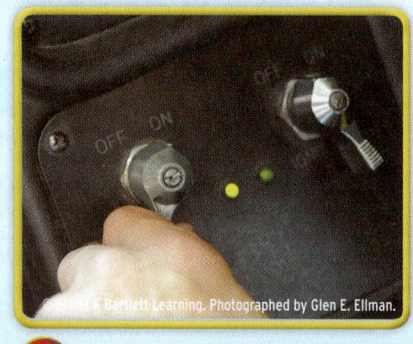

5. Turn on the battery selector switch.

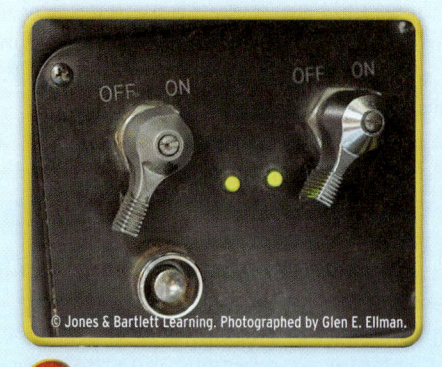

6. Allow the apparatus to complete the system check sequence. Engage the ignition switch.

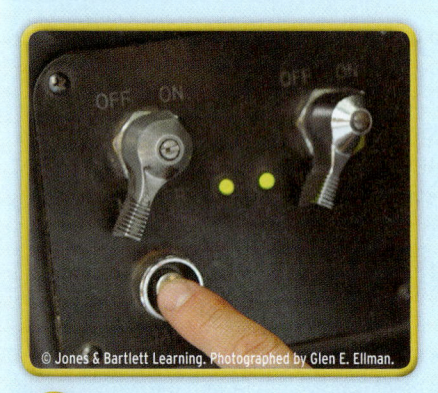

7. Engage the starter switch.

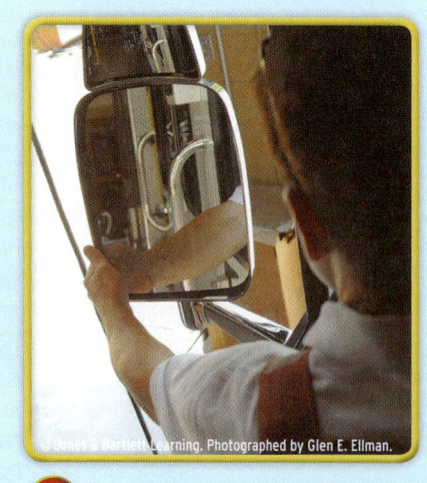

8. Adjust the seat and mirrors, if necessary.

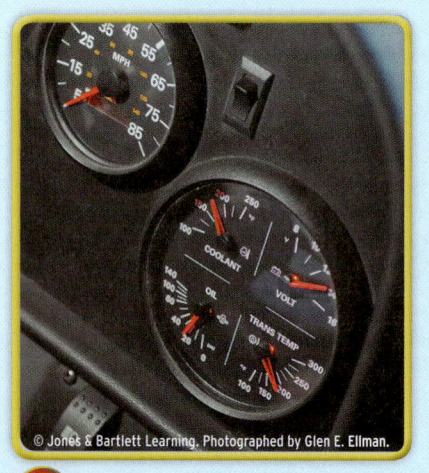

9. Check the gauges: fuel, air pressure, voltmeter, and oil pressure.

(Continued)

SKILL DRILL 9-2   Starting a Fire Apparatus (*Continued*)

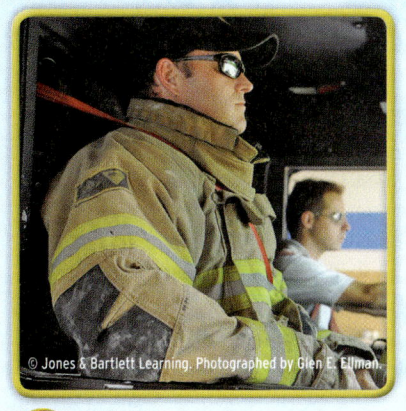

10 Ensure that each crew member is wearing a seat belt before moving the fire apparatus.

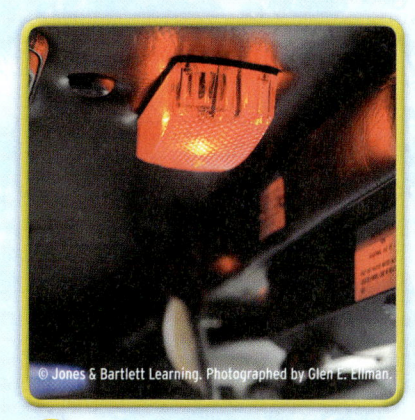

11 Check the compartment-door indicator light, if applicable, to ensure that no compartments are open.

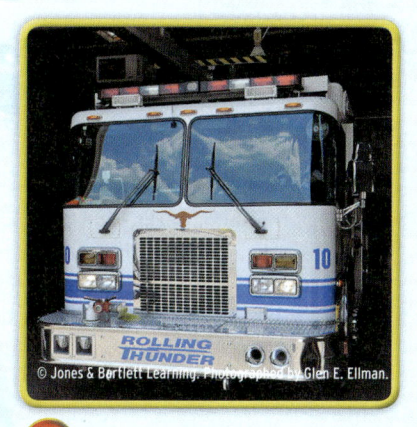

12 Turn on the headlights.

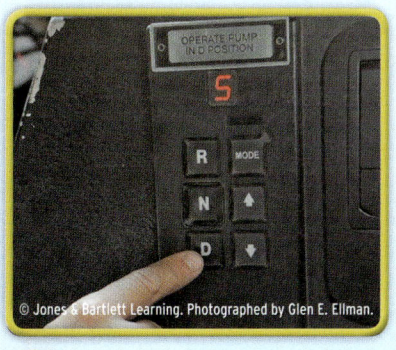

13 Allow the engine to warm up before moving, if applicable. Place the transmission in "drive."

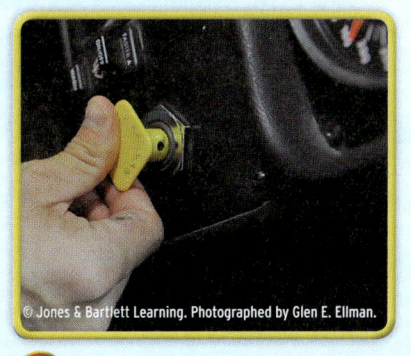

14 Release the parking brake.

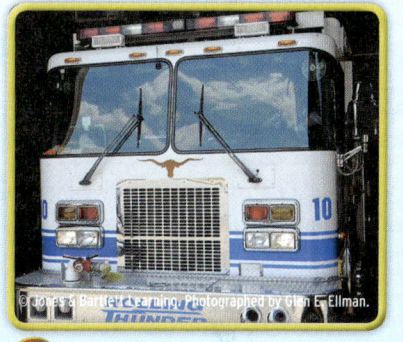

15 Activate the emergency lights and audible warning devices.

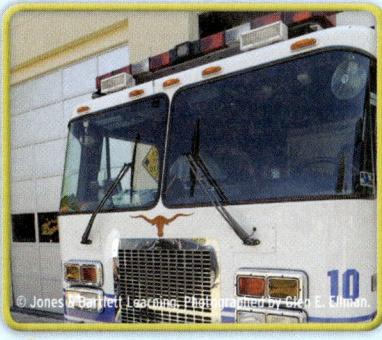

16 Drive the fire apparatus out of the fire station at a speed less than 5 mph (8 km/h). Check the sidewalk to make certain that all pedestrian traffic has stopped.

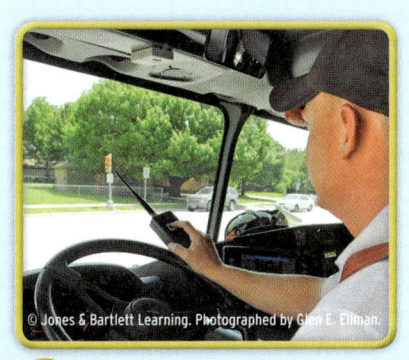

17 Activate any signal control system to stop traffic in front of the fire station.

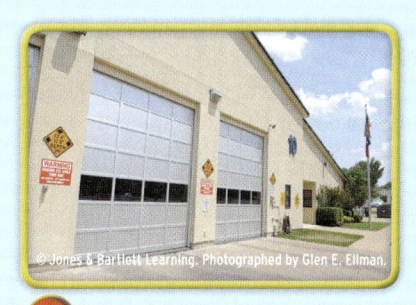

18 Close the fire station doors with the remote control to ensure security.

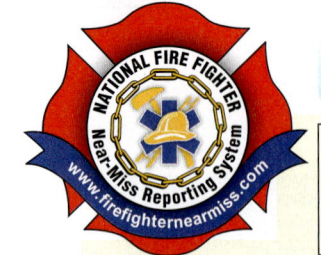

Near-Miss REPORT

Report Number: N/A

Synopsis: Two Fire Apparatus Collide While Backing Up On Scene.

Event Description: My crew was responding to a report of a structure fire in our first due response area. Our driver that day was an "actor," as the normally assigned driver had the day off. Our protocol is that the first due engine secures a water supply and "lays in" to the address of the fire. The driver was instructed as to where the hydrant was, and I asked him to stop so the back step fire fighter could secure the hydrant and get us water for the attack. The driver passed the house on fire and the hydrant we were going to utilize for water. I instructed him to stop the apparatus and back up to the address of the structure fire, and I would radio the next engine to bring us a supply line. When I made the order, I assumed that my back step fire fighter heard me and that he would act as a spotter for the driver to safely back the apparatus. I was wrong. The driver proceeded to back the apparatus without a spotter and ran into another emergency response vehicle, already on scene, delaying our initial attack on the fire.

Lessons Learned: Always use a spotter while backing. There are so many moving parts to a fire scene that we all have to be on our game in order to provide the highest level of safety for one another. I assumed that the spotter was an automatic response and that the driver would not back up without one. Tunnel vision and inexperience dictated an alternate response, and the result was a collision that delayed the initial attack and could have made a negative impact on the fire attack as a whole.

DRIVER/OPERATOR Tip

Driving a fire apparatus while wearing turnout pants and boots can be very cumbersome for some fire fighters. For this reason, some fire departments do not require their driver/operators to dress in turnout gear while driving to the incident. Evaluate your ability to safely operate the fire apparatus while wearing turnout pants and boots. If you do not feel safe operating under these conditions, notify your supervisor and determine the best course of action. Remember—safety always comes first.

Driving Exercises

Riding in a fire apparatus as it is responding to an emergency scene can be very exciting. Driving the fire apparatus to a scene is even more exciting. You may develop a rush of adrenaline while operating the fire apparatus on the roadway. This excitement, however, should not make you lose sight of the task at hand—transporting the fire apparatus and its members to the emergency scene in a safe and efficient manner. The fire apparatus should not be driven faster than existing conditions permit or at a speed greater than can be maintained with safety. At all times, you must be able to maintain control of the fire apparatus. Do not allow the situation or other members of the crew to push you into driving the fire apparatus beyond your abilities. Instead, always use common sense and good judgment. A speedy response is achieved through a safe and efficient means of operation—not by taking unnecessary risks. Never endanger life or property, under any circumstances.

During the emergency response, you may have to maneuver the fire apparatus around objects at the scene or parked vehicles that are blocking access to a preferred location. This type of maneuver is done at a reduced speed with an emphasis on the safety of pedestrians, other objects, and the fire apparatus. NFPA 1002, *Standard for Fire Apparatus Driver/Operator Professional Qualifications*, requires that all driver/operators complete a serpentine exercise that simulates these conditions. The exercise measures the driver/operator's ability to maneuver in close quarters without stopping the fire apparatus.

■ Performing a Serpentine Maneuver

As part of the serpentine maneuver exercise, a minimum of three marker cones are spaced 30 to 38 ft (9 to 12 m) apart in a line. The spacing of the marker cones should be equal to the fire apparatus' wheelbase. The space on the sides of the marker cones must provide adequate space for the fire apparatus to travel freely. To perform the serpentine maneuver, drive the fire apparatus along the left side of the marker cones in a straight line and stop with the fire apparatus just past the final marker cone. You are now in position to begin the exercise. Back the fire apparatus to the left of marker cone 1, to the right of marker cone 2, and to the left of marker 3. Once the front of the fire apparatus is past marker cone 3, drive the fire apparatus forward between the marker cones by passing to the right of marker cone 3, to the left of marker cone 2, and to the right of marker cone 1.

During the entire exercise, the marker cones should not be struck and the fire apparatus should move in a continuous motion, except when required to change direction of travel. A spotter is necessary for this exercise. To perform the serpentine exercise, follow the steps in **SKILL DRILL 9-3**:

1. Position the fire apparatus past marker cone 1. (**STEP 1**)
2. Activate the emergency lights on the fire apparatus. (**STEP 2**)
3. Ensure that a spotter is in position at the rear of the fire apparatus. (**STEP 3**)

CHAPTER 9 Driving Fire Apparatus 201

SKILL DRILL 9-3 Performing the Serpentine Exercise
NFPA 1002, 4.3.3, 4.3.3(B)

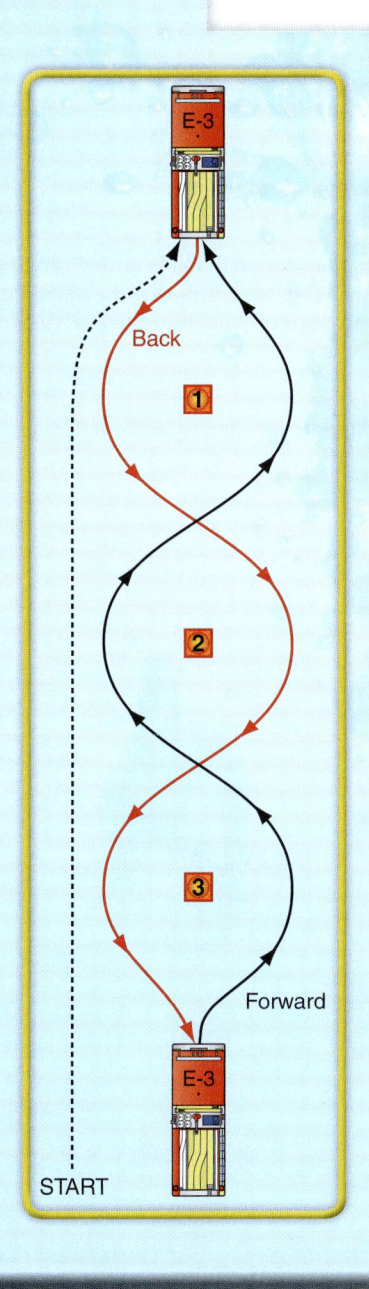

1. Position the fire apparatus past marker cone 1.
2. Activate the emergency lights on the fire apparatus.
3. Ensure a spotter is in position at the rear of the fire apparatus.
4. Place the fire apparatus in reverse.
5. Proceed in reverse through the exercise area, to the left of marker cone 1.
6. Proceed in reverse through the exercise area, to the right of marker cone 2.
7. Proceed in reverse through the exercise area, to the left of marker cone 3.
8. Position the front of the fire apparatus past marker cone 3.
9. Proceed forward through the exercise area, to the right of marker cone 3.
10. Proceed forward through the exercise area, to the left of marker cone 2.
11. Proceed forward through the exercise area, to the right of marker cone 1.
12. Once the rear of the fire apparatus passes marker cone 1, the exercise is complete.

© LiquidLibrary

4. Place the fire apparatus in reverse. (**STEP 4**)
5. Proceed in reverse through the exercise area, to the left of marker cone 1. (**STEP 5**)
6. Proceed in reverse through the exercise area, to the right of marker cone 2. (**STEP 6**)
7. Proceed in reverse through the exercise area, to the left of marker cone 3. (**STEP 7**)
8. Position the front of the fire apparatus past marker cone 3. (**STEP 8**)
9. Proceed forward through the exercise area, to the right of marker cone 3. (**STEP 9**)
10. Proceed forward through the exercise area, to the left of marker cone 2. (**STEP 10**)
11. Proceed forward through the exercise area, to the right of marker cone 1. (**STEP 11**)
12. Once the rear of the fire apparatus passes marker cone 1, the exercise is complete. (**STEP 12**)

■ Performing a Confined-Space Turnaround

When responding to an incident, you may inadvertently pass a street on which you should have turned. When this situation occurs, the best course is to drive the fire apparatus around the block rather than try to turn the fire apparatus around in the confines of a roadway. Other motorists may be confused by your actions as you attempt to move a large fire apparatus around 180 degrees, only to proceed back in the direction

SKILL DRILL 9-4

Performing a Confined-Space Turnaround
NFPA 1002, 4.3.4, 4.3.4(B)

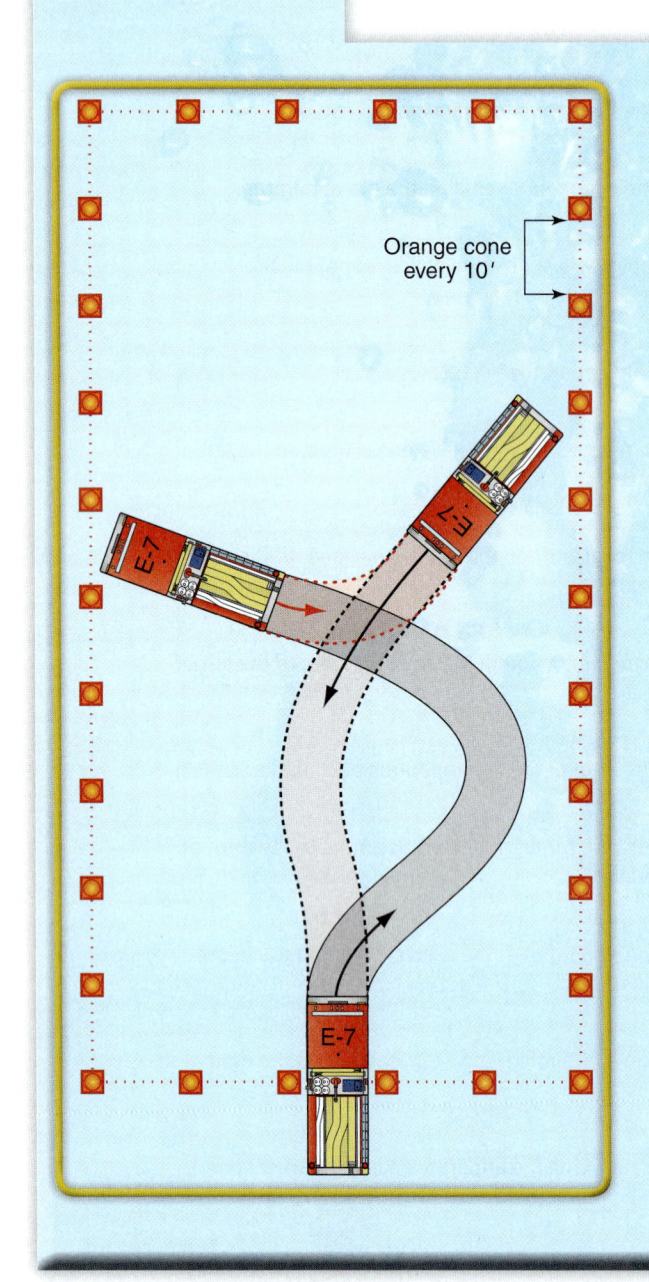

Orange cone every 10'

1 Position the fire apparatus outside the boundary opening.

2 Proceed forward through the opening.

3 Maneuver the fire apparatus so that it is turned 180 degrees. This will require driving forward, swinging the tail of the apparatus almost 90 degrees, and then maneuvering forward. "Forward, swing, forward."

4 Proceed forward through the opening and out of the set boundary.

© LiquidLibrary

---

from which you just came. However, even seasoned driver/operators can go down a wrong road or find themselves in a position where they need to turn around and go the other way.

NFPA 1002 requires that all driver/operators complete an exercise that simulates these circumstances, during which they turn a fire apparatus 180 degrees within a predetermined area where the apparatus cannot complete a U-turn. This exercise, which is called a confined-space turnaround, measures your ability to turn the fire apparatus around in a confined space without going outside a set boundary. It is completed in a 50 ft × 100 ft (15 m × 31 m) area, where marker cones may be used to identify the set boundary. The fire apparatus enters the area through an opening, no more than 12 ft (4 m) wide, in the center of one of the 50-ft (15-m) sides. The fire apparatus proceeds forward, turns around 180 degrees, and returns through the same opening. You may maneuver the fire apparatus forward and reverse as many times as needed to accomplish the task, but the fire apparatus must remain inside the set boundary lines. During the entire exercise, the fire apparatus must remain in the marked boundary and move in a continuous motion, except when required to change direction of travel. A spotter is necessary for this exercise.

To perform the confined-space turnaround exercise, follow the steps in **SKILL DRILL 9-4**:

1 Position the fire apparatus outside the boundary opening. (**STEP 1**)

2 Proceed forward through the opening. (**STEP 2**)

3 Maneuver the fire apparatus so that it is turned 180 degrees. This will require driving forward, swinging the tail of the apparatus almost 90 degrees, and then maneuvering forward. "Forward, swing, forward." (STEP 3)

4. Proceed forward through the opening and out of the set boundary. (STEP 4)

Performing a Diminishing Clearance Exercise

Once at the scene, you may have to operate the fire apparatus in tight quarters. Sometimes other fire apparatus, trees, storefront signs, or buildings can obstruct your path. However, the most common obstruction on an emergency scene is parked cars. Any one of these obstructions may restrict the horizontal or vertical clearance of the fire apparatus and make your task as driver/operator difficult at best. During these situations, you must judge the distance you have available to clear through openings and not cause any damage.

NFPA 1002 requires that all driver/operators complete an exercise that simulates a restricted horizontal and vertical clearance for a fire apparatus. This "diminishing clearance" exercise measures your ability to maneuver the fire apparatus in a straight line and judge the distance of the fire apparatus to an object in front of it. The fire apparatus should proceed at a speed that requires your quick judgment. It moves forward down two rows of marker cones to form a lane 75 ft (23 m) long. The lane's width diminishes from a starting point of 9 ft 6 inches (2.9 m) to a width of 8 ft 2 inches (2.5 m). Marker cones identify the lanes boundary. To perform the exercise successfully, you must proceed forward down the lane without striking the marker cones. Bring the apparatus to a complete stop 50 ft (15 m) past the last marker cone at a predetermined

DRIVER/OPERATOR Tip

When operating the fire apparatus, you must always drive with "due regard for the safety of others." This statement or something similar is found in most state laws that pertain to emergency vehicle operations. An emergency vehicle operator may have the right to disregard certain traffic laws but does not have the right to jeopardize the safety of other motorists or pedestrians. For example, some fire departments and local laws allow emergency vehicles to exceed the speed limit on roads and highways. Usually, certain conditions must be met to do this—namely, light traffic and good weather conditions. If the emergency vehicle operator exceeds the speed limit under adverse conditions, he or she is not "driving with due regard for the safety of others." During the entire response, you must be constantly aware of other motorists and pedestrians as well as your own safety.

DRIVER/OPERATOR Tip

The National Fallen Firefighters Foundation (NFFF) summarizes the issues pertaining to vehicle safety:
- It's not a race.
- Safe is more important than fast.
- Stop at red lights and stop signs! There are no excuses.
- If they do not get out of your way, do not run them over! Think and react carefully.

Safety Tip

The use of sirens during gridlock merely confuses other drivers when they have nowhere to move their cars. Use the public address system and give the drivers directions.

Safety Tip

You should understand that a prompt, safe response is obtained by adhering to the following guidelines:

- Leave the station in a standard manner:
  - Perform a 360-degree walk around the fire apparatus. Check for open compartments.
  - Quickly mount the fire apparatus.
  - Make sure that all personnel are on board and are seated with seat belts on.
  - Make sure the station doors are fully open.
  - Close the fire station doors with a remote control upon leaving.
  - Drive defensively and professionally at reasonable speeds.
  - Know where you are going.
  - Use warning devices to move around traffic and to request the right-of-way in a safe and predictable manner.

Do not:
- Leave your quarters before the crew has mounted safely and before the fire station doors are fully open.
- Drive too fast for the current conditions.
- Drive recklessly or without regard for safety.
- Take unnecessary chances with negative right-of-way intersections.
- Intimidate or scare other drivers.

DRIVER/OPERATOR Tip

According to a National Incident for Occupational Safety and Health (NIOSH) report:

On August 14, 2004, a 25-year-old female career fire fighter (the victim) died when she apparently fell from the tailboard and was backed over by an engine. The victim and her crew had been released from the scene of a residential fire. The road was blocked by other apparatus, so the victim's crew began backing to an intersection approximately 300 ft (90 m) away so as to then proceed forward. The victim took her position on the tailboard as the "tailboard safety member" and signaled the driver to begin backing. A captain acting as the "traffic control officer" guided the backing operation from the road on the driver's side, behind the apparatus, by using hand signals. When the captain turned and walked into the intersection to stop cross-traffic, the victim apparently fell from the tailboard and was run over by the engine. Members on the scene provided advanced life support and the victim was transported to a local hospital, where she was pronounced dead.

You should always be aware of the hazards involved with moving fire apparatus. Even when the situation is not deemed urgent, remain alert to your surroundings. An injury can occur at any time—not just during emergency situations.

SKILL DRILL 9-5 Performing a Diminishing Clearance Exercise
NFPA 1002, 4.3.5, 4.3.5(B)

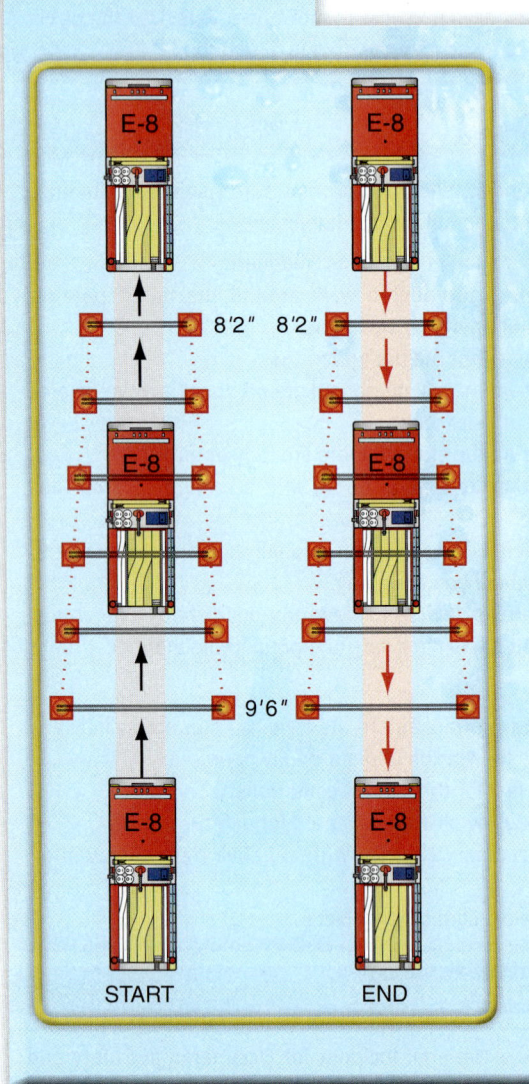

1. Position the fire apparatus at the opening of the diminishing clearance. Proceed forward through the lane. Stop the fire apparatus at the finish line.

2. Proceed in reverse through the lane. Identify any vertical heights on the crossbar that may strike the fire apparatus.

finish line. No portion of the fire apparatus can protrude past this set line. The fire apparatus then proceeds in reverse past the point where it entered the diminishing clearance exercise.

During the course of the fire apparatus moving forward and reversing, a vertical crossbar prop is positioned to determine your ability to judge the height of the fire apparatus. The crossbar may be positioned at several heights, including one that is lower than the fire apparatus. You must be capable of judging the vertical and horizontal clearances of the fire apparatus.

During the entire exercise, the fire apparatus must remain within the marker cones and move in a continuous motion, except when required to change direction of travel. A spotter is necessary for this exercise.

To perform the diminishing clearance exercise, follow the steps in **SKILL DRILL 9-5**:

1. Position the fire apparatus at the opening of the diminishing clearance.
2. Proceed forward through the lane.
3. Stop the fire apparatus at the finish line. (**STEP 1**)
4. Proceed in reverse through the lane.
5. Identify any vertical heights on the crossbar that may strike the fire apparatus. (**STEP 2**)

Returning to the Station

When returning to the fire station, you cannot become complacent. Operating an emergency vehicle on the roadway can be dangerous even when driving back from a call. You may be fatigued and unable to react appropriately. Civilian drivers may think that the fire apparatus is responding to an emergency and unexpectedly stop in front of it. Some civilian drivers, while trying to be courteous, may wave or invite the fire apparatus into traffic ahead of them. While their intentions are good, you must always obey the rules of the road and be cautious of other drivers. Do not allow anyone to force you into traffic.

When the fire apparatus returns to the firehouse, it should be allowed to cool whenever possible. This should take place on the ramp of the firehouse and should not take place inside, as the high exhaust temperatures can cause serious damage to exhaust removal hoses and equipment. This helps extend the life of the engine and transmission. If the fire apparatus is driven hard everywhere it goes and does not have adequate time to cool down before being shut off, damage to the power train may occur over time.

Reversing the Fire Apparatus

For most fire departments, the largest number of fire apparatus accidents are related to backing up fire apparatus. Very few fire departments respond with only one member on the fire apparatus. If two or more members are on the fire apparatus, this type of accident is entirely preventable. Every fire department should have an SOP that covers fire apparatus backing procedures. Each member of the fire department needs to be trained and held accountable for these procedures.

Most modern fire stations are now built with drive-through bays so that fire apparatus do not have to back into the station. While this arrangement may reduce the number of backing-up accidents at the station, it may also contribute to backing-up skills becoming rusty.

Whenever an emergency vehicle is backing up, its emergency lights should be turned on and the driver/operator should use a spotter to assist with the procedure. A **spotter** is a person who guides the driver/operator into the appropriate position while the apparatus is operating in a confined space or in reverse mode. The spotter should always be in the driver/operator's full view **FIGURE 9-5**. No vehicle should be backed into an intersection, around a corner, into the fire station, or in traffic unless emergency lighting is used and a spotter precedes it to safely direct such movement. During poor-visibility conditions, rear apparatus spotlights may be used as necessary. Never hesitate to use more than one spotter to assist with backing-up maneuvers if the situation warrants. If the driver/operator cannot see the spotter at any time, the vehicle should be stopped.

It is your responsibility to ensure that all spotters know in advance what is expected, where you intend to back up the fire apparatus, and which signals will be used. Before backing up the fire apparatus, roll down the windows and turn off any audio equipment to ensure any orders to stop the fire apparatus given by the spotter are clearly heard and understood. The spotter should use a portable radio to communicate with you. Any verbal communication between the driver/operator and the spotter should take place via radio.

The following are some suggested procedures for spotters:
- The rear spotter must stay behind and to the left of the fire apparatus. This spotter should position his or her body as a landmark for you to line up on. The spotter should always be able to see you in the side mirror. If the spotter cannot see you, then you cannot see the spotter. Stop immediately!
- Any spotter can give a loud "Stop!" order directly to you when it is deemed necessary.
- During high noise conditions, one spotter must be equipped with a radio to inform you to stop. Select an appropriate radio channel for this communication.

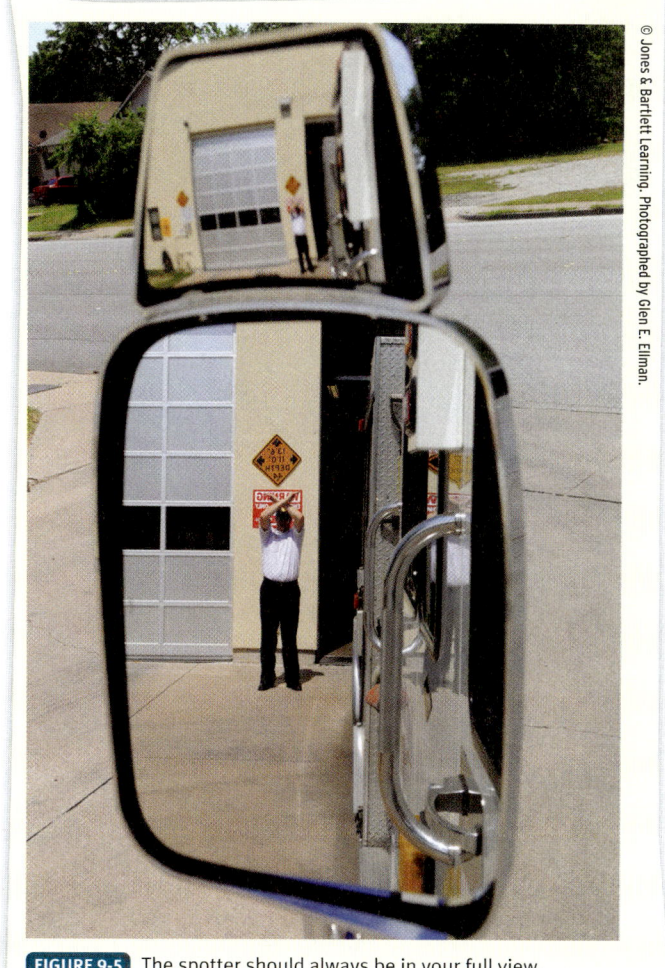

FIGURE 9-5 The spotter should always be in your full view.

- All verbal signals must be loud enough and clear enough to be heard by you.
- All hand signals must be in "large" movements, and as simple as possible. Signals given in front of the body can be difficult to see.
- While the fire apparatus is backing up at night or in limited-visibility conditions, the spotters should use flashlights to illuminate the surrounding area and hand signals.
- When the spotter is directing the fire apparatus backward or forward in a straight line, the spotter should have both arms extended forward and slightly wider than the body, parallel to the ground. The palms should face the direction of desired travel. The spotter will bend both arms repeatedly toward the head and chest to direct the fire apparatus **FIGURE 9-6**.
- When the spotter is directing the fire apparatus either to the right or to the left while it is moving, the spotter should have the directional arm extended from the side of the body, parallel to the ground, indicating the direction in which to travel. The motioning arm should be extended in the opposite direction (palm upward) and repeatedly bent toward the head, indicating the desired direction of travel **FIGURE 9-7**.

FIGURE 9-6 Arm placement when the spotter is directing the fire apparatus in a straight line.

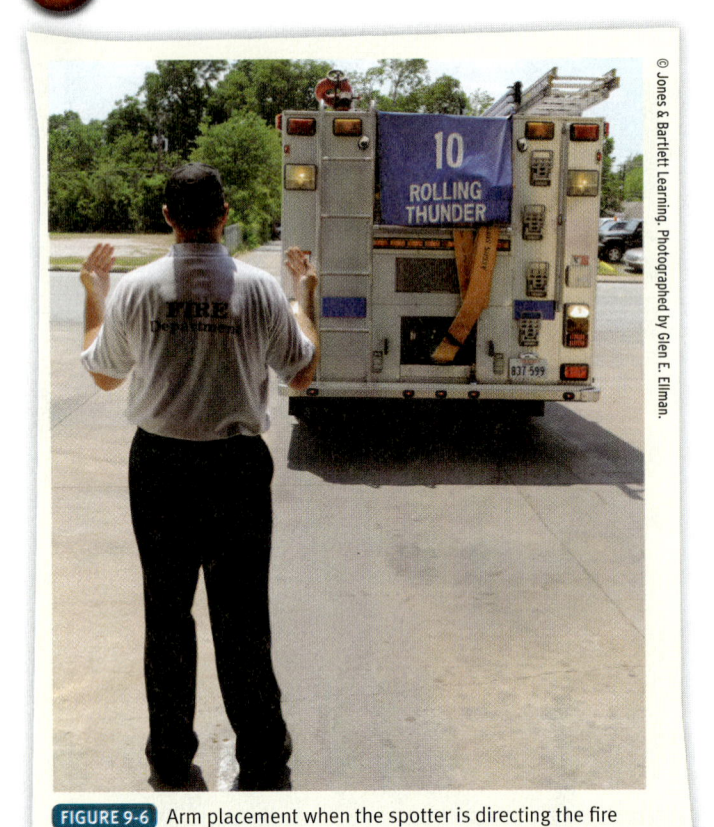

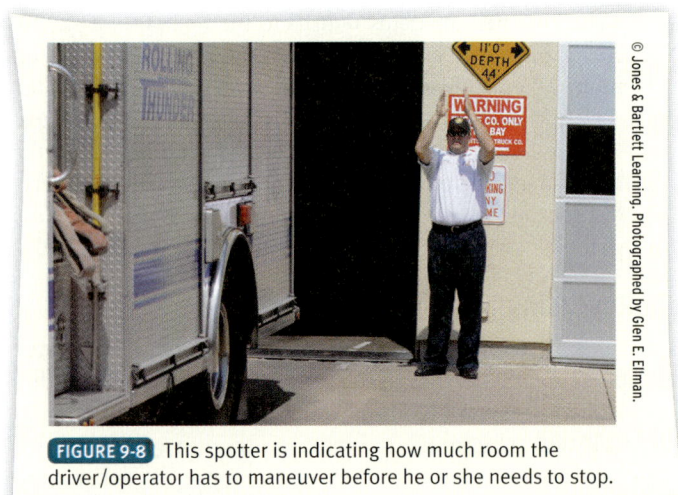

FIGURE 9-8 This spotter is indicating how much room the driver/operator has to maneuver before he or she needs to stop.

- To provide you with a visual reference for the distance to the stopping point, the spotter should have both arms extended sideways with elbows bent upward at 90 degrees. The spotter's palms should face forward, hands above the head, and the spotter should bring the elbows forward as the distance narrows. As the elbows reach the straightforward position, the hands continue coming together above the head to indicate that the stopping point is being reached. Upon reaching the stopping point, the spotter should give a loud "Stop!" signal **FIGURE 9-8**.

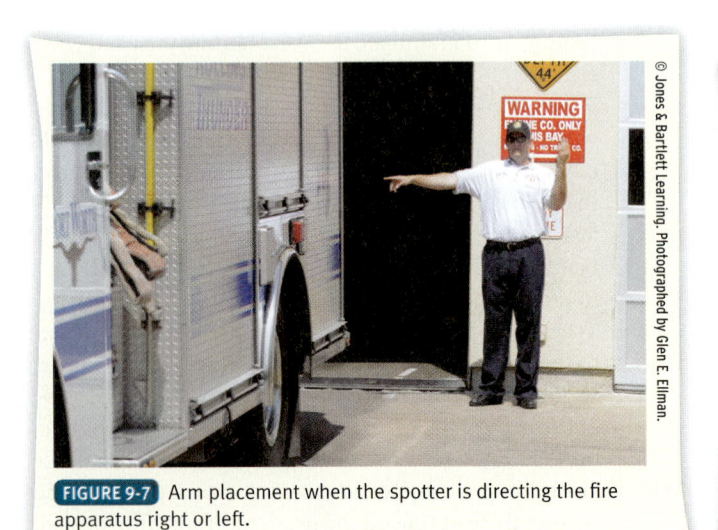

- The spotter may signal to you to stop the fire apparatus when it has reached the desired objective or if the safety of the operation is compromised. To do so, the spotter will cross the arms at the wrist (forearms) above the head, and then maintain this position until the fire apparatus comes to a complete stop. While motioning with the arms, the spotter should also shout as loudly as possible, "Stop!" These actions should catch your attention and cause you to bring the fire apparatus to a halt **FIGURE 9-9**.

The spotter must understand that in most circumstances, you are able to operate the fire apparatus in reverse without direction. In these cases, it is the spotter's responsibility to ensure that you do not hit anything or anyone. Regardless of the number of spotters utilized, you should receive directions only from one spotter in the rear of the vehicle and, if utilized, from one spotter to the front of the fire apparatus. If the fire apparatus is equipped with a rear-mounted camera, it should be used as well **FIGURE 9-10**. This technology should not take the place of an actual spotter, but simply serves to augment your ability to see what is behind you.

NFPA 1002 requires that all driver/operators complete an exercise that simulates backing up a fire apparatus into a fire

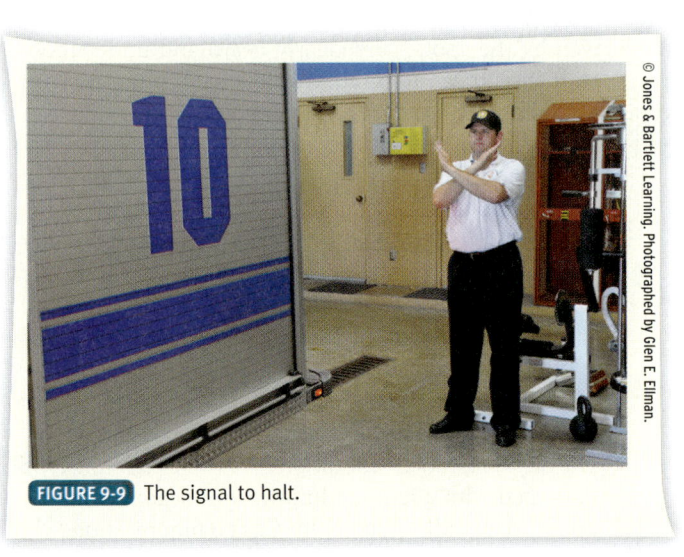

FIGURE 9-7 Arm placement when the spotter is directing the fire apparatus right or left.

FIGURE 9-9 The signal to halt.

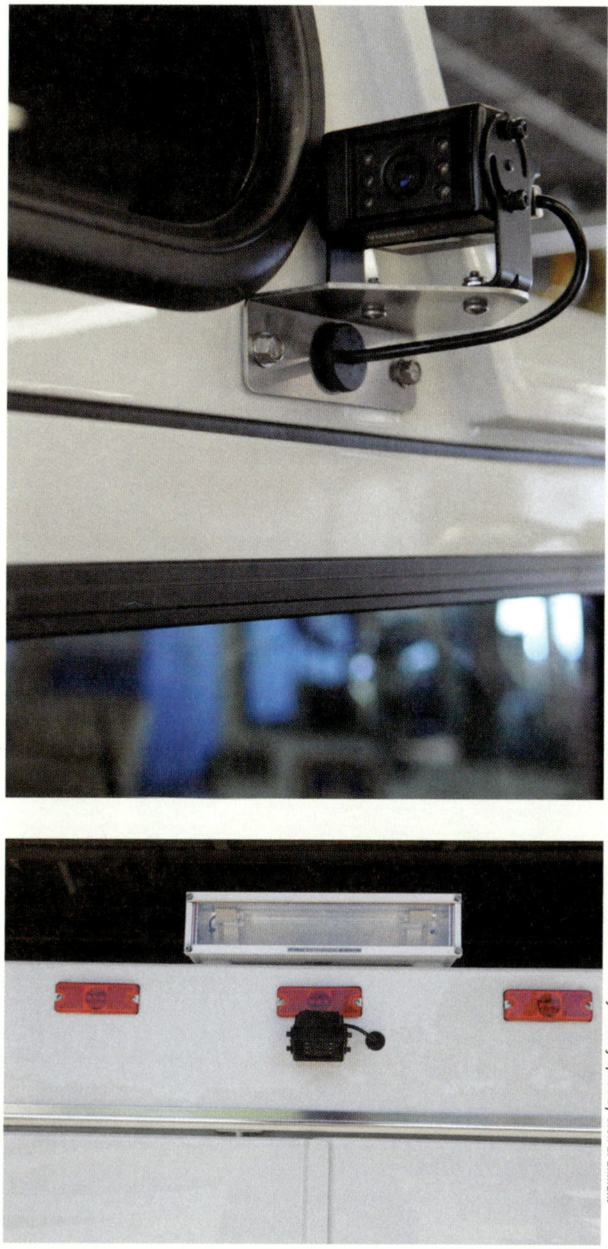

A

B

© Jones & Bartlett Learning. Photographed by Glen E. Ellman.

© Jones & Bartlett Learning. Photographed by Glen E. Ellman.

FIGURE 9-10 A camera is an important piece of safety equipment. **A.** Side-mounted camera. **B.** Rear-mounted camera.

station: the station parking procedure drill. A fire apparatus bay is simulated by allowing for a 20-ft (6-m) minimum setback from a street that is 30 ft (9 m) wide; barricades are placed at the end of the setback, spaced 12 ft (3.7 m) apart to simulate the garage door. The setback distance should accurately reflect those distances found during normal duties. A marker placed on the ground indicates the proper position of the left-front tire of the fire apparatus once stopped and parked. A reference line may be used to facilitate using the fire apparatus mirrors. The minimum depth of the fire apparatus bay is determined by the length of the fire apparatus. During the entire exercise, the fire apparatus must remain within the marked boundary and the fire apparatus should move in a continuous motion, except when required to change direction of travel. A spotter is necessary for this exercise.

To perform the correct procedure for backing a fire apparatus into a fire station bay, follow the steps in **SKILL DRILL 9-6**:

1. Position the rear of the fire apparatus past the fire station bay's opening at a 90-degree angle to the station. Ensure a spotter is correctly positioned behind the fire apparatus. (**STEP 1**)
2. Activate the emergency lights.
3. Turn off any fire apparatus–mounted stereo equipment. (**STEP 2**)
4. Disengage the parking brake, if set. (**STEP 3**)
5. Shift the transmission to reverse. (**STEP 4**)
6. Proceed in a reverse mode and turn the fire apparatus to align it with the objective. (**STEP 5**)
7. Continue backing the fire apparatus until it has reached the desired objective or the spotter signals "Stop." (**STEP 6**)

Although it is not recommended, during an emergency situation a fire apparatus may have to be backed up without a spotter. In this situation, you should do a preliminary inspection; check for obstructions, vertical and horizontal clearances, and power lines; and ensure that all compartments, doors, latches, and gates are closed. Proceed with extreme caution and back the unit just far enough to where it can be turned around and then driven forward.

DRIVER/OPERATOR Tip

Some fire apparatus may be equipped with a 15- to 20-ft (4.5- to 6.1-m) coiled wire and push button for the spotter to use while the fire apparatus is being operated in reverse. This device plugs into the rear of the fire apparatus and allows the spotter to directly communicate with the driver/operator. Wireless intercom headsets are found more commonly with modern apparatus.

Safety Tip

© Photos.com

At night, spotters should use flashlights. You should stop immediately if the spotter disappears from the rear-view mirror.

Shutting Down the Fire Apparatus

Once the fire apparatus is inside the fire station, it should be properly shut down. All of the electrical loads should be turned off first. This includes the headlights, air conditioner/heater, emergency lights, and any other electrical load that has an on/off switch. If these switches are left in the "on" position, the components will put an unnecessary load on the system the next time the fire apparatus is started.

Next, shift the transmission into neutral and engage the parking brake. If needed, allow the fire apparatus to cool down before shutting it off. This is best done with the fire apparatus sitting at an idle rate for 3 to 5 minutes. Allowing the apparatus to cool down is best accomplished on the ramp and not in

SKILL DRILL 9-6 Backing a Fire Apparatus into a Fire Station Bay
NFPA 1002, 4.3.2, 4.3.2(B)

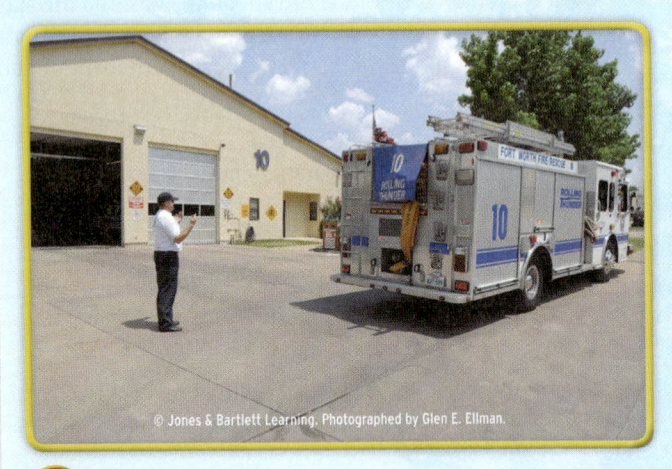

1 Position the rear of the fire apparatus past the fire station bay's opening at a 90-degree angle to the station. Ensure a spotter is correctly positioned behind the fire apparatus. Activate the emergency lights.

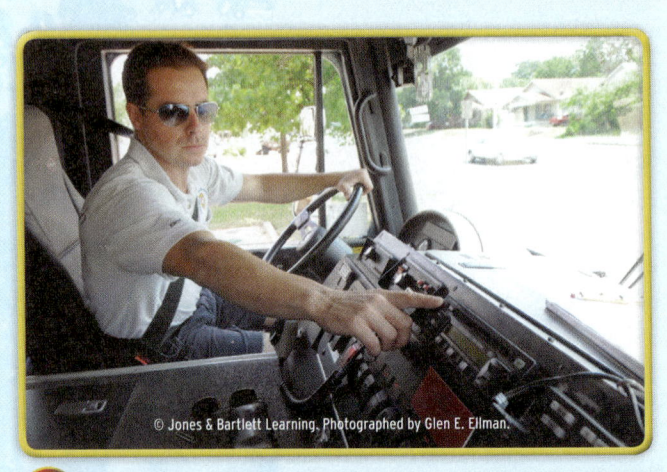

2 Turn off any fire apparatus–mounted stereo equipment.

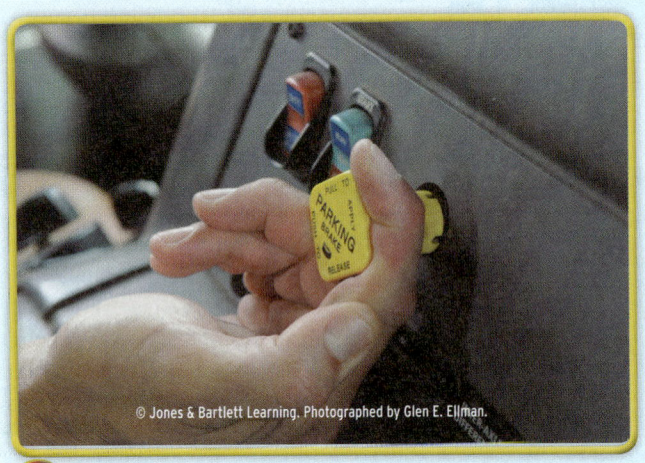

3 Disengage the parking brake, if set.

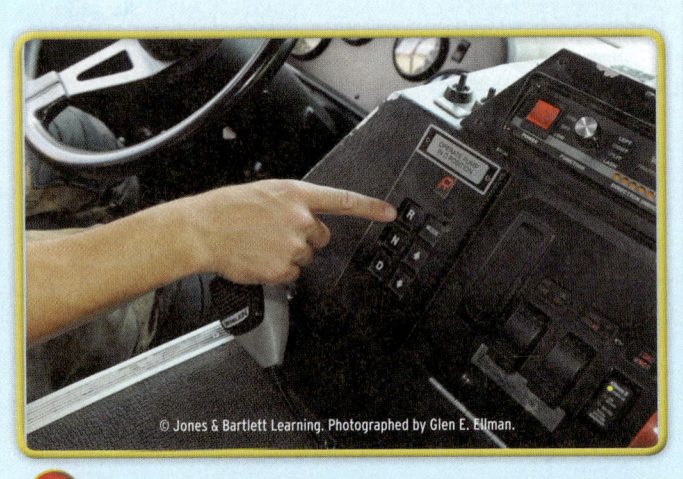

4 Shift the transmission to reverse.

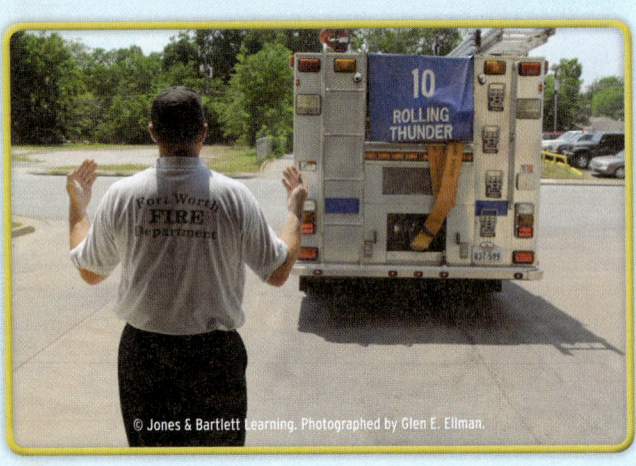

5 Proceed in a reverse mode and turn the fire apparatus to align it with the objective.

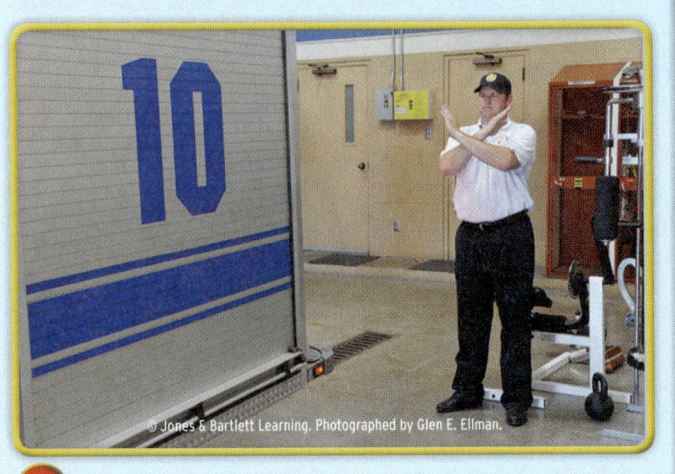

6 Continue backing the fire apparatus until it has reached the desired objective or the spotter signals "Stop."

the firehouse. Repeatedly operating the apparatus in the firehouse can cause damage to the exhaust removal hoses due to excessive temperature (particularly with newer diesel engines). The engine's lubricating oil and coolant fluid are able to carry heat away from the combustion chamber, bearings, shafts, and other engine components when the engine is run at idle speed. This step is particularly important with turbocharged engines, because the delicate bearings and seals inside the turbocharger are subject to the high heat of combustion exhaust gases. This heat is carried away by normal oil circulation while the engine is operating. If the engine is abruptly stopped, however, the turbocharger temperature may increase considerably and perhaps result in seized bearings or loose oil seals. Failure to adequately cool the engine for the proper length of time before shutdown can lead to reduced engine life and engine component failure. Finally, turn the ignition and battery switches to the off position. Reconnect any electrical shore lines, exhaust, and extractor systems.

As the driver/operator, you are responsible for the readiness of the fire apparatus at all times. Before anything else is done at the station, the fire apparatus must be returned to a ready state. Any equipment that was used during the emergency must be replaced, cleaned, or repaired. If the call was EMS related and only a few bandages were used, then replace them. If the fire apparatus returned from a small rubbish fire and the on-board water tank is now low, then fill the water tank **FIGURE 9-11**. If the SCBA and other equipment need to be cleaned after a structure fire, then clean these items and return the equipment to service.

To perform the procedure for shutting down and securing a fire apparatus, follow the steps in **SKILL DRILL 9-7**:

1. Turn off the emergency lights, headlights, and any other electrical loads. (**STEP 1**)
2. Shift the transmission into neutral. (**STEP 2**)
3. Engage the parking brake. (**STEP 3**)
4. Ensure that the apparatus has adequately cooled down before shutting it off. (**STEP 4**)
5. Turn the ignition switch to the off position. (**STEP 5**)
6. Turn the battery to the off position. (**STEP 6**)
7. Reconnect any applicable electrical cords and extractor system. (**STEP 7**)
8. Replace, clean, and repair any used equipment. (**STEP 8**)

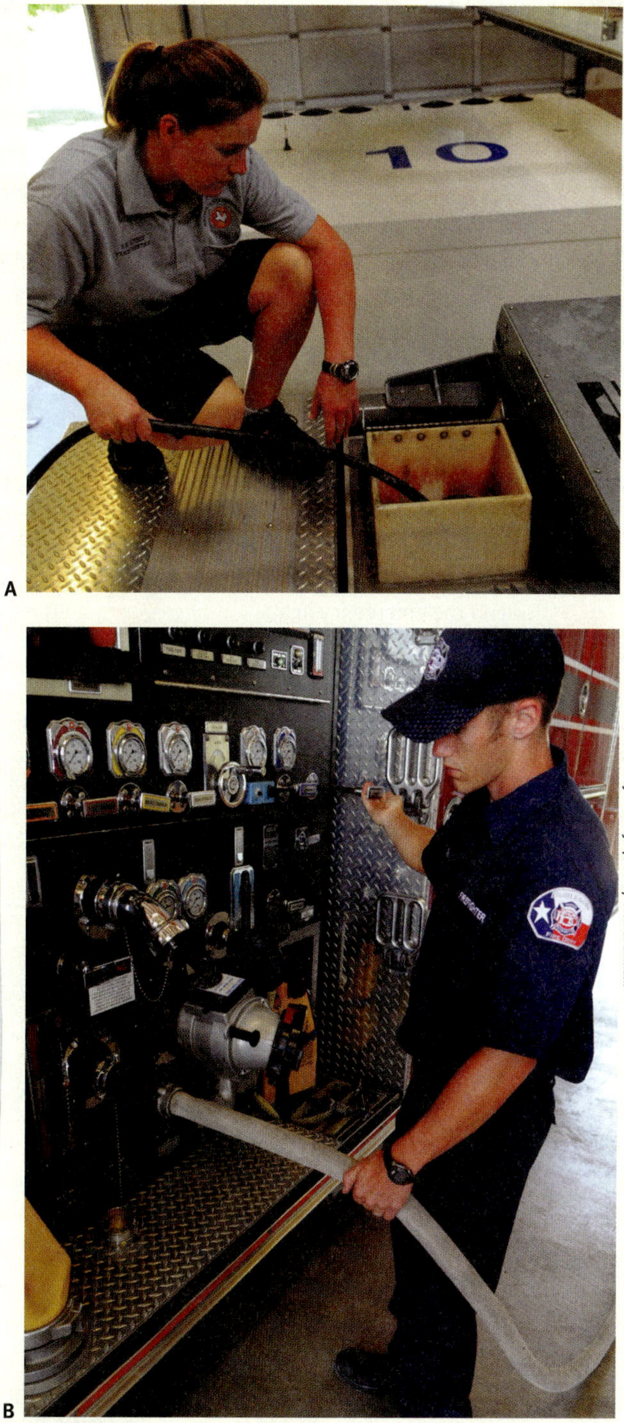

FIGURE 9-11 Fill the on-board tank if it is low. This can be done two ways: **A.** with a garden hose or **B.** with a fire department hoseline.

SKILL DRILL 9-7

Shutting Down and Securing a Fire Apparatus
NFPA 1002, 4.3.1, 4.3.1(B)

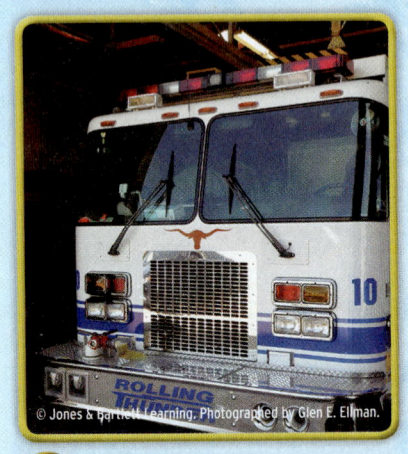

1. Turn off the emergency lights. Turn off the headlights and any other electrical loads.

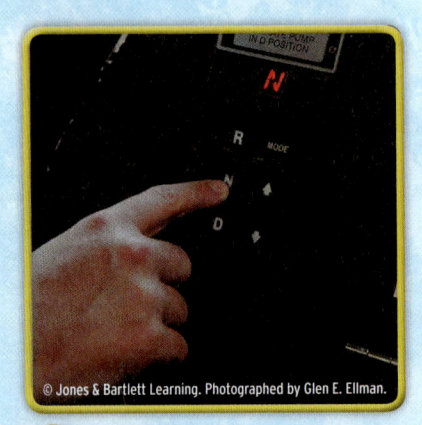

2. Shift the transmission into neutral.

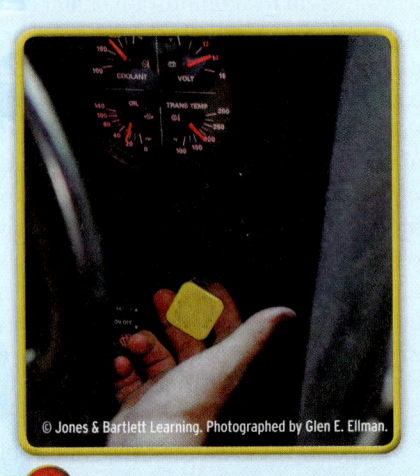

3. Engage the parking brake.

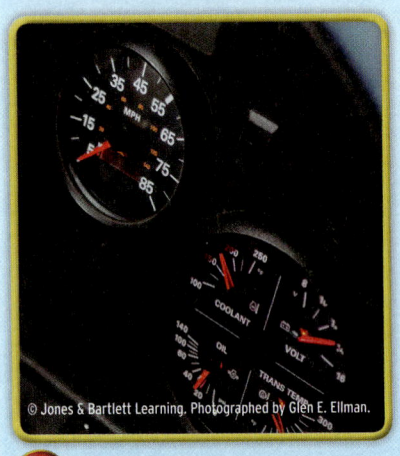

4. Ensure that the apparatus has adequately cooled down before shutting it off.

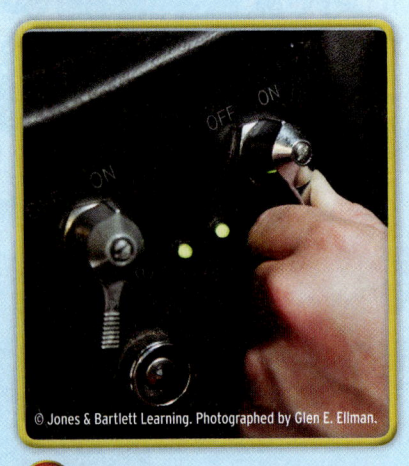

5. Turn the ignition switch to the off position.

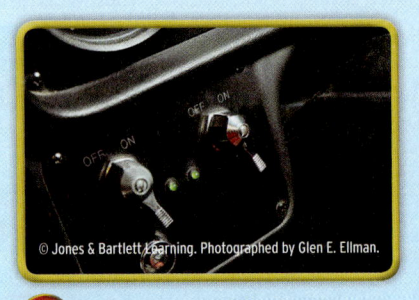

6. Turn the battery to the off position.

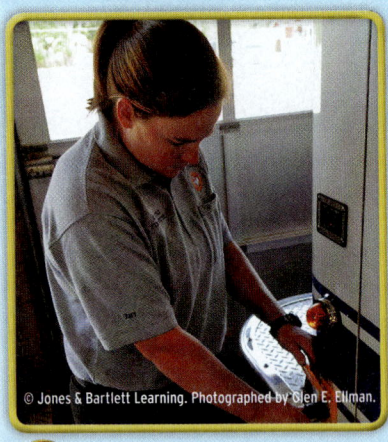

7. Reconnect any applicable electrical cords and extractor systems.

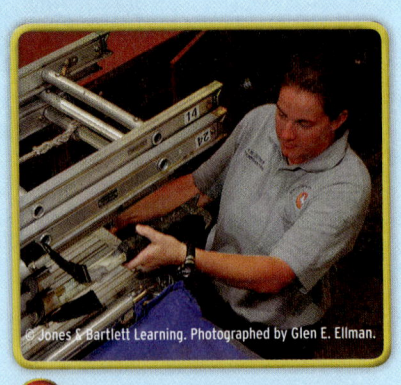

8. Replace, clean, and repair any used equipment.

Wrap-Up

Chief Concepts

- A preliminary inspection must be completed before the fire apparatus is ready to depart for the response.
- The driver/operator should follow the recommended starting sequence for the fire apparatus.
- Before the fire apparatus can get underway, you must ensure that all company members are seated and belted, unless they meet an exception under NFPA 1500.
- While responding to the scene, the driver/operator may need to complete several maneuvers so that the fire apparatus can access the incident. NFPA 1002 requires the driver/operator to complete several exercises to prove his or her skill in managing these situations.
- Do not become complacent when returning to the station.
- Follow safe procedures when backing up the fire apparatus. Always use spotters to assist with backup operations.
- When operating a fire apparatus in reverse, stop immediately if you lose sight of the spotter.
- Follow the standard sequence for shutting down the fire apparatus.

Hot Terms

air pressure gauges Gauges that identify the air pressure stored in the tanks or reservoirs of an apparatus equipped with a pneumatic braking system.

battery selector switch A switch used to disconnect all electrical power to the vehicle, thereby preventing discharge of the battery while the vehicle is not in use.

due regard The care exercised by a reasonably prudent person under the same circumstances.

fuel gauge A gauge that indicates the amount of fuel in the fire apparatus' fuel tank.

ignition switch A switch that engages operational power to the chassis of a motor vehicle.

oil pressure gauge A gauge that identifies the pressure of the lubricating oil in the fire apparatus engine.

parking brake The main brake that prevents the fire apparatus from moving even when it is turned off and there is no one operating it.

spotter A person who guides the driver/operator into the appropriate position while operating in a confined space or in reverse mode.

starter switch The switch that engages the starter motor for cranking.

system check sequence A series of checks that an electrical system completes to ensure that all of the systems are functioning properly before the fire apparatus is started.

voltmeter A device that measures the voltage across a battery's terminals and gives an indication of the electrical condition of the battery.

Wrap-Up, continued

References

National Fire Protection Association (NFPA) 1002, *Standard for Fire Apparatus Driver/Operator Professional Qualifications*. 2014. http://www.nfpa.org/codes-and-standards/document-information-pages?mode=code&code=1002. Accessed March 27, 2014.

National Fire Protection Association (NFPA) 1500, *Standard on Fire Department Occupational Safety and Health Program*. 2013. http://www.nfpa.org/codes-and-standards/document-information-pages?mode=code&code=1500. Accessed April 22, 2014.

National Fire Protection Association (NFPA) 1901, *Standard for Automotive Fire Apparatus*. 2009. http://www.nfpa.org/codes-and-standards/document-information-pages?mode=code&code=1901. Accessed April 9, 2014.

DRIVER/OPERATOR
in action

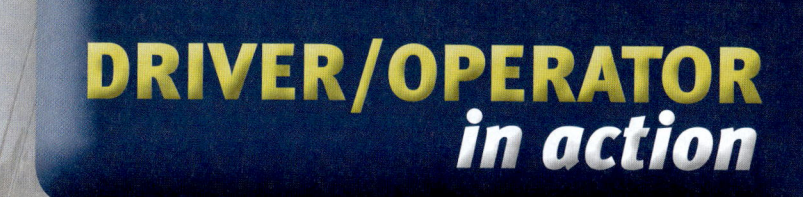

While your company is returning to the firehouse from the last fire, your company officer commends you and the other members of the crew for performing so well. He is pleased with how you maneuvered the apparatus around the rear of the fire building and set the apparatus in a position to adequately perform its task. He asks that you explain some of the training that you received from the department's training division on how to drive a fire apparatus.

1. Which switch delivers operational power to the chassis?
   A. Starter switch
   B. Ignition switch
   C. On switch
   D. Chassis switch

2. NFPA 1901 requires that a fire apparatus be capable of moving within __ seconds of starting up.
   A. 30
   B. 40
   C. 50
   D. 60

3. Who on the apparatus is responsible to ensure all personnel are seated with their seat belts fastened while the apparatus is in motion?
   A. The company officer
   B. The driver/operator
   C. The fire fighter
   D. Everyone on the apparatus

4. Who is responsible for ensuring that the spotters know in advance what is expected when the apparatus is being backed up?
   A. The fire chief
   B. The company officer
   C. The training officer
   D. The driver/operator

5. Whenever possible, you should allow the engine to warm up for ____ minutes.
   A. 1 to 2
   B. 3 to 5
   C. 5 to 7
   D. 7 to 10

Emergency Vehicle Driving

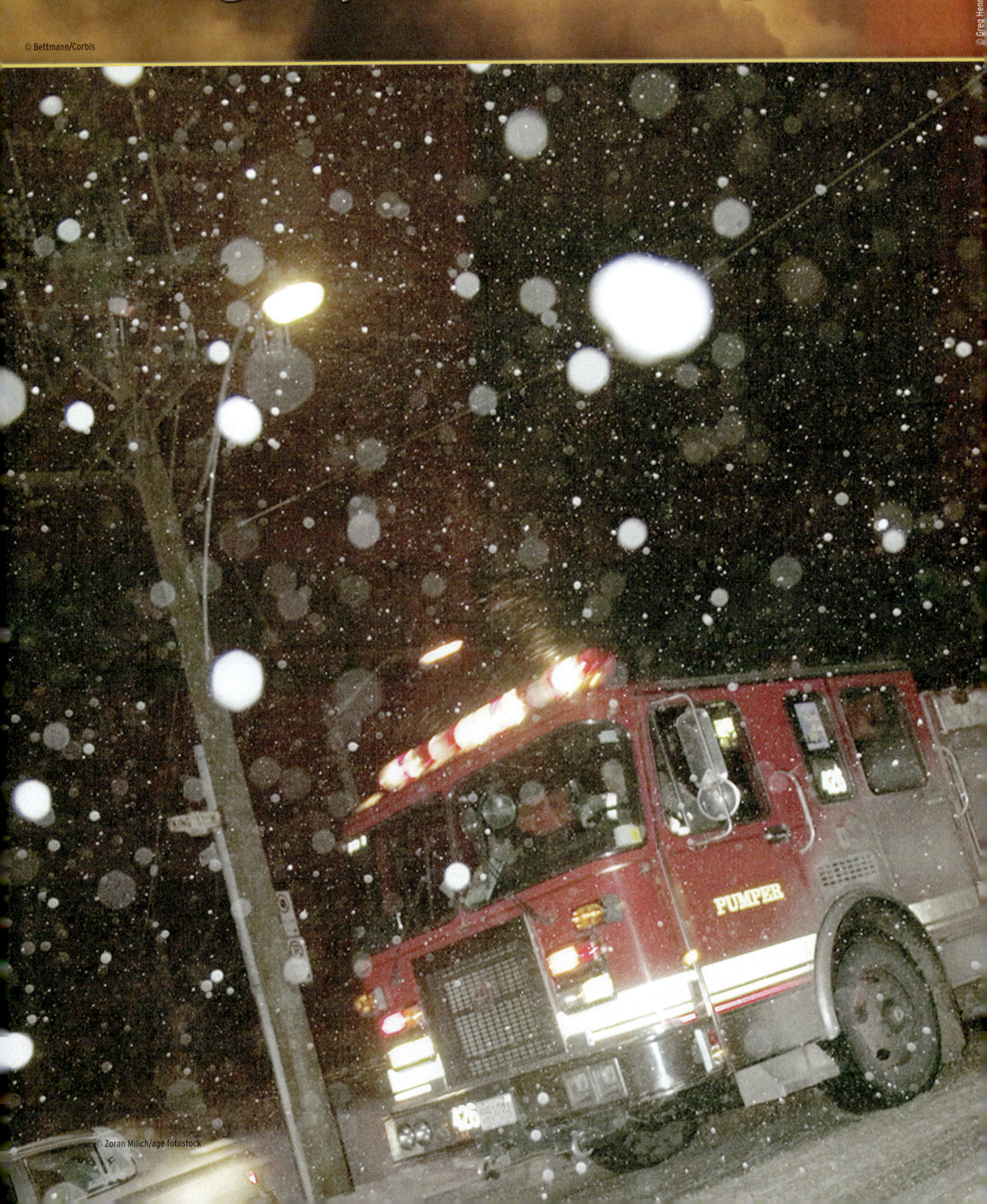

CHAPTER 10

Knowledge Objectives

After studying this chapter, you will be able to:

- Describe pre-emergency response dispatch information. (p 217–218)
- Discuss the various mapping systems used in the fire service. (p 218–219)
- Discuss emergency vehicle operations laws. (p 219–220)
- Describe the effects of vehicle control during a liquid surge on the roadway. (NFPA 1002, 4.3.1, 4.3.1(A), 4.3.6, 4.3.6(A) ; p 220–225)
- Describe the effect of a wet roadway on the braking reaction time. (NFPA 1002, 4.3.1, 4.3.1(A), 4.3.6, 4.3.6(A) ; p 221–222, 224)
- Describe the effect of the fire apparatus' load on the control of the vehicle on a wet roadway. (NFPA 1002, 4.3.1, 4.3.1(A), 4.3.6, 4.3.6(A) ; p 221–224)
- Describe the risk of a fire apparatus roll-over due to the effects of the apparatus' high center of gravity. (NFPA 1002, 4.3.1, 4.3.1(A), 4.3.6, 4.3.6(A) ; p 221–224)
- Describe general steering reactions of a fire apparatus. (NFPA 1002, 4.3.1, 4.3.1(A), 4.3.6, 4.3.6(A) ; p 221–224)
- Describe the effect of speed in controlling a fire apparatus on the roadway. (NFPA 1002, 4.3.1, 4.3.1(A), 4.3.6, 4.3.6(A) ; p 221–224)
- Describe the effect of centrifugal force in controlling a fire apparatus on the roadway. (NFPA 1002, 4.3.1, 4.3.1(A), 4.3.6, 4.3.6(A) ; p 222–223)
- Describe the applicable laws and regulations in operating a fire apparatus. (NFPA 1002, 4.3.1, 4.3.1(A), 4.3.6, 4.3.6(A) ; p 219–220)
- Describe the principles of skid avoidance when operating a fire apparatus. (NFPA 1002, 4.3.1, 4.3.1(A), 4.3.6, 4.3.6(A) ; p 221–223)
- Describe the principles of safe night driving of a fire apparatus. (NFPA 1002, 4.3.1, 4.3.1(A), 4.3.6, 4.3.6(A) ; p 223)
- Discuss proper shifting and gear patterns of a fire apparatus. (NFPA 1002, 4.3.1, 4.3.1(A), 4.3.6, 4.3.6(A) ; p 222–223)
- Describe how to safely cross intersections, railroad crossings, and bridges. (NFPA 1002, 4.3.1, 4.3.1(A), 4.3.6, 4.3.6(A) ; p 223–225)
- Describe the weight and height limitations of a fire apparatus for both roads and bridges. (NFPA 1002, 4.3.1, 4.3.1(A), 4.3.6, 4.3.6(A) ; p 221–224)
- Describe how to control the fire apparatus using defensive driving techniques under emergency conditions. (NFPA 1002, 4.3.6, 4.3.6(A) ; p 220–225)
- Describe your responsibilities as you approach an emergency scene. (p 225–226)
- Describe Level I and II staging procedures. (p 227–229)
- Identify potential hazards while approaching emergency incidents. (p 225–226)
- Describe the driver/operator's role when positioning the fire apparatus to operate at various emergency incidents. (p 226–234)
- Describe how to operate a fire apparatus safely through an intersection. (NFPA 1002, 4.3.1, 4.3.1(A), 4.3.6, 4.3.6(A) ; p 223–225)
- Describe how to operate a fire apparatus across a railroad crossing. (NFPA 1002, 4.3.1, 4.3.1(A), 4.3.6, 4.3.6(A) ; p 225)
- Describe how to operate a fire apparatus on a curve, either left or right. (NFPA 1002, 4.3.1, 4.3.1(A), 4.3.6, 4.3.6(A) ; p 222–223)
- Describe how to operate a fire apparatus on a section of limited-access highway with an entrance and exit ramp. (NFPA 1002, 4.3.1, 4.3.1(A), 4.3.6, 4.3.6(A) ; p 222–223)
- Describe how to operate a fire apparatus while passing other vehicles. (NFPA 1002, 4.3.1, 4.3.1(A), 4.3.6, 4.3.6(A) ; p 220–221)
- Describe how to operate a fire apparatus on a downgrade requiring a down-shift and braking. (NFPA 1002, 4.3.1, 4.3.1(A), 4.3.6, 4.3.6(A) ; p 222–225)
- Describe how to operate a fire apparatus on an upgrade requiring a gear change to maintain speed. (NFPA 1002, 4.3.1, 4.3.1(A), 4.3.6, 4.3.6(A) ; p 222)
- Describe how to operate a fire apparatus and travel safely under either an underpass or a low-clearance bridge. (NFPA 1002, 4.3.1, 4.3.1(A), 4.3.6, 4.3.6(A) ; p 223)
- Describe how to maintain safe following distances when operating a fire apparatus. (NFPA 1002, 4.3.1, 4.3.1(A), 4.3.6, 4.3.6(A) ; p 221–222)
- Describe how to accelerate in a fire apparatus. (NFPA 1002, 4.3.1, 4.3.1(A), 4.3.6, 4.3.6(A) ; p 220–225)
- Describe how to decelerate in a fire apparatus. (NFPA 1002, 4.3.1, 4.3.1(A), 4.3.6, 4.3.6(A) ; p 220–225)
- Describe how to turn in a fire apparatus. (NFPA 1002, 4.3.1, 4.3.1(A), 4.3.6, 4.3.6(A) ; p 222–223)
- Describe how to operate the fire apparatus safely under adverse driving conditions. (NFPA 1002, 4.3.1, 4.3.1(A), 4.3.6, 4.3.6(A) ; p 222)
- Describe the operational limits of the fire apparatus. (p 229–232)

Skills Objectives

After studying this chapter, you will be able to:
- Identify dispatch information. (p 217–219)
- Perform the alley dock exercise with the fire apparatus. (NFPA 1002, 4.3.1, 4.3.1(B), 4.3.6, 4.3.6(B) ; p 238–239)

Additional NFPA Standards

- NFPA 1561, *Standard on Emergency Services Incident Management System*
- NFPA 1620, *Recommended Practice for Preincident Planning*
- NFPA 1901, *Standard for Automotive Fire Apparatus*

You Are the Driver/Operator

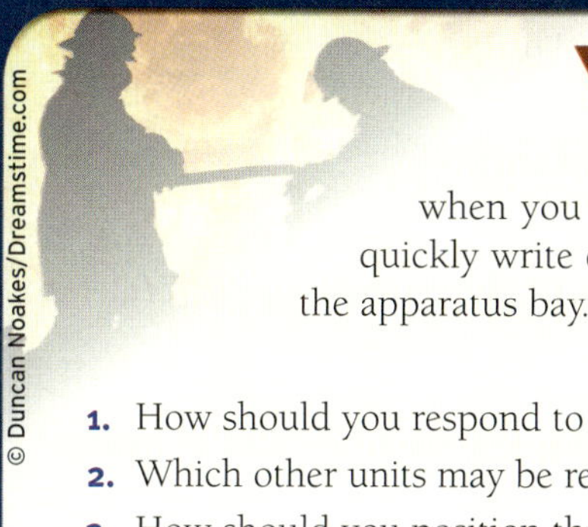

You have been promoted to the position of driver/operator and are working your first shift in a new fire station. It has been a few hours since your shift began. So far, you have checked and washed the apparatus, completed training, and just sat down to eat lunch when you hear the tones go off. As the dispatch comes in at the station, your heart begins to race. You quickly write down the incident address and look up the exact location on the station's map before going to the apparatus bay.

1. How should you respond to this call?
2. Which other units may be responding?
3. How should you position the apparatus upon arrival?

Introduction

Driving a fire apparatus to an emergency is one of the most exciting tasks driver/operators will perform. It can also be one of the deadliest tasks that they will perform. Each year fire fighters are killed and injured while responding to and from emergency incidents. Data trends indicate that fewer fire fighters are dying on the fireground, both in actual numbers and in relative terms; however, more are being killed while responding to emergency incidents or performing duties other than fighting fires. Each time a company rolls out of the station responding to a call, the fire fighters put their lives at risk. This chapter discusses the laws and regulations that pertain to driving the fire apparatus to an emergency scene. It also discusses safe driving practices for driver/operators to follow so that they can do their job—get fire fighters to the emergency scene to help others.

Pre-Emergency Vehicle Response

Most emergency responses start with the dispatch for an emergency. The driver/operator and the rest of the crew will receive a message about the emergency that will indicate the type of emergency, the location of the emergency incident, and the assigned tactical radio frequency. The driver/operator will then locate the emergency scene on a map using the information given during the dispatch and determine the most efficient response route using the department's mapping system. In addition, the driver/operator will determine the fire apparatus response mode for the emergency based on the information in the dispatch.

■ Dispatch

The **communications center** will give the information for the emergency to you in the form of a dispatch. **Dispatch** is the process of sending out emergency response resources promptly to an address or incident location for a specific purpose. This step is usually performed by a telecommunicator at the communications center. Fire departments use a variety of dispatch systems, ranging from telephone lines to radio systems. The communications center must have at least two separate ways of notifying each fire station. The primary method may consist of a hard-wired circuit, a telephone line, a data link, a microwave link, or a radio system.

The majority of fire departments use a verbal message to those units that are responding to the incident. This dispatch may be announced from speakers located in the station or via an apparatus-mounted radio. In some fire departments, response vehicles may be equipped with **mobile data terminals (MDTs)**—that is, computers located on the fire apparatus **FIGURE 10-1**. With this approach, the dispatch can be transmitted to the fire apparatus through both the radio speakers and the MDT. Sensitive information, however, may be transmitted to the MDT without announcing it over a radio frequency, as the radio communications may be monitored by the media.

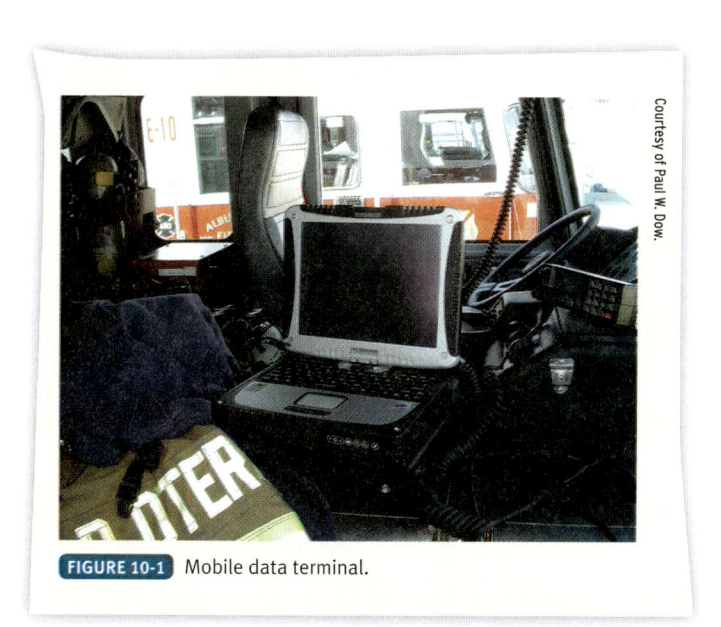

FIGURE 10-1 Mobile data terminal.

When dispatched for an emergency, whether the message is delivered at the fire station or in the fire apparatus, you should always pay attention to the following information:

- **Type of emergency.** This may be a structure fire, emergency medical services (EMS) call, or nonemergency call for service. The information given will determine how you will respond—that is, emergency mode or nonemergency mode. Each fire department should have a predetermined response mode for all types of incidents to which its personnel will respond. For example, when dispatched to a structure fire, the unit may respond to the scene with lights and sirens. If the fire apparatus is dispatched to a call that is not life-threatening, it may respond without lights and sirens. Always follow your local standard operating procedures (SOPs) in determining the mode of response.
- **Location of the emergency.** Each dispatch includes the physical address of the emergency. Usually, the dispatch also contains information such as cross streets, the geographical location of the response district, and possibly grid numbers to locate the incident on a map. These data are used to pinpoint the location of the incident.
- **Description of the incident.** The dispatcher should clearly describe what is happening at the incident. This information may include the victim's condition during an EMS incident or the location of a fire in a multistory occupancy.
- **Other responding units.** You should be familiar with your fire department's normal response to emergencies. If your fire apparatus is dispatched to a structure fire in your response district and the units that normally respond with your company are not dispatched as well, this can be a problem. Perhaps your district's normal backup units are on another call or out of service for training. Although other units may respond in their place, there could be a delay in response time. At the scene of a fire, this factor can drastically change the tactics of the initial units.
- **The assigned tactical radio frequency.** Each fire department should be capable of assigning units to a separate radio channel for on-scene tactical communications. During the initial dispatch to a structure fire or as part of other multicompany responses, most fire departments assign a tactical channel to the responding units. You need to ensure that you are on the correct channel while responding.
- **Additional information from the dispatcher.** Most dispatchers provide some additional information to a responding fire apparatus while the unit is going to the call. This information can be used to determine the appropriate action to take while responding to the incident. For example, if the dispatcher advises that the scene is a violent one, you might adjust your response. In some fire departments, responding units are required to stage several blocks from the scene until it is deemed safe by the local police department. During this type of response, the driver/operator would turn off the emergency lights and siren so that the unit is not identified until the scene is safe to enter.

You should carry a writing utensil and a notepad at all times. When a call goes out, you can then write down the information from the initial dispatch, especially the location of the emergency. Some calls and their locations may become well known to fire fighters. This is no excuse to become complacent, however. Even veteran driver/operators can be stumped with an unusual address or location in their response area. Being prepared can help avoid confusion and ensures that valuable time is not wasted by asking for the communications center to retransmit the information. Write it down the first time!

■ Maps

Because it can take years to learn a response area, you must be familiar with your maps. Some fire departments may not have maps for their response area, but instead rely solely on the fire fighter's knowledge of the response area. While this approach may be effective for some fire departments, most fire departments have a map that driver/operators can use to locate incidents.

Fire department maps may be accessed several different ways. The most common type of map is found at the fire station. Usually it comprises a large paper map, which may be placed in various areas around the station. Most of these maps show details of the fire station's primary response area. Some are color-coded to identify the response districts of other fire stations **FIGURE 10-2**. The maps may utilize a grid system that divides the entire response area into more specific areas.

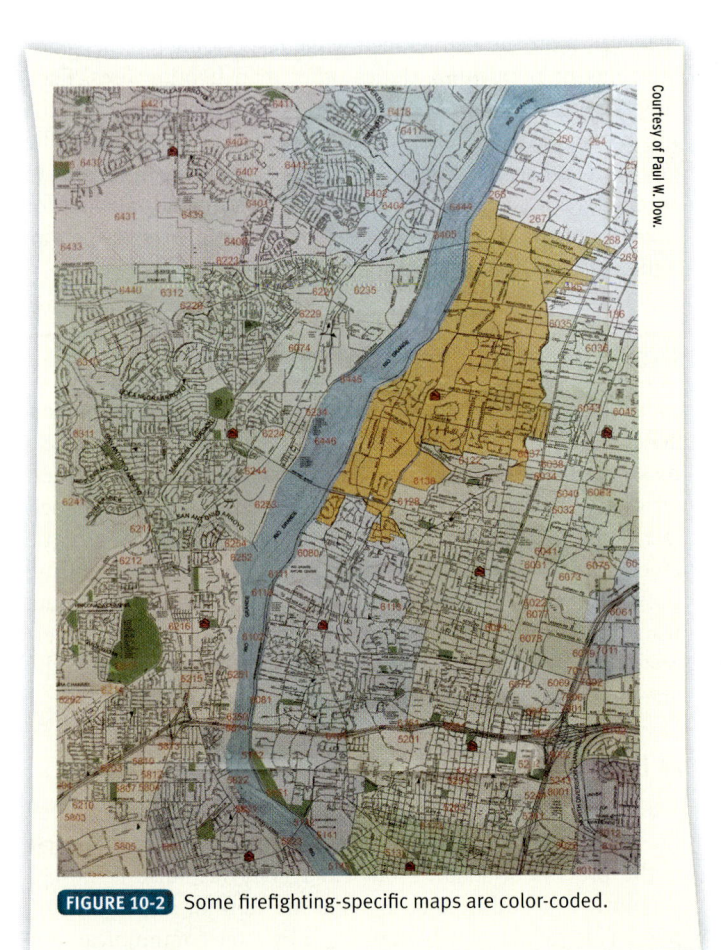

FIGURE 10-2 Some firefighting-specific maps are color-coded.

Courtesy of Paul W. Dow.

These areas may be sectioned off according to the fire station's response area. For example, in the Albuquerque (New Mexico) Fire Department, the entire city and surrounding county are divided into fire boxes. These areas may be several square blocks or several square miles, depending on the density of the area. Each fire station has any number of fire boxes within its response area. When a call is dispatched, the incident's location is identified with an address and a fire box. This practice allows Albuquerque fire fighters to look on the map, locate the station's response area, the fire box, and then the actual street address of the call.

Before you leave the station, you should reference the station-mounted map. Knowing where you are going saves valuable time during the response.

Smaller versions of the station-mounted maps may also be found on the fire apparatus. These maps are sometimes grouped with all of the neighboring districts' response areas. When responding to out-of-station calls, these maps can prove very useful. While such maps may not be as detailed as those found at the fire station, they are still effective.

You should never try to read a map while responding to an emergency. Firefighting is a team concept. Another member of the crew should reference the map and guide you.

Another map that some fire departments are now using is found on the MDT. When used in tandem with a **global positioning system (GPS)**, the MDT may be capable of pinpointing the exact location of the emergency in relation to your location. A GPS device uses satellite technology to locate the fire apparatus anywhere in a specified area. Some fire departments use this technology to dispatch the closest unit to an incident. When a call is dispatched, the information is transmitted to the MDT, so the location of the emergency appears on the screen and aids the driver/operator in locating the scene. Of all of the maps, this one is usually the easiest to update and may be the most current.

All of these maps used by fire fighters may have similar features. Sometimes they identify the sites of hydrants, enabling crews to locate a water supply while en route to the fire scene. The maps may also identify parks, schools, and other important features of the response area.

Whichever type of map your fire department uses, it is important to select a safe and efficient route when responding to each call. The goal is for the fire apparatus to arrive at the correct location in a safe and timely fashion. This responsibility will always fall upon you as the driver/operator.

To identify the critical information received from the dispatch, locate the emergency scene, and determine the proper route on the map and the response mode, follow the steps in **SKILL DRILL 10-1**:

1. Start with the dispatch for an emergency. Using a notepad, document the type of emergency, the location of the emergency incident, and the assigned tactical radio frequency (if applicable).
2. Locate the emergency scene on a map using the information given during the dispatch.
3. From the fire station, determine the most efficient response route using the map.
4. Determine the fire apparatus response mode for this emergency, using the information from the dispatch.

DRIVER/OPERATOR Tip

Never hesitate to reference your station's map!

Emergency Vehicle Laws

No member of any fire department should be allowed to drive an emergency vehicle or fire apparatus until that person has completed a training course approved by the fire department. Simply allowing any member to drive these vehicles without the proper training is irresponsible. Several Emergency Vehicle Operations courses are available, and each fire department should ensure that its members are trained to operate the fire apparatus that they will be driving. The days of allowing any fire fighter with a driver's license to jump into the front seat and pilot the fire apparatus to the emergency scene are behind us. The fire service can and should provide fire fighters with qualified training to ensure that all driver/operators drive safely and act responsibly while operating emergency vehicles.

Each fire department is governed by federal regulations as well as by different state laws and local regulations. Some of these laws and regulations are very detailed and descriptive; others are vague and leave much of their interpretation to the members of the fire department. All members of the fire department should be familiar with applicable federal, state, provincial, and local regulations governing the operation of emergency vehicles, including their department's own procedures. A lack of knowledge regarding the applicable emergency vehicle driving laws is not an excuse for disobeying them. As the driver/operator of a fire apparatus, you must understand that you will be held responsible for your actions while driving an emergency vehicle. Fire fighters who are found to be at fault for an accident involving a fire apparatus may be prosecuted in both criminal and civil court—which can create many problems for those members both at work and at home. As a driver/operator, you must understand the local laws and regulations with which you must comply.

The use of sirens and warning lights does not automatically give the right-of-way to the fire apparatus. These devices simply request the right-of-way from other drivers, based on their awareness of the emergency vehicle's presence. You must take every step possible to make your presence and intended actions known to other drivers, and you must drive defensively so that you will be prepared for unexpected, inappropriate actions of others. The driver/operator of a fire apparatus is not the only person allowed to use the roadway even under emergency conditions: You must follow many of the same laws as any other driver on the road.

Many states provide certain privileges to emergency vehicle driver/operators while they are responding to an emergency. They also specify the conditions under which these privileges are granted. For example, in New Mexico, the motor vehicle code states that the following four privileges may be granted as long as the emergency vehicle sounds an audible signal and the vehicle is operating with its emergency lights activated; all other laws apply during the emergency vehicle's response:

1. **Park or stand irrespective of the provisions of the motor vehicle code.** This privilege allows for the driver/operator to position the fire apparatus in the

roadway to block the scene and provide for the safety of the fire fighters and those involved in the emergency.

2. **Proceed past a red or stop signal or stop sign, but only after slowing down as necessary for safe operation.** The fire apparatus should come to a complete stop before proceeding through the intersection.
3. **Exceed the maximum speed limits as long as the driver/operator does not endanger life or property.** Many fire departments allow fire apparatus to exceed the posted speed limit by only 10 mph (16 km/h) during an emergency response and only in light traffic and good weather conditions.
4. **Disregard regulations governing direction of movement or turning in specified directions.** This provision allows for the driver/operator to drive or position the vehicle against the flow of traffic. This maneuver should be done only in a safe and controlled manner. Some fire departments refer to this practice as "bucking" traffic and strictly prohibit it. Other fire departments allow moves against the normal flow of traffic to be made within one block of an incident and only for the purpose of positioning the fire apparatus.

These laws do not relieve you from the duty to drive with due regard for the safety of all persons, nor do they protect you from the consequences of reckless disregard for the safety of others. Each driver/operator is accountable for his or her own actions.

Other state or local laws that may apply to emergency vehicle operators include the following provisions:

- Comply with any lawful order or direction of any police officer invested by law with the authority to direct, control, or regulate traffic.
- Bring the apparatus to a complete stop and do not proceed until it is confirmed that it is safe to do so, such as at any stop signal (i.e., sign, light, or traffic officer), blind intersections, intersections where the operator cannot see all lanes of traffic, stopped school buses with red warning lights flashing, and unguarded railroad crossings.
- Do not leave the scene of an accident in which you are involved.

DRIVER/OPERATOR Tip

State laws and many other rules and regulations may be defined in greater detail by local fire departments. Each driver/operator is responsible for knowing the state and local laws governing the operation of fire apparatus.

DRIVER/OPERATOR Tip

"Due regard" is a legal term. Would a reasonably careful person performing similar duties under the same circumstances react in the same manner? As the driver/operator of a fire apparatus, you should ask yourself this question. If you are performing in an unsafe manner and putting others at risk, you are not driving with due regard for the safety of others. Be aware that you will be held responsible for your actions. Drive safely or do not drive at all.

Emergency Vehicle Driving

When starting the emergency response, you should accelerate slowly and in a controlled manner. Allow the engine to gradually build up speed instead of flooring the accelerator from a stopped position. Both of your hands should remain on the steering wheel at all times unless you are operating air horns, sirens, or other essential equipment. For this reason, you should check and memorize the position of instruments and controls before moving the fire apparatus. It should never be necessary to search for instruments or controls while the fire apparatus is in motion, as this behavior will draw your attention away from the road. Taking your eyes off of the roadway for too long to search for controls may result in a collision.

■ Level of Response

Local jurisdictions determine which level of response is appropriate for nonemergency and emergency incidents. During an emergency response, the fire apparatus should be driven with both the emergency lights and the sirens activated—a practice commonly referred to as a <u>Code 3 response</u>. When the fire apparatus is operating with only the emergency lights and no audible siren, it is engaging in a <u>Code 2 response</u>. During normal operations or nonemergency responses, the fire apparatus does not have any emergency lights or sirens operating; this situation is considered a <u>Code 1 response</u>. A Code 2 response is usually prohibited in many fire departments because it does not properly alert other drivers to the presence of the fire apparatus. Although some fire fighters might argue that the sirens are unnecessary at 3 a.m. when the streets may be empty of traffic, sirens should still be used to alert others of the fire apparatus' approach and to avoid any potential liability should an accident occur.

During a nonemergency response, the apparatus should be operated in a nonemergency mode (without lights and sirens) and obey all traffic laws. This includes units that are en route to move up or to fill an empty station.

■ Passing Vehicles

The fire apparatus should be driven with the intention of passing other vehicles on the left side. On streets with multiple lanes, the fire apparatus should be driven in the far left lane to provide ample room for the other drivers to pull to the right and stop. Weaving in and out of the other vehicles should be avoided. This action confuses other drivers and may cause a collision with other vehicles as they try to avoid the fire apparatus. Always pass other vehicles on the left side.

When operating the fire apparatus on straight sections of roadway, you must remain in your own lane **FIGURE 10-3**. Some driver/operators have a tendency to occupy parts of two lanes. This practice should be avoided, because it confuses other drivers by not making your intentions clear while traveling down the road. When making lane changes, use your turn signal and try to remain in the far left lane until you need to turn. While performing a two-lane change, make sure that you clear each lane individually before proceeding. Be aware that other vehicles may attempt to race or even pass the fire apparatus while you are responding to the scene.

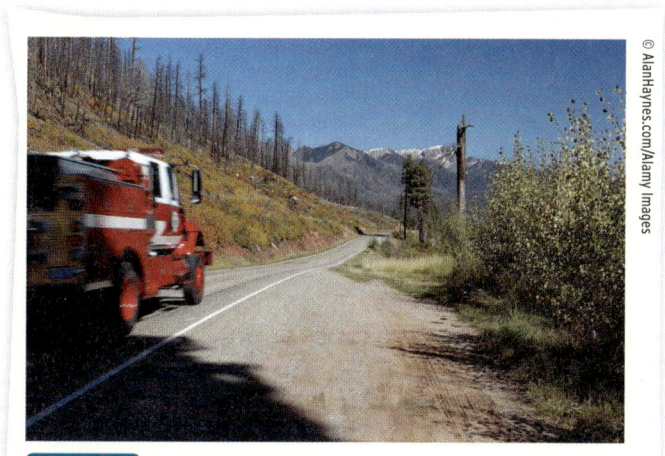

FIGURE 10-3 When operating the fire apparatus on straight sections of roadway, you must remain in your own lane.

Fire apparatus that are following each other to an emergency should maintain an adequate distance to avoid a rear-end collision. Overtaking and passing other vehicles during an emergency response should be attempted with extreme caution and should be done only on the left side.

Defensive Driving Practices

While responding to the incident, you should yourself ask the following questions:

- Can I stop this fire apparatus?
- What will I do if someone pulls in front of me?
- Is another vehicle in my blind spot?
- Am I too close to the vehicle in front of me?

All of these questions relate to the need to operate the fire apparatus in a safe manner and to drive defensively. If you drive cautiously and anticipate that the unexpected may happen, then you will be more prepared when it does. Defensive drivers are safer than aggressive drivers. To drive defensively, you must always be aware of your surroundings. Scan the area in front of the fire apparatus to determine which hazards may lie ahead. Is another vehicle about to pull in front of the fire apparatus? If you are checking the road ahead, then you will see any potential problems and be better prepared to avoid a collision.

While traveling behind other vehicles, consider how close you can safely be to the vehicles ahead. While driving in good weather conditions (during daylight with good, dry roads and low traffic volume), you should ensure a safe distance from the vehicle ahead of you by following the "3-second rule." This distance will change depending on the speed at which the fire apparatus is traveling and the road conditions. To determine the appropriate following distance, first select a fixed object on the road ahead such as a sign, tree, or overpass. When the vehicle that you are following passes the object, slowly count, "One one-thousand, two one-thousand, three one-thousand." If you reach the object before completing the count, then you are following too closely. Making sure that there are at least 3 seconds between the fire apparatus and the car ahead of it gives you enough time and distance to respond to any problems that occur ahead of you. While responding in poor driving conditions (e.g., in inclement weather, in heavy traffic, or at night), you should double the 3-second rule to 6 seconds, for added safety. As the driving conditions worsen, you will, in turn, have to increase the distance that you travel behind other vehicles.

During the response, consider how fast you are going in relation to the street on which you are traveling. Although many fire departments allow fire apparatus to travel faster than the speed limit, it may not always be safe to do so. For example, in a residential neighborhood, the speed limit is usually 25 mph (40 km/h) or less. In such an area, small children and other pedestrians might be present, so you must adjust your speed accordingly.

Being able to control the fire apparatus and stop when required should be your goal. The distance that it takes for you to recognize the hazard, process the need to stop the fire apparatus, apply the brakes, and then come to a complete stop is referred to as the **total stopping distance**. The distance that the fire apparatus travels after you recognize the hazard, remove your foot from the accelerator, and apply the brakes is referred to as the **reaction distance**. The distance that the fire apparatus travels from the time that the brakes are activated until the fire apparatus makes a complete stop is known as the **braking distance**. These distances are very important for you to consider while responding in the fire apparatus, and they will differ for each fire apparatus depending on several factors:

- **The size and weight of the fire apparatus.** The more weight the fire apparatus is carrying, the more energy it will take to bring it to a complete stop. Larger vehicles generally will have a greater total stopping distance than smaller vehicles that are traveling at the same speed.
- **The fire apparatus' overall condition, including brakes, tires, and suspension.** Fire apparatus that are maintained in optimal condition are capable of coming to a complete stop more quickly than fire apparatus that are poorly maintained. Tires should always have adequate tread life and be inflated to the proper pressure. The brakes should be capable of stopping the fire apparatus as required. The suspension system of the fire apparatus should not allow excessive bounce; this will prevent the tires from making the proper contact with the road and delay the braking process.
- **The speed at which the fire apparatus is traveling.** Faster speeds will require the fire apparatus to travel a greater distance before it comes to a stop.
- **The surface condition of the road.** Dry, paved roads provide the best surface for both driving and stopping conditions. By comparison, when roads are wet or covered with ice and snow, they have less friction with the tires of the apparatus. The lower the friction value, the longer it will take for the fire apparatus to come to a complete stop.

Driver/operators must also be aware of the term **liquid surge** and know how it relates to driving, especially for fire apparatus that carry water. Liquid surge is the movement of liquid inside a container as the container is moved. As the fire apparatus accelerates or decelerates, the water carried inside the tank on the fire apparatus will slosh around. This movement can be very hazardous owing to the large amount of water that is carried on many fire apparatus. If the fire apparatus has to brake quickly, then the liquid surge will try to force the fire apparatus forward—putting additional strain on the fire apparatus' braking system and increasing the total stopping distance. To reduce the effects of liquid surge, the water tanks on fire apparatus are designed with baffles inside them. These plates inside the tank slow down the movement of the water and displace some of the energy transferred during the movement of the fire apparatus.

As a driver/operator, you should know how to prevent the fire apparatus from skidding. Skids can happen whenever the tires lose grip on the road. This problem can be caused by slippery surfaces, a too-sudden change in speed or direction, or lack of tire maintenance. A road that is safe under good conditions may, in contrast, be very dangerous when it is wet or covered with snow or ice. Traveling at high speeds even under normal conditions will increase the possibility of a skid if the fire apparatus must complete a turn or stop suddenly. If the fire apparatus is responding in rain or snow conditions, this problem is even more profound. Auxiliary engine brakes can sometimes cause loss of control of vehicles in rain and icy conditions. The activation of the engine brake can cause the vehicle to pull to one side, and the driver/operator could potentially lose control. Most original equipment manufacturers (OEMs) recommend turning secondary braking off in wet and icy conditions. Although adverse weather conditions such as rain and ice contribute to skidding, poor driving skills are the main cause of skidding. If the fire apparatus begins to skid, take the following actions:

- **Stay off the brake.** Until the vehicle slows, your brakes will not work and could cause you to skid more.
- **Steer.** Turn the steering wheel in the direction you want the vehicle to go. As soon as the vehicle begins to straighten out, turn the steering wheel back the other way. If you do not do so, your vehicle may swing around in the other direction and you could start a new skid.
- **Continue to steer.** Continue to correct your steering, left and right, until the vehicle is again moving down the road under your control.

■ Maintaining Control on Hills, Turns, and Curves

While driving down hills, you should rely on the engine and the auxiliary braking device to slow down the fire apparatus. If only the fire apparatus brakes are used to control the speed of the fire apparatus, they may heat up to the point where they become ineffective in stopping the fire apparatus. This situation is commonly referred to as **brake fade**. Brake fade occurs when the brake drums become hot and expand away from the brake shoes, so that the stroke of the slack adjusters becomes less effective. To avoid this problem, you should use the brakes only in short, 5- to 10-second bursts rather than as a continuous application.

Also, while traveling down a steep slope, you may need to use the auxiliary braking system and down-shift the transmission to a lower gear. To complete this action properly, shift into one gear lower than the gear that would be used when going up the hill. Down-shifting will make it easier to control the fire apparatus and will save wear on the brakes.

When traveling up hills, you should avoid over-throttling the fire apparatus. This action will result in a loss of power while the engine works to catch up to the amount of work that is being demanded. Instead, you should slowly build up speed and use the lower gears of the transmission until adequate horsepower is achieved. To do so, you may have to manually shift the transmission into these lower gears while climbing a hill.

When making left or right turns, make sure that you have enough clearance to completely make the turn without striking curbs, trees, and other objects that may be in the blind spot of the fire apparatus. Fire apparatus may be top heavy from aerial ladders, water, and other equipment. To avoid the potential for roll-over owing to the apparatus' load, you must slow down before making the turn—90 percent of braking should be done in a straight line before entering a corner. How fast you take a turn will depend on the road conditions and the type and design of the apparatus. If you are turning right from the far left lane, you may not be able to see whether vehicles on your right have completely stopped. In this case, you should have the fire officer or other crew member in the front seat look out the window into the blind spot and determine if it is clear to proceed with the turn. When you are alone, you will have to slow down, make your intentions very clear to other motorists, and proceed with extreme caution while making such a turn.

When turning to the left, you should turn wide enough to make the turn but not so wide that you travel into an outside lane and strike another vehicle. During the response, you may have to make a U-turn to position the fire apparatus or maneuver down a one-way street. In such a case, you should make sure that the area is wide enough to complete the turn and that adequate clearance for both the front and the rear of the fire apparatus is available. Remember, the back of the fire apparatus will swing out away from the turn. Therefore, if the vehicle is too close to the outside curb, the back end may swing out and strike objects such as poles, trees, and parking meters along the curb. With some fire apparatus, you may not realize you are turning too fast until it is too late. When in doubt, slow down.

Curved roadways are found all over this country—in the mountains, along the coastlines, and in urban areas of major cities. Curved sections can be found on small dirt roads and on highway entrance and exit ramps. No matter where they are, curved roadways can pose a very serious problem for emergency vehicles. Many of these ramps are designed with extreme curves and can be difficult to judge when traveling at normal speeds. As a driver/operator, you must realize that traveling on these curves with a fire apparatus is very different from traveling on the same route with a passenger car.

Driver/operators of fire apparatus should be familiar with the term **centrifugal force**, including how it relates to driving on curved roads. Centrifugal force is the tendency for objects to be pulled outward when rotating around a center. The fire apparatus is subject to this force when making a turn; the centrifugal force will try to keep the fire apparatus going in a straight line while you are making the turn. If it is to avoid losing control, the fire apparatus must have proper traction with the roadway. To keep the fire apparatus in the turn without allowing centrifugal force to pull the vehicle off the road, you should slow down before the curve and brake gently while making the turn.

Driving along curves will also severely affect the weight transfer of the fire apparatus. As with any vehicle, the weight carried on a fire apparatus is usually distributed among all four tires of the apparatus while it travels down the road. The weight on the front axle however is not the same as the weight on the rear axle; typically, one-third of the weight is on the front axle, and two-thirds of the weight is on the rear axle. There is also a 7 percent allowance side to side—meaning the left side weight may be different than the right side weight. This keeps the vehicle's center of gravity in the middle of the vehicle, depending on its height and weight. When the apparatus travels on a curve, however, the center of gravity will shift, causing the weight of the fire apparatus to shift to one side or the other. If this shift of weight is too great, the fire apparatus will roll over. Remember to slow the fire apparatus down well before entering a turn; otherwise, you risk losing control of the vehicle.

Every curve in a road has a **critical speed**. If the fire apparatus is traveling faster than the critical speed, it will not be capable of completing the turn and will go off the road or roll over. Either way, you will lose control of the fire apparatus and wreck. To determine the critical speed, you should know how sharp the curve is and how slippery the road conditions are. As the curve gets sharper and the road more slippery, the critical speed goes down; as a consequence, the fire apparatus must travel around the curve at a slower speed. This does not have to be a complicated process. For example, if it is raining and the roads are slippery, you will not be able to drive around the curve at the same speed as if it were dry. Once the fire apparatus is beyond the critical speed, it is too late to try to correct the problem. Prevention is the key—so slow down **FIGURE 10-4**.

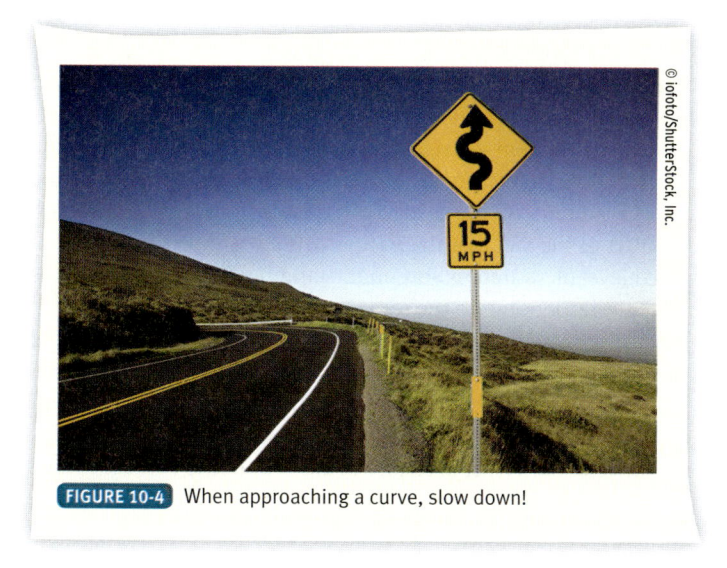

FIGURE 10-4 When approaching a curve, slow down!

Night Driving

Responding to an emergency during the night is usually more difficult than during the day. The streets and landscape are difficult to see, and the reduced visibility makes the response area look dramatically different. Landmarks and street signs that are easily seen during the day may be missed as you respond in darkness. The lights of other vehicles, street lights, and traffic signals can make it difficult to maneuver the fire apparatus along the roadway.

To reduce the risks of responding during the night, follow these guidelines:

- Keep your eyes constantly scanning the roadway. Scan carefully for pedestrians, cyclists, and animals on the road.
- To avoid glare from oncoming lights, glance to the right edge of the road.
- Keep the fire apparatus' front windshield and headlights clean.
- Keep the interior cab lights off and adjust the instrument panel lights to a low setting.
- Many fire apparatus cabs are equipped with red lights inside the cab. These lights should be used during the night because they do not interfere with your vision during the response.
- Stay alert at night. You must be well rested and prepared to operate the fire apparatus.
- Slow down and increase your following distance.

Bridges and Overpasses

Bridges and overpasses are obstacles that you must be aware of before the emergency response begins. Know beforehand which overhead obstructions your fire apparatus can safely pass beneath. Fire apparatus are required by National Fire Protection Association (NFPA) 1901, *Standard for Automotive Fire Apparatus*, to have labels in the cab that identify the height of the vehicle. You should ensure that the fire apparatus is capable of fitting underneath any obstacle before attempting to navigate it. When in doubt, find another access point or use a spotter to prevent damaging both the obstacle and the fire apparatus.

Another potential problem concerning bridges is their weight limitation. Some bridges are not designed to carry the heavy loads associated with certain fire apparatus. You should identify these potential problems and, if they present obstacles to the fire apparatus, access the scene of the emergency from another route or use smaller fire apparatus to respond to the scene. Under no circumstances should you attempt to operate a fire apparatus over a bridge that is not capable of supporting its weight.

Intersections

During an emergency response, intersections present the greatest potential danger to fire apparatus. When approaching and crossing an intersection, you should not exceed the posted speed limit. If you are traveling too fast, you will not be able to stop in time to avoid a collision. Also, do not assume you have the right-of-way simply because you are using the emergency

Safety Tip

Because of their design, diesel engines have very little compression of backpressure to assist in stopping the fire apparatus. Auxiliary braking systems, however, provide braking torque through the driveline to the rear wheels. Use of an auxiliary brake reduces brake wear, reduces brake heat build-up, and can help minimize the occurrence of brake fade during heavy or frequent braking. Be aware that an auxiliary braking system should not be used during slippery road conditions or inclement weather; doing so may cause the rear wheels to lock up, resulting in a loss of control of the fire apparatus.

Several types of auxiliary braking devices are available for diesel-powered engines. The most popular include the following options:

- **Compression brake.** The compression brake is a mechanical system added to the engine valve train that is electronically actuated. This system alters the operation of the engine's exhaust valves so that the engine works as a power-absorbing air compressor.
- **Transmission retarder.** An efficient means of slowing a vehicle down, the transmission retarder utilizes the transmission fluid to create backpressure that assists in slowing the fire apparatus. The application of this type of device will help avoid engine damage. If the transmission fluid is overheated, however, major transmission damage can result.
- **Exhaust brake.** A shutter valve activated in the exhaust system just behind the turbocharger will engage this type of device. The closed valve causes a build-up of pressure in the exhaust system, which then passes back through the turbocharger and the valves and into the combustion chamber of the cylinder. The pressure build-up creates braking horsepower, which is then used to slow the vehicle down. With a transmission that offers the same type of direct interface, this system is quite efficient because the same horsepower used to keep the vehicle in motion can help slow it down. The maximum efficiency is reached at the maximum engine speed (rpm) for which the exhaust brake is rated.
- **Electromagnetic retarder.** This device is the most efficient, but most expensive, means of slowing a fire apparatus. When engaged, the electromagnet around the driveshaft creates an opposing magnetic field around the driveshaft that causes the driveshaft to resist turning, thereby slowing the fire apparatus. The system may be applied in stages either manually or by combinations of brake and accelerator pedal settings. Any heat that is generated by this system is dissipated by cooling fins on the retarder.

---

warning lights and sirens: Other drivers may not see or hear the fire apparatus as you approach the intersection. Scan the intersection for possible hazards such as right turns on red, pedestrians, and vehicles traveling fast or weaving through traffic. Observe the traffic in all four directions: left, right, front, and rear. Proceed through the intersection only when you can account for all lanes of traffic at the intersection. In multilane intersections, you should clear each lane individually before proceeding. In some cases, other vehicles may block your view or the view of other drivers. As a consequence, you might think the lane is cleared and completely miss another vehicle that is proceeding through the intersection. In some cases, you may have to slow down to less than 5 mph (8 km/h) while in the intersection and visually clear each lane of traffic before proceeding.

At all intersections with green lights or where the fire apparatus has the right-of-way, you should slow down as necessary to ensure safe operation by disengaging the throttle and pressing the brake pedal. This strategy ensures that you are ready for any potential hazard—that you are driving defensively. When approaching an intersection where all lanes of traffic are blocked with other vehicles, you should turn off all sirens and horns at least 200 ft (60 m) before the stopped traffic is reached. Leave the emergency lights on and bring the fire apparatus to a stop at least 100 ft (30 m) from the nearest vehicle in traffic. This stance will let the civilian drivers know that you are still there and responding to an emergency, but will not "push" them into the intersection. Never encourage or force traffic to proceed against red lights or to advance into dangerous traffic conditions. Instead, stay in the far left lane so that when the light turns green or the left green arrow is activated, you can proceed with lights and sirens through the intersection. The fire apparatus should come to a complete stop at all uncontrolled intersections, stop signs, and yellow and red lights. Proceed through the intersection only after it has been determined that the other vehicles have stopped and that it is safe to do so.

Many jurisdictions use **traffic signal preemption systems** at intersections to assist fire apparatus during the emergency response. These systems can change the signal from red to green for an emergency vehicle as it approaches the intersection. A flashing light on the fire apparatus, also known as an **emitter**, will trigger a **receiver** on the traffic signal and change the light to allow the fire apparatus to secure the right-of-way through these intersections in as safe and efficient a manner as possible. In jurisdictions using this type of traffic control system, each emergency vehicle is equipped with an emitter, which is usually mounted next to the emergency lights, and which emits visible flashes of light or invisible infrared pulses at a specified frequency. A receiver device is mounted on or near intersection traffic control devices to recognize the signal and preempt the normal cycle of traffic lights. Once the emergency vehicle passes through the intersection and the receiving device no longer senses the remote triggering device, normal operation of the intersection's traffic signals resumes. Such a system provides the fire apparatus with the benefit of a quicker response. You should be alert to the fact that these intersections will require a heightened level of awareness and understanding. Other fire apparatus that are responding to the same emergency scene may also trigger this system from another direction and proceed through the intersection at the same time.

An encounter by the public with an emergency response vehicle en route to an emergency is not a normal, everyday occurrence. This fact is clearly evident from the confusion that is often witnessed when fire apparatus approach civilian traffic at intersections controlled by traffic signal preemption systems.

For example, while the traffic signal preemption system cycles the light through the normal sequence of yellow and then red, an approaching fire apparatus is typically unable to determine how long the light was green for cross traffic. An unusually short green light for cross traffic may appear to that traffic as a malfunctioning light, encouraging the civilian drivers to run a yellow light. Proceed only after ensuring that it is safe to do so: A green light given as a result of traffic signal preemption system activation should not be assumed to be safe until verified visually, in all directions.

When a green light is given to the responding fire apparatus due to a traffic signal preemption system's activation well in advance, the driver/operator must still slow down as necessary to ensure safe operation. If the system is not granted a green light on approach, you should come to a complete stop just before the intersection to ensure safe operation. This delay will provide time for the system to activate the traffic signal, allow the intersection to clear completely, and give those civilian drivers who are either inattentive or prone to running yellow lights a chance to clear through.

As is the case with all intersections, when approaching a traffic signal preemption system–controlled intersection where all lanes are blocked, turn off all sirens and horns but leave the emergency lights on. Depending on your department, the system may only be operational when the vehicle's emergency lights are activated and the **parking brake** is in the off position. When activation has been granted and the green light delay occurs, activate sirens and horns for a few seconds to give the civilian vehicles time to clear the intersection completely.

■ Railroad Crossings

The driver/operator must obey all railroad crossing signals when responding to emergencies. Whenever you approach an unguarded railroad crossing, you should bring the fire apparatus to a complete stop before entering the grade crossing. Do not assume that the track is devoid of any trains in an attempt to continue the response. While stopped at the crossing, turn off all sirens, roll down the windows, operate the fire apparatus at an idle, and listen for the sound of an oncoming train. Railroad crossings must be treated with the same caution as any other intersection. Remember that with the siren activated, it may be difficult to hear a train horn or crossing bells. At intersections with railroad crossbars, you should never proceed between the crossbars in an attempt to continue the response. In this situation, you may have to alert the dispatch center or other responding units of a delayed response due to an inability to cross the railroad tracks safely.

Approaching the Scene of an Emergency

All emergency scenes have one thing in common: they are all dynamic in nature. A scene can go from bad to worse in a matter of seconds. For this reason, fire fighters should always be cautious. As a driver/operator, as you approach the scene, you should slow down, identify the correct address/location, and recognize any potential hazards. If you take all three of these actions, you can make the scene safer for the members of your crew and anyone else in the immediate area.

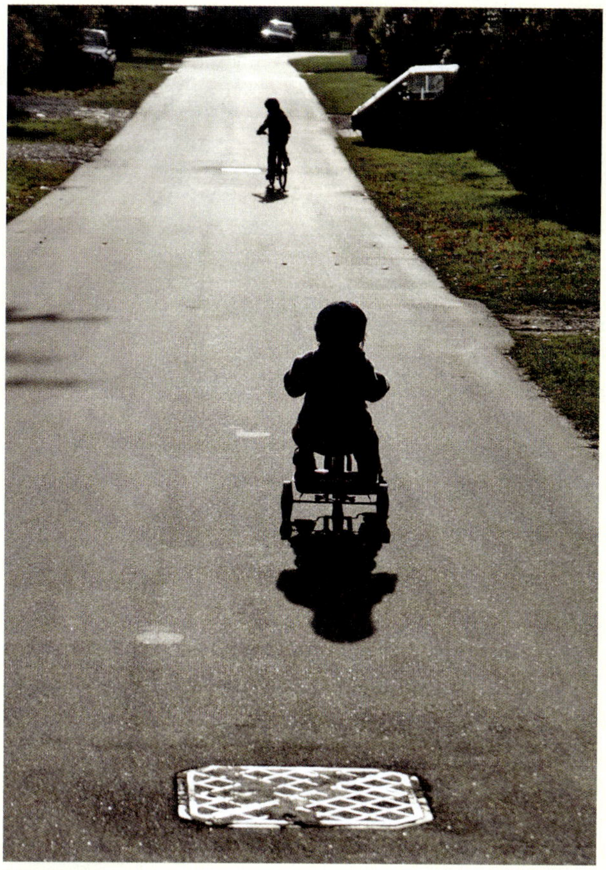

FIGURE 10-5 Slow down as you approach the scene—you never know who else is on the road.

■ Slow Down

When fire apparatus are responding to an emergency, the commotion usually attracts a lot of attention from the public. People are naturally curious about what is going on and may want to help. This is especially true in residential neighborhoods. Children may dart out into traffic, others may try to flag down fire apparatus, or people may stop their cars in the middle of the street. Some individuals even become so preoccupied with watching the emergency that they do not pay attention to their surroundings. This is why it is so essential for you to slow down and proceed with the utmost caution, especially in the last few blocks before reaching the emergency **FIGURE 10-5**.

■ Identify the Address/Location

Responding to the wrong location can not only be embarrassing, but may also lead to loss of property and even lives. This type of mistake may be avoided by writing down the address when the call is dispatched. If you forget the address, you can reference the information that you wrote down earlier. Although some fire departments have onboard computers that can be used to locate the incident, it is always better to have a hard copy as a backup.

Once the apparatus is in the vicinity of the emergency, all crew members aboard the fire apparatus should help in locating the address. In some response areas, identifying the location of

FIGURE 10-6 Not every apartment complex is numbered the same way.

FIGURE 10-7 Smoke can help you in locating the incident.

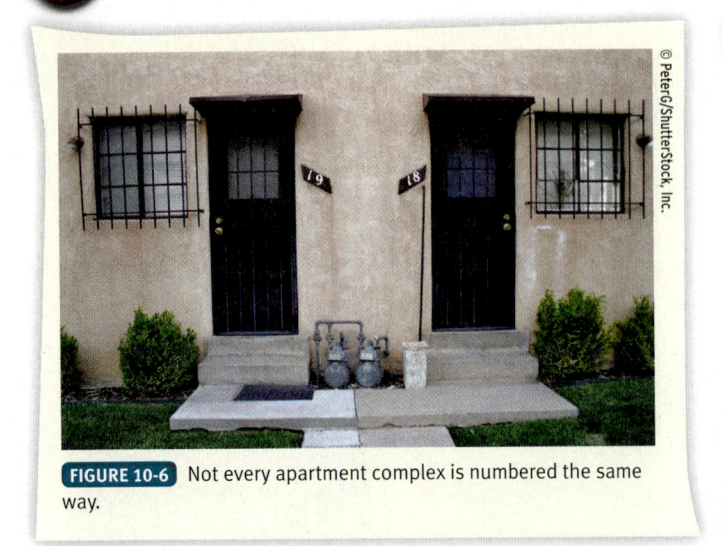

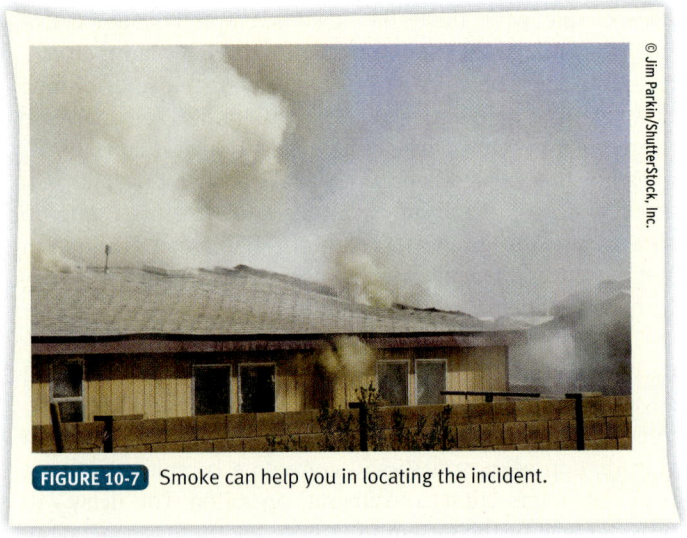

the incident may be difficult to do even during daylight hours. At night, the task is usually even more challenging. That is why everyone on the fire apparatus should be looking for the correct location. Firefighting is a team concept. Although the driver/operator is responsible for delivering the members of the company to the scene, you may need some assistance along the way.

In large apartment complexes, especially garden-style apartments, finding the location can be even more difficult. Unfortunately, not every apartment complex is numbered the same way. While some may have a letter to identify the building and a number for the actual apartment, others use the exact opposite addressing system **FIGURE 10-6**. Knowing the response district and having access to current maps can make all the difference. This information is best obtained before the emergency.

In rural areas, many fire departments rely on the knowledge of the fire department members. They may use local landmarks and old terminology to locate an emergency site. While this approach is not the preferred method to find emergency locations, in some jurisdictions it is the only way. In these situations, it is critical to have someone guide responders from other outside agencies to the scene as they seek the correct location. This may involve staging a unit on a main street to direct others down a dirt road that is not labeled.

Locating the correct location may involve more than just looking for a physical address. Some calls may be dispatched to an area and not a specific address. When trying to locate an emergency scene, the entire crew should look for some of the following signs:

- Civilians attempting to wave them down
- Smoke in the area **FIGURE 10-7**
- Police cars with their emergency lights on
- Large crowds of people
- Congested streets that normally are devoid of traffic
- Residential lights that are flickering on and off during the night
- Headlights from a car that is off the roadway

■ Recognize Potential Hazards

Recognizing potential hazards while approaching the incident can be difficult sometimes. You may respond to the same types of calls over and over. This routine may become monotonous, and it is easy for some members to become complacent. By constantly being on the lookout for hazards, you can ensure the safety of your crew. Some of the hazards that you may encounter include fallen power lines in the area, violent scenes, large amounts of pedestrian traffic, and debris in the roadway from a motor vehicle accident (MVA). While these hazards may be easily mitigated, failure to recognize them could put the crew's safety at risk. Do not become complacent; always be aware of your surroundings.

Fire Scene Positioning

While approaching a fire scene, you should attempt to view at least three sides of the structure. To do so, you may have to drive slightly past the structure. This positioning gives the crew on the fire apparatus a better size-up of the building, including the company officer who may have to share initial size-up information with other responding units.

Every fire department should train its members on proper staging procedures. Always follow your fire department's staging procedures. Some fire departments require that the first engine, ladder, and battalion chief go directly to the fire scene. With only a few necessary units at the scene, the Incident Commander (IC) can begin to orchestrate strategies and tactics without being overwhelmed. Eventually, specific tasks will be assigned to each unit by the IC. If tasks have not been delegated within a reasonable amount of time, the responding fire apparatus should attempt to contact the IC for an assignment.

■ Proper Positioning

As the first-arriving units are approaching the incident, the emphasis should be on the proper positioning of the fire apparatus. This initial placement should allow members to effect an investigation and allow for future operations. In most cases, it requires parking near the main entrance to the building. Stay outside with your fire apparatus, monitor all radio traffic, and await orders from the IC. While the other members of the crew are completing an investigation on the building's interior, you should further size up the incident from the exterior and

FIGURE 10-8 A fire department connection.

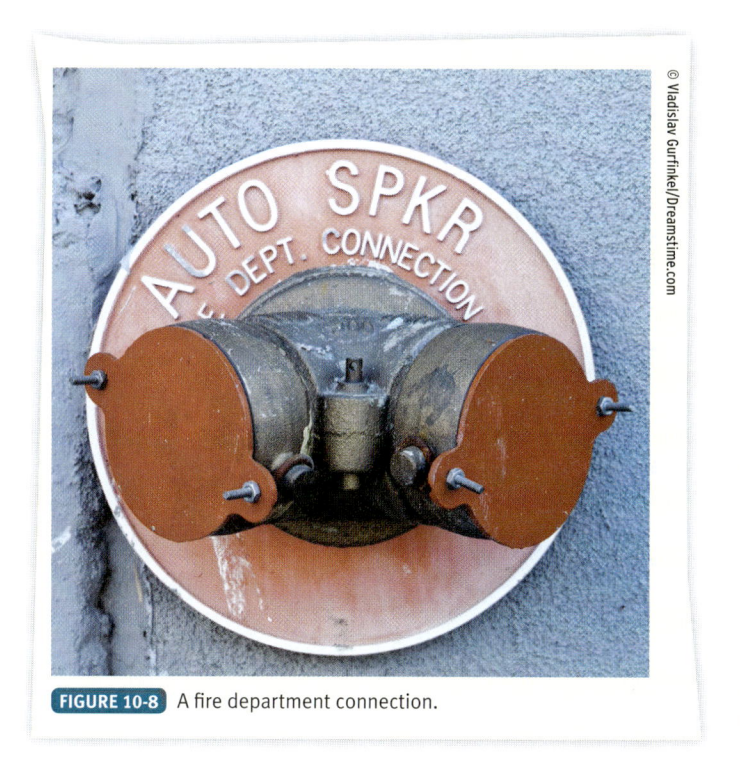

prepare for any needed operations. This effort may include the following steps:

- Determining the best position to spot other incoming fire apparatus
- Locating the nearest hydrant
- Locating the sprinkler system or standpipe connection **FIGURE 10-8**
- Preparing equipment that may be requested by the officer or IC, such as carbon monoxide detectors, thermal imaging cameras, and positive-pressure ventilation fans
- Observing any potential hazards on the scene

Always follow your department's SOPs and chain of command. Do not make decisions or issue orders when you do not have the authority to do so. Obtain information about the incident and relay it through the chain of command.

Working Fire

When the fire apparatus arrives at a working fire, the driver/operator must position it for maximum potential benefit. Unfortunately, there is usually a natural inclination to drive the fire apparatus as close to the fire as possible, which often results in positioning of fire apparatus that is both dysfunctional and dangerous. The placement of all fire apparatus on the fireground should take into account the following considerations:

- Your fire department's SOP
- A direct order from the IC
- A conscious decision on the part of the company officer based on existing or predictable conditions

Efficient fire apparatus placement must begin with the arrival of the first-responding fire apparatus. This vehicle will set the tone for the entire incident. If the initial fire apparatus is placed in the optimal position, then other fire apparatus will follow suit. In contrast, improper placement of the first-arriving units will create a problem that will have to be tolerated for the remainder of the incident. First-arriving fire apparatus should park at maximum advantage and go to work; later-arriving fire apparatus should be placed in a manner that builds on the initial plan and allows for expansion of the operation. Remember that firefighting is a team concept. Driver/operators who are already on the scene should communicate to those who are en route to the emergency and let them know in advance the most advantageous positions in which to place their vehicles. While this decision is usually the responsibility of the IC, all personnel will be affected if later-arriving units are positioned erroneously.

Later-arriving companies should follow their fire departments' staging procedures. Everyone must maintain an awareness of which site access provides the best tactical options and ensure that the immediate fire area does not become congested with fire apparatus. When possible, an access lane should be maintained down the center of the street. Park unneeded units out of the way. Fire apparatus that is not working should be left in the staging area or parked where it will not compromise access. Take advantage of the equipment on fire apparatus already in the fire area instead of bringing in more fire apparatus—many times only additional personnel are needed to address the incident.

When fire apparatus are on a fire scene, they are classified into one of two categories:

- **Working.** These fire apparatus are actually in use on the fire scene. The fire apparatus or the equipment that they carry is actively being used.
- **Parked.** These fire apparatus are not being used on the fire scene. Their only reason for being on scene, for the time being, is to transport personnel to the scene of the fire. No significant amount of tools or equipment from such fire apparatus is actively being used. Given these facts, the fire apparatus should remain in the appropriate staging area or be positioned so that they do not compromise the access route of other incoming units.

Staging

NFPA 1561, *Standard on Emergency Services Incident Management System*, identifies the need to provide a standard system to manage reserves of responders and other resources at or near the scene of the incident. If too many units arrive at the incident without direction, their presence may lead to possible freelancing and confusion. At such a chaotic scene, the IC will have great difficulty controlling the personnel and maintaining discipline. Accountability of all personnel on scene may also be complicated if it is not known when units arrived or who was given an assignment.

To avoid this dilemma, later-arriving fire apparatus should stay in an uncommitted position and await orders from the IC, a practice commonly referred to as **staging**. Staging is the standard procedure used to manage uncommitted resources at the scene of an incident. Its objective is to provide a standard system of initial placement for responding fire apparatus, personnel, and equipment prior to their assignment at tactical incidents **FIGURE 10-9**. Staging also provides a way to control and record the arrival of subsequent resources and eventually their assignment to specific locations or functions within the Incident Management System (IMS).

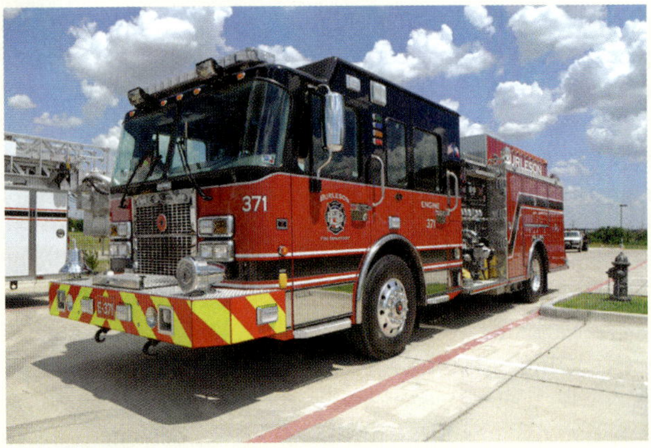

FIGURE 10-9 The objective of staging procedures is to provide a standard system of initial placement for responding fire apparatus, personnel, and equipment prior to their assignment at tactical incidents.

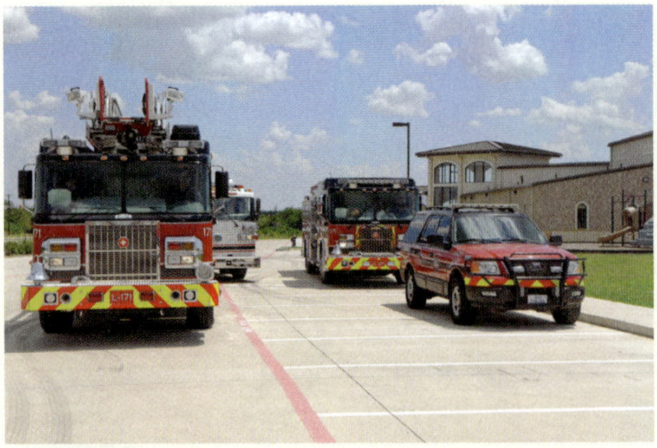

FIGURE 10-10 Level I staging.

When used successfully, proper staging of fire apparatus can accomplish the following goals:

- **Reduce unnecessary radio traffic.** During the first few critical moments of a structure fire, vital information is disseminated to all members who are responding. The IC will give a size-up of the incident. First-arriving units may request a water supply or additional resources to be sent to a specific location. Now is not the time to clutter the radio channel with needless radio traffic.
- **Reduce excessive apparatus congestion at the scene.** When too many fire apparatus are cluttering the scene, matters can become both dangerous and confusing. By placing fire apparatus in an uncommitted location close to the immediate scene, the IC can evaluate conditions prior to assigning companies. This will allow time for command personnel to formulate and implement a plan without undue confusion and pressure.
- **Provide the IC with a resource pool.** The IC may then assign units and resources at his or her leisure. These units should be ready to deploy as required by the IC.

DRIVER/OPERATOR Tip

Once at the scene of the incident, do not place the front of the fire apparatus too close to the rear of another fire apparatus. This will block in fire apparatus and may prohibit some equipment from being accessed, such as ground ladders carried on an aerial apparatus. Most modern aerial apparatus carry their ground ladders in the rear compartment. To remove the ladders, there must be a clear area behind them greater than the nested length of the ground ladder; for a 35-ft (11-m) extension ladder, this can be as much as 20 ft (6 m). Likewise, poor positioning of fire apparatus can cause problems in accessing the hose that is carried on the apparatus. If too many units are confined into a tight space together, the fire fighters will have a difficult time deploying the attack lines around other apparatus. Do not block other operations with your fire apparatus. Remember—hoselines can be extended; ladders cannot.

Level I Staging

Many fire departments use two levels of staging. Generally, **Level I staging** is in effect for all first alarm assignments, or incidents involving three or more units. For example, during a working structure fire response, all units continue responding to the scene until the first-in unit reports its arrival on the scene. Following its arrival and assumption of command, the first-in unit begins the assignment of the remainder of the dispatch. During Level I staging, the only units that proceed directly to the scene of a working structure fire are the first-due engine, ladder, and chief **FIGURE 10-10**. These units respond directly to the scene and initiate appropriate operations as directed by their department's SOPs or by the IC. All other units stage in their direction of travel, uncommitted, approximately one block from the scene. A position that supports the maximum number of tactical options with regard to access, direction of travel, water supply, and other considerations is preferred. Staged units announce their arrival, report their company designation, and identify their staged location/direction (e.g., "Engine Five, South"). These units remain in position until they receive an assignment from the IC.

Level II Staging

Level II staging is utilized on second or greater alarms or when mutual aid units report to an incident. This type of staging places all reserve resources in a central location and automatically requires the implementation of a staging area manager. The **staging area manager** is the person responsible for maintaining the operations of the staging area. The **staging area** is an area away from the incident where units will park until requested to enter the emergency scene **FIGURE 10-11**. This area should allow staged apparatus to access any geographic point of the incident without delay or vehicle congestion.

First alarm units that are already in Level I staging or en route to Level I staging will stay in Level I unless otherwise directed by the IC. All other responding units will proceed to the Level II staging area.

When activating Level II staging, the IC should give an approximate location for the staging area. This area should be some distance away from the emergency scene to reduce site

FIGURE 10-11 Level II staging.

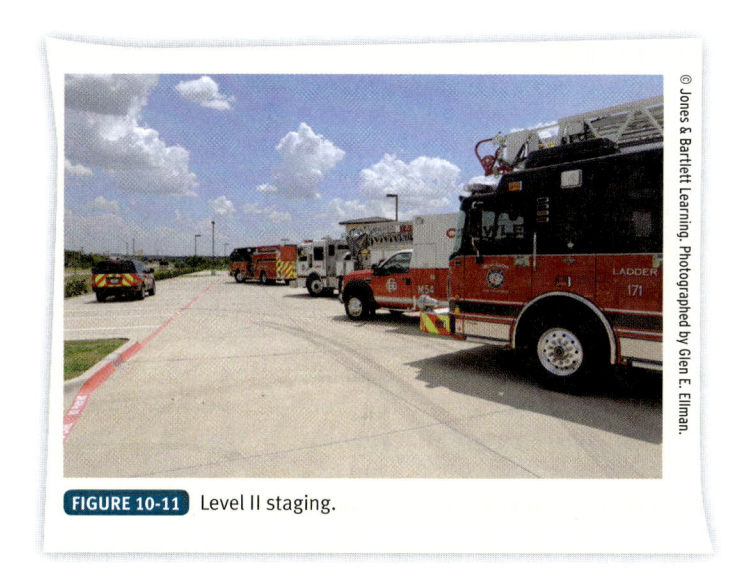

congestion, yet close enough to permit a prompt response to the incident site. Large parking lots or empty fields are excellent choices for a staging area.

The IC may designate a member of the department to serve as the staging area manager. When this position is not designated, the first fire officer to the Level II staging area will assume this role. The staging area manager takes a position that is both visible and accessible to incoming and staged companies. This is accomplished by leaving the emergency lights operating on the fire apparatus. No other fire apparatus positioned in the Level II staging area should leave its emergency lights on. All incoming resources into the staging area are logged and their availability reported to the IC. All subsequent arriving units should report in person to the staging area manager and await assignment, a strategy that reduces unnecessary radio traffic. Within the staging area, like units should be positioned next to one another—for example, all ladders next to each other, and all engines next to each other. This makes the staging area manager's job of identifying resources easier. Only the staging area manager may release resources from the staging area.

■ Engines and Ladders

Engine and ladder companies are the quintessential bread-and-butter apparatus of the fire service. The proper placement of ladders and engines should complement one another so as to rescue civilians and effect total fire extinguishment. Never assume that these two types of units can be positioned in the same way; instead, each unit has a specific function that should be taken into account when positioning the apparatus at a fire scene. Some fire departments have driver/operators who operate both types of fire apparatus on a regular basis. If this is the case, position the fire apparatus according to its function—not in the order in which it arrives on the fireground.

Many fire departments in the United States have both engines and ladders in their fleets. This section focuses primarily on these two indispensable pieces of equipment. Although other fire apparatus are also discussed, their presence on a fire scene is usually not as critical to its outcome.

The placement of the first-arriving engine or ladder should be based on the initial size-up and the fire department's SOPs. If the engine driver/operator arrives on scene first, he or she must choose a setup position that provides for efficient operation of the engine company as well as the first-arriving ladder apparatus. Just because your vehicle is the first fire apparatus to arrive at the scene, that fact does not mean that you are entitled to the best position on the fire scene. Instead, you must look at the big picture and imagine how the scene might unfold. An engine company occupying a spot that would be better suited for a ladder apparatus is an example of poor fire apparatus positioning and inexperience.

Usually, only the engine company responds to the fire scene with hose, water, and a fire pump on board the fire apparatus. As a consequence, the engine's placement depends on the conditions encountered upon arrival. While other responding fire apparatus may assist the engine company, it is ultimately the engine crew's responsibility to provide the water flow for fire extinguishment. This water may be supplied through handlines or master streams. It is imperative that the engine company establish a water supply that will last for the duration of the incident.

The ladder company should be positioned to support the engine company's operations and vice versa—preplanning is the key. When positioning a ladder apparatus on the scene of a fire, the driver/operator must take into account all of the hazards that may plague the engine company as well as some additional hazards that are specific to an <u>aerial device</u> (a generic term used to describe the hydraulically powered aerial ladder or platform that is operated from the top of an aerial apparatus). Aerial ladders and aerial platforms may be used as launching points for rescue, entry, search, and ventilation operations. They may also be used to stretch hoselines to upper floors or the roof, bridge a gap, perform ladder pipe operations, and serve as observation posts from which to assess conditions. When their need is evident upon arrival, aerial devices should be raised immediately. When need for them is anticipated to arise later, these devices should be positioned for rapid setup and future use. In these situations, the driver/operator of the ladder apparatus should remain in the vicinity of the turntable until the fire is under control.

The IC may give specific instructions regarding the placement of fire apparatus and the operations to be performed. As a driver/operator, you must base your decision about placement of the fire apparatus on the following conditions: rescue potential and exposures.

DRIVER/OPERATOR Tip

Each fire department should develop a procedure for the placement of initial fire apparatus that driver/operators should follow upon their arrival at an incident. Always follow your fire department's procedures, and learn the procedures for other jurisdictions covered by mutual aid agreements.

Rescue Potential

Rescue is the first priority for every responding fire apparatus. If civilians are potentially trapped inside the structure upon arrival, you should ensure that the front of the structure is available for access by the ladder apparatus. Position the fire apparatus to assist in or perform this operation. In this scenario, engine apparatus should be out of the way but preparing to go to work. For efficient and safe control, all apparatus driver/operators must work together to ensure that the aerial apparatus is positioned for maximum use and minimum stress to the aerial device. Usually, the front of the building is left available for the first-arriving ladder apparatus regardless of the conditions. It may be necessary or advantageous for ladder apparatus to circle the block and come in from the opposite end of the street, if such action will improve the fire apparatus placement.

Exposures

When exposure protection is necessary upon arrival, do not position the fire apparatus between the fire and the exposure. Doing so may cause the fire apparatus to become an exposure problem itself. Instead, position the vehicle far enough away from the exposure to remain safe, but close enough to deliver fire streams for exposure protection. Regardless of the initial placement, if conditions change (i.e., rapid fire spread that exposes the fire apparatus) and lead to collapse potential, then repositioning may be required and must be accomplished quickly and safely. Proper training and planning are essential in such cases.

As a driver/operator, you must always think ahead and position the fire apparatus with the idea that it might have to be repositioned at some point during the incident. Do not get blocked in or out of the fire area. Consider the collapse potential based on severe fire conditions and building construction. Many fire fighters have been killed and fire apparatus damaged because of failure to recognize a building's collapse potential. To ward off this threat, most fire departments specify a **collapse zone**—that is, a distance of 1½ times the height of the building in which fire fighters and fire apparatus must not be located in case of a building collapse. In buildings with bowstring trusses, identification of an even larger area as the collapse zone may be required. If such a building's walls and bowstring roof assembly fail, they may propel outward greater than 1½ times the height of the building. When tall buildings are involved with fire and a danger of collapse is present, a collapse zone of 1½ times the building's height may not be practical, as it would require positioning fire apparatus so far away that they may not be effective.

In some circumstances, the fire apparatus should be positioned in one of the **corner safe areas** of the fireground. In his book *Safety and Survival on the Fireground*, retired Fire Chief Vincent Dunn describes studying this area by looking at the structure from a bird's-eye view: There are four areas of the fireground that may not be covered by collapsing walls. As the fire progresses, fire fighters must continually reevaluate the potential for building collapse. Positioning the ladder apparatus at the corner safe areas of a building affords coverage on two fronts. This strategy enables coverage of a much wider area, permitting greater access and providing observation points from which to check the stability of the building and other issues.

When positioning the fire apparatus, note the locations of street lights, traffic signals, trees, utility poles, and wires at street corners or other parts of the site. Placement of the aerial device should be oriented toward providing as much effective operating area for the basket/tip as possible on both fronts of the building.

Fire Conditions

The initial engine company needs to be positioned for the efficient deployment of the first attack line—the most important attack line on the fireground. You should not position the fire apparatus with the preconnected attack line directly in front of the building's entrance. While this positioning may simplify the attack line deployment, it will place the engine in a position that compromises the operation of other incoming fire apparatus, especially the ladder apparatus. Instead, the engine should be placed past the structure, with the front of the building being left open for the ladder company. Most engines have an excess of fire hose, whereas aerial devices have a fixed length. Do not render the aerial device useless by blocking it out just to make stretching the attack lines easier.

Water Supply

Dependent upon department procedures, the first-due engine companies approaching the scene with any evidence of a working fire in a structure may secure a water supply. The next-in engine company may be too far away or encounter a delay while responding to perform this task. In some cases, however, securing the water supply may not be the first-arriving engine company's primary task—for example, when there is an obvious critical rescue requiring the entire crew or when the exact location of the fire in a multiple-unit occupancy is unknown. Whenever possible, the supply line should consist of large-diameter hose (LDH), as this type of hose reduces the friction loss and provides an adequate water supply. Always notify other responding apparatus when laying LDH across streets and intersections, as this supply line may block other fire apparatus from reaching the scene of the fire. When laying the hose from the hose bed, always attempt to position it to the same side of the street as the hydrant.

Slope

Positioning the fire apparatus uphill from the incident may prevent future problems, such as those caused by water runoff from the fire scene. The slope of the area will usually not affect normal engine operations. NFPA 1901 requires that fire apparatus have two wheel chocks mounted in readily accessible locations, each designed to hold the fire apparatus when loaded to its maximum in-service weight on a 20 percent grade with the transmission in neutral and the parking brake released. When the pump is engaged, make sure that these wheel chocks are placed in the proper positions. If there is any doubt about the unit's ability to keep from rolling down the hill, chock it or move it!

Some sloping surfaces may not allow for adequate deployment of an aerial device. To operate with 100 percent capacity of the aerial device, some aerial apparatus stabilizers can correct for a slope and grade of only a few degrees. You may be able to park the fire apparatus in an optimal position, but if the aerial device is incapable of operating in that position, this placement is futile. You must know the limitations of the fire apparatus that you are operating and position it accordingly.

Terrain and Surface Conditions

The terrain is the landscape on which the apparatus is positioned. In many cases it may be an asphalt roadway or a concrete driveway, but sometimes it may include areas off the roadway. In these circumstances, you should position the fire

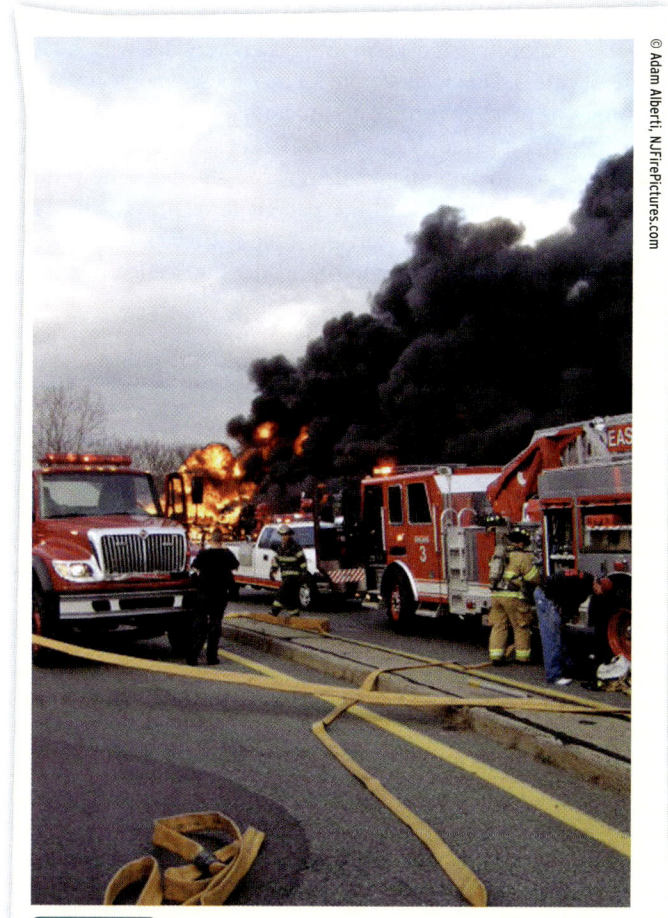

FIGURE 10-12 Too much smoke will starve the engine of fresh air and cause it to shut down.

FIGURE 10-13 Use caution when operating around trees.

apparatus with future pump operations in mind. If possible, leave the fire apparatus on the asphalt roadway or a concrete driveway that can support the weight of the fire apparatus. If this positioning is not feasible, you should prevent significant amounts of water from flowing underneath the fire apparatus if it is positioned on top of soil that is unstable or may become unstable. Otherwise, the fire apparatus may become stuck and the ensuing mess may hamper future operations. Where the ground is of doubtful stability, as is sometimes the case with vacant lots or other unpaved areas that may have hidden voids, and if the terrain is deemed not substantial enough, ladder apparatus should be positioned elsewhere.

Wind Conditions
Upon arrival, note the wind conditions. Place the fire apparatus out of the path of oncoming smoke and heat. Too much smoke will starve the engine of fresh air and cause it to shut down **FIGURE 10-12**. Should the wind shift during the operation and compromise the engine operation, notify the IC. If possible, it may be necessary to reposition the engine at another location. While you are operating the fire apparatus, if you need self-contained breathing apparatus (SCBA) because of the smoke conditions, move the fire apparatus: If you cannot breathe the air, neither can the fire apparatus. Remaining in the original position may cause the fire apparatus to stall and render its pumping operations useless.

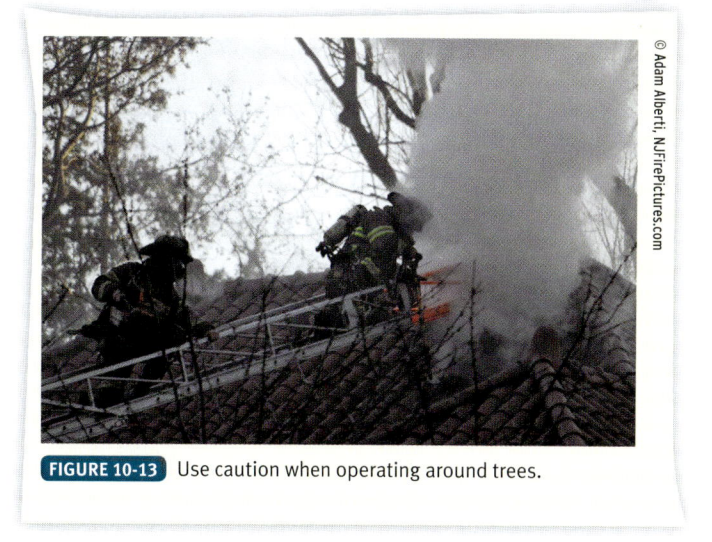

The wind may also affect master stream operations. When deck guns are not reliable because of heavy wind conditions, the use of portable ground monitors may be a better alternative. The wind may also limit the operations of some aerial devices on scene. All aerial devices are designed to be operated in winds from 35 mph to 50 mph (56–80 km/h) without any reduction in tip load, but always refer to the operating manual to determine the recommended operational extremes.

Overhead Obstructions
Overhead wires may interfere with any aerial device's operation. Do not be intimidated by overhead wires when the situation clearly calls for use of the aerial device; rather, exercise caution and be creative in your approach. The IC should have wires removed by the utility company when fire conditions warrant doing so. All aerial devices should remain a minimum of 10 ft (3 m) from all overhead wires. Do not try to guess which wires may be energized; instead, consider all wires to be live until proven otherwise.

When trees obstruct operations, it may be possible to extend or raise the aerial device through light branches. However, retraction or lowering of the boom through branches may present a problem, and some cutting may be required to overcome this obstacle. Use caution when operating around trees, as an electrical hazard should always be suspected **FIGURE 10-13**. Before an incident occurs, you should practice positioning the fire apparatus for operation with overhead obstructions in the area to become familiar with the fire apparatus' limitations and functions under these conditions. Possible alternatives may include placing the fire apparatus on sidewalks, setting it up at corners, and extending the aerial device parallel to the front of a building. The crew should also practice using this device at intersections with light posts, traffic signs or signals, intersecting overhead wires, and other obstacles to enable personnel to judge where and how fire apparatus is to be positioned for maximum coverage under similar circumstances.

Auxiliary Appliances
An <u>auxiliary appliance</u> is a standpipe and/or sprinkler system. The determination of whether a building has one or both of these systems is best made during development of a

preincident plan. A **preincident plan** is described by NFPA 1620, *Recommended Practice for Preincident Planning*, as a document developed by gathering general and detailed data to be used by responding personnel to determine the resources and actions necessary to mitigate anticipated emergencies at a specific facility. When creating such a preincident plan, you should locate the fire department connection, fire pump, standpipe system, and sprinkler system in the building. If this information is not readily available, you will have to rely on other members of the crew to help locate these systems, which may slow down the initial operations and result in more work for the fire fighters on scene. For example, if an engine company responds to a fire in a multistory apartment building, the crew may prefer to use the building's built-in standpipe system to establish a water supply. If you cannot identify the location of the fire department connection, the engine crew will not be able to use the standpipe to connect attack lines and, therefore, will have to stretch additional hoselines up to the fire floor. This delay in water application may cause the fire to progress past the extinguishment capabilities of a single hoseline.

■ Positioning of Other Fire Scene Apparatus

Engines and ladder trucks are not the only fire apparatus required at a fire scene. Depending on the size, construction, occupancy, and involvement of the structure, a multitude of other types of fire apparatus may be needed to mount an effective response.

Specialized Fire Apparatus

Specialized fire apparatus may be equipped with an assortment of specialized equipment, such as that needed for heavy technical rescue, hazardous materials response, or mobile air supply. The personnel assigned to these fire apparatus are required to have specialized training, and their role on the fire scene is usually to provide support operations.

Specialized fire apparatus may need to be positioned close to the incident depending on the conditions. The driver/operators of these vehicles may have to be creative in their approach to the fire scene. Approaching from the same direction as all the other units may not be effective, for example. Instead, these driver/operators must listen to the radio, observe scene conditions, and identify the most efficient position for the task assigned.

Command Vehicles

A **command vehicle** is one that the fire chief uses to respond to the fire scene. This vehicle should be positioned at a location that will allow maximum visibility of the fire building and surrounding area. It should be easily identified at the scene and placed in a logical position. The command vehicle should not restrict the movement or positioning of other apparatus at the fire scene.

Ambulances

An **ambulance** is a specially designed vehicle that is capable of transporting sick and injured patients. It is usually staffed with trained emergency technicians and/or paramedics. These vehicles should be parked in a safe position that will provide the most effective treatment and transportation of fire victims and firefighting personnel, while not blocking other apparatus or interfering with firefighting operations. Ambulance drivers are also responsible for positioning their vehicles with a clear route of egress. During large fire scenes, these emergency vehicles may be staged with other apparatus in a Level II staging area. When requested, they will respond to the scene. Once on the fire scene, the ambulance driver may stay with the vehicle while other personnel load the patient into the vehicle. This practice ensures that the patient is picked up as close to the scene as possible without compromising fire scene operations if the ambulance needs to be relocated.

Positioning at an Intersection or on a Highway

Operating at an emergency scene that is located either on or adjacent to a highway or intersection is extremely dangerous. Personnel should understand and appreciate the high risk that fire fighters are exposed to when they are working in or near moving vehicles. According to the U.S. Fire Administration, the third leading cause of fatal injuries to fire fighters in 2012 was being struck by an object, which includes being struck by a vehicle. Seventeen fire fighters died while responding to or returning from emergency incidents, and 18 fire fighters died as the result of vehicle crashes **TABLE 10-1**. This type of fire fighter fatality is not uncommon; indeed, it happens every year. Each call near a roadway should be treated with caution. Always consider moving traffic to pose a threat to scene safety.

Each day, fire fighters are exposed to motorists of varying abilities, with or without licenses, with or without legal restrictions, and driving at speeds from creeping along to going well beyond the speed limit. Some of these motorists have visual impairments, and some are impaired because of the use of alcohol and/or drugs. On top of everything else, motorists often become distracted by the incident and look at the scene and not the road. Their lack of attentiveness while passing a roadside emergency scene may affect fire fighters' safety as they work at the scene.

TABLE 10-1	Causes of Fatal Injuries to U.S. Fire Fighters, 2012

Eighty-one fire fighters died while on duty in 2012.

- The total breakdown included 42 volunteer, 28 career, and 11 wildland agency fire fighters.
- There were four multiple fire fighter fatality incidents, claiming a total of 10 fire fighters.
- Fifteen fire fighters died in duties associated with wildland fires.
- Activities related to emergency incidents resulted in the deaths of 45 fire fighters.
- Twenty-two fire fighters died while engaging in activities at the scene of a fire.
- Seventeen fire fighters died while responding to or returning from 16 emergency incidents.
- Eighteen fire fighters died as the result of 14 vehicle crashes, six involving personally owned vehicles (POVs), six involving apparatus, and six from two separate incidents involving aircraft.
- Heart attacks were the most frequent cause of death, accounting for 39 fire fighter deaths.
- Eight fire fighters died while engaged in training activities.
- Twelve fire fighters died after the conclusion of their on-duty activity.

Source: U.S. Fire Administration, *Fire fighter Fatalities in the United States, 2012.*

When the fire apparatus arrives at the scene, other members may have a desire to quickly dismount the apparatus and go to work. The driver/operator should not allow personnel to exit the cab until the driver/operator is satisfied with the position of the fire apparatus. To achieve this goal, it may be necessary to angle the fire apparatus off of a roadway. Only when the unit is parked and ready should the other members be allowed to exit the vehicle.

Four actions that all fire fighters can take to protect themselves and the other crew members while operating in traffic conditions include never trusting traffic, engaging in proper protective parking, reducing motorist vision impairment, and wearing high-visibility reflective vests.

■ Never Trust Traffic

Every fire fighter must have a healthy respect for all vehicles. Do not assume that because vehicles are moving around an emergency scene that the danger is gone. Anytime that the scene is located near moving traffic, there is a potential danger to fire fighters. Fire fighters should exit the apparatus on the curb side or the nontraffic side whenever possible. Always look before stepping out of the fire apparatus or into any traffic areas on scene. When walking around fire apparatus parked adjacent to moving traffic, keep an eye on traffic and walk as close to the fire apparatus as possible. Never turn your back to oncoming traffic for extended periods of time.

■ Engage in Proper Protective Parking

This aspect of safety relies on your ability as the driver/operator. As you position the fire apparatus, think about the consequences of your actions. Never allow convenience to compromise safety. Always position your apparatus to protect the scene, patients, and emergency personnel, and to provide a protected work area. When possible, position the fire apparatus at a 45-degree angle away from the curbside to direct motorists around the scene **FIGURE 10-14**. Initial fire apparatus placement should always allow for adequate parking of other fire apparatus and a safe work area for emergency personnel. Allow enough distance between the fire apparatus and the scene to prevent a moving vehicle from knocking fire apparatus into the work areas.

FIGURE 10-14 An example of proper protective parking.

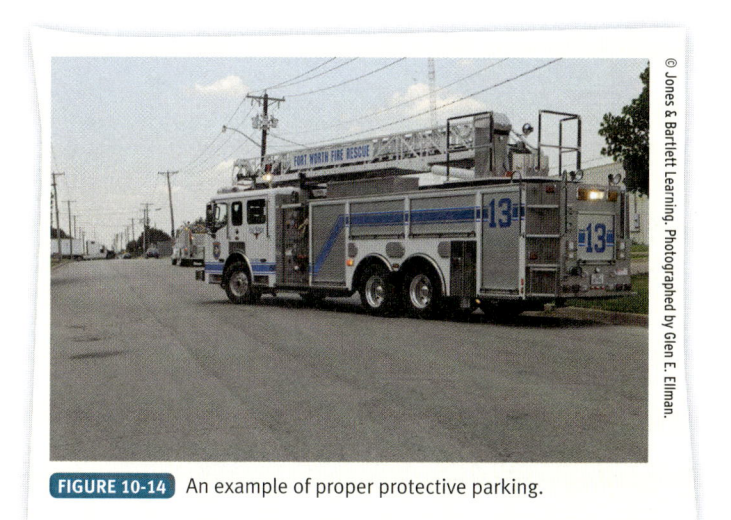

■ Reduce Motorist Vision Impairment

During an emergency, the need for emergency lights is evident. At the incident, the use of emergency lighting may still be needed when the safety of personnel is otherwise compromised. Never hesitate to operate emergency lighting at a scene. However, understand that emergency vehicle lighting provides a warning only and does not ensure effective traffic control; the latter consideration entails protecting the emergency scene from oncoming traffic by redirecting, blocking, or stopping all moving vehicles.

While most state laws require only one lighted lamp exhibiting red light visible under normal atmospheric conditions from a distance of 500 ft (150 m), many fire apparatus exceed this requirement. Unfortunately, the use of too many lights at a scene may create a dangerous situation. An excess of emergency lights flashing can cause a carnival effect and create confusion for motorists. Limit the number of fire apparatus operating emergency lights to only those blocking oncoming traffic—and even these fire apparatus may not need all of their emergency lights to be on.

If provided, use directional arrows at the rear of the apparatus to direct any oncoming traffic **FIGURE 10-15**. It is safer to divert traffic with advanced placement of signs and traffic cones rather than to rely on warning lights on fire apparatus to reroute oncoming vehicles.

DRIVER/OPERATOR Tip

Each colored emergency light on the fire apparatus serves a specific purpose and results in a different reaction from other motorists. The following list identifies the lights' color and reaction:

- **Red.** For most civilians, a red light identifies the need to stop. Unfortunately, it may also attract those drivers who are under the influence of drugs and/or alcohol as well as fatigued drivers.
- **Blue.** A blue light identifies the fire apparatus as being associated with either fire or police. States may have different laws dictating who can and cannot use blue lights on their vehicles. A blue light has good visibility during both daytime and nighttime operations.
- **Amber.** An amber light signals danger or caution. This color is widely used by other services to get drivers' attention. Many experts believe it to be the best warning light for the rear of emergency vehicles. It may deter those drivers who are fatigued or who are under the influence of drugs or alcohol. During foggy conditions, an amber-colored light is more readily visible than other colored lights.
- **Clear.** Clear light is associated with caution. Although it provides good visibility, such a light should normally be shut off at an emergency scene, to prevent blinding other drivers. For the same reason, it should not be used at the rear of the fire apparatus.

■ Wear High-Visibility Reflective Vests

Turnout gear does not adequately identify a fire fighter who is operating in or near traffic conditions. The reflective trim on the turnout gear may be dirty, covered with other equipment, or missing. To effectively identify themselves, fire fighters

FIGURE 10-15 Use of directional arrows to divert the flow of traffic.

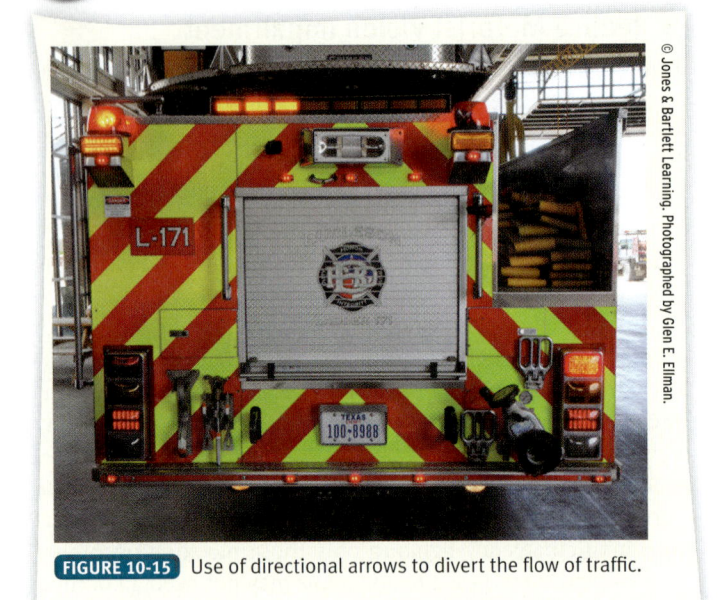

should wear American National Standards Institute (ANSI)-approved reflective vests. These vests should be retroreflective and fluorescent. Each fire department should require all personnel operating under these conditions to wear such vests. Some manufacturers make reflective vests out of flame-retardant material that may be worn over turnout gear.

Safety Tip

The American National Standards Institute has identified three classes of safety vests:

- **Class 1.** This vest has the lowest level of visibility. It is generally worn in environments where speeds do not exceed 25 mph (40 km/h) by parking lot attendants, roadside maintenance workers, delivery vehicle drivers, and warehouse workers.
- **Class 2.** This category includes the most popular style of safety vest. It is commonly worn in environments where traffic is moving in excess of 25 mph (40 km/h) by construction workers, utility workers, school crossing guards, and emergency responders. A fire-retardant Class 2 safety vest is also available for fire fighters; it is constructed of treated fluorescent polyester and carries reflective striping.
- **Class 3.** This vest offers the highest level of visibility. It is worn in environments where the traffic is moving in excess of 55 mph (80 km/h) by roadway construction workers, utility workers, survey crews, and emergency response personnel.

Manual on Uniform Traffic Control Devices

The U.S. Department of Transportation's Federal Highway Administration publishes the *Manual on Uniform Traffic Control Devices for Streets and Highways (MUTCD)*. Under federal law, each state is required to adopt the provisions in this manual. Section 6I, "The Control of Traffic Through Incident Management Areas," applies to all incidents that fire fighters might encounter on or near the roadway. It defines a **traffic incident** as an emergency traffic occurrence, a natural disaster, or other unplanned event that affects or impedes the normal flow of traffic. When traffic incidents occur, some form of **traffic control** must take place.

The goals of traffic control are fourfold:

- To improve responder safety while working at the incident
- To keep the traffic flowing as smoothly as possible around the incident
- To prevent the occurrence of secondary accidents at the scene
- To prevent unnecessary use of the surrounding road system

Within 15 minutes of arriving on the scene of a traffic incident, the IC should estimate the magnitude of the incident, the expected length of the queue of backed-up motorists on the highway or roadway, and the duration of the incident. According to the *MUTCD*, traffic incidents may be classified into one of three general classes of duration, each of which presents its own unique hazards and traffic control needs **FIGURE 10-16**:

- **Major traffic incidents** include fatal crashes involving multiple vehicles, hazardous materials incidents on the highway, and other disasters. They usually require closing all or part of the highway for a period exceeding 2 hours. When this type of incident occurs, fire fighters must request assistance from traffic engineering and law enforcement to divert traffic around and past the incident.
- **Intermediate traffic incidents** are less severe in nature and usually affect the lanes of travel for 30 minutes to 2 hours. Traffic control is required to divert moving traffic around and past the incident. The highway may need to be closed for a short period to allow fire fighters to accomplish their task. Law enforcement personnel usually handle traffic control needs.
- **Minor traffic incidents** may involve minor crashes and disabled vehicles. Lane closures are kept to a minimum and are less than 30 minutes in duration. Traffic control is needed only briefly, if at all. The fire fighters may handle any minor traffic control needs.

MUTCD defines a **traffic incident management area (TIMA)** as an area of highway where temporary traffic controls are imposed by authorized officials in response to a traffic incident, natural disaster, hazardous material spill, or other unplanned incident. This area is further subdivided into the following sections:

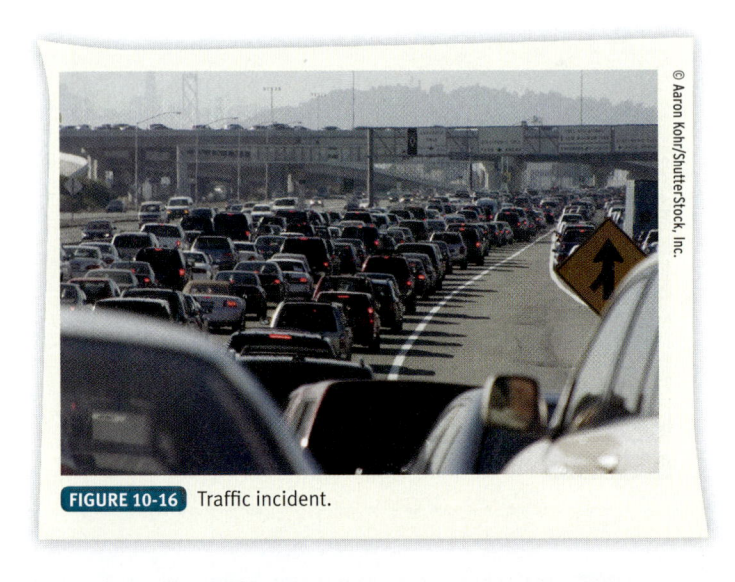

FIGURE 10-16 Traffic incident.

VOICES OF EXPERIENCE

Because some incidents have a greater potential for violence than others, it may not always be a good idea to drive slowly past the address and stage a distance from the scene. All responses are department-specific, but if you are dealing with a potentially violent scene, it is often safer to have the police secure a scene before making your presence known to those involved in the incident.

In our department, we have had numerous occasions where our personnel arrived before the police department, but staged within sight of the scene. Passing or staging within sight of the scene often only creates more tension in a situation that requires more calm. We have had involved parties actually charge at our apparatus because they believe we should be administering care, even though our protocols require for the police to secure such a scene for everyone's safety before we can move in.

At one particular incident several years ago, a subject at such a scene fired a rifle from a second story window. The bullet traveled over half a mile. Had our personnel been staged nearby, they would have easily been in range of the bullets.

As a result of this incident, many of us will stage on a nearby side street, out of sight of the actual scene, until central dispatch advises us that the police have secured the scene. This prevents us from being sighted by the parties involved in the incident until the scene is secured. It also puts a buffer of structures between us and any possible gunfire, and we can quickly retreat from the area if involved parties approach.

Christopher Drake
Muskegon Fire Department
Muskegon, Michigan

- The **advance warning area** is the section of highway where motorists are informed about the upcoming situation ahead. It may be identified by an emergency vehicle with its lights activated or by warning signs. On highways, the advance warning signs should be positioned farther ahead of the actual site because of the high speeds at which vehicles are traveling. When roadways are smaller and have lower speed limits, the distance can be shortened.
- The **transition area** is where the vehicle is redirected from its normal path and where lane changes and closures are made.
- The **activity area** is the section where the work activity takes place. It may be stationary or may move as work progresses.
- The **buffer space** is a lateral and/or longitudinal area that separates motorist flow from the work space or an unsafe area. This area might also provide some recovery space for an errant vehicle.
- The **incident space** is the area where the actual incident is located.
- The **traffic space** is the portion of the highway in which traffic is routed through the activity area.
- The **termination area** is the area where the normal flow of traffic resumes.

By defining these areas, fire fighters gain a better understanding of where fire apparatus should be positioned at the scene. Communicating to incoming apparatus and describing their placement becomes easier when the scene is divided into separate areas.

Safety Tip

On August 5, 1999, two career fire fighters of the Midwest City Fire Department (MCFD) were struck by a motor vehicle on a wet and busy interstate. MCFD Ladder Company 2 and Squad 2 had responded to a single motor vehicle accident on the interstate. The ladder apparatus was positioned approximately 150 ft (45 m) behind Squad 2, near the median wall, with its emergency lights left on.

A few minutes after arriving on scene, Ladder Company 2 was hit from behind by a passenger vehicle. Fire fighters began to attend to the injuries of this driver while other members began to flag traffic away. A fire fighter who was watching the oncoming traffic situation noticed a vehicle coming toward the rear of Ladder Company 2 and the fire fighters. Two warnings were yelled out over the radio. This car hit several fire fighters as they were attempting to flee its path. The vehicle collided with the median wall and wedged into the space between Ladder Company 2 and the wall. Several company members were able to avoid the impact of the vehicle, but two fire fighters and a civilian were not so fortunate. The impact knocked the three individuals approximately 47 ft (14 m), killing one fire fighter and severely injuring the other fire fighter and the civilian. While the fire fighters were attending to the injured, yet another vehicle spun out of control on the interstate and struck the vehicle that had impacted the rear of Ladder Company 2.

Motor Vehicle Accidents

A **motor vehicle accident (MVA)** may involve one or more vehicles, either on or off the roadway. This type of emergency is a very common reason for calling out fire fighters. In metropolitan areas, the majority of these incidents tends to result in only very minor damage to both the vehicles and the passengers. By comparison, MVAs in rural areas and highways may have quite different outcomes; they are usually very serious and result in great damage to both the vehicles and the passengers.

As the fire apparatus approaches the accident scene, traffic is usually backed up behind the MVA. This makes the approach to the scene slower than normal and may be frustrating for the fire fighters, who are ready to go to work. As the driver/operator, you must not get impatient and allow your emotions to get the best of you. Proceed with caution and remain calm. In this situation, you must have a consistent approach to the incident site. Do not weave the fire apparatus in and out of traffic to gain access to the scene, as such maneuvers confuse other motorists about your intentions. Keep the fire apparatus in the far left lane while approaching the scene. If necessary, the fire officer can use the public address system on the fire apparatus to direct the backed-up traffic to the far right and allow the fire apparatus to reach the scene.

Positioning at an Intersection

Based on Coaching the Emergency Vehicle Operator (CEVO) courses, motor vehicle accidents are more likely to occur at an intersection than anywhere else. These accidents usually involve more than one vehicle. A unique hazard that is present with an accident in an intersection is large groups of people attempting to help the accident victims. Traffic control should be the first priority once the fire apparatus arrives at the scene. If the moving traffic is not controlled, then the scene will not be safe for fire fighters. For most incidents, the fire apparatus itself can be positioned to shield the work area for fire fighters and to protect fire fighters from moving traffic.

Whenever possible, police should be called for assistance with traffic control. Police officers are specifically trained to carry out this type of operation. The initial fire apparatus must assess the parking needs of later-arriving units and specifically direct the parking and placement of these vehicles as they arrive to provide protective blocking of the scene. When parking the fire apparatus to protect the scene, be sure to protect the work area as well. Doing so ensures that victims can be extricated, treated, moved about the scene, and loaded into ambulances safely. Do not position the fire apparatus exhaust in the direction of the victims who are entrapped in motor vehicles.

At intersections or at sites where the incident is near the middle of the street, two or more sides of the incident may need to be protected. In such a case, fire apparatus should block all exposed sides. Where fire apparatus are limited in numbers, prioritize the blocking scheme from the most critical sides to the least critical. Once enough fire apparatus have blocked the scene, park or stage unneeded vehicles off the street whenever possible. When ambulances are positioned at a scene, always protect the victim loading areas.

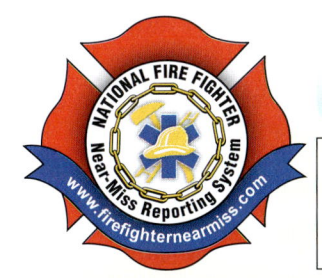

Near-Miss REPORT

Report Number: 09-0001127

Synopsis: Ladder truck slides into intersection on wet road.

Event Description: While driving a ladder company to a possible structure fire in very poor weather conditions (hard, steady rain), I approached an intersection with a traffic light that was red. As I approached, I decided to leave my lane of travel and attempt to go through the intersection in the on-coming lane. This was a four-way intersection. As I approached, a vehicle came from the right hand road headed straight for me. I hit the brakes, began to slide, adjusted my steering, and somehow missed her.

Lessons Learned: We should always approach intersections with extreme caution, particularly in inclement weather. It is impossible to steer while wheels are locked in a slide. You must steer through in order to change direction in wet conditions, no brakes, and low speed.

DRIVER/OPERATOR Tip

If the fire apparatus is equipped with a traffic control device, it may be tied into the emergency lighting system. In such a case, when the emergency lights are activated, so is the traffic control device. While the fire apparatus is positioned at an intersection for the response to an emergency and operating its emergency lights, this may pose a problem: the intersection lights would continue to cycle through at the request of the apparatus' traffic control device. To overcome this problem, the traffic control device is designed to shut off when the fire apparatus' parking brake is set. This system ensures that the fire apparatus can operate its emergency lights while parked and not disrupt the directional lights at an intersection.

Positioning on a Highway

Because speeds are higher, traffic volume is more significant, and civilian motorists have little opportunity to slow, stop, or change lanes, fire fighters must be constantly aware of moving vehicles on highways. Although at times the scene may seem safe, matters can change at a moment's notice.

When approaching an emergency scene on a highway, identify a position that will allow fire fighters to work in a safe area. Sometimes this may involve disrupting the normal flow of traffic or blocking it off completely. The safety of the fire fighters should always be the first priority—not the continuous flow of traffic. When doubt arises about the proper positioning of the fire apparatus, always err on the side of caution: Block the highway to provide a safe working area for fire fighters. For emergencies on a highway, continue to block the scene with the first-arriving fire apparatus to provide a safe working area. Other companies may then be used to provide additional blocking if needed. If possible use the largest, heaviest fire apparatus (usually ladder apparatus) as the first blockers.

Vehicle Fires

Fire fighters respond to more vehicle fires than they do structure fires. In fact, approximately 25 percent of all reported fires in the United States involve vehicles. These types of fires should not be taken lightly. Given the various amounts of plastics, foams, and synthetic materials from which modern-day vehicles are constructed, a vehicle may be consumed quickly by an intense, fast-moving fire. Most often, the vehicle is usually so severely damaged before the fire department arrives on scene that it is a total loss. The majority of vehicle fires results in a total loss.

When responding to a vehicle fire, do not position the fire apparatus where it will become an exposure hazard. **FIGURE 10-17**.

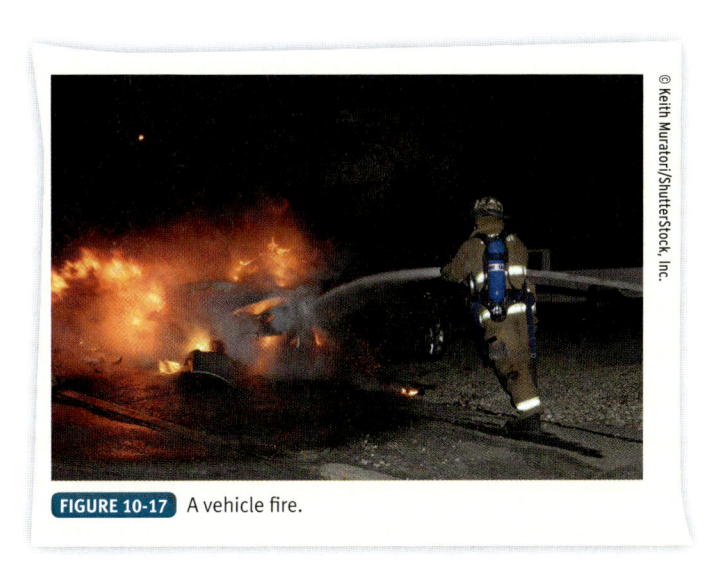

FIGURE 10-17 A vehicle fire.

Try to position the fire apparatus in a location that is uphill and upwind of the burning vehicle. While this may not always be the most advantageous position on the scene, you do not want smoke or flammable liquids to compromise the safe operation of the fire apparatus. If you have to position it downhill from the burning vehicle, create a dike in front of the fire apparatus to pool any flammable liquids. Be aware that the brakes on the burning vehicle may be compromised by the fire conditions and the vehicle may roll downhill; do not place the fire apparatus in a position that might allow the burning vehicle to roll into it.

You should position the fire apparatus at a 45-degree angle to the burning vehicle to protect the area near the pump panel as well as the scene. Most fire apparatus have the fire pump mounted on the driver's side in the middle of the vehicle; this is the location where the driver/operator stands while operating the fire pump. Be aware of where the fire fighters are deploying hoselines at the scene. While the other members of the crew are extinguishing the fire, the driver/operator is responsible for providing adequate water from the pump and ensuring that the crew remains safe. This effort may involve positioning traffic cones or warning devices to alert oncoming traffic to the emergency scene.

Railroads

When positioning the fire apparatus near a railroad track, try to place it on the same side as the incident. This placement will ensure that fire fighters do not have to cross the tracks, thereby risking injury or death from oncoming trains. Every railroad track should be considered active. If possible, contact dispatch and request that the railroad tracks be shut down while on-scene operations continue. Whenever possible, the apparatus should not enter the railroad right of way until confirmation is received from the railroad that train traffic has been suspended. *Never* park the fire apparatus on top of the railroad tracks.

Positioning at the Emergency Medical Scene

An emergency medical scene can be just as dangerous as the other types of incidents to which fire fighters respond. Usually, the danger is not associated with the emergency scene itself, but rather with the people involved. Every day, fire fighters somewhere are surprised by a scene that becomes violent when initially it appeared safe. At a moment's notice, what looks like a routine call can turn into a deadly encounter. Thus the first priority when arriving at an EMS scene is to provide a protected environment for fire fighters to work in. If the fire fighters are not safe, then they cannot provide adequate care. Ideally, the driver/operator should position the fire apparatus either 100 ft (30 m) before or after the address. This placement will allow the entire crew to size up the situation and recognize any potential hazards. Do not position the fire apparatus directly in front of the address, as such placement does not allow the fire fighters adequate time to identify or react to any potential hazards.

Some incidents have a greater potential for violence than others, including assaults, fights, and domestic disputes. When fire fighters are requested to respond to these types of calls, you should turn off the emergency lights and sirens a few blocks away from the physical address of the incident. Fire fighters should enter the scene on their own terms and not rush into an unknown situation. For such calls, you should drive slowly past the address and park the fire apparatus at least 100 ft (30 m) from the building/location.

At EMS scenes, the fire apparatus should be positioned for a quick exit. If necessary, turn it around. This may involve backing the fire apparatus into an alley or side street. NFPA 1002, *Standard for Fire Apparatus Driver/Operator Professional Qualifications*, requires that all driver/operators complete an exercise—called the alley dock exercise—that simulates the process of backing a fire apparatus into an alley or tight space. This exercise measures your ability to drive on a street past a simulated area, and then back up the fire apparatus into the dock provided.

During the alley dock exercise, a street may be simulated by arranging marker cones 40 ft (12 m) from a boundary line. The marker cones should mark off an area 12 ft (4 m) wide and 20 ft (6 m) long, indicating the "dock" the fire apparatus will back into. As part of the exercise, you will pass the marker cones with the dock on the left and then back up the fire apparatus, using a left turn into the dock. This exercise should then be completed with the dock on the right side of the fire apparatus. The minimum depth of the apparatus bay is determined by the length of the fire apparatus. During the entire alley dock exercise, the fire apparatus must remain within the marked boundary and move in a continuous motion, except when required to change direction of travel. A spotter is necessary for this exercise.

To perform the alley dock exercise, follow the steps in **SKILL DRILL 10-2**:

1. Position the rear of the fire apparatus past the dock's opening and at a 90-degree angle to the marker cones. (**STEP 1**)
2. Ensure that a spotter is correctly positioned behind the fire apparatus. (**STEP 2**)
3. Activate the emergency lights. (**STEP 3**)
4. Roll down the windows. (**STEP 4**)
5. Turn off any mounted stereo equipment. (**STEP 5**)
6. Disengage the parking brake, if set. (**STEP 6**)
7. Shift the transmission into reverse. (**STEP 7**)
8. Proceed in a reverse mode and turn the fire apparatus to align it with the objective. (**STEP 8**)
9. Continue backing the fire apparatus until it has reached the desired objective or the spotter signals "stop." (**STEP 9**)

Special Emergency Scene Positioning

Although these incidents occur with less frequency than others, the need for proper scene positioning is always paramount. Special emergency scenes may include anything from a building collapse to a hazardous materials incident. During these incidents, fire fighters should be very cautious and resist the urge to rush into the scene and mitigate the situation. Usually, these incidents unfold slowly at first, until enough information has been gathered to determine the appropriate course of action.

When responding to these incidents and preparing to position the apparatus, the driver/operator must consider the

CHAPTER 10 Emergency Vehicle Driving   239

SKILL DRILL 10-2
Performing the Alley Dock Exercise
NFPA 1002, 4.3.1, 4.3.1(B), 4.3.6, 4.3.6(B)

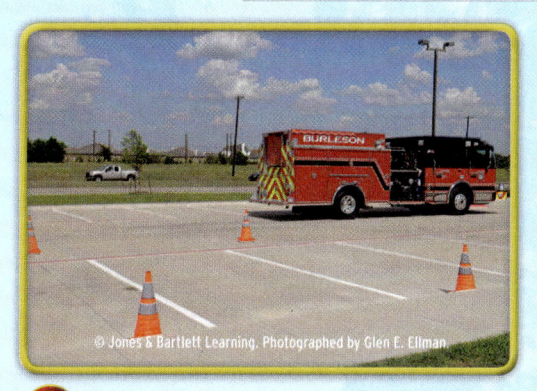

1 Position the rear of the fire apparatus past the dock's opening and at a 90-degree angle to the marker cones.

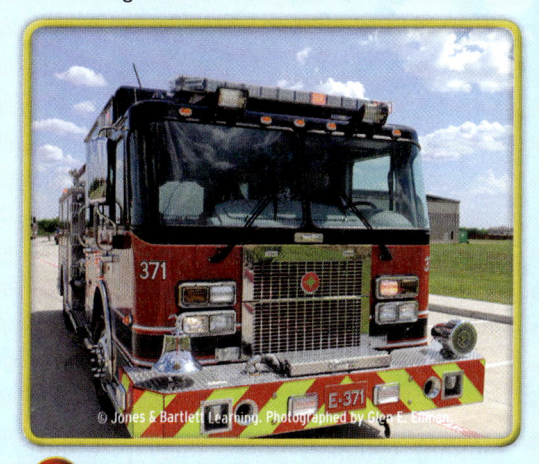

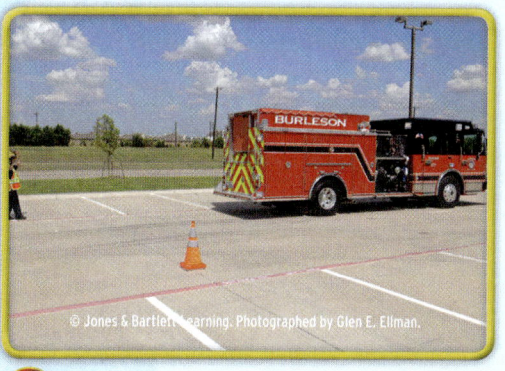

2 Ensure that a spotter is correctly positioned behind the fire apparatus.

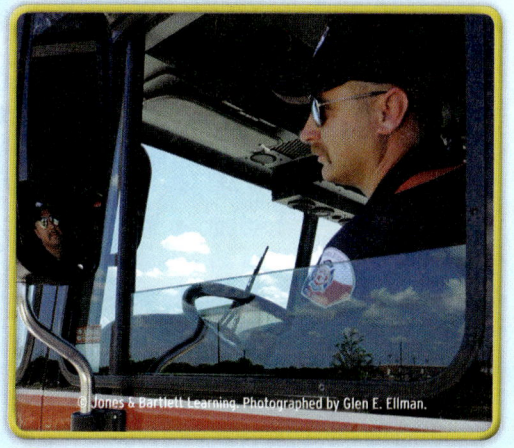

3 Activate the emergency lights.

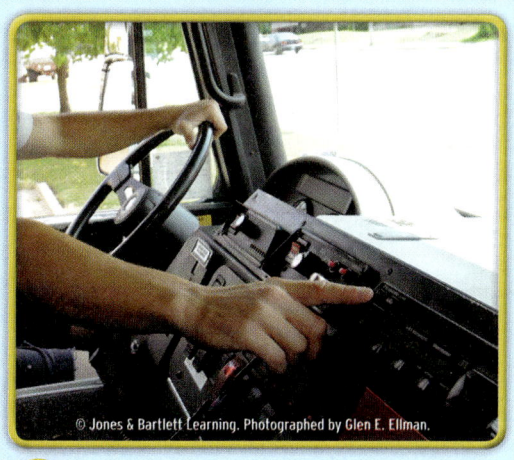

4 Roll down the windows.

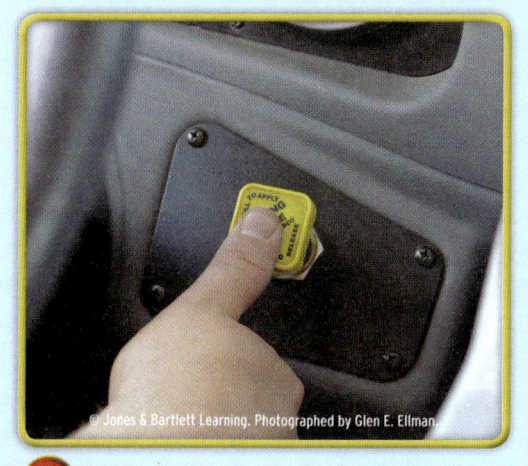

5 Turn off any mounted stereo equipment.

6 Disengage the parking brake, if set.

(Continues)

SKILL DRILL 10-2 Performing the Alley Dock Exercise (Continued)
NFPA 1002, 4.3.1, 4.3.1(B), 4.3.6, 4.3.6(B)

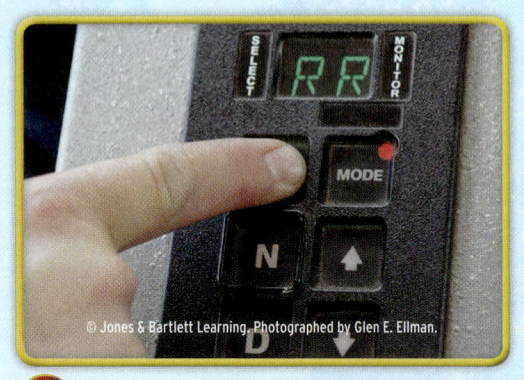

7 Shift the transmission into reverse.

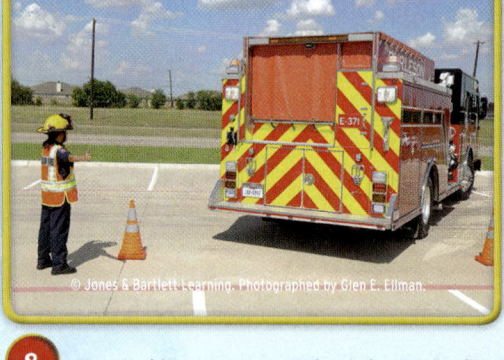

8 Proceed in a reverse mode and turn the fire apparatus to align it with the objective.

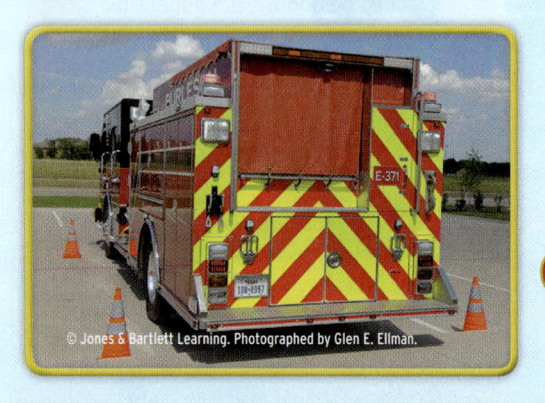

9 Continue backing the fire apparatus until it has reached the desired objective or the spotter signals "stop."

control zones. These areas at an incident—which are labeled "hot," "warm," or "cold" based on the severity of the incident—surround the incident:

- **Hot zone.** The area for entry teams and rescue teams only. This zone immediately surrounds the dangers of the site (e.g., hazardous materials release) and is demarcated to protect personnel outside the zone.
- **Warm zone.** The area for properly trained and equipped personnel only. This zone is where personnel and equipment decontamination and hot zone support take place.
- **Cold zone.** The area for staging vehicles and equipment until requested by the IC. The command post is located in this zone. The public and the media should be kept clear of the cold zone at all times.

The following list identifies some ideas for proper apparatus positioning during these incidents:

- **Hazardous materials incident.** The first course of action at any hazardous materials incident is to isolate the area and prevent anyone from entering it. The first-arriving company may have to position its apparatus to block a highway to prevent anyone from entering the scene. The proper apparatus position for these incidents is uphill and upwind. The material should be identified; once the scene is deemed safe, and if needed, the apparatus may then be driven closer to the scene.
- **Building collapse.** During this type of incident, the primary danger to fire fighters and fire apparatus is secondary collapse. Position the apparatus out of the collapse zone. Heavy equipment such as bulldozers and cranes may be required for on-scene operations. Do not block this equipment from reaching the incident; always leave a path for its entrance and exit.
- **Trench collapse.** Once a trench fails, the probability of secondary collapse is quite high. For this reason, first-arriving units should be positioned no closer than 150 ft (45 m) to the trench. All other incoming nonessential apparatus should stage at least 200 ft (60 m) away from the trench. Only equipment that is needed for a rescue should be brought any closer than the first-arriving units.
- **Terrorism.** These types of incidents may present as an explosion, a building collapse, release of radioactive material, or any other potential hazard. Terrorist incidents have the potential to injure and kill large numbers of people. During a possible terrorist incident, fire fighters should position the apparatus based on the demands of the emergency. Be aware of the potential for future hazards and the possible need for rapid escape, but position the apparatus to best accomplish the tasks at hand.

Wrap-Up

Chief Concepts

- The communications center gives the dispatch to the responding fire apparatus.
- As the driver/operator, you must disseminate the dispatch information and identify which information will aid your crew in locating the emergency and responding to it.
- A variety of maps may be used to locate emergency incidents.
- No member of any fire department should be allowed to drive an emergency vehicle or fire apparatus until he or she has completed a training course approved by the fire department.
- Fire fighters should always be cautious. As the fire apparatus approaches the scene, the driver/operator should slow down, identify the correct address/location, and recognize any potential hazards.
- While approaching a fire scene, the driver/operator should attempt to view at least three sides of the structure.
- Operating at an emergency scene that is located either on or adjacent to a highway or an intersection is extremely dangerous.
- The first priority upon arrival at an EMS scene is to provide a protected environment for fire fighters to work in.
- When responding to a special emergency scene, the driver/operator must consider the control zones (areas at the incident that are labeled "hot," "warm," or "cold" based on the severity of the incident) that surround the incident.

Hot Terms

activity area The area of the incident scene where the work activity takes place; it may be stationary or may move as work progresses.

advance warning area The section of highway where drivers are informed about an upcoming situation ahead.

aerial device An aerial ladder, elevating platform, aerial ladder platform, or water tower that is designed to position personnel, handle materials, provide continuous egress, or discharge water.

ambulance A vehicle designed, equipped, and operated for the treatment and transport of ill and injured persons.

auxiliary appliance A standpipe and/or sprinkler system.

brake fade Reduction in stopping power that can occur after repeated application of the brakes, especially in high-load or high-speed conditions.

braking distance The distance that the fire apparatus travels from the time the brakes are activated until the fire apparatus makes a complete stop.

buffer space The lateral and/or longitudinal area that separates traffic flow from a work space or an unsafe area; it might also provide some recovery space for an errant vehicle.

centrifugal force The outward force that is exerted away from the center of rotation. Also, the tendency for objects to be pulled outward when rotating around a center.

Code 1 response Response in a fire apparatus in which no emergency lights or sirens are activated.

Code 2 response Response in a fire apparatus in which only the emergency lights are activated; no audible devices are activated.

Code 3 response Response in a fire apparatus in which both the emergency lights and the sirens are activated.

collapse zone An area encompassing a distance of 1½ times the height of a building. Fire fighters and fire apparatus must not be located in this area in case of a building collapse.

command vehicle A vehicle that the fire chief uses to respond to the fire scene.

communications center A building or portion of a building that is specifically configured for the primary purpose of providing emergency communications services or public safety answering point (PSAP) services to one or more public safety agencies under the authority or authorities having jurisdiction.

control zones A series of areas at hazardous materials incidents that are designated based on safety concerns and the degree of hazard present.

corner safe areas Areas outside a building where two walls intersect; these areas are less likely to receive any damage during a building collapse.

critical speed Maximum speed that a fire apparatus can safely travel around a curve.

dispatch To send out emergency response resources promptly to an address or incident location for a specific purpose.

emitter A device that emits a visible flashing light at a specified frequency, thereby activating the receiver on a traffic signal.

global positioning system (GPS) A satellite-based radio navigation system consisting of three segments: space, control, and user.

incident space The area where the actual incident is located.

intermediate traffic incident A traffic incident that affects the lanes of travel for 30 minutes to 2 hours.

Wrap-Up, continued

Level I staging Initial staging of fire apparatus in which three or more units are dispatched to an emergency incident.

Level II staging Placement of all reserve resources in a central location until requested to the scene.

liquid surge The force imposed upon a fire apparatus by the contents of a partially filled water or foam concentrate tank when the vehicle is accelerated, decelerated, or turned.

major traffic incident A traffic incident that involves a fatal crash, a multiple-vehicle incident, a hazardous materials incident on the highway, or other disaster.

minor traffic incident A traffic incident that involves a minor crash and/or disabled vehicles.

mobile data terminal (MDT) A computer that is located on the fire apparatus.

motor vehicle accident (MVA) An incident that involves one vehicle colliding with another vehicle or another object and that may result in injury, property damage, and possibly death.

parking brake The main brake that prevents a fire apparatus from moving even when it is turned off and there is no one operating it.

preincident plan A document developed by gathering general and detailed data, which are then used by responding personnel to determine the resources and actions necessary to mitigate anticipated emergencies at a specific facility.

reaction distance The distance that the fire apparatus travels after the driver/operator recognizes the hazard, removes his or her foot from the accelerator, and applies the brakes.

receiver A device placed on or near a traffic signal to recognize a signal from the emitter on an emergency vehicle and preempt the normal cycle of the traffic light.

staging A specific function whereby resources are assembled in an area at or near the incident scene to await instructions or assignments.

staging area A prearranged, strategically placed area, where support response personnel, vehicles, and other equipment can be held in an organized state of readiness for use during an emergency.

staging area manager The person responsible for maintaining the operations of the staging area.

termination area The area where the normal flow of traffic resumes after a traffic incident.

total stopping distance The distance that it takes for the driver/operator to recognize a hazard, process the need to stop the fire apparatus, apply the brakes, and then come to a complete stop.

traffic control The direction or management of vehicle traffic such that scene safety is maintained and rescue operations can proceed without interruption.

traffic incident A natural disaster or other unplanned event that affects or impedes the normal flow of traffic.

traffic incident management area (TIMA) An area of highway where temporary traffic controls are imposed by authorized officials in response to an accident, natural disaster, hazardous materials spill, or other unplanned incident.

traffic signal preemption system A system that allows the normal operation of a traffic signal to be changed so as to assist emergency vehicles in responding to an emergency.

traffic space The portion of the highway where traffic is routed through the activity area of a traffic incident.

transition area The area where vehicles are redirected from their normal path and where lane changes and closures are made in a traffic incident.

References

Dunn, V. *Safety and Survival on the Fireground*. Tulsa, OK: Pennwell Books; 1992.

National Fire Protection Association (NFPA) 1002, *Standard for Fire Apparatus Driver/Operator Professional Qualifications*. 2014. http://www.nfpa.org/codes-and-standards/document-information-pages?mode=code&code=1002. Accessed March 27, 2014.

National Fire Protection Association (NFPA) 1561, *Standard on Emergency Services Incident Management System*. 2014. http://www.nfpa.org/codes-and-standards/document-information-pages?mode=code&code=1561. Accessed April 30, 2014.

National Fire Protection Association (NFPA) 1620, *Recommended Practice for Preincident Planning*. 2010. http://www.nfpa.org/codes-and-standards/document-information-pages?mode=code&code=1620. Accessed April 30, 2014.

National Fire Protection Association (NFPA) 1901, *Standard for Automotive Fire Apparatus*. 2009. http://www.nfpa.org/codes-and-standards/document-information-pages?mode=code&code=1901. Accessed April 9, 2014.

U.S. Department of Transportation, Federal Highway Administration. *Manual on Uniform Traffic Control Devices for Streets and Highways (MUTCD)*. U.S. Department of Transportation; 2009.

U.S. Fire Administration, Federal Emergency Management Agency (FEMA). *Firefighter Fatalities in the United States in 2012*. August 2013. https://www.usfa.fema.gov/downloads/pdf/publications/ff_fat12.pdf. Accessed August 5, 2014.

DRIVER/OPERATOR
in action

During the emergency response, you concentrate on getting the other members of the crew to the scene quickly and safely. While the officer and pipeman are thinking of the tasks they may be assigned, you must stay focused on the road and drive in a defensive manner. As you approach the scene, the Incident Commander assigns your engine company to assist with exposure protection at the rear of the building. Now that you are on scene, it is up to you to assist the other members of the crew and ensure that they have the tools and equipment necessary to perform their job.

1. What is a Code 3 response?
   A. Responding to an emergency without lights and sirens
   B. Responding to a nonemergency with lights and sirens
   C. Responding to an emergency with lights and sirens
   D. Responding to an emergency with lights but not sirens

2. The movement of liquid inside a container as the container is moved is called _____.
   A. Pressure
   B. Centrifugal force
   C. Liquid surge
   D. Critical speed

3. If the apparatus begins to skid, you should do all of the following *except* _____.
   A. Stay off the brake
   B. Steer
   C. Continue to steer
   D. Engage the parking brake

4. At the scene of a trench collapse, the first-arriving apparatus should be positioned no closer than ___ feet (meters) from the trench.
   A. 50 (15)
   B. 75 (25)
   C. 100 (30)
   D. 150 (45)

5. Which traffic safety vest is required for fire department personnel?
   A. Class 1
   B. Class 2
   C. Class 3
   D. Class 4

Fireground Operations

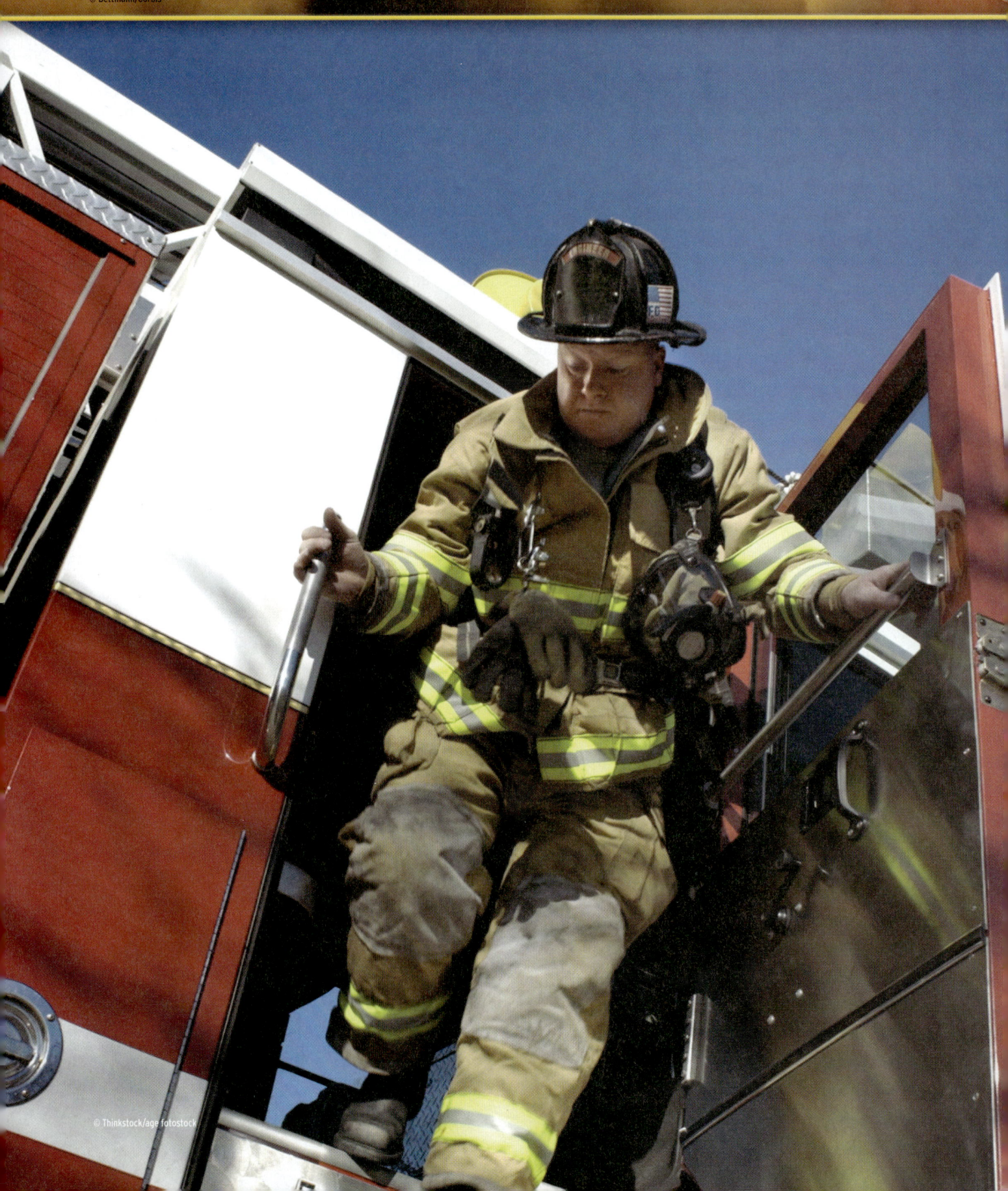

CHAPTER 11

Knowledge Objectives

After studying this chapter, you will be able to:

- Describe securing a water source after arriving on scene. (NFPA 1002, 4.3.7, 4.3.7(A), 5.2.1(1), 5.2.1(2), 5.2.1(3), 5.2.1(4), 5.2.1(A)); p 246–247, 253–254)
- Describe the driver/operator's responsibility with proper hose layouts. (NFPA 1002, 4.3.7, 4.3.7(A), 5.2.1(1), 5.2.1(2), 5.2.1(3), 5.2.1(4), 5.2.1(A)); p 246, 254–255, 257)
- Describe cab procedures when positioning the fire apparatus at the fireground. (NFPA 1002, 4.3.7, 4.3.7(A), 5.2.1(1), 5.2.1(2), 5.2.1(3), 5.2.1(4), 5.2.1(A)); p 246–248)
- Describe the driver/operator's responsibilities prior to exiting the cab of the fire apparatus. (NFPA 1002, 4.3.7, 4.3.7(A), 5.2.1(1), 5.2.1(2), 5.2.1(3), 5.2.1(4), 5.2.1(A)); p 246–248)
- Describe the driver/operator's responsibilities after exiting the fire apparatus. (NFPA 1002, 4.3.7, 4.3.7(A), 5.2.1(1), 5.2.1(2), 5.2.1(3), 5.2.1(4), 5.2.1(A)); p 248–250)
- Describe the driver/operator's responsibility to make connections to a fire department sprinkler and/or standpipe connection. (NFPA 1002, 4.3.7, 4.3.7(A), 5.2.1(1), 5.2.1(2), 5.2.1(3), 5.2.1(4), 5.2.1(A)); p 255, 257–260)
- Describe the driver/operator's role in troubleshooting problems on scene with the fire apparatus or its equipment. (NFPA 1002, 4.3.7, 4.3.7(A), 5.2.1(1), 5.2.1(2), 5.2.1(3), 5.2.1(4), 5.2.1(A)); p 261, 263–264)
- Describe the driver/operator's role in the safe operation of the pump. (NFPA 1002, 4.3.7, 4.3.7(A), 5.2.1(1), 5.2.1(2), 5.2.1(3), 5.2.1(4), 5.2.1(A)); p 260–264)
- Describe the various types of apparatus-mounted equipment found on different fire apparatus. (NFPA 1002, 4.3.7, 4.3.7(A), 5.2.1(1), 5.2.1(2), 5.2.1(3), 5.2.1(4), 5.2.1(A)); p 264–266, 269–272)

Skills Objectives

After studying this chapter, you will be able to:

- Engage the fire pump. (NFPA 1002, 4.3.7, 4.3.7(B), 5.2.1(1), 5.2.1(2), 5.2.1(3), 5.2.1(4), 5.2.1(B)); p 247–250)
- Hand-lay a supply line. (NFPA 1002, 4.3.7, 4.3.7(B), 5.2.1(1), 5.2.1(2), 5.2.1(3), 5.2.1(4), 5.2.1(B)); p 254–255, 257)
- Connect a hose to a fire department connection (FDC). (NFPA 1002, 4.3.7, 4.3.7(B), 5.2.1(1), 5.2.1(2), 5.2.1(3), 5.2.1(4), 5.2.1(B)); p 255, 257–260)
- Perform a changeover operation. (NFPA 1002, 4.3.7, 4.3.7(B), 5.2.1(1), 5.2.1(2), 5.2.1(3), 5.2.1(4), 5.2.1(B)); p 260–262)
- Operate an auxiliary cooling system. (NFPA 1002, 4.3.7, 4.3.7(B), 5.2.1(1), 5.2.1(2), 5.2.1(3), 5.2.1(4), 5.2.1(B)); p 263)
- Disengage the fire pump. (NFPA 1002, 4.3.7, 4.3.7(B), 5.2.1(1), 5.2.1(2), 5.2.1(3), 5.2.1(4), 5.2.1(B)); p 263–264)
- Demonstrate the procedure for operating a PTO-driven generator. (NFPA 1002, 4.3.7, 4.3.7(B), 5.2.1(1), 5.2.1(2), 5.2.1(3), 5.2.1(4), 5.2.1(B)); p 265–268)
- Demonstrate the procedure for operating a PTO-driven hydraulic system. (NFPA 1002, 4.3.7, 4.3.7(B), 5.2.1(1), 5.2.1(2), 5.2.1(3), 5.2.1(4), 5.2.1(B)); p 271–274)

Additional NFPA Standards

- NFPA 1901, *Standard for Automotive Fire Apparatus*
- NFPA 1936, *Powered Rescue Tools*

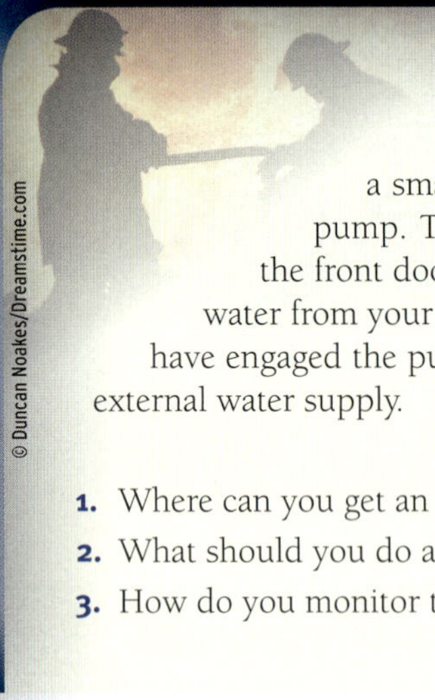

You Are the Driver/Operator

At 2:00 a.m., you wake up to the tones going off in the station. The incident is a structure fire in your district, and you know exactly where it is. As you pull the apparatus around the corner at the scene, you see a single-story residential structure with fire blasting out of a small bedroom window. After passing the building, you stop the apparatus and begin to engage the fire pump. The fire fighters pull the 1¾-inch (45-mm) preconnected attack hose off the engine and stretch it to the front door. After exiting the cab, setting the wheel chocks, and engaging the pump panel, you hear the call for water from your company officer. The hose moves slightly as you charge it, and the fire fighters begin their attack. You have engaged the pump and supplied the attack line with water, but you will soon run out of water unless you secure an external water supply.

1. Where can you get an external water supply?
2. What should you do after the water supply is established?
3. How do you monitor the pump operations?

Introduction

All fire apparatus are operated in two basic ways: in driving operations and in on-scene operations. The focus of this chapter is the on-scene operations in which the driver/operator will play a role at the scene of an emergency. This includes operating the fire pump and other fixed systems and equipment that are mounted to the fire apparatus.

While operating the fire pump, the driver/operator is responsible for producing effective handline and/or master streams, engaging all pressure control and safety devices, setting the rated flow for the fire attack operation, and continuously monitoring the apparatus for potential problems. When operating other fixed systems and equipment, the driver/operator must follow the manufacturer's instructions and department policies and procedures. These fixed systems may include any apparatus-mounted equipment.

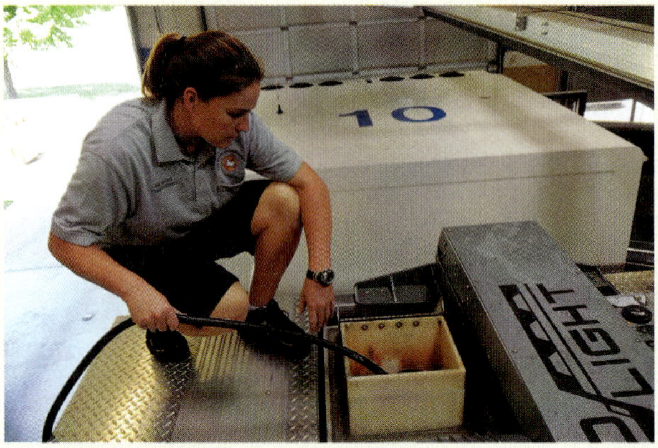

FIGURE 11-1 An internal water tank.

Fire Pump Operations

As the driver/operator, securing a water source upon arrival on scene is one of your primary responsibilities. While on the fireground, you will operate the fire pump from one of three different water sources:

1. **Internal water tank:** This includes the water in the apparatus-mounted water tank. This supply has a limited amount of water and must be supplemented by another source of water before it runs out **FIGURE 11-1**.
2. **Pressurized source:** This includes water from a hydrant or another fire pump. Both will supply water under pressure. The most common pressurized source is the hydrant **FIGURE 11-2**.
3. **Static source:** This includes water sources such as a lake, stream, pool, or water tank. This water must be drawn into the fire pump using hard suction hose. This operation will be covered in the chapter *Drafting and Water Shuttle Operations* **FIGURE 11-3**.

The driver/operator must also be capable of transferring water from an internal water tank supply to an external source, a practice referred to as a **changeover operation**.

In-Cab Procedures

When approaching the scene, you as the driver/operator should position the fire apparatus according to your fire department's policies and procedures and turn the front wheels toward the curb on a 45-degree angle **FIGURE 11-4**. If the fire apparatus should then happen to move for any reason, it will travel in the direction of the curb and stop, making the scene a little safer for all involved. If no curb is present, you should still position the wheels in this manner so that the fire apparatus is not pushed straight ahead or into the other side of the street.

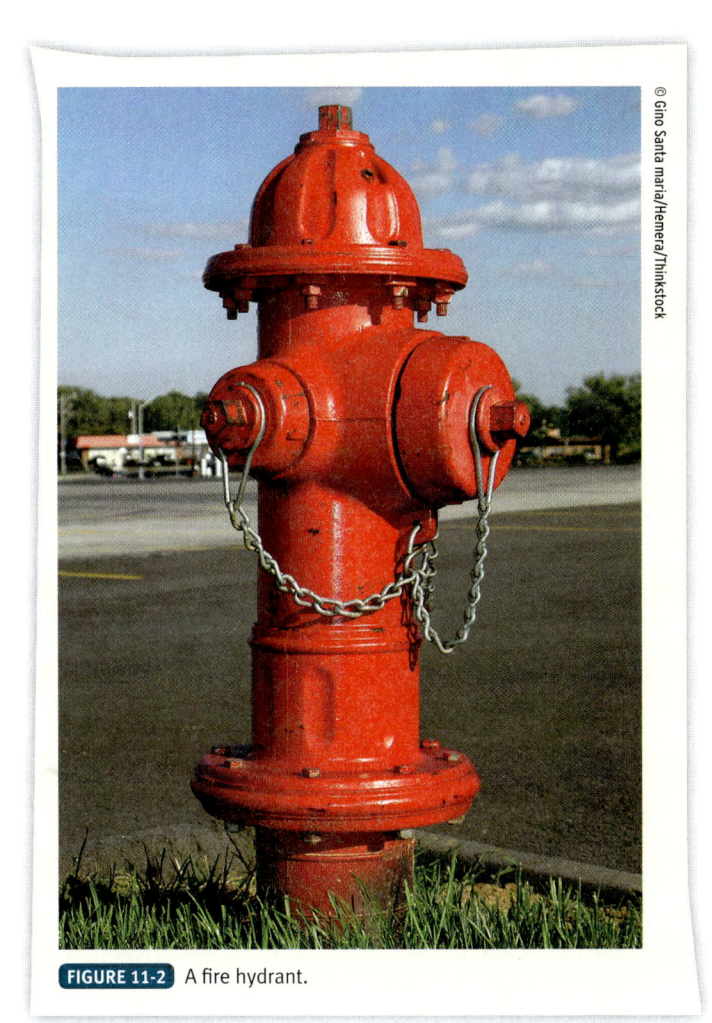

© Gino Santa maria/Hemera/Thinkstock

FIGURE 11-2 A fire hydrant.

DRIVER/OPERATOR Tip

Many department-specific positioning procedures have been developed, such as those dealing with aerial versus engine positioning, the three-sided approach, and avoidance of obstructing aerial devices or other specialized pieces of equipment.

Courtesy of Tom Fields, Douglas Forest Protective Association

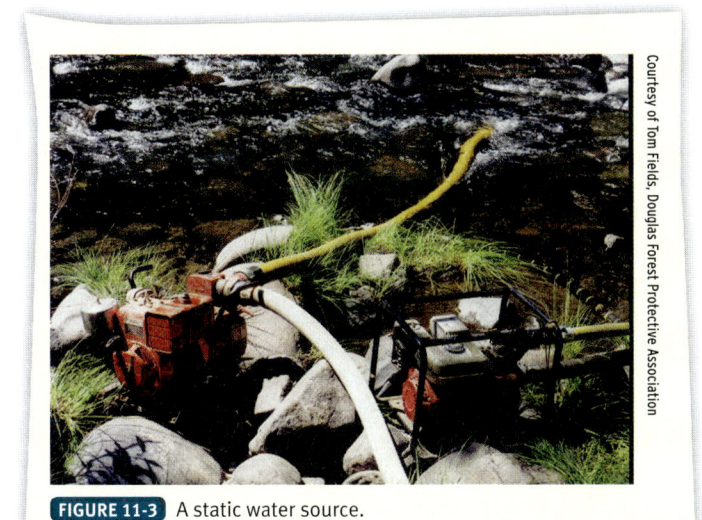

FIGURE 11-3 A static water source.

© Jones & Bartlett Learning. Photographed by Glen E. Ellman.

FIGURE 11-4 Position the wheels of the apparatus at a 45-degree angle toward the curb to prevent the apparatus from moving if the parking brake fails.

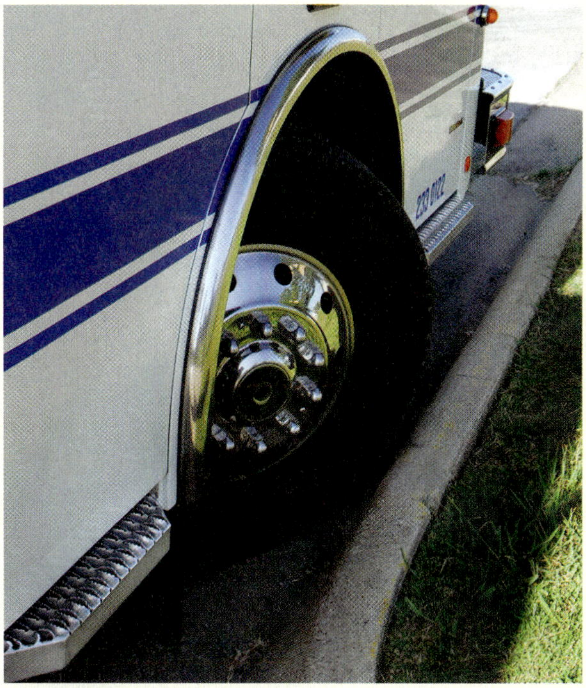

At this point, all unnecessary emergency lighting, such as headlights, should be turned off except what is needed for the protection of personnel working in and around the fire apparatus on scene. For example, if you are the driver/operator of an engine on scene and your fire apparatus is surrounded at both the front and the back by other fire apparatus, it is probably safe to turn off the light bar and leave on the hazard lights.

Leaving all of the emergency lighting on can drain the electrical system of the fire apparatus. Newer fire apparatus have features that automatically change emergency response lighting to "on scene" modes; this is a feature that you would use when operating at the scene of the emergency. On older fire apparatus, you must explicitly choose which emergency lights remain illuminated.

DRIVER/OPERATOR Tip

Radios play an important role in communications on the fireground. Most fire apparatus have radio communications equipment both inside the cab and outside the vehicle near the pump panel. If the fire apparatus is equipped with both types of devices, it may be necessary to transfer the radio communications headset from the cab to the outside radio.

Once you have arrived on scene but before you exit the cab of the fire apparatus, there are several steps that you need to complete. Exiting the cab prematurely can waste valuable time and cause you to overlook an important function in the cab. For example, if the pump is not properly engaged before you exit, you may spend time trying to troubleshoot the problem

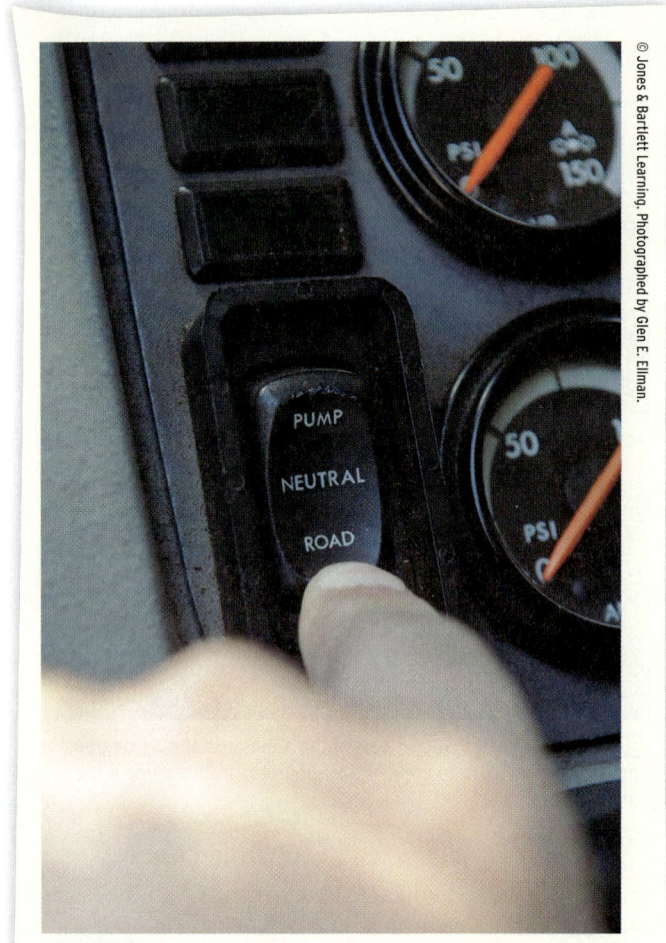

FIGURE 11-5 The pump shift control switch transfers the engine's power from the "road" position to the "pump" position.

at the pump panel instead of getting water to the attack lines. When you are content with placement of the fire apparatus, the first procedure that you must perform is placing the transmission into neutral or park, based on the fire apparatus. Next, apply the parking brake. Failure to apply the parking brake on today's modern fire apparatus will not only cause an unsafe situation, but will also prevent the pump's throttle from working—thus rendering the pump inoperable.

The next step to be completed prior to exiting the cab is to change the fire apparatus' transmission from the "road" position to the "pump" position. In doing so, you are basically transferring the motor's power from the drivetrain to the pump, which allows the pump to operate. A pump shift control switch can be found inside the cab **FIGURE 11-5**; it may be electronic, mechanical, or pneumatic. Place your foot on the brake, and move the pump switch from the "road" position to the "pump" position. It is important to pause in the neutral position between the road and pump positions, as this allows the fork in the transfer case to correctly move from the road to pump position. If the transfer is made too quickly, the fork may not have had enough time to move over correctly. Look for the "Pump engaged" indicator light to ensure that this switch has actually taken place. Next, place the apparatus transmission into drive, which allows the motor to power the pump instead of the drivetrain of the fire apparatus. Upon proper engagement of the pump, a light near the pump shift control switch or in the cab will become illuminated, indicating that the pump is engaged with the transmission and ready to pump. In conjunction with this "Okay to pump" light, you should hear the revolutions per minute (rpm) of the fire apparatus, increase slightly and, depending on the apparatus, you may see a reading of 10 to 15 mph (16 to 24 km/h) on the speedometer. Not all apparatus will show a speed increase on the speedometer however, as some speedometers are disabled when the apparatus is in pump. For push-button transmission selectors, check the transmission selector display to verify that the transmission is in the correct gear (1:1 which is 4th gear) and that the apparatus is in fact in pump (seeing "5" on the selector would indicate that the shift from road to pump did not occur and the apparatus is still in drive). These changes signal that the transmission is now spinning the impeller of the pump.

DRIVER/OPERATOR Tip

If the fire apparatus does not go into the "pump" position after you complete the correct procedures, reverse the procedure to take the fire apparatus out of "pump" mode and try again.

■ Exiting the Cab

Once the pump is engaged, your first task upon exiting the cab of the fire apparatus is to chock the wheels of the fire apparatus. Follow your department's standard operating procedure/guideline (SOP/SOG) as well as the manufacturer's recommendations regarding which wheels are to be chocked. Usually, two wheel chocks are placed against the rear driver's-side tires. This step is necessary in case the fire apparatus moves during the incident—it will be stopped by the wheel's chocks.

Safety Tip

Always place wheel chocks to prevent the fire apparatus from rolling when pumping.

Next, you need to circulate water into the pump. Walk to the pump panel on the fire apparatus and open the "tank to pump" valve. This valve allows water to flow from the onboard tank into the pump. Depending on the manufacturer of the fire apparatus, the label for this valve may use different terminology—for example, "Water" or "Tank to Pump." Becoming familiar with the layout of the pump panel and knowing how the valves operate will greatly enhance your efficiency in operating the pump.

At this point, water is flowing into the pump, but you need to remove any air inside the centrifugal pump for it to operate properly. This small positive-displacement pump draws air and water from the top of the centrifugal pump. Remember, a centrifugal pump can pump only fluids—not air.

Once the pump is primed (no air inside the pump), open the "tank refill" valve. This valve allows water to flow from the pump back into the onboard tank; it is basically a small discharge that directs water only back inside the onboard water tank. The label for this valve may carry any of several names, such as "Recirculation Valve" or "Tank Refill." By completing this procedure, you ensure that water flows from the onboard tank into the pump, and then out from the pump back into the tank. This will help to keep the pump from overheating.

The steps for engaging the fire pump with an automatic transmission are summarized in **SKILL DRILL 11-1**:

1. Shift the transmission into neutral. (**STEP 1**)
2. Set the parking brake. (**STEP 2**)
3. Operate the pump shift control switch.
4. Ensure that the "Pump engaged" light is on. (**STEP 3**)
5. Shift the transmission into the drive position. (**STEP 4**)
6. Identify indicators of pump engagement inside the cab; the "Okay to pump" light should be on, and if you get a speedometer reading, it should be 10–15 mph (16–24 km/h). (**STEP 5**)
7. Exit the cab. (**STEP 6**)
8. Chock the wheels of the apparatus. (**STEP 7**)
9. Open the tank-to-pump valve to allow water to enter the pump. (**STEP 8**)
10. Operate the priming pump to ensure all of the air is out of the pump. (**STEP 9**)
11. Open the tank fill valve to recirculate water until attack lines are ready to be supplied.
12. Charge the attack lines. (**STEP 10**)

DRIVER/OPERATOR Tip

The decision of whether to prime the pump depends on whether your department has a policy to leave its pumps wet or dry. If the pump is always wet, it is probably not necessary to prime the pump, although doing so would not hurt. However, if your department always leaves its pumps dry, there will be air inside that should be pulled out with the primer pump. Each department sets its own policy governing this issue.

DRIVER/OPERATOR Tip

Prior to opening the first discharge valve and charging the attack line, remember to close the tank fill valve. Failure to do so will cause the pump to treat the tank fill as a discharge, causing your pump discharge pressure settings to be incorrect.

Internal Water Tank

Once the fire pump is engaged, the driver/operator is ready to supply the attack lines for firefighting operations using the internal water tank as a water supply. This approach has the advantage of providing for a quick deployment of water but is limited by the amount of water carried on the apparatus. Usually, the internal water tank is used only to fight small fires, such as vehicle fires, dumpster fires, small brush fires, and other nuisance fires and also to start the initial fire attack until a large water source can be obtained. If more water is necessary than the amount carried on the apparatus, then an external water supply from a pressurized water source or a static water source must be established.

Pressurized Sources

It is the driver/operator's responsibility to secure a water source upon arrival on the scene. Fire hose evolutions are critical in the driver/operator's success. Fire hose evolutions are standard methods of working with fire hose to accomplish different objectives in a variety of situations. Most fire departments set up their equipment and conduct regular training so that fire fighters will be prepared to perform a set of standard hose evolutions. As part of hose evolutions, specific actions are assigned to specific members of a crew, depending on their riding positions on the fire apparatus. Every fire fighter should know how to perform all of the standard evolutions quickly and proficiently; that is, when an officer calls for a particular evolution to be performed, each crew member should know exactly what to do.

As the driver/operator, you should know the pressures at which the lines need to be supplied and should ensure that the lines are properly flaked out before they are charged with water pressure. Consequently, you need to know not only how to deploy the hoselines, but also which size, length, and nozzle configurations are required. You will need all of this information to supply the attack lines with the correct water flow for fire extinguishment.

Hose evolutions are divided into supply line operations and attack line operations. Supply line operations involve laying hoselines and making connections between a water supply source and an attack pumper. Attack line operations involve advancing hoselines from an attack pumper to apply water onto the fire.

■ Supply Line Evolutions

The objective of laying a supply line is to deliver water from a hydrant or an alternative water source to an **attack pumper**. In most cases, this operation involves laying a hoseline with a moving vehicle or dropping a continuous line of hose out of a bed as the fire apparatus moves forward. It can be done using either a forward lay or a reverse lay. A **forward lay** starts at the hydrant and proceeds toward the fire; in this case, the hose is laid in the same direction as the water flows—from the hydrant to the fire. A **reverse lay** involves laying the hose from the fire to the hydrant; with this evolution, the hose is laid in the opposite direction to the water flow. Each fire department will determine its own preferred methods and procedures for supply line operations based on available apparatus, water supply, and regional considerations.

Forward Hose Lay

The forward hose lay is most often used by the first-arriving engine company at the scene of a fire **FIGURE 11-6**. While en route to the fire scene, the driver/operator stops the engine at a hydrant close to the fire scene. A fire fighter dismounts the fire apparatus and either wraps the hose around the hydrant or places a strap around it to secure the hose in place. When this step is complete, the fire fighter signals the driver/operator to continue on to the fire by stating, "Driver, go." You then proceed to the fire scene no faster than 15 mph (25 km/h). At the fire scene, you disconnect the supply line from the hose bed, connect it to the pump, and call for the supply line to be charged with water.

250 Fire Apparatus Driver/Operator

SKILL DRILL 11-1
Engaging the Fire Pump with an Automatic Transmission
NFPA 1002, 5.2.1, 5.2.1(B)

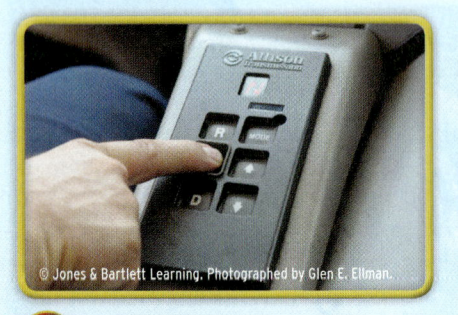

1. Shift the transmission into neutral.
2. Set the parking brake.
3. Operate the pump shift control switch. Ensure that the "Pump engaged" light is illuminated.
4. Shift the transmission into the drive position.
5. Identify indicators of pump engagement.
6. Exit the cab.
7. Chock the wheels of the apparatus.
8. Open the tank-to-pump valve to allow water to enter the pump.
9. Operate the priming pump to ensure all of the air is out of the pump.
10. Open the tank fill valve to recirculate water until attack lines are ready to be supplied. Charge the attack lines.

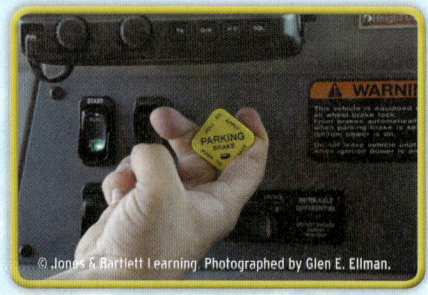

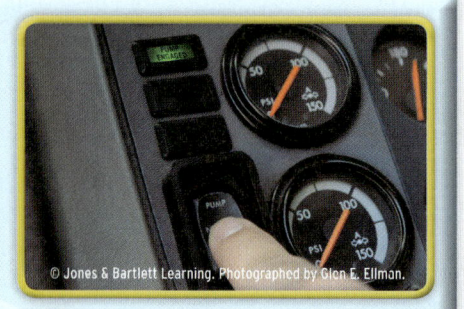

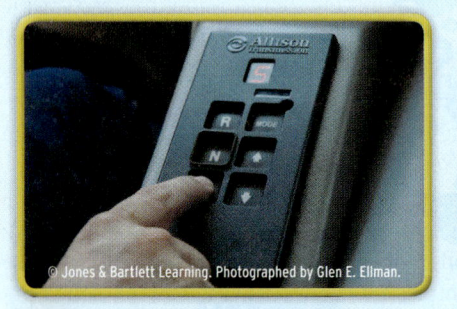

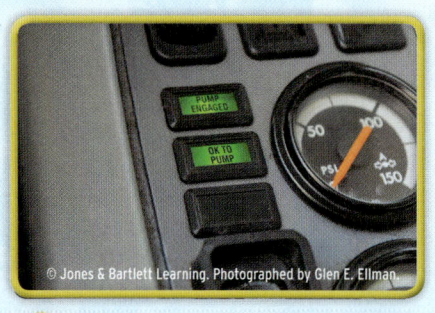

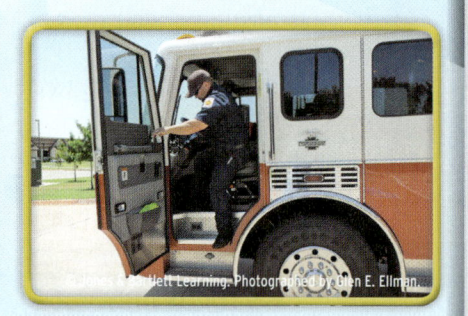

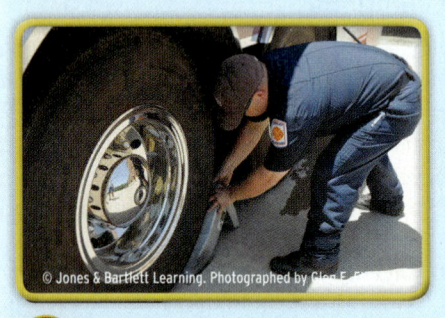

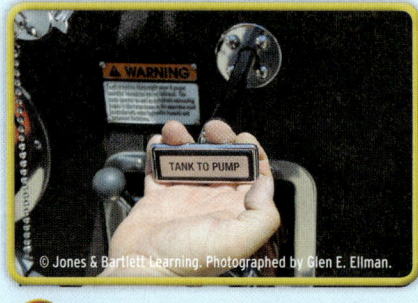

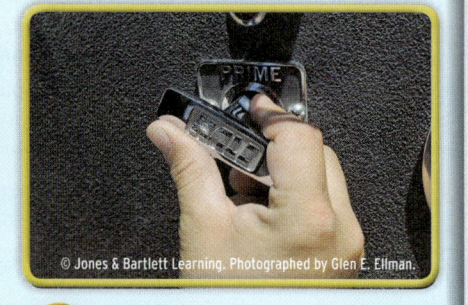

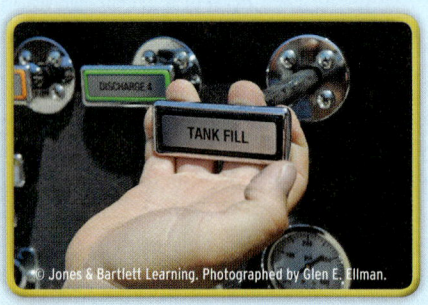

© LiquidLibrary

FIGURE 11-6 A forward hose lay is made from the hydrant to the fire.

FIGURE 11-7 The four-way valve.

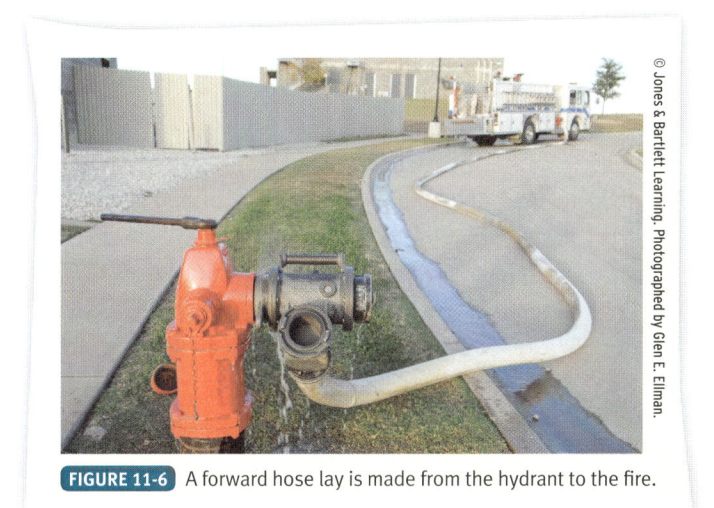

The forward hose lay allows the engine company to establish a water supply without assistance from an additional company. It also places the attack pumper close to the fire, allowing access to additional hose, tools, and equipment that are carried on the fire apparatus.

Safety Tip

When performing a forward lay, the fire fighter who is connecting the hose to the supply hydrant must not stand between the hose and the hydrant. When the fire apparatus starts to move away, the hose could become tangled and suddenly be pulled taut—and anyone standing between the hose and the hydrant could be seriously injured. As the driver/operator, you should not move the apparatus unless you are sure all fire fighters are clear of the fire apparatus and in a safe position. Keep your window rolled down so you can effectively communicate with the fire fighter pulling the hose.

A forward hose lay can be performed using medium-diameter hose (MDH; 2½ inch [65 mm] or 3 inch [77 mm]) or large-diameter hose (LDH; 3½ inch [90 mm] and larger). The larger the diameter of the hose, the more water that can be delivered to the attack pumper through a single supply line. When MDH is used and the beds are arranged to lay dual lines, a company can lay two parallel lines from the hydrant to the fire.

If the fire hydrant is close to the fire, it may supply a sufficient quantity of water to charge the lines (rather than using an interim supply engine to boost the flow). A 5-inch (125-mm) hose can supply 700 gpm (2800 L/min) over a distance of 500 ft (150 m) and lose only about 20–25 psi (140–175 kPa) of pressure due to friction loss.

Four-Way Hydrant Valve

In situations where long supply lines are needed or when MDH is used, it is often necessary to place a supply engine at the hydrant. This supply engine pumps water through the supply line so as to increase the flow to the attack pumper. Some departments use a **four-way hydrant valve** to connect the supply line to the hydrant, thereby ensuring that the supply line can be charged with water immediately, yet still allowing for a supply engine to connect to the line later.

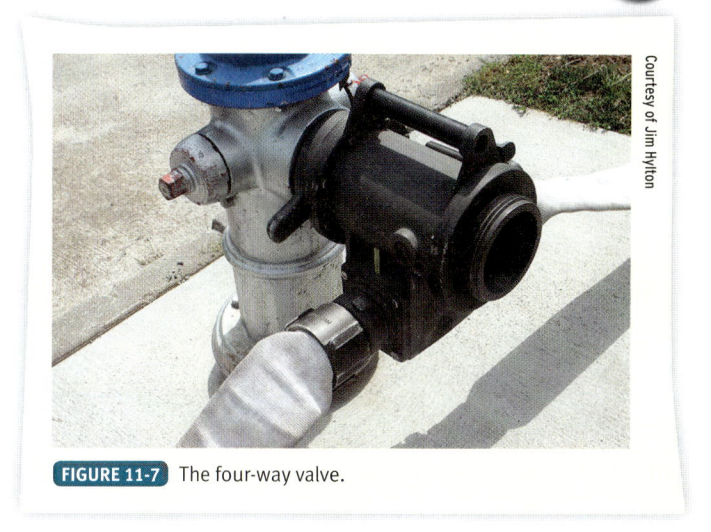

When a four-way valve is placed on the hydrant, the water flows initially from the hydrant through the valve to the supply line, which delivers the water to the attack pumper **FIGURE 11-7**. The second engine can then hook up to the four-way valve and redirect the flow by changing the position of the valve. At this point, the water flows from the hydrant to the supply engine. The supply engine can then increase the pressure and discharge the water into the supply line, boosting the flow of water to the attack pumper. This operation can be accomplished without uncoupling any lines or interrupting the flow.

Safety Tip

When the fire fighter is connecting a supply line to a hydrant, he or she should wait to get the appropriate signal from the driver/operator before attempting to charge the line. If the hydrant is opened prematurely, the hose bed could become charged with water or a loose hoseline could discharge water at the fire scene. Either situation will disrupt the firefighting operation and could cause serious injuries. Make sure that you know your department's signal to charge a hoseline, and do not become so excited or rushed that you make a mistake. Confirm that all of the hose connections are in place before calling for water from the hydrant.

Reverse Hose Lay

The reverse hose lay is the opposite of the forward lay **FIGURE 11-8**. In the reverse lay, the hose is laid out from the fire to the hydrant, in the direction opposite to the flow of the water. This evolution can be used when the attack pumper arrives at the fire scene without a supply line. It is also used to supply the attack pumper directly through the hydrant.

The reverse hose lay may be a standard tactic in areas where sufficient hydrants are available and additional companies that can assist in establishing a water supply will arrive quickly. In this scenario, one company is assigned to lay a supply line from the attack pumper to a hydrant. The first engine arrives on the scene of a fire and begins a fire attack. When the second engine arrives at the scene, it drops off the fire fighters and the fire officer. At this point, the second engine deploys its LDH supply

FIGURE 11-8 A reverse hose lay is made from the fire to a fire hydrant.

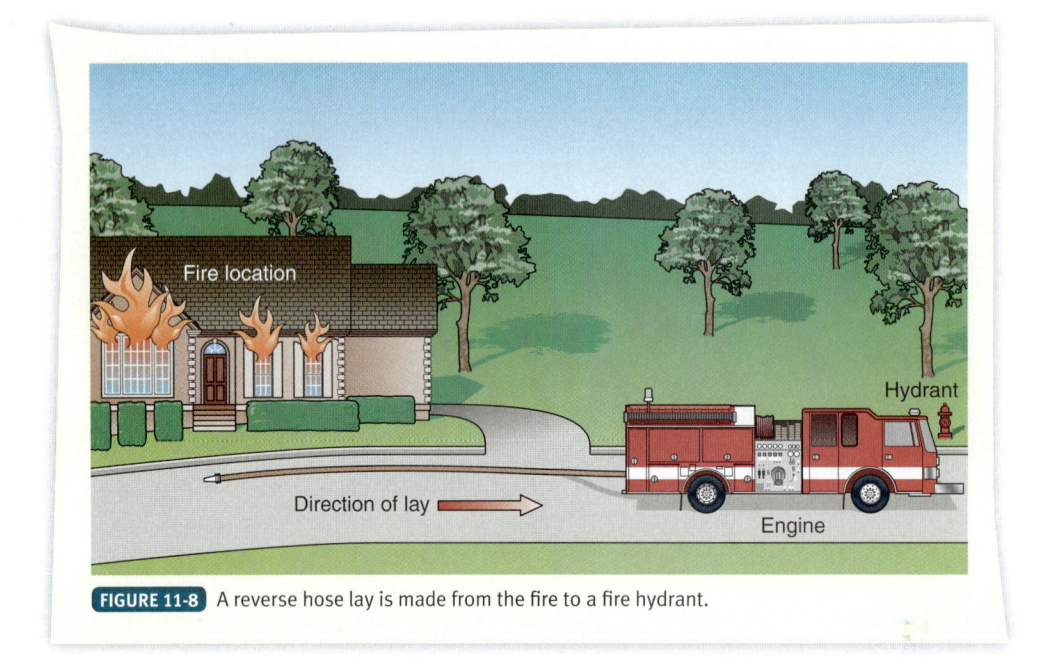

line to the first engine, where it is connected to that engine's intake. The second engine then proceeds to a water source, laying LDH as it drives no faster than 15 mph (25 km/h). When this apparatus arrives at the water source, the driver/operator of the second engine will be operating alone. He or she secures a water supply, connects the supply line to a LDH discharge, and pumps water to the first engine through the supply line. The attack pumper focuses on immediately attacking the fire using water from the onboard tank. The supply engine stops close to the attack pumper, and hose is pulled from the bed of the supply engine to an intake on the attack pumper. The supply engine then drives to the hydrant (or alternative water source) and pumps water back to the attack pumper. Usually the supply engine parks in such a way that hose can be pulled from the supply engine to the inlet to the attack pumper.

DRIVER/OPERATOR Tip

When laying out supply hose with threaded couplings, you may find that the wrong end of the hose is on top of the hose bed. Double-male connectors allow you to attach a female coupling to a female coupling. Whereas double-female connectors allow you to attach a male coupling to a male coupling. A set of adapters (one double-male and one double-female) should be easily accessible to help you manage these situations. In fact, some fire departments place a set of adapters on the end of the supply hose for precisely this purpose.

As the driver/operator, you should know the equipment carried on your fire apparatus as well as—if not better than—the rest of the crew. Think about potential situations that might require the use of the adapters before you have to use them on a fire scene. For example, if your fire apparatus is set up for a forward lay and it is used to deploy hose in a reverse lay at a fire, a double-male adapter will be needed at the nozzle and a double-female adapter will be needed at the pump discharge.

Split Hose Lay

A <u>split hose lay</u> (also called an alley lay) is performed by two engine companies in situations where hose must be laid in two different directions to establish a water supply **FIGURE 11-9**. This evolution could be used when the attack pumper must approach a fire either along a dead-end street with no hydrant or down a long driveway.

To perform a split hose lay, the attack pumper drops the end of its supply hose at the corner of the street and performs a forward lay toward the fire. Normally, the fire fighter would get out of the fire apparatus and secure the supply hose to the hydrant. In this case, however, there is no hydrant in the immediate area. Instead, the fire fighter has to secure the end of the supply line to a fixed object such as a street sign or tree to keep it from dragging behind the attack pumper as the apparatus drives away. When the supply engine gets to the intersection where the end of the attack pumper's supply hose is anchored, it will stop and pull off enough hose to connect to the end of this supply line, and then perform a reverse lay to the hydrant or water source. When the two lines are connected together, the supply engine can provide water to the attack pumper.

A split lay often requires coordination by two-way radio, because the attack pumper must advise the supply engine of the plan and indicate where the end of the supply line is being dropped and anchored. In many cases, the attack pumper is out of sight when the supply engine arrives at the split point.

A split hose lay does not necessarily require split hose beds. It can be performed with or without split beds if the necessary adapters are used.

■ Connecting a Fire Department Engine to a Water Supply

When an engine sets up at a hydrant, supply hose must be used to deliver the water from the hydrant to the engine. This special type of supply line is intended to deliver as much water as possible over a short distance. In most cases, a soft suction

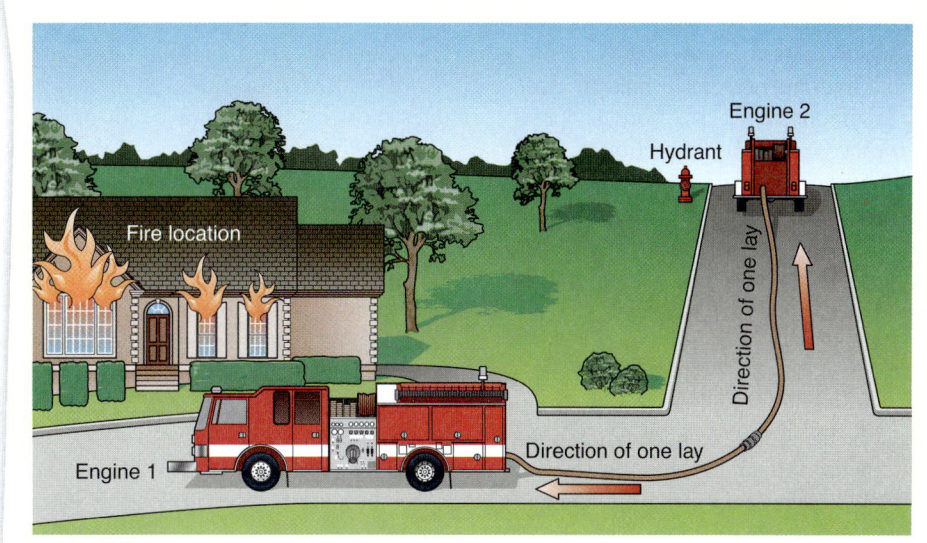

FIGURE 11-9 Engine 1 performs a forward hose lay from the corner to the fire. Engine 2 performs a reverse hose lay from the hose at the corner to a fire hydrant.

DRIVER/OPERATOR Tip

A **split hose bed** is a hose bed that is divided into two or more sections. This division is made for several purposes:

- One compartment in a split hose bed can be loaded for a forward lay (female coupling out), and the other side can be loaded for a reverse lay (male coupling out). This arrangement allows a line to be laid in either direction without the use of adapters.
- Two parallel hoselines can be laid at the same time (called "laying dual lines"). Dual lines are beneficial if the situation requires more water than one hoseline can supply.
- The split beds can be used to store hoses of different sizes. For example, one side of the hose bed could be loaded with 2$\frac{1}{2}$-inch (65-mm) hose that can be used as a supply line or as an attack line; the other side of the hose bed could be loaded with 5-inch (125-mm) hose for use as a supply line. This setup enables the use of the most appropriate-size hose for a given situation.
- All of the hose from both sides of the hose bed can be laid out as a single hoseline. This is done by coupling the end of the hose in one bed to the beginning of the hose in the other bed.

In a variation of the split hose bed known as a combination load, the last coupling in one bed is connected to the first coupling in the other bed. When one long line is needed, all of the hose plays out of one bed first, and then the hose continues to play out from the second bed. If the team needs to lay dual lines, they can uncouple the connection between the two hose beds, and the two hoselines can play out of both beds simultaneously. When the two sides of a split bed are loaded with the hose arranged in opposite directions, either a double-female or double-male adapter is used to make the connection between the two hose beds.

hose is used to connect directly to a hydrant. Alternatively, the connection can be made with a short length of large-diameter supply hose.

Securing a Water Source

As the driver/operator, securing a water source upon your crew's arrival on the scene is one of your primary responsibilities. Before you even leave the fire station to respond to the scene, you should have a working knowledge of water sources at or close to the scene. This can be accomplished by using a map book with hydrant locations in it and by being familiar with water sources within the response area, including lakes, ponds, canals, and drafting hydrants.

DRIVER/OPERATOR Tip

It is not wise to always rely on the fire officer to help you find or spot a hydrant while responding to the scene. Many times the fire officer may be focused on listening to or speaking on the radio, or obtaining information from the onboard computer. Securing a water source is the driver/operator's responsibility, whether that source is a hydrant, draft, or some other source.

Upon your arrival on scene, it is generally the fire officer's call whether you will lay a supply line to the incident. If the fire officer calls for a supply line, follow your fire department's SOP for laying this line. If your crew is the first engine company on scene, the fire officer may decide to forgo laying a supply line and proceed straight into the scene. This tactic is commonly used when the second-due engine is immediately behind the first-due engine. Use of this tactic should be communicated by the officers on both engines so that a water supply is secured regardless of the order in which units arrive on scene.

Sometimes an available hydrant may be located in close proximity to the building on fire. In such a case, you may position the fire apparatus so that you can use a section of hose to connect to the hydrant instead of performing a forward lay. In this kind of <u>hand lay</u>, you position the engine close to the fire scene and deploy the supply hose from the bed of the fire apparatus to the hydrant either yourself or with very little assistance from other fire fighters.

■ Hand Lays

If you find yourself having to create a hand lay to a hydrant, several considerations must be taken into account. First, what is the distance between the fire apparatus and the closest hydrant? Second, what is the best hose to make the connection? Third, how long will this step take to complete?

To determine how far away the closest hydrant is, either reference the map book in your fire apparatus or simply eyeball the estimated distance from your pump intake to the hydrant.

When determining the best hose to make the connection, you may or may not have several options for hose. Suppose the hydrant is approximately 15 ft (5 m) away. If you use LDH in your fire department, it is common practice to carry short lengths of LDH for the purpose of making a connection between the fire apparatus intake and the hydrant. These lengths of hose generally range from 15 ft (5 m) to 25 ft (8 m) and have names such as soft suction hose or pony lines **FIGURE 11-10**. It is important for you to know how long each line found on the fire apparatus is and how many of these lines the fire apparatus carries. This can be accomplished during your morning checkout of the fire apparatus by removing the hose and laying it out for inspection.

Some fire departments may carry reduced-length 3-inch (77-mm) or 2½-inch (65-mm) hose for refilling the onboard tank from a hydrant. Use caution when applying hoselines with these diameters as supply lines during fire operations: You may find that you need to pump more water than these lines can deliver.

If the hydrant is 60 ft (18 m) away, using the shorter LDH lines most likely will not be an option. In most cases, pulling hose from the hose bed is the next choice. If you carry LDH, it is most often available in 100-ft (30-m) lengths. You need to pull a full section from the hose bed and deploy it between the fire apparatus and the hydrant. While pulling it, keep in mind the direction in which you need to go; your goal is to minimize sharp turns and twists in the hose, thereby reducing kinks and severe bends that might reduce the flow. Also, watch out for any oncoming traffic while operating in the roadway. Always wear your traffic safety vest as required by your department.

When considering the third question—How long will this hand lay take to accomplish?—you must take into account several factors:

- The distance from the fire apparatus to the hydrant
- The choice of hose
- Any possible obstacles in the way to deploy the hose, such as vehicles, trees, and bushes

An additional consideration when obtaining a water source is the need to double-tap a hydrant. When connecting to a dry-barrel hydrant during a hose lay or connecting straight in to the hydrant, fire departments often use the largest (i.e., steamer) connection. This leaves two 2½-inch (65-mm) port connections unused. Once the hydrant is opened, however, these additional connections cannot be subsequently used, unless the hydrant is shut down—thereby cutting off the water supply, at least momentarily. The hydrant is capable of delivering additional water through these port connections. If you anticipate that additional water may be needed, place an appliance such as a gated ball valve on the dry-barrel hydrant prior to opening the hydrant. Then, if additional water is needed, a supply line can be connected from the valve to an intake on the fire apparatus **FIGURE 11-11**. Always follow your local SOP when obtaining a water supply.

FIGURE 11-10 Large-diameter hose generally range from 15 ft (5 m) to 25 ft (8 m) in length and have names such as soft suction hose or pony lines.

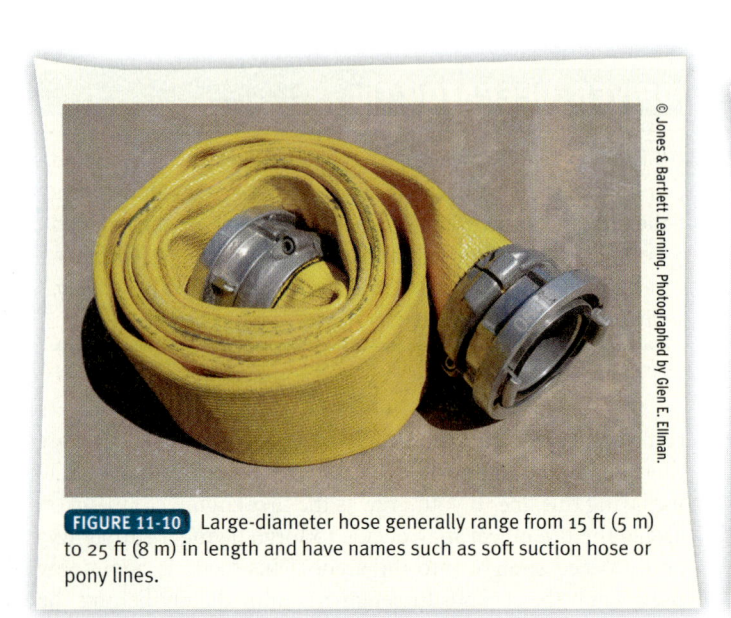

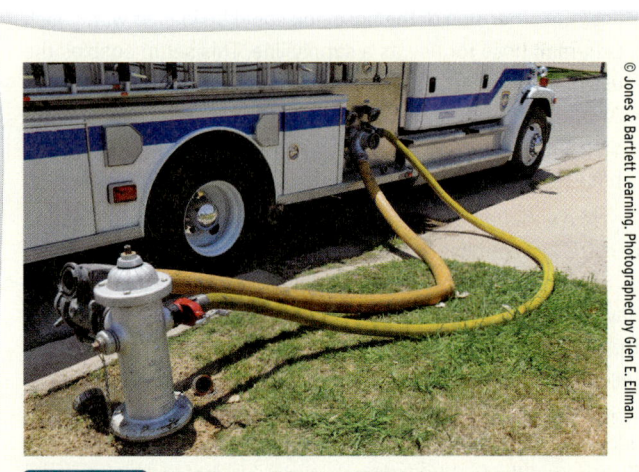

FIGURE 11-11 The more outlets that are used on a dry-barrel hydrant, the more water you will have available to attack the fire.

Only with practice, practice, practice will you build confidence and become more proficient in securing a water source. Follow the steps in **SKILL DRILL 11-2** to hand lay a supply line:

1. Position the fire apparatus for the intake to be used. (**STEP 1**)
2. Roll out or pull the supply line to the hydrant. (**STEP 2**)
3. Connect the supply hose to the hydrant, after properly flushing the hydrant. (**STEP 3**)
4. Connect the supply hose to the pump's intake. (**STEP 4**)
5. Check for any kinks in the supply line. (**STEP 5**)
6. Open the hydrant and charge the supply line. (**STEP 6**)

DRIVER/OPERATOR Tip

When using the soft suction hose for the connection, knowing the length of the hose and the positioning of the fire apparatus is important. If the fire apparatus is too close to the hydrant for the length of the hose used, kinks in the hose can occur, which will reduce the flow (gpm [L/min]) to the pump.

By positioning the fire apparatus a proper distance from the hydrant based on the length of hose used, it should be possible to avoid having kinks in the hose. Knowing the intake locations on the fire apparatus will give you options for the hookup. You should use caution when positioning the fire apparatus to ensure that you do not place the fire apparatus too far into the street. Doing so may make the road impassable for other vehicles—including additional fire apparatus. Understanding of the preferred positioning comes with practice by hooking up to the hydrant from all intakes on the fire apparatus, including the fire officer's side, front, and rear, if the apparatus is equipped to do so.

Deploying the hose in an "S shape" is the best approach, as it will both decrease the chance of blocking the road and minimize or eliminate any kinks in the hose. To do so, you should keep the fire apparatus close to the side of the street that the hydrant is on. This will allow other fire apparatus to drive past your vehicle and position themselves on the fire scene. The last thing the engine apparatus wants to do is to block the scene for any ladder company that needs access.

Stop the engine apparatus with either the front bumper in line with the hydrant or the rear bumper in line with the hydrant. Do not position the intake directly even with the hydrant. Doing so will cause severe kinks in the short section of hose that is used to make this connection. Once the front or rear bumper is lined up with the hydrant, the short section of supply hose is connected to the intake, and the line is charged, it will have an "S shape" to it; one end of the "S" is connected to the hydrant and the other end is connected to the pump's intake.

Standpipe/Sprinkler Connecting

■ Connecting Supply Hoselines to Standpipe and Sprinkler Systems

Another water supply evolution is furnishing water to standpipe and sprinkler systems. Fire department connections (FDCs) on buildings are provided so that the fire department

FIGURE 11-12 A standpipe connection.

can pump water into standpipe and/or sprinkler systems. This setup is considered to be a supply line because it supplies water to standpipe and sprinkler systems. Such a supply line is connected to the discharge side of the attack pumper. The function of the hoseline in this case is to provide either a primary or secondary water supply for the sprinkler or standpipe system. The same basic techniques are used to connect the hoselines to either type of system.

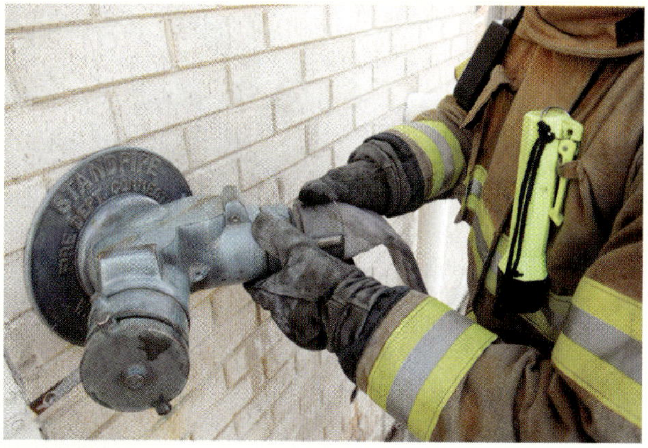

Standpipe systems are used to provide a water supply for attack lines that will be operated inside a building. Outlets are provided inside the building where fire fighters can connect attack lines. The fire fighters inside the building must then depend on fire fighters outside the building to supply the water to the FDC **FIGURE 11-12**.

Two general types of sprinkler systems exist:
- A dry standpipe system depends on the fire department to provide all of the water.
- A wet standpipe system has a built-in water supply, but the FDC is provided to deliver a higher flow or to boost the pressure.

The pressure requirements for standpipe systems depend on the height at which the water will be used inside the building. The fire department connection for a sprinkler system is also used to supplement the normal water supply. The required pressures and flows for different types of sprinkler systems can vary significantly. Unless more specific information is available, sprinkler systems should generally be fed at a pressure of 150 psi (1050 kPa).

Due to certain building characteristics within a response area as well as the height and construction materials used in the building, private fire protection systems may be present in a fire building. As a driver/operator, it is your responsibility to have a complete and thorough understanding of these systems. Preincident planning as well as familiarization with your response area will help you to identify those buildings that have sprinkler systems and standpipes. When performing this planning or during routine driving through your response area, you should be looking for the FDCs, hydrant locations, and sprinkler valves associated with the building **FIGURE 11-13**.

VOICES OF EXPERIENCE

While my company was operating on the scene of a fire in an abandoned structure, a request came in for a mutual aid response in an adjacent county. Additional fire units, including mine, were dispatched to the scene. As we responded to the scene, I could already see the fire from the other side of the river that separated the two counties.

Upon arrival, we found a 5000-ft² (465 m²) structure with 99 percent involvement. The only portion that was not yet on fire was the basement level and garage. The home was located in an affluent neighborhood and was at the edge of the county—the farthest point on the water system.

The initial volunteer department on the scene was working with 2½-inch (65-mm) hoselines on each side of the structure. To quickly suppress this fire, we needed more water. The first responding mutual aid engine laid 1000 ft (300 m) of large-diameter hoseline (LDH) in a reverse hose lay to prepare for an aerial operation. An aerial ladder was set up in front of the burning structure in an attempt to cover the burning building and to protect the exposures: two houses less than 50 ft (15 m) from the burning building.

As the crews began to fight the fire, we learned that the hydrant would not be able to supply enough water to support the aerial operations. We had responded to the mutual aid request with our mostly urban response units, which did not having drafting capabilities. However, the volunteer department that initially responded to the call had two units on the scene equipped with hard suction hose.

The next obstacle was obtaining access to a static water supply to draft from. The closest we could get the engines to a static water supply was approximately 25 ft (8 m). Not a problem: The driver/operators assembled 30 ft (9 m) of drafting hose, and one fire fighter held the strainer down in the water until a weight could be found. The draft was established and the water supply was secure.

Now the fireground operations were able to proceed in full. The aerial ladder company was able to knock down the bulk of the fire to allow crews to save the homeowner's vehicles and property in the basement. The training and knowledge of the driver/operators, as well as the entire response's ability to adapt to the situation, made a difference in being able to save some of the homeowner's belongings.

Brent Willis
Martinez-Columbia Fire Rescue
Martinez, Georgia

CHAPTER 11 Fireground Operations

SKILL DRILL 11-2
Hand Laying a Supply Line
NFPA 1002, 5.2.1, 5.2.1(B)

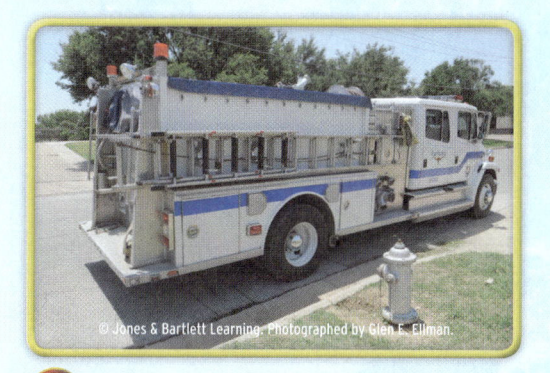

1. Position the apparatus for the intake to be used.

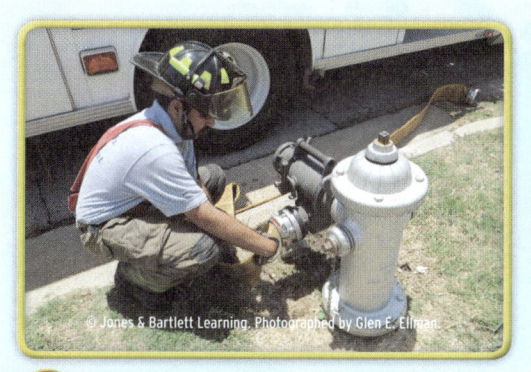

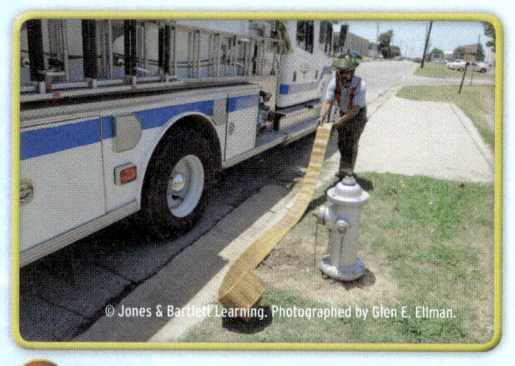

2. Roll out or pull the supply hose to the hydrant.

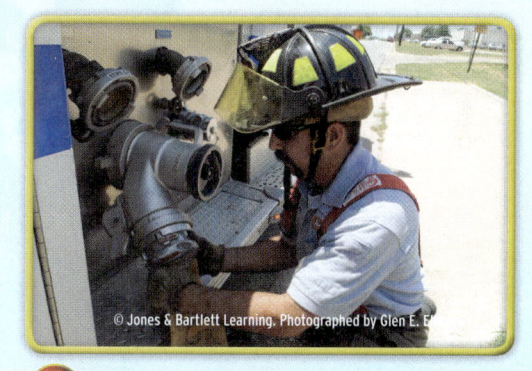

3. Connect the supply hose to the hydrant.

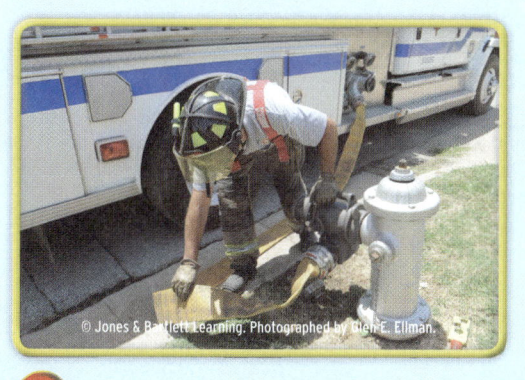

4. Connect the supply hose to the pump's intake.

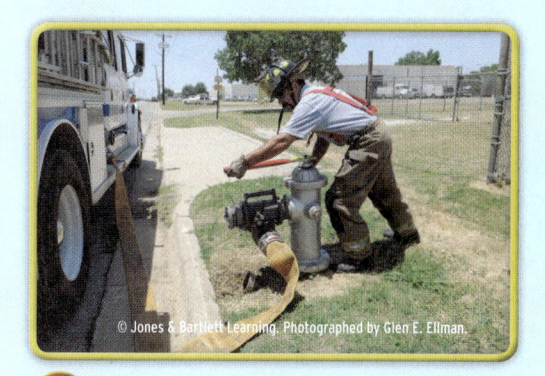

5. Check for any kinks in the hose.

6. Open the hydrant and charge the supply line.

If you are unaware of the locations or cannot find the FDC connection on scene, you become the owner of the problem, with all eyes looking at you for its resolution.

The fire department connection can be either free standing or wall mounted. It generally consists of a Siamese connection with two 2½-inch (65-mm) female connections **FIGURE 11-14**.

Depending on the occupancy, multiple-connection standpipes may be present. Local codes may dictate the number and size of standpipes provided **FIGURE 11-15**.

Each female connection should have a clapper valve inside the Siamese connection that will swing to the closed position on the connection that is not in use **FIGURE 11-16**. This allows

FIGURE 11-13 Signs indicating the location of the FDC can be very helpful.

FIGURE 11-14 **A.** A free-standing FDC is usually located away from the building. **B.** A wall-mounted FDC is located directly on the building itself. Usually, the sprinkler control room is found directly behind this connection inside the building.

FIGURE 11-15 A multiple-connection standpipe.

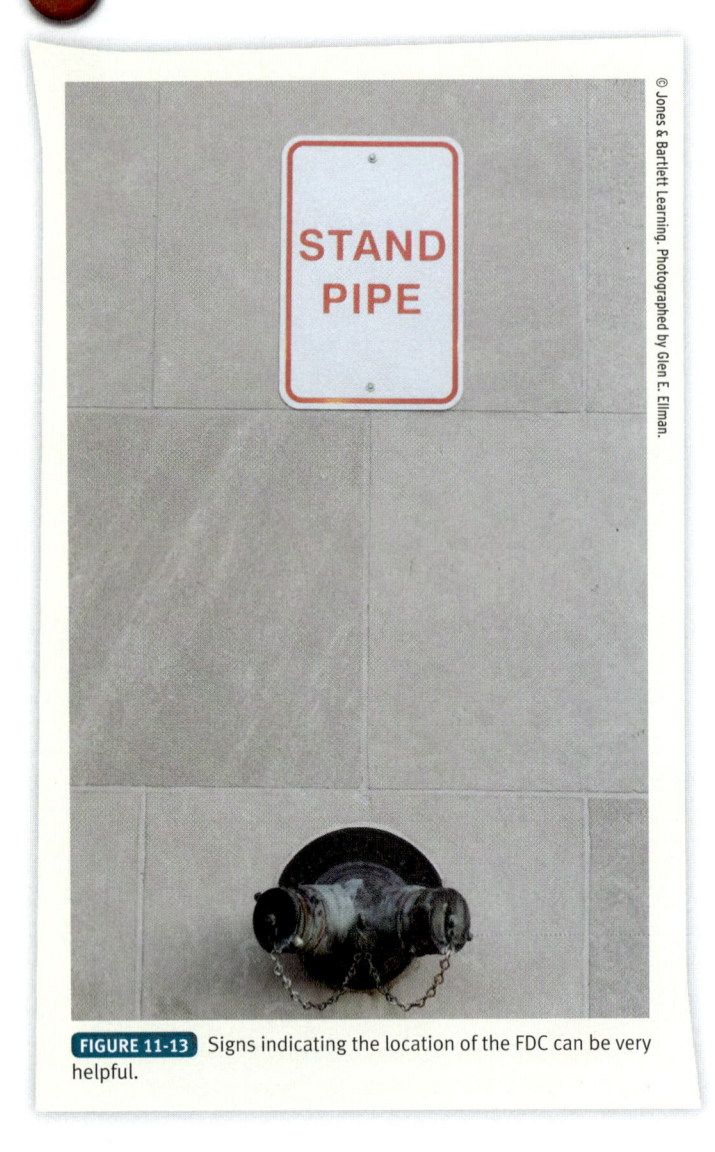

one side of the Siamese connection to be charged without water discharging from the other open intake. Depending on the fire department's SOP, it is generally recommended that both or all connections to the FDC be used when supplying a standpipe.

If the exterior FDC connection is damaged such that a connection to it is impossible, an accepted practice is to hook up to the standpipe discharge on the first floor of the building. This may allow you to connect only one line into the standpipe—but better one line than none at all.

After the engine is connected to a sprinkler/standpipe, the fire department's SOP/SOG may specify when you will supply the standpipe. One factor that may affect this decision is whether the standpipe is a wet or dry pipe system. Whether a system is wet or dry may be dictated by state or local codes. A wet system has water under pressure in the pipe at all times; it is typically supplied by the water utility department having jurisdiction. In contrast, a dry system has no water in the pipe and depends on the fire department to supply the water. Regardless of which system may be present, a supply line must be established.

Follow the steps in **SKILL DRILL 11-3** to connect hose to a fire department connection:

1. Secure a water supply using LDH to ensure the maximum available pressure and volume of water. (**STEP 1**)

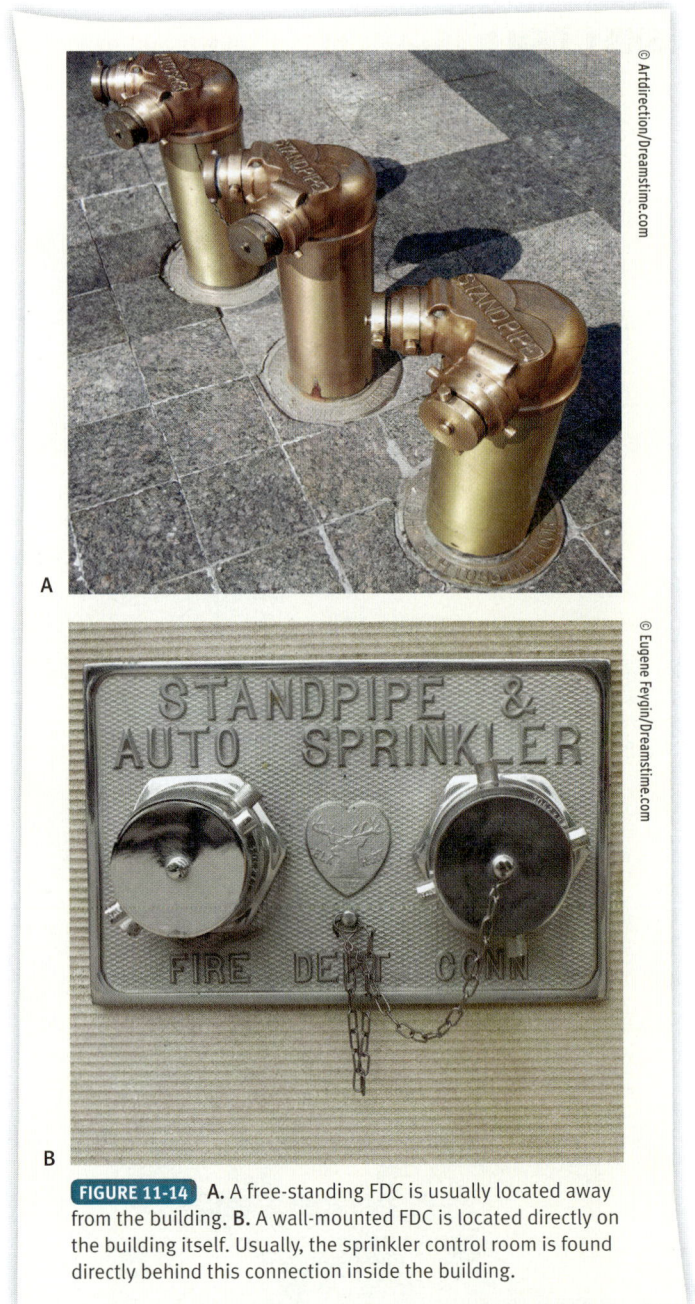

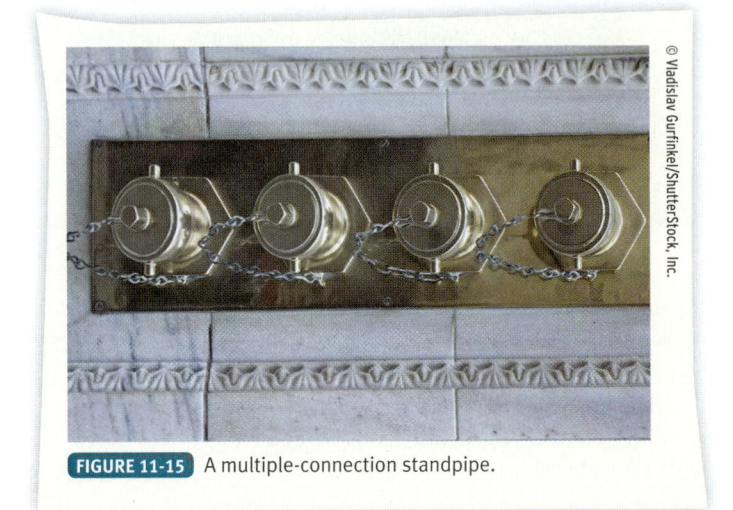

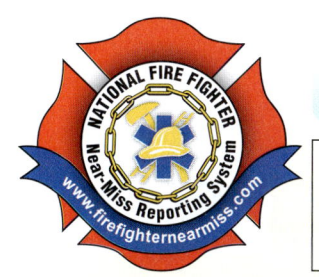

Near-Miss REPORT

Report Number: 10-000004

Synopsis: Cold weather freezes pumper.

Event Description: We are an all-volunteer rural department and respond when paged. A page was received around 03:45am on the coldest day in 10 years for our state with a temperature of 16°F (−9°C) and a wind chill of −6°F (−21°C). The call was for a reburn of a trailer and a new burn of a trailer 70 ft (21 m) away. When we arrived, both trailers were fully involved, so no entry was required. We requested mutual aid for another department and tanker support from a third department. The fire was contained quickly, and one department released with their tanker when our pumper froze up. There was a second pumper on scene for back up from another fire department and no further help was needed. The problem was extreme cold. We had to tarp the pumper and then use a turbo heater to thaw it out. We did not perform winter preparation for our equipment because we did not think it would be a problem.

Lessons Learned: Even though we live in the southern part of the U.S. and do not get the extreme cold that northern states do on a regular basis, we still need to prepare our equipment for hard winters. Drain air tanks and the pump in cold weather and keep water circulating on the scene.

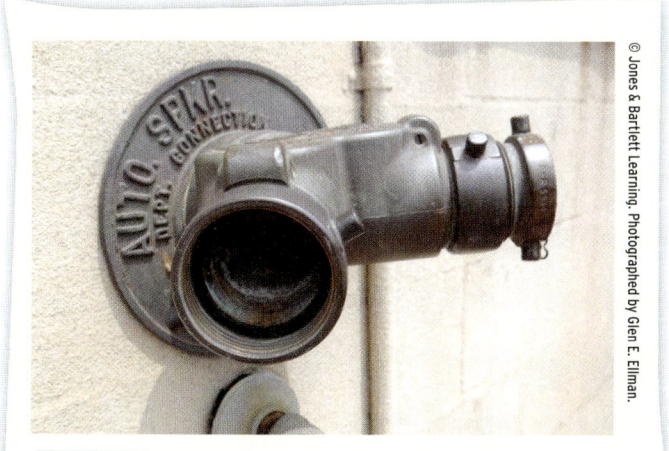

FIGURE 11-16 A clapper on a Siamese connection allows for one hose to be charged while the other side is still being connected.

Performing a Changeover

When you first arrive at the scene, you may initially need to supply attack lines from your onboard tank, and then have a supply line laid to your pump from another fire apparatus or a hand-laid supply line. When supplying attack lines from the onboard water tank, you are limited by the amount of water in the tank. For example, if you are supplying one attack line with 100 gpm (380 L/min) and your water tank contains 500 gal (1890 L), your tank will run dry in approximately 5 minutes. The tank water will last only so long, so a supply line will be needed to sustain a fire attack for a longer period. It is wise to recognize early on that the amount of water flowing through the attack lines is or will be far greater than the amount of water carried in the onboard tank. For this reason, it is important to establish a supply line early, and then perform a changeover operation.

During a changeover operation, you switch from the onboard water tank supply to an external water source. The goal with this task is simple: to make the changeover prior to running out of water in the tank and with the least amount of pressure fluctuation for the firefighting crew on the nozzle. Overpressurizing the attack lines can cause fire fighters to lose control of the handlines, causing an unsafe situation.

As the driver/operator, you need to constantly supply the attack lines with the correct pressure to ensure a safe operation. Two devices that will assist you in this task are the pressure relief valve and the pressure governor **FIGURE 11-17** and **FIGURE 11-18**.

There are several factors you need to keep in mind prior to the changeover. How much water is currently in the tank? What are the flow rate (gpm) and pressure (psi) currently used on the attack line by the firefighting crew? What is the incoming pressure from the supply line? What is the setting of the pressure control device?

2 Position the apparatus in a safe and effective position for the given situation. (**STEP 2**)

3 Engage the pump. (**STEP 3**)

4 Pull enough 2½-inch (65-mm) or 3-inch (77-mm) hose to reach from the pump discharge to the FDC. (**STEP 4**)

5 Remove or break the protective cover for the FDC. (**STEP 5**)

6 Inspect the FDC for debris inside and any signs of damage. (**STEP 6**)

7 Connect the male end to the FDC. (**STEP 7**)

8 Connect the female end of the hose to the pump discharge.

9 Use a double-male adapter if you pull a female coupling off the hose bed and intend to connect it to a FDC. (**STEP 8**)

SKILL DRILL 11-3

Connecting Hose to a Fire Department Connection
NFPA 1002, 5.2.1, 5.2.1(B)

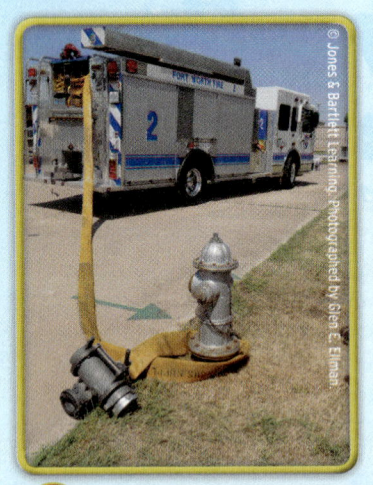

1. Secure a water supply with LDH.
2. Position the apparatus appropriately.
3. Engage the pump.
4. Pull the hose to the fire department connection.
5. Remove or break the protective cover from the fire department connection.
6. Inspect the fire department connection.
7. Connect the male end of the hose to the fire department connection.
8. Connect the female end of the hose to the pump.

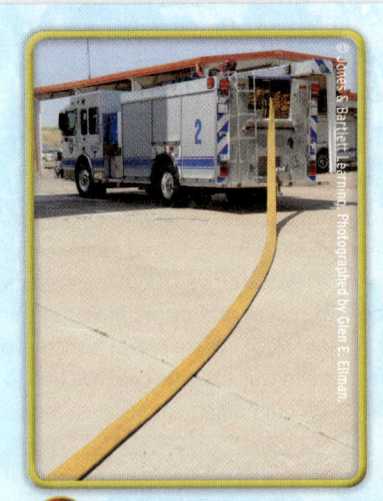

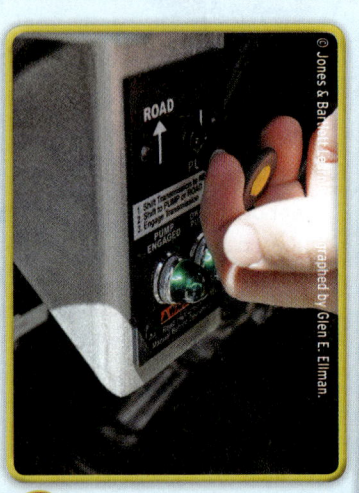

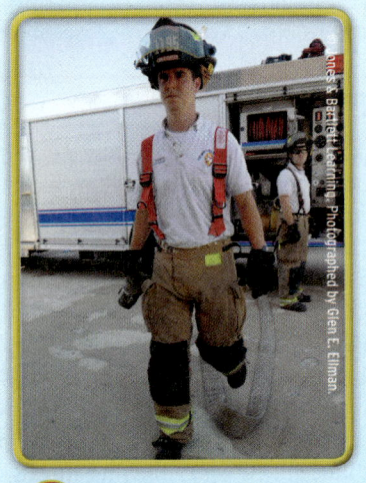

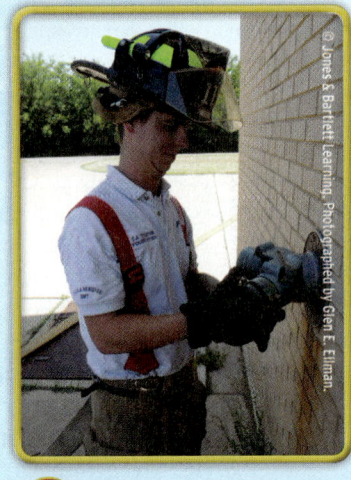

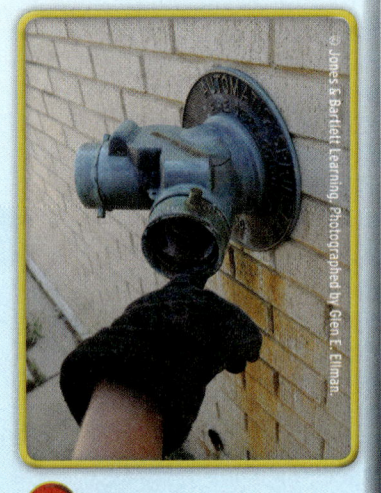

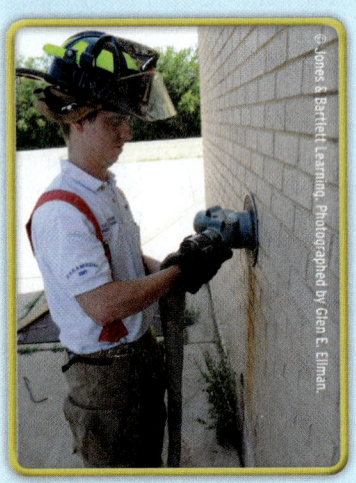

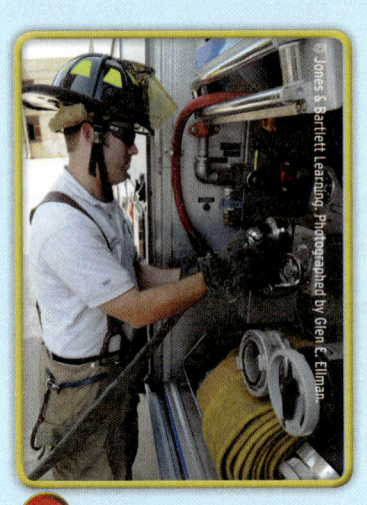

CHAPTER 11 Fireground Operations   261

FIGURE 11-17 A pressure relief valve.

FIGURE 11-18 A pressure governor.

FIGURE 11-19 A transfer valve.

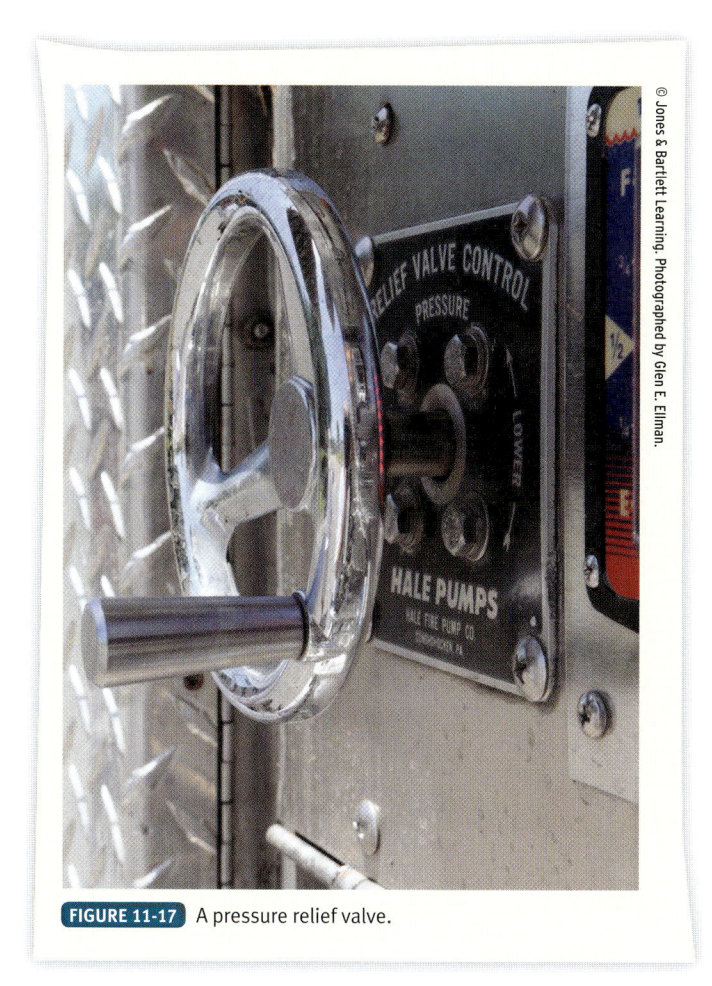

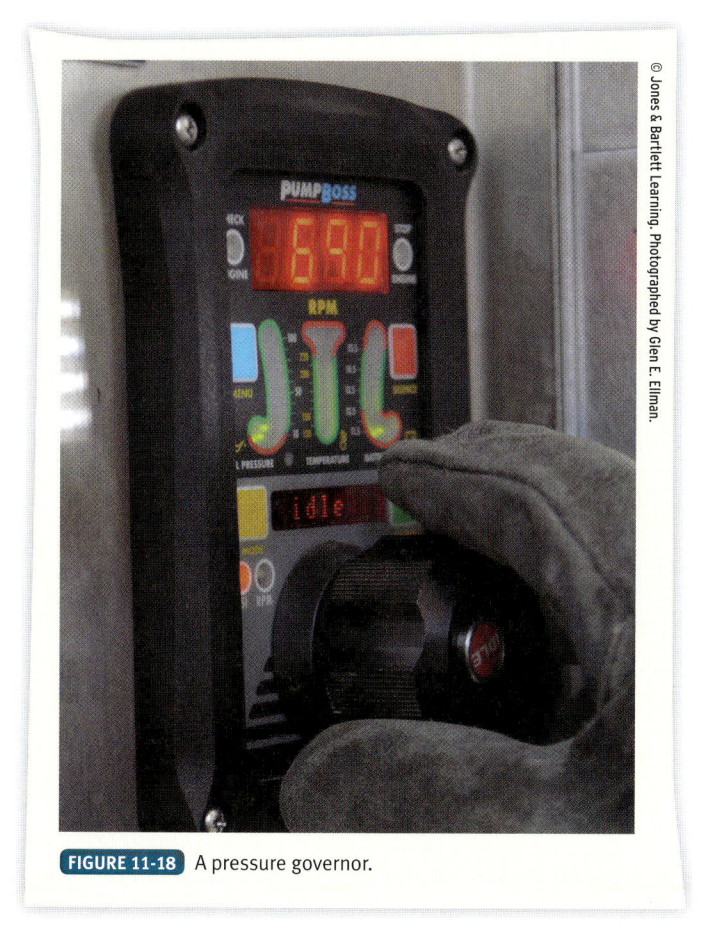

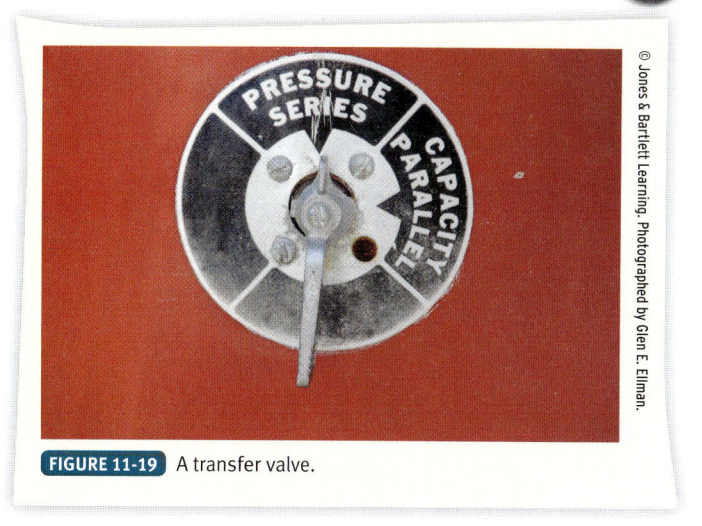

At the beginning of the changeover, keep your eyes on the pressure gauge for the line that the attack crew is using. The goal is ensure the fluctuation does not exceed 10 psi (70 kPa). Slowly open the valve from the external water source, which will introduce water into the pump. Once this valve has been fully opened, close the tank-to-pump valve. The tank-to-pump valve does not need to be closed on the newer apparatus, as a check valve will close so as to not allow water to flow into the pump from the tank once the supply line intake is opened. Many departments leave the tank-to-pump valve open, as an extra safety feature, so that the tank water will automatically flow into the pump if the pressurized supply is lost and the driver/operator is remote from the pump panel for some reason. If the pressure-relieving device is set for a lower pressure than the incoming supply pressure, you will need to increase the setting on the valve above the incoming pressure from the supply line.

Once the changeover has been accomplished, recheck the gauges to ensure that they have the proper settings. If no other additional lines are required for pumping, now is a good time to refill the onboard tank. Slowly open the tank fill valve to allow water to refill the tank. The tank fill valve should be opened just enough to let water into the tank, but not enough to permit fluctuations of pressure for the attack lines.

Follow the steps in **SKILL DRILL 11-4** to perform a changeover operation. Always refer to and follow the manufacturer's recommendations for your department's specific apparatus.

1. Calculate and flow an attack line from a discharge using the onboard water tank. (**STEP 1**)
2. Slowly open the intake valve to allow water into the pump. (**STEP 2**)
3. Attempt to keep the pressure fluctuation from exceeding 10 psi (70 kPa) while using either a pressure governor or pressure relief valve. (**STEP 3**)
4. After opening intake valve fully, close the tank-to-pump valve. (**STEP 4**)
5. Adjust the pump settings as needed. (**STEP 5**)

Monitor the Fire Pump

As the driver/operator, you have additional duties and responsibilities on scene aside from pumping water or foam. Once the pumping operation is under way, you must monitor specific

SKILL DRILL 11-4

Performing a Changeover Operation
NFPA 1002, 5.2.1, 5.2.1(B)

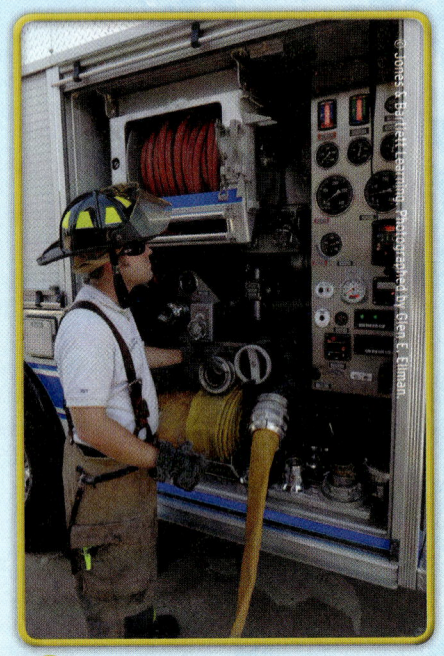

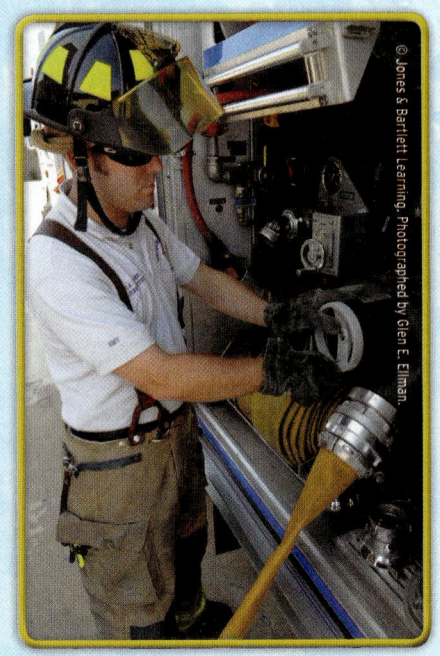

1 Calculate and flow an attack line from a discharge using the onboard water tank.

2 Slowly open the intake valve to allow water into the pump.

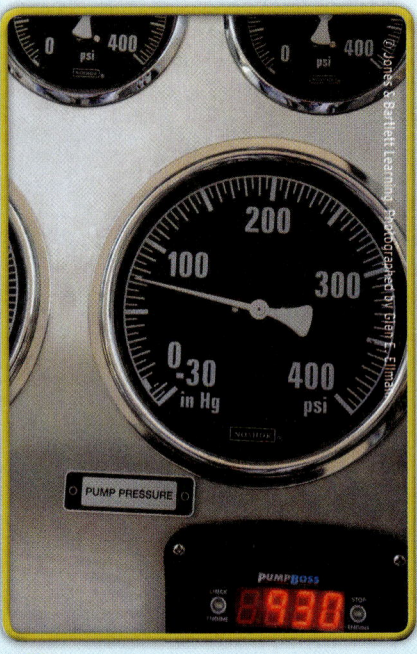

3 Attempt to keep the pressure fluctuation from exceeding 10 psi (70 kPa) while using either a pressure governor or pressure relief valve.

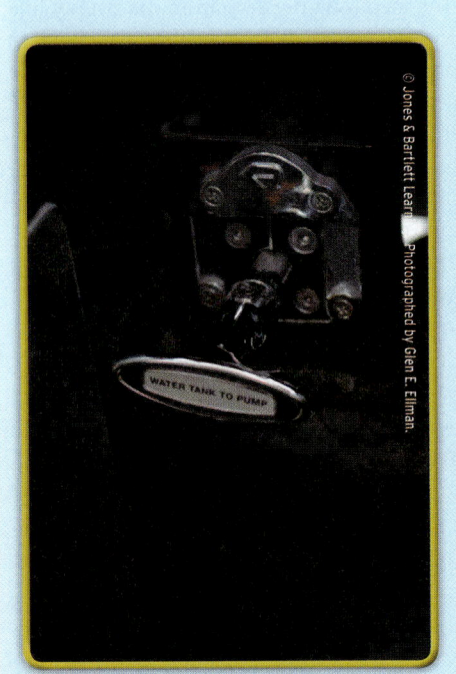

4 After opening intake valve fully, close the tank-to-pump valve.

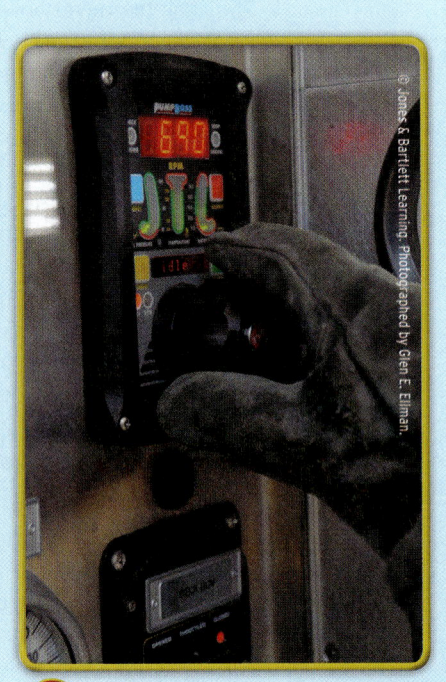

5 Adjust the pump settings as needed.

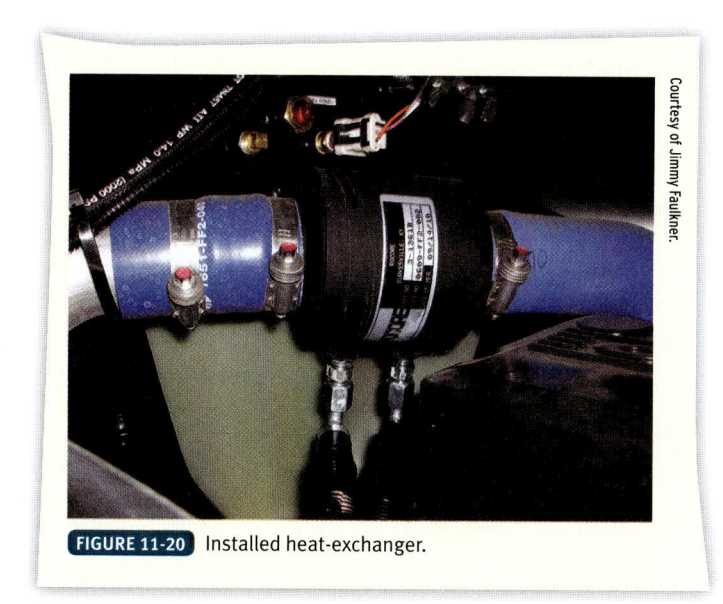

FIGURE 11-20 Installed heat-exchanger.
Courtesy of Jimmy Faulkner.

gauges on the pump panel, such as the oil pressure and engine temperature. During the pumping operation, if you discover that the engine temperature is increasing, you need to take steps to reduce this temperature. First, shut down or turn off all unnecessary loads on the engine, such as the air conditioning system and external lighting. Next, if needed, open the auxiliary cooler on the fire apparatus. The auxiliary cooler is a heat-exchanger system usually installed in the engine radiator hose. The heat-exchanger allows the engine coolant to flow around copper piping in a tube. The copper piping, which has cold pump water from the fire pump flowing through it, reduces the temperature of the engine coolant by conduction in the heat-exchanger **FIGURE 11-20**. In older apparatus, simply opening the cab doors and lifting the engine cover has been known to help reduce engine temperatures, while in newer apparatus this is not necessary. Modern diesel engines, however, are designed to get air to the engine with engine covers in the closed position. Opening the engine covers in diesel engines will change the air flow and could negatively affect the operation of the engine significantly.

Follow the steps in **SKILL DRILL 11-5** to operate an auxiliary cooling system:

1. Ensure the pump is operating at 50 psi (350 kPa) pump discharge pressure or lower.
2. Switch the auxiliary coolant valve open, which allows the pump water to flow through the heat-exchanger. The warmer water exiting the heat-exchanger is then returned to the suction side of the fire pump.
3. When pumping operations are finished, the auxiliary coolant valve should be returned to the closed position.

Of course, your final duty as the driver/operator on the fireground is to disengage the fire pump. Follow the steps in **SKILL DRILL 11-6** to disengage the fire pump with an automatic transmission. Always refer to and follow the manufacturer's recommendations for your department's specific apparatus.

1. Close the discharge valves. (**STEP 1**)
2. Step into the apparatus' cab. (**STEP 2**)
3. Place your foot on the brake pedal and move the transmission selector into neutral. (**STEP 3**)
4. Ensure that the speedometer no longer has a reading of 10–15 mph (16–24 km/h). (**STEP 4**)
5. Move the pump's shift control switch to the "road" position. (**STEP 5**)
6. Confirm that the indicator lights ("Pump engaged" and "Okay to pump") are in the off positions. (**STEP 6**)
7. Exit the cab, and close and drain all valves as necessary. (**STEP 7**)

Operating Other Fixed Systems and Equipment

Upon arrival at the emergency scene, the driver/operator will position the apparatus for effective operations. The chapter *Emergency Vehicle Driving* covers the procedures for placing the apparatus at an incident.

Each apparatus will be equipped with a unique complement of tools and equipment according to its specific function on the emergency scene. The apparatus driver is responsible for knowing how to operate every piece of equipment on his or her apparatus. While most of the time other members of the company may be the ones using the equipment, the driver will support them by preparing it for use and inspecting it before the shift begins.

When positioned at the scene of an incident and operating the emergency lights and/or other electrical appliances, it is advisable to engage the **high idle switch**, which sets the apparatus engine to 900–1100 rpm. High idle will typically be disabled when the apparatus is in pump. This step will help ensure that the alternator is providing its full amperage rating.

National Fire Protection Association (NFPA) 1901, *Automotive Fire Apparatus*, requires that the vehicle's electrical system be monitored by an **automatic load management system**, which is designed to protect the electrical system from needless damage while maintaining the operation of essential devices. Damage to the apparatus' electrical system can occur if the total continuous electrical load exceeds the minimum continuous electrical output. Many new fire apparatus have complex electrical systems whose outputs will exceed the alternator capacity and can be supplied only by the deep discharge of the apparatus batteries. These high-powered batteries experience serious damage when they are deeply discharged. The automatic load management system, therefore, is designed to protect the electrical system from needless damage while maintaining the operation of essential devices.

A system that is protected with an automatic load management system incorporates a **load sequencer**, which is a component that will activate electrical loads in a specific order to prevent overloading the electrical system. The electrical system also has a **load monitor**, a component designed to prevent any additional electrical loads from exceeding the system's capabilities. In these circumstances, the system will perform **load shedding**, in which a component deactivates unnecessary electrical loads in order of necessity and to prevent damage to the system.

The driver/operator must appreciate how the automatic load management system works and learn how to operate it

SKILL DRILL 11-6: Disengaging the Fire Pump with an Automatic Transmission
NFPA 1002, 5.2.1, 5.2.1(B)

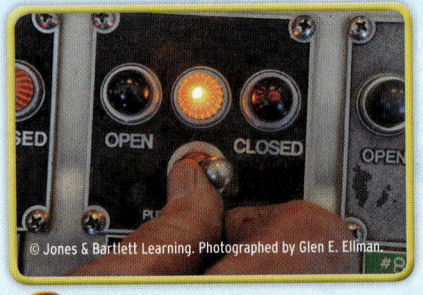

1. Close the discharge valves.
2. Step into the apparatus' cab. 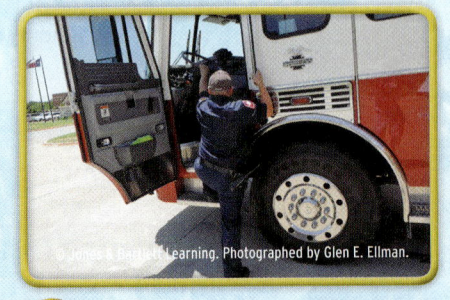
3. Place your foot on the brake pedal and move the transmission selector into neutral. 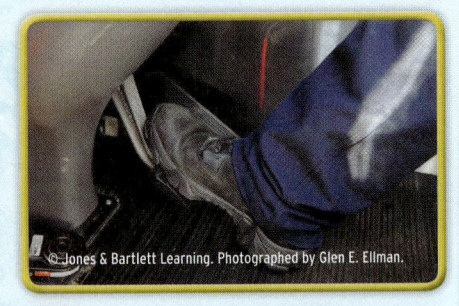
4. Ensure that the speedometer no longer has a reading of 10–15 mph (16–24 km/h). 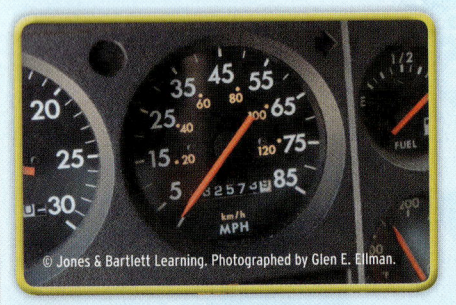
5. Move the pump's shift control switch into the "road" position.
6. Confirm that the indicator lights ("Pump engaged" and "Okay to pump") are in the off positions.
7. Exit the cab, and close and drain all valves as necessary.

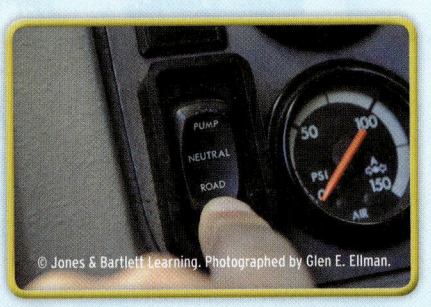

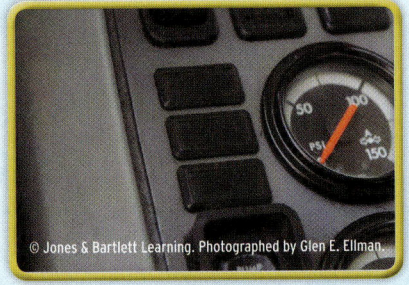

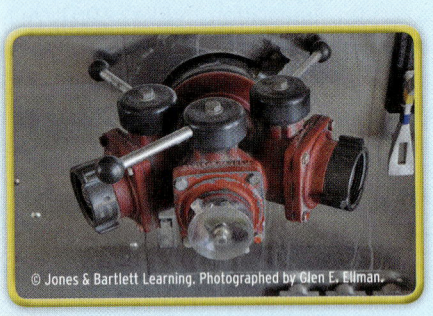

correctly. It is especially important to recognize the difference between load shedding and a possible electrical system failure.

■ Apparatus-Mounted Equipment

Fire apparatus are equipped with a variety of apparatus-mounted equipment. This equipment is not specific to every type of apparatus or fire department. For example, an engine company from one department may have only a fire pump on its apparatus, whereas another fire department may have fire pumps, hydraulic rescue tool systems, and generators mounted on the apparatus. Regardless of which type of equipment is carried on the apparatus, the driver/operator is responsible for its maintenance and safe operation. While each apparatus manufacturer provides different systems and equipment on its apparatus, they all share some common features. The driver/operator should reference the owner's manual to obtain more information about this apparatus-mounted equipment.

FIGURE 11-21 An inverter.

FIGURE 11-22 A portable generator.

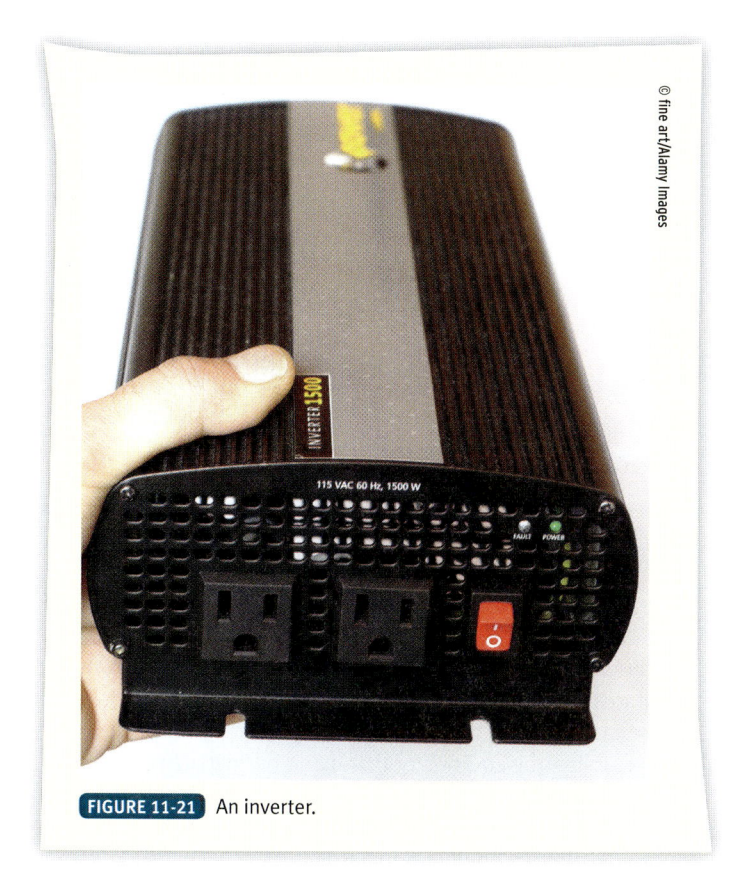

Electric Generators

The fire apparatus driver/operator should not assume that a dependable supply of electrical power will be provided at every emergency scene. Some emergencies may occur in isolated areas that lack power sources, or the involved structure itself may be unable to supply the electrical requirements of the fire department. Therefore it is prudent for the fire apparatus to be self-sufficient and provide its own electrical power—generally a 110-volt alternating current (AC) delivered through electrical cords. This portable electricity can be supplied by a **generator**, which is an engine-powered device that creates electricity, or an **inverter**, which is an appliance that converts 12-volt direct current (DC) from a vehicle's electrical system to 110-volt AC power **FIGURE 11-21**.

An inverter can provide a limited amount of AC current and is typically used to power only a small electric tool or a few small lights. It does not produce enough power to operate the high-powered lights that are usually used to illuminate an emergency scene. Drawing too much current from an inverter can seriously damage it and other electrical components on the apparatus.

Given the limitations of inverters, the most common power source for fire apparatus is the generator. Three types of generators are found on fire apparatus:

1. **Portable generator.** This type of generator is the smallest of the three options. It is usually powered with gasoline fuel. Although it does not offer the high output of the other two types of generators, it makes up for this shortcoming with its light weight and portability. Portable generators can produce up to 6000 watts (6 kilowatts) of power and come in a variety of sizes **FIGURE 11-22**.

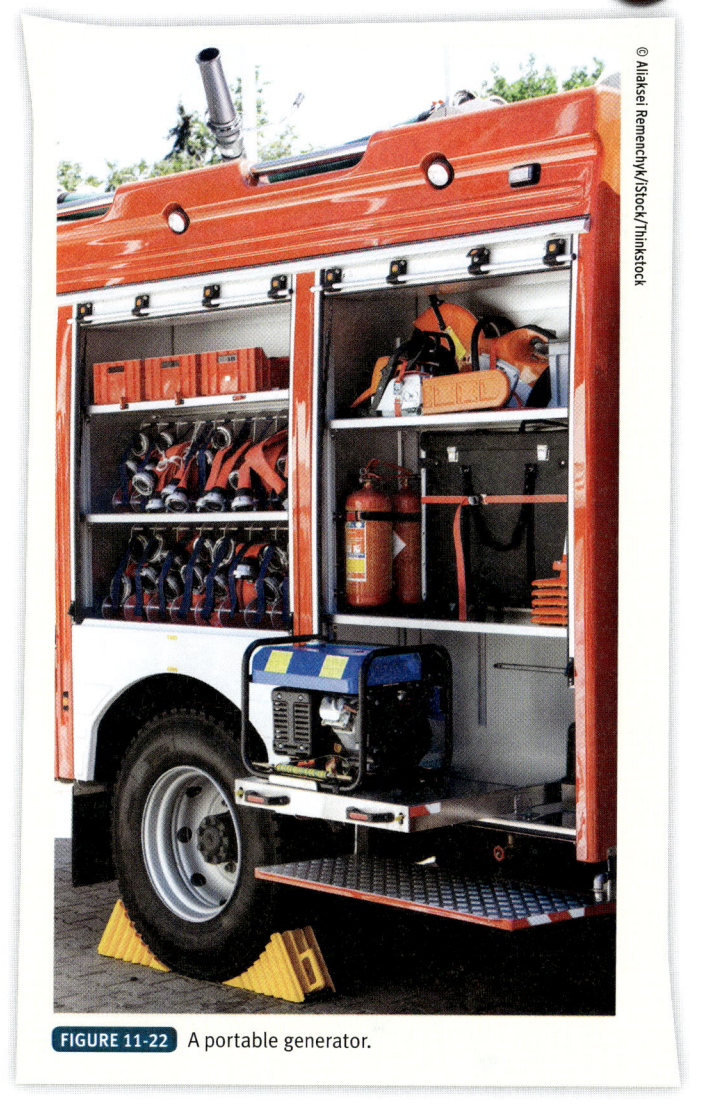

2. **Apparatus-mounted generator.** This type of generator is permanently mounted on the apparatus and has a motor separate from the vehicle that drives it. It may be powered by gasoline or diesel fuel. An apparatus-mounted generator may use the same fuel tank, which is usually diesel fuel, as the apparatus or it may have its own fuel supply **FIGURE 11-23**.

3. **Transmission-driven generator.** This type of generator is powered by the vehicle's motor and is driven by a power take-off (PTO) system. With this type of setup, the apparatus' engine powers the generator and any other system that is connected to its driveline. Transmission-driven generators may produce 25 kilowatts or more.

To engage a generator PTO, follow the steps in **SKILL DRILL 11-7**:

1. Ensure all breakers for the generator are in the off position. (**STEP 1**)
2. Ensure the transmission is in the neutral position. (**STEP 2**)
3. Ensure the parking brake is set to the on position. (**STEP 3**)
4. The engine must be at idle. (**STEP 4**)
5. Activate the in-cab "Generator PTO" switch. (**STEP 5**)

FIGURE 11-23 An apparatus-mounted generator.

FIGURE 11-24 A lantern.

6. Ensure the "Generator PTO engaged" light is illuminated. (**STEP 6**)

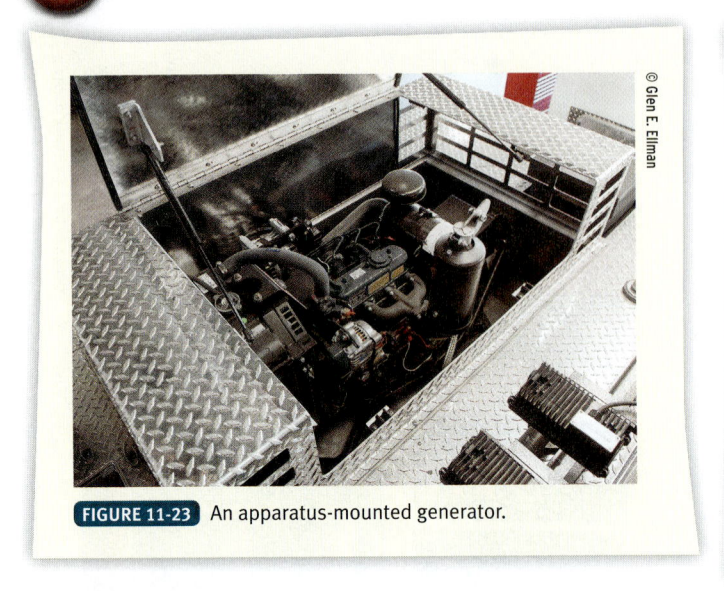

To disengage a generator PTO, follow the steps in **SKILL DRILL 11-8**:

1. Ensure all breakers for the generator are in the off position. (**STEP 1**)
2. Ensure the transmission is in the neutral position. (**STEP 2**)
3. Ensure the parking brake is set to the on position. (**STEP 3**)
4. The engine must be at idle. (**STEP 4**)
5. Deactivate the in-cab "Generator PTO" switch. (**STEP 5**)
6. Ensure the "Generator PTO engaged light" is off. (**STEP 6**)

Scene Lighting Equipment

Because most emergency incidents occur at night, lighting is required to illuminate the scene and enable safe, efficient operations. It is usually the responsibility of the driver/operator to provide for sufficient scene lighting, while other members of the crew are completing tasks at the incident. Departmental SOPs or the incident commander (IC) will dictate responsibility for setting up lighting.

For this purpose, fire apparatus are equipped with a vast assortment of lighting equipment. Some fire departments equip all of their apparatus with the same type of lights that are found in the same location on the apparatus. Other departments may have special apparatus respond to the incident to provide on-scene lighting. Almost all fire apparatus have some capability to illuminate areas around the apparatus. The ability to adequately light up an emergency scene may mean the difference between a safe emergency scene and a dangerous one.

Some lights have a different pattern than others. For example, **spotlights** project a narrow concentrated beam of light, whereas **floodlights** project a more diffuse light over a wide area.

When used incorrectly, these lights may also create a problem. If they are directed improperly at a scene, they can temporarily blind fire fighters or approaching vehicles. The scene lighting should be proportionate with lights positioned above and behind the fire fighters to lessen the chance of any problems.

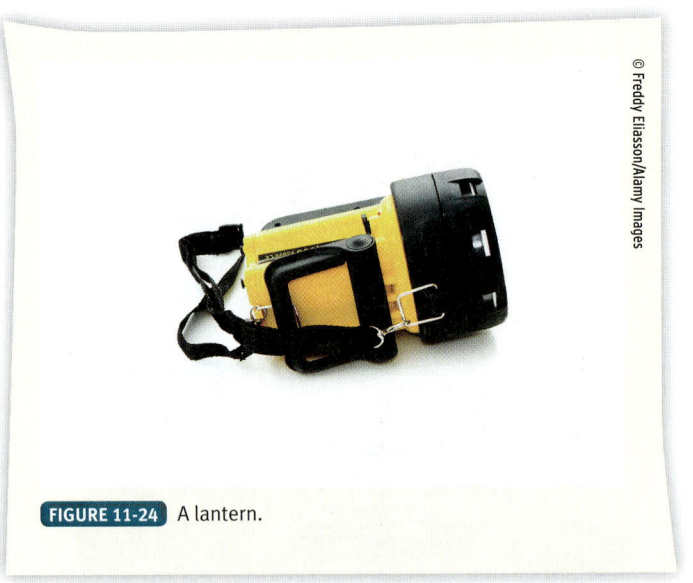

Four types of lighting equipment may be found on the fire apparatus. Not every apparatus will have these types of lights, but the driver/operator should be trained in the operation and location of all lighting equipment that his or her department carries.

1. **Lanterns.** While each fire fighter should carry a personal flashlight to illuminate his or her immediate work area, the fire apparatus is usually equipped with a high-powered lanterns. This type of hand light projects a powerful beam of light and is easily maneuvered on any emergency scene. Lanterns can be equipped with a shoulder strap for easy transportation and may be set up inside a structure to illuminate the work area after the fire is under control or used during the initial stages of vehicle extrication. With the visibility provided by this powerful light, the fire fighters can begin their operation while other, more powerful lights are set up. Lanterns are powered by a rechargeable battery that has a recharging station located on the apparatus **FIGURE 11-24**. When the apparatus engine is operating, the battery is recharging for the next use. Lanterns may provide lights ranging from an 8-watt spotlight to a 20-watt flood beam.

2. **Portable lights.** While crews may begin the operation with hand lights, the work area is further illuminated by portable lights that are powered by a generator and supplied by an electrical cord. Some of these devices are mounted on tripods and can be deployed at various heights **FIGURE 11-25**. Portable lights can be taken into buildings to illuminate the interior or set up outside to light up the emergency scene. These lights usually range from 300 to 1500 watts and can use several types of bulbs, including quartz and halogen bulbs.

3. **Apparatus-mounted lights.** Floodlights or spotlights may be attached to the exterior of the apparatus. Some are mounted to the body of the apparatus and are controlled by a single switch inside the cab **FIGURE 11-26**. These lights provide a quick and effective way to illuminate one side of the work area. When used, they should completely illuminate the scene and eliminate dark shadows. To operate them, the driver/operator must first engage the generator and then control the

CHAPTER 11 Fireground Operations

SKILL DRILL 11-7
Engaging the PTO Generator
NFPA 1002, 5.2.1, 5.2.1(B)

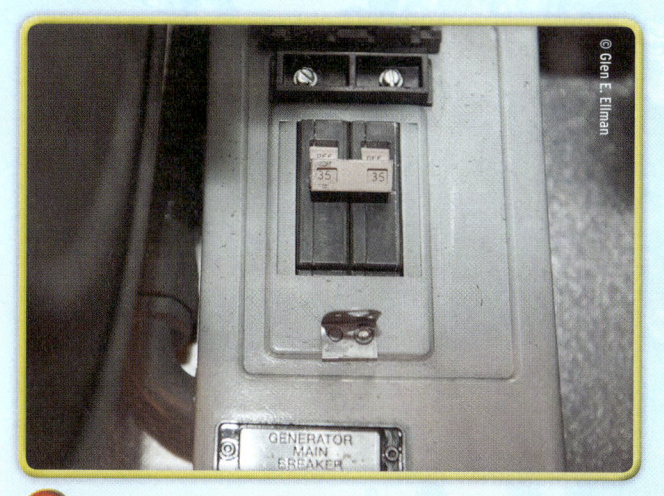

1 Ensure all breakers for the generator are in the off position.

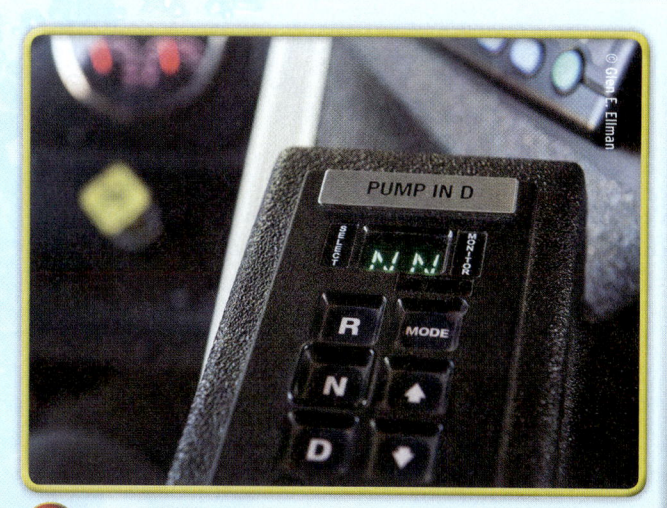

2 Ensure the transmission is in the neutral position.

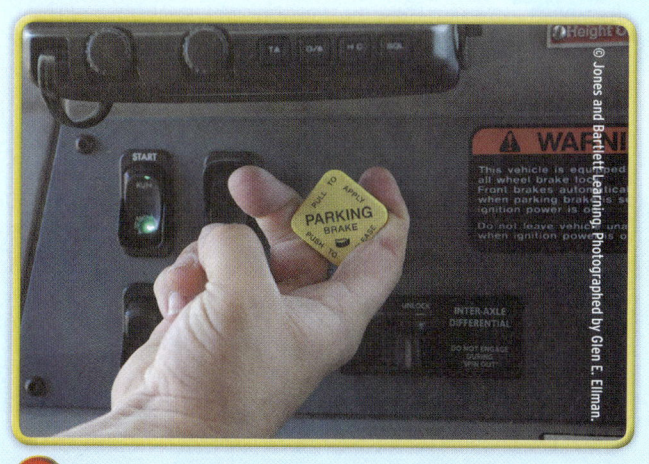

3 Ensure the parking brake is set to the on position.

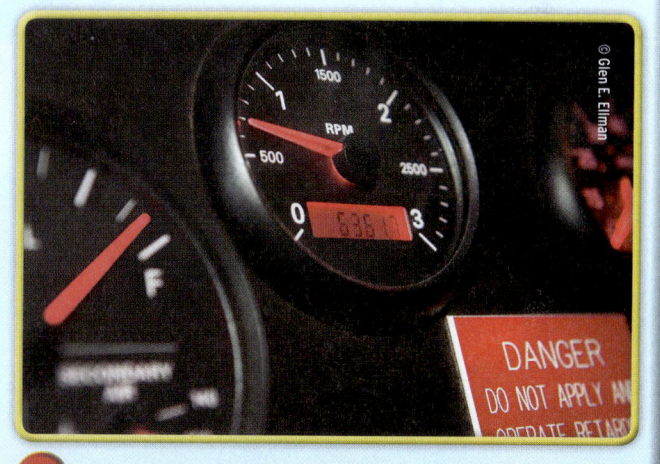

4 The engine must be at idle.

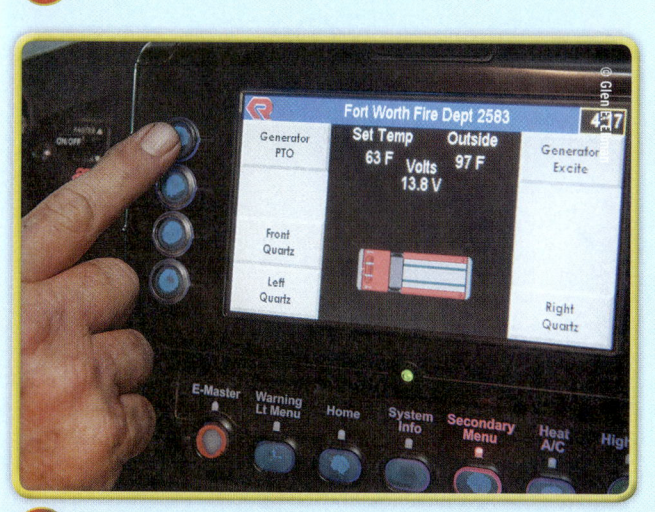

5 Activate the in-cab "Generator PTO" switch.

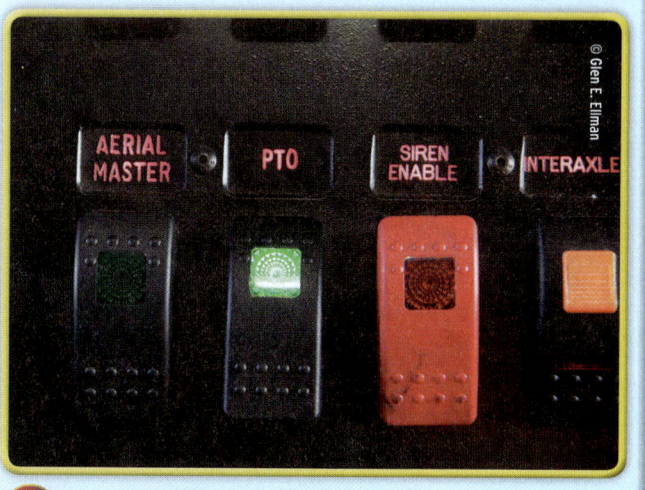

6 Ensure the "Generator PTO engaged" light is illuminated.

© LiquidLibrary

SKILL DRILL 11-8 Disengaging the PTO Generator
NFPA 1002, 5.2.1, 5.2.1(B)

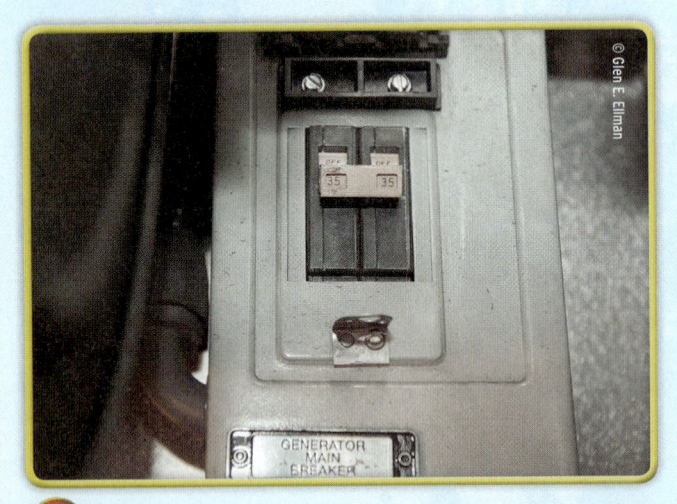

1. Ensure all breakers for the generator are in the off position.

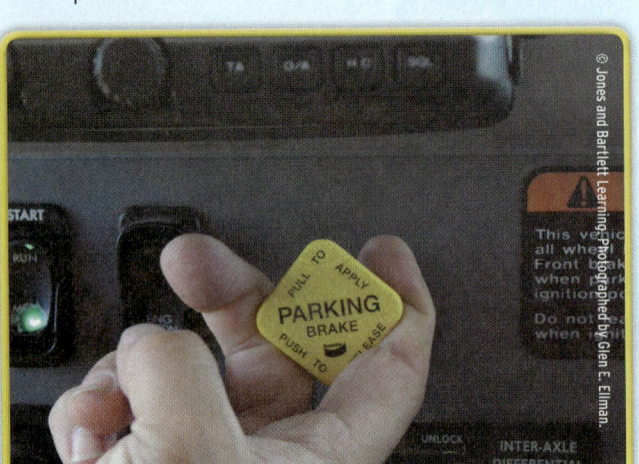

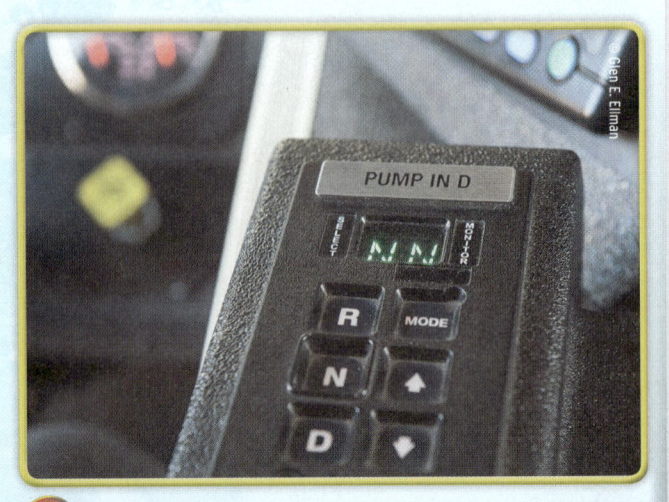

2. Ensure the transmission is in the neutral position.

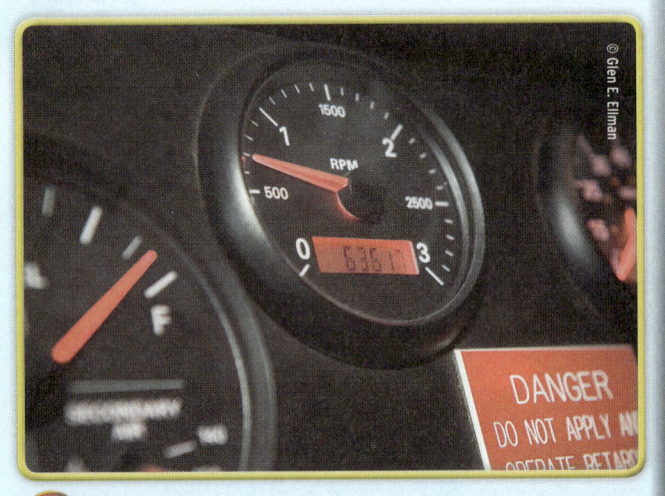

3. Ensure the parking brake is set to the on position.

4. The engine must be at idle.

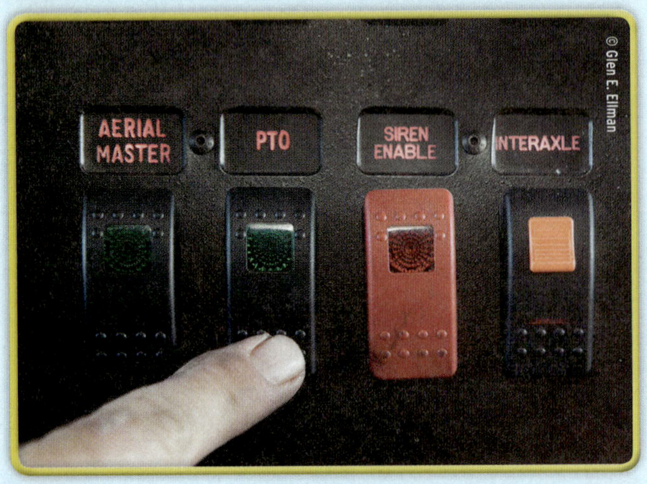

5. Deactivate the in-cab "Generator PTO" switch.

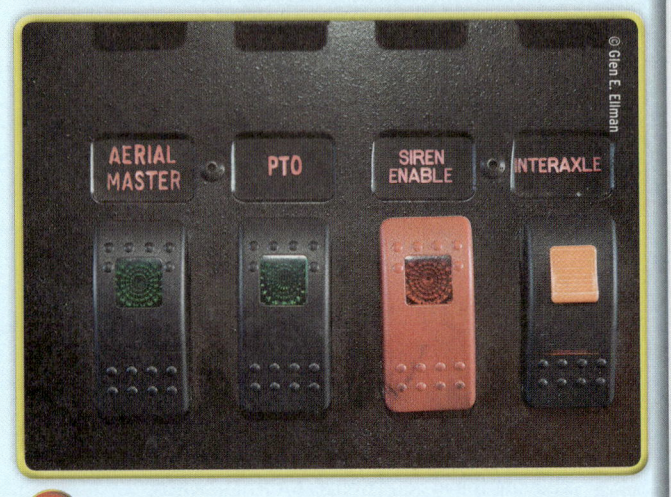

6. Ensure the "Generator PTO engaged" light is off.

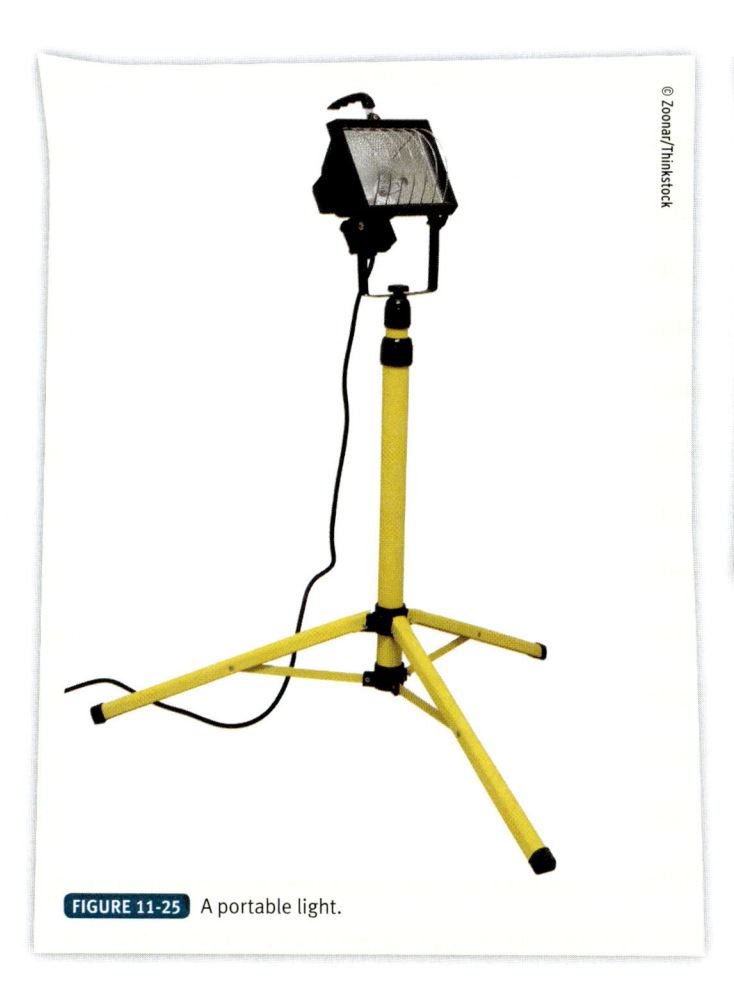

CHAPTER 11 Fireground Operations 269

FIGURE 11-26 A side apparatus-mounted light.

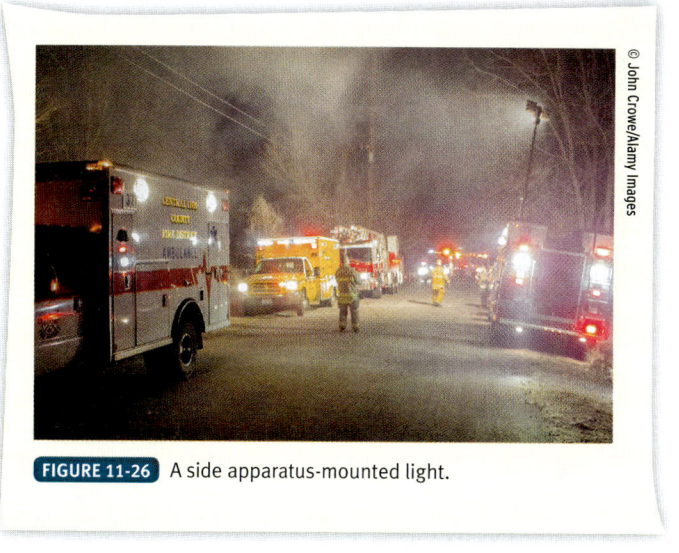

driver/operators that they are in the raised position. Some apparatus are also equipped with sensors to notify driver/operators when the tower light is still in the raised position—a factor that must be taken into account when the apparatus is moved.

Power Equipment Distribution

The power needed to operate the electrical equipment must be supplied through an electrical cable or cord. This cord must

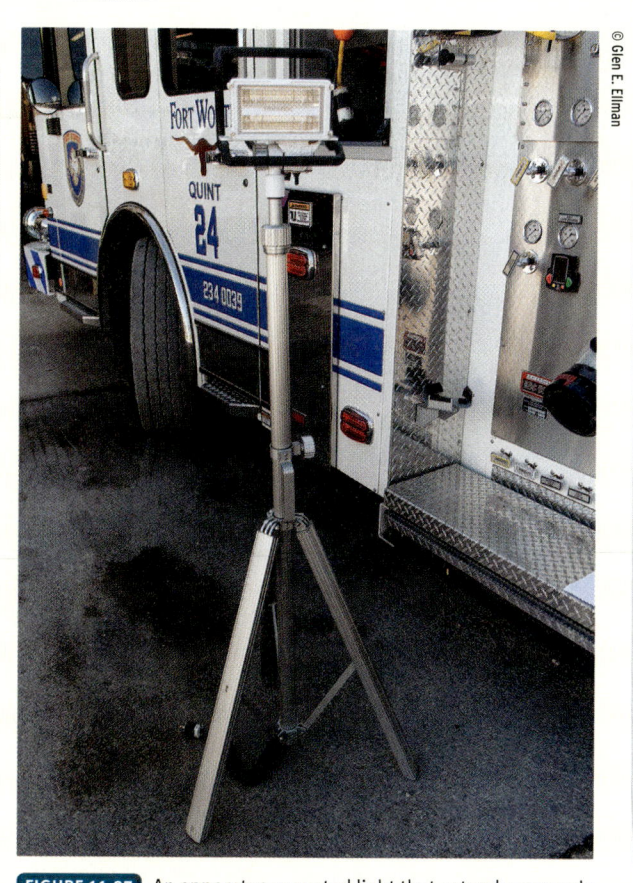

FIGURE 11-25 A portable light.

individual switches for each light at the sides and rear of the apparatus. Do not preset all of the individual light switches to the on position, as turning on all of them simultaneously may place an unnecessary load on the generator and seriously damage it. Some lights may be angled slightly toward the ground to provide better coverage of the emergency scene, while other types of lights are attached to a pole and elevated from different locations on the apparatus **FIGURE 11-27**. These lights may be manually raised from their nested position to better illuminate the emergency scene. Many newer apparatus use LED scene lights that run off of the vehicle's 12-volt system and don't require generator power.

4. **Tower lights.** When the body-mounted lights are insufficient to meet the incident lighting requirements, a tower light may be more appropriate **FIGURE 11-28**. This set of powerful floodlights can be operated above most obstacles and provide the desired on-scene lighting. The lights may be controlled from the ground with a remote control or a control panel in a compartment. They are raised from the top of the apparatus by either a 12-volt motor or a pneumatic-powered system. The tower lights' extended height above the apparatus is usually not more than 15 feet (5 m). Multiple 1500-watt halogen lamps (or LEDs on newer tower lights) are usually mounted at the top and may provide for 360-degree rotation with tilt capabilities. These lights are also illuminated by a 12-volt light to signal to

FIGURE 11-27 An apparatus-mounted light that extends on a pole near the side of the chassis.

FIGURE 11-28 A tower light.

FIGURE 11-29 A junction box.

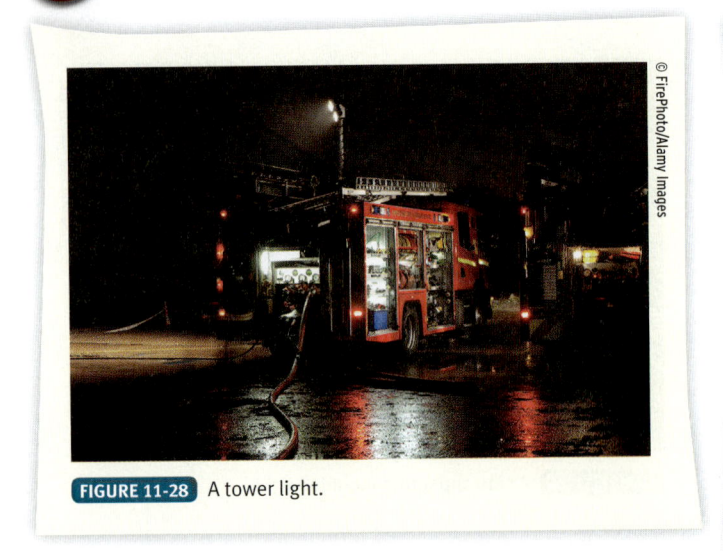

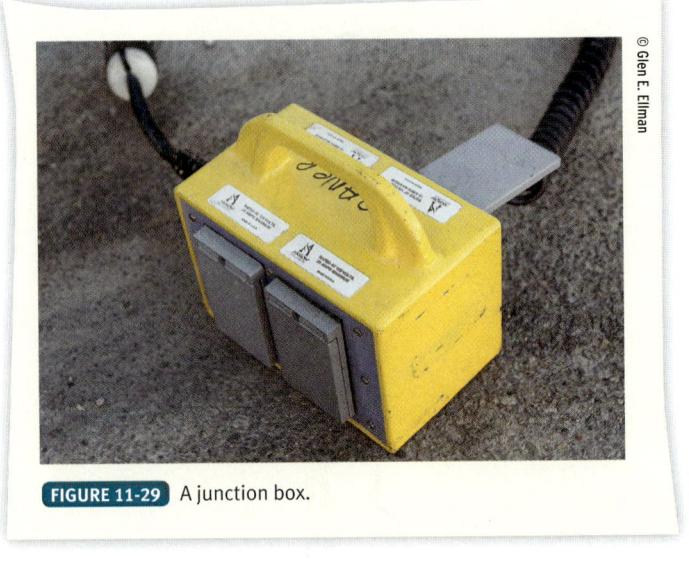

be waterproof and provide a durable insulation. Fire fighters can be hard on their equipment and expect it to perform when needed. The cord that is used in everyday household applications is not suitable for the fireground. Always purchase quality commercial-grade electrical cords and adapters for fire service use.

Most electrical cords will have a three-prong adapter. The most common size of electrical cord is a 12-gauge, 3-wire type. This size cord works well for most 110-volt powered equipment and is usually stored on the apparatus in lengths of 50 and 100 ft (15 and 30 m). For normal operations, these lengths are adequate for operations close to the fire apparatus.

When multiple cords are necessary, a junction box may be used. A **junction box** is a device that attaches to an electrical cord to provide additional outlets **FIGURE 11-29**. It allows several cords or power-operated tools to be supplied by a single electrical cord and may be used as a mobile power outlet. In this case, a single cord is stretched from the apparatus, a junction box is attached to the end, and the other cords or tools are then connected to the junction box. A small light is attached to the top of the junction box to ensure it has power and the crew can locate it in the dark. This light turns on only when the junction box is charged with electricity. Just like the electrical cord, the junction box must be waterproof, be durable, and have flip-up covers lined with soft neoprene rubber at each outlet opening.

When the electrical equipment is required at a location that is a considerable distance from the apparatus or if the equipment operates on 220 volts, a larger cord is needed. For these situations, most departments equip their apparatus with an electrical cord reel. Electrical reels are usually powered with a 12-volt DC rewind motor. The reel holds 100–200 ft (30–60 m) of electrical cord and is sized to the load and circuit breaker rating. Using too small of a cord for a high electrical flow may overload the cord and cause it to overheat. When the correct size of wire for the electrical demand is used, however, the cord will not overheat and cause a potential electrical problem.

The connectors and plugs used for fire department electrical equipment may have special connectors that attach with a slight clockwise twist. This feature keeps the power cord from becoming unplugged during fire department operations.

Powered Rescue Tools

NFPA 1936, *Powered Rescue Tools*, defines the following components that relate to this section of the chapter.

A **power rescue tool** is a tool that receives power from the power unit component and generates energy used to perform one or more of the following functions: spreading, lifting, holding, crushing, pulling, or cutting. These tools are generally powered by a **power unit**, which is a prime mover and principal power output device used to power the rescue tool. Power units rely on either a portable power unit or a PTO-driven system on the fire apparatus.

The **power rescue tool system** generally consists of a reservoir, fluid, a power unit, an enclosed system, and an actuator used to operate a power rescue tool. A **hydraulic reservoir** is the container that stores the hydraulic fluid until it is needed in the system. This reservoir may be equipped with a filter to condition the fluid as it returns through the system. The fluid used in hydraulic rescue tools can be phosphate ester, ethylene glycol, automatic transmission fluid oil, or mineral-based hydraulic oil; the last option is the most common. Each manufacturer may identify a specific type of hydraulic fluid that should be used with its product. Always reference the owner's manual to determine which fluid to use.

The power units for power rescue tools are usually machine powered. Although manual units are still available, their operation is usually limited to an emergency backup role. The two types of power units are described here:

1. **Portable power units.** These units are powered by an independent motor and may be transported away from the apparatus **FIGURE 11-30**. Each unit can weigh anywhere from 26 to 97 lb (12–45 kg) and is usually carried by one or two fire fighters. Such devices can be powered by 120- or 220-volt AC electric, gasoline, diesel, or a manual hand pump, which provides emergency backup power. Gasoline and diesel units may sustain operations for only 20–60 minutes; consequently, the driver/operator must be constantly aware of the fluid levels in these types of units. Some newer portable power units are powerful enough to allow up

FIGURE 11-30 A portable power unit.

FIGURE 11-31 Hydraulic spreaders.

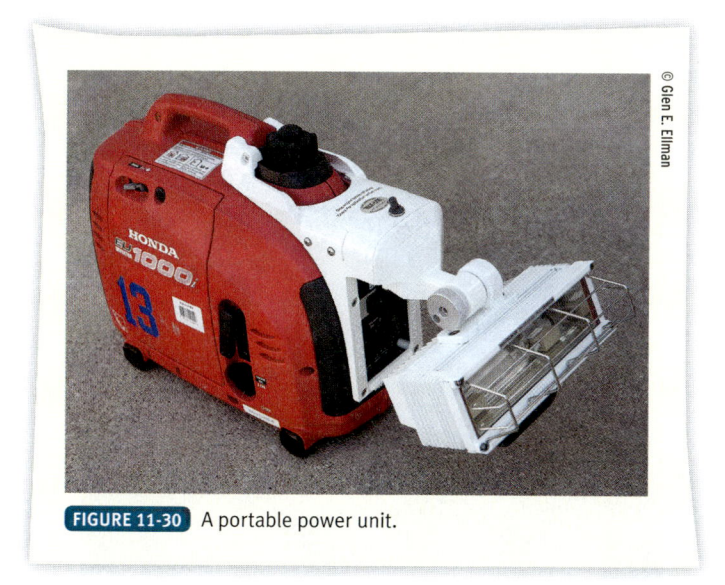

to four tools to be operated at the same time, thereby enabling fire fighters to work on several vehicles or several areas of a single vehicle at the same time. Other units will operate only a single tool at a time.

2. **PTO-driven hydraulic unit.** This system is more powerful than most portable power units. It is powered by the vehicle's engine through a PTO system and activated either by remote controls or by controls mounted inside the vehicle's cab. The apparatus' engine usually must sustain a set rpm to achieve the hydraulic pump's required rpm; in most cases, the engine must operate in a high idle position to meet this demand. Some PTO-driven hydraulic systems are capable of operating up to six tools simultaneously. The driver/operator, however, must be aware of the limitations of the equipment on his or her apparatus. Do not attach and operate more tools than the manufacturer recommends, as this may damage the equipment and delay the response operation.

A positive-displacement pump is used to pressurize the hydraulic fluid in the system. This pump may be either a single-stage or two-stage model. A single-stage pump pumps a constant pressure and flow of fluid. A two-stage pump, in contrast, operates at two different pressure modes. Depending on the apparatus, the system first operates in a low-pressure/high-volume mode (5000 psi [35,000 kPa]) until the tool is under a load. Then, the system's pressure builds and the second mode—a high-pressure/low-volume mode (10,000 psi [70,000 kPa])—is activated to deliver added power. Sometimes this switching of modes can cause a few seconds' delay in the unit's operation. During this gap, the operator must hold the load position until the second mode kicks in and the fluid pressure builds in the system.

During the operation of the tool, the pressurized hydraulic fluid will move from one section of the system to the other through the hydraulic hoselines, pressurizing the system and then returning to the hydraulic fluid reservoir. Hydraulic hoselines are usually kink resistant and electrically nonconductive. They are constructed with several reinforced layers of thermoplastic or rubber material. The methods used to couple the hoselines will differ depending on the manufacturer. Driver/operators should familiarize themselves with the correct method for coupling and uncoupling hydraulic hoselines for their department's equipment.

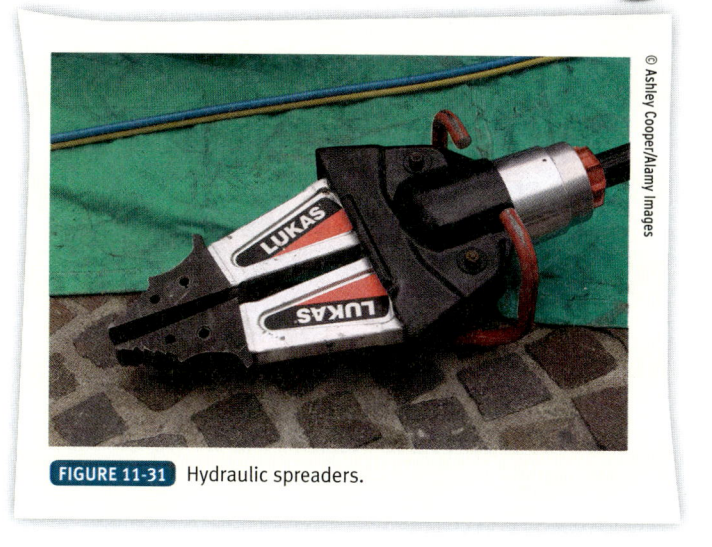

Once the fluid is under pressure and traveling through the system, it operates an actuator. An **actuator** converts the fluid pressure in a hydraulic rescue tool system into a mechanical force. This force is then used to operate one of four types of hydraulic tools:

1. **Spreaders**. A spreader is a powered rescue tool that has at least one movable arm that opens to move material. This tool contains a single piston that connects to two movable metal arms **FIGURE 11-31**.
2. **Cutters**. A cutter is a powered rescue tool with at least one movable blade that is used to cut, shear, or sever material. The design of this tool means that it is intended solely for cutting **FIGURE 11-32**.
3. **Combination tools**. A combination tool is a powered rescue tool that is capable of at least spreading and cutting **FIGURE 11-33**.
4. **Extension rams**. An extension ram is a powered rescue tool with a piston or other type extender that generates extending forces or both extending and retracting forces. Extension rams use the most hydraulic fluid during their

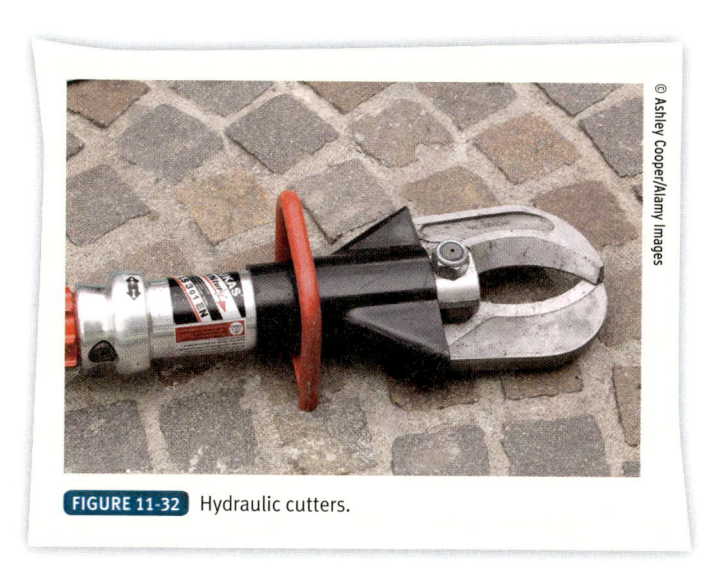

FIGURE 11-32 Hydraulic cutters.

FIGURE 11-33 A hydraulic combination tool.

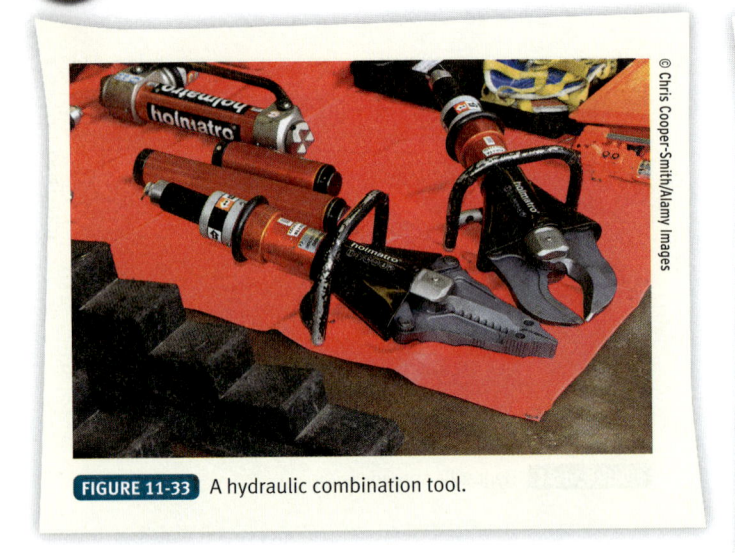

operation, so the pump being used must have enough capacity to allow the ram to reach full extension. During extension, this is a very powerful tool; however, during retraction, an extension ram can produce only approximately half of its full operating force **FIGURE 11-34**.

These tools are extremely powerful and should be used only by fire fighters who are properly trained in their operation. Always reference the manufacturer's and operator's manuals before use. To engage a PTO-driven hydraulic system, follow the steps in **SKILL DRILL 11-9**:

1. Ensure the transmission is in the neutral position. (**STEP 1**)
2. Ensure the parking brake is set to the on position. (**STEP 2**)
3. The engine must be at idle. (**STEP 3**)
4. Activate the in-cab "Hydraulic PTO" switch. (**STEP 4**)
5. Ensure the "Hydraulic PTO engaged" light is illuminated. (**STEP 5**)

To disengage a PTO-driven hydraulic system, follow the steps in **SKILL DRILL 11-10**:

1. Ensure all valves are in the closed position. (**STEP 1**)
2. Ensure the transmission is in the neutral position. (**STEP 2**)

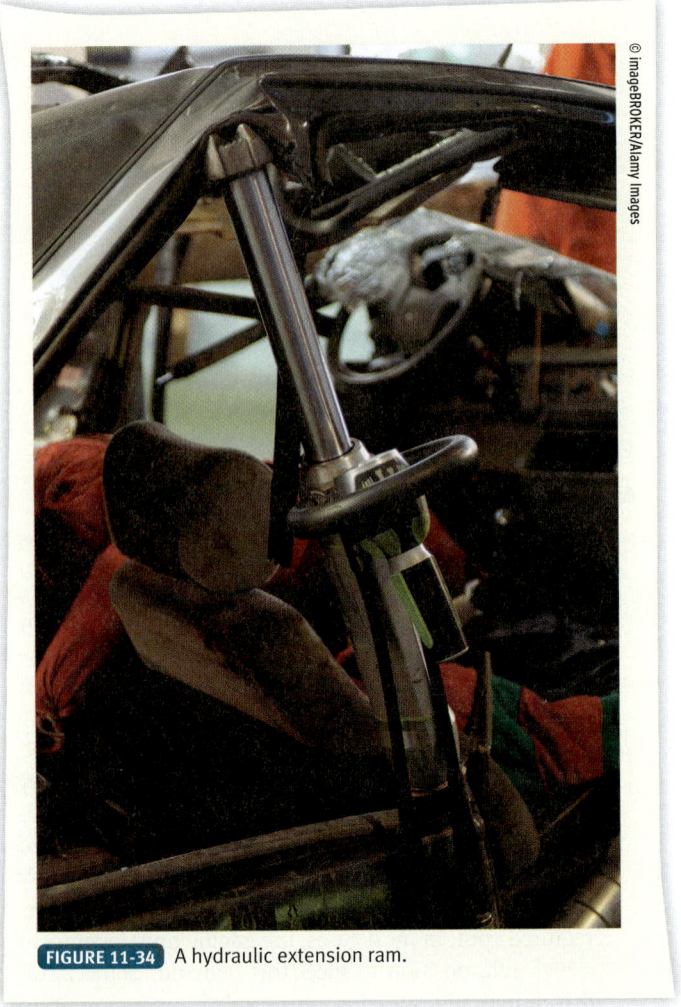

FIGURE 11-34 A hydraulic extension ram.

3. Ensure the parking brake is set to the on position. (**STEP 3**)
4. The engine must be at idle. (**STEP 4**)
5. Deactivate the in-cab "Hydraulic PTO" switch. (**STEP 5**)
6. Ensure the "Hydraulic PTO engaged" light is off. (**STEP 6**)

CHAPTER 11 Fireground Operations 273

SKILL DRILL 11-9
Engaging the PTO-Driven Hydraulic System
NFPA 1002, 5.2.1, 5.2.1(B)

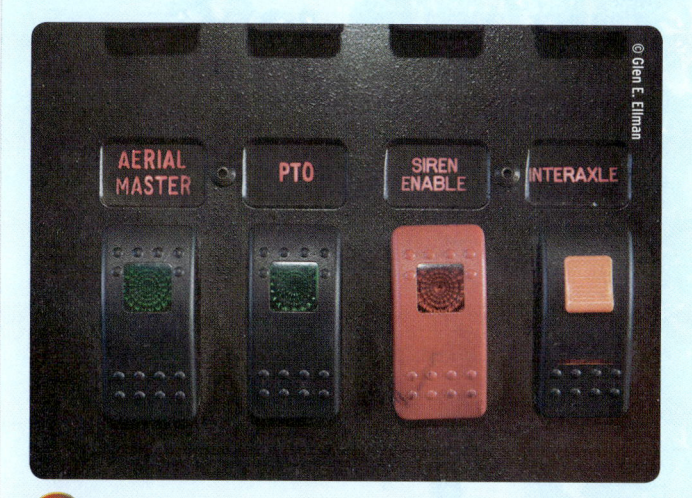

1 Ensure the transmission is in the neutral position.

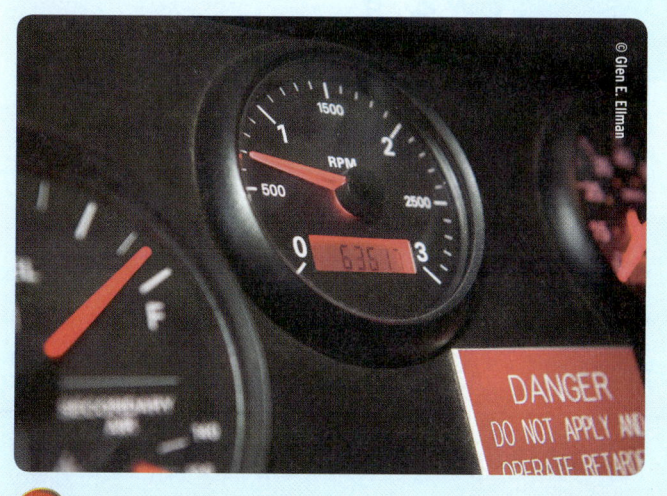

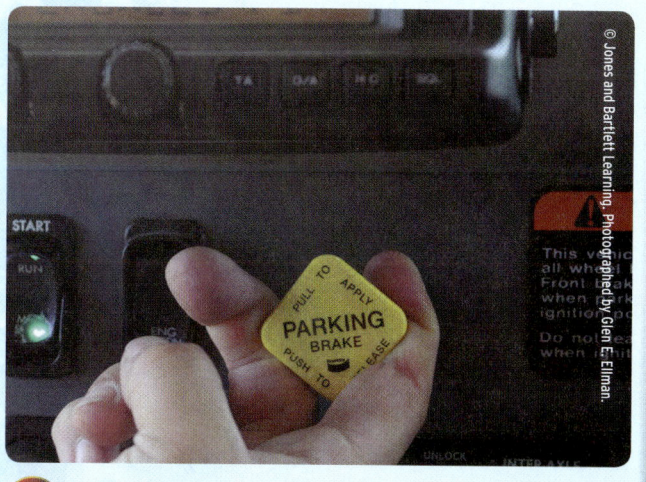

2 Ensure the parking brake is set to the on position.

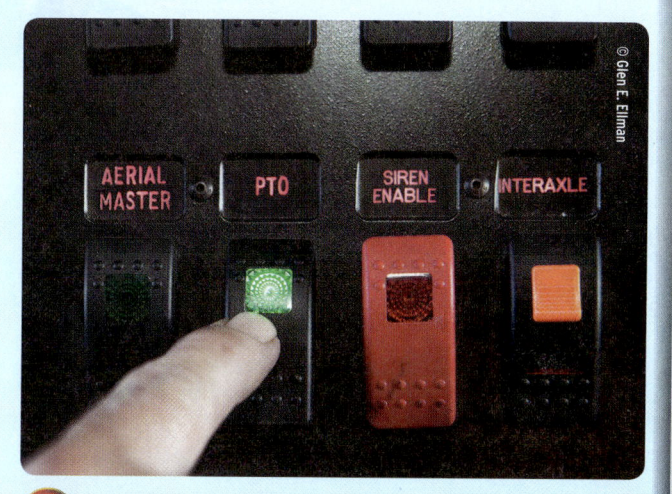

3 The engine must be at idle.

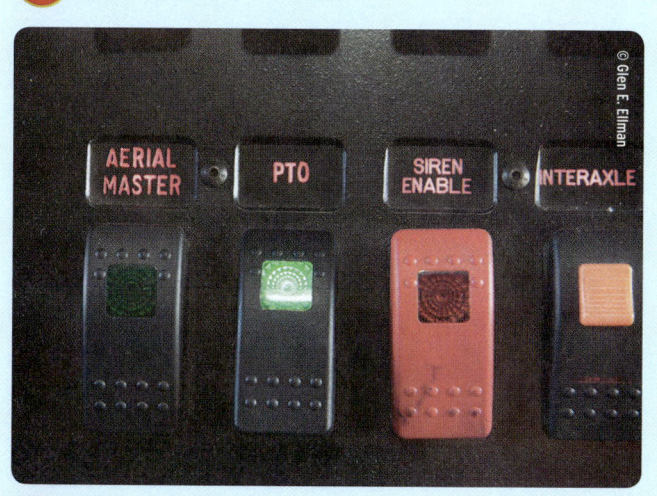

4 Activate the in-cab "Hydraulic PTO" switch.

5 Ensure the "Hydraulic PTO engaged" light is illuminated.

SKILL DRILL 11-10
Disengaging the PTO-Driven Hydraulic System
NFPA 1002, 5.2.1, 5.2.1(B)

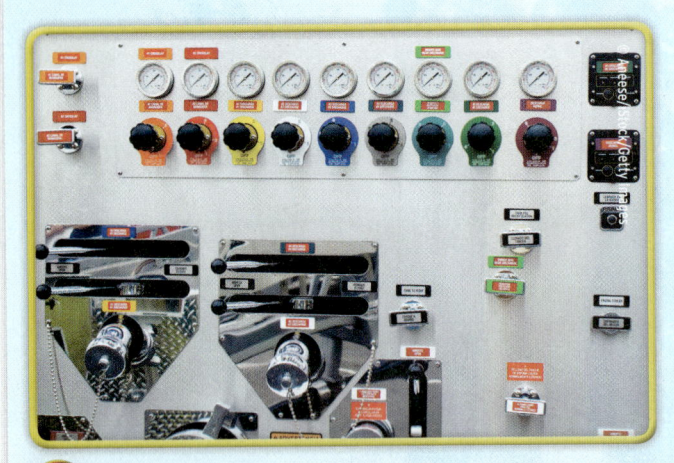

1. Ensure all valves are in the closed position.

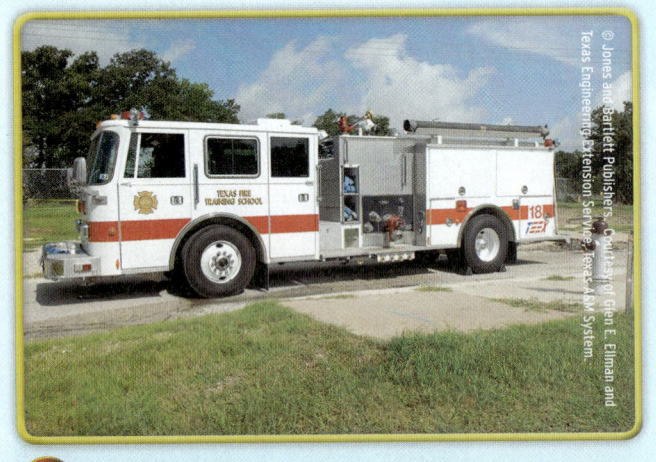

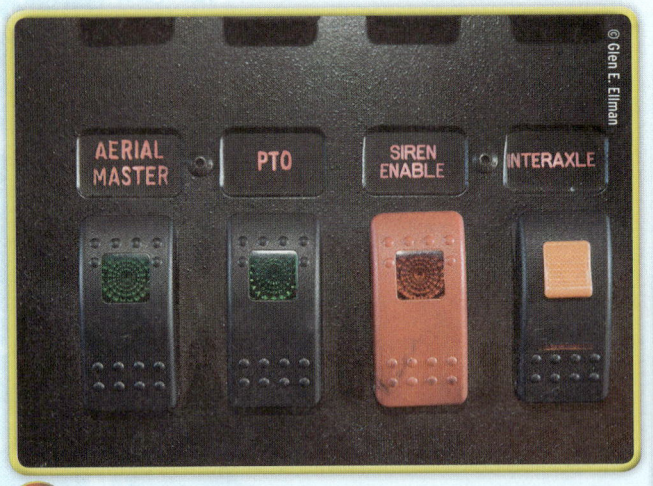

2. Ensure the transmission is in the neutral position.

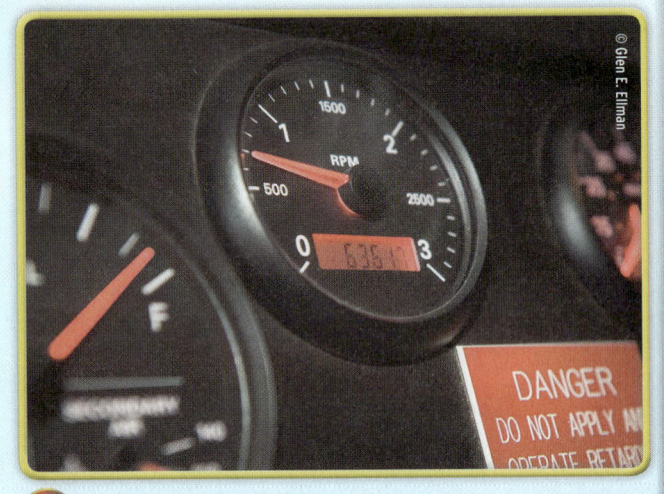

3. Ensure the parking brake is set to the on position.

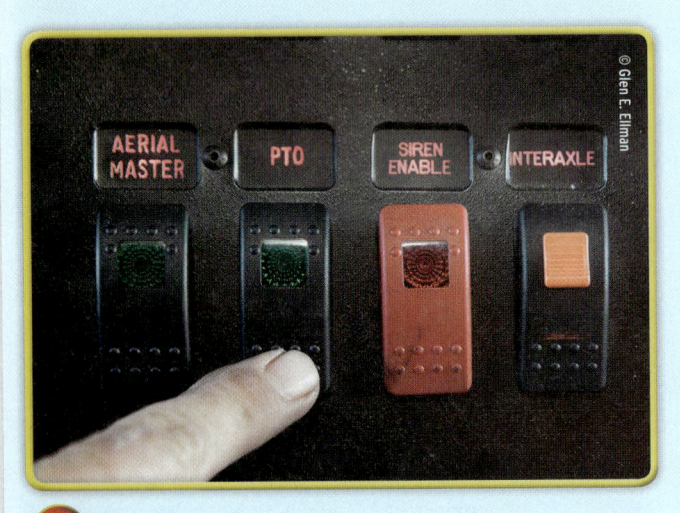

4. The engine must be at idle.

5. Deactivate the in-cab "Hydraulic PTO" switch.

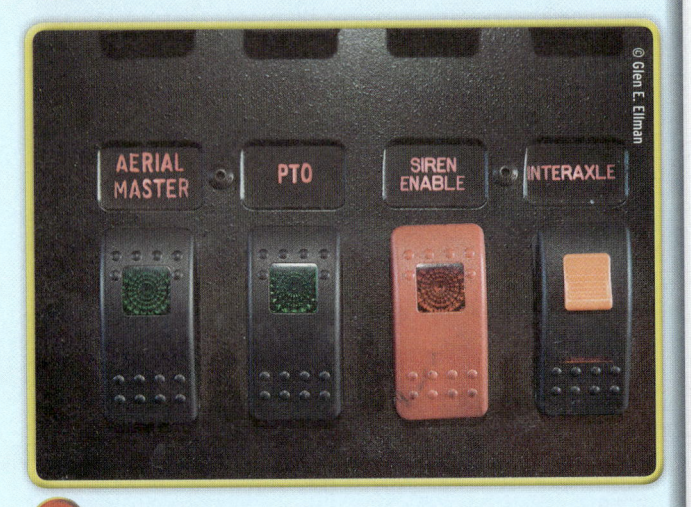

6. Ensure the "Hydraulic PTO engaged" light is off.

Wrap-Up

Chief Concepts

- As the driver/operator, securing a water source upon arrival at the scene is one of your primary responsibilities.
- Potential water sources include the internal water tank, a pressurized source, and a static source.
- Before you leave the fire station to respond to the scene, you should have a working knowledge of water sources at or close to the scene. This can be accomplished by using a map book with hydrant locations in it and by becoming familiar with water sources within the response area, including lakes, ponds, canals, and drafting hydrants.
- When your crew first arrives at the scene, you may initially need to supply attack lines from your onboard tank, but then have a supply line laid to your pump from another fire apparatus or via a hand-laid supply line.
- Once the pumping operation is under way, you must monitor specific gauges on the pump panel to ensure that an adequate supply of water or foam is available for the duration of the incident.
- Fixed apparatus systems include generators to power lights and equipment.
- Hydraulic systems may be powered by the apparatus or a separate power unit.

Hot Terms

actuator A device that converts the fluid pressure in a hydraulic rescue tool system into a mechanical force.

attack pumper An engine from which attack lines have been pulled.

automatic load management system A system designed to protect the electrical system from needless damage while maintaining the operation of essential devices.

changeover operation The process of transferring from use of the pumper's internal water tank to use of an external water source.

combination tool A powered rescue tool that is capable of at least spreading and cutting.

cutter A powered rescue tool with at least one movable blade that is used to cut, shear, or sever material.

extension ram A powered rescue tool with a piston or other type extender that generates extending forces or both extending and retracting forces.

floodlights Lights that project a more diffuse light over a wide area.

forward lay A method of laying a supply line where the line starts at the water source and ends at the attack pumper.

four-way hydrant valve A specialized type of valve that can be placed on a hydrant and is used in conjunction with a pumper to increase water pressure in relaying operations.

generator An engine-powered device that creates electricity.

hand lay A process in which the engine is positioned close to the fire scene and the driver/operator deploys the supply hose from the bed of the fire apparatus to the hydrant either alone or with very little assistance from other fire fighters.

high idle switch A switch that sets the apparatus engine to run at 900–1100 rpm.

hydraulic reservoir A container that stores hydraulic fluid until it is needed in the system.

inverter An appliance that converts 12-volt DC (direct current) from a vehicle's electrical system to 110-volt AC power.

junction box A device that attaches to an electrical cord to provide additional outlets.

load monitor A component designed to prevent any additional electrical loads from exceeding the apparatus electrical system's capabilities.

load sequencer A component that activates electrical loads in a specific order to prevent overloading the electrical system.

load shedding A component that deactivates unnecessary electrical loads in order of necessity and thereby prevents damage to the electrical system.

power rescue tool A tool that receives power from the power unit component and generates energy used to perform one or more of the following functions: spreading, lifting, holding, crushing, pulling, or cutting.

power rescue tool system The combination of a reservoir, fluid, power unit, enclosed system, and an actuator used to operate a power rescue tool.

power unit A prime mover and the principal power output device used to power a rescue tool.

reverse lay A method of laying a supply line in which the line starts at the attack pumper and ends at the water source.

split hose bed A hose bed arranged such that either one or two supply lines can be laid out.

Wrap-Up, continued

split hose lay A scenario in which the attack pumper lays a supply line from an intersection to the fire, and then the supply engine lays a supply line from the hose left by the attack pumper to the water source.

spotlights Lights that project a narrow concentrated beam of light.

spreader A powered rescue tool that has at least one movable arm that opens to move material.

References

National Fire Protection Association (NFPA) 1002, *Standard for Fire Apparatus Driver/Operator Professional Qualifications*. 2014. http://www.nfpa.org/codes-and-standards/document-information-pages?mode=code&code=1002. Accessed March 27, 2014.

National Fire Protection Association (NFPA) 1901, *Standard for Automotive Fire Apparatus*. 2009. http://www.nfpa.org/codes-and-standards/document-information-pages?mode=code&code=1901. Accessed April 9, 2014.

National Fire Protection Association (NFPA) 1936, *Powered Rescue Tools*. 2010. http://www.nfpa.org/codes-and-standards/document-information-pages?mode=code&code=1936. Accessed April 30, 2014.

DRIVER/OPERATOR
in action

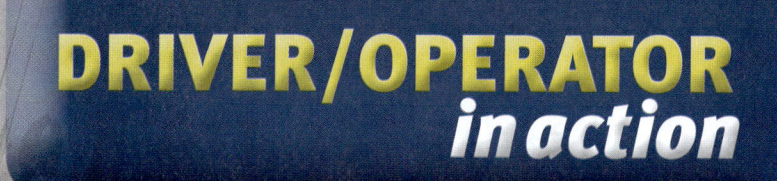

When you are flowing water from the onboard water tank, you have to react quickly. From the moment that you pull the discharge for the first attack line, you will be losing water from the onboard water tank. Your next objective is to obtain a sustainable water supply before the onboard water supply runs out. Achieving this goal is not as easy as it might seem at first glance. You need to be an expert on how the fire pumper works and how the water supply in the onboard tank should be managed. Test your expertise by answering the following questions.

1. When engaging the fire pump, you shift the transmission into the _____ position.
   A. neutral
   B. reverse
   C. drive
   D. first gear

2. Which type of hose lay starts at the fire scene and is laid to the water source?
   A. Forward lay
   B. Reverse lay
   C. Split lay
   D. Open lay

3. What is a "changeover operation"?
   A. Switching from the internal water tank supply to an external water source
   B. Switching from the external water source to the internal water tank
   C. Switching from a hydrant to a drafting operation
   D. Switching from a drafting operation to a hydrant

4. Which component on fire apparatus is designed to deactivate unnecessary electrical loads in order of necessity, thereby preventing damage to the electrical system?
   A. Load sequencer
   B. High idle
   C. Load monitor
   D. Load shedding

5. In general, sprinkler systems should be fed at a pressure of _____ psi, unless more specific information is available.
   A. 75
   B. 100
   C. 150
   D. 175

Drafting and Water Shuttle Operations

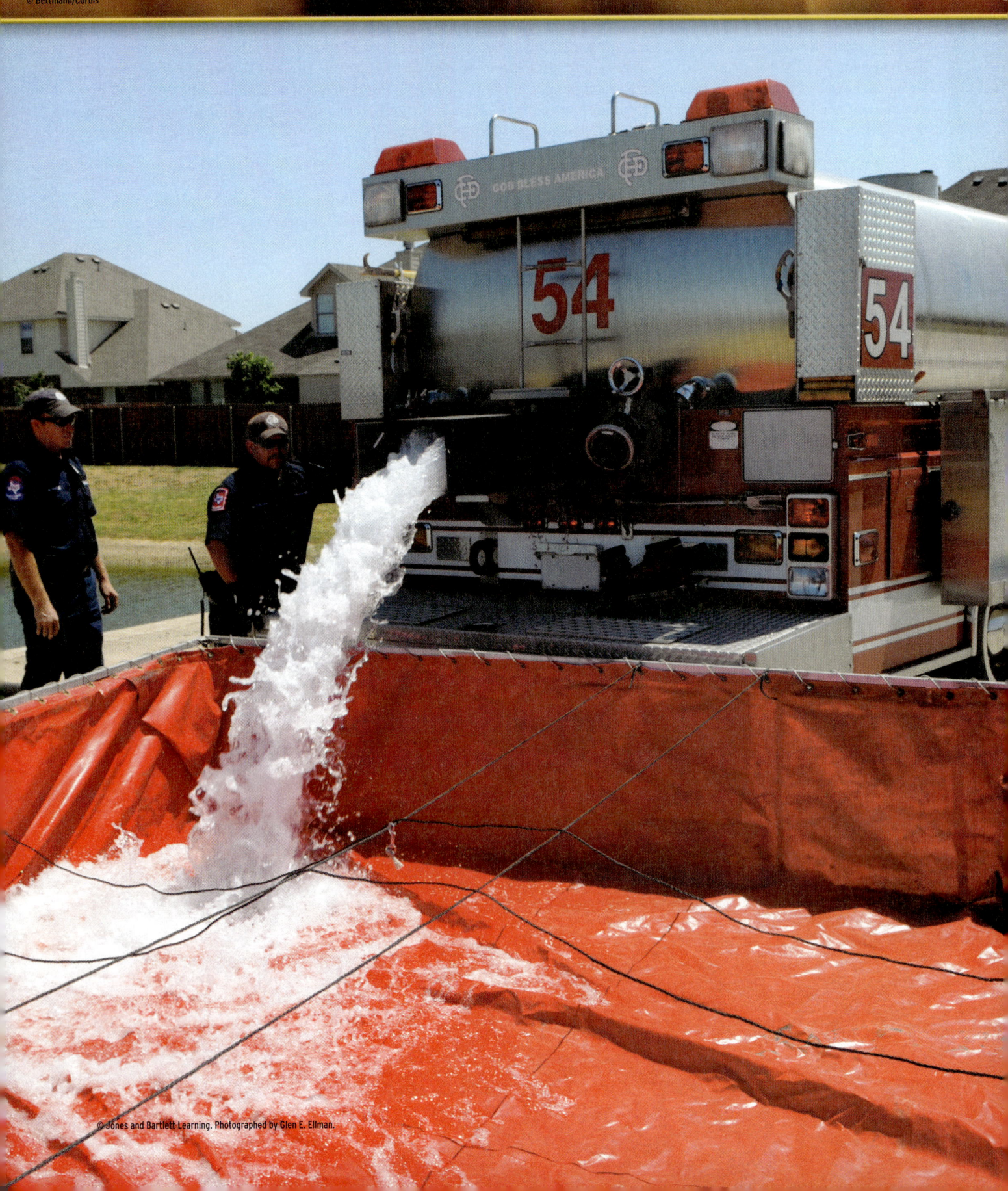

CHAPTER 12

Knowledge Objectives

After studying this chapter, you will be able to:

- Describe the mechanics of drafting. (NFPA 1002, 10.2.1, 10.2.1(A) ; p 280)
- Describe how to verify the operational readiness of the pump. (NFPA 1002, 10.2.1, 10.2.1(A) ; p 281–284)
- Describe water supply management within the Incident Management System. (p 284)
- Describe the process for selecting a suitable site for water drafting. (NFPA 1002, 10.2.1, 10.2.1(A) ; p 284–289)
- Describe how to position a fire pumper for drafting. (NFPA 1002, 10.2.1, 10.2.1(A), 10.2.2, 10.2.2(A) ; p 287–292)
- Describe the process for establishing a pumping operation from a draft. (NFPA 1002, 10.2.1, 10.2.1(A), 10.2.2, 10.2.2(A) ; p 289–293)
- Describe how to perform drafting operations. (NFPA 1002, 10.2.1, 10.2.1(A), 10.2.2, 10.2.2(A) ; p 293–295)
- Describe complications of drafting operations. (NFPA 1002, 10.2.1, 10.2.1(A), 10.2.2, 10.2.2(A) ; p 294, 296–297)
- Describe how to provide an uninterrupted water supply. (NFPA 1002, 10.2.1, 10.2.1(A), 10.2.2, 10.2.2(A) ; p 297)
- Describe water shuttle operations. (NFPA 1002, 10.2.1, 10.2.1(A), 10.2.2, 10.2.2(A) ; p 297–298, 300–302)
- Describe dump site operations. (NFPA 1002, 10.2.3, 10.2.3(A), 10.2.3(B) ; p 302–306)
- Describe water shuttle operations in the Incident Management System. (p 306–307)

Skills Objectives

After completing this chapter, you will be able to:

- Perform the vacuum test. (p 284–285)
- Position the hard suction hose into the water. (NFPA 1002, 10.2.1, 10.2.1(B), 10.2.2, 10.2.2(B) ; p 290–292)
- Draft from a static water source. (NFPA 1002, 10.2.1, 10.2.1(B), 10.2.2, 10.2.2(B) ; p 293–295)
- Provide water flow to handlines, master streams, and supply lines. (NFPA 1002, 10.2.1, 10.2.1(B), 10.2.2, 10.2.2(B) ; p 294, 296)

Additional NFPA Standards

- NFPA 1901, *Standard for Automotive Fire Apparatus*
- NFPA 1911, *Standard for the Inspection, Maintenance, Testing, and Retirement of In-Service Automotive Fire Apparatus*

You Are the Driver/Operator

You are the driver/operator of the second engine responding to an alarm for a structure fire located just outside of town. The first engine has arrived on the scene and is using its tank water to attack a single-story house fire. There is no one in the structure, and crews are commencing a defensive operation to protect exposures. The incident commander (IC) has assigned several water tenders to establish a water shuttle operation. The IC requests that you establish a fill site and draft from the large creek beside the road to supply the water tenders. The whole operation depends on your ability to establish a water supply from the creek: Are you ready?

1. How should you position the apparatus to draft from the creek?
2. How much water do you need to supply the water shuttle operation?
3. What are some of the problems you may encounter while performing this operation?

Introduction

At most fire incidents, a driver/operator pumps water from the tank onboard the fire apparatus or from a pressurized water source such as a fire hydrant or a relay supply line. In many rural fire areas and other emergency situations or disasters, however, the usual water supplies either are not available or are inadequate. The ability to **draft** water from a static source makes your fire apparatus a versatile resource. These occasions—when you are called upon to draft and supply an uninterrupted flow of water from a static water source—present some of the most challenging operating conditions that you and your fire pumper will face. Success in these conditions will be achieved if you make sure that the pump on your fire apparatus is in good operating condition, if you understand and apply the principles involved in drafting, and if you can deliver water to the incident from a static water source.

The Mechanics of Drafting

A closer look at the drafting process will reveal what is actually taking place during this operation. **Atmospheric pressure**, which is pressure created by the weight of the atmosphere, is 14.7 pounds per square inch (psi) (equivalent to 101 kilopascals [kPa]) at sea level. As you move up in elevation from sea level and the atmosphere thins or lessens, this supply pressure decreases: the pressure drops approximately 0.5 psi (3.45 kPa) for every 1000 ft (305 m) of elevation above sea level. The atmospheric pressure at your drafting site is the maximum supply pressure for drafting. Thus, if the atmospheric pressure at your drafting site is 14.1 psi (101 kPa), then the vacuum pressure required to draft will not exceed 14.1 psi (101 kPa). Essentially, without atmospheric pressure, you would not be able to draft.

When you engage the primer, you begin pumping air out of the fire pump. This process creates a **vacuum**, which is any pressure less than atmospheric pressure. A vacuum must be contained inside some type of airtight vessel (the hard-sided supply hose, for example); otherwise, air would simply rush in to refill the vacuum. As the vacuum increases inside the hose, the atmospheric pressure in the hose decreases, which results in greater pressure on the outside of the hose. This difference in pressure can be used to support a column of liquid.

Mercury was chosen as the liquid used to measure vacuum in the laboratory because its density makes it more convenient to use than water for this purpose. Thus, pressure is commonly measured in units of inches or millimeters of mercury (Hg). **TABLE 12-1** lists the conversion factors used to convert inches (mm) of Hg to feet (cm) of water or to pounds per square inch (psi) or kilopascals (kPa) of pressure.

A fire pumper must be able to develop a vacuum equal to about 22 inches Hg (507.8 mm Hg). This equates to the ability to lift water approximately 24.8 ft (7.5 m) at sea level. While it is possible to lift water 20 ft (6 m) or more, the discharge capacity of the fire pump is severely restricted due to the amount of vacuum being created on the supply side of the pump **FIGURE 12-1**. As you lift water to a greater height, more atmospheric pressure is required to support the weight of the water, which reduces the available pressure to move it. Stated simply, the higher you must lift the water, the less water you will be able to pump. **Dependable lift** is the height that a column of water can be lifted in a quantity considered sufficient to provide reliable fire flow; it is generally considered to be 15 ft (4.5 m).

The pumps found in fire apparatus have their capacity ratings established by pumping from a draft. For example, a pumper must lift water—10 ft (3 m) through 20 ft (6 m) of hard-sided supply hose for pumps up to 1500 gpm (5678 L/min), 8 ft (2.5 m) for pumps up to 1750 gpm (6624 L/min), and 6 ft (2 m) for pumps up to 2000 gpm (7570 L/min), and larger—and deliver its rated capacity at a discharge pressure of 150 psi (1000 kPa), as measured at the pump panel.

TABLE 12-1	Vacuum to Water Column and Pressure Conversions
U.S. Measurement System	
1 inch Hg = 1.13 ft of water	
1 inch Hg = 0.49 psi	
1 psi = 2.31 ft of water	
Metric System	
1 mm Hg = 1.36 cm of water	
1 mm Hg = 0.13 kPa	
1 kPa = 10.20 cm of water	

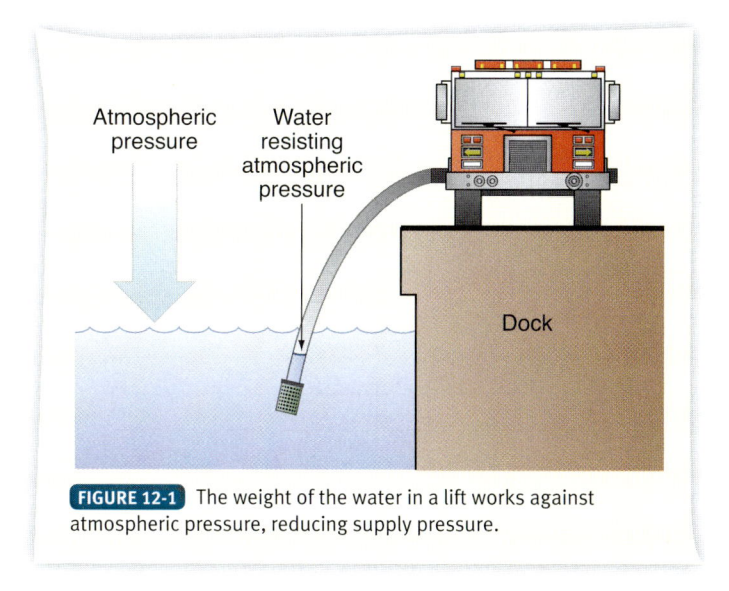

FIGURE 12-1 The weight of the water in a lift works against atmospheric pressure, reducing supply pressure.

Inspections, Routine Maintenance, and Operational Testing

Fire departments generally have a prescribed process for performing inspections, routine maintenance, and operational testing. In fact, many fire departments have created a written report form for this process **FIGURE 12-2**. Such a form is intended to help you perform the equipment inspection and operational testing in a consistent manner and to prevent items on the checklist from being missed. Fire apparatus inspection and routine maintenance are discussed fully in the chapter *Performing Pumper Check-Out and Maintenance*. Nevertheless, a few items on the checklist must be given special attention to ensure the operational readiness of the fire apparatus for drafting from a static water source. For example, you need to check the operational readiness of the priming system and the overall condition of the fire pump on your fire apparatus on a periodic basis.

■ Inspecting the Priming System

Priming is the process of removing air from a fire pump and replacing it with water. The priming pump is a positive-displacement pump used to remove the air from the fire pump during priming. This pump must be lubricated and sealed as it turns if it is to efficiently pump air **FIGURE 12-3**. The primer oil reservoir is a small tank that holds the lubricant for the priming pump. It is generally located slightly higher than the pump and often is enclosed behind an access panel on the side or the top of a fire apparatus. Be sure to check the level of oil in the primer oil reservoir **FIGURE 12-4**. If the priming pump runs out of lubricating oil, you will not be able to prime the pump. You may also severely damage the priming pump by running it without lubrication. Refill the reservoir to the full mark if needed, using the correct type and weight of oil recommended by the manufacturer.

When you check the primer oil level in the reservoir, you should also confirm that the anti-siphon hole is not clogged. This very small hole is found in the fitting on top of the primer oil reservoir or in the top of a loop in the lubrication line leading to the priming pump **FIGURE 12-5**. If the anti-siphon hole becomes plugged, air will not be able to enter the lubrication line following operation of the priming pump. This can cause the oil in the primer reservoir to continue to be siphoned into the priming pump even after the priming pump stops running. The excessive flow of oil may create an oil spill on the floor of the fire apparatus bay, which can present a serious safety hazard. It will also drain the primer oil reservoir, which may result in no oil being available the next time you attempt to prime the pump.

Next, you will need to check the operation of the primer valve. It is located on the pump panel and is usually labeled "Primer" **FIGURE 12-6**. The apparatus should be running to develop full potential (voltage and amperage). The primer should not be operated off of the batteries alone. Pull out on the primer valve handle firmly until it stops, and hold it in that position for several seconds—30 seconds maximum on a 1000 gpm (3785 L/min) pump and 45 seconds maximum over 1000 gpm rating (3785 L/min) pump. You should hear a whirring sound and see a small amount of water discharged onto the floor under the fire apparatus (if the pump is primed). Return the valve handle to its closed position. The valve should move freely and the primer motor should start and stop as you move the valve handle out and back in.

DRIVER/OPERATOR Tip

Primers have evolved from the electric rotary vane, through the oil-less phase, to the Venturi-style air primers. The original primer used an electric starter-style motor to drive a rotary vane pump that was used to evacuate the air from the pump and allow atmospheric pressure to get the water to the pump. The pump required an oil reservoir that lubed the vanes of the primer pump and created a seal. The exhaust of the primer was a mixture of frothy oil and water that became an environmental problem, necessitating a better solution. The "oil-less" primer was a hybrid of the original that had closer tolerances and worked essentially the same way as the oil primer without the oily spill at every incident. The electric oil-less primer was still a severe electrical draw when operating, however, and had a limited run time as well as an adverse effect on some of the new electronic systems in the Environmental Protection Agency (EPA)-compliant engines.

The answer was to use an air-operated Venturi-style primer very similar to the foam eductor. Air from the chassis' compressed air system for the brakes was used. The primer is set up to have air blow through a Venturi-style primer with the pump primer port open, allowing the primer air to act as a suction for the main pump. The suction from the air pump blowing through the air primer decreases the atmospheric pressure inside the pump and facilitates lift. The engine is running, so the air supply is practically limitless. The system will not overheat or cause other problems to the engine, because it does not consume electricity needed for other systems. An additional advantage is that it does not have cavities for water, so it is not susceptible to freezing if any water is left in the primer. The air primer is also quieter, and the driver/operator does not have to worry about run times, electrical loads causing problems, or overheating the drive motor. Proven to be very reliable and efficient, this system may be installed on new apparatus or retrofitted for use on older ones.

DAILY ENGINE INSPECTION SHEET

Week of _____   Unit I.D. _____
                                         Shop # _____

Date:							
	Mon.	Tues.	Wed.	Thurs.	Fri.	Sat.	Sun.
Name:							
Knox box serial number							
Fuel level							
Motor oil							
Radiator							
Wipers							
Gauges							
Brakes							
Starter							
Lights/siren							
Generator							
Mirrors							
Body condition							
Water level							
Pump controls/gauges							
Press control device							
Hydrant tools							
Hose/nozzles							
Appliances							
Tools/ladders							
SCBA—PPE							
Radios							
Box-lights							
Map books/computer							
Keys							
Accountability							
Clipboard							
Tire pressure							
Batteries							
Transmission fluid							
Bleed air tanks							
Primer fluid							
Drain valves							
Tool box							
Power tools							

Comments:
_____
_____
_____
_____
_____
_____

FIGURE 12-2 The printed inspection form ensures that nothing is overlooked on your fire apparatus.

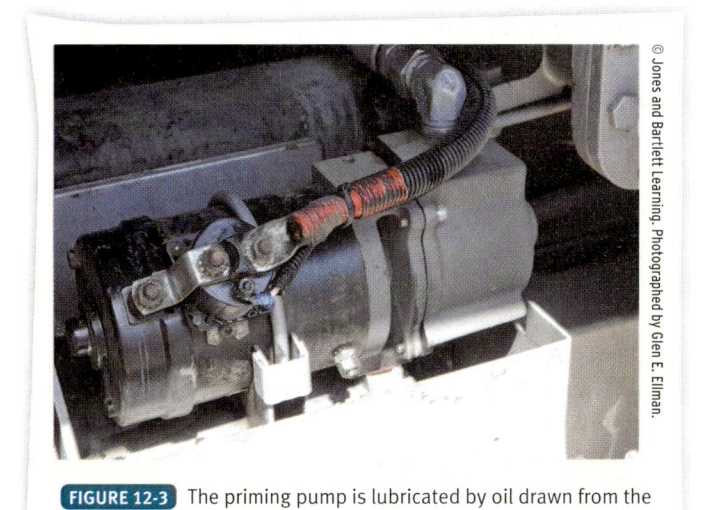

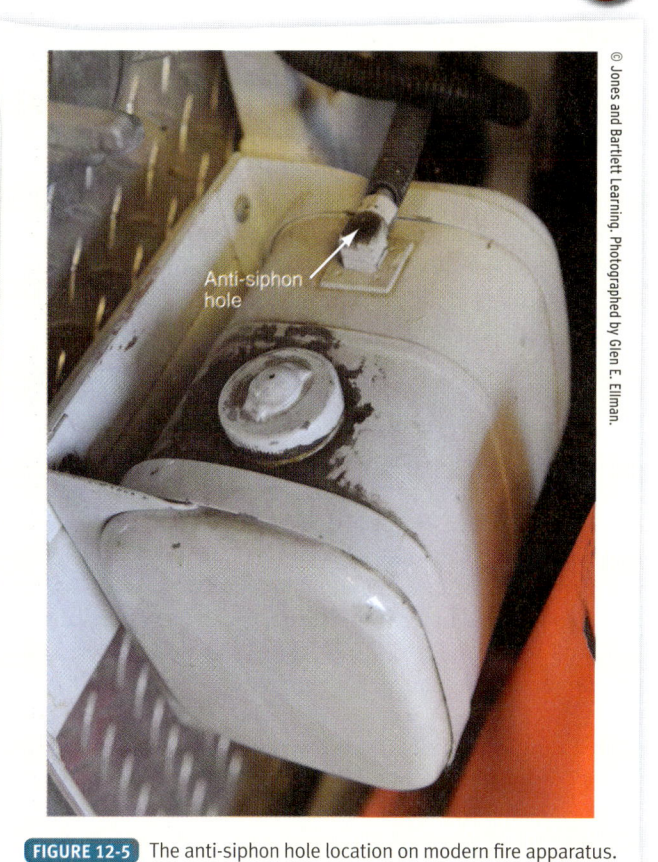

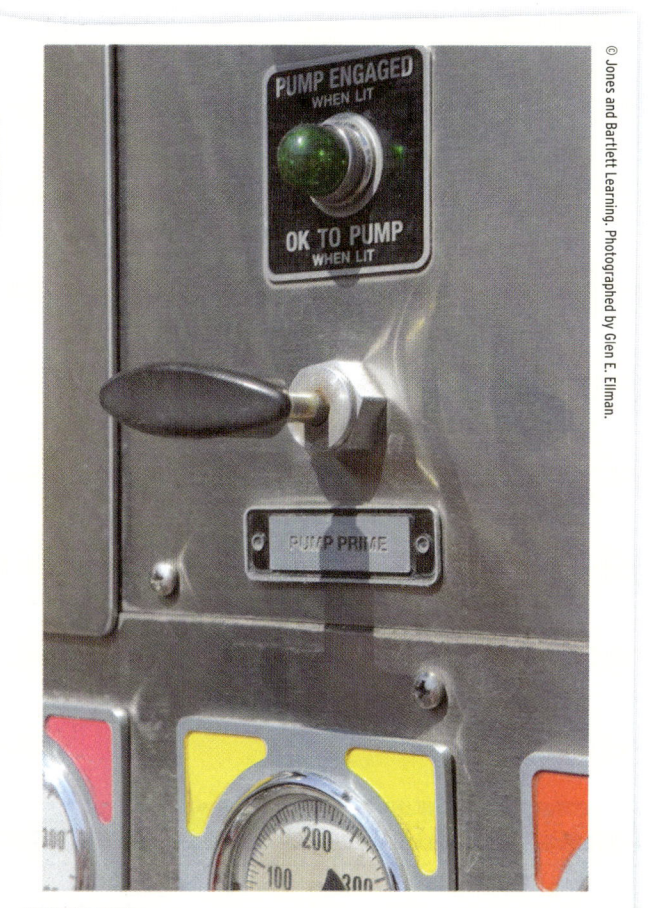

CHAPTER 12 Drafting and Water Shuttle Operations   283

FIGURE 12-3 The priming pump is lubricated by oil drawn from the primer oil reservoir.

FIGURE 12-5 The anti-siphon hole location on modern fire apparatus.

FIGURE 12-4 Check the primer oil reservoir for the proper oil level.

FIGURE 12-6 The primer control handle operates the priming pump and the primer valve at the same time.

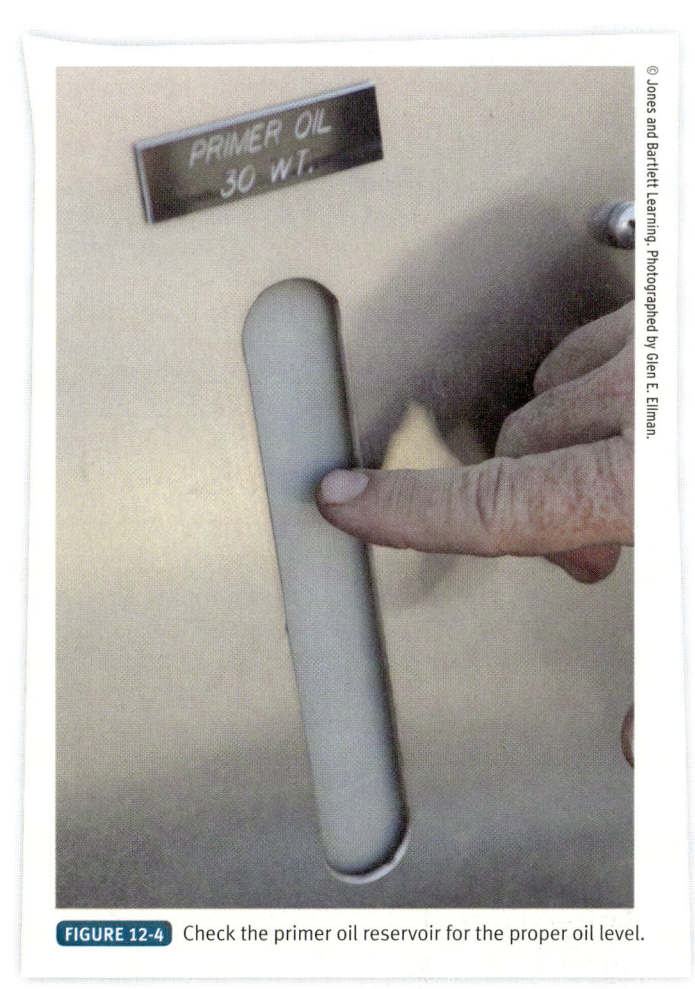

Safety Tip

Always chock the wheels of the fire apparatus when working around it.

Performing a Vacuum Test

The best way to assess the operational readiness of the priming system is to conduct a vacuum test periodically. This is part of annual pump testing and not part of a routine check performed by a driver/operator. To conduct this test, a separate calibrated gange set muct be used. This test also gives you a good indication of the general condition of the fire pump and all its valves and plumbing. National Fire Protection Association (NFPA) 1911, *Standard for the Inspection, Maintenance, Testing, and Retirement of In-Service Automative Fire Apparatus*, lists the very specific conditions for this test when it is performed for the certification of a new fire pump. While the most important of these conditions are presented here, it is not necessary to exactly replicate the certification test conditions during a periodic vacuum test.

Before performing the vacuum test, take the time to remove all discharge caps and drain the booster tank. Failure to do so may mask the effects of vacuum leaks due to worn or damaged valves in those components. Leaking valves and pump packings could effect your ability to draft and/or maintain maximum capacity white drafting.

Follow the steps in **SKILL DRILL 12-1** to perform the annual vacuum test on a pump:

1. Chock the wheels of the fire apparatus to prevent movement while you are working on it. (**STEP 1**)
2. Drain the water from the fire pump and the booster tank. (**STEP 2**)
3. Close all drains, discharge valves, intake valves, cooler lines, and any other possible sources of vacuum leaks. Place caps on all suction or external intake fittings. (**STEP 3**)
4. Remove the caps from all discharge fittings. (**STEP 4**)
5. Turn the battery isolation switch to the "on" position. It is not necessary to start the engine. (**STEP 5**)
6. Pull the primer control handle out firmly until it stops, and hold it in that position. This will engage the primer motor and open the primer valve. (**STEP 6**)
7. Continue to hold the primer control handle in the fully engaged position until the maximum vacuum is achieved (usually 15 to 20 seconds). You should see a vacuum reading of 22 inches Hg (560 mm Hg) on the supply master gauge on the pump panel. (**STEP 7**)
8. Return the primer control handle to the fully closed position. (**STEP 8**)
9. Record the vacuum reading from the supply master gauge on your inspection report form. Wait 5 minutes and record the reading again. The reading should not drop more than 10 inches Hg (250 mm Hg) in 5 minutes. If the reading drops excessively, you should note this fact on your inspection report form and have the fire apparatus scheduled for maintenance to repair the vacuum leak. (**STEP 9**)

DRIVER/OPERATOR Tip

Do not forget to refill the booster tank and prime the fire pump before placing the fire apparatus back in service!

Finding a Vacuum Leak

A fire pump that retains any vacuum for 5 minutes should prime and draft water easily in most situations. Vacuum leakage in excess of the amount specified by NFPA 1901, *Standard for Automotive Fire Apparatus*, may cause problems during the process of obtaining or maintaining a prime when you are attempting to lift water more than 10 ft (3 m), or when you are pumping a relatively small volume of water.

To find a suspected vacuum leak, place an EMS glove over the uncapped discharge and pull the primer. If the glove sucks in, there is a leak. If the driver/operator cannot verify the location of the leak, an evaluation must be performed by a qualified mechanic.

Water Supply Management in the Incident Management System

Water supply management is a vital part of any fire incident and can become a major part of the Incident Management System (IMS) in scenarios where a reliable public or private water system is not available. Drafting operations, relay pumping, water shuttles, and nurse tanker operations will become the responsibility of the water supply officer in these situations. The water supply officer position reports to the operations section chief and is responsible for ensuring that an adequate supply of water is available to mitigate the incident. In smaller incidents, if no operations section chief is designated, then this officer reports directly to the IC. Water supply officers should be given a priority on any scene, but particularly if a water shuttle is established. In those circumstances, both a dump site and a fill site will be incorporated into the IMS organization.

Selecting a Drafting Site

Ensuring that fire fighters have a steady supply of water is critical to the success and safety of the incident response. When drafting water is the chosen method for providing that supply, the reliability of the static water source becomes a primary consideration in the process of selecting an appropriate drafting site. Once this reliability has been established, operational requirements such as accessibility, purpose of the site, and positioning of the fire apparatus may influence site selection.

Determining the Reliability of Static Water Sources

It is very important to evaluate the reliability of a static water source before committing a fire pumper to draft from it. Failure to determine the reliability of a static water source can seriously affect your ability to support fireground operations and may even result in damage to the fire pumper. Several factors must be considered when you are determining the reliability of a static water source—namely, accessibility, quantity of water available, and quality of the water in the static water source.

SKILL DRILL 12-1 Performing an Annual Vacuum Test

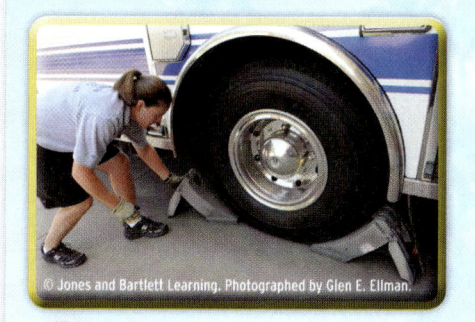

1 Chock the wheels.

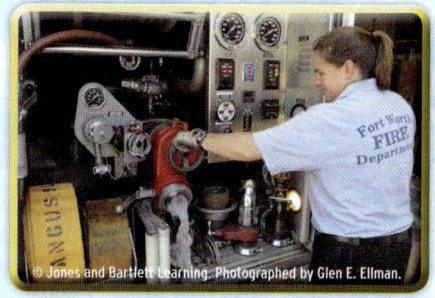

2 Drain the fire pump and booster tank.

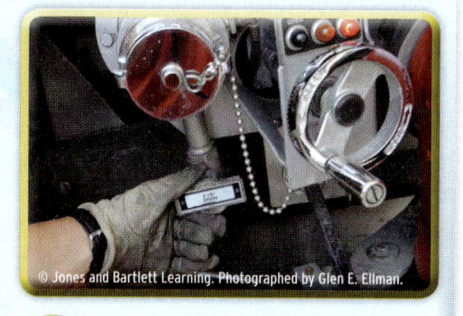

3 Close all drains, valves, and other possible vacuum leaks to isolate the fire pump.

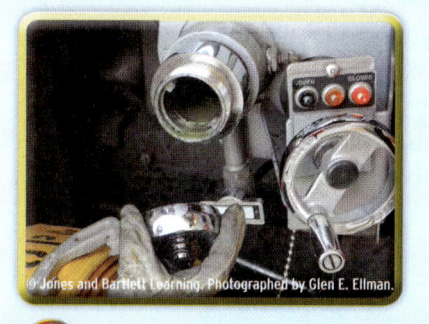

4 Remove the caps from all discharge fittings.

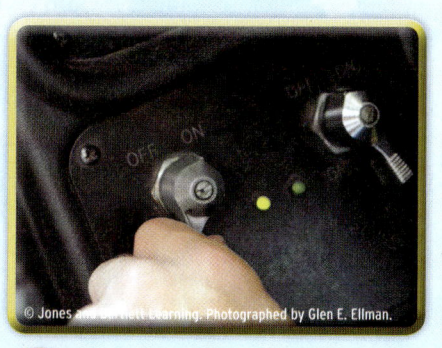

5 Turn the battery switch to the "on" position.

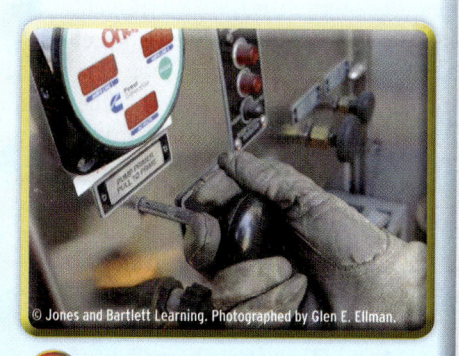

6 Firmly pull the primer control handle to the fully open position, and hold it in that position.

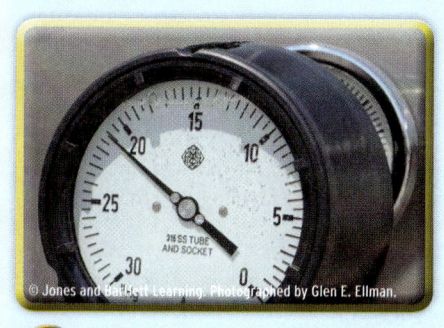

7 Continue to operate the priming pump until the maximum vacuum is achieved. The master supply gauge should show a reading of 22 inches Hg (560 mm Hg).

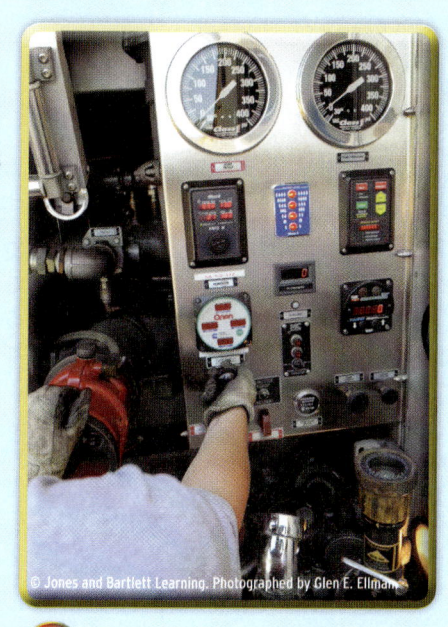

8 Close the primer control handle.

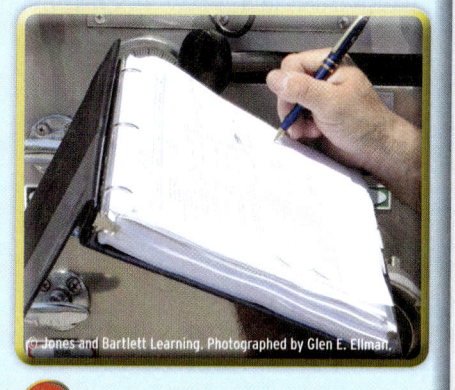

9 Record the vacuum reading from the master supply gauge, wait 5 minutes, and record the reading again. The vacuum should not drop more than 10 inches Hg (250 mm Hg). Report the excessive leakage by following your department's policy, because fire pump maintenance or repair is indicated.

© LiquidLibrary

Estimating the Quantity of Water Available

The first consideration in determining the reliability of a static water source is to estimate the quantity of water available. This should occur during preplanning and not while on scene. When considering a lake or large river for drafting purposes, there is usually no question that an adequate supply of water will be available. In contrast, smaller static sources such as small rivers, streams, cisterns, and ponds require careful evaluation. These supplies may also be affected more dramatically by seasonal fluctuations in stream flows. In your role as driver/operator, you must be able to calculate the estimated amount of water available in both moving and nonmoving water sources.

Calculating Available Water in a Nonmoving Source

To calculate the amount of water available in a nonmoving source, you must determine the dimensions of the pond, cistern, or swimming pool. The length, width, and depth must be known or estimated. Multiplying the length (L) times the width (W), times the depth (D), times a constant (C), yields the quantity of water (Q) that is available. The constant is 7.5 for the U.S. system of measurement, reflecting the fact that there are 7.48 gallons in 1 cubic foot of water. The constant is 1000 for the metric system of measurement, reflecting the fact that there are 1000 liters in 1 cubic meter of water.

Formula 1: Calculating Available Water in a Nonmoving Source (U.S. Measurement System)

$$Q = L \times W \times D \times C$$

where:

- Q = gallons of water available
- L = length of static source in feet
- W = width of static source in feet
- D = depth of static source in feet
- C = a constant, 7.5 (7.48 gal in 1 cubic foot of water)

Example

Calculate the amount of water available in a small pond that is 100 ft long and 80 ft wide. You estimate the depth of the pond to be 4 ft.

$$Q = L \times W \times D \times C$$
$$Q = 100 \text{ ft} \times 80 \text{ ft} \times 4 \text{ ft} \times 7.5$$
$$Q = 240{,}000 \text{ gal water available}$$

Formula 2: Calculating Available Water in a Nonmoving Source (Metric System)

$$Q = L \times W \times D \times C$$

where:

- Q = liters of water available
- L = length of static source in meters
- W = width of static source in meters
- D = depth of static source in meters
- C = a constant, 1000 (1000 L in 1 cubic meter of water)

Example

Calculate the amount of water available in a small pond that is 30 m long and 10 m wide. You estimate the depth of the pond to be 2 m.

$$Q = L \times W \times D \times C$$
$$Q = 30 \text{ m} \times 10 \text{ m} \times 2 \text{ m} \times 1000$$
$$Q = 600{,}000 \text{ L water available}$$

Calculating Available Water in a Moving Source

To calculate the amount of water available in a moving source, you must determine the dimensions of the stream, canal, or river. The width (W) and depth (D) must be known or estimated. Because this water source is moving, use velocity (V) in place of length in the formula. Velocity can be determined by measuring the distance the water travels in 1 minute. Multiplying the width (W) times the depth (D), times the velocity (V), times a constant (C), yields the quantity of water (Q) that is available. The constants are the same ones used in the previous examples.

Formula 3: Calculating Available Water in a Moving Source (U.S. Measurement System)

$$Q = W \times D \times V \times C$$

where:

- Q = gallons of water available
- W = width of source in feet
- D = depth of source in feet
- V = velocity (distance traveled in 1 minute) in feet
- C = a constant, 7.5 (7.48 gal in 1 cubic foot of water)

Example

Calculate the amount of water available in a stream that is 10 ft wide and 2 ft deep. The water is traveling 15 ft/min.

$$Q = W \times D \times V \times C$$
$$Q = 10 \text{ ft} \times 2 \text{ ft} \times 15 \text{ ft/min} \times 7.5$$
$$Q = 2250 \text{ gpm}$$

Formula 4: Calculating Available Water in a Moving Source (Metric System)

$$Q = W \times D \times V \times C$$

where:

- Q = liters of water available
- W = width of source in meters
- D = depth of source in meters
- V = velocity (distance traveled in 1 minute) in meters
- C = a constant, 1000 (1000 L in 1 cubic meter of water)

> ### Example
> Calculate the amount of water available in an irrigation ditch that is 2 m wide and 1 m deep. The water is traveling at a speed of 6 m/min.
>
> $$Q = W \times D \times V \times C$$
> $$Q = 2\,m \times 1\,m \times 6\,m/min \times 1000$$
> $$Q = 12{,}000\ L/min$$

Evaluating Water Quality of a Static Source

The next step in determining the reliability of a static water source is to consider the quality of the water in the static source. The water should be free of aquatic weeds, moss, algae, and other trash or debris. Whether it is floating or submerged, this type of foreign material tends to plug the strainer on the supply hose and hinder your ability to deliver a reliable water supply for firefighting operations **FIGURE 12-7**. Even small pieces of debris that may pass through the strainer can cause problems by plugging the nozzles on attack lines. Obviously, clean water is preferred over muddy or murky water, which contains sand or silt that can clog nozzles, damage the wear rings inside the pump, and even cause pump failure.

> #### DRIVER/OPERATOR Tip
> Always thoroughly flush and refill the fire pump and booster tank with clean water following any drafting operation. Leaving contaminated water in the pump can lead to a variety of maintenance problems, including premature pump failure.

Accessibility of the Static Water Source

You must be able to safely position your fire apparatus close enough to the water source to completely submerge the strainer of the hard-sided supply hose in the water once it is connected to the fire pump. Soil conditions and site-specific obstructions can affect your ability to get the fire apparatus close enough to the external water source to draft from it.

In preparing for drafting, you must check the soil near the edges of the water source, especially when it is a lake, river, or stream. Make sure that it is dry and solid enough to support the weight of the fire apparatus, especially for extended wet operations. Unstable soils and conditions may cause the vehicle to tip, slide, or roll over. If the soil is saturated, it may be too soft or muddy to support the fire apparatus. You must avoid driving a fire apparatus on soil in this condition because the vehicle will sink into the ground and may become stuck. This would render the fire apparatus unusable, causing a delay to the operation. In addition, a large tow truck may be required to free the fire apparatus, and the towing operation may itself damage components on the pump or the chassis.

> #### Safety Tip
> Be especially careful when considering driving a fire apparatus on a dirt-fill bank, levee, dike, or dam. These surfaces often appear to be firm and dry, but may hide a deeper layer of saturated soil. This layer of saturated soil may give way under the weight of a modern fire apparatus, causing the fire apparatus to slide or roll into the water.

Once you have determined that the soil will support your fire apparatus, you should identify a drafting site that is relatively level and free of trees, bushes, rocks, fences, and other obstructions that may limit access to the static water source. Obstructions not only limit your ability to access the site, but also create safety concerns. Rocks and other ground debris can cause trip hazards when you try to get through them to access the water. Operating on too steep of a slope can make the fire apparatus prone to shifting or rolling. It may also affect the cooling and lubrication systems of the fire apparatus, by robbing the engine of horsepower and possibly causing premature mechanical failures.

Obtaining access to static water sources can be especially difficult during winter weather conditions. Snow can hide possible hazardous conditions, so be careful as you approach the water. Ice covering the water presents an access problem and a potential life-safety situation. You may have to chop a hole in the ice with an axe, a chainsaw, or an ice auger to gain access to the water source. If a hole is needed in the ice to place the hard suction nose, then a second vent hole will also be needed. Always firmly tap or "sound" the ice carefully to determine whether it is safe to walk on. Never walk on ice without a personal flotation device and safety line unless you know for certain that the water is less than waist deep.

Special Accessibility Considerations

Drafting from a bridge is one possible solution to accessibility problems. You must be sure that the bridge is designed to support the weight of the fire apparatus, however. You should also

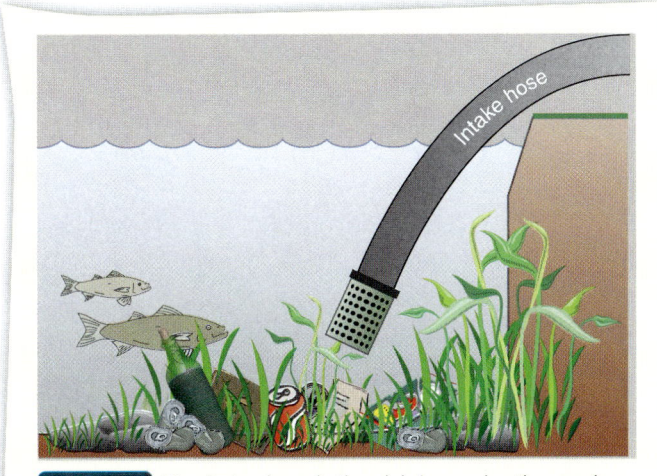

FIGURE 12-7 Weeds, trash, and other debris can clog the supply strainer and attack line nozzles.

evaluate the height of the <u>lift</u>—that is, the vertical distance from the water level to the center of the fire pumper. Lifting water more than 15 ft (4.5 m) is not practical for most fire pumpers. The effects of restricting or blocking traffic also should be considered, along with the obvious safety hazards for personnel and equipment when they are operating near moving traffic.

Clearly, it is a good idea to identify drafting sites during preplanning efforts rather than waiting for a fire to force you to find one in an emergency situation. Because determining water availability from both static and moving sources can be complicated, it is best to perform these calculations when you are not under the pressure of working in an actual emergency incident.

During preplanning, you will be able to determine which sources will and will not work for your operation. Problem areas can be identified and noted before the emergency operation, and predetermined drafting sites can be located. The fire department can improve these drafting sites by clearing obstructions and installing gravel or pavement, if necessary, to provide a solid surface on which to drive the fire apparatus.

The installation of dry hydrants should be considered in areas where access is difficult or when a location would make an ideal drafting site that could be used frequently. Dry hydrants can be required, in local fire prevention codes, to be installed by the property owner to provide quick access to static water supplies **FIGURE 12-8**. Once installed, their maintenance can be required as part of the code to ensure that they remain accessible and in good working condition. Otherwise, maintenance may be the responsibility of the fire department that installed them.

Consider placing **portable pumps** near static water sources whenever accessing these sources with a fire pumper is not possible. These pumps can deliver water through a hose to another spot that offers better accessibility for fire apparatus. For example, if a deep spring pond is located 20 ft (6 m) off the roadway but cannot be directly accessed by a vehicle, while not an ideal drafting option, multiple pumps may be used to supply larger volumes of water when needed.

Floating pumps may be used when the water is not deep enough to allow the use of conventional hard-sided drafting supply lines **FIGURE 12-9**. Floating pumps have intake ports and strainers that go below the surface of the water and do not draw air into the pump. The use and operation of portable and floating pumps are discussed in more detail later in this chapter.

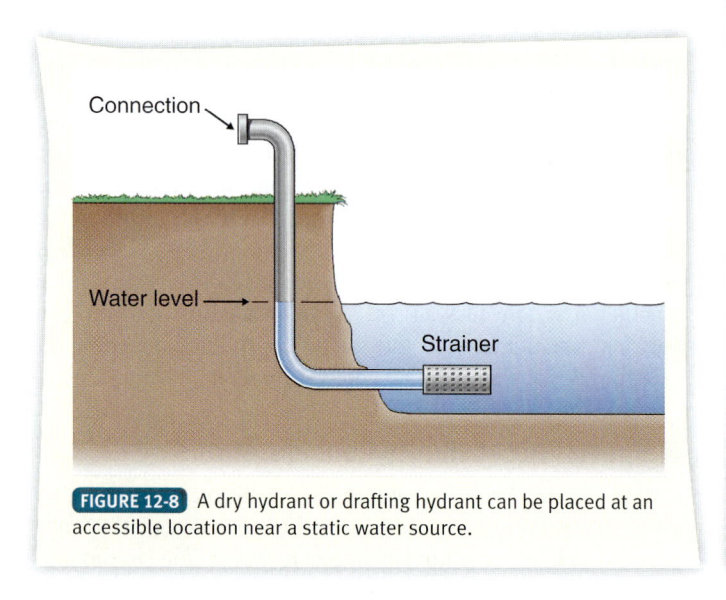

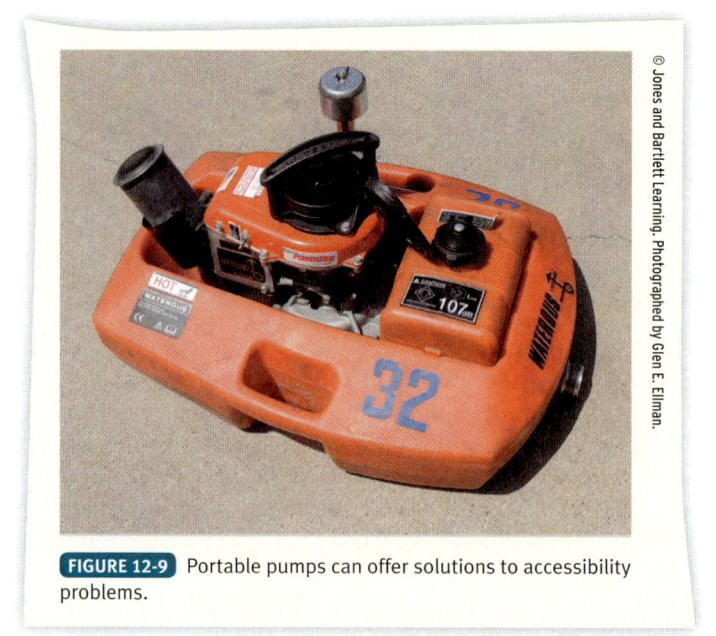

Another option for drafting from relatively shallow flowing water sources is to place a dam in the streambed **FIGURE 12-10**. You can use fallen trees, rocks, soil, a ladder wrapped in a salvage cover, or anything else that will block the flow of water in the flowing stream. This should be considered an option of last resort, because extreme caution must be used to ensure that the following conditions are met:

- The water source, once dammed, will provide adequate quantities of water.
- Creating a dam will not have a negative effect downstream.

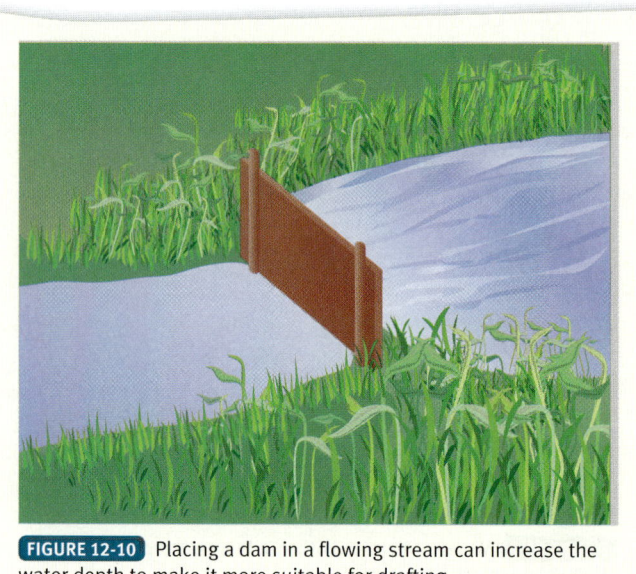

FIGURE 12-9 Portable pumps can offer solutions to accessibility problems.

FIGURE 12-8 A dry hydrant or drafting hydrant can be placed at an accessible location near a static water source.

FIGURE 12-10 Placing a dam in a flowing stream can increase the water depth to make it more suitable for drafting.

- The dam is strong enough to remain in place for the duration of the operation.
- Once the operation is completed, releasing the water will not have a negative effect downstream.

Operational Considerations for Site Selection

Whenever you have multiple, strong options for possible drafting sites, the best choice is determined by the location and the purpose of the drafting operation. If you are directly supplying water for firefighting operations that are nearby, then the closest available drafting site is usually the preferred option. Its use generally requires little coordination with other companies, but you must be mindful of fire apparatus movement in and out of the scene because hoselines will be extended from the pumper to the incident site.

As the distance from the incident increases, your water supply options become somewhat limited. You may have to consider other possible methods for obtaining water to supply your pumper. Consider a water shuttle, relay pumping, or a nurse tanker operation as a source for water. You may have to lay a supply line from an access point that can easily be extended from or connected to by another pumper without interfering with the operations of the incident. The other pumper(s) will finish establishing the supply line for you. In such cases, designating a water supply officer can be beneficial in coordinating the supply operation.

If your purpose for drafting is to supply a water shuttle or to be the source pumper in a relay pumping operation, operational considerations will apply to the site selection, in addition to the other considerations that have already been discussed. Try to select a drafting site whose use will not block access to the fireground for any additional equipment that may respond to the incident. It is also wise to select a drafting site that allows water tenders in a shuttle operation to be filled without having to back up or turn around. Ultimately, these water sources should be as close as possible to the incident to aid in the quick delivery of water and eventual fire extinguishment.

Pumping from a Draft

The next step in the process of obtaining a water supply from a static water source is establishing a pumping operation from a draft. Once you have found a suitable location with an adequate water source that is close enough to reach, you are ready to set up your pump to draft. This task requires teamwork, and you should be assisted by two or more fire fighters in completing it. Hard-sided supply hose (also called hard suction hose or suction hose) is heavy and can be very awkward to handle when fewer than two fire fighters are available. Becoming proficient in this skill through regular drills will help your company provide a water supply quickly, which may mean reduced property damage and saved lives.

Making the Connection

The first step in establishing a drafting operation is to locate an appropriate water source. If the location allows, you should place the fire apparatus in its final position before making any connections, while ensuring that you have adequate space to work around the pump panel and to connect the hose to the intake valve of the pump. If the space is limited, you may have to connect the hard suction hose away from the final position and then slowly move the fire apparatus with fire fighters carrying the hose as you advance toward your final position. This procedure can be very dangerous for the fire fighters as they walk alongside a moving fire apparatus and should not be the first choice for making suction hose connections.

> **Safety Tip**
>
> Be very careful when moving the fire apparatus into the final position for drafting. Fire fighters will be very close to the fire apparatus, carrying the heavy suction hose, and the footing may be very slippery. It is a good idea to have a spotter available to stop you at the first sign of a problem.

> **DRIVER/OPERATOR Tip**
>
> The pump transmission should not be engaged until after all hose connections have been made. Engaging the pump transmission and allowing a dry pump to rotate prior to priming may result in undue wear on the pump, which may lead to damage to the pump, seals, and bearings as a result of water not flowing.

Before any connections are made, the gaskets will need to be inspected for proper placement, cracks, and any debris that might affect your ability to create a vacuum and obtain a draft. Many times a hand-tight connection will be sufficient. Using a rubber mallet to tighten the connections, however, will provide a strong seal and ensure that they do not loosen when they are being moved around during placement. Regardless of the positioning constraints, the hard suction hose must be connected to the pump intake; in fact, it may take multiple sections to properly submerge the hose into the water.

Once you have determined the length of hose needed, place a strainer on the hose's end. The strainer will prevent large debris such as trash, rocks, weeds, small twigs, and animals/fish from entering the pump, which may cause pump failure and possibly permanent damage. It is important to ensure that the connection between the strainer and the hose is just as tight as the connection between the hard suction hose and the pump intake valve.

Three types of strainers are typically used for drafting operations, each with a specific function. The barrel strainer **FIGURE 12-11** is most commonly used for deep water sources in which you are confident that the strainer will not be able to contact the bottom of the source or large debris fields. Barrel strainers are cylindrically shaped, generally 10 inches (250 mm) to 16 inches (400 mm) long, and made of aluminum.

The low-level strainer **FIGURE 12-12** is designed for use in clean, shallow water sources. This square-shaped, flat strainer

FIGURE 12-11 The barrel strainer is used for deep water sources.

FIGURE 12-13 The floating strainer is used to prevent debris on the surface and from the bottom of the water source from entering the pump.

FIGURE 12-12 The low-level strainer is used primarily for drafting operations from a portable tank.

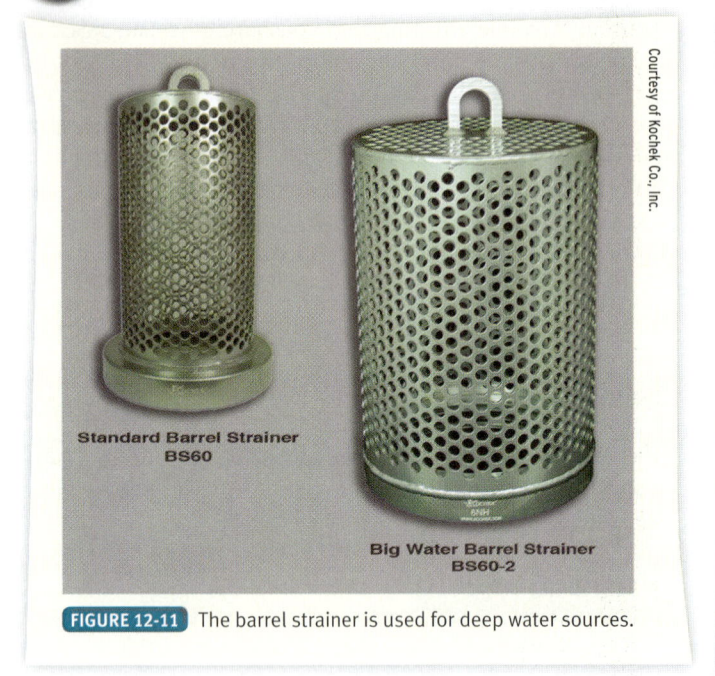

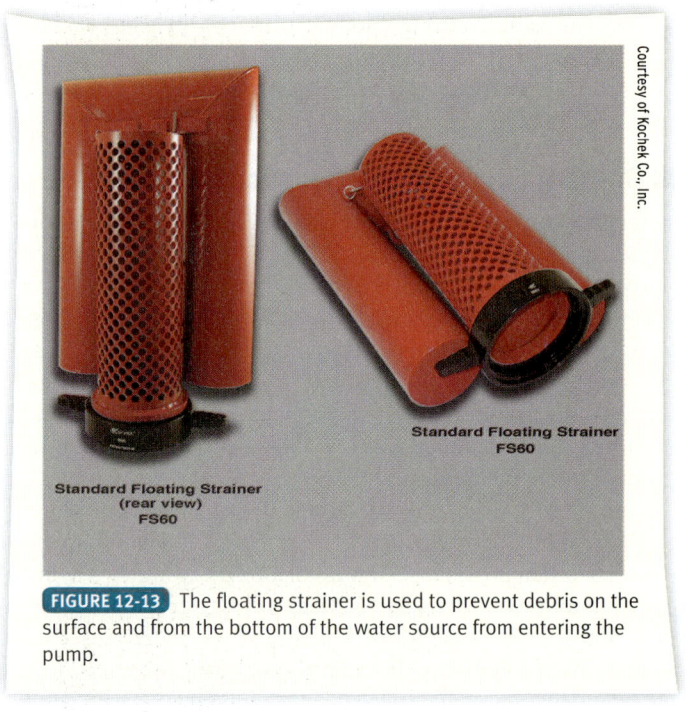

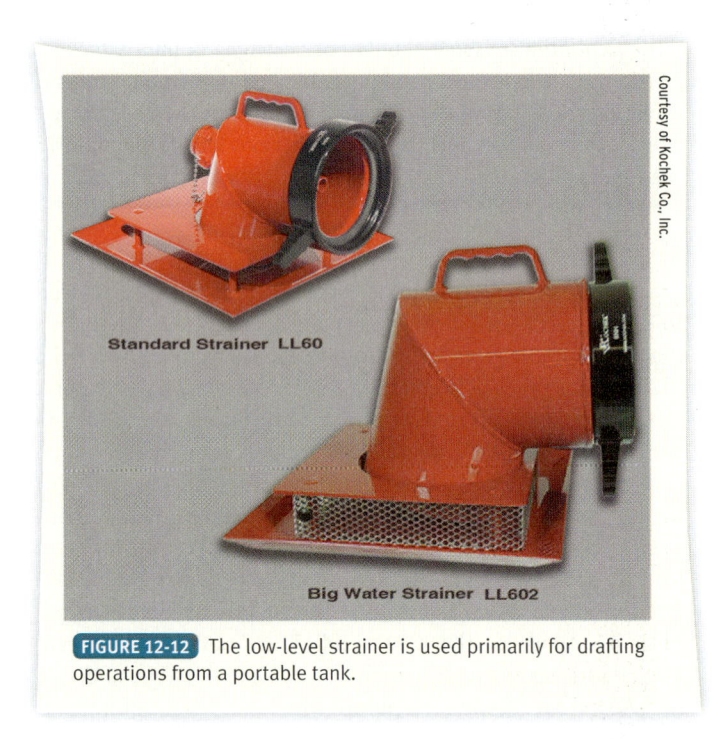

has an opening between two flat plates of aluminum, typically with a 2-inch (50-mm)-wide gap between the 16-inch (400-mm) plates on the top and bottom of the strainer. This device is generally considered a lower-flow strainer because the intake opening is slightly smaller than the diameter of the hose, so as to avoid creating a strong draft that can draw in debris. A low-level strainer is used primarily when drafting from portable tanks because the water is free from debris and the strainer can touch the bottom without fear of dirt or silt entering the pump.

The floating strainer **FIGURE 12-13** is designed to operate below the surface scum and above the weeds, dirt, and silt in the water source. This type of strainer is ideal for water sources in which the depth or the bottom quality is unknown. They may be made out of aluminum or polyethylene and contain a large, hollow chamber that allows them to float. As with the floating pump, the intake port is equipped with a strainer that is placed below the surface of the water and will not draw air into the pump.

Once all of the connections are made, you should be ready to place the hard suction hose and strainer into the water. Before doing so, however, you should tie a rope to the strainer to help you move the hose if that step becomes necessary once it is in the water, and to secure the hose once you start drafting water. Make sure that the strainer is completely immersed in the water so that air will not be drawn into the pump. When you are using a barrel strainer, there should be at least 24 inches (0.5 m) of water in all directions around the strainer. The low-level and floating strainers are designed to operate in shallow conditions and require only 24 inches (0.5 m) of water depth. You may wish to use a straight ground ladder to support the hard suction hose as it enters the water and to keep it off the shore line **FIGURE 12-14**. If you are drafting from a moving water source, you can use a straight ground ladder to weave the strainer over and under two rungs to prevent it from drifting along with the current of the water **FIGURE 12-15**.

Now that you have the connections made and the strainer securely placed, you are ready to begin the drafting operation. Follow the steps in **SKILL DRILL 12-2** to position the hard suction hose in the water:

1. Stop the fire apparatus just short of where you expect to draft from. Leave plenty of room to connect the suction hoses first together and then to the fire pump. Remember that these hoses are heavy and do not bend very easily, so allow enough room for your hose team to work. (**STEP 1**)

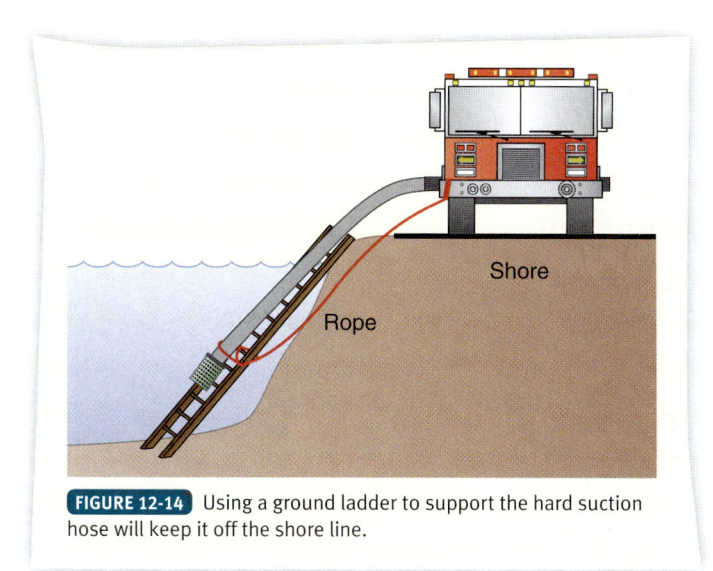

FIGURE 12-14 Using a ground ladder to support the hard suction hose will keep it off the shore line.

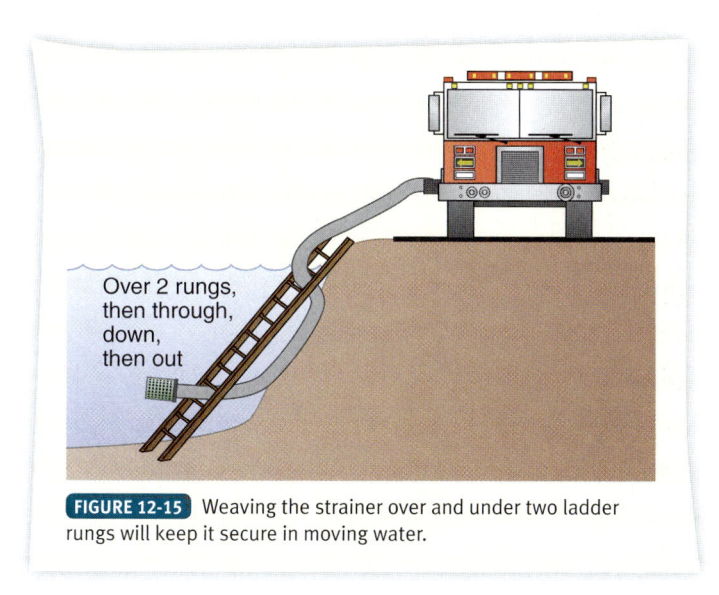

FIGURE 12-15 Weaving the strainer over and under two ladder rungs will keep it secure in moving water.

2. Inspect the gasket in the female coupling for damage or debris. The gasket should be pliable enough to make an airtight seal. (**STEP 2**)
3. Connect the sections of suction hose together and install the strainer on the end that is placed in the water. The couplings should be made tightened as much as possible by hand and then tightened slightly more by striking the tightening lugs smartly two or three times with a rubber hammer. This action ensures an airtight seal, and it prevents the couplings from working loose as the hoses are moved into position. Do not overtighten the connections, as this can cut the gasket in the coupling, causing an air leak and preventing you from priming the fire pump. (**STEP 3**)
4. Connect the suction hose to the fire pump. If necessary, connect the suction hose assembly and prepare for advancement. (**STEP 4**)
5. Advance the suction hose assembly while moving the fire apparatus into position. Use extreme caution when operating around moving fire apparatus. (**STEP 5**)
6. Once the fire apparatus is in its finishing position, set the parking brake and chock the wheels. (**STEP 6**)
7. Ensure that the strainer assembly does not touch the bottom of the water source. There should be 24 inches (0.61 m) of water in all directions around the strainer for drafting. (**STEP 7**)
8. The suction hose assembly is ready to draft. Engage the pump at this time (**STEP 8**)

DRIVER/OPERATOR Tip

Some situations may require ingenuity on your part to create a solution that will allow you to draft successfully. For example, in shallow water you may need to dig a hole in the bottom of the static water source or dam up the stream with a ladder and a tarp to provide sufficient water depth for drafting. Securely fastening a scoop shovel, pointed downward, underneath the strainer will prevent it from lying directly on the bottom of the static water source.

Preparing to Operate at Draft by Priming the Pump

The first step in preparing to draft from a water source is to find the water source. Then, once the suction hose has been connected and placed into the water source, air is drawn from the pump using the priming pump. Activation of the priming pump lowers the atmospheric pressure within the fire pump, making it lower than the outside atmospheric pressure. The two pressures will try to equalize, and water will be drawn into the pump. The atmospheric pressure outside the pump presses down on the water source, which in turn causes water to rise inside the hard suction supply hose and replace the air being pumped out. This process continues until all of the air is removed from the pump and replaced with water.

The steps involved in priming a fire pump are very similar to those used to test the priming pump or conduct a vacuum test. Before you begin, ensure that all of the drains and valves are closed. This will prevent air from entering the pump while you are trying to remove the air already in it. Depending on the apparatus, firmly pull (or push if it is an air primer) the priming pump handle out until it stops and hold it out; you will hear a loud whirring sound as the air is pumped out. Water and air will also be discharged under the fire apparatus as the residual water in the pump mixes with the air being pumped out. As you hold the handle out, a vacuum reading will appear on the supply master gauge, indicating that a draft is starting. More water will start to flow out of the priming pump and be discharged under the apparatus when the air is pumped out. Do not stop operating the priming pump until you note pressure on the discharge side; at that point, you can slightly advance the throttle. Care should be taken however to not operate the primer longer than 30 or 45 seconds.

SKILL DRILL 12-2

Positioning the Fire Apparatus for Drafting Operations
NFPA 1002, 10.2.1, 10.2.1(B), 10.2.2, 10.2.2(B)

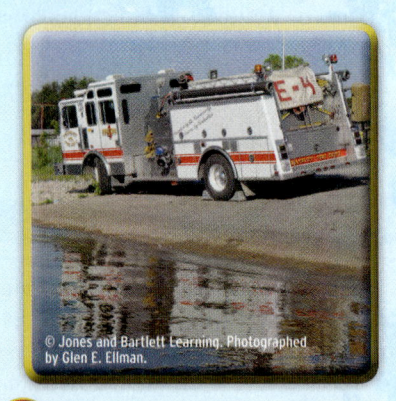

1. Allow plenty of room at the draft site to connect the suction hoses.

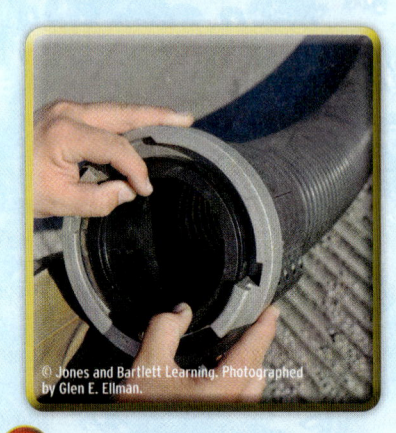

2. Inspect the gasket.

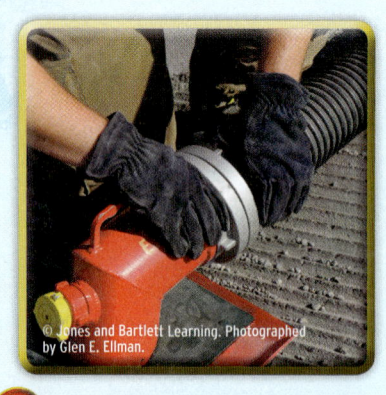

3. Assemble the suction hose and strainer.

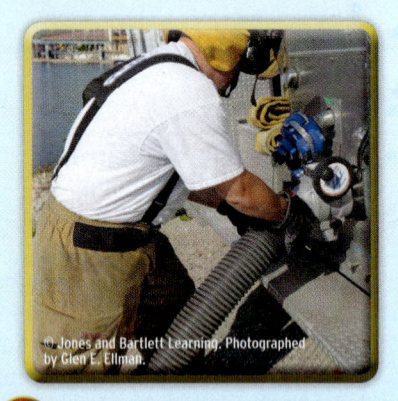

4. Connect the suction hose to the fire pump. Connect the suction hose assembly and prepare for advancement if necessary.

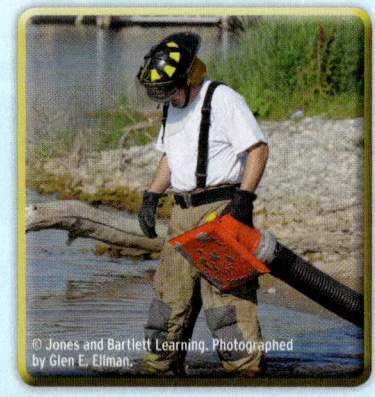

5. Advance the suction hose assembly while moving the fire apparatus into position. Use extreme caution when operating around moving fire apparatus.

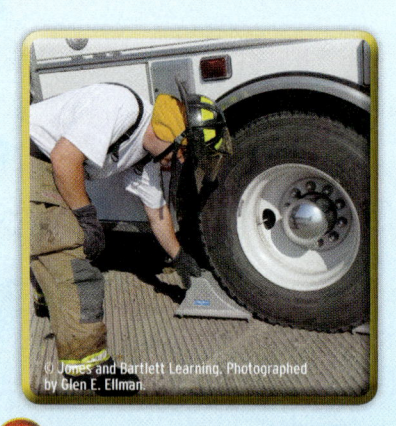

6. Once the fire apparatus is in its final position, set the parking brake and chock the wheels.

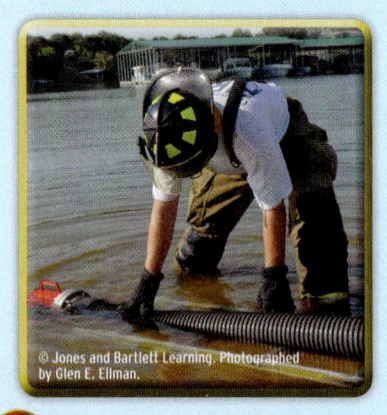

7. Ensure that the strainer assembly does not touch the bottom of the water source. There should be at least 24 inches (0.5 m) of water in all directions around the strainer for drafting.

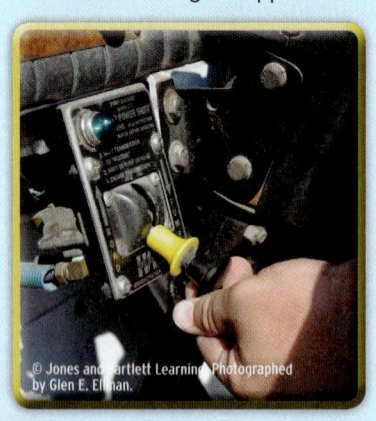

8. The suction hose assembly is ready to draft. Engage the pump at this time.

DRIVER/OPERATOR Tip

Most modern fire apparatus in use today are equipped with single-stage pumps. If you are drafting with a two-stage pump, it is recommended that you switch to the "volume" or "parallel" stage before you begin any drafting operation. This will allow the priming pump to completely evacuate all of the air that may become trapped in the "pressure" or "series" stage.

DRIVER/OPERATOR Tip

If you must flow water onto the ground, make sure you discharge the water far enough away from the fire apparatus and drafting site that it will not saturate the soil under the fire apparatus. Otherwise, the instability of the ground may cause the fire apparatus to sink, slide, or tip over.

Drafting Operations

Once you have primed the pump, you are ready to start drafting water and producing discharge pressures **FIGURE 12-16**. Before you start supplying water to handlines, master streams, or a relay pumping operation, you will need to establish a dump line. A **dump line** is a small-diameter hoseline (booster line, 1¾-inch [45-mm] hose, or 1½-inch [38-mm] hose) that remains in the open position and continues flowing water during the entire drafting operation. This line will help to maintain the draft even if your discharge pressures are low because it is constantly flowing water that has been drafted from the water source to start the flow of water. Slowly open the corresponding discharge valve for the dump line and begin flowing water. If you open this valve too fast, you may cause a loss of vacuum and break the draft of the pump. You may have to slightly increase the engine speed (rpm) to maintain the draft.

The water from the dump line should be discharged back into the water source, away from the strainer, to avoid introducing air into the hard suction hose; an inflow of air may lead to loss of the vacuum and end the pump's draft. If you cannot discharge the dump line back into the water source, you will have to discharge the water onto the ground, away from your drafting site. Always check and follow your department's standard operating procedures/standard operating guidelines (SOPs/SOGs) for establishing a dump line. Some departments, especially if you are in a location where water sources are in short supply, recommend discharging the water back into your tank, thereby not wasting any water on the ground.

Once a sustained stream of water flows through the dump line, you can begin to attach the hoselines that you will be supplying; these lines may differ depending on the purpose of your drafting operation. Your operation will go faster if other crew members can make these connections while you are establishing the draft and dump line. Once water is flowing from the dump line and the lines being supplied are attached, you are ready to increase the amount of water that will flow.

To provide water to the operation or to master streams and handlines from a static water source, follow the steps in **SKILL DRILL 12-3**:

1. Prepare the pump for drafting. Close all discharge valves and cap any suction fittings not being used.
2. Close all drain valves and tank valves.
3. Close the auxiliary cooler line.
4. Move the transfer valve to the "volume," "parallel," or "capacity" position if the pump is a two-stage pump.
5. Always provide water to the fire first, then establish a dump line. This line will be used to flow a small amount of water to cool the pump while you are drafting but not otherwise flowing water. Make sure the water from this line will not run under the fire apparatus, as it may soften the ground and cause the fire apparatus to sink. (**STEP 1**)
6. Place the pump in gear by following the pump manufacturer's recommended procedure. Depending on your specific apparatus, confirm that the pump is correctly engaged by checking the shift indicator light or checking the reading on the speedometer.
7. Engage the shift lock mechanism (if the pump is equipped with one). (**STEP 2**)
8. Prime the pump. Advance the hand throttle to the manufacturer's recommended setting (generally 1200 to 1500 rpm).
9. Pull (or push, depending on the apparatus) the primer control handle out firmly until it stops, and hold it in that position. You will hear a loud whirring sound as the priming pump begins pumping air from the fire pump.
10. Notice that the suction hose begin to settle as it fills with water and gets heavier.
11. Look at the master supply gauge on the pump panel, which should begin to show a pressure reading on the negative side of zero. This measurement, which is

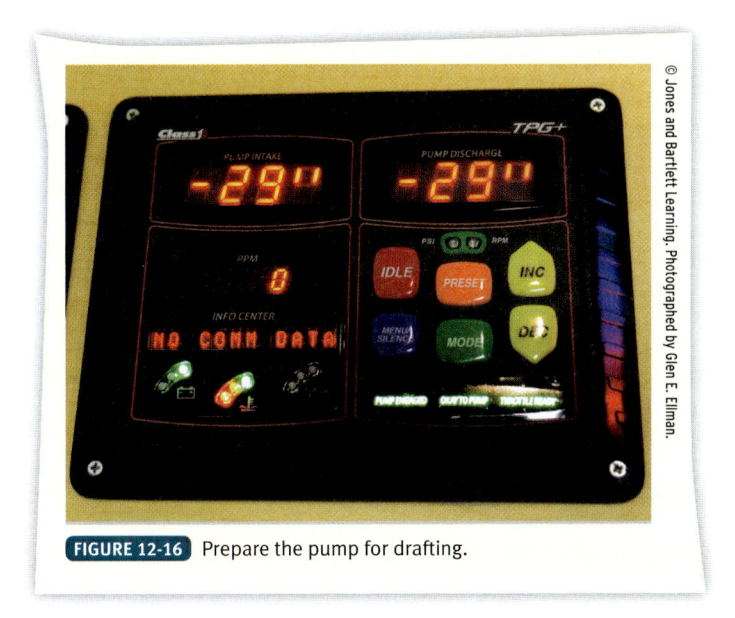

FIGURE 12-16 Prepare the pump for drafting.

given in inches (or millimeters) of mercury, is another indication that the priming pump is developing a vacuum within the fire pump.

12. Continue holding the primer control handle in the fully engaged position (30–40 seconds) until the whirring sound changes to a gurgling sound, and you see water being discharged from the priming pump onto the ground. You should also see some indication on the master discharge gauge of pressure being developed by the fire pump.

13. Push the primer control handle all the way in to the fully closed position (30–40 seconds). The fire pump is now primed and ready to begin delivering water. (**STEP 3**)

Note: Some manufacturers recommend priming the fire pump before placing the pump into gear. This step is taken because some newer pumps have a mechanical seal on the pump shaft; this seal will not tolerate operating without water to cool and lubricate it. If you have this type of equipment, simply reverse the steps described here. The only difference is that you will not see a pressure indication on the master discharge gauge when the pump is primed because the fire pump is not turning; all other indicators will appear the same during the priming process. Always follow your department's SOPs and the manufacturer's recommendations for your specific apparatus.

14. Adjust the discharge pressure. Adjust the hand throttle or computer governor to obtain the desired discharge pressure.

15. Slowly open the discharge valve for the hoseline that is serving as the dump line. Opening the valve quickly may lead to a loss of the vacuum and cause the pump to lose draft.

16. Begin flowing a small amount of water back into the water source or tank through the dump line for pump cooling purposes. (**STEP 4**)

17. Begin the water delivery. The fire pump is now ready to begin delivering water to attack handlines, supply lines for an attack pumper, a relay pumping operation, a master stream appliance, a sprinkler system, or a standpipe system. You may begin supplying water according to your fire department's SOPs as soon as the hoses are connected and you receive the order to do so. (**STEP 5**)

Note: Operation of the fire pump from this point will be very similar to pumping operations utilizing a pressurized source. These pumping operations are covered in detail in Chapter 9, *Driving Fire Apparatus*. Be sure to continuously monitor the fire apparatus for potential problems during the drafting operation.

Producing the Flow of Water

Whether you are supplying attack lines or water for the fire attack pumper, make sure the crews know that you are ready to start flowing water before you open the discharge valve. This notification can be made over the radio, through face-to-face contact with the crew, or through hand signals as established by your department's SOPs.

Slowly open the corresponding discharge valve for the hoseline and begin flowing water. As with the dump line, if you open the hoseline too fast, you may cause a loss of vacuum and end the pump's draft. Continue to increase the throttle until you have reached the desired discharge pressure; then set the pressure relief valve or governor to prevent sudden spikes in pressure.

Once the draft has been accomplished, do not drop the draft until the operation is completed and either the water supply officer or the IC gives the order to do so. Establishing a drafting operation takes time, and the incident should not be left without a water supply unless directed through the incident command structure.

Following the steps in **SKILL DRILL 12-4** will help you provide the needed flow to handlines, master streams, and supply lines:

1. Ensure the receiving hoselines or pumpers are ready to receive water.
2. Slowly open the corresponding discharge valve for the hoseline and begin flowing water. If you open the valve too fast, you may cause a loss of vacuum and end the pump's draft. (**STEP 1**)
3. Increase the engine's speed (rpm) to maintain the draft and provide adequate discharge pressure. Open the discharge valve and increase the throttle simultaneously until you have reached the desired discharge pressure. (**STEP 2**)
4. Set the pressure-regulating mechanism by adjusting the pressure governor or the pressure relief valve after achieving the desired flow. (**STEP 3**)

Complications During Drafting Operations

You must be able to recognize some of the common problems that you may encounter while attempting to draft or during the operation itself. While you are operating on the shore of a static water source during an emergency incident is not the time to have to call in a mechanic to help diagnose a common problem. As a driver/operator, it is your responsibility to know what the problem is and how to correct it. This section highlights a few of the problems more commonly encountered during drafting operations and describes the actions needed to identify and correct them.

The driver/operator must continuously observe the intake pressure while drafting. If you see any drop in this pressure, check the strainer for the presence of debris. If you are flowing large volumes of water, you will be drafting large volumes of water from your water source—and this action may draw debris from areas that you did not see when you initially set up the operation.

SKILL DRILL 12-3

Drafting from a Static Water Source
NFPA 1002, 10.2.1, 10.2.1(B), 10.2.2, 10.2.2(B)

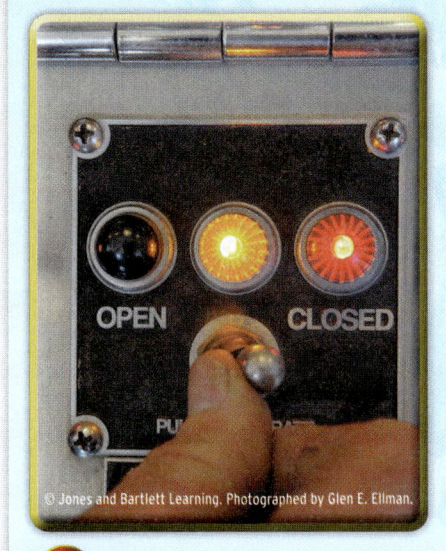

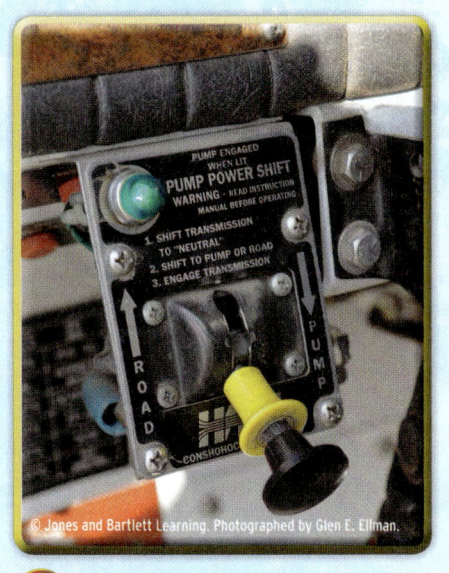

1 Prepare the pump for drafting.

2 Place the pump in gear.

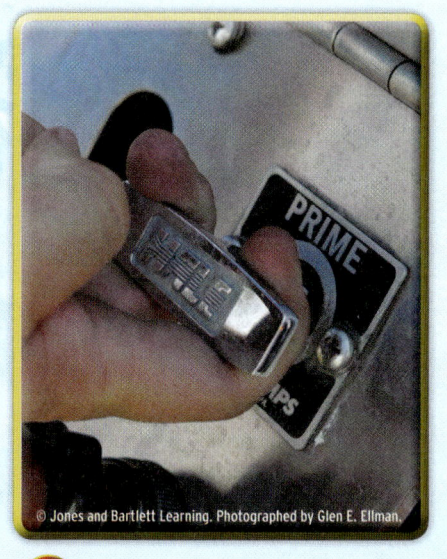

3 Prime the pump. (Note: Steps 2 and 3 may be reversed if the pump manufacturer recommends priming the pump prior to shifting it into pump gear.)

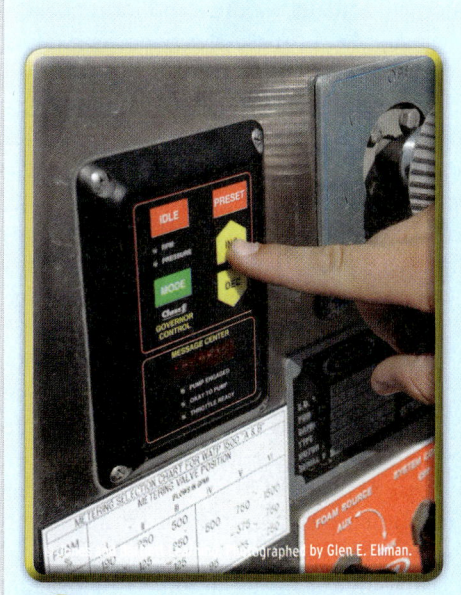

4 Adjust the discharge pressure.

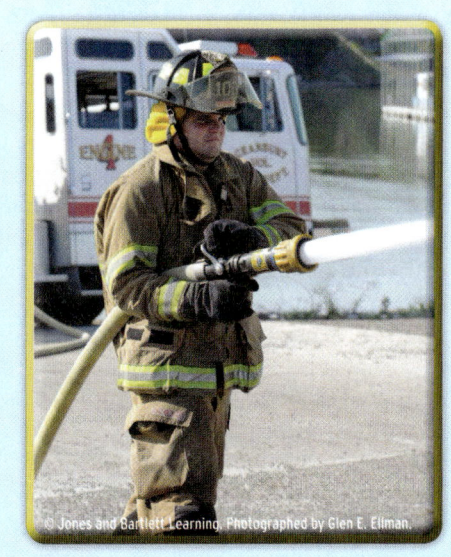

5 Begin the water delivery.

SKILL DRILL 12-4: Providing Water Flow for Handlines and Master Streams
NFPA 1002, 10.2.1, 10.2.1(B), 10.2.2, 10.2.2(B)

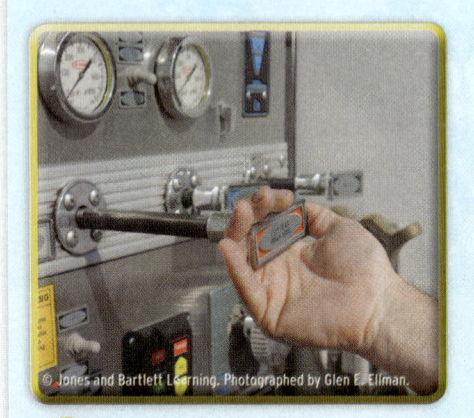

1. Ensure that hoselines or pumpers are ready for water. Open the corresponding discharge valve slowly.
2. Increase the engine's speed (rpm) to achieve desired pressure.
3. Set the pressure-regulating mechanism.

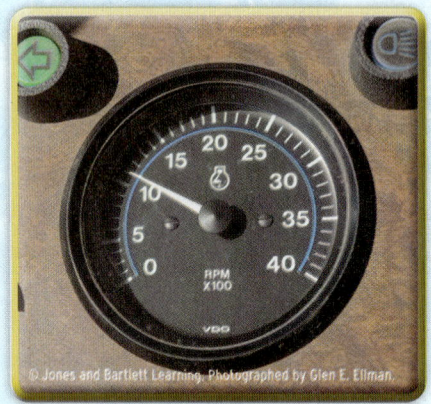

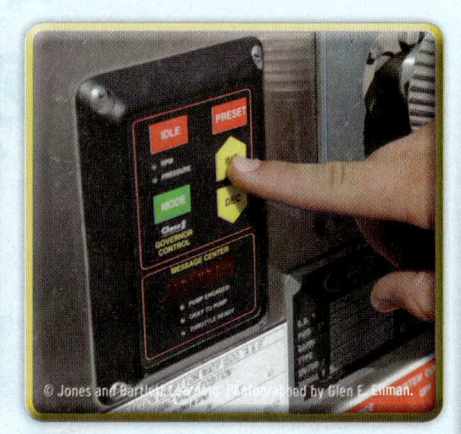

You must also continuously observe the engine and pump temperature gauges. Drafting operations require these components to work hard; sometimes, not enough water will flow to keep them cool. Remember, if you are simply supplying a dump line while you wait to fill a tanker shuttle operation, your flow will be less than 100 gpm (400 L/min). Open and close the cooling lines as recommended by your fire apparatus' manufacturer to prevent engine or pump overheating conditions.

If not enough water covers the strainer or if the draft is strong as a result of flowing large volumes of water, a whirlpool may form as a vacuum draws in water—just like in your kitchen sink when you release the stopper to drain the water. This whirlpool allows the pump to suck in air, which can break the vacuum and cause a loss of water supply. To avoid this problem, you can place an inflatable ball into the whirlpool, which acts to seal the whirlpool and prevent air from being sucked into the pump.

Another problem you may encounter during drafting operations is **cavitation**, which occurs when you attempt to flow water faster than it is being supplied to the pump. Cavitation during drafting operations is usually caused by a vacuum leak, which introduces air into the intake water supply. As the air flows through the pump, it creates small water hammers along its path through to the discharge point. Simply correcting the vacuum leak will correct the cavitation problem.

A more technical explanation of cavitation requires us to follow the path of water through the fire pump. As water is being drawn into the pump, the supply pressure is reduced owing to lift, friction loss, and/or flow restrictions. When the supply pressure is reduced to the point it registers as a vacuum, the boiling point of the water is reduced. When the boiling point is reduced sufficiently to match the ambient temperature of the water, the water will actually vaporize and form pockets of steam in the water supply. As these steam pockets travel through the pump to the discharge side, they are subjected to the discharge pressures; as a consequence, the steam pockets instantly collapse and re-form as water, creating a slight water hammer. The more severe the cavitation becomes, the more severe each water hammer will be.

Cavitation affects a fire pump's ability to deliver water and, if allowed to continue, can actually damage the pump. This problem is fairly easy to diagnose because it causes the discharge pressure reading on the pump panel to fluctuate significantly. Ultimately, the fluctuations become so severe that you cannot determine what the actual discharge pressure is. You will also hear a rattling noise that sounds like gravel is going through the pump. When a pump is cavitating, its discharge pressure does not respond to an increase in the throttle (rpm) as it does under normal operations. In fact, increasing the throttle setting during cavitation will make it worse.

If you suspect cavitation during a drafting operation, follow these steps:

1. **Check the water around the intake screen on the hard supply hose.** It has been our experience that a significant cause of cavitation is trying to discharge more water than what is being taken in. This problem occurs when a sufficient water level is not maintained above the intake. To alleviate this problem, lower the intake deeper into the water, construct a dam to back up the water in a stream, use a low-level strainer in portable drop tanks, or place a beach ball or similar round object in the whirlpool to stop it from introducing air in the supply intake.

2. **Check the vacuum reading on the master intake gauge.** This reading should indicate approximately 1 inch Hg (250 mm Hg) of pressure for each 1 foot of lift under normal operating conditions. If the vacuum reading is at or near normal, suspect that a vacuum leak is allowing air to enter the water supply, causing cavitation. If the vacuum reading is significantly higher than normal, suspect cavitation due to supply restrictions.
3. **If you have a near-normal vacuum reading**, check for vacuum leaks by confirming the tightness of all supply hose couplings. Next, recheck all valves at the pump panel. Also check the water level in the booster tank, and gradually refill the booster tank if it is not full. If signs of cavitation persist, there may be a problem requiring the fire apparatus to be taken out of service for repairs. It is possible to continue drafting in most cases even with a vacuum leak, if doing so is necessary to maintain support of fireground operations. The key is to keep water moving through the pump at all times, which prevents the accumulation of air in the pump housing and avoids loss of the vacuum (prime). You can accomplish this by flowing water through the dump line whenever you are not supplying water through your discharge lines. You need to advise your IC and your hose teams of the problem if you are supplying attack lines. Also, you need to advise the attack pumper if a relay operation is under way.
4. **If you have a higher than normal vacuum reading**, check the intake screen: The second leading cause of cavitation is a plugged intake screen. An obstruction will restrict the ability of water to enter into the intake hose and cause the vacuum on the supply side of the pump to increase. In such a case, you must clean the screen to allow the drafting operation to return to normal. If the screen is clean and the supply vacuum reading is still high, then confirm that the suction valve is fully open (if one is being used). If everything checks out and the vacuum reading is still high, try reducing the throttle slightly or gating down the discharges slightly; you are probably attempting to pump water faster than it can be supplied to the pump. You should notice an immediate improvement in the cavitation situation once the pump's discharge is lowered slightly.

Failure of the pump to prime is one of the most common problems that occurs during drafting operations. Many times the cause of this problem is driver/operator error—in many areas, pumping from draft is not a routine operation. Make sure that you are not the cause of the problem by double-checking the steps required for priming a pump. The fire pump on your fire apparatus should prime in 30 seconds or less in most cases.

Inability to prime the pump may be caused by any of several factors. Performing these diagnostic steps will help you identify the problem and quickly find a solution:

1. Note the vacuum reading on the master intake gauge after holding the primer valve fully open for 20 to 30 seconds.
2. If the vacuum reading is less than 12–15 inches Hg (310–380 mm Hg), recheck all valves on the pump control panel to verify that they are in the closed position. This includes the supply, discharge, recirculation, and drain valves. The only valve that should be open is the one to which the hard suction line is connected (if you are using a gated suction). Recheck the couplings on the hard suction line to make sure they are tight. Confirm that the suction strainer is completely submerged. Try priming the pump again. Often a worn tank-to-pump valve will be the source of a vacuum leak. If you can cover it with water, you can generally obtain a prime. Depending on your specific apparatus, you should also check the primer oil reservoir to make sure sufficient lubrication oil is available for the efficient operation of the priming pump. If you still cannot obtain a prime, you may have other vacuum leaks, or mechanical problems with the pump or the primer system. These problems are generally not correctable on the fireground and require that the fire apparatus be taken out of service for repairs.
3. If the vacuum reading is greater than 12–15 inches Hg (310–380 mm Hg), make sure the intake screen is clean and you are not attempting to lift water too high. You should not attempt to lift water more than 15 ft (4.5 m). Reposition the fire pump so the lift is 10–15 ft (3–4.5 m), which is a more practical height. Make sure the suction valve is open (if one is being used). Try to prime the pump again. If you are still unsuccessful and the vacuum reading is high, remove the suction hose from the pump and check both the inlet strainer on the fire pump and the inside of the suction hose for an obstruction. Reconnect the hard suction hose, and try to prime the pump again. If you are still unsuccessful and the vacuum reading is high, replace the hard suction hose with another hose and try again. It is possible you have a defective suction hose, which is collapsing internally when vacuum is applied.

Uninterrupted Water Supply

Establishing an uninterrupted water supply is one of the most important objectives for any IC. In areas where municipal water supplies are not readily available or static water supplies are not available close to the incident, the IC must establish a plan to obtain an uninterrupted water supply through a relay pumping operation (see the chapter *Relay Pump Operations*), a tanker shuttle, or a nurse tanker operation. These operations can be labor and equipment intensive. Appointing a water supply officer to oversee them will ease the burden on the IC.

Water Shuttle

Although an uninterrupted water supply is essential for all firefighting operations, a water source may not always be close enough to the scene of the fire. In many rural and remote areas of a jurisdiction, water must be carried to the fire scene in an operation called a <u>water shuttle</u>. A specialized vehicle called a tanker or a tender is used for this operation: While the National Incident Management System (NIMS) uses the term "tender," the "tanker" label is still widely used in the fire service on a national basis. For our purposes, we will refer to these specialized vehicles as tankers.

A water shuttle does not just consist of the tankers, but also includes <u>fill sites</u> and <u>dump sites</u>. A fill site is a location where the tankers can get their water tanks filled; a dump site is where the tanker can offload the water. Water shuttles can become very large and complex operations. In such cases, a water supply officer is generally assigned to coordinate the required activities. In contrast, if the incident is small or quickly mitigated, the water shuttle may be quite simple and short in duration.

■ Fill Sites

A fill site is any location at which a tanker can be filled, such as a hydrant, a pond, a lake, or a river. Fill sites are not always readily available, however, and they can often be located great distances from the incident and beyond the limits for a practical relay operation. It is wise to select a drafting site that, if possible, allows tankers in the shuttle operation to enter and exit without having to back up or turn around. This will improve safety at the fill site, as personnel will not need to walk in the area as backing spotters while vehicles are entering and exiting. A fill site utilizing a static water source has the same characteristics and hazards as the locations used for a drafting operation. In fact, the only difference between a fill site and a static water source for drafting is the distance from the incident. Fill sites utilizing a hydrant are often the most reliable due to their unobstructed access and the quantity and quality of the water that they offer.

FIGURE 12-17 Screw-type gate valve in place on a hydrant.

DRIVER/OPERATOR Tip

Preplanning in regard to fill site locations is highly important, as they are likely to be very few and far between. The time to start looking for suitable fill sites is not when a fire needs to be extinguished, but rather long before an incident occurs. Consider making the preplanning excursion serve as a departmental training exercise.

Establish a Fill Site Using a Hydrant

Using a hydrant as a fill site can be a very simple operation, especially if you find a suitable hydrant that has a flow pressure of at least 50 psi (350 kPa). This pressure will allow the tanker to be filled quickly and without the help of a pumper. There are only a couple of ways that you can use a hydrant as a fill site. Regardless of which approach you use, however, you must flush the hydrant until the water runs clear before connecting any hoselines.

If you choose to use the 2½-inch (65-mm) outlets on the hydrant, first connect a control valve—either a quarter-turn hydrant valve or a screw-type gate valve **FIGURE 12-17**—to the outlets. You can then connect two 2½- or 3-inch (65- or 77-mm) medium-size hoselines to the control valves.

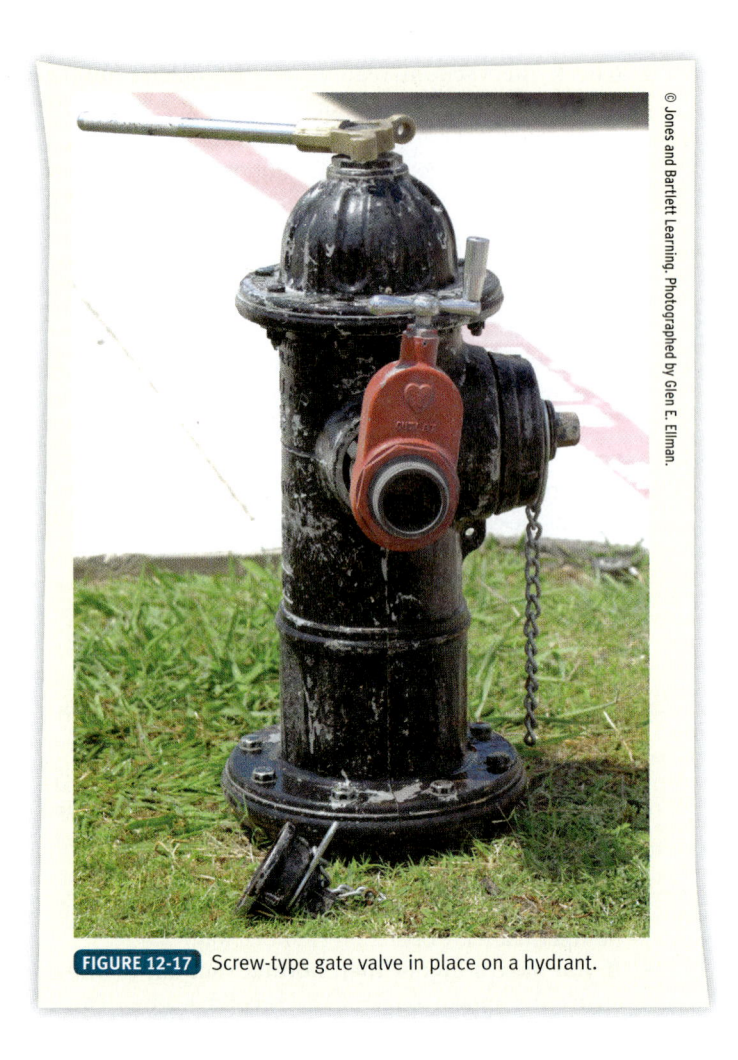

Using a control valve on each outlet allows you to supply two tankers simultaneously without having to shut down the hydrant between filling operations. It also allows you to use both outlets at the same time to fill one tanker more quickly. Both options improve your flexibility to adapt to whatever circumstances may arise. First make sure that the control valves are closed, and then open the hydrant fully; your fill site is now ready. Having the hydrant open and the hoses already connected will speed up the process of filling a tanker in a shuttle operation. If control valves are not available, consider using hose clamps on the hoselines to stop the flow of water. As a last resort, you can simply shut the hydrant down between filling each tanker.

Large-diameter hose (LDH) can also be used at a fill site from a hydrant. If the hydrant is located far off the road or another hard surface, attach a short section of LDH from the steamer connection of the hydrant to a manifold. You can attach as many as four medium-size hoselines to a manifold, thereby enabling you to fill either one or two tankers at a time with ease and at the speed that you prefer. If the hydrant is located close to the road or another hard surface, you can simply connect the LDH to the steamer connection and supply the tanker directly if it has a large-diameter intake connection.

VOICES OF EXPERIENCE

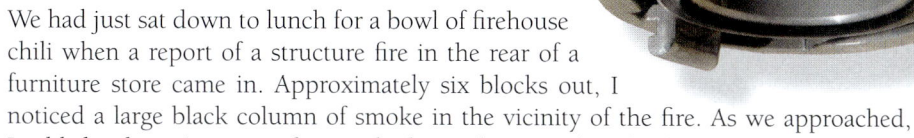

We had just sat down to lunch for a bowl of firehouse chili when a report of a structure fire in the rear of a furniture store came in. Approximately six blocks out, I noticed a large black column of smoke in the vicinity of the fire. As we approached, I told the driver/operator that we had "good water" (i.e., high water pressure in the hydrants) in the area and that there was a hydrant just south of the address.

As the acting lieutenant, I assumed command at the scene. After the size-up, I transmitted a second alarm due to the size of the building and the amount of fire showing. This fire would have to be fought defensively.

We secured an uninterrupted supply of water using 200 ft (60 m) of 5-inch (125-mm) hoseline. The first fire attack line placed into operation was a 2½-inch (65-mm) hose. The second fire attack line placed into operation was an elevated master stream supplying 3-inch (77-mm) hose. Finally, I ordered the use of the deck gun. The defensive suppression operations began flooding the structure with water.

Suddenly, the driver/operator appeared with a fretful look on his face. I immediately inquired, "What's wrong?"

"The pumper is making a weird noise and it is throttling up and down," he said. "And now the 5-inch (125-mm) supply is bouncing violently!"

I ran with great haste to the fire apparatus and began shutting all nonessential fire attack lines down. There was no residual water left in the single water main that was supplying this entire firefighting operation. We were attempting to supply more water to fight the fire than the domestic water system could afford.

That day I learned these lessons:

- Know the water main size within your response area.
- Driver/operators must watch their gauges vigilantly.
- Be mindful of fire apparatus using the same water main for their water supply.
- Consider notifying the water department to increase the water flow to the water grid, if necessary.
- High water pressure does not equate to high water flow.

Michael Washington
Cincinnati Fire Department
Cincinnati, Ohio

If you do not have a manifold and the tanker is not equipped with a large-diameter intake connection, you can use a wye to split the LDH into two medium-size hoselines and supply the tanker. Using LDH will increase the flow (gpm [L/min]) and fill the tanker faster, but this approach requires that the hydrant be closed between filling operations unless you are using a manifold.

If possible, leave a fire fighter (or two) at the hydrant fill site to fill incoming tankers and to monitor the site. While this may be a good task to assign to junior personnel, an experienced and knowledgeable crew member may be able to manage the entire fill site, make the connections, and complete the filling operations without the tanker driver/operator ever having to leave the cab of the truck. If fire personnel cannot be spared for this task, leave the hose next to the hydrant for the next incoming tanker to speed up the operation. In this circumstance, you should call for the police to monitor the site, as you will have a lot of equipment left unattended and the apparatus movement in the area could become a traffic hazard or a danger to bystanders.

Establishing a Fill Site at a Static Water Source

Establishing a fill site from a static water source entails following the same procedures discussed earlier in this chapter. The location of the fill site should be chosen after considering how other fire apparatus will access the incident; ideally, you should select a site that will not block egress to the fire scene. Other factors that must be taken into account during the process of determining the reliability of a static water source include accessibility of the supply, quantity of available water, and quality of the water.

Once you have selected the best location, simply follow the steps outlined in Skill Drills 12-2, 12-3, and 12-4 to start flowing water through the dump line. Remember, water must be constantly flowing during a drafting operation to prevent the loss of draft (vacuum) in the pump and to avoid overheating. You can discharge the dump line back into the static water source.

After establishing a flow of water, you can use your pumper as a sort of "hydrant": Use either two medium-size hoselines to supply the tankers, a LDH line if the tanker is equipped with one, or both methods if you need to supply multiple tankers simultaneously. As with all drafting operations, start the flow through the discharge valves slowly, while simultaneously increasing the throttle, to avoid breaking the vacuum and the draft of the pump. When the tanker is full, slowly throttle down and close the discharge valves, while keeping the dump line open during the entire operation.

The benefit of establishing a fill site at a static water source is that the pumper drafting the water can supply the tankers being filled at a remote location that is better suited for tanker movement. For example, the pumper might be set up at the shore of a small lake, but provide fill hoses to a location on a roadside, several hundred feet away. This type of operation allows the tankers to drive up, fill their tanks, and drive away, all without turning around or backing.

Fill Sites in Inaccessible Areas

Sometimes you may not be able to get a pumper close to the static water source because the area is blocked by trees or surrounded by undeveloped roadway or pathways. In these situations, you may have to consider using portable pumps as a way of getting the water to the tankers. Establishing a suitable drafting site for a portable pump requires 24 inches (0.5 m) of water in all directions around the strainer and enough hose to get the water to the fill site.

As when you establish a drafting site for a pumper, you must ensure that the quantity of water available is large enough to support drafting with the portable pump. If the source is large but not deep enough, you can use a floating strainer for the portable pump hard suction hose; this strainer is exactly like the one used with the hard-sided hoses used by a pumper, only smaller. If a floating strainer is not available, you may need to dig a hole in the water to provide the depth needed for the strainer or create a dam in a creek using a ladder wrapped in a salvage cover. Before undertaking any such damming operation, consider how changing the stream might affect the surrounding areas.

> **DRIVER/OPERATOR Tip**
>
> Consider putting a washtub in the bottom of the hole to prevent any sediment from getting into the strainer. This step will keep the water relatively clean and may help to prevent damage to the pumps that use the water from this source. (This tip has saved many buildings.)

Once you have the area ready for the portable pump to start drafting, connect the hard-sided suction lines to the pump, and place a strainer on the intake end of the hose. You can use a ladder to secure these smaller hard-sided suction hoses in moving water sources, just as you can with the hoses from a pumper. Connect the discharge lines to the pump and determine where you will discharge the water once it starts flowing. Most portable pumps will flow water at a maximum rate of only 250 gpm (1000 L/min), so using a dump line will not be possible. In addition, you will not be able to use control valves to stop the flow of water at any point while the pump is running, so you should consider putting the hoselines into a **portable tank**; otherwise, you can supply a pumper directly. Start the portable pump and obtain a draft by following the manufacturer's guidelines to start flowing water. Once the portable tank contains water, a pumper can draft from the portable tank and supply the tankers without having to shut down the portable pump. You may want to use multiple portable pumps to supply multiple portable tanks in an operation, given that portable pumps cannot provide large quantities of water at any time. Set one portable pump up at a time to increase the effectiveness of the operation.

Portable floating pumps have become a very popular option for obtaining water in inaccessible areas in recent years. These devices are very good choices for use at a fill site at a static water source. Depending on the flow (gpm [L/min]) you need to supply, you might consider using multiple floating pumps. When placing a floating pump into service, follow the manufacturer's guidelines for operating the pump, and make sure the fuel tank is full of fuel.

Once in the water, portable floating pumps are difficult to turn on and off and reposition, so make sure that they are ready for a long-duration operation before launching them. Attach the hose to the discharge port of the portable floating pump, and tie off the pump with a rope to a secure place on the bank or shore of the static source. You must first place the floating pump in the water before you start it, because it will automatically prime, begin to draft, and start pumping water through the hoseline very quickly. Given this fact, it is important to have personnel in place to direct the flow into a portable tank or have the hose attached to an engine to serve as its water supply. Consider using multiple floating portable pumps to fill multiple portable tanks because, like portable pumps, these devices have limited discharge capabilities.

Whether you are using a floating or stationary portable pump, you must monitor the pump to ensure that it is functioning properly and flowing water. Check for clogged strainers if the flow is reduced, as this problem is the most common source of flow restrictions.

When an inaccessible area will serve as a fill site, the use of some type of portable pump that discharges the water into a portable tank is a highly practical means of obtaining a water supply. This portable tank operation must be supported with a pumper so that incoming tankers do not have to establish a draft each time they arrive to obtain water, which would significantly slow down the operation. Once the portable tank is filled, the pumper drafting from that static water source can flow water through a dump line while waiting to fill the tankers as they arrive. The key consideration is for the pumper to slowly fill the tankers so that it does not drain the portable tank faster than it can be supplied by the portable pumps.

DRIVER/OPERATOR Tip

At no time should portable tanks and pumping operations be left unattended. The fill area can pose a danger to bystanders owing to the constant flow of water and the attractive nuisance that a full portable tank can present to children as a drowning hazard.

■ Filling Tankers

Whether the fill site is being supplied by a hydrant or a pumper (i.e., a static water source), the procedure for filling the tanker (tender) is the same. When filling tankers, you should fill only one at a time when you are using medium-size hoselines. Trying to fill more than one tanker at a time will certainly slow down the water supply operation, although you have the flexibility to fill two tankers at one time if the situation dictates it. For example, if you are filling a 1500-gal (6000-L) tanker and a 3000-gal (12,000-L) tanker, you can get the smaller tanker back to the scene more quickly if you fill both tankers simultaneously. You will have to judge whether sacrificing speed is worth the increased efficiency. Without question, you can fill more than one tanker at a time when you are using a LDH hydrant manifold or a pumper from draft.

Having two hoselines ready with control valves and personnel at the ends ready to connect to the tankers will increase the speed of the operation and reduce turnaround times for the operation. When you arrive to fill your tanker, simply attach one hose at a time from the control point—that is, the control valves on the hydrant, the hose clamps, the manifold from a LDH connection at the hydrant, or the pumper being used to supply the fill site from a draft—to the tank fill valves on the tanker. Make sure the tank fill valves are open on the tanker before you open the control point valves to fill the tank. It is easy to overlook the step of opening these valves, but by doing so you will waste valuable time.

Once the tank is completely full on the tanker, close the control point valve before closing the tank fill valve on the tanker. Following this sequence allows you to disconnect the hose from the tanker more easily, because the line will have less pressure in it. Remove the hoselines and advise the driver/operator of the tanker that it is safe to drive away from the fill site. Repeat this operation for each tanker until the operation is terminated through IMS by either the IC or the water supply officer.

DRIVER/OPERATOR Tip

On some tenders, it is critical to not attempt too many connections when filling the tank, because possible structural damage can occur based on tank vent sizes.

■ Safety for Water Shuttle Operations

Water shuttle operations present the same risks that are encountered in relay pumping operations. The purpose of both operations is to provide an uninterrupted water supply for the firefighting efforts. The water shuttle operation relies on a fill site to obtain the water and a dump site to deliver it to the attack pumper; a relay pumping operation uses a source pumper to provide the water to the attack pumper. A water shuttle, however, requires the frequent movement of apparatus. Thus the safety concerns associated with this type of water supply should be identified before the components of the operation are considered.

Steps that can be taken to improve incident safety include preplanning locations for obtaining the water, being trained in the use and operation of the equipment, and knowing which equipment you have to use. Communication between the tankers and the fill sites may require assignment of a separate radio frequency, which avoids problems on the main tactical channel as tankers report their locations or indicate that they are returning for refilling. Personnel operating at the fill sites will need to wear the same level of personal protective equipment (PPE) as is worn during a relay operation to protect these crew members from falling equipment, catastrophic equipment failures, and traffic in and around the fill site.

A water shuttle operation involves moving tankers full of water from the fill site to the dump site, with the empty tankers then returning to the fill site. Tankers are specialized types of fire apparatus that carry several hundred or several thousand gallons of water, which can weigh more than 80,000 pounds (36,000 kg). Many of the vehicles being used as tankers may have previously served the jurisdiction in another capacity before being converted to fire department use. Put simply, they were never intended to be driven under emergency conditions and at high rates of speed. Unfortunately, most personnel are not familiar with the handling characteristics of these large vehicles and do not make adjustments to their driving habits when at the wheel of these apparatus. These two circumstances alone have caused too many fire fighters to lose their lives.

Extreme caution must be emphasized while driving tankers, because they do not handle in the same manner as a standard pumper. The ability to maneuver is greatly reduced with tankers, due to their size and weight. Driver/operators should be well trained in driving these vehicles both full and empty before they attempt to operate one during an emergency incident. At no time should these vehicles be operated beyond the posted speed limit, regardless of what is allowed by the state's motor vehicle laws or codes.

> **Safety Tip**
>
> Never drive a tanker that is not completely full or completely empty. Driving such a vehicle with a partially full tank can cause dangerous weight shifting, which can result in the tanker rolling over.

Establishing Dump Site Operations

The location at which the shuttled water will be offloaded is called a dump site. Establishing the dump site location to create a static water source for the firefighting operation takes practice and forethought. This site should be on relatively level ground, be firm, and not be susceptible to significant changes as a result of fire apparatus movement or getting wet from the water. It must be large and strong enough to support the weight of the water and the weight of the incoming tankers, and it should provide enough room for the movement of the tankers in and out of the site. Large parking lots and fields that are flat and smooth can make excellent locations for dump sites.

The ideal dump site location is close enough that the source pumper can supply the attack pumper(s) without a relay pumper, but not so close that the tankers cannot access it. For example, if the attack pumper is positioned just past the building and a ladder truck is in the front, the dump site might be located down the street at an intersection that would allow for the tankers to approach and depart in different directions. While space may be available in the street that is closer to the incident, the dump site should be located farther away to maintain the efficiency of the operation. As in the case of a long driveway, the attack pumper may be located near the building but be supplied by a source pumper located on the main roadway.

In cases where no intersections or large parking lots are available for use as a dump site, care must be taken not to obstruct the flow of additional responding apparatus or the tanker shuttle by placing the portable tanks in the roadway. Thought should be given as to which way a tanker will offload its water: does the tanker offload from the rear or can it dump from the side? Once you have determined that you have a good site, you are ready to set up the portable tanks and create a static water source for a source pumper.

■ Using Portable Tanks

Portable tanks are usually carried on tankers and should hold as much water as the capacity of the tanker will allow. For example, a 3000-gal (12,000-L) tanker usually carries a portable tank that can hold 3000 gal (12,000 L). If the tanker cannot offload its entire tank at one time, it will slow the operation because the tank's contents must be offloaded incrementally or the tanker will have to dump any water that it has left before leaving for the fill site. Using portable tanks at a dump site can be very easy, and personnel should be able to set up such a system quickly and safely. Portable tanks provide a source of water that is free from debris and not subject to the effects of stream currents and unknown shore soil conditions.

When using portable tanks, thought should be given to the possibility of expanding the operation. The area selected for this kind of dump site should be big enough to hold two to three portable tanks connected together in addition to the source pumper, which will be drafting from these tanks.

Before deploying any portable tank, place a salvage cover or tarp on the ground in the area where the tank will be positioned to prevent any damage to the tank by rocks, sticks, or glass that may be present on the ground. Once the salvage covers are in place, remove the portable tank from the fire apparatus and place it on the salvage cover. A self-expanding type of portable tank can be laid flat on the salvage cover and is ready for water. If you are using a metal frame type of portable tank, open the portable tank by completely unfolding the frame outward and pushing the lining into place until it touches the frame all around the edges. If you are setting up multiple portable tanks, start with the tank at the high point of the ground and work downward. Ensure that the portable tank's drain is on the low side of the tank, and check that the drain is closed or secure before filling the tank.

The tank is initially filled by a tanker before it enters the water shuttle operation. Once the tanks are in place, the tanker positions itself to offload the water through a dump valve on the tank. The **dump valve** is a large opening—sometimes as large as 12 to 16 inches (300 to 410 mm)—that is connected directly to the tank and allows it to be emptied quickly, in some cases within 1 minute **FIGURE 12-18**. The portable tank should not overflow while it is being filled, so initially fill the tank slowly. If multiple portable tanks are being used, once the first tanker has emptied its tank and moves out of the way, the next tanker can get into position to repeat the steps until all of the portable tanks are full.

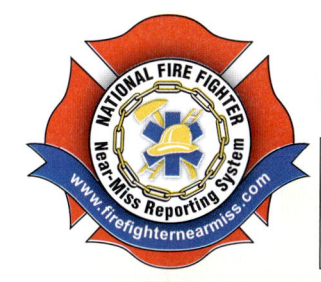

CHAPTER 12 Drafting and Water Shuttle Operations

Near-Miss REPORT

Report Number: 10-0001205

Synopsis: Crew loses water pressure during fire attack.

Event Description: When entering a structure fire, I was the guy on the nozzle pushing a fire down a narrow hallway with my officer behind me. We had a good knock on the hallway and were approaching the room that was fully involved. I hit the main fire and then my officer used our thermal-imaging camera (TIC) to try to find the source, because our vision was completely obscured. As the fire began to roll over our heads, I went to hit the roll and got one spurt of water out of the hose and then there was only a trickle of water available. The heat quickly began to bank down on us, and my helmet face shield melted down over my face mask. My officer told me to hit the fire, and I showed him the limp hose. He quickly grabbed me, and we backed down the hallway to our point of entry at the front door. I stayed at the door to observe the fire, and my officer went straight to the engineer who had lost the prime on the pump for an unknown reason. We regained prime and attacked the fire again pushing it back down the hallway and put out the fire pretty quickly. We later found out that there was an error in hydrant changeover procedures. After this incident, training was reinforced and mandated for the engineer. I gave him my melted helmet as a good reminder!

Lessons Learned: The lesson learned was that we had a protected egress and used it quickly and effectively. Stay low and if it is too hot, you are probably not the only one who thinks this. Keep in good communication and proximity with your team and be aware of your surroundings at all times.

■ Offloading Tankers

When offloading a tanker, the driver/operator must review the dump site characteristics upon arrival to ensure that his or her specific tanker can access the location. Despite the best of intentions, not all of the personnel who set up the dump site may know what your tanker requires or how it maneuvers. As the driver/operator, you should know your vehicle better than anyone. Once again, consider how much room you have to maneuver, whether the area will support the weight of your tanker, how you will offload the tanker, and in which direction you must travel to exit the site. If a dirt area is being used as the dump site, consider what happens when the water is splashed on the ground: If the dirt turns into mud, the tankers may sink and become stuck.

Once the tanker is positioned at the dump site, unloading it through a dump valve is the easiest strategy to implement **FIGURE 12-19**. These valves may be located on each side of the vehicle as well as at the rear; they are found directly on the tank and allow the water to exit or dump from the tank very quickly. Some newer tankers are equipped with in-cab electric or air-actuated controls to open the dump valves, meaning that the driver/operator does not have to get out of the cab to operate the valves. Once the tanker is in position and has been given approval to start dumping water, you simply activate the switch and the valve opens, which releases the water from the tank.

In older tankers, the water is released manually by personnel at the dump tank. This is one of the most common methods used to offload a tanker. Using these valves does not require any changes to the procedure: The tanker must still be positioned at the portable tank, but the dump valve (5–6 square inches [3–4 mm²]) is opened manually by a fire fighter at the portable tank.

Another method of offloading a tanker when large dump valves are not installed on the fire apparatus is to attach medium-size lines (2½ to 3 inches [65 to 77 mm]) to the pump of the tanker and place the other end of the lines into the portable tank. A commercially made device must be attached to the tank to free up personnel in the dump site from performing this task. The driver/operator of the tanker should pump water through these hoselines at a maximum pressure of 50 psi (350 kPa).

■ Use of Multiple Portable Tanks

The use of multiple portable tanks has become a standard practice in rural firefighting operations. When the tanks are set up, they are positioned starting at the high point of the ground and then going down slope. Remember, the main objective is to keep the water moving toward the tank being used for drafting.

Even if the ground appears flat, there is usually a slightly noticeable slope. If there is not, simply hook the tanks together using the rings on the drains if they are so equipped. Many tanks are equipped with two "drains" so that they can be hooked together; otherwise, a **jet siphon** may be used to move the water from one tank to another.

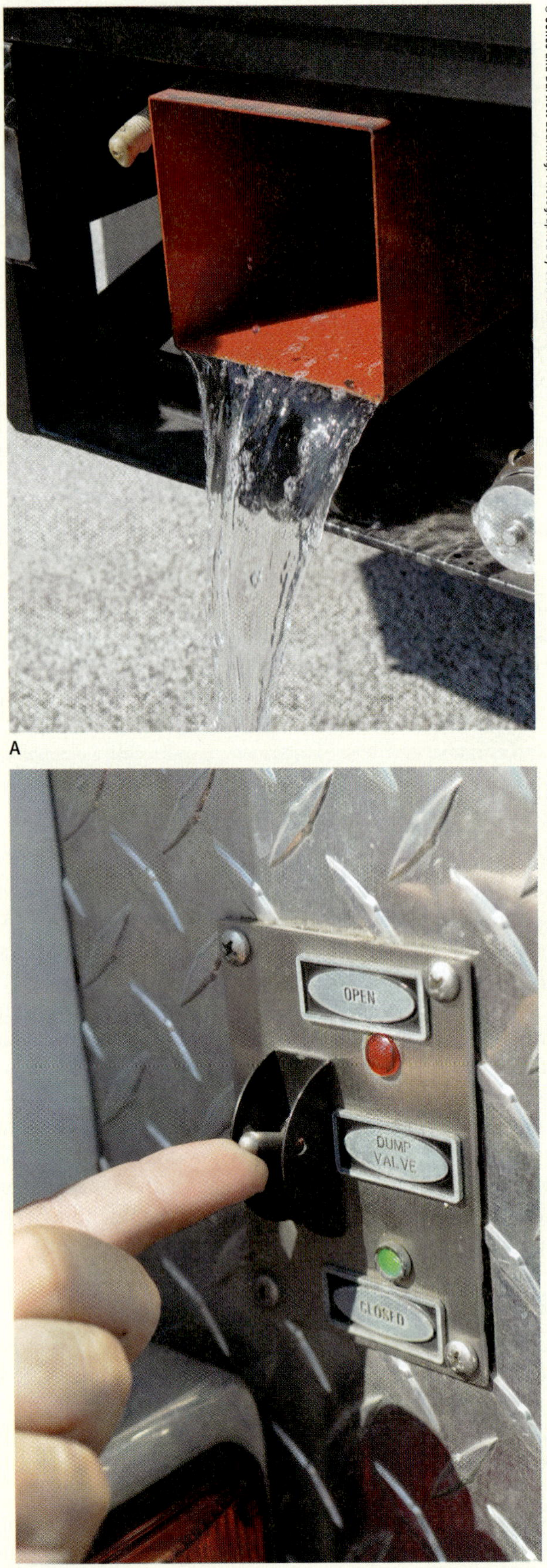

FIGURE 12-19 Unloading water through a dump valve.

FIGURE 12-18 **A.** A manually operated dump valve. **B.** A dump valve from a pneumatic valve.

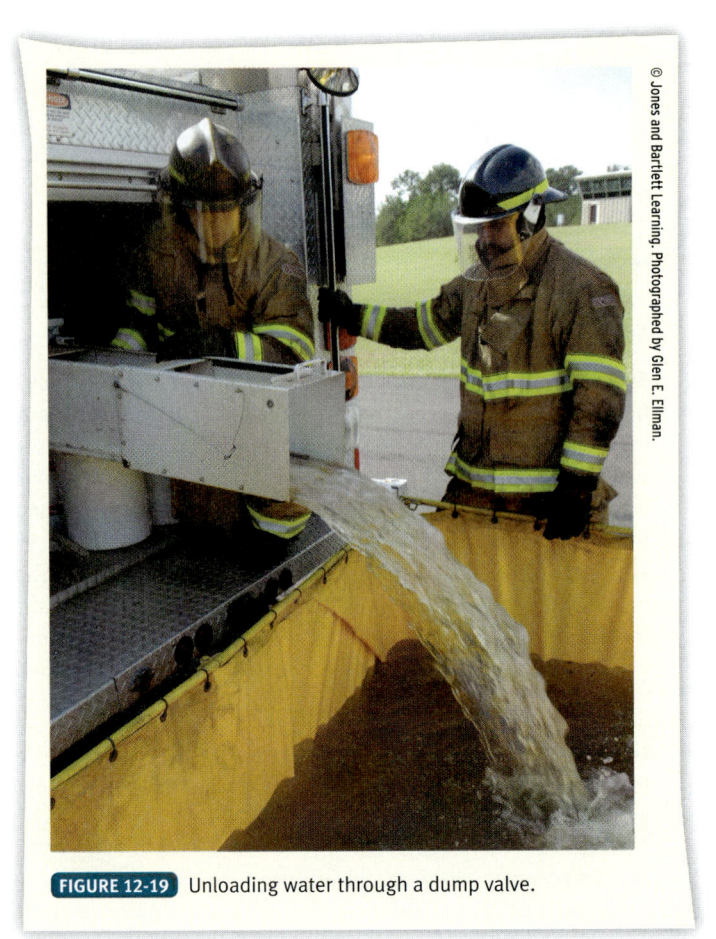

Jet siphon adapters use the hard suction hose as a pathway for flowing water that is being forced through the hose by Venturi forces. The jet siphon has a connection for a 1½- or 1¾-inch (38- or 45-mm) hose to flow water through the hose, which will create the Venturi forces needed to draw the water from the tank up through the hose and then discharge it into the second tank. The jet siphon is connected to one end of a loose hard suction hose in the tank from which you wish to remove water; the other end of the hose is secured to the top of the tank that you want water to flow into. A 1½- or 1¾-inch (38- or 45-mm) hose is attached to the jet siphon device and placed into the tank once it is full. The source pumper connects the hose to a discharge port and pumps it at a pressure of 100 to 125 psi (700 to 875 kPa).

Do not use the dump line to supply the jet siphon, as it may not always be in operation and the dump line must constantly flow water. Multiple jet siphons can be used to move the water between tanks, depending on how many tanks you have in operation.

■ Source Pumper Considerations for Portable Tank Operations

The main objective in moving water from one tank to another when using multiple tanks is to keep the main portable tank full. Obviously, when only one tank is being used, it represents the main tank—the one being used by the source pumper for its water supply.

After the source pumper has established a draft from this static water supply, all efforts should be taken to prevent air from being introduced into the pump—which explains why it is preferred that dumping operations are done in one tank while the drafting takes places in another tank. When only one tank is being used, the tanker operator must use care not to dump the water on or near the strainer, as introduction of the water creates air turbulence when it enters the tank. Using a blow-up ball is very important in portable tank operations because the size of the water "container" is much smaller and whirlpools are created easily in shallow water.

The main tank should not run low on water during the operation if the tanker shuttle is working as designed. If it does run out, the incident will lose its water supply, putting fire fighters at risk if they are operating in interior positions at the fire scenario. If the main tank continues to run low, the incident commander or the water supply officer must be notified of the situation and may consider adding more tankers to the shuttle operation to keep up with the water demands.

DRIVER/OPERATOR Tip

Use a low-level strainer when drafting from portable tanks. This approach will allow you to get the maximum volume out of the tank without worrying about drawing in debris or silt, as might occur in a pond, stream, or lake.

■ Traffic Flow Within a Dump Site

The movement of tankers into and out of the dump site can cause significant congestion, which may result in slow water delivery to the portable tanks. This congestion can be prevented with a little foresight during the layout of the dump site and the portable tanks. Consideration must be given to how the tankers will offload their contents: Will two tankers offload their water at the same time? How will they approach the portable tanks to dump the water? In which direction will the tankers depart the dump site to return to the fill site? Establishing a smooth traffic pattern will improve efficiency and increase safety around the dump site—the tankers will need to make fewer movements if they do not have to back up to reposition themselves for offloading.

DRIVER/OPERATOR Tip

Using two members for a crew on a tanker will improve fire fighter safety by providing a fire fighter to act as a backing guide whenever the vehicle operates in reverse at the fill or dump site. The second crew member can act as a spotter as the tanker approaches the portable tank to offload its water.

Most modern tankers have the ability to offload from the sides and the rear of the vehicle, which gives the driver/operator greater freedom in deciding the direction of travel into the dump site and determining how to approach the portable tank. Some older tankers can offload only from the rear of the vehicle, which means that backing the vehicle into position is unavoidable. Once you know how the tankers will be offloaded, you can determine the best direction of approach to the portable tanks.

The portable tanks should be placed in as open an area as possible so that you can easily maneuver around the site. If both sides of the tanks are accessible and offloading into two tanks will not disrupt the source pumpers' drafting operation, then two tankers can offload their contents at the same time. This will significantly improve the efficiency of the operation.

All tankers should travel the same path to enter and then exit the dump site. These vehicles are large and difficult to maneuver, especially in scenarios characterized by heavy congestion. Once you determine the entry and exit directions to the site, be sure to communicate the traffic plan to all driver/operators of the tankers. A traffic plan that flows in a semi-circular direction will be the most efficient because the vehicles will not be traveling on the same roadway in opposite directions. For example, have the tankers approach the dump site from the north, enter from the east, and travel in a westerly direction to the portable tanks for offloading. Once completely unloaded, the tankers can exit the dump site on the west side and travel north again toward the fill site. If a circular traffic pattern is not possible, try to have the tankers back into position at the portable tank(s). The roads that lead into and out of the fill site should also be different to prevent congestion there **FIGURE 12-20**.

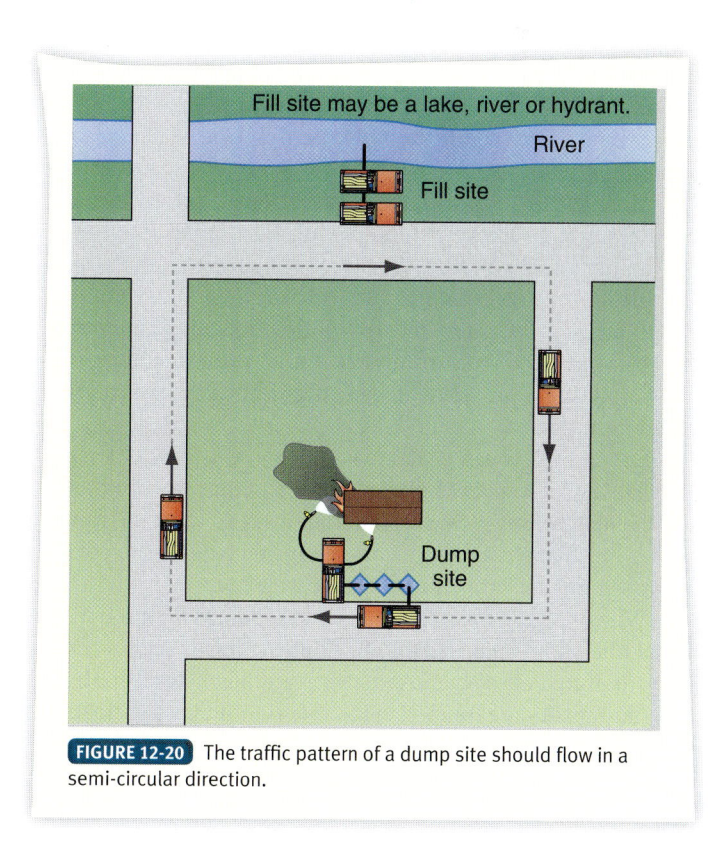

FIGURE 12-20 The traffic pattern of a dump site should flow in a semi-circular direction.

> **DRIVER/OPERATOR Tip**
>
> Vehicles that are parked along the travel routes and fire apparatus that are parked and not being used increase the risk of an accident with a tanker. If police assistance is available, have the police department shut down the roads on which the tankers are traveling for added safety.

Nurse Tanker Operations

The operation of offloading a tanker into another tanker or into a pumper as a form of a water source is called a **nurse tanker operation**. Its name derives from what happens as a mother nurses her child: This type of operation eliminates the use of portable tanks (bottle), as the attack pumper is supplied directly by the nurse tanker (mother). A nurse tanker operation is set up when there is no room to establish a dump site, a relay operation, or a combination of the two. Such operations can also be used when the size of the fire is small enough that establishing such a detailed supportive water supply mechanism is not practical. The nurse tanker operation can be performed at the start of an incident as a way to provide water to the attack pumper while the relay or fill-and-dump operation is being established. In this sense, it represents a stopgap measure that creates the needed time to set up a longer duration water supply and provides water to support the fire attack until an uninterrupted water supply is established.

The ideal nurse tanker is the largest tanker that is available, as it will serve as the primary source of water for the fire attack operation. Tractor-trailer tankers, which can carry as much as 6000 gal (24,000 L) of water, are very good choices for this operation because they can be supplied by smaller tankers through a second nurse tank operation. The nurse tanker must have a fire pump to supply the water to the attack pumper.

Most tractor-trailer tankers have a small pump located on the trailer to assist with offloading. The larger the pump on the tanker, the more water it will be able to supply and the greater the pressure it can deliver. The nurse tanker essentially can function like a combination of a contained portable tank and source pumper if it is positioned near the attack pumper, provided it can meet the demands of the attack pumper.

Other tankers can supply, via nursing, this new "source"; alternatively, it can be supplied by the source pumper at a dump site that was established farther away to keep the nurse tanker full. The availability of fire pumps on tankers can create many options for providing a reliable water supply.

When you are filling a nurse tanker, do not fill it too fast. Remember, you want to avoid or limit the introduction of air into the water. Also, because tankers are filled from the bottom, air bubbles are trapped in the water until they can float to the top. Using two medium-size hoselines at 50 psi (350 kPa) should be sufficient to fill the nurse tanker.

■ Communication for Tanker Operations

Communication plays a vital role on the fireground; likewise, it needs to be a vital part of the water supply and tanker shuttle operations. A number of tankers may be operating around an emergency scene in addition to traveling to the fill site and back to the dump site. Driver/operators need to communicate with one another effectively, especially if the fill or dump sites are located off a narrow roadway or in a tight area. The water supply officer should request from the IC that all tanker operators be assigned to a tactical channel. This practice will eliminate important but nonemergent radio traffic on the main tactical channel, in which communications between the IC and fire attack crews must have priority. The tanker driver/operators must be able to communicate their locations within the shuttle flow and indicate whether they are filling or returning to the dump site so that command officers can make decisions based on the time it takes to sustain a steady flow of water to the attack pumper.

Staying in touch via effective communication is also a way of maintaining accountability for each tanker and its personnel. If a tanker and crew have not been in contact with a member of the water supply team, having these communication capabilities in place will allow members of the command structure to reach them and determine if a problem exists. If a tanker and crew are out of contact, this situation would constitute an emergency for the IC and would be treated as a missing fire fighter Mayday.

> **DRIVER/OPERATOR Tip**
>
> Many fire departments operate on different radio frequencies, which can cause complications at an emergency. Planning an exercise with neighboring fire departments to work out any communication issues prior to an incident will help things run smoothly during an actual mutual aid call.

Water Shuttle Operations in the Incident Management System

Having a sustainable water supply is a vital part of any fire incident scene. Water supply officers should be given a top priority at any scene; if this position is not officially assigned, however, the IC assumes the responsibility for this function. Once a water shuttle operation is established, then a water supply officer should be established as part of the IMS, which may also include a dump site officer and a fill site officer.

The dump site officer is responsible for establishing the dump site, creating the traffic patterns, and ensuring that the source pumper at the site has a sustained water supply. If the incident is complex and includes multiple dump sites, several of these officers may be collectively responsible for all of them and will have to coordinate the larger flow between the fill site and each dump site depending on the demands of each location. They will need to communicate with each dump site to ensure that the water is routed to where it is needed.

The fill site officer is responsible for establishing the fill site location(s), ensuring that the water source for filling the tankers will meet the demand, and creating the traffic patterns in and out of the fill site. Filling two tankers at a time requires a strong water source such as a pumper at draft or a hydrant with a LDH manifold. If these options are not available and the fill operation is the cause of slower dumping cycles, fill site officers may consider establishing multiple fill sites. This will require the same level of communication between multiple fill sites as is necessary between multiple dump sites. The ultimate goal is to provide an uninterrupted water supply to the fire incident.

Wrap-Up

Chief Concepts

- The ability to draft water from a static source makes your fire apparatus a versatile resource.
- Fire departments generally have a prescribed process for performing inspections, routine maintenance, and operational testing of water supply apparatus and mechanisms.
- Water supply management is a vital part of any fire incident and can become a major part of the Incident Management System (IMS) in the event that a reliable public or private water system is not available.
- The water supply officer takes responsibility for drafting operations, relay pumping, water shuttles, and nurse tanker operations.
- Once you as the driver/operator have found a suitable location with an adequate water source that is close enough to reach, you are ready to set up your pump to draft. This task requires teamwork, and the driver/operator should be assisted by two or more fire fighters.
- The first step in preparing to draft from a water source is to prime the pump.
- Once the suction hose has been connected and placed into the water source, air is drawn from the pump using the priming pump.
- Once the pump is primed, you are ready to start drafting water and producing discharge pressures.
- Whether you are supplying attack lines or supplying water for the fire attack pumper, make sure that the crews know that you are ready to start flowing water before you open the discharge valve—either over the radio, through face-to-face contact with the crew, or through hand signals as established by the organization.
- Slowly open the corresponding discharge valve for the hoseline and begin flowing water.
- Establishing an uninterrupted water supply is one of the most important objectives for any incident commander.
- In many rural and remote areas of a jurisdiction, water must be carried to the fire scene in an operation called a water shuttle, utilizing a specialized vehicle called a tanker (tender).
- Establishing the dump site location to create a static water source for the firefighting operation takes practice and forethought.
- The location at which the shuttled water will be offloaded is called a dump site.
- In a nurse tanker operation, a tanker is offloaded into another tanker or into a pumper that serves as a water source for on-scene operations.
- Having a sustainable water supply is a vital part of any fire incident scene.

Hot Terms

anti-siphon hole A very small hole in the fitting on top of the primer oil reservoir or in the top of the loop on the lubrication line leading to the priming pump.

atmospheric pressure Pressure caused by the weight of the atmosphere; equal to 14.7 psi (101 kPa) at sea level.

cavitation A condition caused by attempting to move water faster than it is being supplied to the pump.

dependable lift The height that a column of water can be lifted in a quantity considered sufficient to provide reliable fire flow.

draft The pressure differential that causes water flow.

dump line A small-diameter hoseline that remains in the open position and flowing water during the entire drafting operation.

dump site A location where a fire apparatus can offload the water in its tank.

dump valve A large opening from the water tank of a mobile water supply apparatus that is used for unloading purposes.

fill site A location where the fire apparatus can get water tanks filled.

jet siphon An appliance that connects a 1½- or 1¾-inch (38- or 45-mm) hose to a hard-sided hose coupling and creates a pathway for flowing water that is being forced through the hose by Venturi forces.

lift The vertical height that water must be raised during a drafting operation, measured from the surface of a static source of water to the center line of the pump intake.

nurse tanker operation The process of supplying water to an attack engine directly by a supply engine.

portable floating pump A small fire pump that is equipped with a flotation device and built-in strainer, capable of being carried by hand and flowing various quantities of water depending on its size.

portable pump A type of pump that is typically carried by hand by two or more fire fighters to a water source and used to pump water from that source.

portable tank Any closed vessel having a liquid capacity in excess of 60 gal (240 L), but less than 1000 gal (4000 L), which is not intended for fixed installation.

primer oil reservoir A small tank that holds the lubricant for the priming pump.

priming The process of removing air from a fire pump and replacing it with water.

vacuum Any pressure less than atmospheric pressure.

water shuttle The process of moving water by using fire apparatus from a water source to a location where it can be used.

References

National Fire Protection Association (NFPA) 1002, *Standard for Fire Apparatus Driver/Operator Professional Qualifications.* 2014. http://www.nfpa.org/codes-and-standards/document-information-pages?mode=code&code=1002. Accessed March 27, 2014.

National Fire Protection Association (NFPA) 1901, *Standard for Automotive Fire Apparatus.* 2009. http://www.nfpa.org/codes-and-standards/document-information-pages?mode=code&code=1901. Accessed April 9, 2014.

National Fire Protection Association (NFPA) 1911, *Standard for the Inspection, Maintenance, Testing, and Retirement of In-Service Automotive Fire Apparatus.* 2012. http://www.nfpa.org/codes-and-standards/document-information-pages?mode=code&code=1911. Accessed April 3, 2015.

DRIVER/OPERATOR in action

While operating at the fill site, you are isolated from the other members of the department. While they are working at the scene of the fire, you are stationed miles from the scene. As a driver/operator, there is quite a bit of weight resting on your shoulders in such a scenario. You have to be prepared to troubleshoot the pumping operation and ensure that the water supply demands of the incident can be met for the duration of the incident.

1. What is the height that a column of water can be lifted in a quantity considered sufficient to provide reliable fire flow called?
   A. Vacuum
   B. Dependable lift
   C. Desirable lift
   D. Fire flow

2. The _____ is most commonly used for deep water sources.
   A. low-level strainer
   B. barrel strainer
   C. floating strainer
   D. mid-level strainer

3. _____ occur(s) when you attempt to flow water faster than it is being supplied to the pump.
   A. Complications
   B. Consequences
   C. Cavitation
   D. Calculations

4. All tankers should travel the same path to enter and then exit the dump site.
   A. True
   B. False

5. What is the most common source of flow restrictions when performing a drafting operation?
   A. Lack of pressure
   B. Clogged strainer
   C. Broken primer pump
   D. Air leaks

Relay Pump Operations

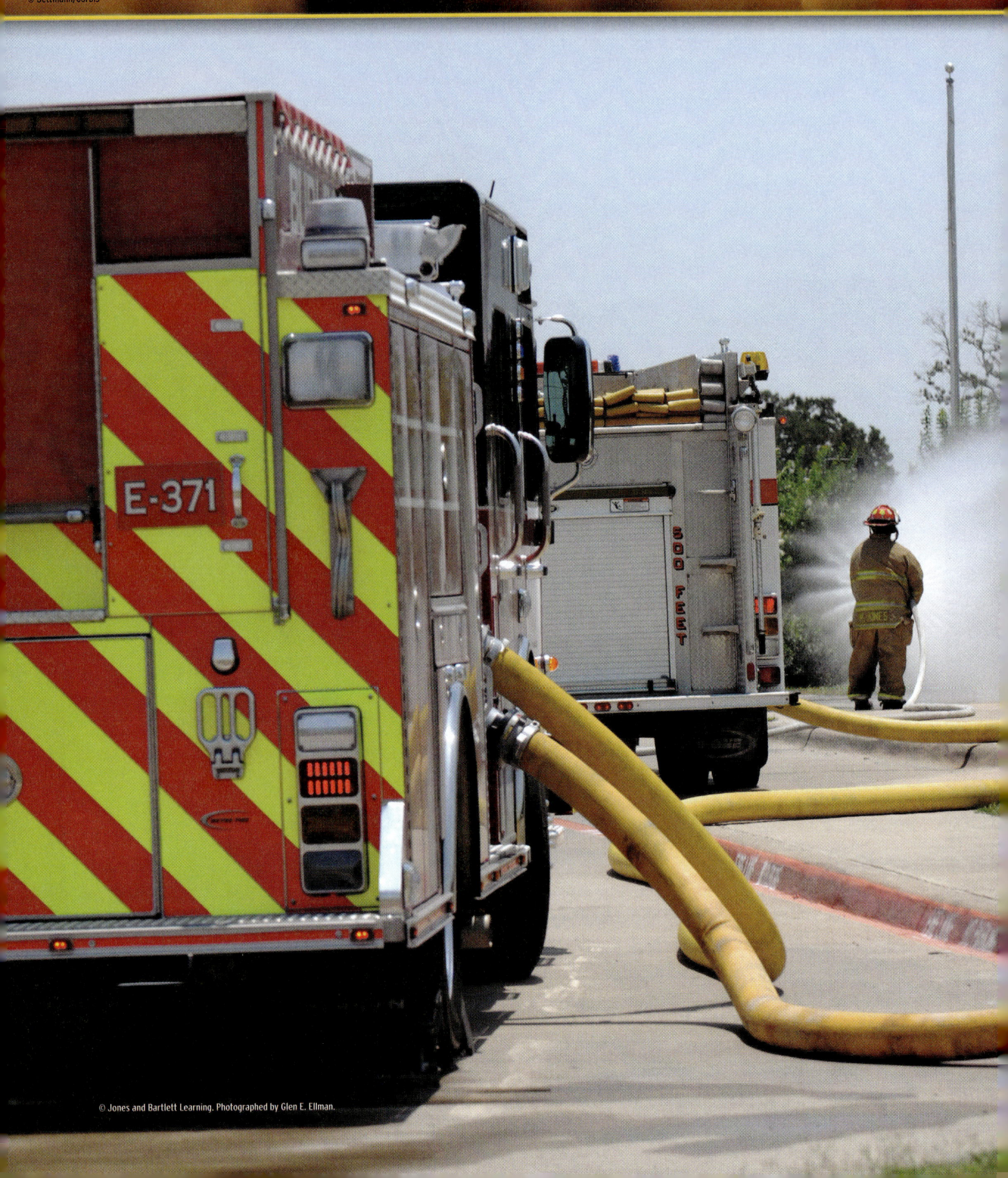

CHAPTER 13

Knowledge Objectives

After studying this chapter, you will be able to:

- Describe relay pumping operations. (NFPA 1002, 5.2.2, 5.2.2(A), 5.2.2(B); p 312–321)

Skills Objectives

There are no skills objectives for Driver/Operator candidates. NFPA 1002 contains no Driver/Operator Job Performance Requirements for this chapter.

You Are the Driver/Operator

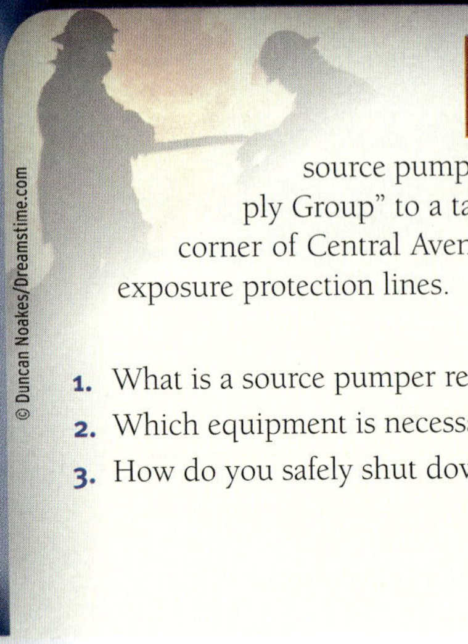

It is your second shift as the driver/operator, and you have been extremely busy. During the night, your engine company is dispatched to yet another run. As you arrive at the scene of a large commercial structure fire, the incident commander (IC) designates your apparatus as the source pumper in a relay pump operation. The IC assigns you and all other units operating in the "Water Supply Group" to a tactical channel and asks that you complete a split lay from the attack pumper to a hydrant at the corner of Central Avenue and Main Street. He needs a flow of 400 gallons per minute (1600 L/min) to supply several exposure protection lines.

1. What is a source pumper responsible for?
2. Which equipment is necessary in a relay pump operation?
3. How do you safely shut down the relay pump operation?

Introduction

Establishing an uninterrupted water supply is one of the most important objectives for any incident commander (IC). In areas where municipal water supplies are not readily available or static water supplies are not available close to the incident, the IC must establish a plan to obtain an uninterrupted water supply through a relay pumping operation, a tanker shuttle, or a nurse tanker operation. These operations can be labor and equipment intensive. Appointing a water supply officer to oversee them will ease the burden on the IC.

Relay Pumping Operations

A <u>relay pumping operation</u> can be one of the most complex of these options because it requires at least two pumpers, and sometimes multiple pumpers, to form a relay. In this process, water is pumped from a water source (hydrant or static) through hose under pressure to the apparatus engaged in fire suppression efforts **FIGURE 13-1**. Relay operations can be as simple as one fire pumper at a pond or lake and the other fire pumper at the fire scene, or as complex as the use of multiple pumpers to supply water over a long distance to the fire operation.

FIGURE 13-1 A relay pumping operation.

Components of a Relay Pumping Operation

To establish any type of relay, you must have a minimum of two fire pumpers, hoselines, and personnel. One fire pumper is located at a water source; it is called the source pumper **FIGURE 13-2**. The other fire pumper is positioned at the fire scene; it is called the attack pumper **FIGURE 13-3**. Any other fire pumpers that are between these two apparatus and are positioned to maintain flow pressure in the relay are called relay pumpers. Two medium-size or large-diameter hoselines are used to supply water in this scenario. Relay pumping operations will demand the use of personnel as they are being established, especially at the source pumper. Once the relay is established, generally the only crew member who needs to remain with the fire apparatus is the driver/operator, as long as the area around the fire apparatus is safe from traffic flow. If it is not, a second member should be left behind to assist the driver/operator; all other crew members could be used as resources if the IC chooses to do so.

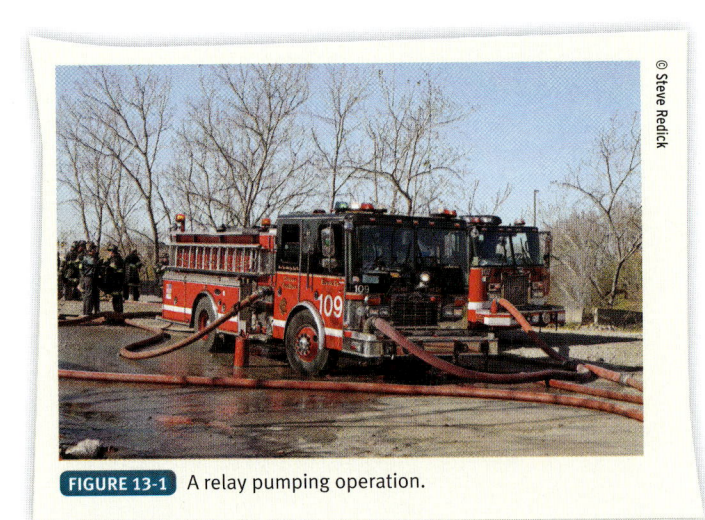

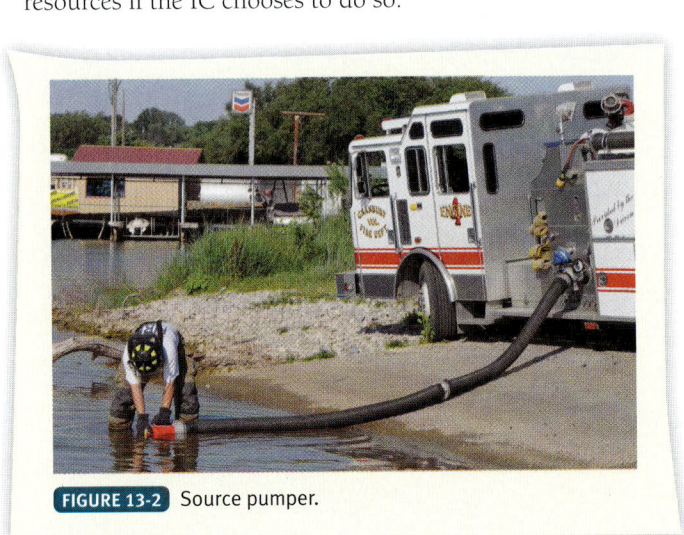

FIGURE 13-2 Source pumper.

CHAPTER 13 Relay Pump Operations

is generally recommended that a supply line be laid down from an open area to the limited access point. Another responding engine should then complete the connection and provide a water supply to the attack pumper.

Upon its arrival at the incident, the attack pumper will start supplying hoselines while operating from its water tank; it will then switch over to the relay supply line when it is ready. This two-step process presents a challenge to both the driver/operator and the initial IC, as the fire attack is initially limited by the capacity of the attack pumper's water tank. The attack pumper will be able to support additional hoselines only if the incoming water supply from the relay operation will support them. The amount of flow available is valuable information for the IC and must be identified so that the IC can make tactical adjustments to the overall strategy until the water supply can be improved.

Ultimately, the attack pumper serves as the "workhorse" at the incident; it provides water to all of the hoselines that are attacking the fire. If the attack pumper does not have water, then no attack on the fire can take place.

Relay Pumpers

Relay pumpers are the fire apparatus that are placed in the middle of the relay pumping operation FIGURE 13-4. They obtain their water from the source pumper and increase the pressure to the next fire pumper in the relay. In essence, these pumpers act like booster pumps to maintain pressure throughout the length of the relay. A relay pumper cannot increase the volume of water being pumped; it can only increase the pressure because the source pumper provides the flow (quantity) based on the volume being discharged by the attack pumper. For example, if the source pumper is flowing 800 gpm (3200 L/min) at 80 psi (560 kPa), the relay pumper will receive a flow of 800 gpm (3200 L/min), but due to friction loss in the hoselines, the water will be at a pressure of only 50 psi (350 kPa). The relay pumper will increase the pressure back to 80 psi (560 kPa) and continue to flow 800 gpm (3200 L/min) to the next pumper, which will then increase the pressure again to overcome the friction loss until, ultimately, the 800-gpm (3028-L/min) flow reaches the attack pumper.

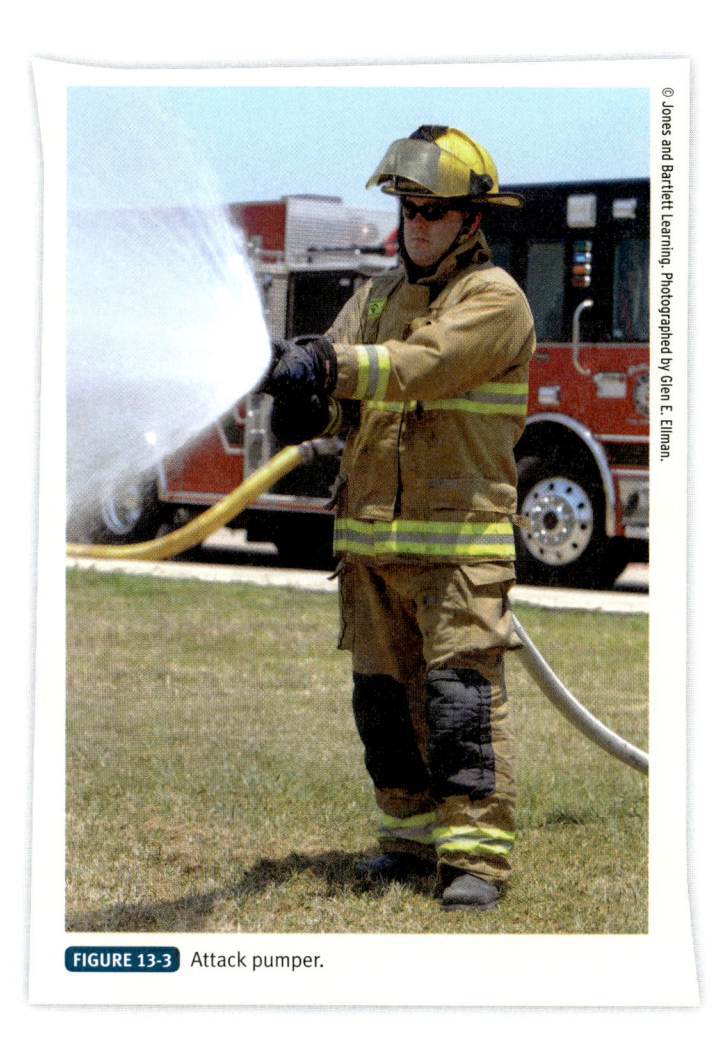

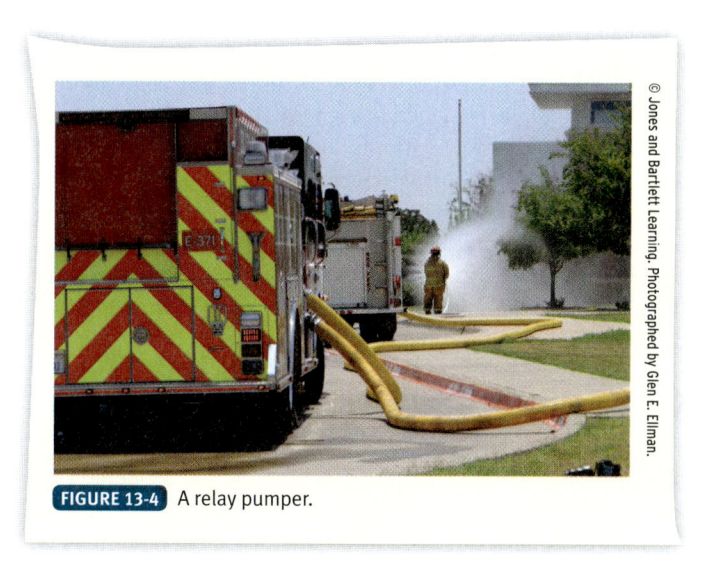

FIGURE 13-3 Attack pumper.

Source Pumper

The source pumper is the most important pumper in a relay because it is located at a water source and supplies the water to the entire incident. The source of the water is either a fire hydrant or a static water source. The source pumper should consist of the largest fire pump of the units assigned to the relay pumping operation, thereby ensuring that it can provide the maximum amount of water. For example, if the source pumper has a 1500-gallon/minute (gpm) (6000-L/min) pump, it should supply the 1000-gpm (4000-L/min) pump on the relay pumper; this setup ensures that the 1000-gpm (4000-L/min) pump can be supplied with enough volume of water to meet its capacity if needed. If the reverse were the case, then the larger pump would not be supplied its capacity because the incoming flow would be less than 1500 gpm (6000 L/min).

Attack Pumper

The attack pumper is usually the first unit on the scene of an incident, and its operation will dictate how much water will be needed, based on how many gpm (L/min) the fire attack requires. If the attack pumper cannot establish its own water supply, it may lay a dry supply line into the scene to be filled later by the source pumper or a relay pumper. If the attack pumper is being positioned in an area that has limited access, it

FIGURE 13-4 A relay pumper.

Equipment for Relay Pumping Operations

Fire hose is the primary path of travel for the water to get from one fire pumper to another in a relay operation. The hose can consist of a single <u>large-diameter hose (LDH)</u>, which is 4, 5, or 6 inches (100, 125, or 152 mm) in diameter, or multiple <u>medium-size hoses</u>, which are 2½ or 3 inches (65 or 77 mm) in diameter. Single lines of LDH, by their design, have a very low friction loss variable—7 psi (48 kPa) per 100 ft (30 m) when flowing 1000 gpm (4000 L/min) in a 5-inch (125-mm) hoseline. Compare this to a single 3-inch (77-mm) medium-size hose, which has a friction loss variable of 21 psi (145 kPa) per 100 ft (30m) for just 500 gpm (2000 L/min). To overcome the higher friction loss associated with use of medium-size hoselines, it is recommended to use two hoses for a water supply. To avoid this issue altogether, it is highly recommended that LDH be used whenever possible.

To determine the friction loss for a relay pumping operation, you must know how much fire hose is in the part of the relay that you are supporting once it is established, the gpm (L/min) as well as the elevation. You can then calculate the friction loss for your part of the relay operation and adjust your discharge pressure accordingly.

Relay pumping operations may require some other standard equipment, such as hose adapters to connect hoses with different types of threads, a Siamese hose (which merges two medium-size hoselines into a single LDH), a manifold (which splits a single LDH into two or three medium-size hoselines), and reducers (which connect larger single hoselines with smaller single hoselines). In addition, no matter which size hose you are using to supply water from the source pumper, each pumper in the relay operation and the attack pumper must be equipped with an intake relief valve. Most modern pumpers are equipped with these valves at the time they are built, but older pumpers may need to be retrofitted with external valves. An intake relief valve will prevent the incoming water supply from reaching an excessively high pressure, which might damage the pump and possibly interrupt the relay operation. Relief valves discharge the excessive pressure through a port located on the valve.

Personnel for Relay Pumping Operations

A safe relay pumping operation requires that you have adequate personnel for the operation. A minimum of two crew members should be assigned to each fire pumper if the pumper will be exposed to moving traffic and other hazards around the fire apparatus. As the driver/operator, it is your responsibility to operate the pump and manage the intake and discharge pressures. The second fire fighter is responsible for managing the area around the fire apparatus so as to ensure the safety of the members by monitoring vehicle movement around the fire pumper and warning you of possible dangers.

Preparing for a Relay Pumping Operation

The length of a relay pumping operation is primarily determined by the distance between the water source and the incident. The amount of water required by the attack pumper and the size of the supply line can also affect whether a relay pumper is required and, if so, how many of these apparatus are needed. As

FIGURE 13-5 Forward lay.

discussed earlier, smaller-diameter supply hoselines decrease the flow capacity and increase the friction loss. Generally, LDH represents the best option for relay pumping operations.

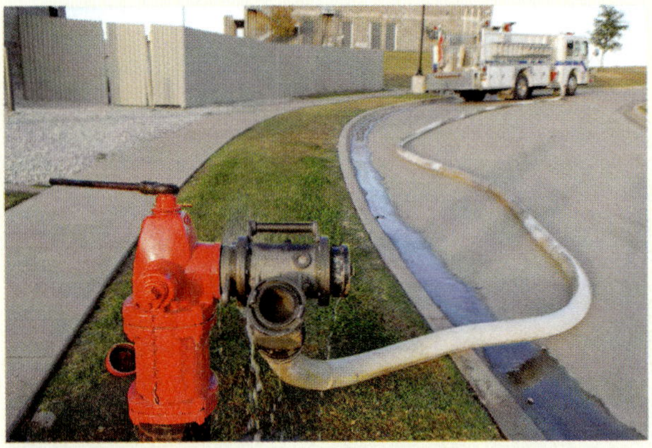

Given that supply hose is critical for a successful relay pumping operation, it must be in place before water can be flowed. A <u>forward lay</u> is a supply hoseline that is brought to the scene by a fire pumper from the water source **FIGURE 13-5**. An engine that connects to a fire hydrant and then proceeds to the fire scene is an example of a forward lay. Hose can also be laid backward from the attack pumper to a water source or to another fire pumper in the relay line; both are examples of the <u>reverse lay</u> technique **FIGURE 13-6**. Alternatively, one fire pumper may lay hose into the scene while another fire pumper lays hose out from the first engine's coupling to the water source; this approach is called a <u>split lay</u> **FIGURE 13-7**. Another type of split lay involves laying a line from an open area to the pumper when there is limited access and having a second pumper connect to that hose and move to the water source.

Once you have the hose in place for the relay, you can determine whether a relay pumper is needed by calculating the amount of friction loss for the length of the hose lay. A good rule of thumb to follow is, if the discharge pressure will exceed 80 psi (560 kPa) for LDH or 175 psi (1225 kPa) for medium-size hoses, a relay pumper is needed to boost the water pressure. Although a good rule of thumb is that no relay operation should extend for more than 800 ft (240 m), it can be longer as long as you keep adding pumpers. Maintaining relay operations over a shorter distance will keep the pump discharge pressures manageable while ensuring the proper quantity of water flows to the attack pumper. Keep in mind that the attack pumper's needs are the deciding factor in terms of the pressure and flow necessary.

Adapters, reducers, manifolds, and appliances may also be used in a relay pumping operation. When two fire pumpers use different threads on their couplings for hose, <u>adapters</u> allow for both pumpers to connect to the same hose. When the sizes of the hoselines differ, <u>reducers</u> are needed to connect the mismatched lines together. <u>Manifolds</u> greatly increase the effectiveness of relays by allowing one LDH to supply two to four medium-size lines with water. When a LDH is split into multiple hoselines in

FIGURE 13-6 Reverse lay.

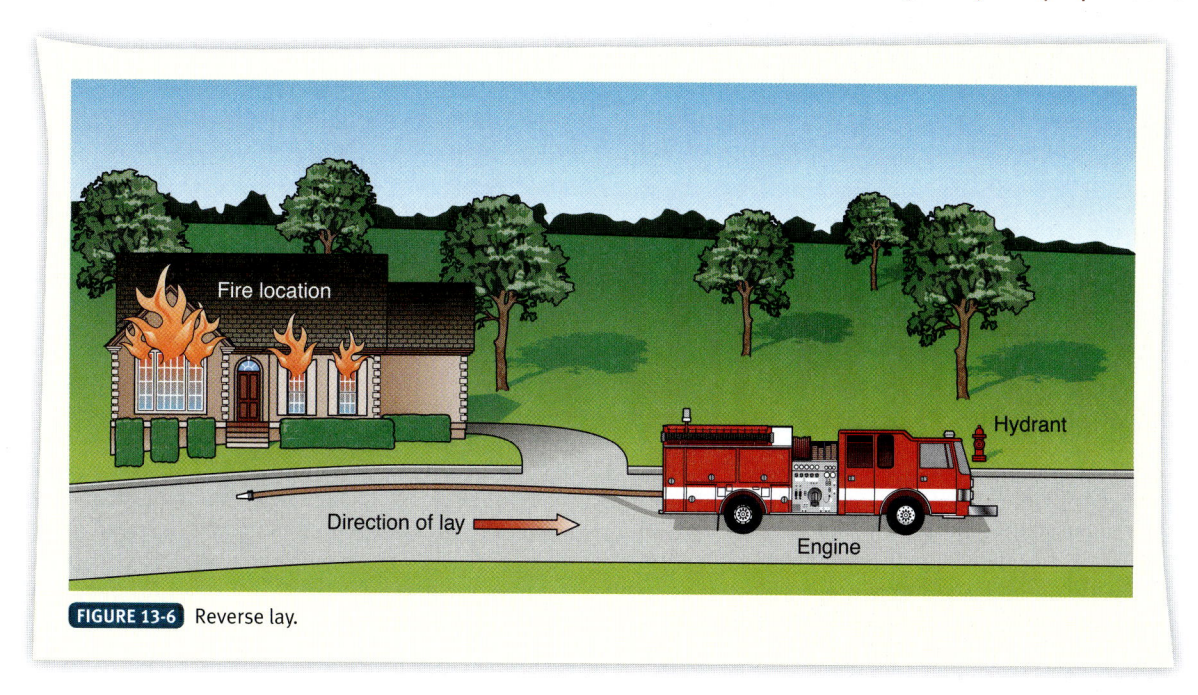

this way, however, the overall friction loss increases due to the restriction of the water back into smaller vessels in addition to the flow restriction within the appliance itself. An appliance is any other component that you can flow water through. The Siamese connection and manifold are examples of appliances that, when used in a relay pumping operation, must be taken into account when calculating the friction loss.

■ Calculating Friction Loss

As stated earlier, the attack pumper's needs drive the relay pumping operation. For this reason, the attack pumper's driver/operator must communicate to the source pumper's driver/operator how much water (gpm [L/min]) is flowing now or is planned to flow. The attack pumper driver/operator can determine his or her flow quickly by adding together the flow of each handline or master stream that the attack pumper is discharging. For example, if the attack pumper were flowing 500 gpm (2000 L/min) from three handlines, the driver/operator would communicate to the source pumper that he or she needs 500 gpm (2000 L/min).

The driver/operator of the source pumper would then calculate the distance between the two pumpers in hose. For this example, assume that two lines of 3-inch hose are laid out over 400 ft. To calculate the friction loss, you would divide the flow in gpm by the number of hoselines being used—two lines, in this case. Each line will flow half of the water required; 500 gpm divided by 2 equals 250 gpm. A 3-inch hoseline at that flow has a friction loss factor of 6 psi per 100 ft, which is multiplied times the number of feet in hundreds (4, in this example), which gives a total friction loss of 24 psi. Once you have calculated

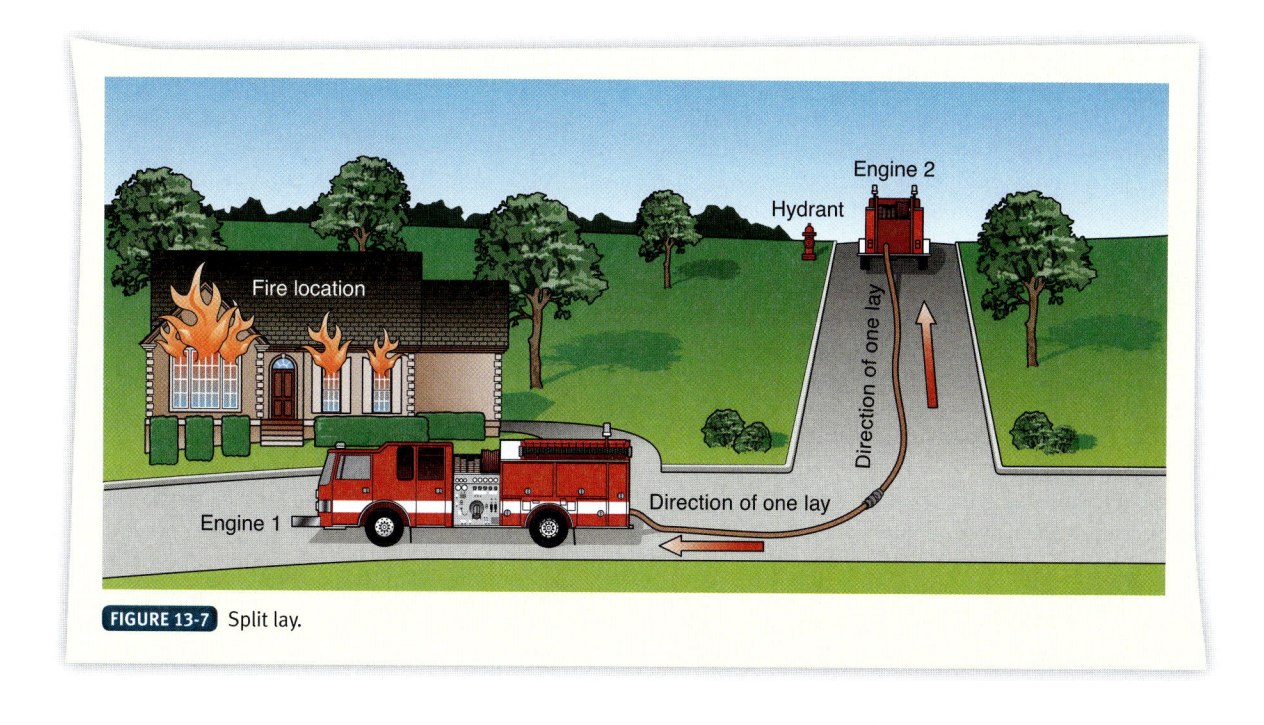

FIGURE 13-7 Split lay.

the friction loss, you would add 20 psi for residual pressure to prevent cavitation, for a total discharge pressure of 44 psi.

In summary, assume the attack pumper is flowing 500 gpm; the source pumper is 400 ft away and has connected to the attack pumper with two 3-inch lines:

> 500 gpm ÷ 2 (number of lines) = 250 gpm
> Friction loss for 3-inch hoseline for every 100 ft = 6 psi
> 6 psi × 4 (number of feet in hundreds) = 24 psi +
> 20 psi − (residual pressure) = 44 psi pump discharge pressure

■ Relay Pumping Operations

One type of relay pumping operation is called a calculated flow relay. It requires the driver/operator of the source pumper to obtain from the attack pumper the flow required for the fire operations; the driver/operator must then calculate the friction loss for each hose layout in the relay and add 20 psi (140 kPa) for residual pressure at the attack pumper. This type of relay is the most common, as it uses actual flow calculations to determine the quantity of water required.

Many fire departments have standardized the supply pressures that they use for constant pressure relays, based on prior experience. The pumper driver/operator in this type of relay sets the pump discharge pressure to 175 or 80 psi (1225 or 560 kPa), depending on the size of the supply line, and maintains this pressure for the duration of the relay pumping operation. Setting the pressure relief valve or pressure governor will maintain the desired pressure in the event of any changes at the attack pumper and will prevent overpressurizing of hoselines or damage to the pump.

■ Operating the Source Pumper

The relay pumping operation starts at the source pumper and is where the largest fire pump should be located. The hose between the pumpers should be placed through either a forward, reverse, or split hose lay. Remember, LDH provides the highest efficiency for relay pumping operations. Once at the water source, the source pumper begins a drafting operation from a static water source (see the "Drafting From a Static Water Source" Skill Drill in the chapter *Drafting and Water Shuttle Operations*) or connects to a fire hydrant.

When setting up a source pumper at a static water source, you must consider the maximum amount of water available for the operation. Once you have established the draft and water is flowing through the dump line, connect the hoselines to be supplied and notify the receiving driver/operator that you are ready to start flowing water. To determine the gpm (L/min) needed, you will need to calculate the friction loss for the supply hose based on the gpm (L/min) rate to be supplied, the length of the relay, the size of the hose being used, plus a residual pressure of 20 psi (140 kPa). If the next pumper is not ready, then wait until it is set up before initiating the flow. If you are supplying the attack pumper, advise its driver/operator that you are ready to begin flowing water; the attack pumper crew will then tell you when to send the water.

Whether you are supplying the next pumper in a relay operation or the attack pumper, the order of the steps remains the same. Open the corresponding discharge valve and slowly begin flowing water while simultaneously advancing the throttle as you are opening the discharge valve; you do not want to lose the draft of the pump (i.e., interfere with the pump's vacuum strength) by flowing more water out than is being supplied to the pump. When you reach the desired pressure, set the pressure relief valve or the pressure governor to prevent damage to your pump if the flow is stopped or interrupted by a relay pumper or the attack pumper.

Establishing a relay pumping operation from a hydrant works in the same way as using a hydrant as a source of water for your own supply; the only difference is that you are supplying another pumper and not the handlines attacking the fire. Select a suitable hydrant that is as close to the incident site as possible. Flush the hydrant before connecting to it with a soft-suction supply hoseline or LDH. If neither of these types of hose is available, you can connect to the hydrant using two medium-size hoselines to establish a water supply. Contact the receiving driver/operator to notify him or her that you are ready to start supplying water. If the next pumper is not ready, wait until it is set up before you begin to flow water. If you are supplying the attack pumper, advise its driver/operator that you are ready to begin the flow; the attack pumper crew will then tell you when to send the water. Fill the supply lines slowly by opening the discharge valves. Advance the throttle to the desired pressure (calculated or constant) and monitor the residual pressure from the hydrant. You will need to set the pressure relief valve or the pressure governor to prevent damage to your pump if the flow is stopped or interrupted by a relay pumper or the attack pumper.

■ Operating the Attack Pumper

The attack pumper is generally the first pumping apparatus to arrive on the scene of a fire. It establishes the hoselines that attack the fire: for example, two 1¾-inch (45-mm) hoselines flowing at 100 gpm (400 L/min) each, requiring a total water flow of 200 gpm (800 L/min) from the pumper. If you start and continue flowing water from the tank on the fire pumper until the relay operation is set up, you will have to monitor your tank level closely to ensure that interior fire crews do not run out of water. Most fire pumpers have 500- to 1000-gal (2000- to 4000-L) water tanks, which allow them to supply the two 1¾-inch (45-mm) hoselines for 2½ to 5 minutes before running out of water.

Getting the water from the source pumper, whether directly or through a relay, is critical to continued operations and fire fighter safety. Once the supply lines are charged, bleed off the air in the hoseline from the bleeder valve located on the pumper's intake valve, until a steady stream of water comes out of the bleeder **FIGURE 13-8**. This air is present as a result of the hose being filled with water; the water displaces this air as it flows into the hose, with the air being forced to the end of the line. It is always a good practice to bleed your supply lines; this action prevents air from entering the pump and causing it to cavitate. The longer the hose lay, the more air that will be displaced.

Slowly open the intake valve while backing down the throttle until the intake valve for the supply line is fully open.

FIGURE 13-8 Bleeder valve on the intake valve.

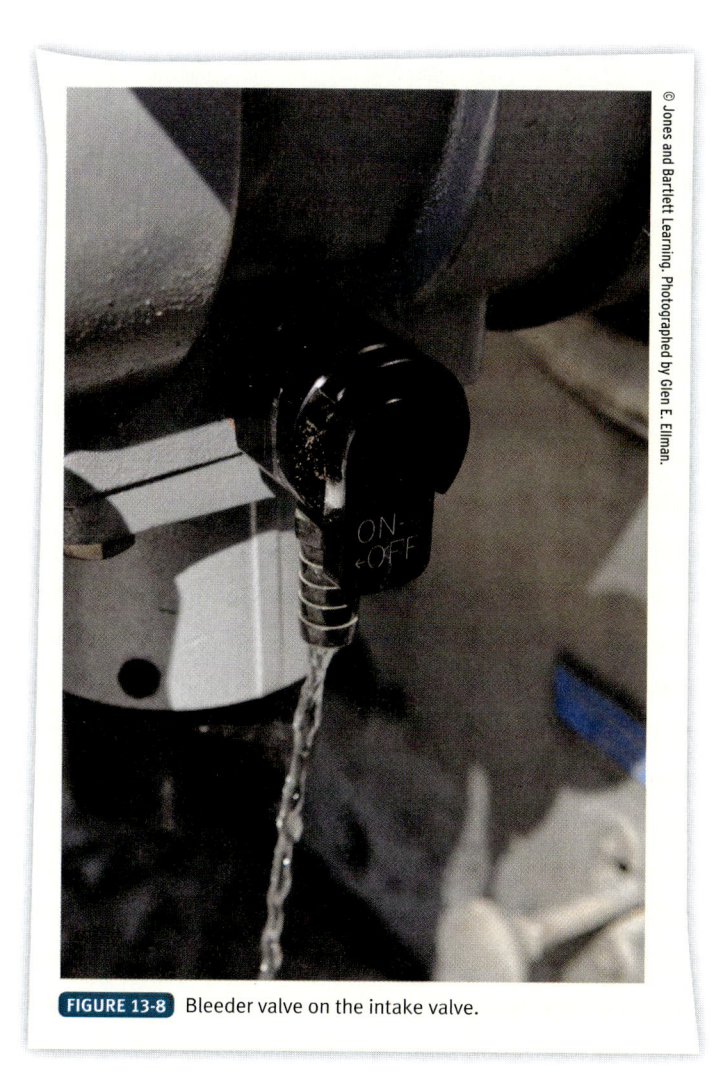

The pressure from the incoming water supply will increase the discharge pressure to the hoselines unless you decrease the throttle rate. The tank-to-pump valve should then be closed in older apparatus, but can remain open in the newer pumps because of the check valve. Then slowly open the tank fill valve; this action will prevent the pump from creating a vacuum in the tank and drawing air into the pump through the open valve into a tank containing little or no water. Open the tank fill valve to only a slight extent; creating too large an opening will take away most of the incoming pressure, so that the handlines will not receive the required pressure and flow. Fill the tank on the attack pumper. When it is full, close the tank fill valve. From this point forward, the attack pumper will be running solely off the relay or source pumper(s).

Advise the source pumper of how much water you need and indicate whether the incoming pressure is sufficient to maintain at least 20 psi (140 kPa) of residual pressure. If you need more flow, contact the personnel providing the supply quickly to communicate your needs, but do not try to flow more water than the source pumper is supplying, as this will cause your own fire pump to cavitate. It is important to notify the crews operating those lines of the situation so that they can make tactical adjustments or retreat to a safe location until the water supply issue is resolved.

Operating the Relay Pumper

The operation of the relay pumper can be quite simple—all you are doing is laying out hose between the next pumper and your location and then supplying the required pressure and volume to the next pumper in line or to the attack pumper. A relay pumper may receive its supply from the source pumper or another relay pumper, depending on the distance between the water source and the attack pumper. If you participate in establishing the relay operation, you will need to provide hose to the receiving pumper, another relay pumper, or the attack pumper through a forward, reverse, or split hose lay. Remember, LDH is the most efficient choice of hose for relay pumping operations. You will need to calculate the friction loss for the supply hose based on the flow rate to be supplied, the length of the relay, the size of the hose being used, plus a residual pressure of 20 psi (140 kPa). Once the hose is in place, the source pumper will contact you to advise that the water flow is ready to start.

A relay pumper is considered ready when the supply hose to the pumper and the discharge hose to the next pumper are connected. When the water fills the supply hose, you should bleed off the air in the hoseline from the bleeder valve located on your pumper's intake valve, until a steady stream of water comes out of the bleeder. Remember, your supply line will contain more air if the hose lay is long. Slowly open the intake valve to allow the water to enter the pump. The tank-to-pump valve on your apparatus should be closed and the pump recirculating valve should be open, which will help prevent the pump from overheating until you start flowing larger quantities of water. Open the discharge valve(s) for the corresponding discharge port(s) to begin flowing water, and adjust the throttle to increase the flow to the desired pressure based on your calculations for friction loss or the predetermined pressure for the relay.

As the driver/operator of a relay pumper, you must monitor the incoming residual pressure from either the source pumper or another relay pumper; your goal is to maintain 20 psi (140 kPa) of residual pressure. To increase the residual pressure, you can either contact the source pumper to request an increase in pressure or decrease your own flow pressure, which may negatively affect the lines supplied by the attack pumper. If the flow or pressure to the attack pumper is ever affected, you must communicate that fact to the driver/operator of the source pumper immediately.

Once the flow is stabilized, set the pressure relief valve or the pressure governor to prevent damage to the fire pump if the flow is stopped or interrupted by either the supply or discharge side of the pump. Remember that you are part of a relay operation and, therefore, are affected by the actions of others supplying your pumper or those receiving your supply.

DRIVER/OPERATOR Tip

If you will be operating for extended periods of time without flowing large volumes of water, consider establishing a dump line away from the fire apparatus so you can continue to flow water without overheating the pump.

VOICES OF EXPERIENCE

It has been my experience that relay pumping operations can be among the most complex tasks that you will have to perform on the fireground. In every relay pumping situation in which I have ever been involved, a number of people and apparatus have had to work together to get the job done.

Although it has long been a long-held belief that relay pumping is a skill that only rural fire departments will need, my experience has been just the opposite. I can recall a number of cases where we had to resort to relay pumping in the Newark (New Jersey) Fire Department. This kind of operation can be as simple as having the source pumper at a hydrant feed an attack pumper in front of a burning building. However, I can recall a situation where a much more complex operation had to be mounted to control a major fire.

I was serving as the acting deputy chief (shift commander) for Tour #3. A call came in for a fire in a major wood-chipping, mulch-making operation in the Port Newark area of the city. Because I was normally the chief of the battalion where the call was happening, I knew that the hydrants were widely spaced and somewhat sparse in that area. The first-due pump arrived on location and reported a heavy fire condition in a large pile of mulch, with possible extension to an office area. Shortly thereafter, the acting battalion chief arrived and called for the working fire signal. I was rolling in under a heavy smoke condition and called for the second alarm prior to my arrival.

As I was arriving on location, a number of the pumper units were working to establish a relay operation to the nearest fire hydrants. After a report of a dead hydrant, I knew that we would need more units and called for a third alarm to be transmitted. To establish this water supply, our personnel had to set up two separate relay operations coming from opposite directions. Each relay consisted of a source pumper, an in-line relay pumper, and an attack pumper receiving the incoming water and applying it through master stream devices.

After using these relay-flow operations for a number of hours, we were able to bring the fire under control with the aid of some large-scale machinery. The key to our success involved being able to move the water from the hydrants, through the source pumpers, through the in-line pumping units, and on to the attack pumpers. We were fortunate to have the skill, capability, and equipment to get the job done in this extraordinary situation.

That day I learned and affirmed a number of important facts:

1. You need to know your hydrant locations.
2. You must be aware of the main sizes in your operational area.
3. Your personnel must be trained to perform this type of operation.
4. The ability to take water into pumpers and move it out effectively and efficiently is not something people will simply know; rather, they must be taught how to move water.
5. The incident commander must have the patience to understand that it will take quite a bit of time to set up relay operations.
6. Yelling and screaming are not a substitute for patience and perseverance.

Dr. Harry Carter
Battalion Chief (ret.)
Newark, New Jersey Fire Department

CHAPTER 13 Relay Pump Operations

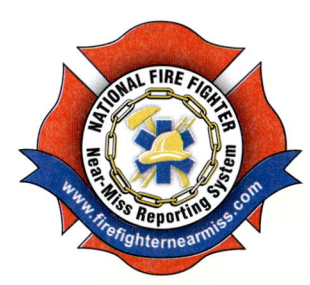

Near-Miss REPORT

Report Number: 12-0000235

Synopsis: Water hammer results in burst 5-inch (127-mm) hose.

Event Description: During a pump operation evolution, a 5-inch (127-mm) supply line suffered a severe water hammer. The attack engine was flowing lines with the supply engine supporting the operation via a humat valve. The attack operator had to ask for more pressure due to the size of the evolution. The attack operator finished the evolution and began to shut everything down on his end. He did not communicate with the supply engine that he was completing his evolution. Instead of communicating with the supply operator regarding decreasing the supply pressure, he went ahead and closed the piston intake. When this happened, the supply operator was boosting the pressure at over 120 psi (827 kPa). This is not normal supply pressure; however, due to the size of the evolution, it was needed. When the pressure reached the closed piston intake, the water hammer could be seen and heard traveling down the 5-inch (127-mm) line until it reached the weakest point, where it burst. Three fire fighters were in close proximity to the line and could have been injured. Also, when the supply line burst, it moved a steel structure that is attached to a six-story drill tower, indicating the seriousness of the water hammer.

Lessons Learned: The main lesson learned is that communication is just as important on the training ground as it is on the fireground. To prevent another occurrence of this type, training officers must ensure students understand the seriousness of water hammer and how easy it can happen if the pump operator does not pay attention to detail.

■ Water Relay Delivery Options

Depending on the nature of the relay pumping operation, the last pumper in the series may supply two attack pumpers. If this is the case, then the last pumper may use a manifold—that is, one LDH that is split into four or five medium-size hoselines that provide the water supply for multiple attack pumpers **FIGURE 13-9**.

To use the manifold as one option in a relay pumping operation, the last relay pumper would provide a supply line to the manifold via a LDH from a discharge port. If two attack pumpers are being used at different locations within the incident, each can be supplied with two medium-size hoselines through the manifold. Once the medium-size hoselines have been attached, contact the attack pumpers to advise them that you are ready to flow water. At that point, the valves on the manifold can be opened to start the flow of water. The pumper supplying the manifold will need to account for the additional friction loss of the appliance plus the residual pressure for the attack pumpers to maintain the correct pump discharge pressure.

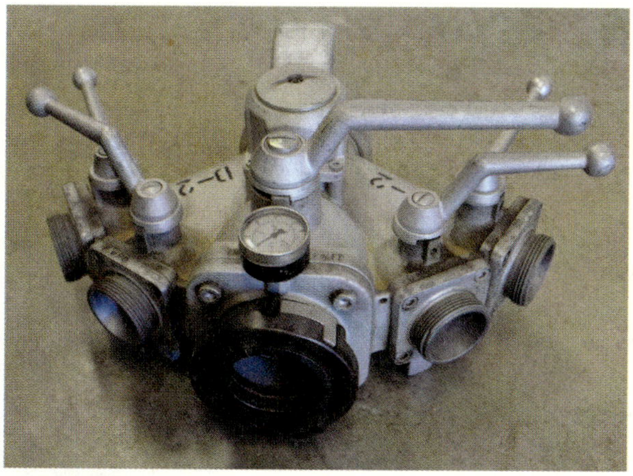

■ Joining an Existing Relay Pumping Operation

Most relay pumping operations are completely set up at the beginning of the incident, because adding a pumper to an existing relay operation usually requires that the flow of water be stopped. Depending on the size of the relay pumping operation, this step could involve a number of pumpers. If you are called to assist with a relay pumping operation and your fire apparatus is not part of the initial setup of the relay, then you need to be able to hook up your pumper to the hoselines that are already in use. Pumpers are generally added to an existing relay pumping operation when there is not enough pressure or flow to meet the demands of the attack pumper.

Many fire departments that regularly use relay pumping operations because of issues related to limited water supply will use a **relay valve** in long hose lays **FIGURE 13-10**. A relay valve lets you hook up into the relay without shutting down the entire relay operation. With this approach, you simply hook up both the supply line and the discharge line to your fire apparatus before opening the relay valve **FIGURE 13-11**. Slowly open the intake valve to your fire apparatus to obtain a water supply. Once the valve is completely open, slowly open the discharge valve from your pump to the hoseline that is connected

FIGURE 13-9 Manifold.

FIGURE 13-10 Relay valve.

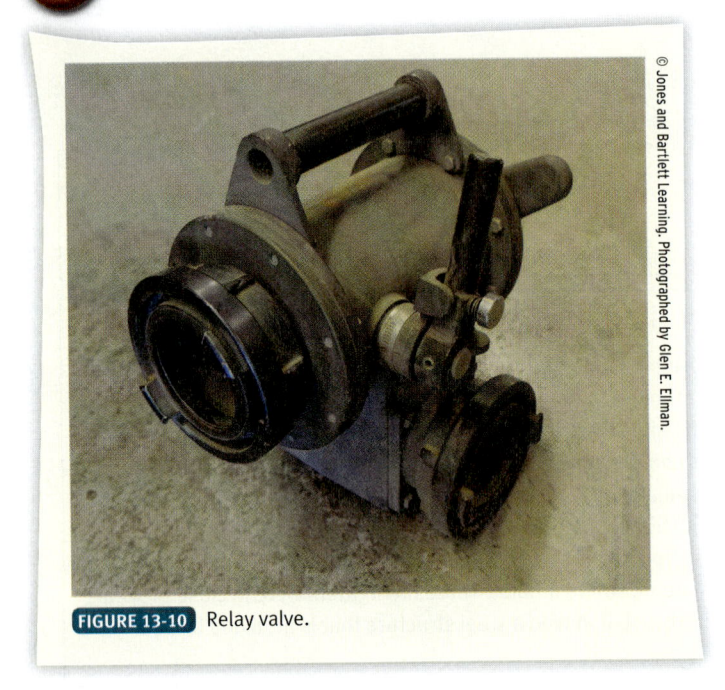

to the relay valve. Observe the incoming supply pressure, and increase the discharge pressure to provide the gpm (L/min) and pressure required by the attack pumper. Monitor the incoming pressure to maintain 20 psi (140 kPa) of residual pressure, and set the pressure relief valve or the pressure governor to prevent damage to your pump if the flow is stopped or interrupted.

If a relay valve is not present or has not been used, then the task of hooking into an existing relay operation is more complex. If you must hook up to an existing relay, get all of your equipment ready and place your fire apparatus in the proper position. Once you have calculated the required discharge pressure based on the length of your hose lay, advise command, or the water supply officer, and the attack pumper that you are ready to hook into the relay. The source pumper and any other relay pumpers in the supply line will then shut down their supply lines while the attack pumper switches from the supply line of the relay to tank water. Attach the incoming line from the source or other relay pumper to your intake valve first, and then attach the discharge line to the discharge valve.

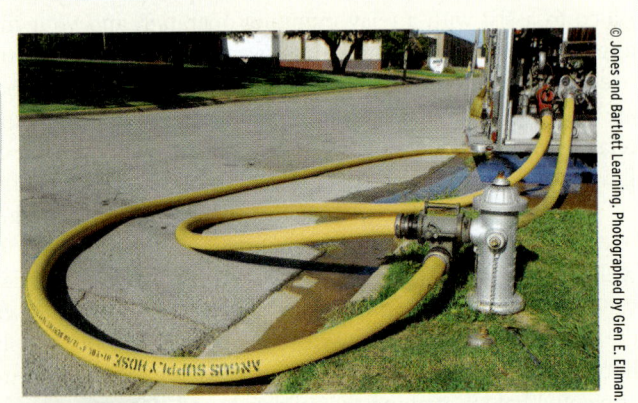

FIGURE 13-11 If you are hooking into a relay valve, hook up both the supply line and the discharge line to your fire apparatus before opening the valve.

Contact the source pumper and inform its crew that you are ready for water, and bleed off the air in the line as this flow enters the intake valve. Contact the next pumper in the relay or the attack pumper to advise its crew that you are flowing water again, and increase the discharge pressure to meet the required gpm (L/min) and pressure flow. After you have water flowing, set the relief valve or gpm (L/min) needed to prevent any sudden surges.

DRIVER/OPERATOR Tip

You need to be quick when hooking into a relay pumping operation that is already flowing water. The attack pumper may have only 2½ to 5 minutes of water in its tank to supply the hoselines and crews operating at the fire.

Pressure Fluctuations in a Relay Pumping Operation

As mentioned previously, the needs and capacity of the attack pumper affect all of the other fire pumpers in the relay operation. The driver/operator of the attack pumper determines the gpm (L/min) needed and notifies the driver/operators of the relay and/or source pumpers of its supply requirements. Unfortunately, should something change suddenly, there may not be time to communicate the need to modify the operation. Mechanical failures or an increase or decrease in hoseline flows, for example, can cause pressure fluctuations. These generally do not have a large effect on the operation and can be handled by the pressure relief valves or the pressure governors.

At other times, you must manually adjust the pump pressures. During an operation, if the attack pumper were flowing 500 gpm (2000 L/min) and a 200-gpm (800-L/min) nozzle was shut down, all of the pumpers in the relay would see an increase in pressure. This event should not be a concern unless the pressure fluctuation is greater than 200 psi (1400 kPa)—a magnitude of change that could cause hoseline failure or pump damage. In such a scenario, the driver/operator of the attack pumper would need to decrease the pump discharge pressure; each pumper in the relay would then need to do the same.

Should the attack pumper open an additional line that results in an increase of flow, all pumpers in the relay will need to ensure that their supply lines do not drop below 20 psi (140 kPa) residual pressure to maintain proper flow. The driver/operator should reduce the discharge flow, notify the next driver/operator in the relay and request additional flow and pressure from the supplying pumper. If additional pressure or flow is not available, the attack pumper must be notified.

Shutting Down a Relay Pumping Operation

The order to terminate or shut down a relay pumping operation is given by the IC or the water supply officer only after careful consideration; relays are difficult to establish and, once in place, should be maintained as long as necessary. Shutting down a relay pumping operation is a simple process, but all pumpers participating in the operation must act in a coordinated fashion.

When shutting down the relay pumping operation, the attack pumper acts first. The driver/operator of the attack pumper must ensure that the tank of the fire apparatus is full and then slowly throttle down. It is important to keep the hoselines flowing water while you shut down a relay, as this will prevent fluctuations in water pressure throughout the entire relay pumping operation. The next pumper in the relay then makes sure that its tank is full and slowly throttles down, while still flowing water. This sequence continues until all pumpers have completed this step, ensuring that their tanks are full. When the source pumper is reached, it contacts the attack pumper to begin closing the intake valve; all pumpers in the relay then begin closing the intake and discharge lines until all pumpers are no longer flowing water, including the dump line from the source pumper. The hoselines can then be disconnected and drained before being reloaded or rolled up. This systematic approach to terminating a relay pumping operation prevents pump damage by keeping the water flowing at low levels before it is finally shut down completely.

The source pumper can then close the hydrant to stop the flow of water into this pump. Alternatively, if it is providing water from a static water source, simply stopping the flow of water through the pump will break the vacuum and draft of the pump. This action will stop the flow of water through the hard suction hose into the pump. If that interruption does not occur immediately, disengage the pump, remove a cap from an unused discharge port, and open the valve. This move should allow the water to drain back through the hard suction hoseline and back into the static water source. The setup steps are simply reversed, all equipment and hose are placed back onto the fire apparatus, and the pumper is ready to return to service.

Safety for Relay Pumping Operations

Safety is the utmost concern in any operation and cannot be overlooked when conducting relay pumping operations. It is an understatement to say that water is critical to the success of any firefighting operation. In areas where an uninterrupted water source is not available and must be established, knowing where and how you will obtain a water supply starts with planning before the incident begins. Identifying large static water sources, dry hydrants, or potential drafting sites before an incident occurs will help improve the efficiency of the incident response.

Incident safety is improved when crew members have the appropriate training, knowledge of how the equipment works, and practice in using it. Which equipment does your company have available? Which appliances are needed for the operation? Do your crew members know how to use them? Make sure that you fully understand the role played by each position within a relay pumping operation, and practice those roles regularly. An effective driver/operator will know which equipment he or she will need or use to provide water to the scene of a fire through a relay pumping operation.

Communication is another area that must be addressed as part of any relay pumping operation. Contact the IC for a tactical channel to which all pump operators can be assigned. With this communications setup, all pump operators can talk to one another directly when making requests for additional water or other pressure adjustments without distracting the fire attack operations personnel who are communicating on the main tactical channel. In addition, constant communication between the pump driver/operators will help prevent situations that might otherwise cause pump damage.

Fire hose is another source of safety concerns during a relay pumping operation. Watch for any signs of damage to or possible trouble with the hose. If a catastrophic failure were to occur in the hoselines of a relay pumping operation, the safety of the fire fighters on the handlines at the fire scene will be compromised. If you can identify defects and replace the hose section before it is used, you will save time later and have a safer operation. If you do see a defect after the operation has begun, simply get the replacement hose in place and follow the shutdown procedures used for entering an existing relay pumping operation, in which the attack pumper switches to tank water before stopping the flow of water from the relay.

The last area of concern regarding safety focuses on the personnel working around a relay pumping operation and their use of personal protective equipment (PPE). The pump driver/operator is at risk for injury if he or she is not wearing some type of protective gear. At a minimum, personnel should wear turnout pants and boots, a helmet, and gloves. This PPE will protect the driver/operator's hands, feet, and head from injury caused by falling equipment or catastrophic failure of a hoseline. If crew members will be operating in or around the street and moving traffic, they must wear reflective vests as well, even during daytime operations.

> **Safety Tip**
>
> The safety of both firefighting personnel and the public should be on your mind at all times. When you have laid hose down in a roadway, have the police close the road to vehicle traffic. If the police are not present at the time, then have a support vehicle block the road.

Wrap-Up

Chief Concepts

- Establishing an uninterrupted water supply is one of the most important objectives for any IC.
- Having a sustainable water supply is a vital part of any fire incident scene.
- A relay pump operation consists of a least two pumpers.
- The source pumper is located at the water source.
- The attack pumper is located at the fire scene.
- The relay pumpers are placed between the source and attack pumpers.
- A relay pump operation may be completed with LDH or multiple medium-size hoses.
- Various hose lays may be used to lay the hose between pumpers.
- Two basic types of hose relay pumping operations are calculated flow and constant pressure relay.
- Relay valves may be used so that the pumping operation does not have to be shut down when a new pumper hooks into the system.
- Constant communication between the driver/operators is necessary for a safe operation.

Hot Terms

adapter Any device that allows fire hose couplings to be safely interconnected with couplings of different sizes, threads, or mating surfaces, or that allows fire hose couplings to be safely connected to other appliances.

forward lay A method of laying a supply line in which the line starts at the water source and ends at the attack pumper.

large-diameter hose (LDH) A hose of 3½ inches (90 mm) size or larger.

manifold An appliance that allows a large-diameter hoseline to be split into four or five medium-size hoselines.

medium-size hose Hose that is 2½ or 3 inches (65 or 77 mm) in diameter.

reducer A device that connects two hoses with different couplings or threads together.

relay pumping operation The process of moving water from a water source through hose to the place where it will be needed.

relay valve A specialized type of valve that can be placed on a hydrant and is used in conjunction with a pumper to increase water pressure in relaying operations.

reverse lay A method of laying a supply line in which the line starts at the attack pumper and ends at the water source.

split lay A scenario in which the attack engine lays a supply line from an intersection to the fire, and the supply engine lays a supply line from the hose left by the attack engine to the water source.

References

National Fire Protection Association (NFPA) 1002, *Standard for Fire Apparatus Driver/Operator Professional Qualifications*. 2014. http://www.nfpa.org/codes-and-standards/document-information-pages?mode=code&code=1002. Accessed March 27, 2014.

DRIVER/OPERATOR
in action

You soon realize that as the source pumper, your apparatus is the most important pumper in this short relay. If you are unable to obtain and flow an adequate amount of water, that failure may affect the ability of the other units to protect the exposures. After making the correct connections, communicating with the other driver/operator at the attack pumper, and determining the correct pressure, you have assured an adequate water supply for the operation.

1. A _____ is a supply hoseline that is brought to the scene by a fire pumper from the water source.
   A. Reverse lay
   B. Fast lay
   C. Forward lay
   D. Split lay

2. Which type of relay pumping operation eliminates the need for pump calculations?
   A. Fire flow relay
   B. Constant pressure relay
   C. Calculated relay
   D. Direct relay

3. A _____ lets a pumper connect into the relay without shutting down the entire relay operation.
   A. Relay adapter
   B. Hydrant valve
   C. Relay manifold
   D. Relay valve

4. To establish any type of relay, you must have, at a minimum, a water source, hoselines, personnel, and _____ pumping apparatus.
   A. 1
   B. 2
   C. 3
   D. 4

5. During a relay pump operation, the source pumper should be the largest fire pump available.
   A. True
   B. False

Foam

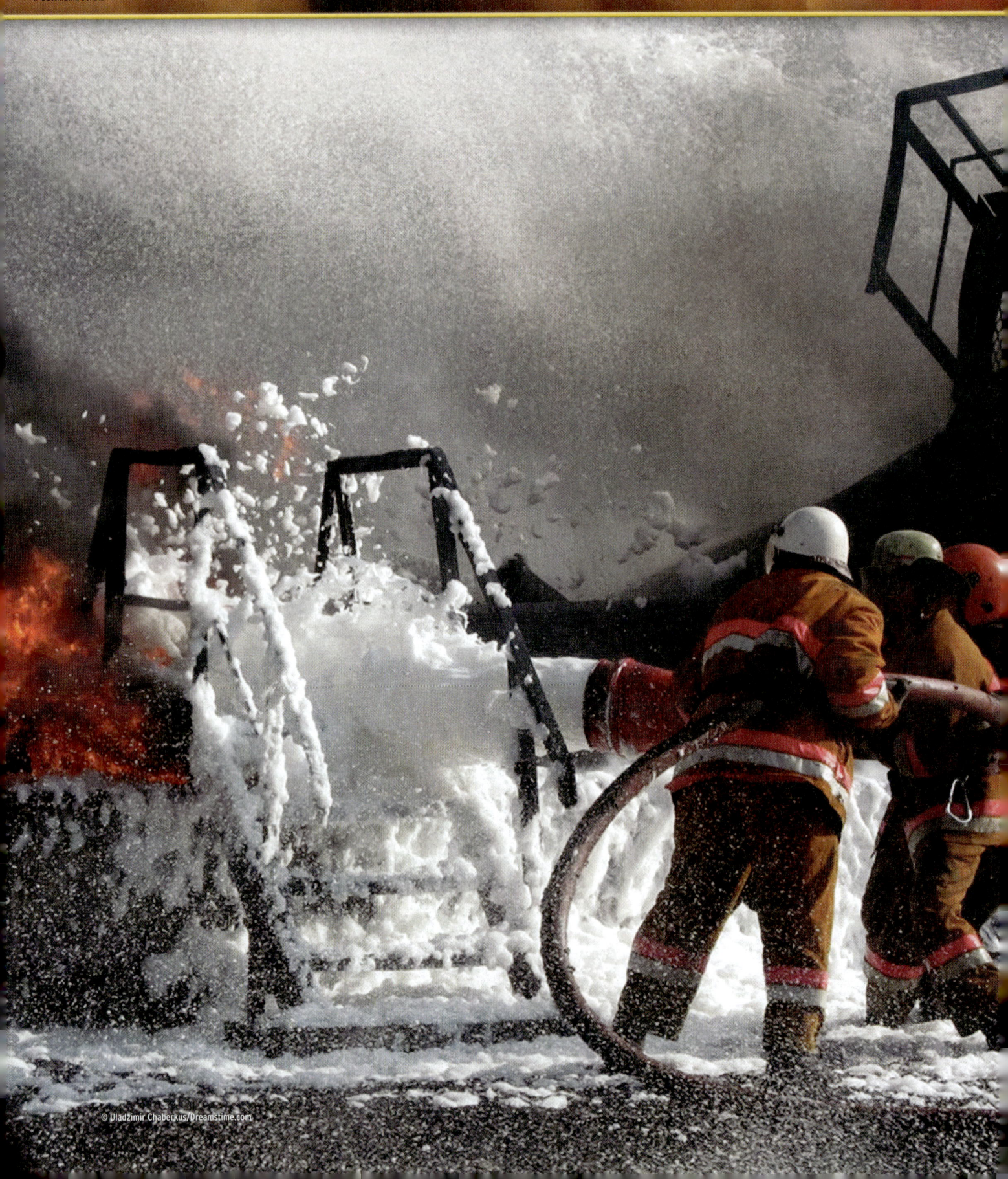

CHAPTER 14

Knowledge Objectives

After studying this chapter, you will be able to:
- Describe how foam works. (5.1.1(3), 5.2.3, 5.2.3 (A); p 327–350)
- Describe the foam tetrahedron. (5.1.1(3), 5.2.3, 5.2.3 (A); p 328)
- Describe foam characteristics. (5.1.1(3), 5.2.3, 5.2.3 (A); p 328–329)
- Describe the different types of foam concentrates. (5.1.1(3), 5.2.3, 5.2.3 (A); p 333)
- Describe foam expansion rates. (5.1.1(3), 5.2.3, 5.2.3 (A); p 333–334)
- Describe foam percentages and their importance. (5.1.1(3), 5.2.3, 5.2.3 (A); p 334–343)
- Describe foam guidelines and limitations. (5.1.1(3), 5.2.3, 5.2.3 (A); p 329–333)
- Describe the different types of foam application systems. (5.1.1(3), 5.2.3, 5.2.3 (A); p 345–350)

Skills Objectives

After studying this chapter, you will be able to:
- Batch-mix foam. (5.2.3, 5.2.3 (B); p 334–335)
- Operate an in-line eductor. (5.2.3, 5.2.3 (B); p 335–338)
- Operate an around-the-pump proportioning system. (5.2.3, 5.2.3 (B); p 337, 339)
- Operate a balanced-pressure proportioning system. (5.2.3, 5.2.3 (B); p 340)
- Operate an injection foam system. (5.2.3, 5.2.3 (B); p 340–341)
- Operate a compressed-air foam system (CAPS). (5.2.3, 5.2.3 (B); p 341–343)
- Apply Class A foam on a fire. (5.2.3, 5.2.3 (B); p 345–347)
- Apply foam with the roll-on method. (5.2.3, 5.2.3 (B); p 346, 348)
- Apply foam with the bankdown method. (5.2.3, 5.2.3 (B); p 348–349)
- Apply foam with the raindown method. (5.2.3, 5.2.3 (B); p 349–350)

Additional NFPA Standards

- NFPA 11, *Standard for Low-, Medium-, and High-Expansion Foam*
- NFPA 18 A, *Standard on Water Additives for Fire Control and Vapor Mitigation*
- NFPA 1403, *Standard on Live Fire Training Evolutions*

You Are the Driver/Operator

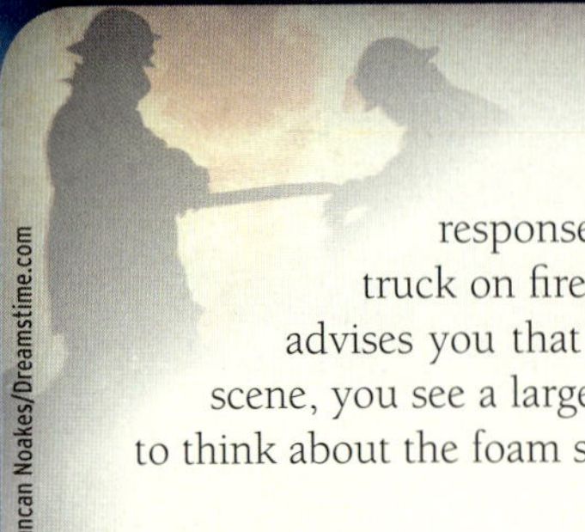

As the driver/operator of an engine company, you take great pride in knowing the capabilities of your assigned apparatus. While working an extra shift, you are assigned to another engine company located on the other side of the city. This is not your usual apparatus or response district. Before you can finish checking the apparatus over, you are dispatched to a reported semi-truck on fire in the middle of a busy freeway. While your company is responding to the call, the dispatch center advises you that the semi-truck was carrying flammable liquids and has caught fire. As you are driving to the fire scene, you see a large column of black smoke and realize that your fire apparatus will be the first on the scene. You start to think about the foam system, including how it operates. The following questions pop up in your mind:

1. What is the procedure to operate the onboard foam system?
2. Which type of foam is appropriate for this situation?
3. Will you have enough of the correct type of foam to knock down this fire?

Introduction

Water has been the main means of suppressing fires for many years. Water is effective, bountiful, and relatively inexpensive to use. While water is certainly effective, foams have added a new dimension to fighting fires. Among the many hazards that fire fighters must contend with today are a wide variety of incidents involving **combustible liquids** and **flammable liquids**. Successful control and extinguishment of these incidents require not only the proper application of **foam** on the fuel surface, but also an understanding of the physical characteristics of foam. A full understanding of foam and its application is imperative to a safe and successful suppression operation. Lack of familiarity with the chemical characteristics of foam and its application can cause severe problems for both you and your crew—so you must know your equipment and operate safely.

With improvements in, and greater simplicity of, application techniques and the versatility of foam concentrates, the use of foam for all types of fires is becoming more common. The National Institute of Standards and Technology (NIST) has determined that foam is three to five times more effective than plain water in extinguishing fires, which can justify its use and its added expense at an incident site.

History

Foam has been available for firefighting for many years. In the 1800s, it was introduced as an extinguishing agent for flammable liquid fires. This foam was produced by mixing two powders—aluminum sulfate and sodium bicarbonate—with water in a foam generator. This method was used for chemical foam extinguishers as well. Inside the fire extinguisher, the two chemicals were stored separately. To operate the fire extinguisher, a seal was broken and the extinguisher was inverted, allowing the aluminum sulfate and sodium bicarbonate to mix and create the foam.

In the 1940s, a foam concentrate based on liquid protein was introduced. This foam, which was made from natural animal protein by-products, was produced by mechanically mixing the protein foam concentrate with water in a **foam proportioner**. A foam proportioner is a device that mixes the foam concentrate into the fire stream in the proper percentage. Protein-based foam was primarily used to fight flammable liquid fires aboard Navy ships **FIGURE 14-1**.

In the 1960s, fluoroprotein foam (FP) and aqueous film-forming foam (AFFF) were introduced. These foams were more versatile and performed better than protein foam. In particular, they were able to knock down fires faster than protein foam and had a longer blanket life.

In the 1970s, alcohol-resistant foams became available. Such foams could be used for fires involving hydrocarbon or polar solvent fuels. The introduction of alcohol-resistant foams allowed flexibility in dealing with the many types of fuels that fire fighters encounter on a daily basis.

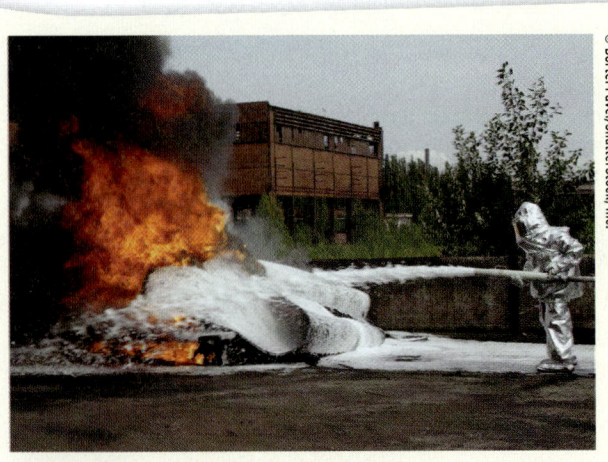

FIGURE 14-1 The protein foam first used on Navy ships in the 1940s is still used in the fire service today.

While the use of foam has been limited in the past for many reasons, the technological improvements made to foams and the equipment associated with their application have made these agents' use more common and acceptable in today's fire service. As more fire apparatus have been equipped with foam systems, operation and maintenance of these systems have emerged as important skills for the driver/operator. The knowledge necessary to properly operate and maintain these systems can come only from learning about and training with the systems.

DRIVER/OPERATOR Tip

Training with foam concentrates and foam systems is critical to being able to properly operate the system when you are at "the big one." Many fire departments do not like to use foam concentrate for training because of the cost factors involved. Even so, the only way to make absolutely sure that you know how to operate the foam system and that it is operating properly is to train as if you are at a real incident. Training foams are available and offer an inexpensive alternative to using regular foam concentrates during such exercises.

Overview

Why is foam used for firefighting? What are the reasons for equipping fire apparatus with foam systems? What are the benefits that make firefighting with foam so popular that fire departments are willing to spend thousands of dollars to add this equipment to their fire apparatus? Is it a fad, or does firefighting with foam truly make a difference?

With the introduction of the automobile and the use by industry of petroleum products, fire fighters soon realized that water was not effective for extinguishing fires involving these products. Because water is heavier than petroleum, its application to petroleum-fueled fires caused more problems than it solved. In fact, water would actually spread the fire and make the situation worse. A method was needed to deal with the growing use of petroleum products and the resulting incidents that occurred when those products ignited. Firefighting foam was one of the methods available to deal with these issues.

■ What Is Foam?

The foam used for firefighting purposes is a stable mass of small, air-filled bubbles. It has a lower density than oil, gasoline, or water, meaning that it will float on top of the fuel. The way that foam works to help extinguish a fire is very simple **FIGURE 14-2**. Once applied to the burning fuel, the foam will float and form a blanket on the surface. This blanket, if applied correctly, will stop or prevent the burning process by separating the fuel from the air, lowering the temperature of the fuel, and/or suppressing the release of flammable vapors.

Foam is created through the application of four components: water, foam concentrate, mechanical agitation, and air. First, water is mixed with the foam concentrate in various

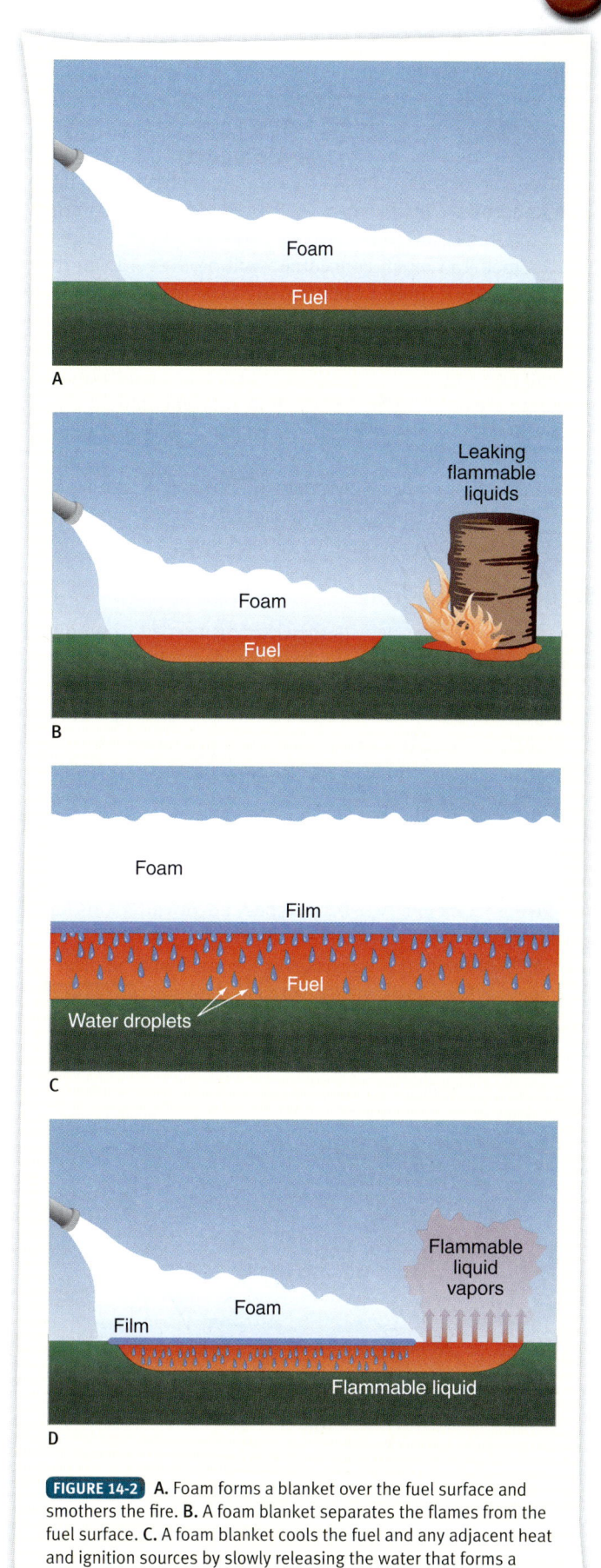

FIGURE 14-2 **A.** Foam forms a blanket over the fuel surface and smothers the fire. **B.** A foam blanket separates the flames from the fuel surface. **C.** A foam blanket cools the fuel and any adjacent heat and ignition sources by slowly releasing the water that forms a major portion of the foam. **D.** A foam blanket suppresses the release of flammable vapors that can mix with air.

ratios to produce a **foam solution**. This solution must then be mixed with air by some form of mechanical agitation. In firefighting, this mechanical agitation usually takes the form of a nozzle that mixes the air and foam solution to form the final product, which is referred to as **finished foam**.

The ratio of water to foam concentrate is critical. Too little foam concentrate in the water will produce a foam solution that is too thin (lean) to be effective and may quickly dissipate into the fuel. Too much concentrate will produce a foam that may be too thick (rich) to be properly expanded or aspirated when mixed with air.

The expansion of foam solution depends on good mechanical agitation and effective **aeration**, the process of introducing air into the foam solution. When an insufficient amount of air is introduced into the solution stream, the solution is poorly aerated. This results in foam with few bubbles; fewer bubbles cause the foam to break down quickly so that it does not suppress vapors effectively. Poorly aerated foam will also break down quickly when exposed to heat and flame.

■ Foam Tetrahedron

A **foam tetrahedron** depicts the elements needed to produce finished foam **FIGURE 14-3**. If any of the elements of the tetrahedron is missing or not present at the proper concentration, foam production will be affected. The result can range from a poor-quality, ineffective foam to no foam produced at all. The foam tetrahedron includes four components:

1. Water
2. Foam concentrate
3. Air
4. Mechanical agitation

Foams come in two basic types: **chemical foams** and **mechanical foams**. Chemical foams are produced through a reaction between two chemicals, like the one that took place in the chemical foam extinguishers used in the 1800s **FIGURE 14-4**. Today, this type of foam is rarely used because it requires the combination of two different chemicals before the foam can be made, which may be difficult to carry out at a fire scene. Also, because of the large amount of powders required, this type of foam has become obsolete in today's fire service.

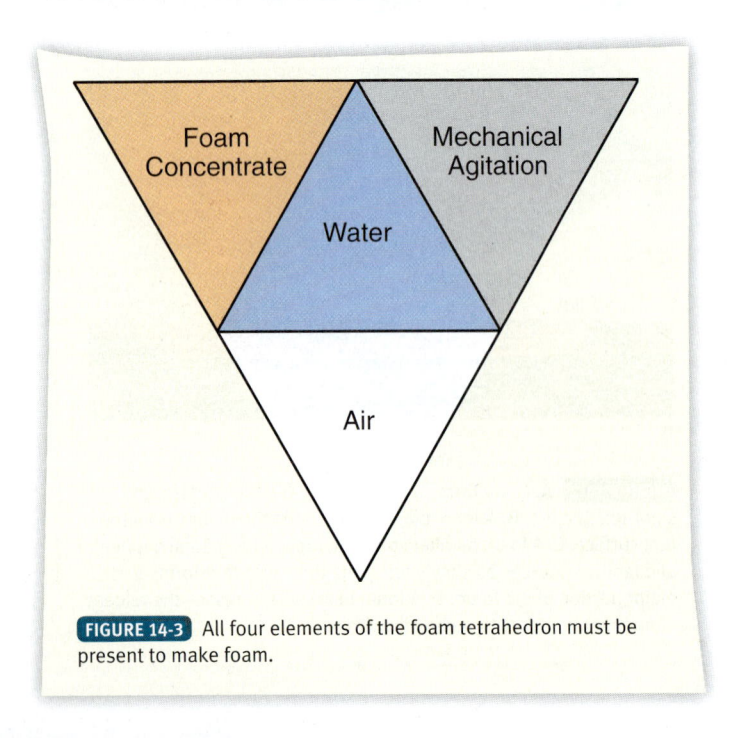

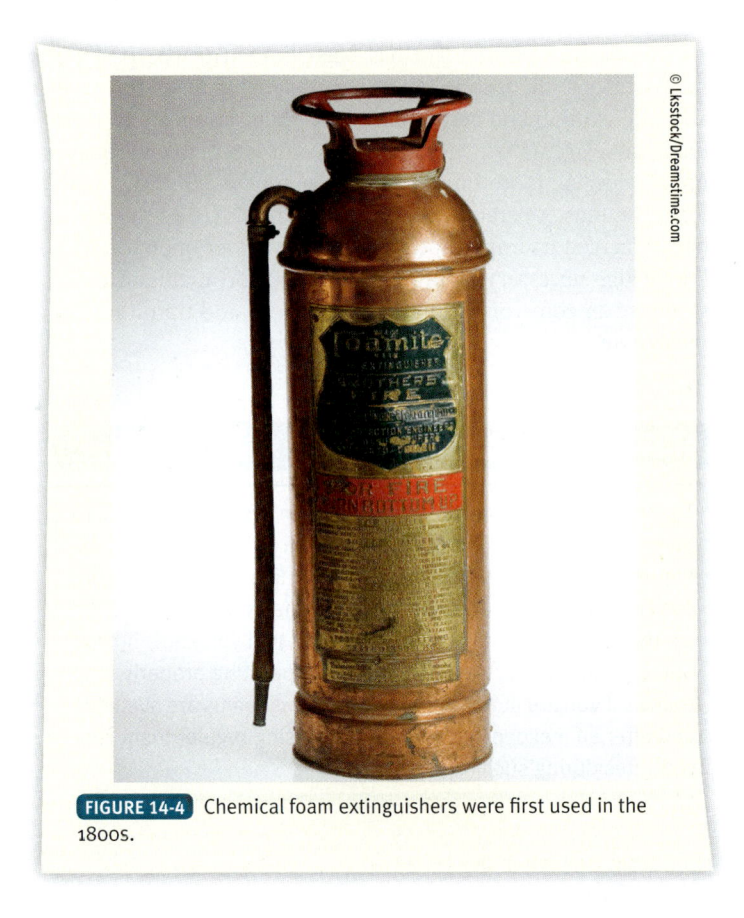

Mechanical foams are produced when water and foam concentrate are mixed in the appropriate amounts (**proportioned**). The ratio of foam concentrate to water must be correct to ensure that the foam-creation operation is effective. The class of materials involved in the spill or fire, which dictates the type of fire, determines the percentage of foam needed.

Hydrocarbon fuels, such as gasoline, jet fuel, and kerosene, have a lower **surface tension** than water. When these types of fuels and water are mixed, the two fluids quickly separate; the fuel rises to the top and the water remains on the bottom. When **foam concentrate (foam liquid)** is mixed with water, the surface tension is reduced, allowing the foam solution to float on the surface of the fuel. Its presence will suppress the vapors both by separating the fuel from oxygen and the ignition source and by cooling the fuel below its ignition temperature.

Producing finished foam has become a very common task for operators of fire apparatus. The modern foam systems are user friendly, and the easy setup and application steps have made foam an important tool for fire fighters to have at their disposal.

■ Foam Characteristics

Good foam must have the right combination of physical characteristics if it is to be effective. Specifically, it must have good knockdown speed and flow as well as good fuel resistance.

Knockdown speed and flow comprises the time required for a foam blanket to spread out across a fuel surface. The foam must also be able to flow around obstacles to achieve complete extinguishment and vapor suppression.

FIGURE 14-4 Chemical foam extinguishers were first used in the 1800s.

FIGURE 14-3 All four elements of the foam tetrahedron must be present to make foam.

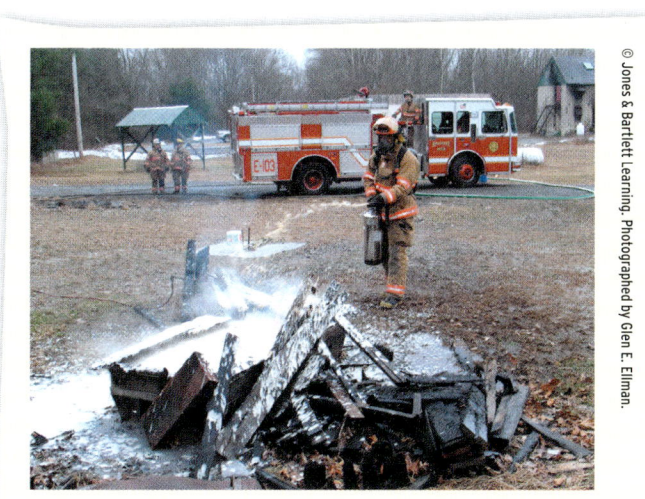

FIGURE 14-5 A good vapor-suppressing foam blanket is needed to prevent re-ignition.

Foam must have good heat resistance so that it can avoid breakdown from the effects of direct flame contact with burning fuel vapors or the heat generated from metal objects. **Fuel resistance** is foam's ability to minimize **fuel pick-up**, which is the absorption of the burning fuel into the foam itself. This **oleophobic** (ability to shed hydrocarbons) quality reduces the amount of fuel saturation in the foam and prevents the foam blanket from burning.

Ideally, foam will produce a good vapor-suppressing blanket. A vapor-tight foam blanket reduces the generation of flammable vapors above the fuel surface and minimizes the chance of reignition **FIGURE 14-5**. When used on polar solvent fuels, foam must also be alcohol resistant. Given that alcohol readily mixes with water and that foam is mostly water, a foam blanket that is not alcohol resistant will quickly dissolve into the fuel and be destroyed.

DRIVER/OPERATOR Tip

Operating foam lines that produce poor-quality foam or no foam at all can prevent the desired results of the operation from being achieved and endanger the fire fighters who are managing the hoselines. It is the driver/operator's responsibility to make sure that foam is being produced at the proper ratio. Know your foam system!

Foam Classifications

Firefighting foams are classified as either Class A or Class B. Understanding the difference in classes of foam as well as the advantages and disadvantages of each class will help you to safely and effectively handle an incident where foam is needed.

Class A Foams

Class A foams are used on ordinary combustible materials such as wood, textiles, and paper; they are also effective on organic materials such as straw and hay. Class A foams, which are sometimes referred to as wetting agents, are very effective because they improve the penetrating effect of water and allow for greater heat absorption. According to foam manufacturers, these wetting agents can extinguish fires involving Class A materials as much as 20 times faster than water **FIGURE 14-6**.

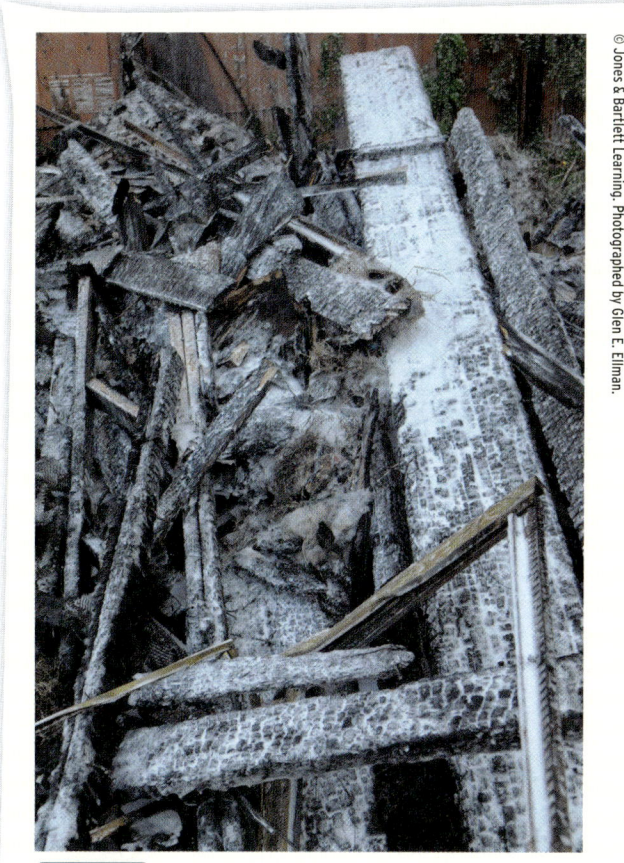

FIGURE 14-6 Class A foam improves the penetrating effect of water.

Class A foam is particularly useful for protecting buildings in rural areas during forest and brush fires when the water supply is limited. It can also be used as a **fire barrier**—that is, an obstruction to the spread of fire. A thick blanket of Class A foam applied to an exposure can provide adequate protection for that exposure, thereby preventing the spread of fire **FIGURE 14-7**. Many fire departments use Class A foam while performing initial attack and overhaul of fires.

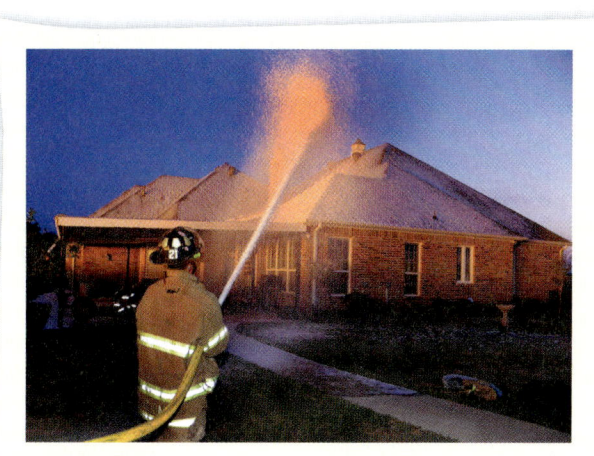

FIGURE 14-7 A thick blanket of Class A foam applied to an exposure can provide adequate protection to that exposure, thereby preventing the spread of fire.

Class A foam increases the effectiveness of the water as an extinguishing agent by reducing the surface tension of the water. As a result, the water penetrates dense materials instead of running off the surface; in addition, more heat is absorbed by the water. The foam also keeps water in contact with unburned fuel to prevent its ignition. Class A foam can be added to water streams and applied with various nozzles.

Class B Foams

Class B foams are used on hydrocarbon, combustible fuels, or polar solvent fires TABLE 14-1. A hydrocarbon is a chemical compound that contains the elements carbon and hydrogen; fuel oil is an example. Polar solvent and water-miscible fuels, such as acetone, mix readily with water and will degrade the effectiveness of ordinary Class B foam.

Class B foams are divided into the following categories:
- Protein foams
- Fluoroprotein foams
- Alcohol-resistant film-forming fluoroprotein foam (AR-FFFP)

Wetting Agents and Foams

There has been a significant amount of discussion over the years regarding nearly every wetting agent, additive, water additive, and foam. Most of these discussions have been and continue to be clouded with misinformation and misunderstanding about each extinguishment medium. It is common for fire fighters to make the mistake that a wetting agent is a foam, because they are very similar by sight (the containers may be the same and they have a similar appearance upon application); however, they are very different in chemical make-up.

- A wetting agent reduces the surface tension of water and enhances penetration into the fuel that is burning.
- A foam creates a stable mass of small, air-filled bubbles with a lower density than oil, gas, or water and will float on top of the burning fuel, creating a blanket that separates the fuel from air, lowering the temperature and suppressing the vapors.

When choosing a wetting agent or a foam, make sure the foam or wetting agent is listed by a national recognized listing agency, and always make sure you follow the manufacturer's specifications on the foam or wetting agent. Always use caution when using foam or wetting agents on the following types of fires:
- Flammable and combustible liquids
- Cooking media, such as vegetable oil or animal fats

Over the past 35 years, there have been some significant scientific advancements for both wetting agents and foams. For a well-trained driver/operator, however, it is wise to always ensure that the product is listed by an independent testing firm and meets the current National Fire Protection Association (NFPA) standards. Moreover, it is just as important to read and understand the manufacturer's specification and have a clear understanding of the limitations of both wetting agents and foams. The future may bring such wetting agents that can handle both Class A and Class B fires with the recent development of NFPA 18A, *Standard on Water Additives for Fire Control and Vapor Mitigation*, and testing criteria designed to test water additives to suppress both classifications of fires with one extinguishing agent.

> **Safety Tip**
>
> According to the *NFPA Fire Protection Handbook*, fire fighters should always exercise caution when using wetting agents described in NFPA 18, *Standard on Wetting Agents*, for Class B situations. The testing criteria used to classify the wetting agent for use on Class B fires may be significantly different from the testing criteria used to classify AFFF, fluoroprotein, and protein foams.

Protein Foams

Protein foams are used to extinguish Class B fires involving hydrocarbons. These agents can protect flammable and combustible liquids where they are stored, transported, and processed. Protein foams contain naturally occurring proteins—that is, animal by-products—as the foaming agent. They are based on keratin protein derived from sources such as chicken feathers or animal hooves that has gone through the process of hydrolysis. Protein foams also include stabilizers and inhibitors, which prevent corrosion and control viscosity. They produce highly stabilized mechanical foam with good expansion properties, excellent heat and burnback resistance, and good drainage characteristics.

Regular protein foams may be created using either fresh or salt water. These foams must be properly aspirated, however; thus they should not be used with non-aspirating structural fog nozzles. Regular protein foams have slower knockdown

TABLE 14-1 Class B Foams and Their Properties

Property	Protein	Fluoroprotein	AFFF	FFFP	AR-AFFF
Knockdown	Fair	Good	Excellent	Good	Excellent
Heat resistance	Excellent	Excellent	Fair	Good	Good
Fuel resistance	Fair	Excellent	Moderate	Good	Good
Vapor suppression	Excellent	Excellent	Good	Good	Good
Alcohol resistance	None	None	None	None	Excellent

AFFF, aqueous film-forming foam; FFFP, film-forming fluoroprotein foam; AR-AFFF, alcohol-resistant aqueous film-forming foam.

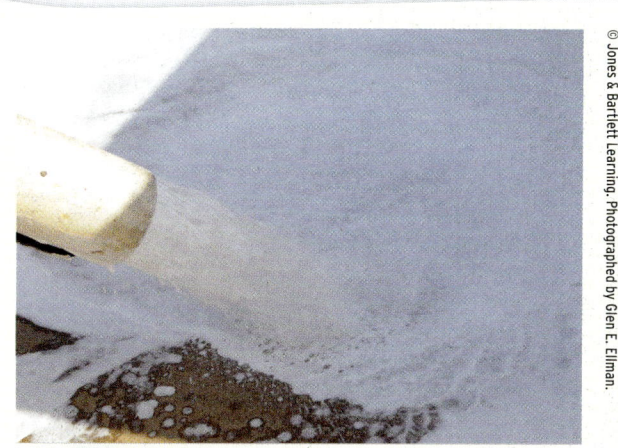

FIGURE 14-8 Regular protein foams have slower knockdown characteristics than other concentrates, but they provide a long-lasting foam blanket after the fire is extinguished.

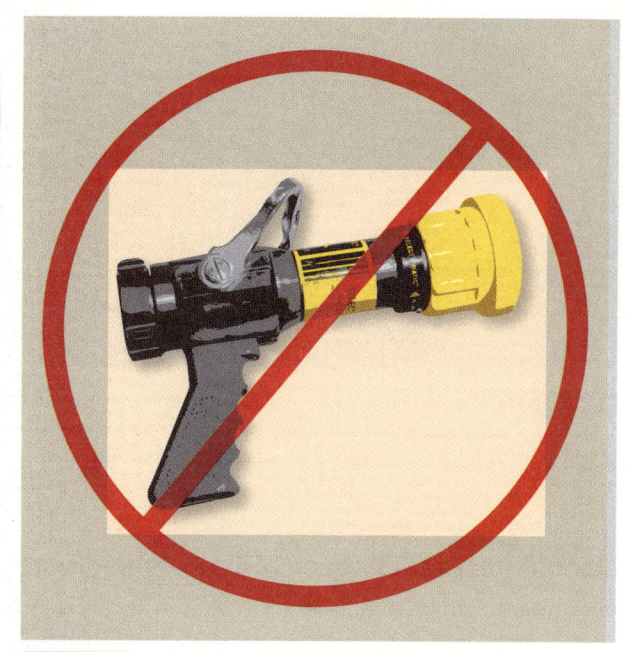

FIGURE 14-9 Fluoroprotein foams must be properly aspirated and should not be used with non-aspirating structural fog nozzles.

characteristics than other concentrates, but they provide a long-lasting foam blanket after the fire is extinguished **FIGURE 14-8**.

Fluoroprotein Foams

<u>Fluoroprotein foam (FP)</u> consists of hydrolyzed protein, stabilizers, preservatives, and synthetic fluorocarbon surfactants. This type of foam is used for hydrocarbon vapor suppression and extinguishment of fuel-in-depth fires. Notably, FP is effective for subsurface application to hydrocarbon fuel storage tanks.

Fluoroprotein foams are intended for use on hydrocarbon fuels and some <u>oxygenated</u> fuel additives. They have excellent heat and burnback resistance, and they maintain a good foam blanket after extinguishment of the fire. The addition of surfactants makes the foam more fluid, which increases the knockdown rate and provides better fuel tolerance than is possible with protein foam.

Fluoroprotein foams may be created using either fresh or salt water. Because they must be properly aspirated, these foams should not be used with non-aspirating structural fog nozzles **FIGURE 14-9**.

<u>Film-forming fluoroprotein foam (FFFP)</u> includes protein and fluorochemical surfactants. With these foams, the fluorochemical surfactants are generally present in higher <u>concentrations</u> than in standard FP. FFFP is able to form a vapor-sealing film on nonpolar solvents. Knockdown performance is improved because the foam releases an aqueous film on the surface of the hydrocarbon fuel.

Alcohol-Resistant Film-Forming Fluoroprotein Foams

Alcohol-resistant film-forming fluoroprotein foam (AR-FFFP) can be used on both hydrocarbon and water-soluble fuels. On hydrocarbon fires, the film-forming ability of this foam allows for rapid fire knockdown and excellent burnback resistance. On water-soluble fuels, its resistance to water-soluble solvents arises because a cohesive polymeric membrane forms on the fuel surface, which protects the foam from contact with polar fuels. AR-FFFP is basically FFFP with a polysaccharide <u>polymer</u> additive. Whereas polar solvents will destroy FFFP, the polymer in AR-FFFP forms a membrane to separate the polar solvent from the foam blanket.

■ Synthetic Foams

<u>Aqueous film-forming foam (AFFF)</u> is based on combinations of fluorochemical surfactants, hydrocarbon surfactants, and solvents. AFFF requires a low-energy source to produce high-quality foam. This foam can be applied using a variety of foam application systems. Because of the versatility of AFFF, it is used by the majority of municipal and airport fire departments in North America. AFFF is also used at refineries, manufacturing plants, and other operations involving flammable liquids.

AFFF is very fluid and quickly flows around obstacles and across the fuel surface. Its ability to flow quickly allows AFFF to achieve a very fast knockdown of hydrocarbon fires. This foam can be used as a premixed solution, is compatible with dry chemical agents, and can be created using either fresh or salt water.

AFFF consists of a mixture of synthetic foaming agents and fluorochemical surfactants. It extinguishes fire by forming an aqueous film on the fuel surface. This film comprises a thin layer of foam solution, which quickly spreads across the surface of a hydrocarbon fuel, creating an extremely fast fire knockdown **FIGURE 14-10**. The surfactants found in AFFF reduce the surface tension of the foam solution, which allows it to remain on the surface of the hydrocarbon fuel. The aqueous film is formed by the action of the foam solution draining from the foam blanket.

Aspirating foam nozzles should be used to apply AFFF to ensure maximum performance. Nozzles that will be used for foam application must be tested for compatibility with the foam system being used.

FIGURE 14-10 The film formed by application of AFFF comprises a thin layer of foam solution, which quickly spreads across the surface of a hydrocarbon fuel, creating an extremely fast fire knockdown.

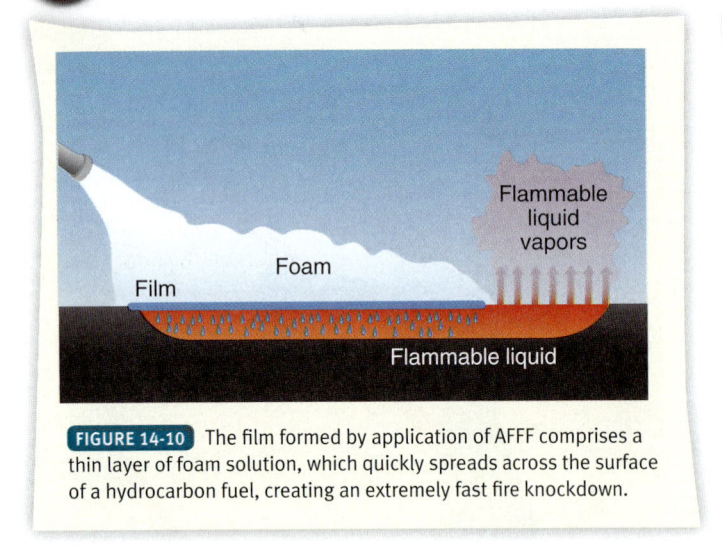

Alcohol-Resistant Aqueous Film-Forming Foams

Alcohol-resistant aqueous film-forming foam (AR-AFFF) comprises a combination of synthetic detergents, fluorochemicals, and high-molecular-weight polymers. Neither polar solvents nor water-miscible fuels are compatible with non-alcohol-resistant foams. Common polar solvents include solutions of the following compounds:

- Alcohols: isopropyl, methanol, ethanol
- Esters: butyl, acetate
- Ketones: methyl ethyl ketone
- Aldehydes: cinnamaldehyde, tolualdehyde

When non-alcohol-resistant foam is applied to the surface of a polar solvent, the foam blanket quickly breaks down into a liquid and mixes with the fuel. By comparison, AR-AFFF acts like a conventional AFFF on hydrocarbon fuels, forming an aqueous film on the fuel surface. When applied to polar solvents, however, AR-AFFF forms a polymeric membrane on the fuel surface. This membrane separates the fuel from the foam and prevents destruction of the foam blanket **FIGURE 14-11**.

AR-AFFF is one of the most versatile types of foam. It provides good knockdown and burnback resistance, and it has a high fuel tolerance on polar solvent and hydrocarbon fires.

> **Safety Tip**
>
> Today, alternative fuels—including ethanol, natural gas, propane, hydrogen, and methanol—are used in a variety of vehicles. Fuel mixtures composed of gasoline and ethanol have become quite common, for example. Gasoline mixtures containing more than 10 percent ethanol are polar solvents and will mix with water. Alcohol-resistant foams should be used for fire incidents involving these types of fuels.

Synthetic Detergent Foams (High-Expansion Foams)

High-expansion foams are highly effective in confined-space firefighting operations and in areas where access is limited or entry is dangerous to fire fighters, such as basements, shipboard compartments, warehouses, aircraft hangers, and mine shafts. These types of foams can be used in both fixed generating systems and portable foam generators.

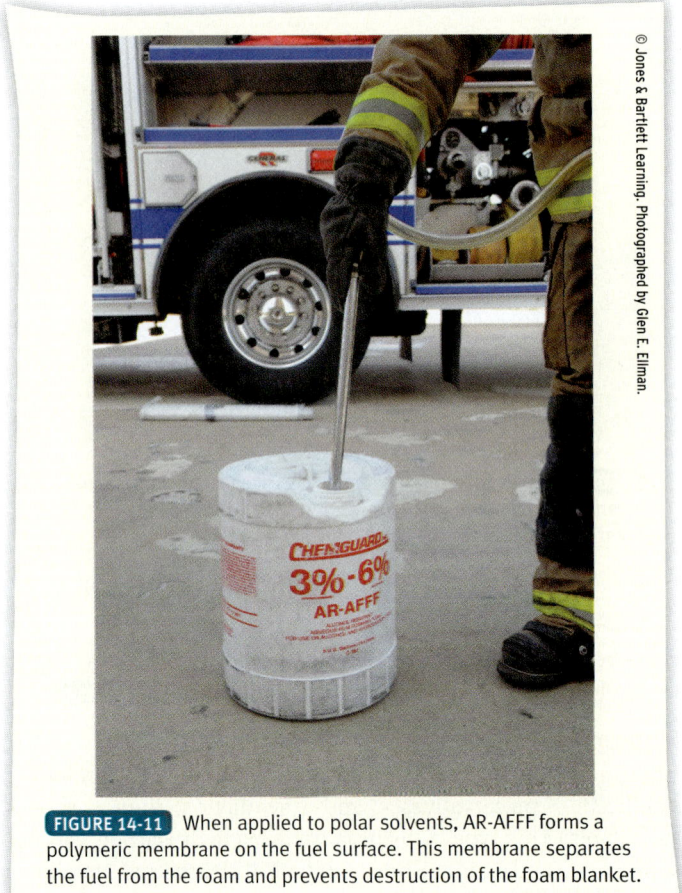

FIGURE 14-11 When applied to polar solvents, AR-AFFF forms a polymeric membrane on the fuel surface. This membrane separates the fuel from the foam and prevents destruction of the foam blanket.

High-expansion foams can be used on either Class A or Class B fires. Each foam manufacturer offers a different product, however, and it is your responsibility as a driver/operator to determine which foam can be used on the fire. High-expansion foams are based on combinations of hydrocarbon surfactants and solvents. They are useful on fuels such as liquefied natural gas for vapor dispersion and control. In certain concentrations, these foams are effective extinguishing agents for flammable liquid spill fires of most types. The foam concentrates are normally proportioned in ratios between 1 percent to 3 percent for these uses **FIGURE 14-12**.

> **Safety Tip**
>
> Make sure that the foam concentrate you are using is designed for the product and the application method being used. Serious injuries or death can occur if the appropriate foam is not applied properly.

Fire control and extinguishment are achieved by rapid smothering and cooling of the fire. High-expansion foams have a tremendous smothering and steam generation effect because the water contained in them is divided into such fine particles, which enhances the heat absorption quality of the water. This factor also presents a potential hazard: Care must be taken

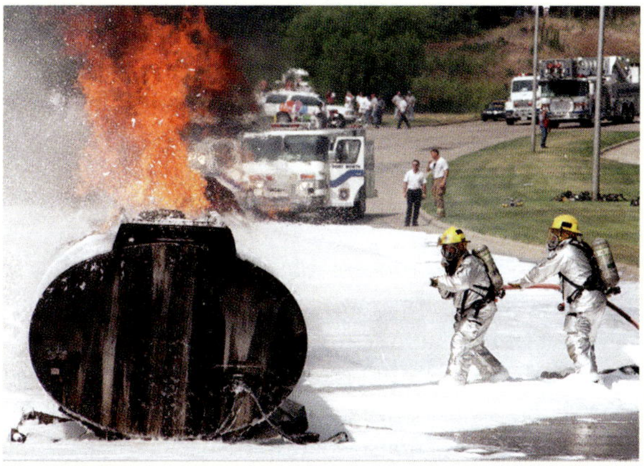

FIGURE 14-12 Synthetic detergent foam is an effective extinguishing agent for flammable liquid spill fires of most types.

with regard to electrical power sources in the area when this type of foam is applied. Remember that foam is mostly water and presents the same electrical shock potential to fire fighters as does water application.

Foam Concentrates

Foam concentrates are designed to be mixed with water at specific ratios **TABLE 14-2**. Foam concentrate ratios vary from 0.1 to 1 percent for Class A foams and from 1 to 6 percent for Class B (i.e., 1 to 6 percent foam concentrate-to-water ratio in the final foam product). The amount of concentrate varies depending on the manufacturer, the type of application, and the type of fuel. For example, when using Class A foam for initial fire attack on a vehicle fire, you might use a 0.3 or 0.5 percent ratio of foam concentrate to water. This ratio allows the foam to help extinguish the fire without creating too much foam. If you were supplying a hoseline that was spraying foam on a house to protect it during a brush fire, you might increase the ratio to 3 percent, thereby creating a thicker foam that would last longer and protect the house for an extended period, depending on your department's standard operating procedures/standard operating guidelines (SOPs/SOGs) and the manufacturer's recommendations.

The foam concentrate must be proportioned at the percentage listed by its manufacturer. Each foam is tested and approved for certain types of fires and at specific ratios—so you should always follow the manufacturer's guidelines when using this product. The foam concentrates are manufactured at different percentages for a variety of reasons. Thus the product's components include the concentrate (a unique chemical compound) plus any freeze protection additives. Military-use specifications and cost are some of the basic factors that determine the percentage of concentrate used in any particular situation.

The current trend is to keep foam concentrate percentages as low as possible, for several reasons. First, lower proportioning rates mean less bulk in storage for fire departments. Second, they mean that you can double your firefighting capacity by carrying the same volume of foam concentrate or you can cut your foam supply in half without reducing the company's fire suppression capabilities. Third, lower proportioning rates can reduce the cost of fixed foam system components and concentrate transportation costs. Historically, foam concentrates were manufactured for use at ratios between 3 percent and 6 percent. Today, however, foam concentrates are produced for uses at ratios as low as 0.1 percent and as high as 6 percent, depending on the liquid fuel and the manner in which the foam is to be used. Remember, the foam concentrate percentage must match the fuel to which the foam is being applied; if a mismatch occurs, the foam may not be effective in controlling the fire.

As mentioned earlier, alcohol-resistant foams can be used effectively on both hydrocarbon and polar solvent fuels. AR-AFFF is a commonly used concentrate for this purpose; it is available in a variety of percentages. For example, AR-AFFF concentrate is available as a 3 percent/3 percent product, which means that it can be used at 3 percent for incidents involving either hydrocarbon fuels or polar solvents. It is also available as a 3 percent/6 percent mixture, which means that foams for hydrocarbon-based incidents are proportioned at a 3 percent concentrate ratio, and foams for incidents involving polar solvents are proportioned at a 6 percent concentrate ratio. Another option available is AR-AFFF 1 percent/3 percent, which means foams for hydrocarbon-based incidents are proportioned at 1 percent and foams for polar solvent–based incidents are proportioned at 3 percent or lower for newer concentrates.

Given the many types of foam concentrates available, the selection of the right concentrate is critical to the safe and effective handling of an incident. Knowledge of the foam types and systems available will assist incident commanders (ICs) in their ability to mitigate an incident. The importance of preplanning and training for these types of incidents cannot be stressed strongly enough.

Foam Expansion Rates

The foam expansion rate is the ratio of finished foam to foam solution after the concentrate is mixed with water, agitated, and aspirated through a foam-making appliance. For example, a low-expansion foam has an expansion ratio of 20:1, which means that 20 parts of finished foam are produced for every 1 part of foam solution. The air inside the bubbles makes up the expanded part of the finished foam. NFPA 11, *Standard for*

TABLE 14-2	Foam Concentrate-to-Water Ratios
Protein foam	3–6%
Fluoroprotein foam	3–6%
Aqueous film-forming foam (AFFF)	1–6%
Film-forming fluoroprotein foam (FFFP)	3–6%
Alcohol-resistant aqueous film-forming foam (AR-AFFF)	3–6%
Class A foam	0.1–1%

Low-, Medium-, and High-Expansion Foam, classifies foam concentrates into three expansion ranges:
- Low expansion
- Medium expansion
- High expansion

Low-Expansion Foam

Low-expansion foam has a foam expansion ratio of up to 20:1. This type of foam is primarily designed for use on flammable and combustible liquids. Low-expansion foam is effective in controlling and extinguishing most Class B fires. Special low-expansion foams are also used on Class A fires where the penetrating and cooling effect of the foam solution is important.

Medium-Expansion Foam

Medium-expansion foam has a foam expansion ratio in the range of 20:1 to 200:1. This kind of foam is used primarily to suppress vapors from hazardous chemicals. Foams with expansion ratios between 30:1 and 55:1 have been found to produce the optimal foam blanket for vapor mitigation of highly reactive chemicals and low-boiling-point organics.

High-Expansion Foam

High-expansion foam has a foam expansion ratio in the range of 200:1 to 1000:1. This type of foam is designed for confined-space firefighting. The foam concentrate consists of a synthetic, detergent-type foam used in confined spaces such as basements, mines, shipboard, and aircraft hangars.

Foam Proportioning

Foam cannot be produced if it is not proportioned properly. Several types of foam application systems are available for this purpose, ranging from basic operations to more advanced foam systems. With the proper training, these systems are user friendly and will produce good-quality finished foam.

Proportioning Foam Concentrate

The application of foams at the proper percentage depends on the foam concentrate being mixed at the proper percentage with water. This percentage of concentrate may be introduced into the water stream by any of several methods. It is imperative that you become familiar with the type of equipment that is used in your agency's foam operations.

As the driver/operator, you have the responsibility to produce effective foam streams. You must have knowledge of all aspects of foam operations so that the foam produced will do what it is intended to do. Foam that is not mixed at the proper percentage or is used on a material or product for which it was not intended will not only be ineffective, but could also put the fire fighters on the hoselines in danger.

To produce finished foam, the water, air, and foam concentrate must be mixed at the proper ratio. In other words, foam concentrate must be added to the water that is flowing from a discharge line to form the proper mixture. This mixture or percentage is based on the type of foam concentrate used, the type of material involved in the incident, and the type of equipment used to produce the finished foam.

Foam Proportioning Systems

The foam proportioner is the device that mixes the foam concentrate into the fire stream in the proper percentage. The two types of proportioners—eductors and injectors—are available in a wide range of sizes and capabilities. Foam solution can also be produced by batch mixing or premixing.

Batch Mixing

Batch mixing is the process of pouring foam concentrate directly into the fire apparatus water tank, thereby mixing a large amount of foam at one time. The proper amount of foam concentrate must be poured into the onboard tank to produce the desired percentage in the finished foam FIGURE 14-13. While this method requires no special appliances, some problems may arise with batch mixing:

- The foam solution is corrosive to the apparatus' pipes, pump, and water tank.
- It is difficult to adjust and maintain the correct application rate, especially if additional water is supplied for an external source.
- The addition of foam solution may cause the gauges to become inaccurate, such that the water tank overflows with foam when the pump is recirculating the mixture.

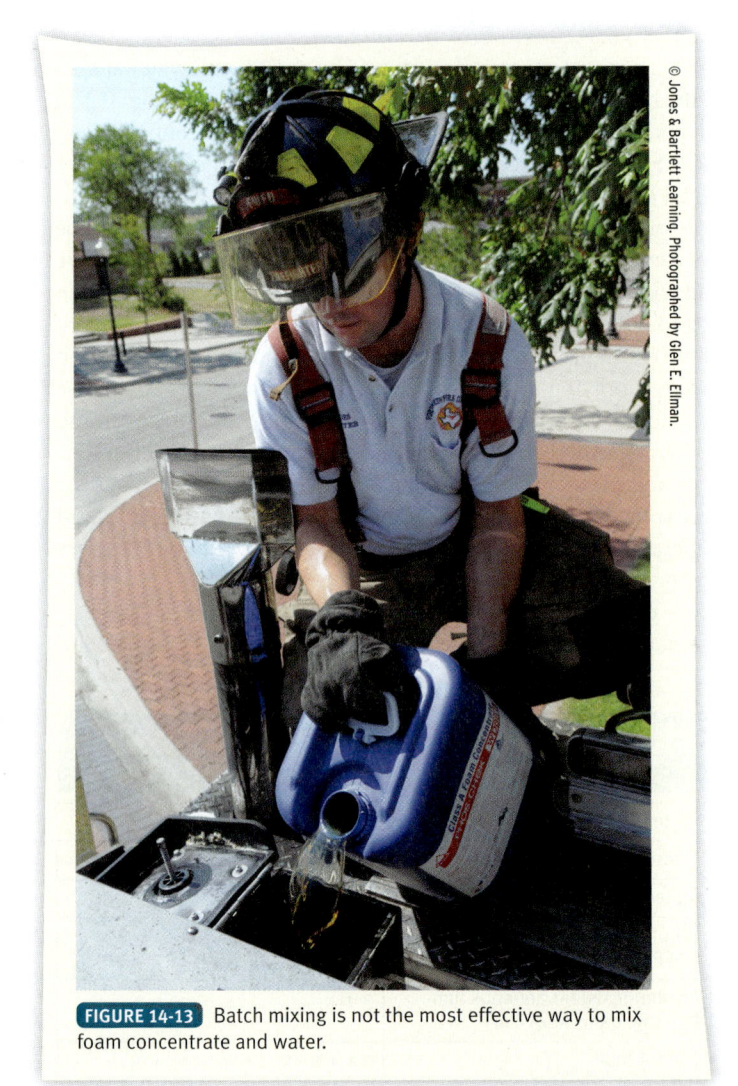

FIGURE 14-13 Batch mixing is not the most effective way to mix foam concentrate and water.

SKILL DRILL 14-1
Batch Mixing Foam
NFPA 1002, 5.2.3, 5.2.3(B)

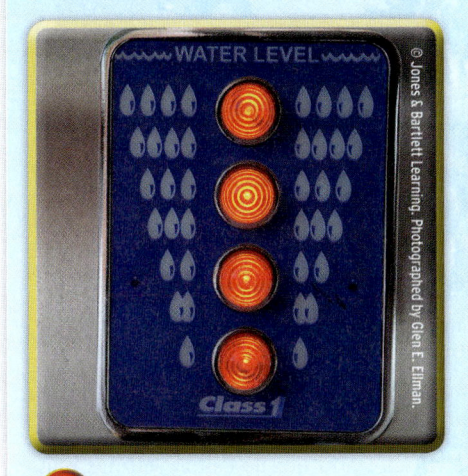

1 Determine the amount of water inside the fire apparatus water tank.

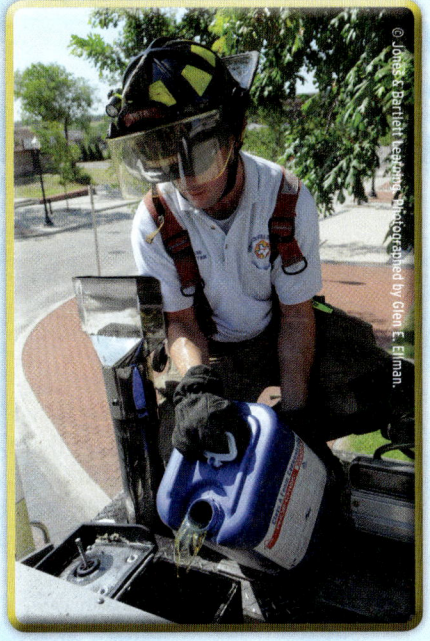

2 Determine the correct percentage of foam required. Add the correct amount of foam concentrate to the water tank.

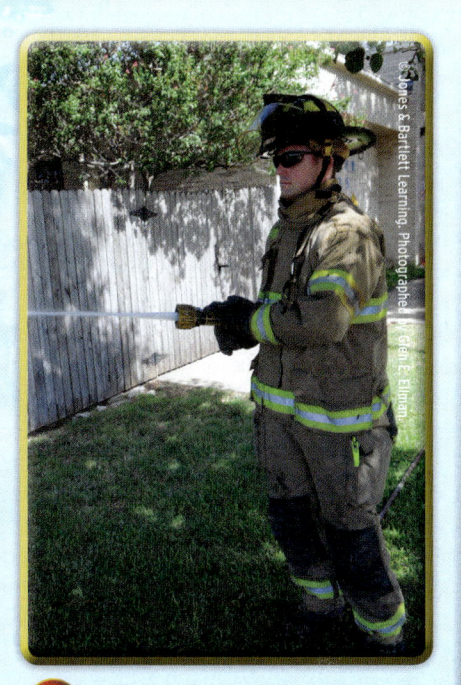

3 Apply the foam on the fire.

Class A foam concentrates that are batch mixed must be used within 24 hours if they are to be effective. As with some of the other systems used to create foam, all discharges will deliver foam when it is supplied from the onboard tank. When the water tank is empty, however, there is no longer any foam available—a new batch has to be mixed. As long as you know the amount of water in the onboard water tank, then you can simply add the foam concentrate to achieve the desired foam solution percentage. For example, if the water tank on the fire apparatus holds 500 gallons of water and you want to use Class A foam at 1 percent, you would add 5 gallons of foam concentrate with an in-line foam eductor.

To prepare foam through batch mixing, follow the steps in **SKILL DRILL 14-1**:

1. Determine the amount of water in the fire apparatus water tank. (**STEP 1**)
2. Determine the correct percentage of foam required for the fire.
3. Add the correct amount of foam concentrate directly into the top of the water tank's fill port. (**STEP 2**)
4. Discharge the foam through the attack lines. (**STEP 3**)

Premixing
Premixing of foam solutions is a technique that is usually reserved for portable fire extinguishers. Many fire departments use these extinguishers filled with premixed foam solutions for small flammable liquid spills at the scene of a motor vehicle accident. They are quick and easy to deploy but contain a limited amount of foam and should be applied only to small fires or fuel spills. Always refer to the foam manufacturer's recommendations regarding how long the foam concentrate should be used after mixing it with water.

Foam Eductors
Induction involves the use of an eductor to introduce the appropriate amount of foam concentrate into a stream of water flowing from a discharge. An **eductor** is an appliance that uses the Venturi principle (i.e., suction effect) to introduce foam concentrate into the water stream. An eductor can be built into the plumbing of an engine, or a portable eductor can be inserted in an attack hoseline. A foam eductor is usually designed to work at a predetermined pressure and flow rate; its metering valve can be adjusted to set the percentage of foam concentrate that is educted into the stream. For example, a simple in-line foam eductor has a small pick-up tube that is submerged in foam concentrate. As the water travels through the in-line eductor, it draws foam concentrate into the water at the desired percentage using the Venturi principle.

Two types of eductors are used in the fire service today: in-line eductors and bypass eductors. In-line eductors have long been used to proportion foam FIGURE 14-14. These appliances may be mounted permanently on the apparatus; alternately, they may be portable and connected anywhere along the hose lay. In-line eductors should be used only for the application of foam. Those mounted permanently to the fire pump are dedicated to one foam discharge; such **pump-mounted eductors** are in-line devices dedicated to producing foam only. By comparison, **bypass eductors** are permanently mounted appliances that can be used for water or foam application, depending on what is required at the incident scene.

As mentioned earlier, eductors use the Venturi principle to mix a specific amount of foam concentrate into the water stream. Specifically, a suction effect is created at the narrow inlet to the eductor. This narrow passage increases water velocity, which reduces the water's pressure as it flows into the larger induction area. Foam concentrate is introduced into the eductor using a metering valve, which allows the driver/operator to adjust the percentage of foam concentrate being added to the water stream.

Most eductors are calibrated to flow the rated capacity at 200 pounds per square inch (psi) (1400 kilopascals [kPa]) inlet pressure. An eductor inlet pressure of 200 psi (1400 kPa) is necessary to overcome friction loss through the eductor as well as the friction loss between the eductor and the nozzle.

Eductors are available for delivering flow rates of 30, 60, 95, 125, and 250 gallons per minute (gpm; 114, 227, 360, 473, and 946 liters per minute [l/min], respectively). The nozzle used with the system must match the flow rating of the eductor.

FIGURE 14-15 The metering device controls the amount of foam concentrate educted into the water.

It is critical that the eductor and nozzle gallon settings match, because the eductors need certain velocities of water flowing through them to allow proper mixing of the foam concentrate. Mismatched equipment can result in either too rich or too lean foam in the fire stream. Always follow the manufacturer's recommendations when selecting nozzles to use with foam eductors.

Metering Device
The **metering device** controls the flow of concentrate into the eductor FIGURE 14-15. The amount of foam concentrate introduced into the water stream is controlled by adjusting the metering valve. As the driver/operator, you should adjust the metering valve to the desired percentage to handle the situation at hand. Metering valves have adjustable settings that range from 0 (the closed position) to 6 percent.

The percentage set on the metering valve will be achieved only if the inlet pressure at the eductor matches the manufacturer's recommended inlet pressure. If the eductor is operated at less than the recommended inlet pressure, a lower flow of water will go through the eductor. This lower flow of water will, in turn, result in a higher percentage of foam concentrate being introduced into the water stream. Depending on the available supply of foam concentrate, unnecessary wastage of foam concentrate will occur and the driver/operator could run out of foam before the fire is extinguished.

The opposite will occur if the inlet pressure to the eductor exceeds the pressure recommended by the manufacturer. A higher inlet pressure at the eductor will cause the foam solution to have a lower percentage of concentrate, which could affect the company's ability to handle the situation in which the foam is being applied.

Operating the In-Line Eductor
The in-line eductor is a very simple, efficient, and inexpensive type of foam proportioner. Many fire departments still use it as standard equipment to create foam at their fire scenes. These devices are constructed out of rugged brass alloys and, if properly maintained, can last for many years. An in-line eductor is attached to the hoseline no more than 150 ft (45 m) from the nozzle and no more than 6 ft (2 m) above the surface of the foam concentrate—a placement that makes it easy to set up and take down. Although this type of device is simple to

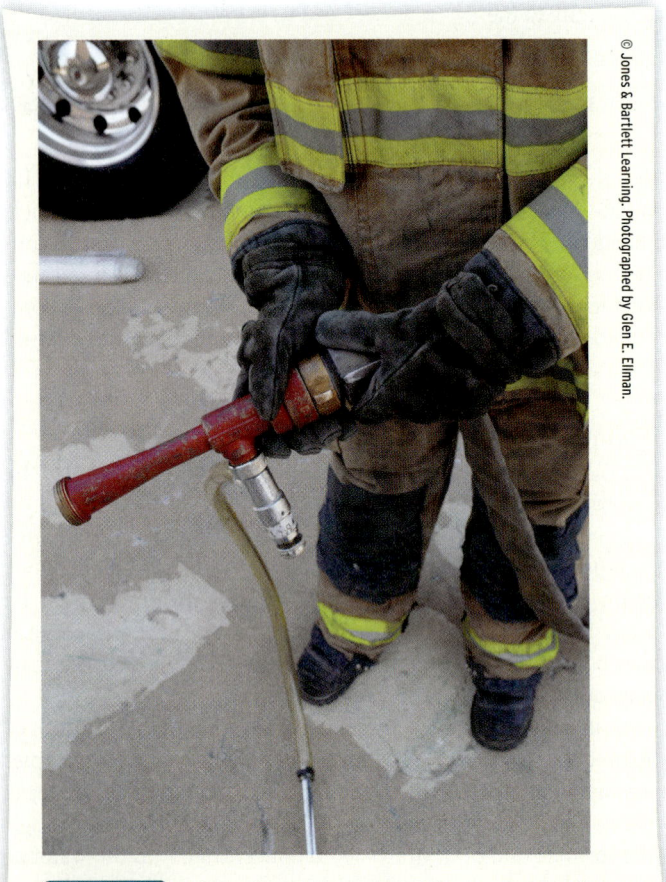

FIGURE 14-14 In-line eductors are very simple to operate and are found in many fire departments.

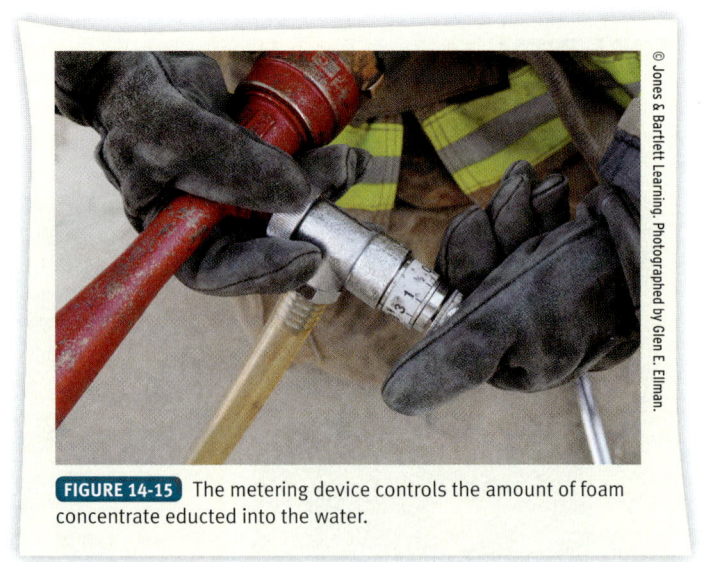

operate, some very specific instructions must be followed to ensure its proper use.

To operate an in-line eductor, follow the steps in **SKILL DRILL 14-2**:

1. Make sure that all necessary equipment is available, including an in-line foam eductor and air-aspirating nozzle. Ensure that there is enough foam concentrate to suppress the fire and that it is the correct type of foam for the job. (**STEP 1**)
2. Don all personal protective equipment (PPE). (**STEP 2**)
3. Procure an attack line, remove the nozzle, and replace it with the air-aspirating nozzle if necessary. (**STEP 3**)
4. Place the in-line eductor on a discharge to the hoseline no more than 150 ft (45 m) from the nozzle. (**STEP 4**)
5. Place the foam concentrate container next to the eductor, check the percentage at which the foam concentrate should be used (this information can be found on the container label), and set the metering device on the eductor accordingly. (**STEP 5**)
6. Place the pick-up tube from the eductor into the foam concentrate, keeping both items at similar elevations to ensure sufficient induction of foam concentrate. (**STEP 6**)
7. Charge the hoseline with water, ensuring there is a minimum pressure of 200 psi (1400 kPa) at the eductor. Flow water through the hoseline until foam starts to come out of the nozzle. The hoseline is now ready to be advanced onto the burning material. (**STEP 7**)
8. Apply the foam using one of the three application methods (sweep technique, bankshot technique, or raindown technique—discussed later in this chapter) depending on the situation. (**STEP 8**)

■ Around-the-Pump Proportioning System

An **around-the-pump proportioning (AP) system** operates on the same principle as the in-line or bypass eductor system. The AP system diverts a portion of the water pump's output from the discharge side of the pump and sends it through an eductor. A vacuum is created at the eductor's foam concentrate inlet, which draws foam concentrate through the metering valve and into the eductor. The foam solution (water/concentrate) is then sent to the suction side of the water pump, where it mixes with the incoming water and is distributed throughout the discharge piping.

The AP system offers several advantages over other foam-creation methods:
- The process used for engaging the pump is the same for water or foam operations.
- The variable flow discharge rate allows for adjustment of the foam depending on the specific application.
- Variable pressure operations are possible, usually within a range of 125 to 250 psi (875–1750 kPa).
- There are no backpressure restrictions, because the system is not affected by hose length or elevation loss.
- There are no nozzle restrictions because the system will operate with any size or type of fixed-gallon nozzle.

Like any other foam system, AP systems also have certain limitations with which you must be familiar. Knowing these limitations will enable you to use the system in an efficient and safe manner. All discharges will have *either* foam *or* water available at the same time. You will not be able to supply some lines with water and other lines with foam simultaneously: Either one or the other mode must be chosen.

DRIVER/OPERATOR Tip

The foam solution is discharged from the around-the-pump eductor to the intake side of the water pump. Thus, when you are using foam, all outlets will be discharging foam when they are opened. Along with the discharges used for firefighting, the following sources will also discharge foam:
- Tank fill
- Pump cooler
- Engine cooler
- Operation of the primer pump

Be aware of the potential problems with sending foam solution into these areas.

The maximum inlet pressure to the water pump cannot be more than 10 psi (70 kPa). Any pressure greater than 10 psi (70 kPa) will affect the operation of the eductor. Some manufacturers' systems are designed to operate with an inlet pressure of as much as 40 psi (280 kPa), however, so check your system's operating instructions for the proper inlet pressure.

AP systems are intended to operate with water supplied from the onboard tank or from draft. As a consequence, use of a pressurized source (hydrant or relay) will affect the operation of the system. Most fire apparatus with AP systems have a direct tank fill that does not go through the pump. In such systems, the tank is filled directly from the pressurized source, and the water pump supply comes from the onboard tank.

Safety Tip

As the driver/operator, you must monitor the tank water level. If you run out of water, firefighting operations will come to a halt. Conversely, overfilling the tank can cause the water to overflow and possibly run down into the foam blanket.

All discharges must be flushed after the foam operation has ended, even if they were not used. When using automatic nozzles, the flow must be determined to ensure that you set the metering valve correctly. The appropriate setting for the metering valve depends on the type of concentrate being used, the percentage needed for the incident, and the rate of flow (in gpm [L/min]). When the flow rate changes, such as when a line is shut down, the metering valve needs to be adjusted to accommodate the new flow.

SKILL DRILL 14-2 Operating an In-Line Eductor
NFPA 1002, 5.2.3, 5.2.3(B)

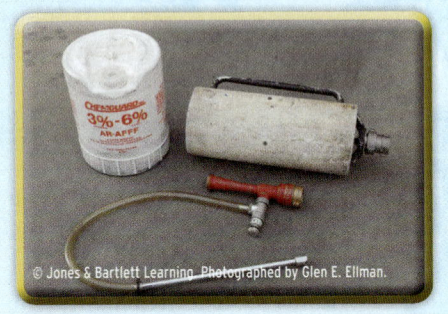

1 Ensure all equipment is available, including the air-aspirating nozzle, foam concentrate, and in-line eductor.

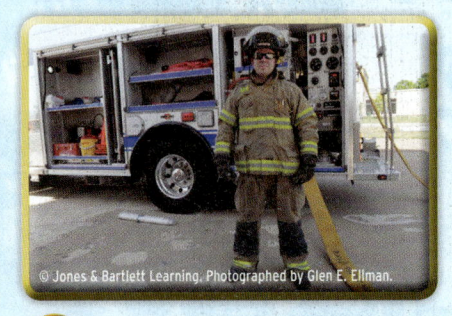

2 Don PPE.

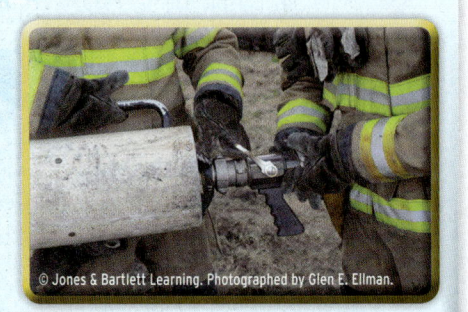

3 Add the air-aspirating nozzle to the attack line.

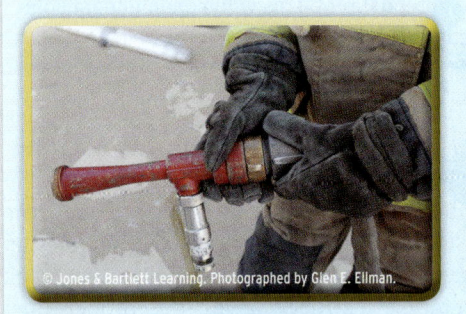

4 Place the in-line eductor no more than 150 ft (45 m) from the nozzle.

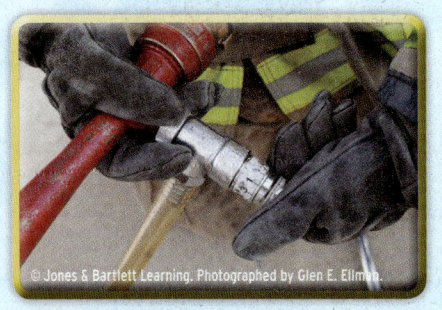

5 Place the foam concentrate next to the eductor, check the percentage for the foam, and set the metering device.

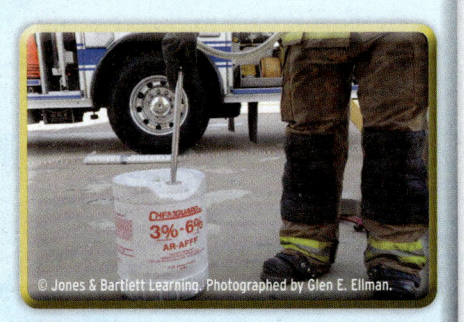

6 Place the pick-up tube into the foam concentrate.

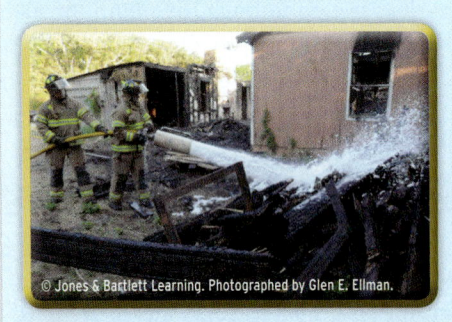

7 Charge the hose with a minimum pressure of 200 psi (1400 kPa) at the eductor. Flow water through the hose until foam begins and the hose is ready to advance on the fire.

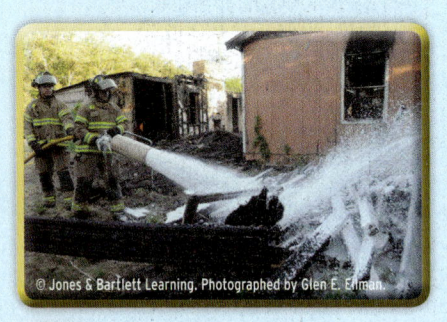

8 Apply the foam.

CHAPTER 14 Foam

To operate an AP system, follow the steps in **SKILL DRILL 14-3**:

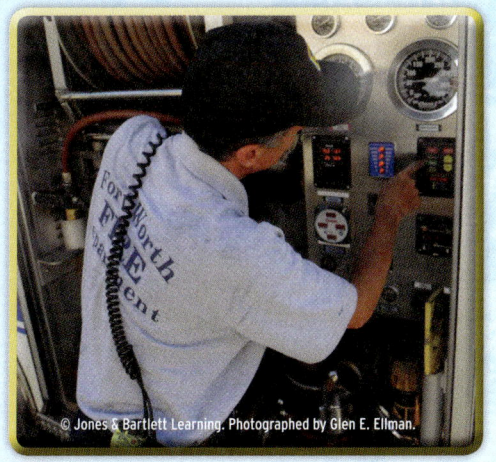

1. With the system engaged, operate the fire pump as you would during normal water pump operations (**STEP 1**)
2. Push the "on" button at the pump panel display to turn the foam system on. (**STEP 2**)
3. Set the desired percentage of foam for the fire using the up/down arrow buttons. (**STEP 3**)
4. Open the foam discharge valve, if required, and set the desired pressure.
5. Discharge the foam through the attack lines. (**STEP 4**)

DRIVER/OPERATOR Tip

Do not operate the AP system for extended periods of time with the discharges closed. Even though these outlets are closed, the system will continue sending water through the eductor, and foam concentrate will continue to be discharged into the water pump. The water pump will become rich with concentrate; as a result, concentrate will be wasted and the water pump may overheat. Some driver/operators have run out of foam concentrate because they operated the foam system with the discharge closed.

SKILL DRILL 14-3
Operating an Around-the-Pump Proportioning System
NFPA 1002, 5.2.3, 5.2.3(B)

1. With the system engaged, operate the fire pump as you would during normal water pump operations.

2. Push the "on" button at the pump panel display to turn the foam system on.

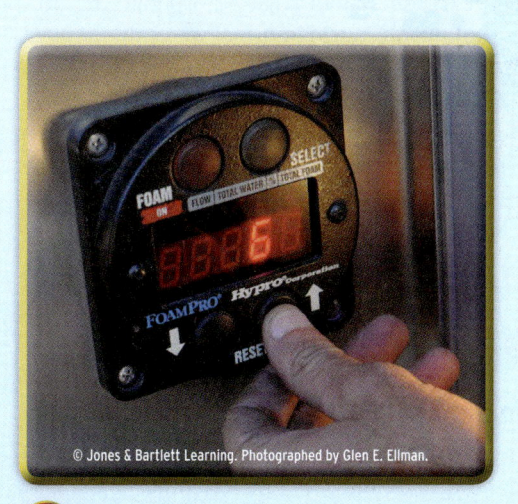

3. Set the desired percentage of foam for the fire using the up/down arrow buttons.

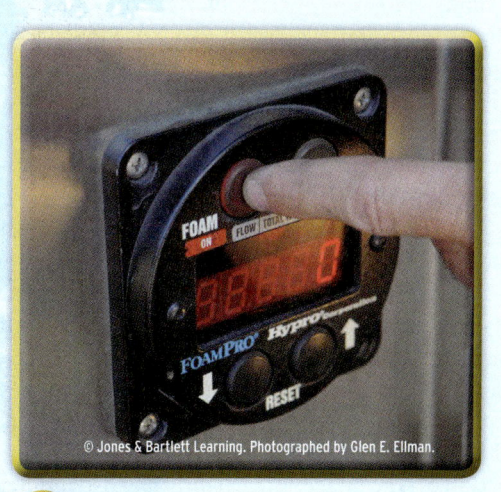

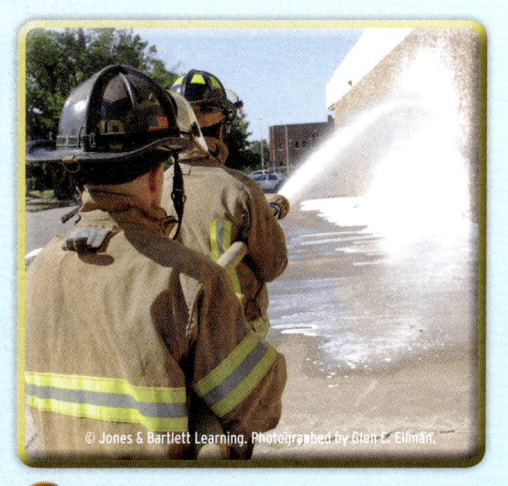

4. Open the foam discharge valve, if required, and set the desired pressure. Discharge the foam through the attack lines.

Balanced-Pressure Proportioning Systems

Balanced-pressure systems are extremely versatile and accurate means to deliver foam. This system uses a diaphragm-type pressure control valve to sense and balance the pressures in the foam concentrate and water lines to the proportioner. The valve keeps the foam concentrate and the water pressure in balance by allowing excess foam concentrate to return to the foam concentrate storage tank **FIGURE 14-16**. This proportioning occurs automatically for flows within the operating limits of the foam concentrate pump and the discharges.

The foam concentrate pump is a separate pump that supplies foam concentrate to the pressure control valve and the ratio controller. The pressure control valve act as a balancing valve: It maintains equal foam concentrate and water pressures at the ratio controllers. Thus the pressure control valve automatically maintains equal pressure within the foam-creation system. Unused foam concentrate from the foam pump discharge is returned to the foam concentrate storage tank.

A **ratio controller** is a device required for each foam outlet to proportion the correct amount of foam concentrate into the water stream over a wide range of flows and with minimal pressure loss. This modified Venturi device provides a metered pressure drop for controlled injection of foam concentrate into a reduced pressure zone.

Metering valves receive foam concentrate from the foam pump and, in turn, discharge the concentrate to the individual ratio controllers. Put simply, these devices function as a concentrate shut-off. They also allow you to adjust the foam percentage for each discharge. The metering valve settings available usually range from "off" to 6 percent. Foam solution can be produced at any ratio controller/discharge connection by opening the corresponding foam solution metering valve to the desired percentage rate. Plain water is simultaneously available at the remaining discharge connections.

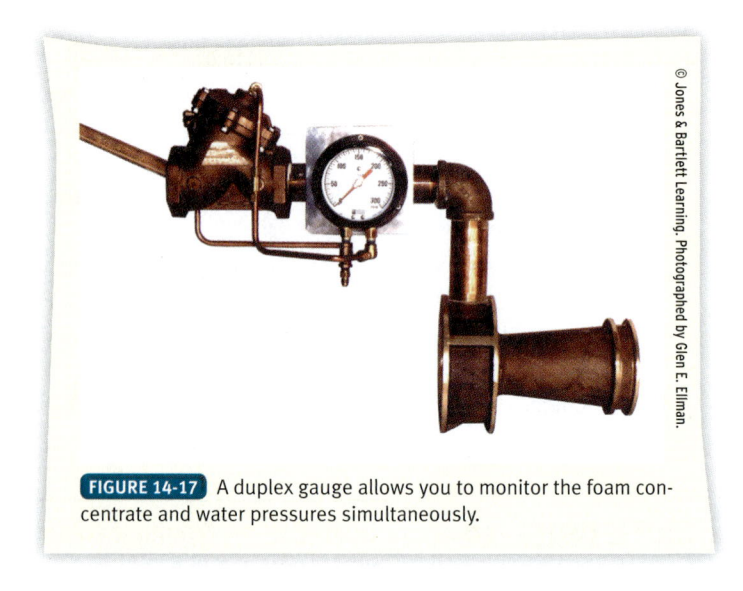

FIGURE 14-17 A duplex gauge allows you to monitor the foam concentrate and water pressures simultaneously.

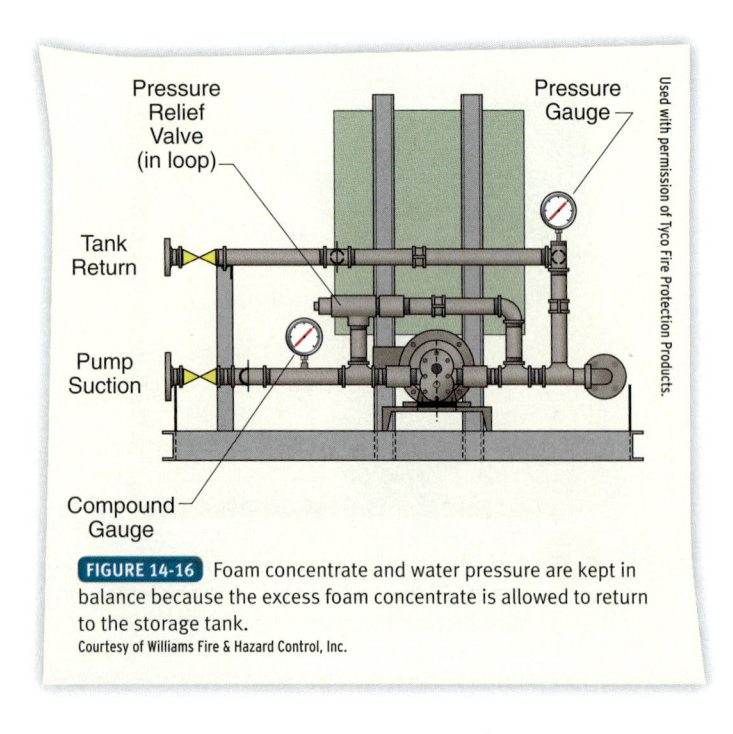

A **duplex gauge** at the pump panel allows the driver/operator to monitor the foam concentrate and water pressures **FIGURE 14-17**. These pressures should be "balanced" (equal)—a feat that is achieved automatically by the balanced-pressure system. For example, if the flow of water into the pump increases, the system will rebalance itself to compensate for the additional pressure to maintain an accurate flow of correctly proportioned foam solution. A manual throttling control valve located at the pump panel enables the driver/operator to override the automatic system by increasing or decreasing foam concentrate pressure, in case a problem occurs within the system.

Many balanced-pressure systems are equipped with a **foam heat exchanger**. The heat exchanger uses water as its cooling source and prevents the foam concentrate from overheating.

To operate a balanced-pressure proportioning system, follow the steps in **SKILL DRILL 14-4**:

1. With the system engaged, operate the fire pump as you would during normal water pump operations.
2. If not electric, engage the foam pump's power take-off (PTO) unit.
3. Push the "on" button at the pump panel display to turn the foam system on.
4. Set the desired percentage of foam for the fire using the up/down arrow buttons.
5. Open the foam discharge valve, if required, and set the desired pressure.
6. Discharge the foam through the attack lines.

Injection Systems

Injection systems use an electrically operated, variable-speed foam concentrate pump that directly injects foam concentrate into the discharge side of the pump manifold. Injection systems are the most common type of system in use today and are designed for use with Class A foam concentrates and with many Class B foam concentrates, depending on the viscosity of the concentrate.

FIGURE 14-16 Foam concentrate and water pressure are kept in balance because the excess foam concentrate is allowed to return to the storage tank.
Courtesy of Williams Fire & Hazard Control, Inc.

Injection systems depend on the water flow for their operation. They will adjust the amount of foam concentrate being injected into the discharge manifold depending on the flow rate (gpm [L/min]) and the percentage set by the driver/operator. The foam concentrate pump will also adjust its operating speed (rpm) depending on the amount of water flowing.

Injection systems are not affected by changes in suction and discharge pressure. The only limitation on such a system is the rated capacity of the foam concentrate pump. Many different sizes of foam concentrate pumps are available, so it is imperative that you know the limits of the specific pumps used on your fire department's apparatus.

DRIVER/OPERATOR Tip

A foam concentrate pump rated at a maximum output of 5 gpm (19 L/min) would be able to supply concentrate at the following flow rates:

- 0.5 percent foam concentrate produces 1000-gpm (3785-L/min) foam solution.
- 1 percent foam concentrate produces 500-gpm (1893-L/min) foam solution.
- 3 percent foam concentrate produces 167-gpm (632-L/min) foam solution.
- 6 percent foam concentrate produces 84-gpm (318-L/min) foam solution.

Direct-injection systems are very user friendly. A control unit located at the pump panel allows the driver/operator to operate the foam system. This control unit has an on/off button that starts and secures the foam operations. It also allows the driver/operator to monitor the water flow rate, concentrate injection percentage, total amount of water flowed, and total amount of concentrate used.

With injection systems, the driver/operator can adjust the foam concentrate percentage while the system is in operation. Concentrate injection rates can be set anywhere in the range of 0.1 to 10 percent. These percentages, which can be changed in 0.1-percent increments, are selected using a button on the control unit.

Injection foam systems can be used with standard nozzles, aspirating nozzles, and a compressed-air foam system. These systems can be set up to supply multiple discharges on the water pump. Depending on the apparatus, the foam concentrate is injected into the discharge manifold at only one injection point, so all discharges that are piped from the foam discharge manifold will be capable of delivering foam. Although other discharges not piped to the foam manifold will be capable of discharging water, all discharges from the foam manifold will produce foam.

To operate an injection foam system, follow the steps in **SKILL DRILL 14-5**:

1. With the system engaged, operate the fire pump as you would during normal water pump operations.
2. Push the "on" button at the pump panel display to turn the foam system on.
3. Set the desired percentage of foam for the fire using the up/down arrow buttons.
4. Open the foam discharge valve, if required, and set the desired pressure.
5. Discharge the foam through the attack lines.

Compressed-Air Foam System

A compressed-air foam system (CAFS) combines compressed air and a foam solution to create the finished foam. It is designed for a quick and effective fire attack and exposure protection. This type of system is generally used to generate Class A foam—specifically, to create a high-quality finished foam that clings to vertical surfaces **FIGURE 14-18**. This foam holds moisture on the fuel's surface, where it either evaporates or penetrates, thereby cooling and lowering the fuel's temperature.

The production of finished foam depends on the correct mixture of water, foam concentrate, and air within the CAFS. This kind of system uses a fire pump, a foam concentrate injection system, and an air compressor to produce high-quality finished-foam streams inside the fire apparatus piping. The foam aeration on the CAFS takes place at the pump discharge—that is, air is introduced at the pump. Thus the foam solution is mixed with air prior to reaching the end of the hoseline. This type of system allows for a more uniform bubble structure and better finished foam.

A CAFS has some key benefits for firefighting operations:

- The quality of the foam is greatly improved due to its consistently smaller bubble structure.
- The foam produced by the CAFS works four to five times faster than water in suppressing fire.
- A CAFS uses less water, thereby reducing the extent of water damage.

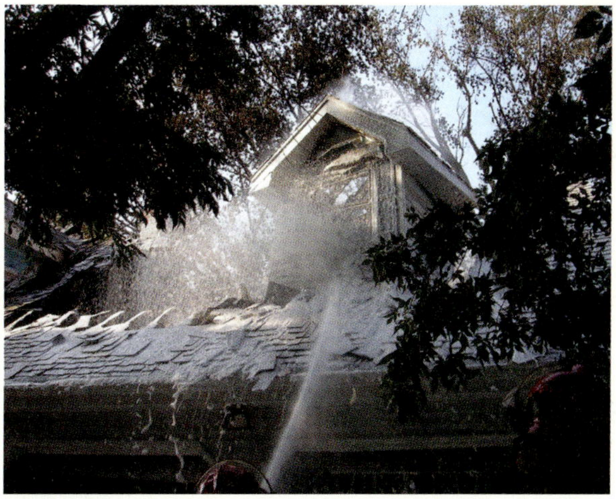

FIGURE 14-18 A compressed-air foam system creates foam that has the consistency of shaving cream, which enables it to cling to a building's surface.

- The quick knockdown, fast fire suppression, and less extensive water damage associated with this type of foam system may help fire investigators in determining the cause of the fire.
- The reach of the fire stream is improved. The foam discharged will be lighter than water because the discharging foam is a mixture of foam solution and air.
- The improved stream reach allows for making the initial fire attack from a greater distance, which reduces the risk of injury to fire fighters.
- The weight of the attack line is less than that of a line containing just water. CAFS hoselines are typically filled with approximately 30 percent compressed air. Fire fighters will be able to move the line more easily, which will reduce their fatigue.
- Because the hose is filled with air, friction loss is insignificant.
- There is not the normal pressure loss with elevation.

Driver/operators should also be aware of some potentially problematic issues related to the CAFS:

- The driver/operator needs to be familiar with the operation of the air compressor.
- Water and air are incompressible. Foam solution must be present in the water stream prior to injecting compressed air. If foam concentrate is not present, unmixed water and air will be discharged in an erratic manner, called slug flow, and the hoseline could be "jerked" out of the hands of the fire fighters.
- A CAFS burst hoseline will react more erratically due to the air in the line.
- Nozzle reaction is greater due to air in the CAFS hose, so nozzles should be opened slowly.

Operating a CAFS is dependent on your apparatus-specific system. Always refer to the manufacturer's recommendations and procedures for your system's make and model. In general, to operate a CAFS, follow the steps in **SKILL DRILL 14-6**:

1. With the system engaged, operate the fire pump as you would during normal water pump operations. (**STEP 1**)
2. Set the desired discharge pressure for the attack line. (**STEP 2**)
3. Push the "on" button at the pump panel display to turn the foam system on (if not already activated). (**STEP 3**)
4. Select either "wet" or "dry" foam to be delivered to the discharge by setting the desired percentage of foam for the fire using the up/down arrow buttons. (**STEP 4**)
5. Open the discharge valve. (**STEP 5**)
6. Discharge the foam through the attack lines. (**STEP 6**)

Safety Tip

A CAFS should be operated at the water flow rates that would be used if just water was being applied. While this type of foam system will extinguish the fire more quickly than a water-based foam system, proper flow rates are still needed to protect fire fighters.

Nozzles

Nozzles are an important part of all foam operations. The proper nozzle is needed for fire fighters to be able to produce a good-quality foam blanket. The following types of nozzles are available:

- Medium- and high-expansion foam generators
- Master stream foam nozzles
- Air-aspirating foam nozzles
- Smooth-bore nozzles
- Fog nozzles

■ Medium- and High-Expansion Foam Generators

Foam generators produce medium- and high-expansion foams. These devices usually consist of either a mechanical blower or a water-aspirating appliance. A water-powered aspirating type of generator uses a water-motor-driven fan to produce the required air flow. Some water-powered high-expansion generators are designed to achieve expansion rates of as much as 1000 gal (3785 L) of finished foam for every 1 gal (3.785 L) of foam solution. The final expansion ratio achieved depends on the generator used, the solution flow rate, and the operating pressure.

<u>Mechanical generators</u> operate similarly to a water-aspirating generator **FIGURE 14-19**. The difference is that the mechanical generator is electrically powered by a fan, which forces the air flow through the unit. High-expansion foam systems are designed for use in total flooding applications and are effective at the following locations:

- Mines
- Warehouses
- Aircraft hangars
- Basements
- Storage buildings
- Paper warehouses
- Machinery spaces
- Hazardous waste facilities
- Wildland fire breaks

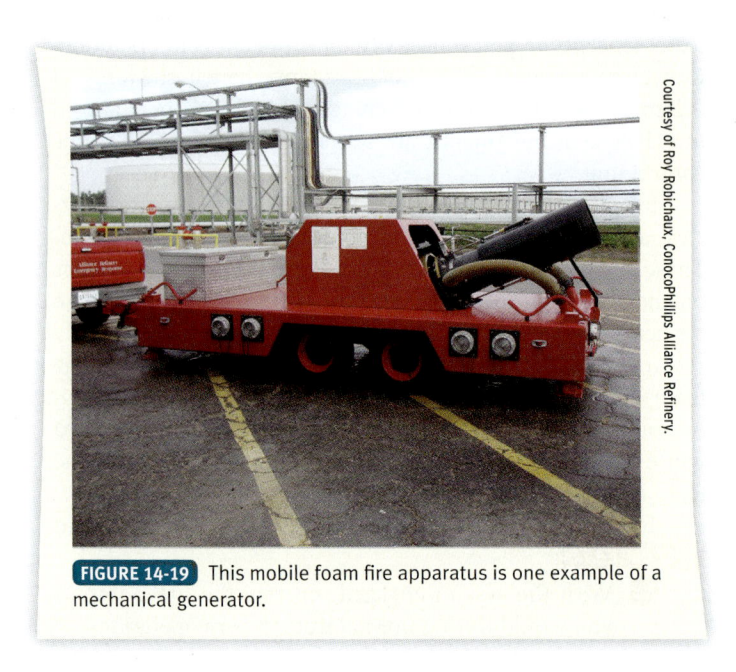

FIGURE 14-19 This mobile foam fire apparatus is one example of a mechanical generator.

CHAPTER 14 Foam 343

SKILL DRILL 14-6
Operating a Compressed-Air Foam System
NFPA 1002, 5.2.3, 5.2.3(B)

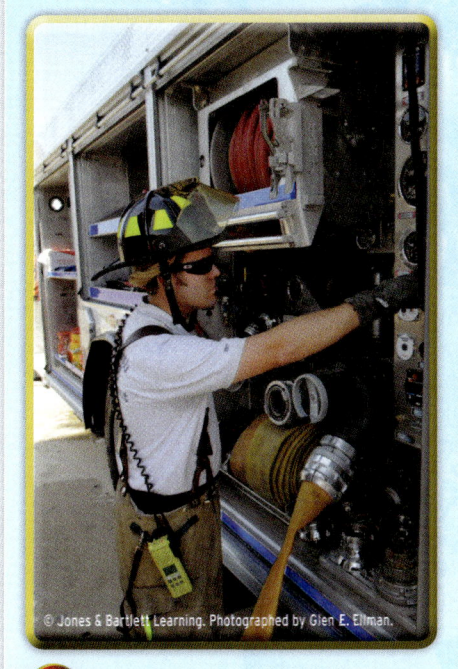

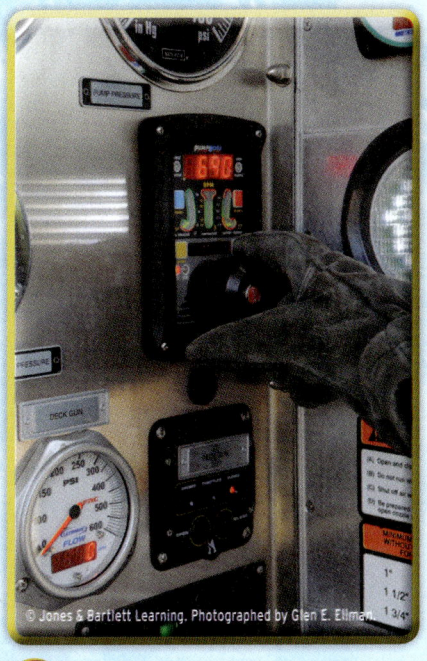

1 With the system engaged, operate the fire pump as you would during normal water pump operations.

2 Set the desired discharge pressure for the attack line.

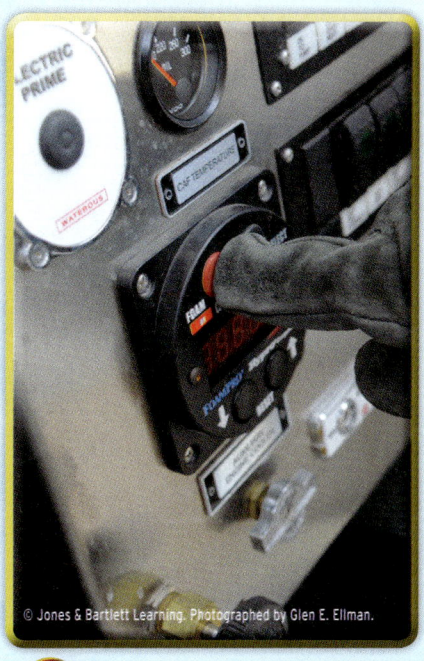

3 Push the "on" button at the pump panel display to turn the foam system on (if not already activated).

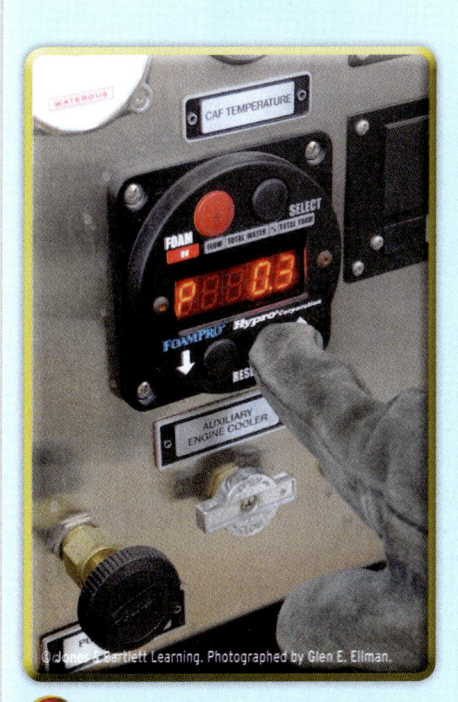

4 Select either "wet" or "dry" foam to be delivered to the discharge by setting the desired percentage of foam for the fire using the up/down arrow buttons.

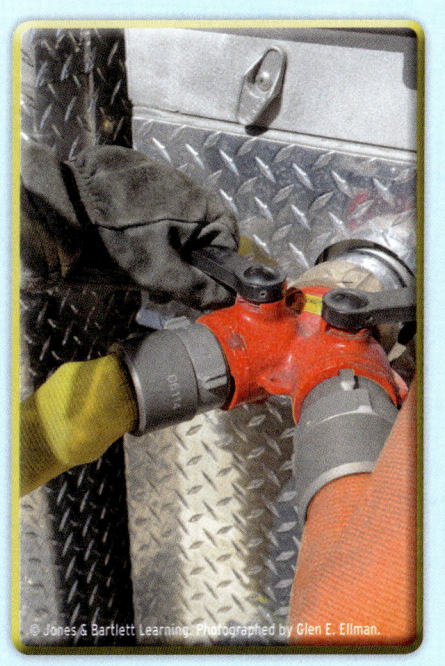

5 Open the discharge valve.

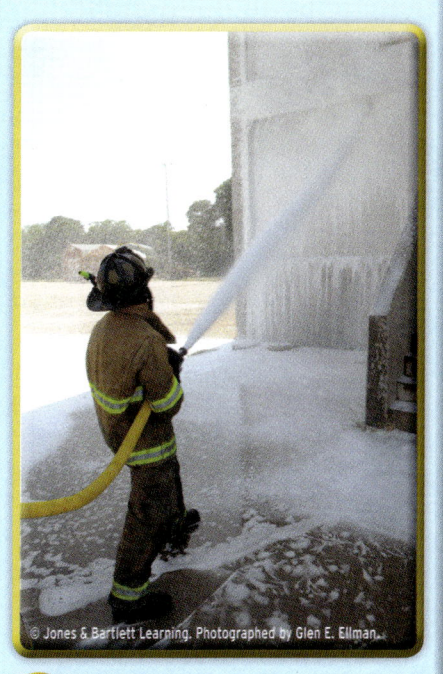

6 Discharge the foam through the attack lines.

VOICES OF EXPERIENCE

While working as a volunteer fire fighter in a rural area, our department used foam on several occasions. Our rural county had a large number of oil field pumping stations. These pumping stations would pump crude oil out of the ground and into holding tanks. These tanks averaged 30 ft (9 m) tall and 15 ft (5 m) in diameter. The tanks would fill and then pump oil into an oil refinery. The tops of these tanks were only tack welded, and the tanks had a single vent pipe to allow for pressure changes and liquid level changes.

The vent stack constantly gave off flammable vapors. When storms would come through the area, lighting would inevitably strike the vent stack. This would ignite the flammable vapors in the tank, blowing off the top of the tank, and setting the oil on fire. Our volunteer department would get the call of an "oil tank on fire."

On arrival, we would be presented with a flammable liquid fire at the top of a tall tank. Our standard procedure was to set up a foam operation to extinguish the fire. We would establish a 95-gpm (360-L/min) foam eductor and a 200-ft (75-m), 1½-inch (38-mm) attack line with a red foam tube. This tube was 4 ft (1 m) long with air inlets near the valve. It mixed air into the foam solution to make the finished foam (the big, bubbly, fluffy, white stuff).

We would use the raindown technique to apply foam to the burning oil surface fire. The fire officer would stand out away from the two crew members on the hoseline and direct the foam stream onto the target. With the raindown technique, the foam is aimed up into the air, the stream arcs over the fuel, and the stream breaks up into large flakes of foam. The fire officer would give the command to the hose team to adjust the position of the nozzle to get the flakes of foam to land where he wanted them to. The fire officer would use the wind to help with the fall of the foam. As the foam flakes begin to hit the surface of the fire, the aqueous film-forming foam (AFFF) properties would begin to start to suppress the flammable vapors. As the foam began to take effect, the fire officer would direct the line to move across the surface to complete extinguishment.

Depending on the wind and rain, it would take approximately 10 gal (38 L) of foam concentrate at a 3 percent concentration to achieve full extinguishment. The more volatile the oil in the tank, the more foam concentrate required to put out the fire. We got very good at this operation, sometimes repeating it three to four times a month. The better we got, the less foam we had to use. Practice make prefect!

Roger Westhoff
Houston Fire Department
Houston, Texas

High-expansion foams produce large volumes of foam that exclude oxygen from the incident area. In addition, the low water content of this type of foam reduces water damage.

Master Stream Foam Nozzles

Master stream foam nozzles allow operators to deal with large incidents where handline nozzles are not able to handle the demands for foam suppression. These master stream nozzles can be supplied from the fire apparatus' onboard systems (injection); alternatively, they can have an eductor as part of the nozzle. A **pick-up tube** draws the foam into the master stream nozzle; this tube is placed into the foam concentrate supply and operated as an eductor system. Master stream foam nozzles can be mounted permanently on the fire apparatus, can be removable so that they can be used as a portable unit, or can be strictly portable devices.

Air-Aspirating Foam Nozzles

Aspirating foam nozzles are designed to mix air with the foam solution as it is discharged. This effect is achieved without having to add a clamp-on tube to a fog nozzle. These foam nozzles are designed to aspirate the foam solution to produce good-quality finished foam.

Smooth-Bore Nozzles

Smooth-bore nozzles are the nozzle of choice when using a CAFS. Because the aeration of the foam solution takes place in the piping and hose, the finished foam will be discharged at the nozzle. Application—not aeration—is the major concern when a smooth-bore nozzle is used with a CAFS.

Fog Nozzles

Fog nozzles can be used to produce finished foam. When the incident involves polar solvent fuels, for example, fog nozzles may not deliver a foam quality that is able to extinguish the fire. Foam aeration tubes are available that can be easily and quickly clamped onto the end of a fog nozzle to aerate the foam solution more efficiently.

Foam Supplies

Foam concentrate is stored in containers that range in size from 5-gal (19-L) pails to 55-gal (208-L) drums **FIGURE 14-20**. Totes and trailers of foam concentrate are available in different sizes as well, ranging from 100 to 1000 gal (378.5–3785 L) of foam concentrate. Foam may be stored in its container without any change in its original physical or chemical characteristics. Freezing and thawing usually will not have any effect on modern foam concentrates, but it is important to check with the concentrate manufacturer for technical information on the concentrate's properties.

The shelf life of foam concentrate will vary depending on the type of concentrate. Typically, protein concentrate has a shelf life in the range of 7 to 10 years. Synthetic concentrates and high-expansion concentrates have a shelf life of 20 to 25 years.

The environmental impact of foam use has been a concern for many years. Many types of foam have undergone testing to assess their effects on the environment. Information regarding the toxicity of foam concentrates is usually available from product environmental data sheets, material safety data sheets, product technical bulletins, and toxicity summary sheets. The manufacturer/supplier of the foam concentrate is a primary resource for researching this information.

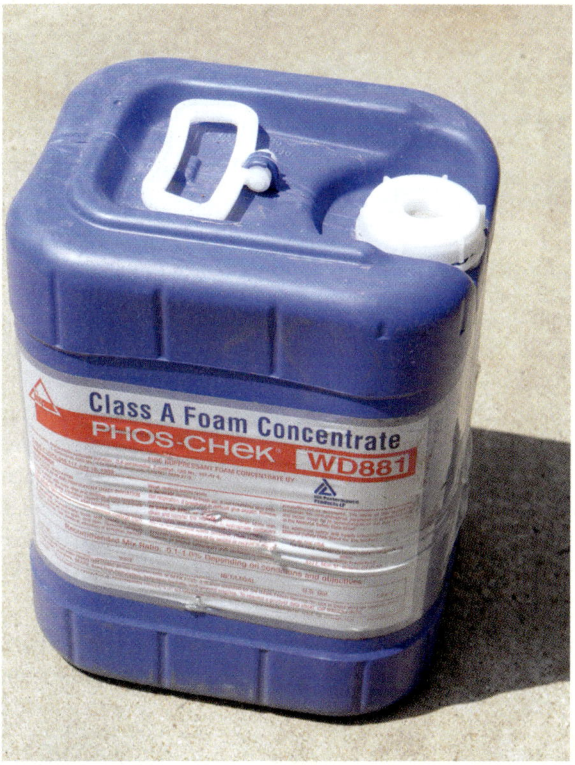

FIGURE 14-20 The standard size of foam concentrate container is a 5-gal (19-L) pail.

Foam Application

Knowing the accepted methods for foam application is important for driver/operators. After all, you may have to use a handline to apply foam or you may need to assist other fire fighters in the application method. Consequently, you need to be the expert on all aspects of foam operation.

Applying Foam

Class A Foam

The use of Class A foam for structural firefighting is becoming a more common practice. The benefits of using foam to extinguish Class A fires or in incidents involving three-dimensional fuels have been proven through testing done by manufacturers and fire departments. The use of Class A foam for firefighting is similar to the use of water. Although the application methods are the same, the results will probably be better with the foam. Training and experimentation with Class A foam in actual fire situations is not recommended due to safety concerns. Instead, the confidence and experience needed in operating foam systems can best be achieved with live fire training.

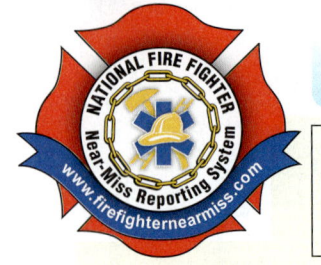

Near-Miss REPORT

Report Number: 10-0000930

Synopsis: Foam supply creates problem during incident.

Event Description: Our department responded to a HazMat incident involving ethyl alcohol. Approximately 2000 gallons (7571 L) of product were spilled onto the ground when the tanker truck rolled onto its side, damaging the man-way cover and rupturing the tank. We used an in-line inductor due to the fact that the on-truck foam tanks contained aqueous film-forming foams (AFFF). I was placed in charge of the in-line foam inductor on our main suppression line. We only had 15 gallons (57 L) of alcohol-resistant aqueous film-forming foams (AR-AFFF) available, so a call for more foam was placed to other departments in the area. When the foam arrived, it was in 5-gallon (19-L) containers. There was a mixture of new, old, and several different types and concentrations of AR-AFFF. When switching from an empty bucket to a fresh one, the inductor plugged, causing a loss of foam on the line and interrupting vapor suppression tactics. The problem was brought to the attention of our operations chief, and due to the lack of materials, we continued to use the foam and clear the plugged inductor as was needed for the duration of the call.

Lessons Learned: This had no detrimental effect on the overall outcome of the situation. After the debriefing, we were able to start the process to order and maintain a reserve of AR-AFFF and reeducate ourselves on foam compatibility and recognition of possible problems.

To apply a Class A foam on a fire, follow the steps in **SKILL DRILL 14-7**:

1. Open the nozzle and test to ensure that foam is being produced. (**STEP 1**)
2. Move within a safe range of the target and open the nozzle. (**STEP 2**)
3. Direct the stream of foam onto the burning surface or the exposure that you are protecting. (**STEP 3**)
4. Be aware that the fire fighters may have to change positions around the structure so as to adequately cover the entire surface. (**STEP 4**)

DRIVER/OPERATOR Tip

All live fire training should be conducted in compliance with NFPA 1403, *Standard on Live Fire Training Evolutions*. While live burns can be an effective teaching tool, the safety of the personnel involved must be the number one priority. **Safety first.**

Class B Foam

The methods for using Class B foam on Class B fires differ from those used when applying Class A foam on Class A fires. Directing a Class B foam stream into a Class B fire can disrupt the fuel and cause the fire to spread. Plunging the stream into an existing foam blanket will allow vapors to escape, which can result in spreading, reignition, or flare-up of the fire. To avoid these problems, three methods are used to produce foam blankets on Class B fires:

- Roll-on method
- Bankdown method
- Raindown method

Sweep (Roll-on) Method

The <u>sweep (roll-on) method</u> should be used only on a pool of flammable product that is located on open ground. With this technique, foam is placed on the fuel surface by directing the foam stream onto the ground in front of the product involved. The foam will then roll onto the surface of the material involved. It may be necessary to move the hoseline to a different position to achieve total coverage. You may also need to use multiple lines to cover the material. If the crew uses multiple hoselines, they need to maintain awareness of the positions of other fire fighters operating in the area. A coordinated attack should be conducted by the IC, and a safety officer should be on the scene.

To perform the roll-on method, follow the steps in **SKILL DRILL 14-8**:

1. Open the nozzle and test to ensure that foam is being produced. (**STEP 1**)
2. Move within a safe range of the target and open the nozzle. (**STEP 2**)
3. Direct the stream of foam onto the ground just in front of the pool of product. (**STEP 3**)
4. Allow the foam to roll across the top of the pool of product until it is completely covered.
5. Be aware that the fire fighters may have to change positions along the spill so as to adequately cover the entire pool. (**STEP 4**)

CHAPTER 14 Foam 347

SKILL DRILL 14-7
Applying Class A Foam on a Fire
NFPA 1002, 5.2.3, 5.2.3(B)

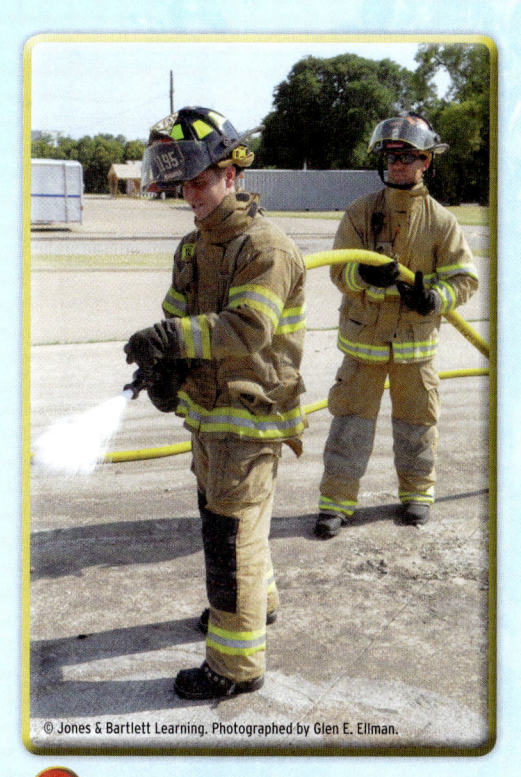

1 Open the nozzle and test to ensure that foam is being produced.

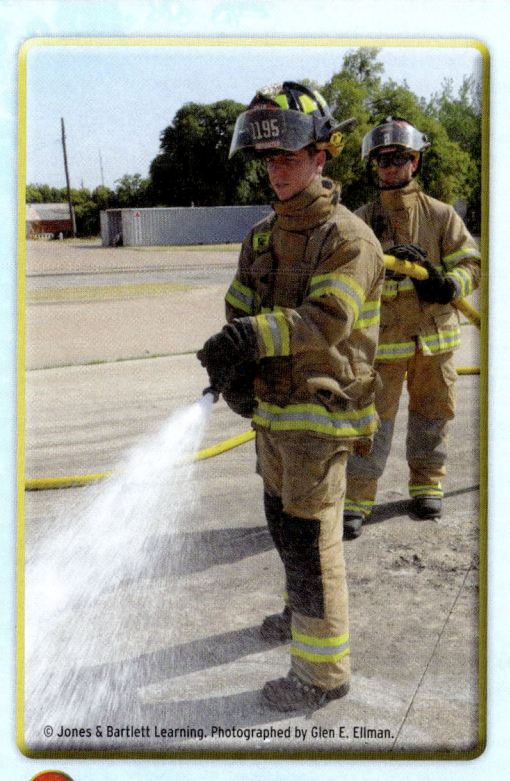

2 Move within a safe range of the target and open the nozzle.

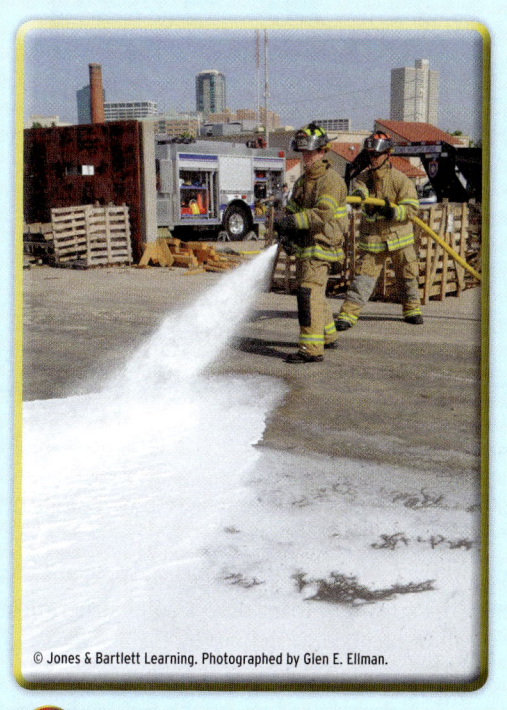

3 Direct the stream of foam onto the burning surface or the exposure that you are protecting.

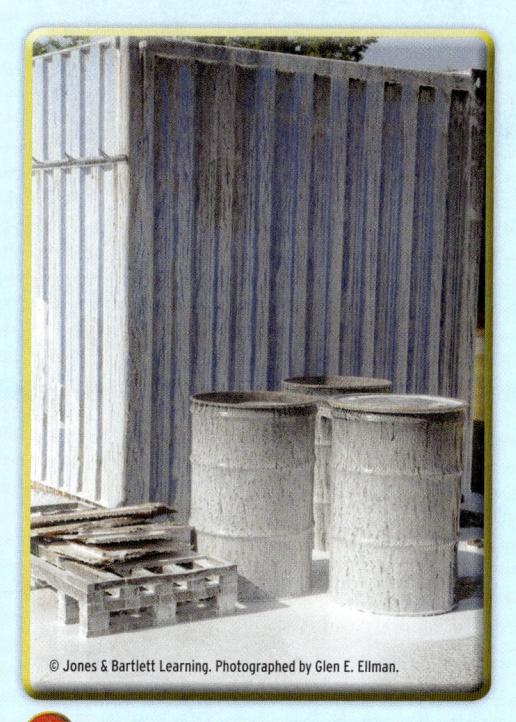

4 Be aware that the fire fighters may have to change positions around the structure so as to adequately cover the entire surface.

© LiquidLibrary

SKILL DRILL 14-8 Applying Foam with the Roll-On Method
NFPA 1002, 5.2.3, 5.2.3(B)

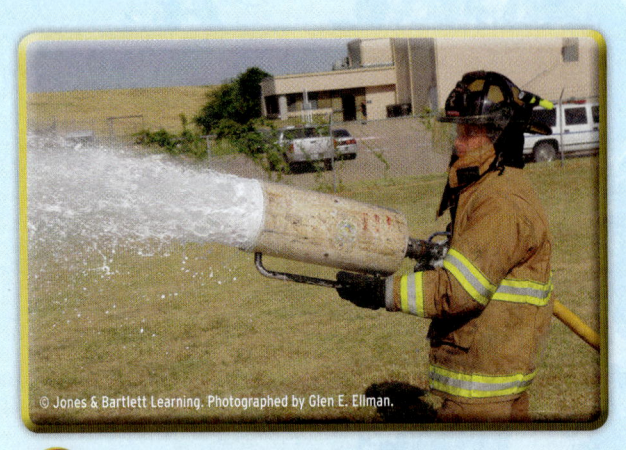

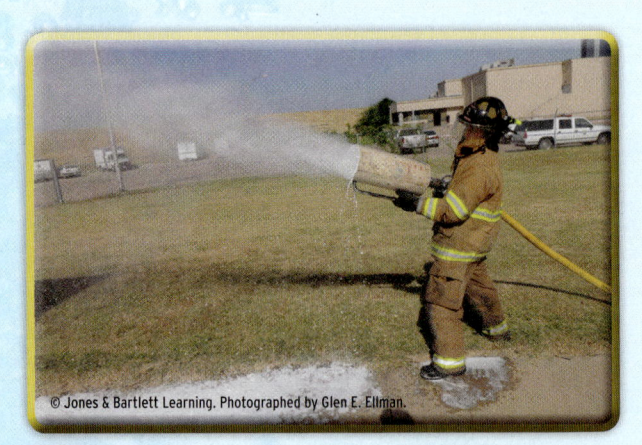

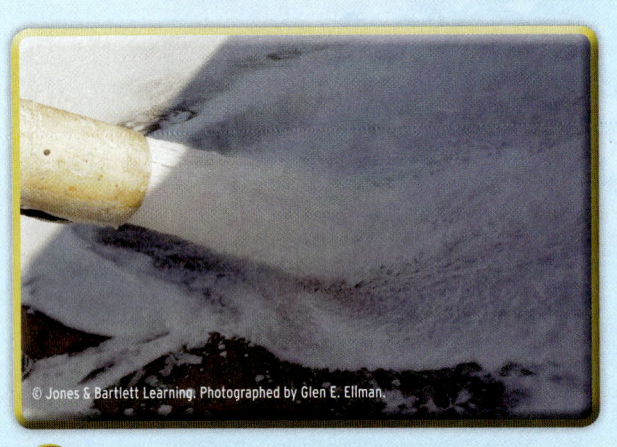

1. Open the nozzle and test to ensure that foam is being produced.
2. Move within a safe range of the target and open the nozzle.
3. Direct the stream of foam onto the ground just in front of the pool of product.
4. Allow the foam to roll across the top of the pool of product until it is completely covered. Be aware that the fire fighters may have to change positions along the spill so as to adequately cover the entire pool.

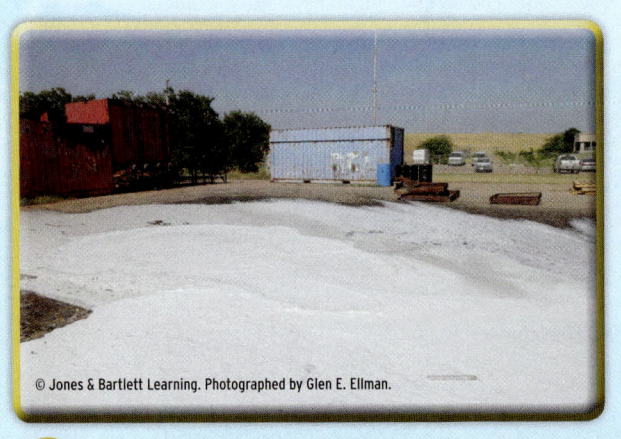

Bankshot (Bankdown) Method

The **bankshot (bankdown) method** is employed at fires where the fire fighter can use an object to deflect the foam stream and let it flow down the burning surface. This application of foam should be as gentle as possible to avoid agitating the material involved. If the material is located in an area where there is a wall, a tank, or other vertical object, then the foam can be directed at and allowed to run down that object. This approach will allow the foam to spread over the material and form a foam blanket.

To perform the bankdown method of applying foam, follow the steps in **SKILL DRILL 14-9**:

1. Open the nozzle and test to ensure that foam is being produced. (STEP 1)
2. Move within a safe range of the target and open the nozzle.
3. Direct the stream of foam onto a solid structure such as a wall or metal tank so that the foam is directed off the object and onto the pool of product.
4. Allow the foam to flow across the top of the pool of product until it is completely covered.
5. Be aware that the fire fighters may have to bank the foam off several areas of the solid object so as to extinguish the burning product. (STEP 2)

SKILL DRILL 14-9 Applying Foam with the Bankdown Method (FF2)
NFPA 1002, 5.2.3, 5.2.3(B)

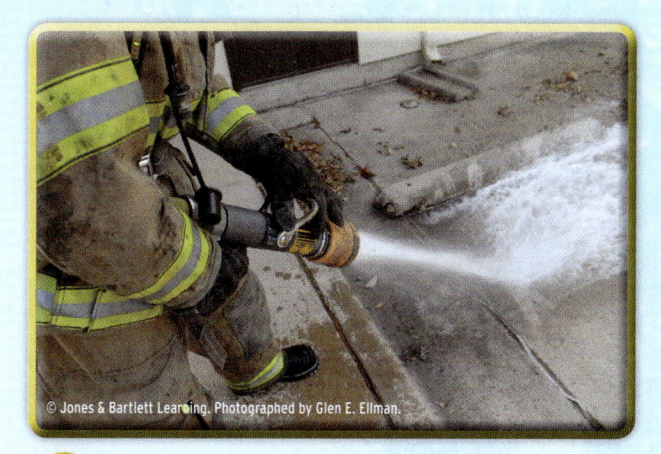

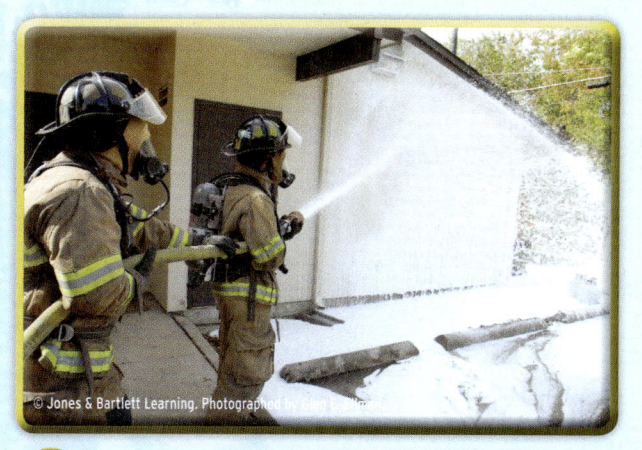

1 Open the nozzle and test to ensure that foam is being produced.

2 Move within a safe range of the target and open the nozzle. Direct the stream of foam onto a solid structure such as a wall or metal tank so that the foam is directed off the object and onto the pool of product. Allow the foam to flow across the top of the pool of product until it is completely covered. Be aware that the fire fighters may have to bank the foam off several areas of the solid object so as to extinguish the burning product.

Raindown Method

The **raindown method** can be used when there is no vertical object to use for a bankshot and it would be too dangerous to get close and use the roll-on method of foam application. This foam application technique consists of lofting the foam stream into the air above the material and letting it fall gently down onto the surface. It can be an effective method as long as the foam stream can completely cover the material involved. Two caveats apply: this method might not be effective when wind conditions are unfavorable, and the coverage of the foam needs to be monitored. The fire itself may vaporize the foam stream producing reduced results.

To perform the raindown method, follow the steps in **SKILL DRILL 14-10**:

1. Open the nozzle and test to ensure that foam is being produced. (**STEP 1**)
2. Move within a safe range of the target and open the nozzle. (**STEP 2**)
3. Direct the stream of foam into the air so that the foam breaks apart in the air and falls onto the pool of product. (**STEP 3**)
4. Allow the foam to flow across the top of the pool of product until it is completely covered.
5. Be aware that the fire fighters may have to move to several locations and shoot the foam into the air so as to extinguish the burning product. (**STEP 4**)

Foam Compatibility

Class A concentrates and Class B concentrates are not compatible. Mixing these different classes of concentrates may cause the concentrate to gel and hinder the operation of foam proportioning equipment. Likewise, Class B foam concentrates may not be compatible with each other. Check with the foam manufacturer for information on compatibility of particular types of foam.

Also make sure that onboard tanks on fire apparatus are properly marked. Many fire apparatus carry onboard water, Class A foam concentrate, and Class B foam concentrate tanks. In some instances, foam concentrate has been poured into the wrong tank—with undesirable results.

SKILL DRILL 14-10 Applying Foam with the Raindown Method
NFPA 1002, 5.2.3, 5.2.3(B)

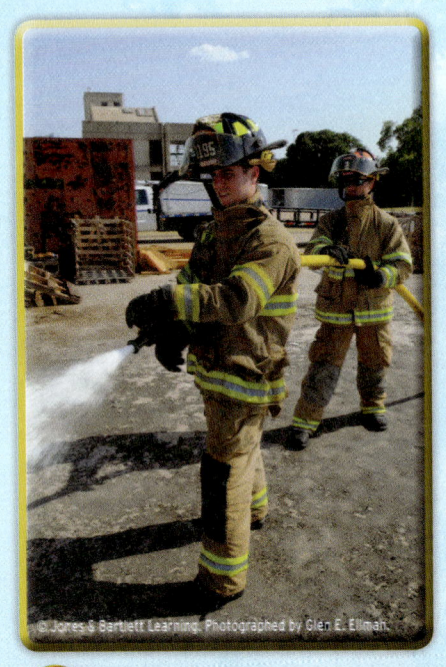

1 Open the nozzle and test to ensure that foam is being produced.

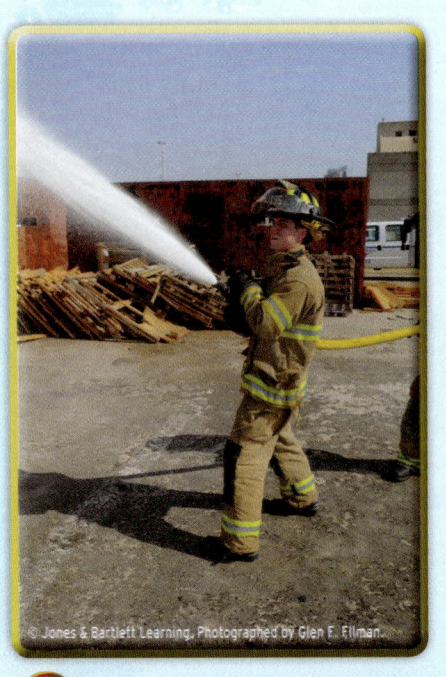

2 Move within a safe range of the target and open the nozzle.

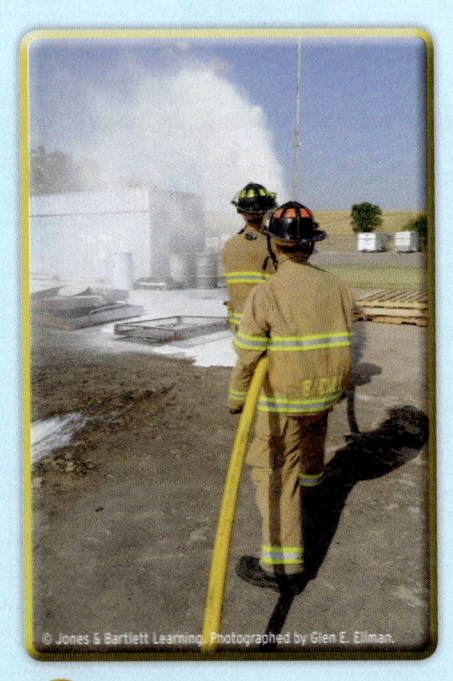

3 Direct the stream of foam into the air so that the foam breaks apart in the air and falls onto the pool of product.

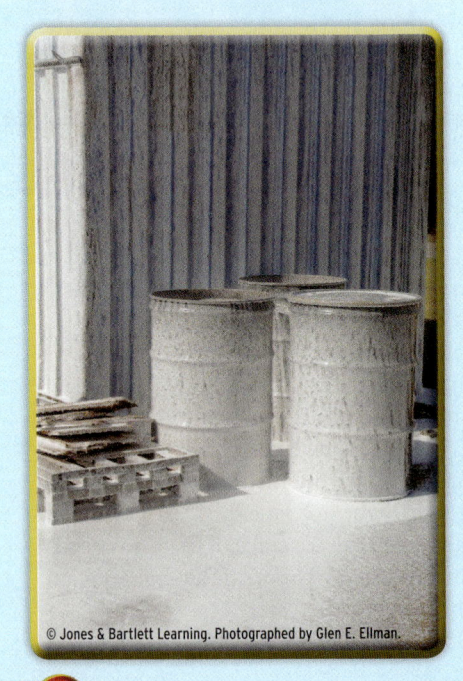

4 Allow the foam to flow across the top of the pool of product until it is completely covered. Be aware that the fire fighters may have to move to several locations and shoot the foam into the air so as to extinguish the burning product.

Wrap-Up

Chief Concepts

- While water is effective in suppressing fires, foams have added a new dimension to firefighting strategies.
- Foam for firefighting consists of a stable mass of small air-filled bubbles. It has a lower density than oil, gasoline, or water and will float on top of the fuel.
- The way that foam works to help extinguish a fire is very simple:
  - Once applied to the burning fuel, the foam will float on top of it, forming a blanket on the surface.
  - This blanket, if applied correctly, will stop or prevent the burning process by separating the fuel from the air, lowering the temperature of the fuel, and/or suppressing the release of flammable vapors.
- Foam is made up of four components: water, foam concentrate, mechanical agitation, and air.
- Firefighting foams are classified as either Class A or Class B.
- Foam concentrates are designed to be mixed with water at specific ratios, ranging from 1 percent to 6 percent.
- The foam expansion rate quantifies the ratio of finished foam to foam solution after the mixture is agitated and aspirated through a foam-making appliance.
- Foam cannot be produced if it is not proportioned properly.
  - Several types of foam application systems are available, ranging from basic operations to more advanced systems.
  - With the proper training, these systems can be very user friendly and will produce good-quality finished foam.
- The proper nozzle is needed for fire fighters to be able to produce a good-quality foam blanket.
- Foam concentrate is stored in containers of various sizes, including 5-gal (19-L) pails, 55-gal (208-L) drums, totes, and trailers.
- Knowing the several accepted methods for applying foam is important for driver/operators because they may have to use a handline to apply foam or may need to assist other fire fighters in the application method.
- Class A concentrates and Class B concentrates are not compatible; mixing these different classes of concentrates may cause the concentrate to gel and hinder the operation of foam proportioning equipment.

Hot Terms

additive A liquid such as foam concentrates, emulsifiers, and hazardous vapor suppression liquids and foaming agents intended to be added to the water.

aeration The process of introducing air into the foam solution, which expands and finishes the foam.

aqueous film-forming foam (AFFF) A concentrated aqueous solution of fluorinated surfactant(s) and foam stabilizers that is capable of producing an aqueous fluorocarbon film on the surface of hydrocarbon fuels to suppress vaporization.

around-the-pump proportioning (AP) system A fire apparatus–mounted foam system that diverts a portion of the water pump's output from the discharge side of the pump and sends it through an eductor to discharge foam.

balanced-pressure system A fire apparatus–mounted foam system that uses a diaphragm-type pressure control valve to sense and balance the pressures in the foam concentrate and water lines to the proportioner.

bankshot (bankdown) method A method that applies the foam stream onto a nearby object, such as a wall, instead of directly at the fire.

batch mixing Pouring foam concentrate directly into the fire apparatus water tank, thereby mixing a large amount of foam at one time.

burnback resistance The ability of a foam blanket to resist direct flame impingement.

bypass eductor A foam eductor that is mounted to the pump and can be used for application of either water or foam.

chemical foam Foam produced by mixing powders and water, where a chemical reaction of the materials creates the foam.

Class A foam Foam intended for use on Class A fires.

Class B foam Foam intended for use on Class B fires.

combustible liquid Any liquid that has a closed-cup flash point at or greater than 100°F (37.8°C) as determined by the test procedures and apparatus set forth in Section 4.4. Combustible liquids are classified according to Section 4.3.

compressed-air foam system (CAFS) A foam system that combines compressed air and a foam solution to create firefighting foam.

concentration The percentage of foam chemical contained in a foam solution.

duplex gauge A gauge at the pump panel that simultaneously monitors both the foam concentrate and water pressures.

eductor A device that uses the Venturi principle to siphon a liquid in a water stream. The pressure at the throat of the device is below atmospheric pressure, allowing liquid at atmospheric pressure to flow into the water stream.

film-forming fluoroprotein foam (FFFP) A protein-based foam concentrate incorporating fluorinated surfactants, which forms a foam capable of producing a vapor-suppressing, aqueous film on the surface of hydrocarbon fuels. This foam may have an acceptable level of compatibility with dry chemicals and may be suitable for use with those agents.

Wrap-Up, continued

finished foam The homogeneous blanket of foam obtained by mixing water, foam concentrate, and air.

fire barrier A continuous membrane or a membrane with discontinuities created by protected openings with a specified fire protection rating. Such a membrane is designed and constructed with a specified fire resistance rating to limit the spread of fire, which also restricts the movement of smoke.

flammable liquid Any liquid that has a closed-cup flash point less than 100°F (37.8°C), as determined by the test procedures and apparatus set forth in Section 4.4, and a Reid vapor pressure that does not exceed an absolute pressure of 40 psi (276 kPa) at 100°F (37.8°C), as determined by ASTM D 323, *Standard Test Method for Vapor Pressure of Petroleum Products (Reid Method)*. Flammable liquids are classified according to Section 4.3.

fluoroprotein foam (FP) A protein-based foam concentrate to which fluorochemical surfactants have been added. The resulting product has a measurable degree of compatibility with dry chemical extinguishing agents and an increased tolerance to contamination by fuel.

foam A stable aggregation of small bubbles of lower density than oil or water, which exhibits a tenacity for covering horizontal surfaces. Air foam is made by mixing air into a water solution containing a foam concentrate, by means of suitably designed equipment. It flows freely over a burning liquid surface and forms a tough, air-excluding, continuous blanket that seals volatile combustible vapors from access to air.

foam concentrate (foam liquid) A concentrated liquid foaming agent as received from the manufacturer.

foam heat exchanger A device that uses water as its cooling source and prevents the foam concentrate from overheating.

foam proportioner A device or method to add foam concentrate to water so as to make foam solution.

foam solution A homogeneous mixture of water and foam concentrate added in the proper proportions.

foam system A system provided on fire apparatus for the delivery of a proportioned foam and water mixture for use in fire extinguishment. The system includes a concentrate tank, a method for removing the concentrate from the tank, a foam-liquid proportioning system, and a method (e.g., handlines or fixed turret nozzles) of delivering the proportioned foam to the fire.

foam tetrahedron A geometric shape used to illustrate the four elements needed to produce finished foam: foam concentrate, water, air, and mechanical aeration.

fuel pick-up The absorption of the burning fuel into the foam itself.

fuel resistance A foam's ability to minimize fuel pick-up.

high-expansion foam Any foam with an expansion ratio in the range of 200:1 to approximately 1000:1.

hydrocarbon A chemical substance consisting of only hydrogen and carbon atoms.

hydrolysis Decomposition of a chemical compound by reaction with water.

induction The use of an eductor to introduce a proportionate amount of foam concentrate into a stream of water flowing from a discharge.

injection system A foam system installed on a fire apparatus that meters out foam by pumping or injecting it into the fire stream.

knockdown speed and flow The time required for a foam blanket to spread out across a fuel surface.

low-expansion foam Any foam with an expansion ratio up to 20:1.

mechanical foam Foam produced by physical agitation of a mixture of water, air, and a foaming agent.

mechanical generator An electrically powered fan used to aerate certain types of foams.

medium-expansion foam Any foam with an expansion ratio in the range of 20:1 to 200:1.

metering device A device that controls the flow of foam concentrate into the eductor.

miscible Readily mixes with water.

oleophobic Oil hating; having the ability to shed hydrocarbon liquids.

oxygenated Treated, combined, or infused with oxygen.

pick-up tube The tube from an in-line foam eductor that is placed in the foam bucket and draws foam concentrate into the eductor using the Venturi principle.

polar solvent A combustible liquid that mixes with the water contained in foam. Such solvents include non-petroleum-based fuels such as alcohol, lacquers, acetone, and acids.

polymer A naturally occurring or synthetic compound consisting of large molecules made up of a linked series of repeated simple monomers.

proportioned Descriptor for a combination of foam concentrate and water used to form a foam solution.

protein foam Foam created from a concentrate that consists primarily of products from a protein hydrolysate, plus stabilizing additives and inhibitors to protect against freezing, to prevent corrosion of equipment and containers, to resist bacterial decomposition, to control viscosity, and to otherwise ensure readiness for use under emergency conditions.

pump-mounted eductor An in-line eductor dedicated to the production of foam.

raindown method A method of applying foam that directs the stream into the air above the fire and allows it to gently fall onto the surface.

ratio controller A device required for each foam outlet to proportion the correct amount of foam concentrate into the water stream over a wide range of flows and with minimal pressure loss.

surface tension The elastic-like force at the surface of a liquid, which tends to minimize the surface area, causing drops to form.

sweep (roll-on) method A method of applying foam that involves sweeping the stream just in front of the target.

viscosity A measure of the resistance of a liquid to flow.

water additive An agent that, when added to water in proper quantities, suppresses, cools, mitigates fire and/or provides insulating properties for fuels exposed to radiant heat or direct flame impingement.

wetting agent A concentrate that when added to water reduces the surface tension and increases its ability to penetrate and spread.

References

National Fire Protection Association (NFPA) 11, *Standard for Low-, Medium-, and High-Expansion Foam*. 2010. http://www.nfpa.org/codes-and-standards/document-information-pages?mode=code&code=11. Accessed July 11, 2014.

National Fire Protection Association (NFPA) 18A, *Standard on Water Additives for Fire Control and Vapor Mitigation*. 2011. http://www.nfpa.org/codes-and-standards/document-information-pages?mode=code&code=18A. Accessed October 7, 2014.

National Fire Protection Association (NFPA) 1002, *Standard for Fire Apparatus Driver/Operator Professional Qualifications*. 2014. http://www.nfpa.org/codes-and-standards/document-information-pages?mode=code&code=1002. Accessed March 27, 2014.

National Fire Protection Association (NFPA) 1403, *Standard on Live Fire Training Evolutions*. 2012. http://www.nfpa.org/codes-and-standards/document-information-pages?mode=code&code=1403. Accessed July 11, 2014.

Scheffery, J.L. Foam Extinguishing Agents and Systems, In *National Fire Protection Handbook, Twentieth Edition*. Quincy, MA; p17-49: 2008.

DRIVER/OPERATOR in action

When you arrive at the scene, you see that the semi-truck has overturned and its spilled fuel has ignited. The officer has determined that the fire fighters will knock down the fire with the foam on the apparatus before it can ignite the tank. You quickly recall the procedures to operate the onboard foam system and deliver foam to the fire fighters at the end of the hoseline. With the correct type and percentage of foam, the fire is quickly controlled and the hazardous materials team later plugs the tank up, stopping the flow of flammable liquid. Understanding the capabilities of the foam system and the foam itself is critical for the driver/operator.

1. Which device mixes the foam concentrate into the foam stream in the proper percentage?
   A. Foam device
   B. Foam proportioner
   C. Around-the-cab pump
   D. Foam applicator

2. Which of the following is not one of the four elements of the foam tetrahedron?
   A. Water
   B. Air
   C. Mechanical agitation
   D. Foam concentrate
   E. All are correct

3. What does AFFF stand for?
   A. Alcohol firefighting foam
   B. Advanced firefighting foam
   C. Aqueous film-forming foam
   D. Always fresh fire foam

4. Compressed-air foam system (CAFS) hoselines are usually filled with approximately ____ percent compressed air.
   A. 5
   B. 10
   C. 20
   D. 30

5. Which of the following is not one of the three methods used to produce foam blankets on Class B fires?
   A. Bankdown
   B. Roll-on
   C. Raindown
   D. Bankshot

353

Apparatus Equipped with an Aerial Device

CHAPTER 15

Knowledge Objectives

After studying this chapter you will be able to:

- Describe the function of aerial apparatus in the fire service. (p 356–357)
- Describe the types and features of aerial apparatus. (p 358–359)
- Describe the construction of aerial apparatus. (p 359–363)
- Describe the aerial apparatus hydraulic system. (NFPA 1002, 6.1.1(2), 6.2.2.(A), 6.2.3(A), 6.2.4(A)); p 359–360)
- Describe the aerial device inspection requirements and process. (NFPA 1002, 6.1.1, 6.1.1(1), 6.1.1(2), 6.1.1(3), 6.1.1(4), 6.1.1(5), 6.1.1(6), 6.1.1(7), 6.1.1(A)); p 363)
- Identify the capabilities and limitations of an aerial device related to reach, tip load, angle of inclination, and angle from chassis axis, as well as the effects of topography, ground, and weather conditions as they apply to safe deployment. (NFPA 1002, 6.2.1(A), 6.2.2(A)); p 363–367)
- Determine the correct position for an aerial apparatus, maneuver the apparatus into that position, and avoid obstacles to operations. (NFPA 1002, 6.2.1(A)); p 363–367)
- Describe how to maneuver and position an aerial apparatus. (NFPA 1002, 6.2.1, 6.2.1(A), 6.2.3, 6.2.3(A)); p 364–367)
- Describe how to recognize system problems and how to correct any deficiency noted in accordance with department policies and procedures. (NFPA 1002, 6.1.1(A)); p 363)
- Describe the stabilization requirements and effects of topography and ground conditions on stabilization. (NFPA 1002, 6.2.2, 6.2.2(A)); p 367–371)
- Describe the safe operating practices for aerial apparatus. (NFPA 1002, 6.2.3(A)); p 371–375, 377–380)
- Describe the considerations and requirement for the deployment of an elevated stream. (NFPA 1002, 6.2.5, 6.2.5(A)); p 384–389)
- Describe the aerial device's emergency operating system(s). (NFPA 1002, 6.2.4, 6.2.4(A)); p 388)

- Transfer power from the vehicle's engine to the hydraulic system and operate vehicle stabilization devices. (NFPA 1002, 6.2.2(B)); p 367–371)
- Stabilize an aerial apparatus for deployment. (NFPA 1002, 6.2.2(B)); p 368–371)
- Raise, rotate, extend, and position an aerial device to a specified location, as well as lock, unlock, retract, lower, and bed the aerial device. (NFPA 1002, 6.2.3(B)); p 371–375, 377–380)
- Use the aerial apparatus to affect rescues. (NFPA 1002, 6.2.3(B)); p 378, 380–382)
- Use the aerial apparatus to perform ventilation. (NFPA 1002, 6.2.3(B)); p 382–384)
- Lower an aerial device using the emergency operating system, so that the device is lowered to its bedded position. (NFPA 1002, 6.2.4, 6.2.4(B)); p 388)
- Deploy and operate an elevated master stream. (NFPA 1002, 6.2.5(B)); p 384–389)
- Connect a water supply to a master stream device, and control an elevated nozzle manually or remotely. (NFPA 1002, 6.2.5(B)); p 384–389)

Additional NFPA Standards

- NFPA 1071, *Standard for Emergency Vehicle Technicians Professional Qualifications*
- NFPA 1901, *Standard for Automotive Fire Apparatus*
- NFPA 1911, *Standard for the Inspection, Maintenance, Testing, and Retirement of In-Service Automotive Fire Apparatus*
- NFPA 1983, *Standard on Life Safety Rope and Equipment for Emergency Service*

Skills Objectives

After studying this chapter, you will be able to:

- Inspect the aerial device to identify system problems. (NFPA 1002, 6.1.1, 6.1.1(B)); p 363)
- Determine the correct position for aerial apparatus and maneuver the apparatus into that position. (NFPA 1002, 6.2.1(B)); p 363–367)

You Are the Driver/Operator

On September 11, 2013, the Glenview (Illinois) Fire Department responded to a reported fire on the ninth floor of a 16-story apartment building. Upon arrival, fire fighters observed a working fire with two occupants on a balcony exposed directly to the fire and smoke. The aerial ladder company took a position adjacent to the building, with the turntable centered at the victims' location. The stabilizers were set, and the aerial ladder was maneuvered nearly vertical to the two victims. The victims were then assisted in climbing down the aerial device by fire fighters.

1. How would you determine exactly where to stop and park the apparatus so that the aerial device could reach the victims?
2. Would it ever be acceptable to use the sidewalk between the building and the curb to set the stabilizers?
3. With two victims who appear uninjured and able-bodied, which circumstances might impact your ability to have them climb down safely?

Introduction

The aerial apparatus is a tool, and a new aerial apparatus can cost more than $1 million. Given this high price, a fire department cannot afford to use such apparatus incorrectly or inadequately. Fire fighters assigned to drive and operate the aerial cannot wait until the incident commander (IC) determines a need for this apparatus. That is, optimal positioning of the aerial apparatus must be a key consideration upon arrival. Positioning must occur based on the current conditions, the occupancy, and what is known—not what may be learned later **FIGURE 15-1**. The aerial apparatus is a tool just like a saw or an axe—that is, it is something that allows fire fighters do their jobs better, faster, and safer. As with a saw, however, if they do not train with and know the capabilities and limitations of the aerial device, fire fighters will not be better, faster, or safer with its use.

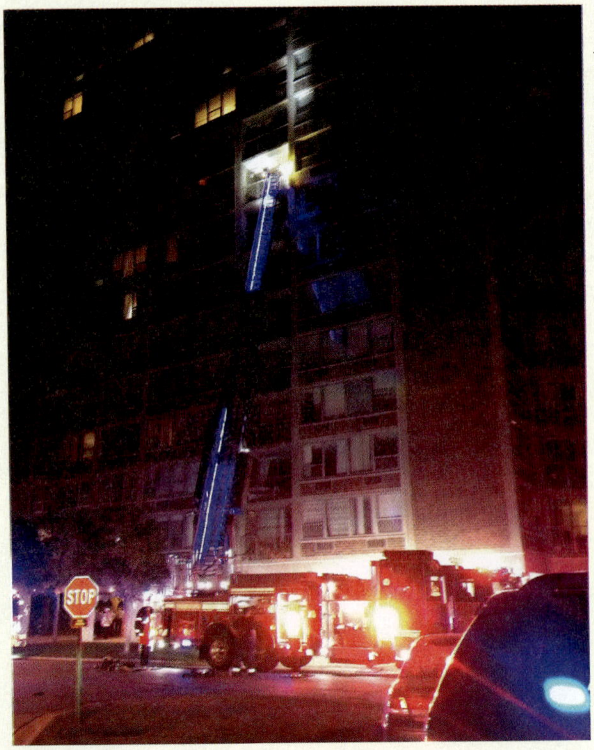

History of Aerial Apparatus

Aerial apparatus has evolved over the past 100-plus years. As the United States entered the 20th century and buildings in the urban environment began to rise past a few stories, fire fighters soon realized they needed additional capabilities to deal with fires in these multistory structures. Portable extension ladders could reach a maximum of only 50 ft (15 m) before the construction necessary for them to reach farther made their use impractical due to the added weight and bulk. The space that these ladders occupied, the number of fire fighters necessary to carry the ladder, and the weight of the fly section made raising them nearly impossible.

Over time, to affect rescues and to apply water to upper stories, innovators developed the vehicle-mounted aerial ladder and the water tower. These apparatus remained separate until the mid-20th century, when advances in construction and manufacturing made it possible for the aerial ladder to support the weight and stress of the elevated stream. In the 1950s, then-Chicago Fire Commissioner Robert J. Quinn modified the **articulating platform** for firefighting use. By the 1970s, apparatus manufacturers had designed aerial apparatus with heavy-duty ladders, attached platforms, and telescoping waterways creating the modern aerial apparatus.

The traditional, most obvious role for aerial apparatus on the fireground remains the rescue of trapped persons. While other functions can also be performed from these devices, the rescue of human life is always the top priority for fire fighters, and all aerial operations must first address this need.

Tactical Priorities

As the aerial apparatus approaches and arrives at the incident, the driver/operator must consult rapidly with the apparatus' officer to determine the tactical priority for the company. It is

FIGURE 15-1 An aerial apparatus reaching the ninth floor.

this priority that will aid the driver/operator in making decisions about placement, positioning, setup, and operation of the aerial apparatus. The order of the tactical priorities remains the traditional one:

1. Rescue
2. Exposures
3. Confinement
4. Extinguishment

■ Rescue

Rescue is accomplished first either by removing victims from the fire's threat or by extinguishing or at least knocking down the fire, thereby making removal of the victim less dangerous. This is accomplished using a variety of tactics. Once adequate resources are assigned to accomplish rescue, fire fighters must then address the threat of fire spreading to exposure property. Exposures may consist of areas attached to the fire building or detached structures, vehicles, or materials.

Along with managing exposures comes the challenge of preventing the spread of fire to uninvolved areas of the fire building or other combustibles by confining the fire. Only once these priorities are accomplished can the idea of extinguishing the fire be addressed. Ventilation is not placed in this order of operations, as it should be used to support one or more of the previously mentioned priorities. At one fire, ventilation may need to be performed early on to support a rescue, whereas at a different fire, this step may be able to wait until time of extinguishment. The skilled and competent driver/operator uses his or her training and experience to work with the company officer to address these tactical priorities.

Fire fighters, of course, are human beings with all-too-human attitudes and behaviors. Emergencies, especially those with victims needing rescue, will affect and potentially alter those attitudes and behaviors. Fire fighters have an obligation to save lives and property to the best of their ability and circumstances. It is their duty to do so in a manner that will achieve success. Damaging equipment so that it can no longer participate in such rescues or, even worse, killing or seriously injuring fire fighters so that they can no longer participate in such rescues, does not allow fire fighters to carry out their duty and fulfill that obligation. Put simply, fire fighters must know their job and their equipment so that they may save lives and property.

■ Aerial Deployment Priorities

The priorities for the use of the aerial apparatus are as follows:

1. Rescue
2. Exposure protection
3. Ventilation
4. Elevated streams

These priorities complement and support the overall tactical priorities identified by the IC.

Priority 1: Rescue

When victim removal via ladder is required above the third floor, it is the aerial ladder that is usually needed for this operation. Most portable ladders carried on fire apparatus will be of insufficient length for operations at heights greater than the third floor. When victim removal is not immediately needed, a secondary means of egress for fire fighters operating in a fire area above the third floor becomes a priority. Again, it is the aerial ladder that is usually needed to fulfill this need.

Priority 2: Exposure Protection

As with any fire, before efforts are directed at extinguishment, the IC must ensure that the fire will not spread. When faced with a large fire and no immediate need for the aerial device to perform rescue work, the apparatus may be called upon to provide an elevated stream. In such a case, the driver/operator must identify exposures upon approach of the incident scene. Past experience and prefire planning will aid in this identification.

Priority 3: Ventilation

With the need for rescue and exposure protection addressed, the aerial may then be used to perform horizontal or vertical ventilation. Providing a safe and rapid method for accessing the windows of upper floors or roofs is a job for the aerial device. As with exposure protection, the driver/operator must identify optimal positioning locations upon approach to the incident scene based on his or her past experience and prefire planning.

Priority 4: Elevated Stream Operations

When called for by the IC, the application of an elevated stream by the aerial apparatus can be an effective tactic in the suppression of heavy fire. The adage that "When the aerial goes up, the building comes down" could not be further from the truth; it is not the position of the elevated stream, but rather the purpose of the stream that supports an offensive or defensive firefighting effort. Commonly used hand lines provide fire flows of 125–180 gpm (500–700 L/min) or 250–325 gpm (1000–1300 L/min); elevated streams can multiply these flows to 500–1200 gpm (2000–5000 L/min). Therefore, application of such streams should be considered when stopping the forward progress of the fire is beyond the capabilities of deployable hand lines. If the apparatus is to perform this operation, the driver/operator must be versed in the expedient setup and application of the elevated stream.

While a hand line can be advanced up and off the tip of an aerial, another elevated stream operation entails deployment of a stream fed by a standpipe. In buildings without standpipes or buildings under construction, however, it may be more expedient to use the aerial's prepiped waterway to deploy a hand line. Depending on how the aerial device is configured, a hand line may be connected to a discharge at the tip specifically for this purpose; removal of the master stream's nozzle and connection of a wye, water thief, or other device may be required; or the hose may be connected directly to the waterway. In all of these situations, the waterway should be equipped with a pressure relief valve to prevent damage should the waterway be retracted while the nozzle is shut. Pump discharge pressure calculations must take into account and combine the aerial's loss of pressure, the elevation, and the hose lay components, including any appliance, the hose itself, and the nozzle.

Whenever a hoseline is deployed in this manner and advanced into a structure, the ability of the aerial to serve other functions is impaired. The apparatus may not be maneuvered to another location as long as the hoseline is connected. Also, the ability of the ladder to support persons in need of evacuation is reduced. Consult the aerial manufacturer's operator's manual for details on these practices and limitations.

Aerial Apparatus Types and Features

Within the fire service, aerial apparatus is known by a variety of names, some of which are specific to certain regions of North America. In this chapter the terms *truck*, *ladder*, and *tower* are used to refer to aerial apparatus. In more specific terms, there are three main types of aerial apparatus:

- Straight ladders
- Elevated platforms
- Articulating platforms

This chapter addresses **straight ladders** and **elevated platforms**. Other chapters consider the unique features and considerations of other tiller aerial; however, the unique features and considerations of articulating platforms are not addressed in this text.

In 1991, the National Fire Protection Association (NFPA) adopted a new standard on aerial apparatus that improved the design and load requirements of such apparatus. That standard has since been incorporated into NFPA 1901, *Standard for Automotive Fire Apparatus*, and has been revised multiple times. Aerial apparatus—particularly aerial ladders—constructed prior to 1991 may not meet the current safety expectations. For more information on older aerial apparatus, refer to the U.S. Fire Administration's Technical Report Series, *Aerial Ladder Collapse Incidents* (USFA-TR-081), published in April 1996.

All aerial apparatus have a turntable, referring to the location where the aerial device attaches to the chassis. There are two locations on the apparatus where this connection is made: the middle of the chassis and the rear of the chassis. When the aerial device is attached at the rear, it is referred to as a rear-mount device. When the aerial device is attached to the middle of the chassis, it is referred to as a midship device.

■ Three Main Types of Aerial Devices

The three main types of aerial devices are aerial ladders, aerial platforms, and articulating platforms **FIGURE 15-2**.

Aerial Ladder

The aerial ladder without any basket or platform is a straight ladder. Straight ladders may be referred to by a number of terms, including *truck*, *ladder truck*, or *aerial ladder*, although some fire departments may use these terms to describe aerial platforms as well.

Straight ladders have a truss construction. NFPA 1901 requires a minimum tip load capacity of 250 pounds (113 kg). By comparison, elevated platforms require a minimum tip load of 750 pounds (340 kg). It is essential for the driver/operator to understand the maximum tip load for the straight ladder he or she will be operating. Generally, apparatus manufacturers produce medium-duty and heavy-duty designs, each of which will have different weight-carrying capabilities. Not knowing these capabilities and overloading the aerial can lead to catastrophic events that not only damage the aerial apparatus, but also result in the injury or death of both fire fighters and civilians. Midship-mounted aerial ladders that utilize a tractor-trailer combination are referred to as tiller apparatus and are covered elsewhere in this text.

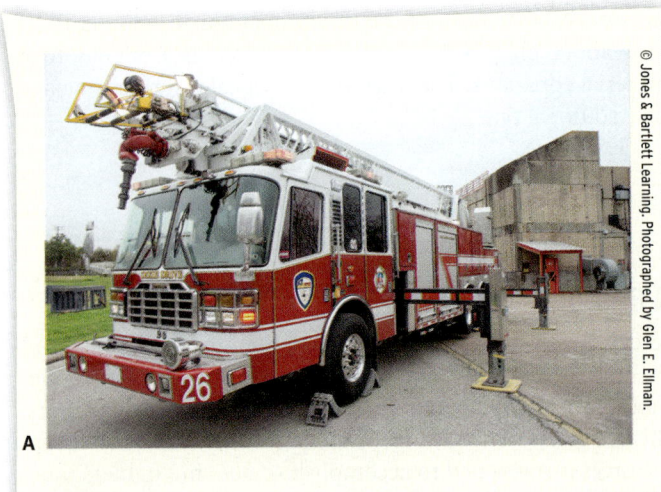

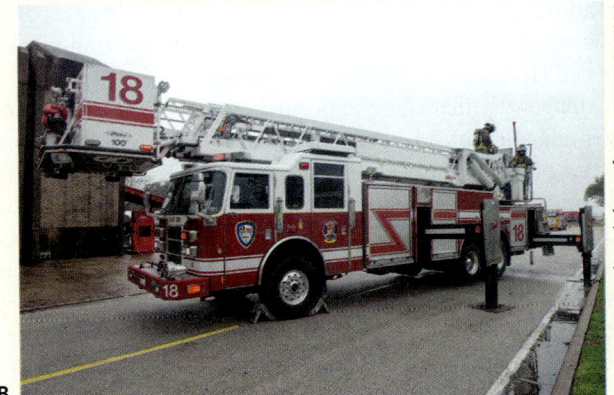

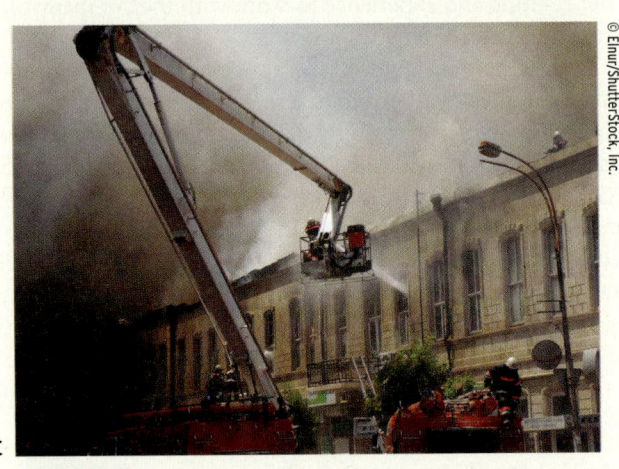

FIGURE 15-2 The three main types of aerial devices: **A.** aerial ladders, **B.** aerial platforms, and **C.** articulating platforms.

Aerial Platform

Aerial platforms can be referred to as tower ladders or ladder towers, depending on the region of the country. In general, platforms have a telescoping boom that does not articulate and is equipped with a bucket, basket, or platform from which fire fighters can operate. The lengths of aerial platforms may vary, just as the lengths of aerial ladders may vary. The boom may or may not serve as a ladder, although the ladder-type boom is most common. All telescoping booms that serve as ladders are of a heavy-duty design by necessity. With such a device, the ladder will be required to hold the weight of the platform plus two to four fire fighters or victims carried on the ladder. Aerial platforms with a boom of the non-ladder design, in contrast, may be outfitted with an extension ladder that is permanently affixed to the boom. Whether these ladders are intended for emergency egress by fire fighters or use in the rescue of civilians is taken into account in the manufacturer's design.

Articulating Platform
The articulating platform consists of a boom with a hinge or knuckle joint in its midsection; the boom is not constructed with a ladder truss design. Such booms may or may not telescope like aerial platforms. Articulating platforms may range from 50 ft (15 m) to more than 100 ft (30 m) in length. Articulating platforms are not covered in this text.

Aerial Ladder Construction
Aerial ladders and aerial platforms may be constructed of either aluminum or steel. Both aerial ladders and aerial platforms of all lengths are manufactured from both materials. When aluminum is used as the base material, it is generally not painted but rather finished with a brushed appearance **FIGURE 15-3**. Steel construction, in contrast, is painted or may also be galvanized **FIGURE 15-4**. Whether a ladder is built using aluminum or steel depends on the manufacturing process used and the fire department's preference. The advantages and disadvantages of each material type are beyond the scope of this chapter.

■ Aerial Ladders and Platforms
Aerial ladders and aerial platforms of aluminum and steel can be constructed using welded, riveted, or bolted connections. Some manufacturers may employ more than one method in the construction of their aerial; however, a discussion of the advantages and disadvantages of each construction method is beyond the scope of this chapter.

The most common construction technique for an aerial device is truss construction. This method is used for both aerial ladders and aerial platforms. As with all trusses, there is a top cord and a bottom cord. On the aerial, the top cord is loaded under tension and the bottom cord is loaded under compression. The truss carries the load of the aerial and any live load to the turntable and into the torque box, where it is transferred first to the **stabilizers** and ultimately into the earth.

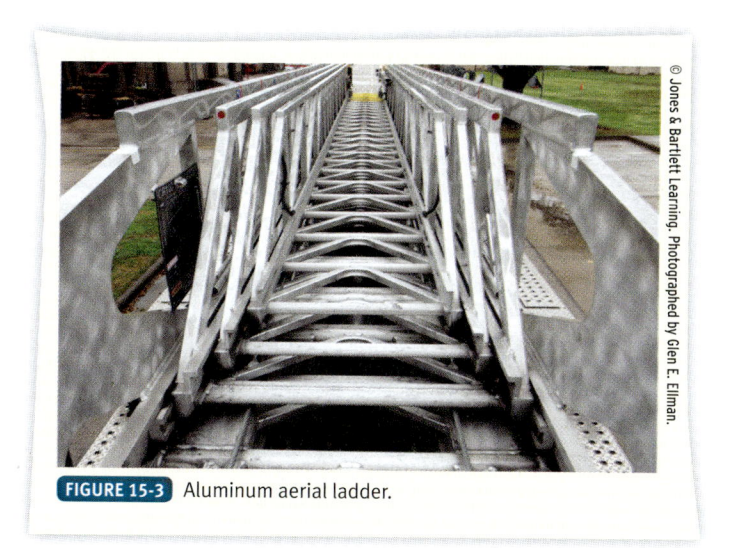

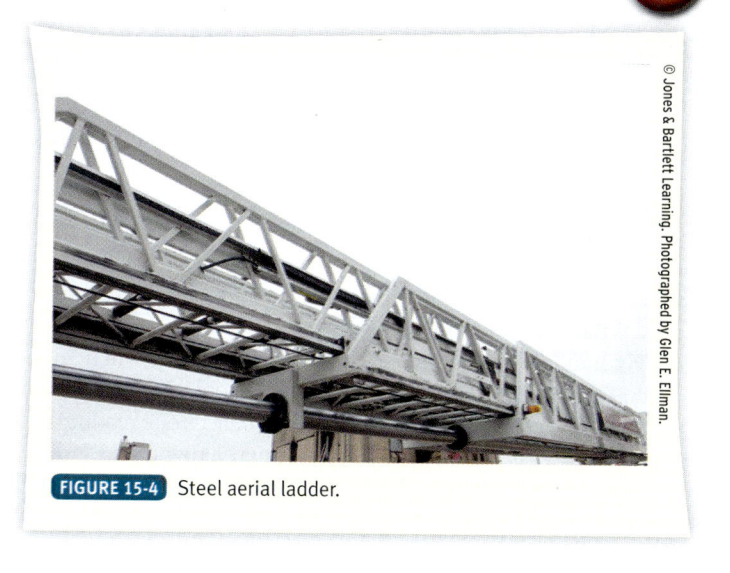

Regardless of the material or construction method used, all aerial apparatus should meet the requirements of NFPA 1901. In the 2009 edition of NFPA 1901, Chapters 8 and 19 specifically apply to aerial apparatus, while Chapters 1 through 4 and 12 through 15 apply to all fire apparatus. A number of other chapters may apply depending on the features desired by the local fire department.

The specific maintenance requirements for aerial apparatus are specified by the manufacturer as well as in NFPA 1911, *Standard for the Inspection, Maintenance, Testing, and Retirement of In-Service Automotive Fire Apparatus*. All aerial apparatus should have an annual inspection conducted by following the manufacturer's requirements and NFPA 1911. At intervals of no more than once every 5 years, each aerial apparatus should also undergo nondestructive testing (NDT) of its complete system, to be performed by a certified third-party who adheres to the requirements of NFPA 1911 and the apparatus manufacturer's specifications.

■ Hydraulic and Electrical Systems
Although there are still many aerial devices that utilize true hydraulic controls, the modern aerial is stabilized and maneuvered using hydraulic systems that are operated by electronic controls. Commonly referred to as "electric over hydraulic" arrangements, these controls regulate the movement of the hydraulic fluid from its reservoir through the hydraulic pump and to the hydraulic cylinders. The cylinders themselves may be called rams, jacks, struts, or some other locally preferred term.

The hydraulic pump is generally powered by a **power take-off (PTO)** unit from the chassis power train. Such a pump can operate at either full or reduced engine speed. To engage the PTO, the driver/operator typically uses an electronic control switch. The hydraulic fluid reservoir then supplies the hydraulic pump.

FIGURE 15-4 Steel aerial ladder.

FIGURE 15-3 Aluminum aerial ladder.

A separate, electrically powered pump is typically used to supply emergency power to the aerial in the event that the chassis motor, PTO, or hydraulic pump fails. Such pumps are designed to run for short intervals. Indeed, excessive operating times can lead to damage and failure.

Hydraulic cylinders are used in three general lifting points on every aerial apparatus: to set the stabilizers, to elevate the aerial from the turntable, and to extend and retract the aerial ladder. On aerial platforms, hydraulic cylinders are also used to keep the basket level FIGURE 15-5.

Hydraulic fluid levels should be checked only when the aerial is completely stowed and the fluid is cool. Checking the levels in other circumstances may produce inaccurate readings. When the fluid is warm, for example, it may expand and indicate a false full or overfull condition. When the aerial is raised from the bedded position, the reservoir level tends to indicate that the reservoir is less than full. The addition of hydraulic fluid at this time will result in an overfull condition and possible spill when the aerial is lowered and stowed.

Depending on the aerial apparatus, the aerial hydraulic pump and the electronic controls may be operated by a single switch or by separate switches. These switches may be located in the cab near the driver's position, near the turntable, or in both locations. Consult the aerial apparatus' operator's manual to determine when it is permissible to engage these switches.

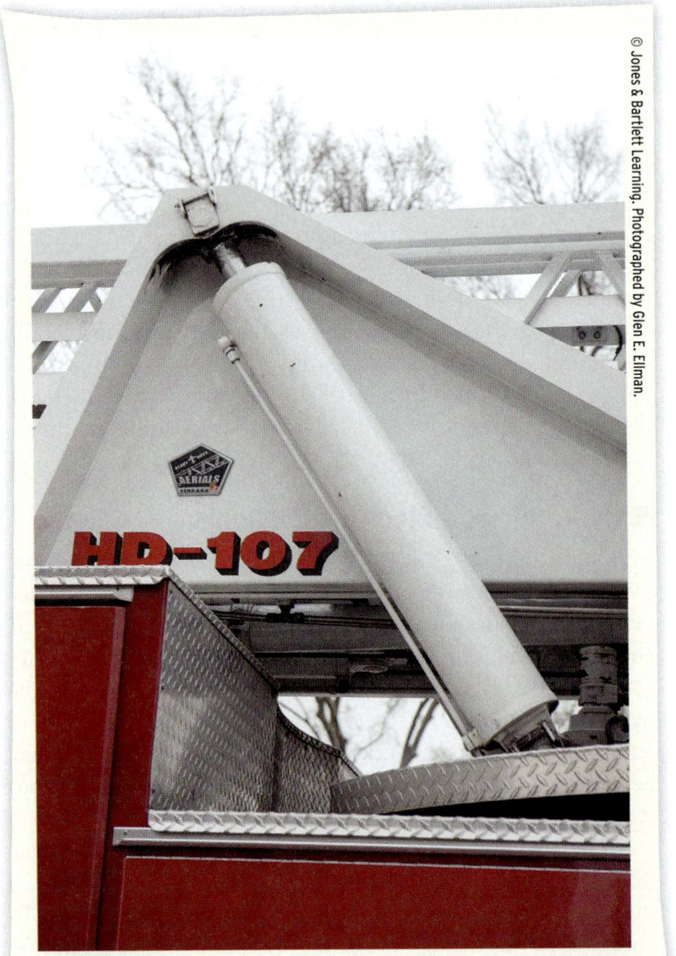

A series of cables attached to sheave and hydraulic cylinders connect the sections of the aerial, permitting it to extend and retract. Older aerial apparatus may use cables woven through sheaves and a winch located at the turntable for this purpose.

The sections of the aerial extend and retract along a series of slides and/or rollers. Each manufacturer engineers this system to achieve maximal efficiency. Slides are made of metal or synthetic materials designed to reduce friction and ensure minimum wear over the life of the aerial. Rollers are similarly constructed. Each of these components may require periodic cleaning and lubrication.

■ Stabilizers (Jacks, Outriggers, and Downriggers)

All aerial apparatus must be stabilized prior to elevation, extension, and rotation of the aerial device to prevent the entire apparatus from overturning. Failure to properly stabilize can result in not only extensive and possibly irreparable damage to the apparatus, but also injury or death to those persons on or near the apparatus. Stabilization is accomplished using stabilizers, also as **jacks**, **outriggers**, or **downriggers**. As with the selection of construction materials and techniques, the type of stabilizer used depends on the manufacturer's design and the preference of the local fire department. However, most manufacturers use a single stabilizer design for each particular model aerial. Thus the stabilizer type is determined by the fire department's selection of a particular manufacturer for this equipment. Whether the apparatus has two, three, four, or more stabilizers is also part of the manufacturer's design. No manufacturer will include stabilizers whose use is optional; that is, all stabilizers are needed for the maximum safe operation of the aerial.

For both aerial ladders and aerial platforms, there are four basic types of stabilizers:

- H-type
- A-type
- Fold-down
- Drop-down

H-Type Stabilizers

H-type stabilizers are the most common type. With the H-type, the stabilizer is first extended horizontally to achieve a maximum width for the footprint, then extended down vertically to take the chassis load off the suspension. As a result, the load is firmly and evenly transferred to the earth FIGURE 15-6. On some aerial devices, this is a multistep process and can be used to short-jack the apparatus (i.e., to set up the apparatus such that only the stabilizers on the working side of the aerial are fully extended). On other apparatus, the "out and down" setting of the stabilizers is a single action. This means by which the H-type stabilizers are engaged is also determined by the manufacturer's design.

A-Type Stabilizers

A-type stabilizers, also referred to as X-type stabilizers, extend out and down from the chassis in a single action. Some manufacturers will describe these stabilizers as "X" or scissors, as the mechanics of these stabilizers perform as such underneath the body of the apparatus FIGURE 15-7. These "behind the scenes" actions are irrelevant to the apparatus operator. A-type

FIGURE 15-5 Hydraulic cylinders.

CHAPTER 15 Apparatus Equipped with an Aerial Device   361

FIGURE 15-6 H-type stabilizers.

FIGURE 15-8 Fold-down stabilizers.

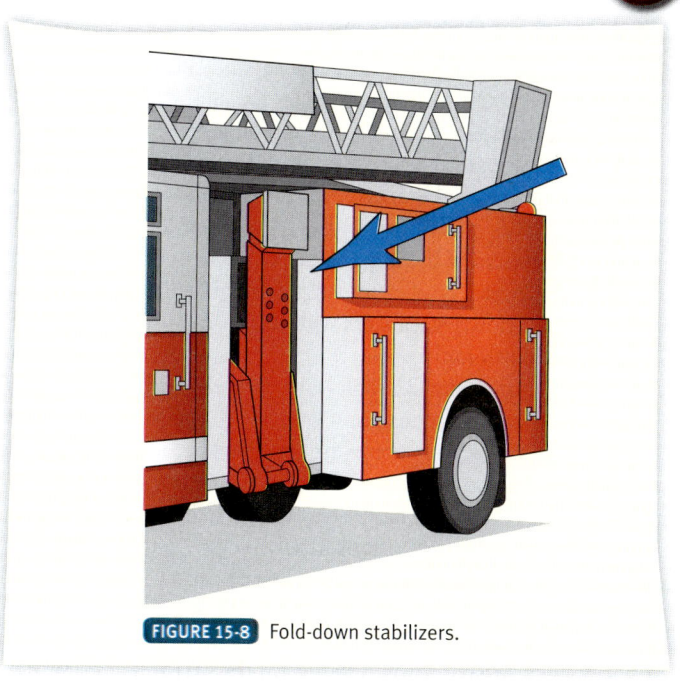

one of the other stabilizer types. Simply put, and as implied by their name, they come straight down from the underside of the chassis and contact the earth to increase the footprint of the aerial apparatus **FIGURE 15-9**.

Jack Locations
While the manufacturer's design will dictate stabilizer locations, the common locations for rear-mount turntable aerials are as follows:
- Two A- or H-type stabilizers, one on each side of the apparatus, may be placed near the turntable.

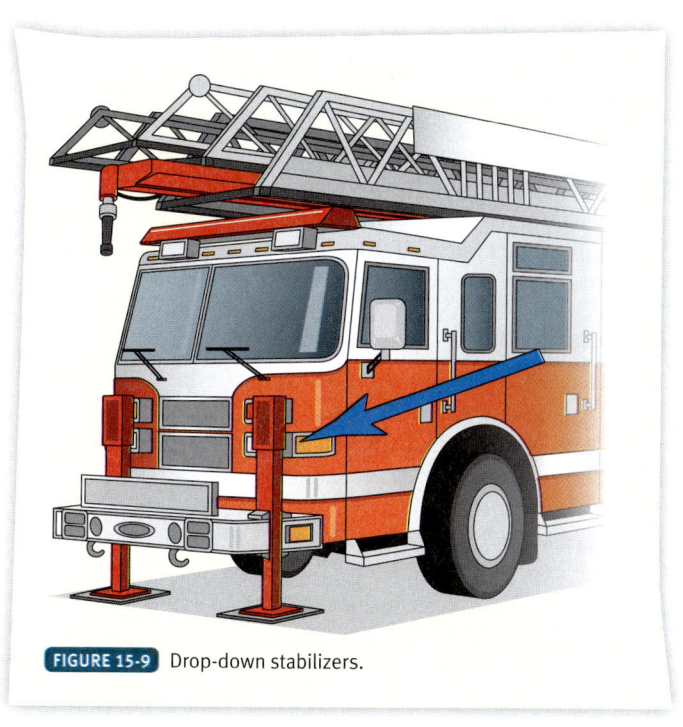

FIGURE 15-7 A-type stabilizers.

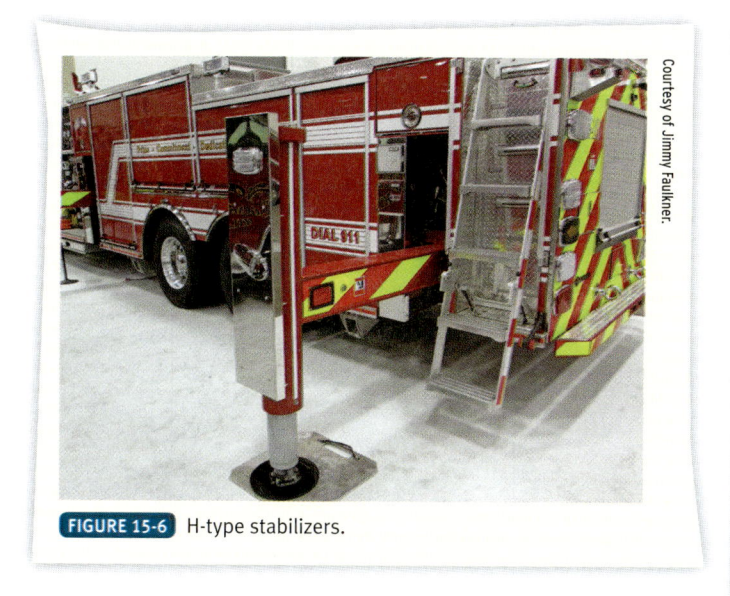

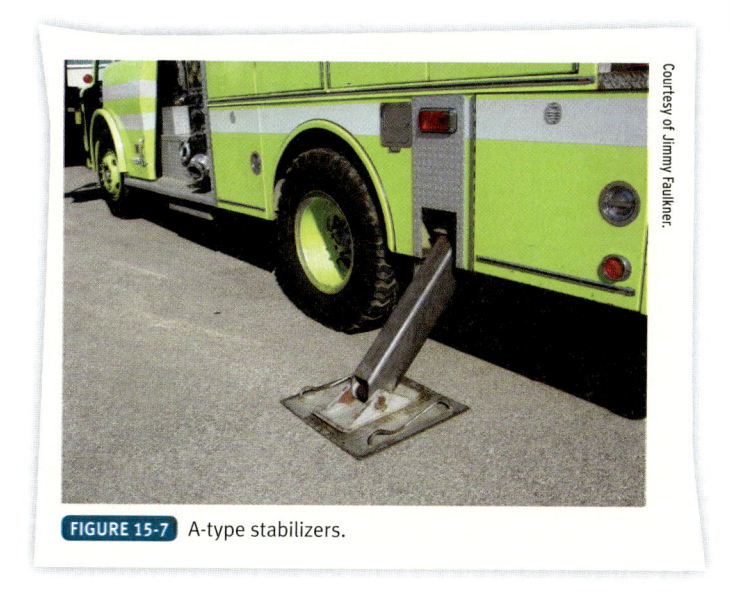

stabilizers cannot be short-jacked and must firmly contact the earth. However, for aerials of the same type and length, the typical width of fully extended A-type stabilizers is often less than the width of the typical H-type stabilizer when short-jacked.

Fold-Down Stabilizers
Fold-down stabilizers extend out following an arc, similar to the arc that might be created if you extended your arms above your head and then lowered them to your side without bending your elbow. Some fold-down stabilizers will then telescope once they touch the ground. Of the four types of stabilizers, fold-downs need the most room to be deployed **FIGURE 15-8**. Such stabilizers require a footprint similar to the H-type stabilizers to deploy but—unlike H-type stabilizers—cannot be short-jacked.

Drop-Down Stabilizers
Drop-down stabilizers do not have horizontal extension. These stabilizers are usually designed to perform in conjunction with

FIGURE 15-9 Drop-down stabilizers.

- Four A- or H-type stabilizers, two on each side of the apparatus, may be placed with one set ahead of and one set behind the rear axles for aerial ladders more than 90 ft (27 m) in length and all aerial platforms.
- If the apparatus is equipped with fold-down stabilizers, there may be only one stabilizer on each side of the apparatus and multiple drop-down stabilizers used on the corners of the apparatus.
- If the aerial is of a midship turntable design, H-type or fold-down stabilizers with drop-down stabilizers are most commonly used.

Aerials more than 20 years old may demonstrate variations of these common designs.

While all of the commonly used stabilizers can lift an apparatus off the ground by 12 to 24 inches (30.5 to 61 cm), a particular apparatus should be raised only as high as required by the manufacturer's specifications to achieve proper stabilization. Some manufacturers' instructions state that the aerial should be raised until the bulge is out of the tires; others indicate that the tires should be raised off the ground by as much as 1 to 2 inches (2.5 to 5 cm). In fact, some manufacturers offer different guidance for different models or types of aerials. Thus it is important to learn and know the manufacturer's requirements as contained in the operator's manual, rather than relying on word-of-mouth advice from others. Failure to adhere to the manufacturer's specifications and exceeding the equipment's limitations may result in damage to the apparatus and/or aerial structure.

An integral part of the stabilization system is rotation interlock and overload protection. The rotation interlock prevents the aerial device from being raised from its bedded position unless all stabilizers are properly set. Many aerials are equipped with an override feature that can be used as its name implies. This feature is useful when a well-trained operator must short-jack an aerial. Once the device is raised from its bedded position while short-jacked, the rotation interlock will prevent the aerial from being rotated onto the short-jacked side of the apparatus. Depending on the manufacturer, however, there are still some trucks in use that would allow rotation to the short-jacked side.

Overload protection is another feature of the stabilization system. Using pressure transducers or other technology, the load imposed onto the chassis by the aerial device is monitored, with an alarm sounding if the load exceeds the capabilities of the stabilization system. If this alarm is ignored, damage to the aerial or chassis, including catastrophic failure, may occur.

■ Aerial Reach

Vertical reach of the aerial ladder or platform is rated by the manufacturer and generally based on the apparatus being set up on level ground with the aerial device raised to its maximum extension at a 75° angle. At other angles of elevation, the vertical reach may be greater or less than this baseline rating. The first 7 to 9 ft (2 to 3 m) of vertical reach for any aerial is obtained from the turntable being mounted on the chassis. As the reach of the aerial expands horizontally, the vertical reach is reduced.

The horizontal reach should be measured following NFPA 1901, which specifies that the distance reached is measured from the middle of the turntable to the last rung of the fly section

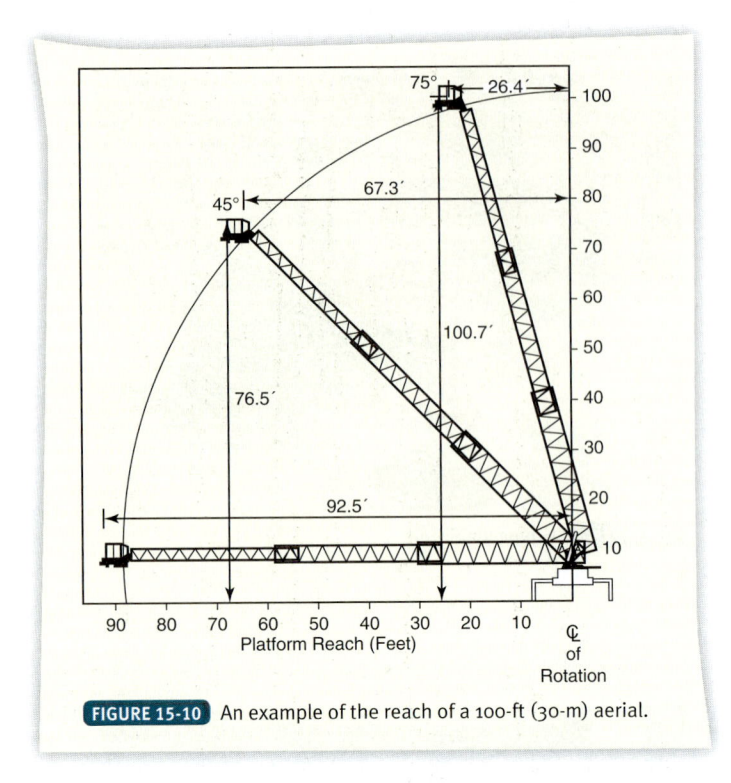

FIGURE 15-10 An example of the reach of a 100-ft (30-m) aerial.

of the aerial ladder or the outermost rail of the aerial platform. While the turntable height aids in obtaining some vertical reach, it reduces horizontal reach. Additionally, the width of the stabilizer footprint reduces the effective reach of the aerial, as it requires the centerline of the turntable to be set back from the operating surface by 7 to 10 ft (2 to 3 m). For an aerial rated at 100 ft (30 m), the effective horizontal reach when perpendicular to the chassis may only be 82 ft (25 m) due to the loss of the turntable elevation and stabilizer footprint **FIGURE 15-10**.

All aerial apparatus should be provided with lights that allow the driver/operator to position and maneuver the aerial in conditions of darkness. These lights are typically provided at the turntable and at the tip of the bed section. Some fire departments may specify the placement of additional lights near the tip of the fly section or on the aerial platform. Besides this lighting, lighting should be provided to help fire fighters climb on and operate from the aerial ladder or platform. Increasingly, small LED fixtures are being used to meet this requirement, thereby reducing the space needed for lighting components.

Equipment Mounting at Tip

On platforms and particularly on aerial ladders, the mounting of equipment such as floodlights, the intercom, breathing air systems, and portable equipment such as tools, portable ladders, and hose should be evaluated to ensure it will not interfere with the ability of the driver/operator to maneuver the aerial into position. In particular, such equipment should be positioned so that it not will catch on windows, balconies, and roofs as the aerial apparatus approaches them.

An intercom system must be provided between the aerial tip or platform, the turntable operator's position, and, if the device is equipped with a fire pump, the pump operator's position. These systems must allow for a hands-free response by the member located at the tip or platform. The driver/operator as well as fire fighters assigned to the aerial apparatus should be well versed in the operation of these devices.

A breathing air system may also be provided, especially on aerial platforms. Such a system will consist of air storage cylinders, a pressure-reducing regulator, hoses and tubing to transfer the breathing air to the aerial tip or platform, and an air pressure or volume monitoring system. At the very least, the monitoring system should notify users when the air cylinders are nearly empty. More elaborate systems will display the actual pressure or volume remaining, thereby enabling fire fighters to better plan their work. All aspects of these systems should be inspected and calibrated as recommended by the manufacturer. Likewise, all members should be training on their operation and use. The air storage cylinders should be inspected internally and hydrostatically tested per Department of Transportation regulations.

Inspection of Aerial Apparatus

Regular inspections should occur daily or weekly, after each use by the aerial operator, and after repairs, using recommendations and practices of the aerial's manufacturer. These inspections should focus on the aerial device, its stabilizing system, and its components, with the member looking for obvious damage, wear, deficiencies, and unsafe conditions. These inspections require a working knowledge of the aerial apparatus and the manufacturer's operator's manual. Specialized training and tools should not be required.

Whenever the aerial PTO or stabilization system will not engage or operate or the aerial device will not perform one of the five basic maneuvers (i.e., raise, lower, extend, retract, rotate), it should be removed from service. Until repairs are made, the aerial apparatus is not useful and may be unsafe. In some jurisdictions, the vehicle may remain in service but be relegated to duty that excludes aerial operations. Provided the chassis itself is safe and operational, it may be necessary to use the vehicle for transportation of personnel, equipment and tools, and ground ladders until such time as repairs can be undertaken. If any components of the aerial device are damaged, frayed, leaking, deformed, or missing parts, supports, or fasteners, the apparatus should not respond to any emergency and should be driven only as necessary to facilitate the needed repairs. Doing otherwise may exacerbate the issue at hand.

Annually, qualified personnel who are certified emergency vehicle technicians (NFPA 1071, *Standard for Emergency Vehicle Technicians Professional Qualifications*) should perform a detailed inspection of the apparatus and aerial device. At least once every five years, whenever a visual inspection indicates an issue, or after major repairs have been performed, the aerial apparatus should be subject to a nondestructive test (NDT) as well as a detailed inspection. The NDT should be performed by an accredited third-party testing firm. Generally, fire departments are not capable of conducting such inspections, nor do they possess the sophisticated equipment necessary to do so. NFPA 1911 contains out-of-service criteria and outlines inspection procedures in detail.

The annual inspection and nondestructive test should examine all welds, fasteners, and bolts; the hydraulic system and its components; the turntable, torque box, suspension, and rotation bearing; and the elevation, rotation, and extension interlocks. The hydraulic system and PTO should be operated to ensure pressure output is adequate and that cylinders, hoses, valves, and related parts do not leak, operate correctly, and are free of damage or excessive wear.

Aerial Apparatus Positioning

To position the aerial apparatus to best advantage, four priorities must be addressed:

1. **Rescue:** Is a physical rescue needed that requires an aerial apparatus?
2. **Exposure protection:** Does fire spread require application of an elevated stream?
3. **Ventilation:** Will access to upper floors or the roof for ventilation require use of an aerial apparatus?
4. **Elevated streams:** Does fire spread require application of an elevated stream? While this may seem similar to the second priority, aerial apparatus placement will not be similar.

Based on the direction provided by the company officer, the driver/operator's knowledge of the structure or complex and surrounding geography, and assessment of conditions, the apparatus must be positioned at the best vantage point. What will this be? The driver/operator must use his or her experience regarding how to park, so the apparatus can be used to support the operation, either immediately or when called for by the IC. This decision may differ for each department. It may also be different for each driver/operator based on his or her length of service and the other factors described previously. How long has the driver/operator been driving and operating this particular aerial? Has the driver/operator been to this structure before? For a working fire in this structure? What is the driver/operator expected to do based on department standard operating procedures (SOPs) or standard operating guidelines (SOGs)?

In any case, parking the aerial apparatus away from the fire never allows it to become a useful resource. Early placement is essential.

■ Residential Structures

For most one- and two-family private dwellings, placement of the apparatus will usually be front and center relative to the structure. Sweeping the A side of the structure will be easily accomplished from this position. If necessary or if conditions warrant, the turntable could be positioned on the A/B or A/D corner of the structure to allow for access to two sides. Local conditions, topography, and SOPs will dictate the best placement. In many cases, the <u>setback</u> from the curb or shoulder may make the horizontal reach a challenge. Increasingly, the capabilities of aerial apparatus are being used on these one- and two-family homes for roof work, overhaul, and application of elevated streams in both offensive and defensive conditions **FIGURE 15-11**. Of course, an unpositioned aerial cannot be used to support the suppression effort or to create a safe work platform for fire fighters working at elevation.

As the structure increases in height, the ability to sweep each higher floor will be reduced. Knowledge of the fire building,

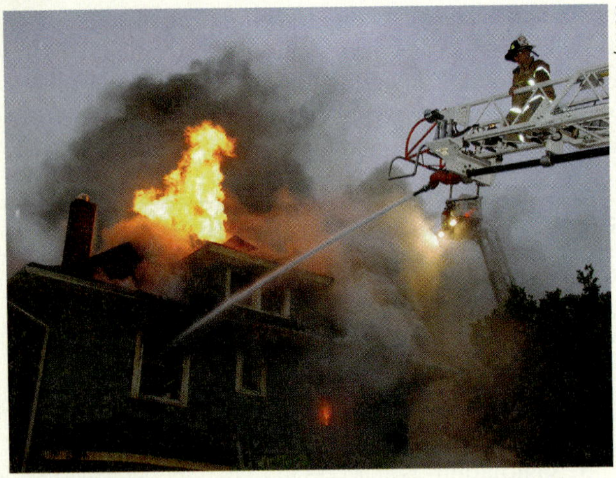

FIGURE 15-11 Use of an aerial apparatus at a private dwelling. 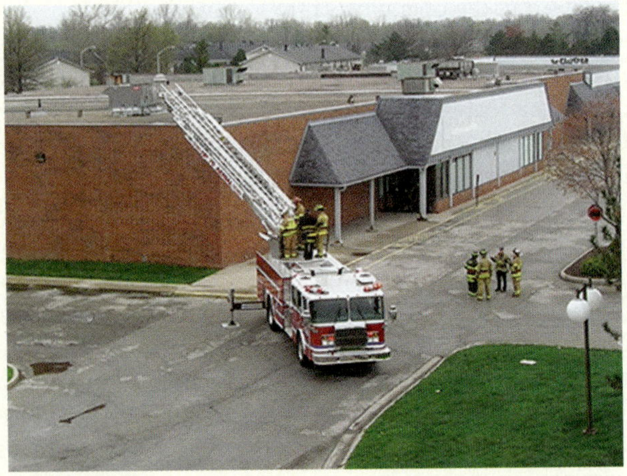
Courtesy of Scott M. Peterson.

FIGURE 15-12 Positioning the aerial at the corner of a commercial structure.
Courtesy of Drew Smith.

therefore, will allow for better positioning at taller structures. At these taller structures, there is less need for the aerial to aid in roof work, so early efforts will be focused on **physical rescue**. By actually setting up at these structures before there is a fire, the driver/operator can gain insight and experience into the challenges, thereby improving his or her positioning ability.

Commercial/Industrial Structures

The prime concern at commercial or industrial structures is usually not rescue, but rather collapse. Even if fire conditions on arrival do not indicate a collapse potential, the driver/operator should consider this possibility. With some exceptions (usually in older communities), commercial and industrial properties are often single-story structures that contain high ceilings and open floor plans, creating the potential for large fire volumes. Lightweight building construction, including those structures that utilize trusses, are another concern for consideration. In buildings with these types of construction, fires may progress rapidly and increase collapse potential. The conventional wisdom calls for positioning the aerial apparatus at a corner in such cases **FIGURE 15-12**. Positioning must take safety into account, but must also allow for the aerial to be used effectively to support the suppression operation. As with residential structures, an unpositioned aerial cannot be used to support the suppression effort or to create a safe work platform for fire fighters working at elevation.

When a second aerial apparatus is dispatched on the initial alarm, it should usually stage unless otherwise instructed by SOP or SOG or given an order by the IC. In some departments with a two-aerial response on the initial alarm, the second aerial positions opposite of the first aerial. This location may be at the rear of the structure or the opposite side or corner. In these cases, this positioning needs to be preplanned.

Positioning and Spotting Considerations

Each driver/operator must address a number of considerations in a matter of seconds—he or she does not have minutes to ponder the decisions to be made. As the driver/operator approaches the scene, enters the block of the fire, hears reports on the radio, observes the area and fire conditions, and converses with the company officer, training and experience come into play. It is the training, education, and simulations prior to an actual emergency that improve success. Here are the questions that the driver/operator must ask and answer at each incident:

- In hilly areas, is there an incline in the roadway that will cause the apparatus to face down or up beyond the limits recommended by the aerial's manufacturer?
- Is there excessive pitch in the roadway that will cause the apparatus to lean to the side up beyond the limits recommended by the aerial's manufacturer?
- Is the roadway wide enough for the aerial to be positioned and the stabilizers fully extended so they can then be set up on solid ground? Will other apparatus be able to pass the setup aerial?
- Will a curve in the road or parked autos affect positioning and setup or access by other apparatus?
- Are there underground structures such as sewers, manholes, parking garages, and tunnels that might reduce the load-bearing capacity where stabilizers must be set **FIGURE 15-13**?
- Is the roadway surface itself suitable to accept the stabilizers **FIGURE 15-14**?
- What are the wind conditions that might affect the aerial apparatus?
- Is there a lightning event that will affect the safety of those persons on or near the aerial?
- Are there snow or ice conditions that might affect the aerial apparatus?
- Are there electrical wires overhead or other overhead obstructions or hazards? If so, can the aerial be set up to operate while maintaining a minimum clearance from the wires of 10 ft (3 m), or even farther for distribution or transmission wires?
- Will trees prohibit the aerial from being raised from its bedded position? If not, will treetops yield to the aerial and not damage it?

FIGURE 15-13 Underground structures may reduce the load-bearing capacity of the aerial's stabilizers.

FIGURE 15-14 An unsuitable roadway surface for an aerial stabilizer.

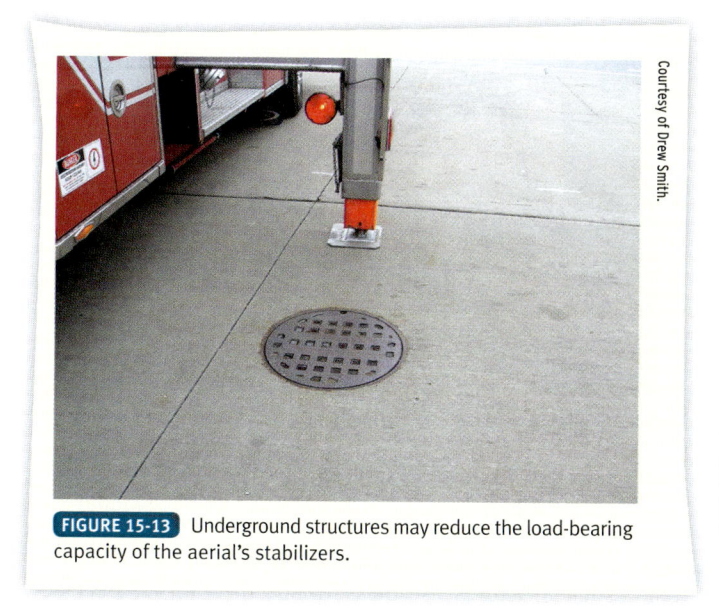

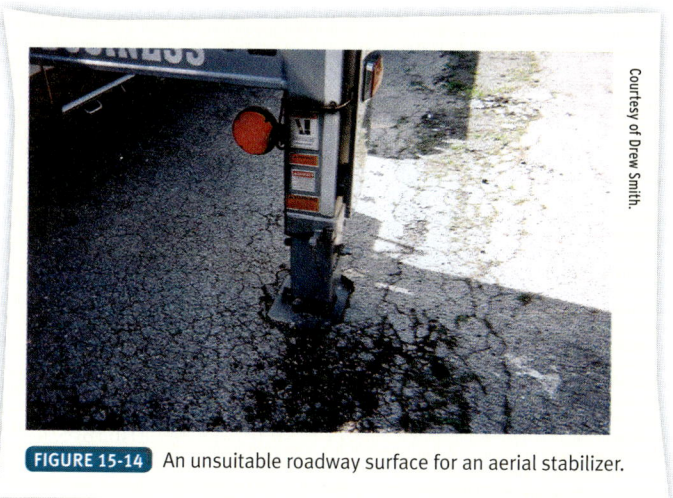

FIGURE 15-15 A low-rise apartment building with parking and landscape setback.

- How far off the side will the aerial have to operate? 30 degrees off center? 45 degrees off center? 90 degrees off center? An aerial device that is extended more perpendicular than parallel to the apparatus may require the driver/operator to reduce the load placed on the ladder or platform.

■ Building Type and Height

When evaluating where to position and set up the aerial apparatus, building type and height are major considerations. The width of the lot, the setback from the paved road or parking lot, the number of stories and general construction type, and the function (occupancy) of the structure will aid the driver/operator in decision making.

Residential Structures

In developed residential areas, the lots will generally have standard widths. Roads and streets that are laid out in a grid and are predominately straight are a significant aid to the driver/operator. Standard urban lot widths may be 25–30 ft (8–9 m) or 50 ft (15 m). In suburban areas, lot widths may be 50–100 ft (15–30 m). Wider lots may exist in some areas, but generally all lots in a subdivision will have similar widths.

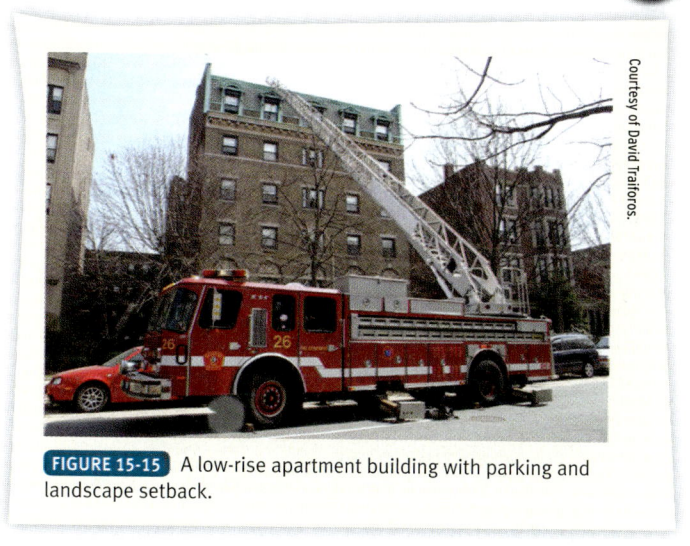

In developed areas, most residential structures will also have a standard setback from the road. Sometimes referred to as the "building line," this distance is helpful to the driver/operator, as it allows him or her to know just how far the aerial apparatus will reach horizontally. While structures may extend into the rear of the lot at varying distances, the building line setback is usually uniform.

In developments with rowhouses or townhouses, similar conditions may exist, but exceptions may be found where roadways curve or terminate in courts or cul-de-sacs. In these locations, the road may end and a driveway may continue. Such driveways may not be constructed to support the weight of an aerial or its stabilizers.

At low-rise apartments, parking or landscaping may increase the setback and affect the positioning and reach of the apparatus **FIGURE 15-15**. At mid-rise apartments, the need for vertical reach will be greater than at other structures. The driver/operator will need to preplan these locations—an effort that should include setting up the aerial at the structure to determine its actual reach.

Commercial Structures

At most commercial structures, the need for the aerial to perform or support a physical rescue is very low. Instead, the more typical role of the aerial apparatus is to support roof operations or elevated stream application. For the taxpayer-type structure or **strip mall**, which is usually a single- or multiple-story commercial building, many of the same considerations that arise with private residences also apply **FIGURE 15-16**. These structures will generally not have a large setback, will occupy much if not all of the lot width, and may be an exposure risk should heavy fire conditions be present. Positioning of the apparatus in such cases should not only address the fire building but allow for operation on adjoining exposures. Some taxpayer structures may allow for rear access.

Strip Malls

Strip malls present with unique considerations. The locations of entrances and exits, particularly those with raised islands or "pork chops," may limit ingress. Parking lot arrangement may impair turning or maneuvering. In some cases, a traffic lane at

© Jones & Bartlett Learning. Photographed by Glen E. Ellman.

FIGURE 15-16 A typical taxpayer structure.

© Jones & Bartlett Learning. Photographed by Glen E. Ellman.

FIGURE 15-17 A strip mall with a tall parapet wall.

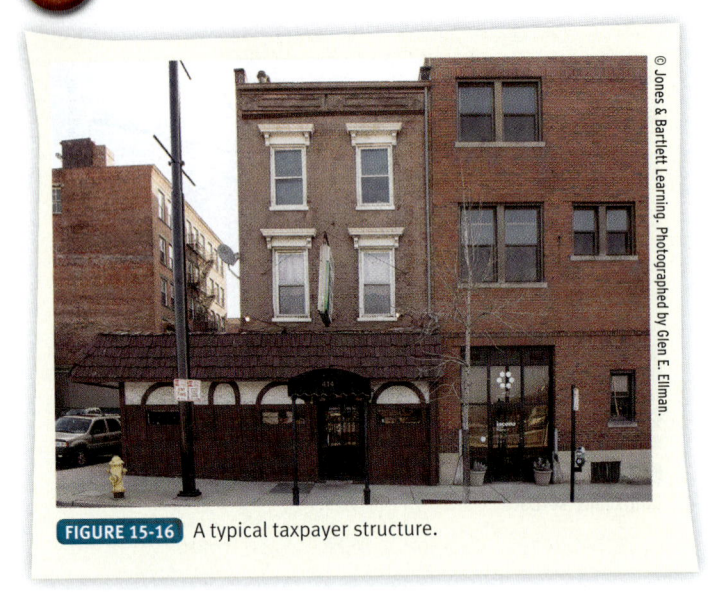

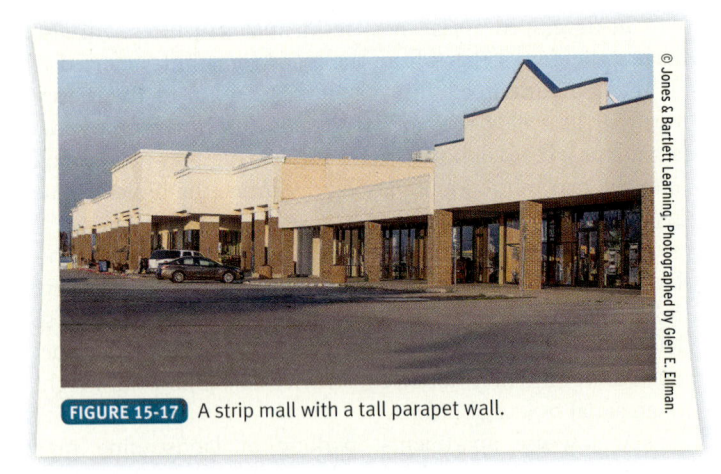

the front of the structure may actually position the aerial in the collapse zone if the driver/operator has not preplanned the complex. The height and the depth of the front façade or parapet may impair roof access FIGURE 15-17. When such difficulties are suspected, the rear of the structure may offer a better option for apparatus positioning. When deciding on which side of the strip mall the aerial should be placed, the evaluation should include the potential for fire spread. Looking at the front of the building, the driver/operator and the company officer should quickly determine the likely direction of fire spread and identify which side of the strip mall has the most uninvolved structure. It is this side that may have the greatest loss or fire spread potential.

Big-Box Structures

At **big-box** structures, setback is usually not an issue, and access to all sides of the structure is usually possible FIGURE 15-18. Usually the biggest question for the aerial driver/operator is "Where is the fire, and how close to it can I get?" Many modern big-box structures use tilt-slab construction. Under defensive fire conditions, wall failure upon roof collapse should be expected at these sites.

Industrial Structures

Industrial structures will present with a combination of access and positioning challenges. Many of these structures have undergone multiple additions or had separate buildings joined

© Jones & Bartlett Learning. Photographed by Glen E. Ellman.

FIGURE 15-18 A big-box structure.

together. The variety of construction types and materials present in such structures, as well as the specific internal processes, can affect fire spread. Preplanning is essential in these cases to ensure effective fire response.

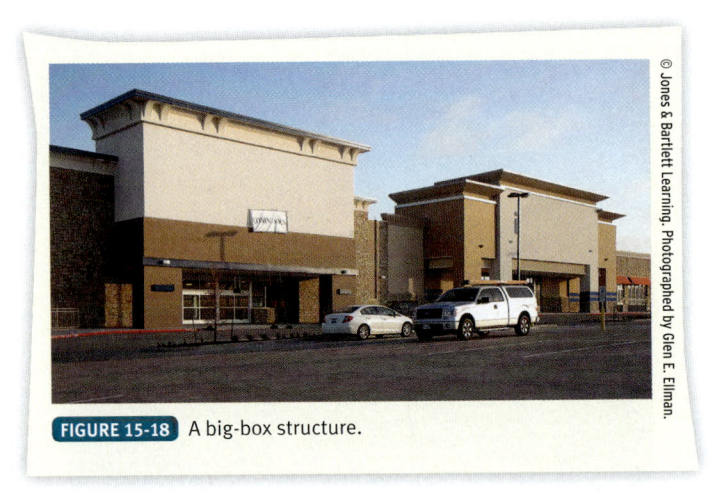

Approach to the Scene

As the aerial apparatus driver/operator begins to approach the scene, he or she should dramatically slow down the vehicle's speed at least 500 ft (150 m) before the reported fire location. This will allow the driver/operator to observe fire conditions; account for parked cars that will affect jack spread; calculate room needed for other apparatus to pass; scan for overhead obstructions such as electrical wires and surface encumbrances such as speed bumps, manhole covers, curbs, and poor pavement; check for victims in need of physical rescue; and perhaps locate the likely location of fire inside the structure.

Collapse Zone

The **collapse zone** is defined as the horizontal separation distance between the wall of a structure and the positioned apparatus. This distance must be equal to or greater than the height of the structure, including all features such as parapets, decorative finishes, and signs. The distance should include a safety factor one-half the structure's height. The tip of the aerial ladder or the aerial platform must remain out of the structure's collapse zone; this distance is equal to or greater than height of the structure above the tip or platform's position plus the safety factor.

Turntable Positioning for Rescue Sweep/Scrub Area

Wind direction and fire and smoke conditions are indicators of the desired turntable location, which determines the **scrub or sweep area** for the aerial. The best-case scenario occurs when the aerial can reach all affected areas of the structure. This is not always possible, particularly at larger structures. As the aerial apparatus approaches the scene, the driver/operator will make his or her size-up of the structure and fire conditions. Also to be noted are the height, width, and depth of the structure and its affected area. Past experience at these structures, even in nonfire incidents, will aid the driver/operator in assessing the situation and making positioning decisions.

Other than big-box stores and industrial properties, most structures will present with either a wide front and a shallow depth or, conversely, a narrow front and a significant depth into the lot. When faced with the wide but shallow arrangement, the driver/operator will be forced to decide exactly where is the best position for maximum sweep/scrub based on fire conditions, wind, any presenting need for physical rescue, and ventilation needs. When presented with the narrow front but deep structure, a corner placement is usually best, as it allows maximum sweep/scrub of the structure and can often address any need for physical rescue, roof access, or elevated stream application. Unless faced with a physical rescue or an immediate need for an elevated stream on the main body of fire, positioning front and center is best left to low-rise residential structures such as private homes or small two- to six-unit apartment buildings three or fewer stories tall.

Rescue Profile

The driver/operator must work with the company officer to create a **rescue profile** of the structure at each working fire. Besides the many factors already discussed, key considerations should include the height of the structure and the location of the fire. While the apparatus should always be positioned to go to work at any fire, whether the aerial device is needed for rescue is based on the rescue profile. The rescue profile will tell the officer whether ground ladders or the aerial is needed and which is the best choice. Generally speaking, fires on the second and perhaps third floors can be handled more quickly with portable extension ladders, whereas higher floors can rarely be reached without the use of an aerial.

Making Up for Poor Placement

Even when a driver/operator attempts best positioning of the aerial apparatus, that choice can come up short. In these cases, some corrective action will be needed. Such instances include circumstances in which the aerial cannot be set up where it can access the structure as needed or in which the ground surface will not provide for proper stabilization. The aerial apparatus should not be driven over unimproved surfaces that will not support its gross vehicle weight. Conversely, leaving the aerial in a poor position renders it useless. In these situations, the driver/operator, in consultation with his or her company officer, must make a risk–benefit analysis of the situation and then proceed.

When a stabilizer cannot be fully deployed and it is allowable per the operator's manual, the apparatus may be short-jacked on the non-operational side. A short-jacked stabilizer on the non-operational side of the apparatus will be safer and stronger than a fully deployed stabilizer placed on unstable surfaces such as grass, earth, noncompacted gravel, or curbs. These surfaces should be avoided, as should manholes, sewers, and other underground vaults where the visible cover or opening may be far smaller than the space beneath.

Setup and Stabilization of Aerial Apparatus

Proper stabilization of the aerial apparatus relies on the driver/operator understanding not only the functioning of his or her vehicle and the information in the manufacturer's operator's manual, but also basic concepts of physics as they apply to weights and load. Before the aerial can be raised and lowered safely, however, the apparatus' chassis must be stabilized. Understanding how this is accomplished enables the driver/operator to safely adapt the setup and stabilization of the unit when unfavorable or unusual conditions are present. Apparatus stabilization is the most critical aspect of preparing the aerial for operation, and proper stabilization broadens the base of vehicle to prevent it from tipping over. Commonly, stabilization widens the footprint of the aerial's chassis to beyond that of its wheels.

The outriggers (also called downriggers or stabilizers) are designed to keep the aerial and its chassis from tipping left to right, front to back, or both. The outriggers act like a load and a lever on a fulcrum. If both are extended an equal length and have an equal force applied, the equation will be equal. Adjusting the degree of extension, rotation, and/or elevation of the aerial acts to increase the force applied to the outrigger on whichever side it is on and decrease the force applied to the opposite side. As the aerial ladder is rotated from the centerline of the chassis and off the side, an increasingly greater load is imposed on the fulcrum. More force is then needed on the opposite side of the chassis to keep the outrigger's foot firmly on the ground. Understanding these concepts and gaining knowledge in and experience with the selection of suitable surfaces for setup will allow the driver/operator to safely use modified procedures, such as short-jacking, when required.

In-Cab Procedures

Each aerial apparatus utilizes a somewhat different setup procedure. These procedures may vary not only among manufacturers, but also among different models of aerials produced by the same manufacturer or the same model produced in different years. It is vital that each driver/operator knows and follows the manufacturer's procedure for the make and model he or she is assigned to operate. Relying on generic procedures or procedures from different makes or models can have disastrous consequences.

When the pump and the aerial are both needed, it is faster to set up the aerial device first, and then place the pump in gear. Once the pump is engaged, the high idle speed used by the aerial becomes disabled, such that the aerial operates at a reduced speed. If necessary to overcome this constraint once the aerial is set up, the driver/operator can throttle above the needed pump pressure and gate down any pump discharges being used.

Setup and stabilization of all apparatus follow at least some common in-cab procedures, which include bringing the apparatus to a complete stop, shifting the transmission to neutral, and setting the parking brake. The aerial controls and power are engaged using various electrical or mechanical switches. Some manufacturers permit the driver/operator to engage these switches before shifting the transmission to neutral and setting the parking brake. Before doing so on your aerial, however, ensure that the manufacturer's operating instructions allow these steps. Finally, understand any safety features that are specific to the particular aerial apparatus. Once the in-cab procedures are completed, the driver/operator can exit the cab and proceed with stabilization.

Setting Stabilizers

As the driver/operator exits the cab, he or she should look around and above the aerial apparatus to check for surface or overhead obstructions or hazards. This is best accomplished by walking around and observing all sides of the aerial apparatus. The driver can exit the cab, look in front and up, and then proceed back toward the rear and then check the opposite side of the apparatus; alternatively, the driver can exit the cab, look up and down the side, and then proceed to the front and around and down the opposite side. Either way, a check of all four sides for surface and overhead obstructions and hazards is required. During this walk-around, the driver/operator can place the wheel chocks, if required. The walk-around should note any manholes, sewers, potholes, or deteriorated pavement unsuitable for stabilizer placement and any overhead electrical wires, flag poles, signs, or banners that would impair or impede the safe operation of the aerial.

Full-Jacking

Full-jacking is the complete extension of all stabilizers and is always the desired action **FIGURE 15-19**. The driver/operator should always strive to use full-jacking. To position and stabilize an apparatus on a level surface, follow the steps in **SKILL DRILL 15-1**.

1. Drive to the fireground location, select an appropriate place, and position the apparatus for the best possible utilization of the aerial device. (STEP 1)
2. Perform in-cab procedures per manufacturer and department policy. This usually includes setting the parking brake and activating the electrical and hydraulic systems used by the aerial.
3. Exit the cab and make a 360-degree walk-around of the apparatus, observing for overhead hazards, such as electrical wires or obstructions; surface obstacles, such as parked vehicles, light poles, or signs; and subsurface hazards, such as sewers, manholes, vaults, and parking structures. Relocate the aerial apparatus if obstructions or hazards are encountered and cannot be compensated for. (STEP 2)
4. Set the wheel chocks and stabilizer ground pads per the manufacturer's instructions or manual and department policy. (STEP 3)
5. Deploy the stabilizers. Depending on the manufacturer and the particular apparatus, there may be two, four, or more stabilizers to deploy, and some may require a two-step process, such as out and then down. In general, extend outward all stabilizers and then make contact with the ground, and then lower the stabilizers in the order specified by the manufacturer. (STEP 4)
6. Level the apparatus side-to-side and front-to-back. Depending on the manufacturer and the particular apparatus, this may be a multiple-step process or may be performed by the use of a single switch. (STEP 5)
7. Before moving to the turntable to operate the aerial, perform any necessary steps to secure the stabilizer controls and to redirect power from the stabilizer controls to the aerial controls. (STEP 6)

Short-Jacking

Short-jacking is an apparatus-specific procedure and must be permitted by the manufacturer's requirements; otherwise, the driver/operator should not seek to short-jack the device. With short-jacking, the stabilizers are not fully extended on the side of the aerial apparatus where the aerial will not be raised, lowered, or rotated to **FIGURE 15-20**. Only aerial apparatus with H-type stabilizers can be short-jacked, but not all H-type stabilizers can accommodate this procedure. With most short-jacked apparatus, the load capacity of the aerial must be reduced as specified in load charts posted on the apparatus and contained in the operator's manual. Failure to comply with these load restrictions or purposefully overriding safety interlocks intended to prevent the aerial from moving into short-jacked positions can and usually will result in a catastrophic event that may damage the aerial and result in serious injury or death to fire fighters.

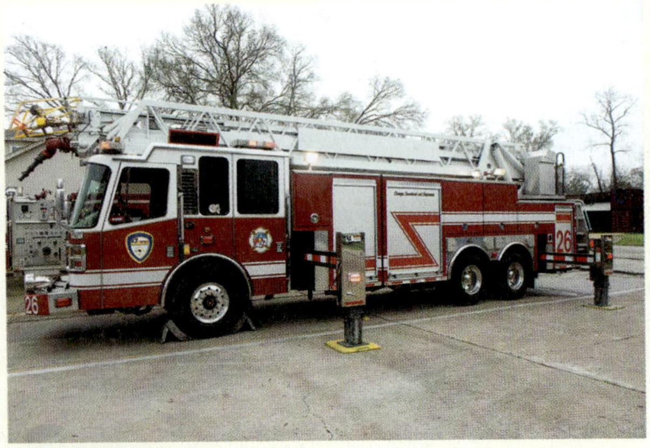

FIGURE 15-19 When full-jacking, all stabilizers are fully extended and set.

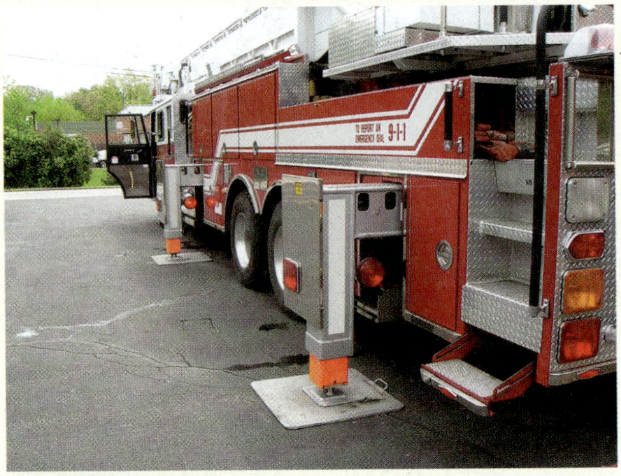

FIGURE 15-20 When short-jacking, only the stabilizers on the working side of the aerial are fully extended and set. The opposite-side stabilizers are set but not fully extended. Use extreme caution if short-jacking is used.

CHAPTER 15 Apparatus Equipped with an Aerial Device 369

SKILL DRILL 15-1
Positioning and Stabilizing an Apparatus on a Level Surface
NFPA 1002, 6.2.1, 6.2.1(B)

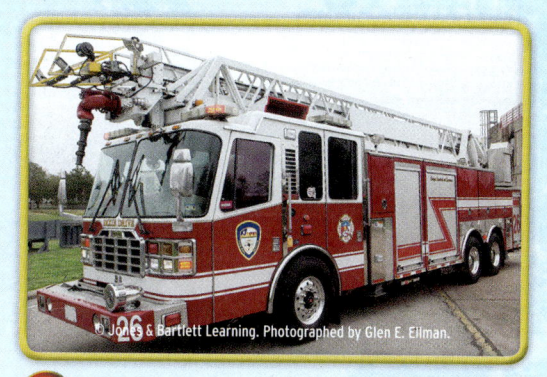

1. At the fireground, select an appropriate place, and position the apparatus for the best possible utilization of the aerial device.

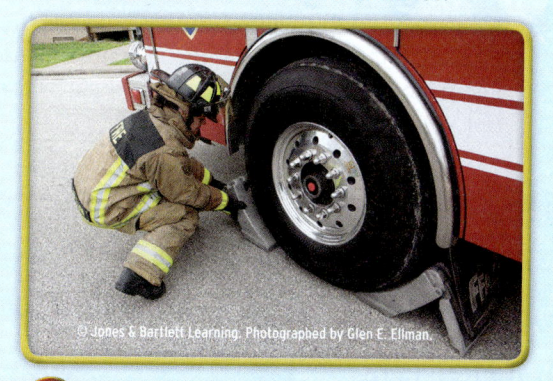

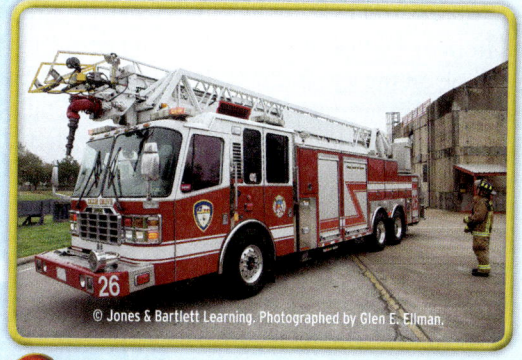

2. Exit the cab and make a 360-degree walk-around of the apparatus, observing for any hazards.

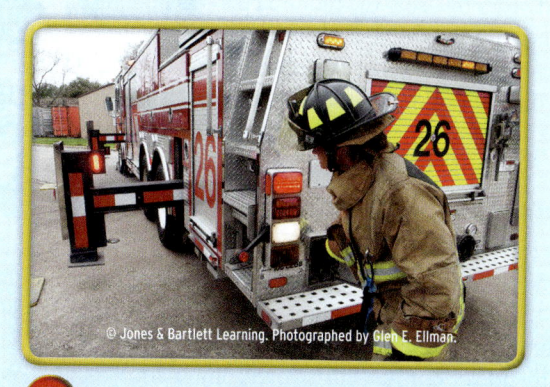

3. Set the wheel chocks and stabilizer ground pads.

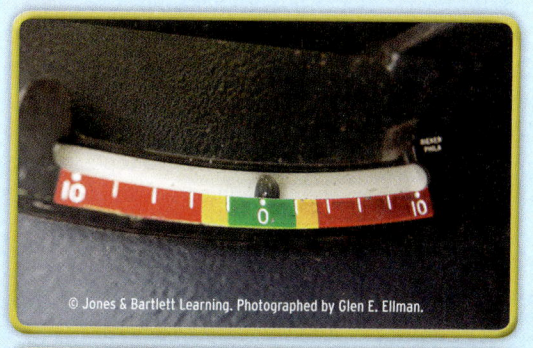

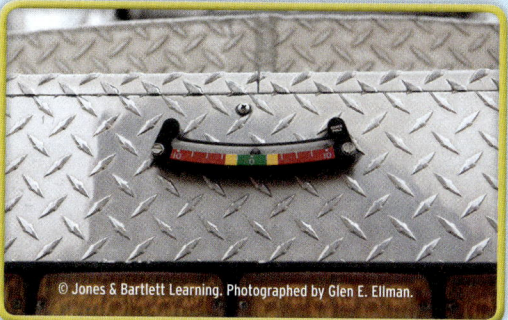

4. Deploy the stabilizers.

5. Level the apparatus side-to-side and front-to-back.

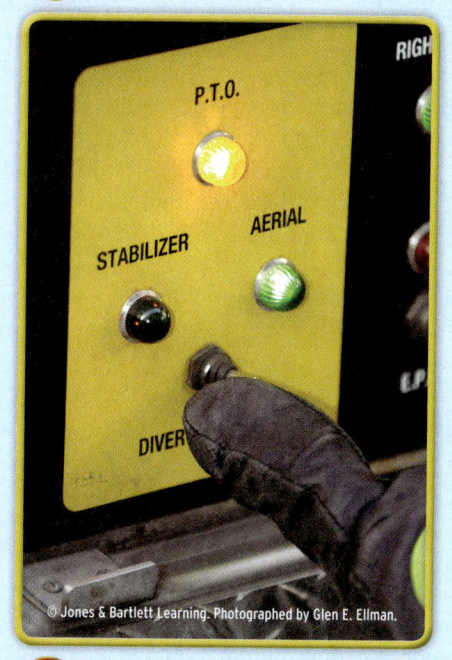

6. Secure the stabilizer controls and redirect power from the stabilizer controls to the aerial controls.

© LiquidLibrary

Modern aerial apparatus are equipped with an aerial rotation interlock that prevents the aerial from being moved into a position in which the stabilizers are not fully deployed. This interlock will prevent the aerial from being raised from the bedded position in such a case. This constraint can be overridden, however; if short-jacking is used, doing so may require raising the aerial from its bedded position. Once the device is raised, and depending on the age and manufacturer of the apparatus, the interlock may then prevent the aerial from being moved onto the short-jacked side. This is not always case, though—so know your apparatus.

The decision to use a short-jacking procedure must be based on a risk–benefit analysis. Convenience should not be a justification. A mission-critical need that can be safely accomplished is the only justification for the use of short-jacking. When this technique is applied, the stabilizers must be fully extended on that side of the apparatus where the aerial will operate.

Following the manufacturer's procedure specific to the aerial, the driver/operator should set all the stabilizers in the prescribed order by using the required pads as intended and setting any pins supplied. Once properly set, the stabilizer interlock system will indicate that the aerial may be raised. Do not rely solely on rules of thumb, such as how high the tires should be raised or how many pin holes on a stabilizer need to be viewed.

■ Compensating for Uneven Grades

When the terrain is even and level, maximum stabilization can be achieved. In contrast, when the terrain is uneven, the stability of the aerial will be compromised. Uneven terrain can be longitudinal (in line with the chassis frame or roadway), lateral (side-to-side or curb-to-curb), or a combination of both. When the unevenness exceeds 6 percent (a 6-inch [15-cm] drop over 100 ft [30 m]), compensation for excessive grade is usually necessary. Six percent is equal to 3.5 degrees of angle and can be measured by the use of apparatus-mounted angle or slope indicators **FIGURE 15-21**. These protractors with a bubble level are usually installed as standard equipment by aerial manufacturers. Angle or slope indicators can also be electronic, appearing as part of a comprehensive load distribution display. While some aerials can operate at greater grades than others, always follow the limitations in the operator's manual. Exceeding these limits may cause a catastrophic failure.

Ideally, the apparatus should be positioned where it can be stabilized on level ground.

When there is a significant difference in lateral grade, follow **SKILL DRILL 15-2** unless the specific apparatus manufacturer's operator's manual states otherwise:

1. Lower the high-side (up-slope) stabilizers until they contact the pad(s). Only make contact with these stabilizers. Do not raise the apparatus at this time. **(STEP 1)**
2. Lower the low-side (down-slope) stabilizers until they make full contact with the pad(s); then continue raising the apparatus until it is leveled to less than 3.5 degrees. **(STEP 2)**
3. If the apparatus is leveled to 3.5 degrees, but the tires or other chassis components are not yet in compliance with operator's manual requirements (such as taking the bulge out of the tires or raising the tires off the ground), use both side stabilizers to achieve compliance.
4. If the apparatus is equipped with automatic or self-stabilizing features, consult the operator's manual for instructions on how to compensate or adjust the controls. **(STEP 3)**

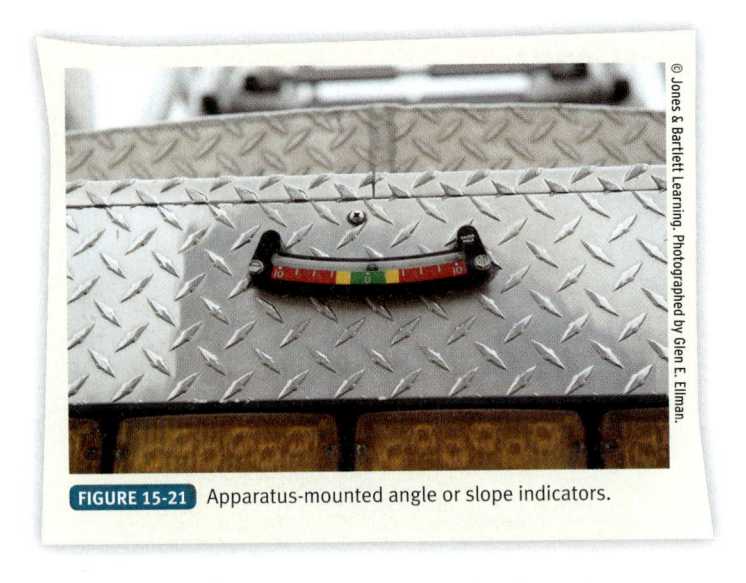

FIGURE 15-21 Apparatus-mounted angle or slope indicators.

Safety Tip

Stabilizing apparatus as required by manufacturer specifications optimizes safety and best use of the aerial device.

Stabilizing on Curbs

Do not set the stabilizers on top of a curb **FIGURE 15-22**. Applying force to the top of a curb with a stabilizer results in a lever. In such a case, the top of the curb becomes the fulcrum, the curb becomes a load, and the stabilizer applies the force. In this situation, the curb could heave from the ground, resulting in an unsupported aerial, particularly if the affected curb is on the operating side of the apparatus. It is best to reposition the apparatus so the stabilizer can be placed on a firm and level surface.

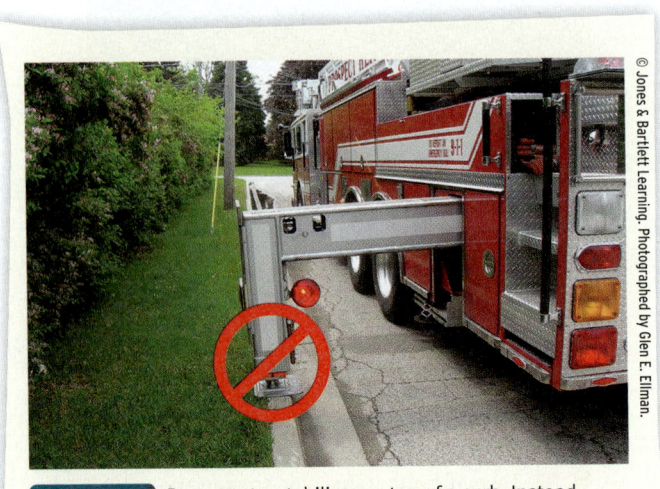

FIGURE 15-22 Do not set a stabilizer on top of a curb. Instead, reposition the apparatus when possible.

SKILL DRILL 15-2
Compensating for Uneven Grades
NFPA 1002, 6.2.2, 6.2.2(B)

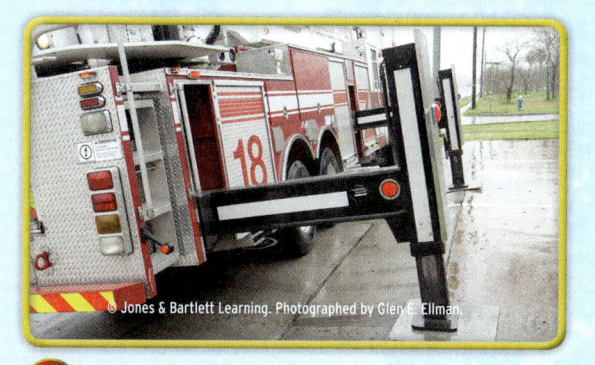

1 Lower the high-side (up-slope) stabilizers until they contact the pad(s). Only make contact with these stabilizers. Do not raise the apparatus at this time.

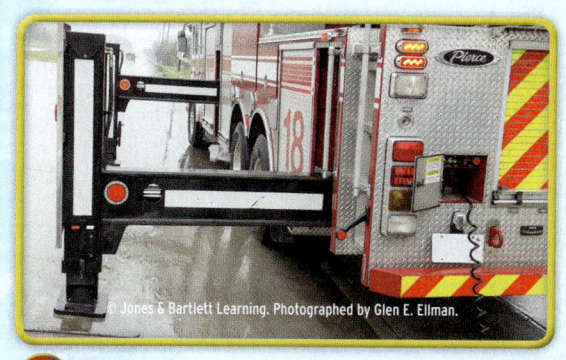

2 Lower the low-side (down-slope) stabilizers until they make full contact with the pad(s); then continue raising the apparatus until it is leveled to less than 3.5 degrees.

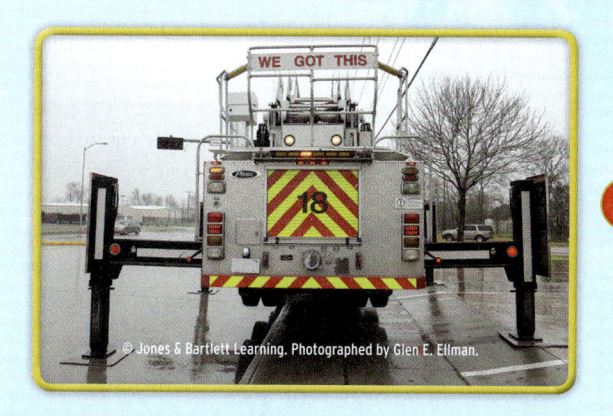

3 If the apparatus is leveled to 3.5 degrees, but the tires or other chassis components are not yet in compliance with operator's manual requirements (such as taking the bulge out of the tires or raising the tires off the ground), use both side stabilizers to achieve compliance. If the apparatus is equipped with automatic or self-stabilizing features, consult the operator's manual for instructions on how to compensate or adjust the controls.

Operation of Aerial Ladder or Platform Controls

Once the stabilizers are fully set and the apparatus has been leveled both longitudinally and laterally, the aerial ladder or platform can be raised, rotated, and extended. Some aerials will have controls at the turntable and at the tip or in the platform to accomplish these operations. There are some platform controls that are fully hydraulic, and some controls are electronic and operate hydraulic valves in the turntable pedestal **FIGURE 15-23**. Inside the pedestal are hydraulic controls. In most cases, the turntable controls override the tip or platform controls, while the hydraulic controls in the pedestal override the electronic controls. Every driver/operator should be familiar with the hydraulic controls and how to operate them. As part of periodic checks and training, these controls should be operated.

The turntable electronic controls and the tip/platform controls are the usual and customary controls operated **FIGURE 15-24**. The driver/operator typically utilizes the turntable controls, while fire fighters operate the tip/platform controls. Most aerials allow for operation of the turntable controls at two speeds: (1) slow, when the motor is at idle, and (2) fast, when the throttle is set to high. The controls at the ladder tip or in the platform generally operate only at a reduced speed regardless of whether the high idle is activated. This is a safety feature to prevent damage to the apparatus and injury to the crew.

As the aerial approaches the work site, the driver/operator should reduce the motor speed to idle and communicate to the tip/platform fire fighter to take over final placement. Excellent communication is essential to safety and efficient operations. Keep the high idle off when the device is located in close proximity to structures, hazards, or people. To guard against the tip/platform fire fighter accidentally maneuvering the aerial device into wires, obstructions, or other hazards, it is best for the driver/operator to stay positioned at the turntable, constantly observing the actions of the tip/platform and maintaining one hand on the turntable controls. In the event of a hazardous maneuver by the tip/platform fire fighter, the driver/operator can override the action.

Jerking or sudden movements of the aerial can be dangerous and can result in damage to the apparatus. The skilled and practiced driver/operator should be able to combine the maneuvers of raising/lowering, rotating, and extending/

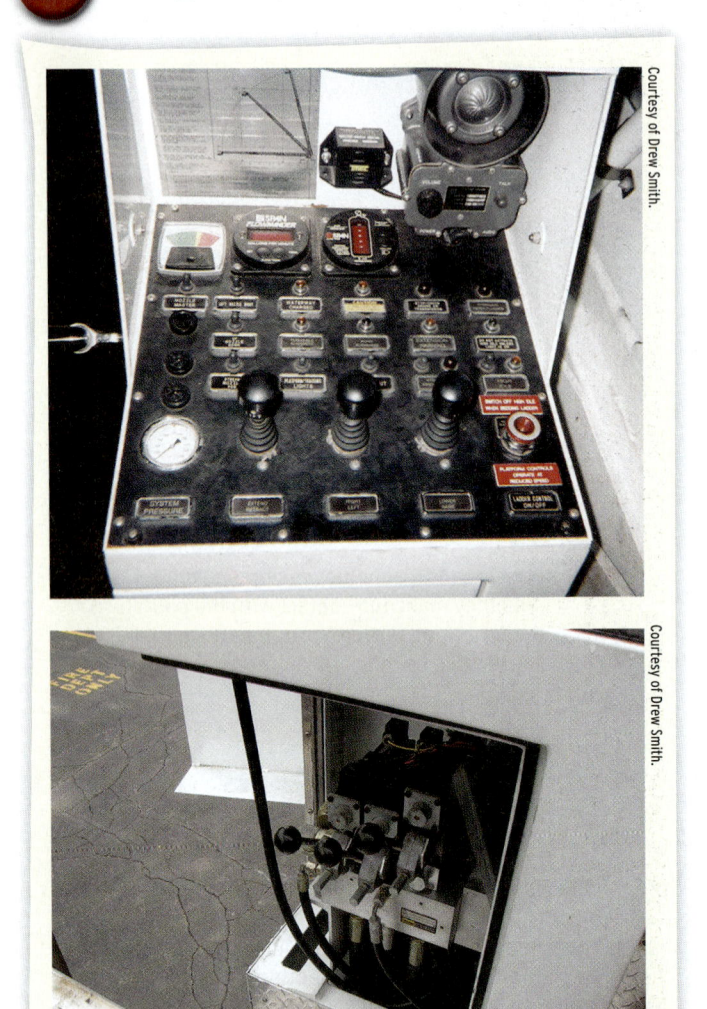

FIGURE 15-23 Aerial turntable controls.

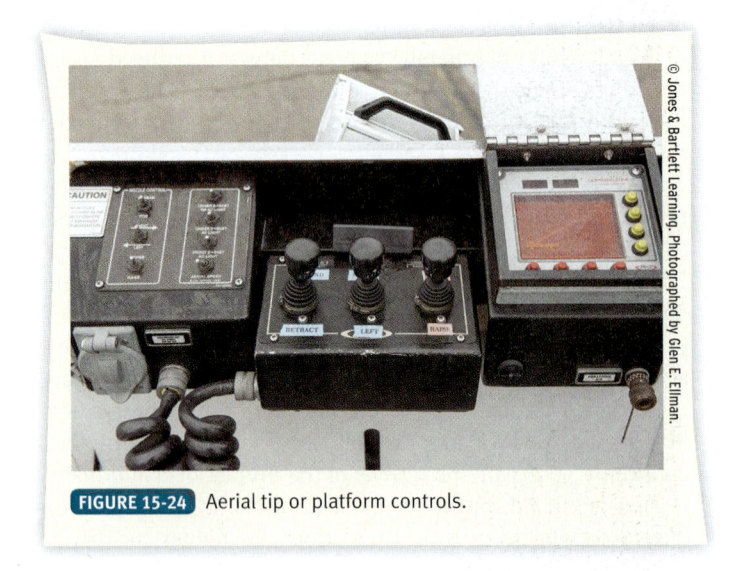

FIGURE 15-24 Aerial tip or platform controls.

retracting the aerial with feathering of the controls to avoid "fly fishing." Doing so increases safety. As part of periodic checks and training, operation of controls in this manner should be practiced.

Safe Aerial Practices

Even though the driver/operator should have checked for overhead obstructions and electrical wires before positioning the apparatus, he or she should check again before raising the aerial device from its bedded position. Pay particular attention to the locations of any overhead wires and treat all wires as if they are electrically charged. Use caution when maneuvering the aerial device, and maintain a minimum separation distance of at least 10 ft (3 m)—and preferably even farther—for distribution wires. To avoid electrocution, the driver/operator of any pump on a raised aerial should stand on the provided slide-out tray, and fire fighters should not touch the aerial apparatus whenever the aerial device is being maneuvered. Before getting on or off the vehicle, fire fighters and driver/operators should make sure that the aerial apparatus is clear of any overhead electrical wire.

The driver/operator should manage the loads placed on the aerial. Shock loads are equivalent to multiplied loads, which the apparatus may not be designed to handle. Loads should be positioned perpendicular—not lateral—to rungs, whenever possible. In particular, fire fighters should climb in the center of the ladder, rather than to the side. Both fire fighters and civilians are considered loads when assessing loads placed on the aerial. Every aerial will have a chart dictating the maximum number of persons who can occupy each section of the aerial; these limits must be respected. Ensure that when the aerial is operated at low angles that any necessary reduction on loading occurs. On platforms, occupants should be evenly distributed and not clustered to one side. Fire fighters climbing onto or off of the tip/platform should avoid shock-loading the aerial and prevent it from bouncing up and down or side to side. Stop movement of the aerial before permitting fire fighters or victims to get on or off.

As part of positioning and during maneuvering of the aerial, the more in line with the chassis the aerial is extended or retracted, the more stable the apparatus will be because the force of the aerial is applied more evenly to all stabilizers. When the aerial is more perpendicular to the chassis, only half of the stabilizers carry the load.

■ Operation in Supported Versus Unsupported Positions

The modern aerial is not designed to have its ladder or boom rest upon a structure. Consequently, the driver/operator should never support the extended ladder or boom against building. The design of the modern aerial is based on the truss construction of the ladder and relies on the use of a Class 3 lever. The point where the bed section attaches to the turntable serves as the fulcrum. The live (humans) and dead (aerial) loads represent a force to the bed section near the fulcrum. This force applies compression to the bed section base rails while the top rails experience tension. Resting the aerial against a structure reverses this loading; that is, the top force changes to compression while the base force changes to tension. Because the aerial is not designed for this reverse loading, it could result in damage or a catastrophic failure **FIGURE 15-25**. Additionally, any waterway underneath the ladder may be damaged if rested against a structure.

FIGURE 15-25 **A.** Supported loading versus **B.** unsupported loading of the aerial structure.

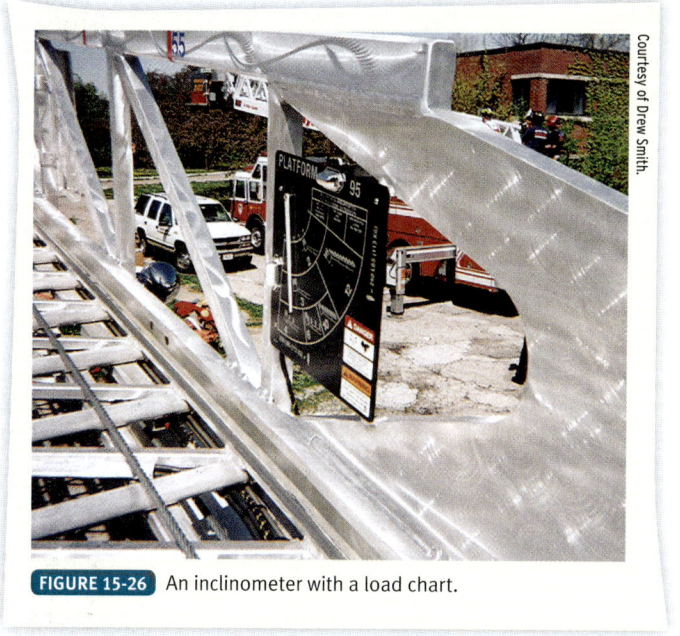

FIGURE 15-26 An inclinometer with a load chart.

FIGURE 15-26. The maximum load may need to be reduced based on whether the waterway is charged, which additional equipment is being supported by the aerial, and/or which other environmental factors are considerations FIGURE 15-27.

Prior to allowing fire fighters to climb the ladder, the driver/operator should ensure that the rungs for each section are in alignment with each other. The maneuvering power should also be disengaged until fire fighters reach the tip or platform. This will improve safety for the climbing fire fighters. In general, no more than two fire fighters should occupy the extreme tip of an aerial ladder and no more than three fire fighters should occupy the platform unless the manufacturer's specifications allow for additional fire fighters. Fire fighters climbing an aerial should be spaced out as evenly as possible to distribute the weight load evenly on each section of the aerial. Fire fighters should avoid bunching up in groups. The driver/operator at the turntable can help manage against this activity by directing when each fire fighter can begin to climb. The weight of equipment must also be accounted for. If an aerial can be loaded with a maximum of four fire fighters, but each member is carrying heavy loads such as saws, hose packs, or additional self-contained breathing apparatus (SCBA), the weight should be estimated by the driver/operator and the loading managed accordingly.

When a prepiped waterway is charged or a ladder pipe is affixed to the tip and charged with a hoseline, there is additional load on the ladder. One hundred feet (30 m) of 3½-inch (90-mm) pipe or hose will hold more than 600 pounds (272 kg) of water. This load cannot be ignored. The driver/operator must know if the aerial is designed to support this water weight plus the normal human load or if the human load must be reduced in such circumstances. This information is usually contained in the operator's manual and also appears on the load plate at the turntable and platform operator's positions.

Environmental conditions are the final load consideration. Snow, ice, and wind all place loads on the aerial and must be

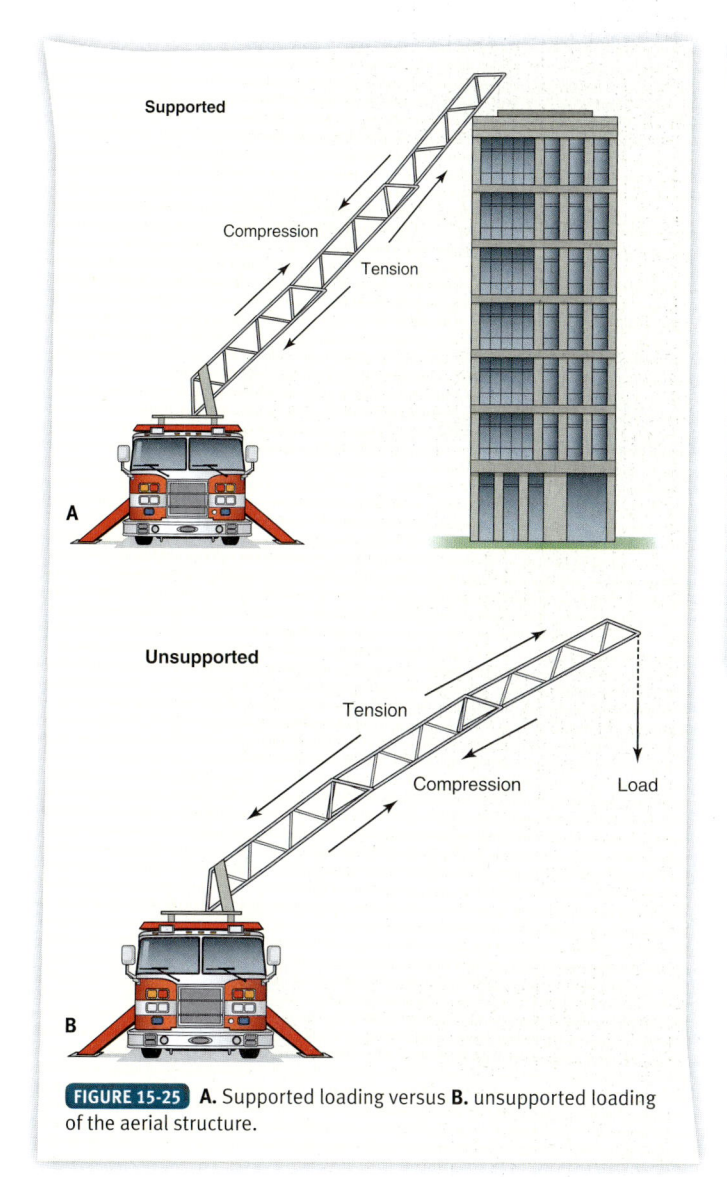

According to the U.S. Fire Administration's Technical Report Series, *Aerial Ladder Collapse Incidents* (USFA-TR-081), in Brooklyn, NY, in November 1994, while attempting a rescue with a 100-ft (30-m) aerial ladder, the driver/operator rested the tip of the ladder on a window sill. Only one rail of the ladder was set on the sill due to the ladder being at an angle to the wall. The ladder was unable to support the weight of the victims due to the tension and compression of the truss having been reversed. This factor, coupled with the torsional effect on the beam, resulted in a collapse that injured both fire fighters and victims and led to the death of one victim.

■ Load Placed on the Aerial

The aerial will need to support a number of loads, including humans, equipment, water, and environmental conditions. Every aerial is rated to support a maximum number of persons regardless of whether they are fire fighters or victims. The driver/operator, in turn, must know the rated capacity of the aerial. This information is contained in the operator's manual and is usually published on a plate or sign affixed to the turntable operator's position and at the platform operator's position

AERIAL LOAD CHART WATERWAY DRY 20 MPH WIND NO ICE BUILD-UP				
DEGREES OF ELEVATION	−5 TO 30	30 TO 40	40 TO 50	50+
PLATFORM	1000#	1000#	1000#	1000#
FLY	ZERO	ZERO	250#	500#
MID	ZERO	250#	500#	750#
BASE	250#	500#	750#	1000#

Disclaimer: For illustration purposes only. Not for actual use with any aerial device.

AERIAL LOAD CHART WATERWAY CHARGED 20 MPH WIND NO ICE BUILD-UP				
DEGREES OF ELEVATION	−5 TO 30	30 TO 40	40 TO 50	50+
PLATFORM	600#	600#	600#	600#
FLY	ZERO	ZERO	250#	500#
MID	ZERO	250#	500#	500#
BASE	250#	500#	500#	750#

Disclaimer: For illustration purposes only. Not for actual use with any aerial device.

AERIAL LOAD CHART WATERWAY DRY 20 MPH WIND UP TO ¼-INCH ICE BUILD-UP				
DEGREES OF ELEVATION	−5 TO 30	30 TO 40	40 TO 50	50+
PLATFORM	750#	750#	750#	750#
FLY				
MID	ZERO	ZERO	ZERO	ZERO
BASE				

Disclaimer: For illustration purposes only. Not for actual use with any aerial device.

AERIAL LOAD CHART WATERWAY CHARGED 20 MPH WIND UP TO ¼-INCH ICE BUILD-UP				
DEGREES OF ELEVATION	−5 TO 30	30 TO 40	40 TO 50	50+
PLATFORM	500#	500#	500#	500#
FLY				
MID	ZERO	ZERO	ZERO	ZERO
BASE				

Disclaimer: For illustration purposes only. Not for actual use with any aerial device.

AERIAL LOAD CHART WATERWAY DRY 50 MPH WIND NO ICE BUILD-UP				
DEGREES OF ELEVATION	−5 TO 30	30 TO 40	40 TO 50	50+
PLATFORM	800#	800#	800#	800#
FLY	ZERO	ZERO	250#	500#
MID	ZERO	250#	500#	750#
BASE	250#	500#	750#	1000#

Disclaimer: For illustration purposes only. Not for actual use with any aerial device.

AERIAL LOAD CHART WATERWAY CHARGED 50 MPH WIND NO ICE BUILD-UP				
DEGREES OF ELEVATION	−5 TO 30	30 TO 40	40 TO 50	50+
PLATFORM	500#	500#	500#	500#
FLY	ZERO	ZERO	ZERO	250#
MID	ZERO	ZERO	250#	500#
BASE	ZERO	250#	500#	750#

Disclaimer: For illustration purposes only. Not for actual use with any aerial device.

FIGURE 15-27 Typical load charts from an operator's manual.

Courtesy of Drew Smith.

accounted for. Many aerials, for example, require reduced loading when faced with winds over a certain speed or the accumulation of snow or ice on the aerial. This information is usually contained in the operator's manual and also appears the load plate at the turntable and platform operator's positions. Under ice and snow conditions, it is best to not extend the aerial past 95 percent of its total length. Doing so will allow the driver/operator to maneuver the aerial periodically to prevent ice build-up. If the waterway has been charged, do not shut off the flow until the water can be immediately drained.

Improper Aerial Operations

The driver/operator must guard against improper or unsafe aerial operations. These can include unnecessary exposure to heat and fire conditions, improper use of the aerial as a crane or other platform, and allowing fire fighters to ride the aerial ladder when it is moving.

The driver/operator should position the apparatus to prevent the aerial from being subjected to excessive heat or flame. Such conditions can damage the aerial and render it inoperable. At the least, the aerial may become damaged and require expensive repairs. At the most, the heat or flame may damage the aerial, preventing it from moving and trapping fire fighters at the tip in or above the fire area. The driver/operator should know which protective features, such as platform sprinklers and heat shields, exist on his or her aerial, how to operate these features, and when these features should be deployed **FIGURE 15-28**.

Do not use aerial as a crane, as it is not intended for this purpose. Objects should not be supported or hauled in such a manner. The lifting of victims in litter baskets affixed to the aerial tip or platform is acceptable, provided the aerial is rated to do so. The weight of the victim and any accompanying fire fighters must be calculated as part of load management.

If fire fighters or technical rescue personnel desire to use an aerial as a high anchor point for a haul/lower system, this activity needs to be preplanned. Only rated anchors should be used for this purpose. These anchors should be appropriate for general use as defined by NFPA 1983, *Standard on Life Safety Rope and Equipment for Emergency Services*. Aerial rungs should be used as anchor points only when such activity is permitted by the apparatus manufacturer. A single beam of the aerial should not be used as an anchor point; however, doing so will impose an eccentric load onto the aerial structure.

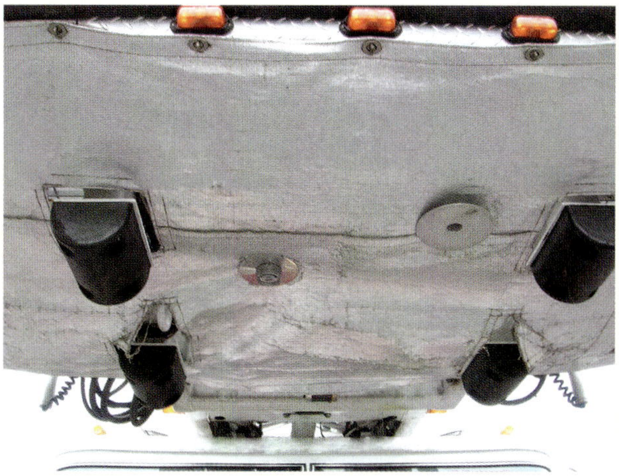

> **Safety Tip**
>
> Just because the apparatus will perform a certain function (e.g., allow you to lower or raise the ladder at full extension at a 90-degree angle to the apparatus with a full platform or ladder load), that does not mean you have to use that capability. Be safe!

In January 2012, an aerial ladder operating an elevated stream collapsed, killing a fire fighter who had climbed to its tip to operate the ladder pipe. An investigation revealed that the load capacity for the 1975-manufactured aerial was unknown. Also, in addition to the weight of the fire fighter, a single 3-inch (77-mm) hoseline was supplying the ladder pipe. Taken together, the weight of the fire fighter and the hose with water was in excess of 600 pounds (272 kg). The aerial had not been tested with a load more than 400 pounds (181 kg). Newer aerials must support at least 250 pounds (113 kg) at the tip with a 2:1 safety factor. In the 2012 case, investigators concluded that the load was more than double that minimum figure; they emphasized that fire fighters should know their aerial apparatus' limitations. Had the same aerial been used by a fire fighter to make a physical rescue, similar results might have occurred.

Personal Protective Equipment Needed

The driver/operator should be training the way he or she would be expected to perform on the fireground. During nonlive fire training or when operating at a structure fire, the driver/operator at the turntable and the fire fighters climbing the aerial ladder or operating at the tip or from the platform should wear full structural firefighting personal protective equipment (PPE). When fire fighters operating from the tip or platform need to use SCBA, there should be a safety evaluation to determine if those operating positions can function unstaffed.

Fall Protection

Whether in training or at a structure fire, any fire fighter climbing the aerial ladder or occupying the tip or platform of an aerial, even for brief periods, should wear and use a ladder belt meeting the requirements of NFPA 1983 **FIGURE 15-29**. Ladder belts should be connected to a ladder rung or to anchors in the platform. Failure to wear and use a ladder belt can result in serious injury or death of fire fighters.

In 2009, while conducting training on a new aerial, two fire fighters who were not using ladder belts were ejected from their aerial platform. The new aerial had become snagged on the top of the structure. When the fire fighters were able to free the aerial, it sprung loose and whipped violently. The two fire fighters fell 83 ft (26 m) to their death. Had ladder belts been worn and properly secured to designated anchors, these deaths may have been prevented.

FIGURE 15-28 Typical under-platform sprinkler.

VOICES OF EXPERIENCE

Regular practice is crucial and needs to occur with daily and weekly rig checks and on incidents that are not working fires. Waiting for those few instances each year where the aerial is needed will not make you ready for its use, let alone proficient. The following are some ideas I have seen work well, along with a few of dubious value.

Besides setting up the aerial behind the fire station, seek out actual locations to practice positioning, stabilization, and operation of their aerial apparatus. Anyone can set up in a wide-open space such as an empty parking lot behind the firehouse. For commercial and industrial areas, visit an office asking if it would be okay for the fire department to practice setup before or after normal business hours. A simple explanation that the department would like to know it can reach certain areas and maneuver the vehicle into position is easily sold. A similar conversation can be had with the owners association or management at apartment complexes. The challenge here is to ensure all occupants receive notice of the drill date and time to prevent panic and unnecessary calls to 911 asking if there is a fire.

In addition to seeking out permission to use actual sites, the IC and company officer can position, set up, and operate the aerial on actual incidents that do not become full working fires. For example, suppose the aerial responds as part of a multiple-company dispatch for an activated fire alarm. The first engine company reports a smoke detector alarm in a roof-top unit of the HVAC system and states that it will be proceeding to the stairs to investigate. Best practices say to provide two ways off any roof. Having the aerial apparatus position, stabilize, and raise itself to the roof offers valuable experience. Company members may learn that what they believed will work is far from what is actually possible.

Finally, some training actually sets us up for failure when it matters most. Two common practices used during inspections and maintenance should cause driver/operators and company officers to reflect on how we can do better. First, is using the manual override always necessary or even warranted? Suppose your aerial has some top-mounted equipment that is stored under the aerial ladder. As part of the weekly comprehensive inspection and maintenance, this equipment is usually accessed by raising the aerial from its bedded position by activating the stabilization override rather than with full deployment of the stabilizers. Why? What is the benefit? Are we giving ourselves an excuse to not do the operation properly?

A second frequently observed practice during these maintenance and inspection tasks is the "setup by committee" method, where all company members participate in the placement of wheel chocks, ground pads, and deployment of the stabilizers. In this case, tasks are not performed following a set procedure, but rather by the participant who gets to the task first. Is this the expectation on the fireground, or is it expected that the driver operator will handle all of these steps.

Seeking out opportunities and then conducting operations as desired is the best way to prepare for when it counts.

Drew Smith
Deputy Fire Chief
Prospect Heights (Illinois) Fire District

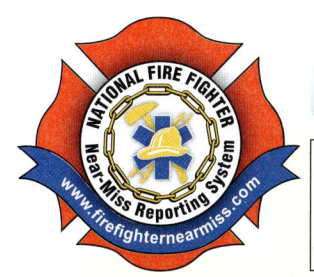

CHAPTER 15 Apparatus Equipped with an Aerial Device   377

Near-Miss REPORT

Report Number: 12-0000036

Synopsis: Crews endangered by lack of communication.

Event Description: My department was called for mutual aid in a nearby district. While we were working on the scene, another mutual aid department was operating an elevated master stream from their tower ladder no more than 15 ft (5 m) to our left. The tower was about 6 ft (2 m) from power lines, and the stream was being directed between the primary and secondary power lines. The fire fighters that were operating the stream would direct it as needed to fight the fire, occasionally hitting the power lines.

My crew and I knew it was a matter of time before one or all of the lines would break. Crews were operating in the D side exposure no more than 5 ft (1.5 m) from the fire building next to a utility pole was 5 ft (1.5 m) from the D exposure as well. The tower did break a secondary line as fire fighters were on the porch. Luckily, when the line broke, the charged end landed into the fire building where no one was operating, instead of the exposure or the street where my team was standing in water from all the master streams in operation.

Shortly after that, the crew that was operating the tower was overcome by smoke due to wind shift and the fact that they were not wearing their self-contained breathing apparatus (SCBA). They backed out, shifted the tower without redirecting the stream or shutting it down, and hit the porch on the D side exposure building. The crew that was operating there had to dive into the exposure, and one fire fighter had to retreat by jumping off of the 5-ft (1.5-m) porch. The stream knocked the door from its hinges. Luckily no one was hurt. My crew and I tried to let the tower crew know what was going on by yelling and signaling. There was no way to radio them due to the fact they are a distant department and we do not carry their frequency on our radios.

I am not sure if they realized what was going on around them, and they should have been wearing SCBAs. This could have been avoided, and luckily no one was injured—just a slight scare.

Lessons Learned: The lesson learned is to always be aware of your surroundings and to obtain a way to communicate with other departments if possible. The tower that was operating was from a volunteer department, and their level of training was not known. Hopefully they went back to their department and critiqued themselves in order to improve.

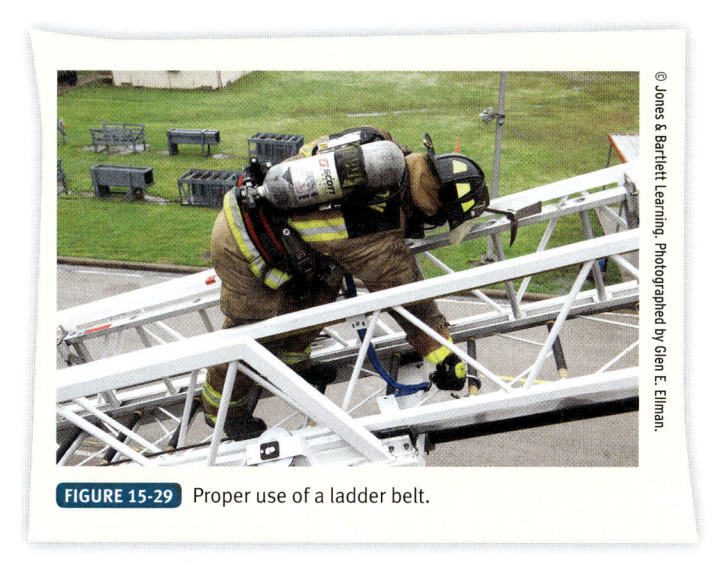

FIGURE 15-29 Proper use of a ladder belt.

Climbing or Riding a Moving Aerial Ladder

When the aerial ladder is being extended, retracted, or otherwise moved, fire fighters should not be in any location other than the platform. Doing otherwise is extremely dangerous. As the ladder is extended or retracted, the ladder rungs of one section pass those of another section, creating areas that can be pinched. A caught foot, hand, arm, or leg could be seriously injured or severed. In one documented fatality that occurred in Illinois, a fire fighter was crushed by two rungs on a moving aerial ladder. Whenever fire fighters climb on the aerial ladder, the rungs must be aligned, all power to the ladder should be shut off, and the driver/operator must remain vigilant at the turntable to ensure these conditions are maintained **FIGURE 15-30**.

Safety Tip

Always wear a ladder belt that is clipped to a rung or a platform anchor. Just as with a seat belt, do not signal the operator to move the aerial until you are belted in and clipped in. Your life is in the balance in such cases. Remember: A dead or seriously injured fire fighter cannot help anyone!

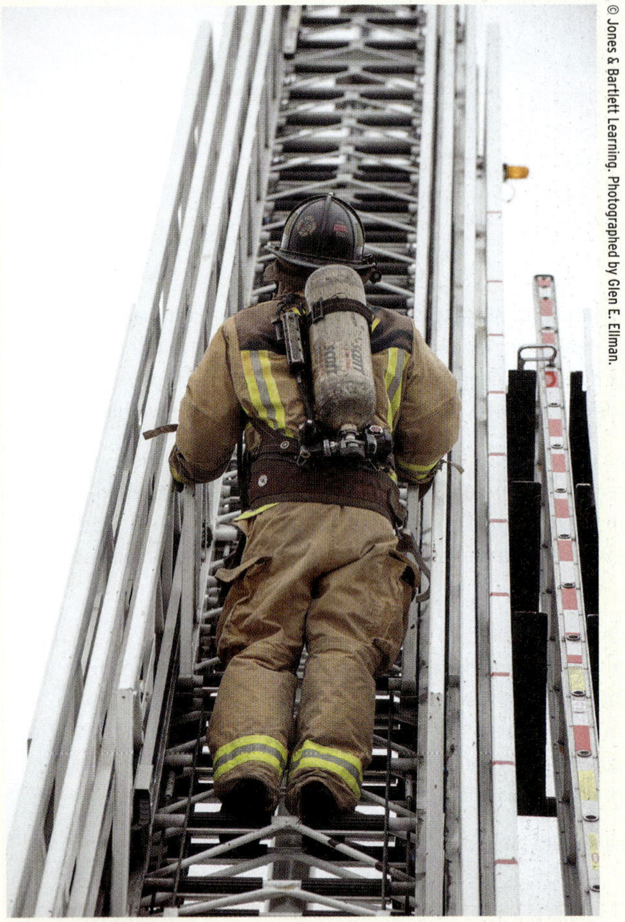

FIGURE 15-30 Climb only when rungs are aligned and maneuvering controls are de-energized.

Allow Space for Deflection

When the aerial is raised to its objective and fire fighters get on or off, such as through a window or via a roof, the aerial platform will move when load is added or removed. That is, fire fighters getting off will lighten the load, so that the basket will rise. Fire fighters or victims getting on to the aerial platform will increase the load, which will lower the basket. In both cases, the skilled driver/operator will ensure that any deflection does not create an unsafe condition such as the aerial resting against the structure or the aerial being too high to safely disembark or be reboarded.

Maneuvering Aerial Device

To practice maneuvering the aerial device, the driver/operator should select a location that is free of hazards and any obstructions. When the aerial apparatus is appropriately positioned and stabilized, the driver/operator should follow the steps in **SKILL DRILL 15-3** to practice maneuvering the aerial device. With aerial apparatus positioned and stabilized at a given location:

1. Access the turntable. (**STEP 1**)
2. Look up and around for overhead hazards, such as electrical wires or obstructions, and for surface obstacles, such as light poles and signs. (**STEP 2**)
3. If members are to occupy the platform, have them do so and verify their position and readiness for the aerial device to be operated.
4. Energize the turntable controls (**STEP 3**).
5. Raise the aerial up from the bedded position (**STEP 4**).
6. Stop raising the aerial and then rotate the aerial left or right. (**STEP 5**)
7. Stop rotation of the aerial and then extend the aerial out. (**STEP 6**)
8. Lower the aerial. (**STEP 7**)
9. Rotate the aerial. (**STEP 8**)
10. Retract the aerial. (**STEP 9**)
11. Return the aerial to the bedded position. (**STEP 10**)

Note: For steps 5, 6, and 7, be sure not to exceed the manufacturer's restrictions and departmental policy.

With the aerial movement speed reduced (typically by using a control at the turntable), the driver/operator can develop proficiency by practicing to combine the following maneuvers:

- Rotate while raising
- Extend while rotating or raising
- Retract while lowering or rotating
- Any combination of the three controls as permitted by the specific aerial's manufacturer

Using the Aerial to Effect a Rescue

When the decision is made to conduct a rescue using the aerial apparatus, the driver/operator must position and stabilize it before deploying the ladder or platform to the victim. When the need for rescue is known, the aerial should be positioned to best effect the rescue while recognizing that other, as-yet-unknown victims may be present and that the aerial may be needed in the future for ventilation or elevated streams. Even though rescue is the top priority, exposure of the aerial to heat and flame that can hinder its operation and safety must be avoided.

Skill in raising, rotating, and extending the aerial simultaneously and in a smooth manner is the sign of a skilled driver/operator. When possible, a rescue should follow the steps in **SKILL DRILL 15-4**:

1. The driver/operator positions, stabilizes, and raises the aerial from the bed, while other company members prepare for the rescue.
2. Once the aerial is ready to be elevated from the bed, the required company members then occupy the platform. Once the apparatus is securely placed into position, the driver/operator elevates, extends, and rotates the aerial to within 10 ft (3 m) or so of its desired position.
3. At this point, a fire fighter can access the tip, or from the platform, performs the final approach and positioning for the rescue. This fire fighter is in a better position to maneuver toward the victim's location and to bring the tip or platform into the needed location.

As the tip of the ladder or the platform approaches the victim, the driver/operator should keep it to the upwind side and raised above the victim's location to prevent this individual

CHAPTER 15 Apparatus Equipped with an Aerial Device 379

SKILL DRILL 15-3 Maneuvering the Aerial Device
NFPA 1002, 6.2.3, 6.2.3(B)

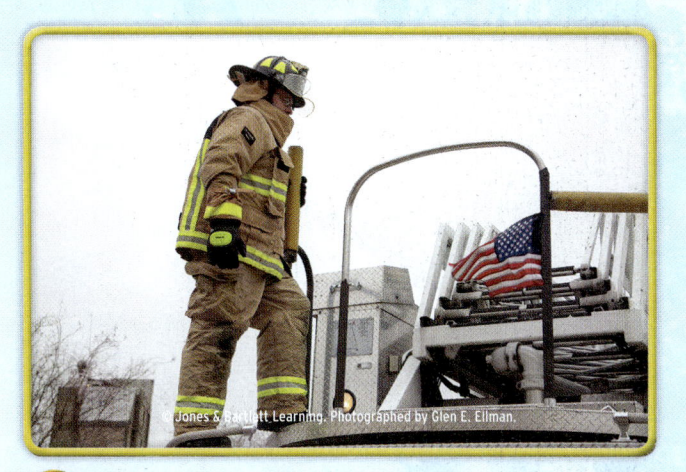

1 Access the turntable.

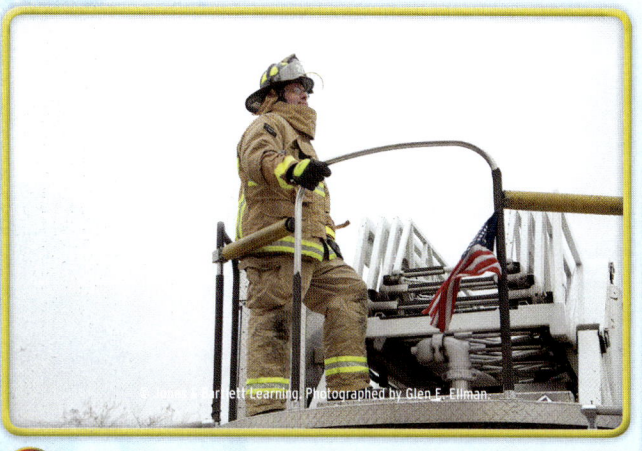

2 Look up and around for overhead hazards, such as electrical wires or obstructions, and for surface obstacles, such as light poles and signs.

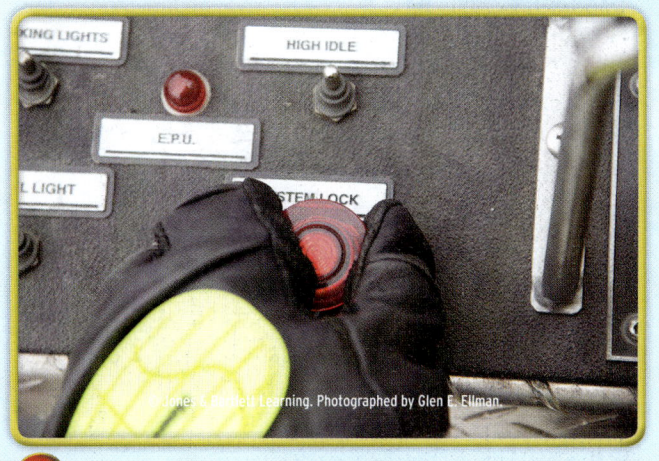

3 Energize the turntable controls.

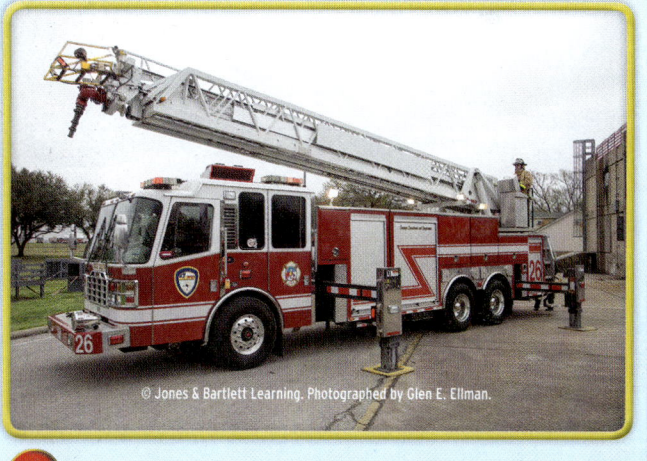

4 Raise the aerial up from the bedded position.

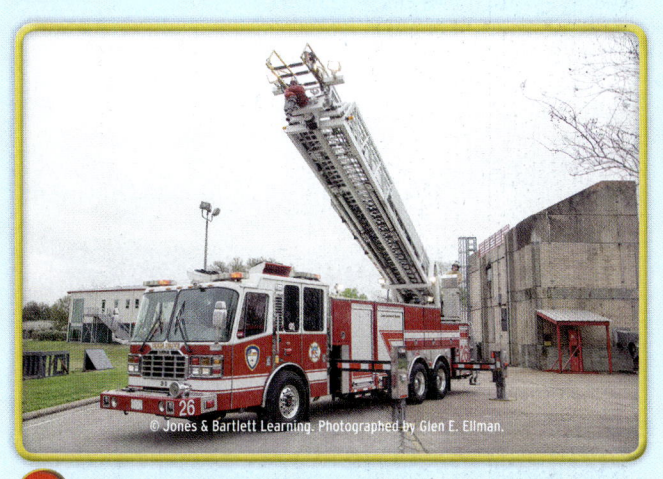

5 Stop raising the aerial and then rotate the aerial left or right.

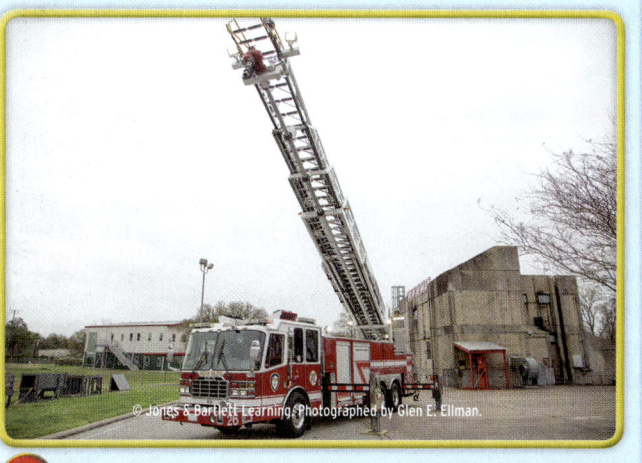

6 Stop rotation of the aerial and then extend the aerial out.

© LiquidLibrary

(Continues)

SKILL DRILL 15-3 Maneuvering the Aerial Device (*Continued*)
NFPA 1002, 6.2.3, 6.2.3(B)

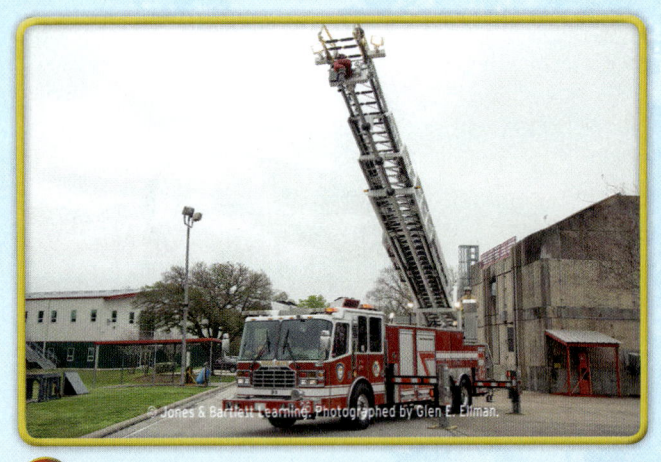

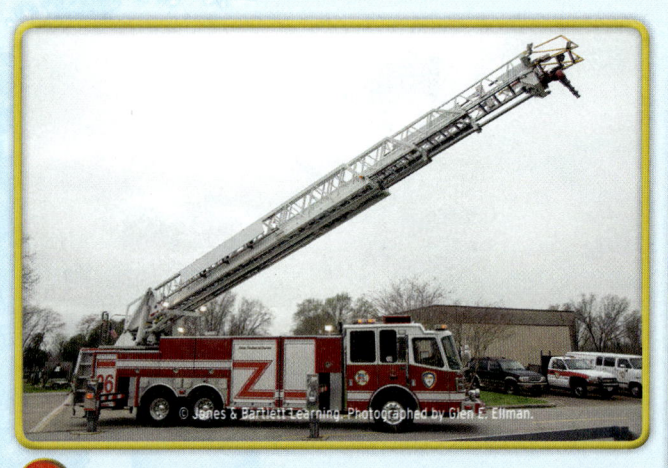

7 Lower the aerial.

8 Rotate the aerial.

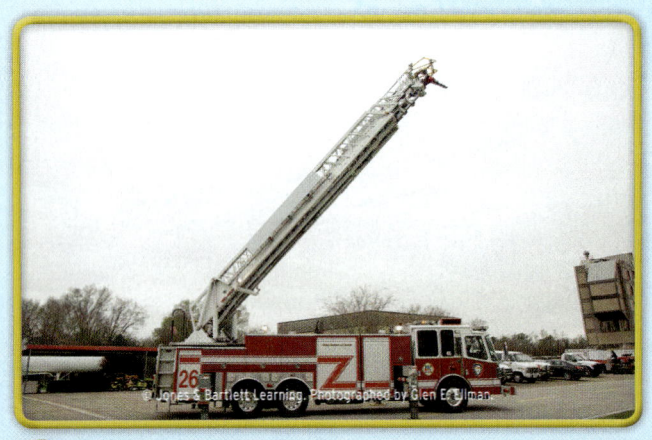

9 Retract the aerial.

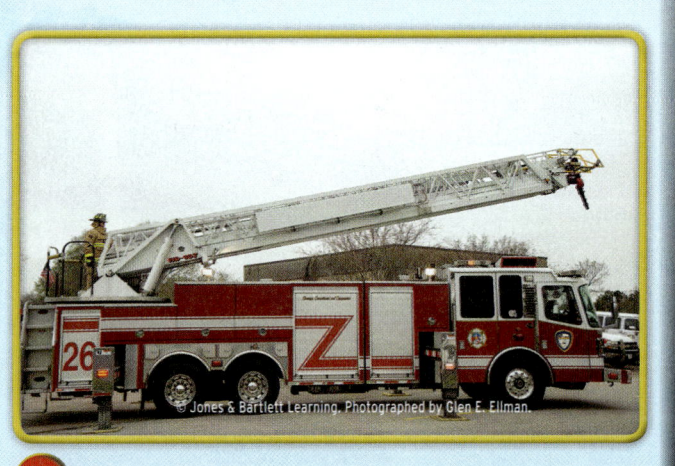

10 Return the aerial to the bedded position.

from accessing the ladder prematurely **FIGURE 15-31**. If a victim were to jump onto the aerial, the shock load might be too much and could result in damage rendering the aerial inoperable or, even worse, leading to a catastrophic failure. A 150-pound (68-kg) person jumping down just 5 ft (1.5 m) will impact with more than 750 pounds (340 kg) of force on the tip already loaded with the weight of the fire fighter(s).

DRIVER/OPERATOR Tip

Approach the victim from above, and then lower the ladder or platform down to the victim.

■ Tip Positioning

When rescuing victims from a window, place the ladder tip or platform at the sill **FIGURE 15-32**. Some fire fighters prefer to

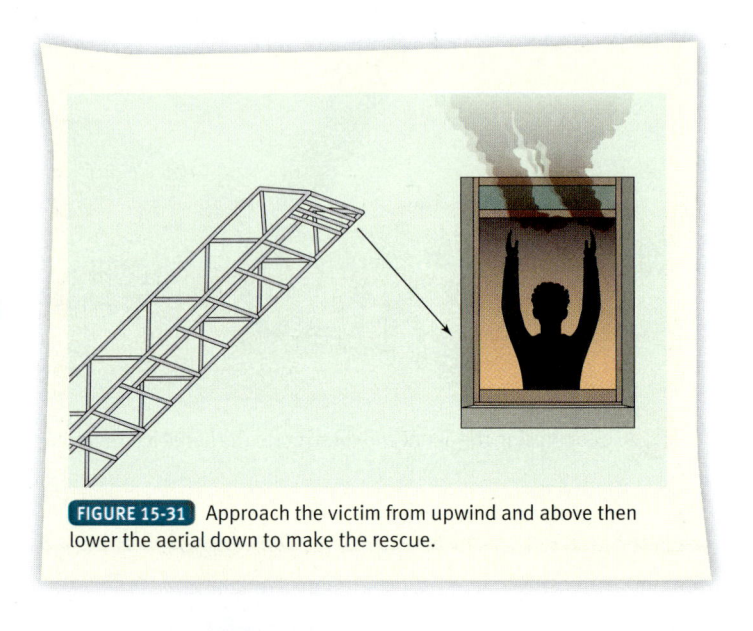

FIGURE 15-31 Approach the victim from upwind and above then lower the aerial down to make the rescue.

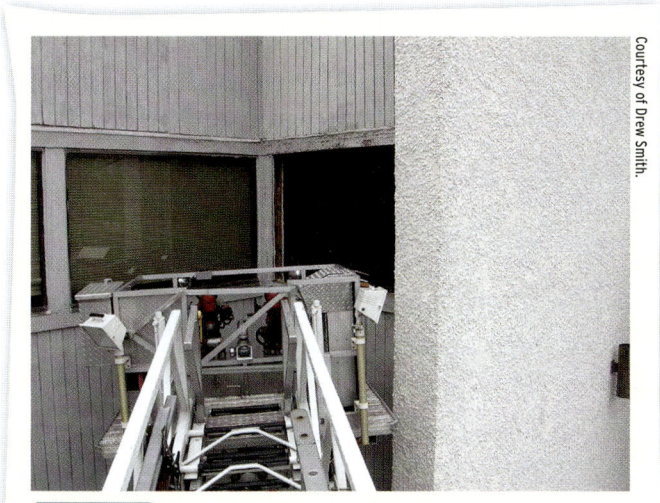

FIGURE 15-32 Position the aerial at the window sill to achieve maximum access into the structure.

position the floor of a platform at sill or balcony railing height instead. If there are multiple victims, fire fighters should go through the window to assist the victims onto the aerial as well as to prevent overloading of the aerial. Before entering the window, the fire fighter should probe the area inside and below the sill to ensure the floor is intact and that he or she will not step on a collapsed person. The aerial can hold only so many people, whether they are fire fighters or civilians. Because fire fighters have PPE and SCBA, they should be able to stay in the structure longer than the unprotected victims. This condition is not absolute, however: Obviously, the specific fire conditions will dictate the level of risk to which the fire fighters should be exposed.

If victims are on a roof or balcony, attempt to position the tip or platform over the edge as much as possible. If victims or fire fighters then slip and fall, they will drop only a few feet versus all the way to the ground **FIGURE 15-33**. Unlike when using a portable extension ladder, it is not usually possible for the ladder or platform to be positioned square or perfectly perpendicular to the structure, resulting in less than ideal conditions for the fire fighter who must climb off the aerial into the structure and any victims who must then climb onto the aerial.

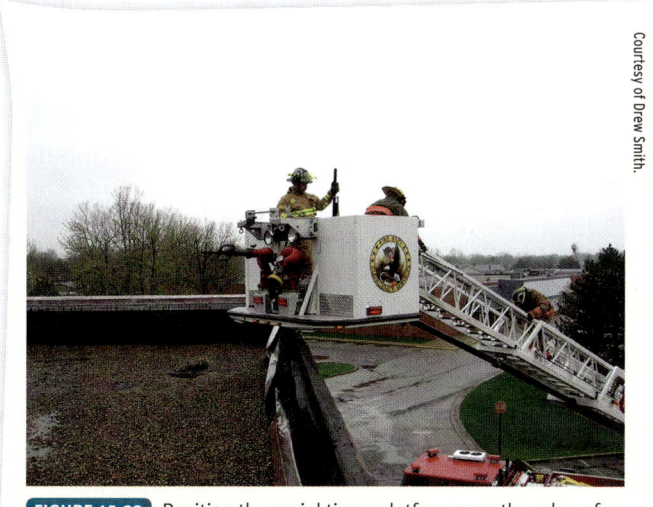

FIGURE 15-33 Position the aerial tip or platform over the edge of the roof or balcony as much as possible to reduce fall hazards.

When victims are able to climb down on the ladder, care must be exercised to avoid overloading it. Follow the aerial manufacturer's recommendation for the number of persons who should occupy each ladder section at specific elevations or under various environmental conditions. When using an aerial platform, it is often quicker to lower the platform to the ground and offload the victims from it and then return the platform for another load of victims, versus letting the individual victims climb down the ladder.

■ Rescue Priorities

Rescue priorities are the same when an aerial apparatus is used as they are without an aerial operation. First, a decision needs to be made as to whether the victim will be removed from the hazard or the hazard will be removed from the victim. In other words, is it best to rescue the person or to cut off the fire or smoke that is causing harm? If you are faced with one or two victims who need minimal assistance, perhaps removing them is the best option. However, if there are multiple victims in one or more locations, it might be best to focus on controlling and containing the fire to reduce the urgency of the situation. Training and experience are the only way to prepare for making this decision.

Multiple Victims

When faced with multiple victims in multiple locations, the driver/operator and company officer must decide who will be rescued first, then second, and so on. As with rescues via ground ladder, the level of threat and proximity to the fire are key considerations. Those individuals who are directly exposed to fire conditions are the top priority. It is not necessary to see flames to be exposed to fire conditions. Heavy, turbulent smoke that obscures or pushes the victim is also indicative of threatening fire conditions. Once these victims are managed, then those victims in groups or clusters are managed. Finally, all others can be aided.

When evaluating those victims in areas other than the immediate fire area, it may be best to have the aerial company shelter these people in place or direct them to use building features to isolate smoke. For example, a fourth-floor fire in a 10-story building results in occupants of the sixth floor being unable to use the stairs. The aerial company may be presented with these people waving from a balcony. Because the aerial company knows the location of the fire and recognizes that the fire has not spread, the officer might decide it is less risky to keep these people in place with the balcony door shut than to have them attempt to climb down a 75-ft (23-m) ladder.

Physical Rescue

Victims will present as unconscious or conscious. Unconscious victims will obviously need a physical rescue. Conscious individuals may need a physical rescue due to their injuries or a chronic condition, may need limited assistance with accessing the aerial or direction on how to climb down, or may need only simple directions on where to go and how to proceed. In any case, the driver/operator and the company officer will need to ensure an adequate number of fire fighters are available to effect the rescues.

Rescue Carries

With any victim, conscious or unconscious, who requires a physical rescue, a variety of carries may be used in conjunction with an aerial operation. Generally, one fire fighter grasps the victim from above the head and another fire fighter grasps the legs from below. The victim is then carried down the ladder feet first. Regardless of the technique used, carrying a victim down the aerial ladder requires at least three fire fighters: two for the carry and one more below the carrying team providing direction and guidance. A basket litter makes handling and maneuvering the victim easier and safer. However, when the victim is in the hazard area, fire fighters should not wait for the basket litter to become available when they are otherwise able to move the victim. Those conscious victims who do not require physical rescue will still need assistance or guidance. Victims who have injuries but can walk or those who are very young, are very old, have special needs, or are simply scared may need a fire fighter to coach them or steady them as they climb onto the aerial or down the ladder.

Whether the company is using an aerial ladder or a platform, it is safer and faster to move the victim onto the aerial and then lower the tip or platform to the ground versus trying to carry the victim or letting the person climb down. If victims are allowed to climb down, the possibility of an individual slipping and falling briefly or panicking would result in the operation coming to a halt for an undetermined period of time. Regardless of whether the victims are carried down, walked down, or lowered, the load on the aerial must be anticipated and managed to prevent overloading.

Ventilation Positioning

Similar to rescue positioning, the driver/operator, in consultation with his or her company officer, must evaluate and size up the fire, smoke, and environmental conditions as they impact the performance of ventilation. When roof work is anticipated or ordered, the positioning of the aerial should aid in not only access but also rapid egress.

■ Horizontal Ventilation via Windows

When performing horizontal ventilation via windows, position the aerial upwind of the ventilation location. The entire aerial does not need to be upwind, but certainly the tip or platform should be. The chassis should be positioned to avoid any falling glass or other debris. Consideration should be given to whether one or multiple windows must be broken out, as this decision may dictate positioning of the aerial apparatus. Finally, once the immediately needed horizontal ventilation is completed, the driver/operator must consider what will be the next priority and whether the aerial's placement will allow for it.

Vertical Ventilation via Rooftop Operations

For vertical ventilation, the aerial should be positioned such that fire fighters accessing the roof will be able to escape rapidly should conditions deteriorate or the IC so orders them to do so. Rapid egress is not always accomplished by positioning the tip or platform close to the work area. In some cases, it may be better to position the aerial away from the fire area. When fire fighters get onto the roof, they should do so in an area where the fire is less likely to spread. This will allow them to assess roof conditions before approaching the work site. In the event of deteriorating conditions, these fire fighters can

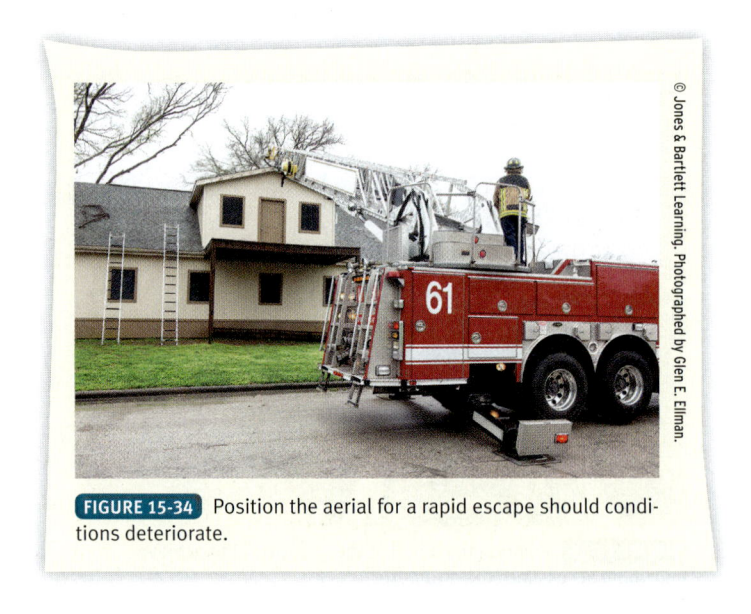

FIGURE 15-34 Position the aerial for a rapid escape should conditions deteriorate.

then travel back, horizontally, to a safer area where they can then board the aerial **FIGURE 15-34**. If the aerial is positioned too close to the work site, these same fire fighters will need to wait for each other to board, thereby prolonging their exposure to the fire conditions.

Regardless of whether initial roof access is via ground or aerial ladder, fire fighters should be provided with two ways off this site. This could be a combination of ground and aerial ladders or all aerial devices. In either case, these means of egress should be opposite each other, such as with aerial apparatus positioned in the front and rear or on each side of the structure. Each aerial apparatus or ladder must be in a useful position and easily located by operating fire fighters.

Many structures will present with a tall parapet wall or false roof on one or more sides. Modern apartment complexes and strip malls with anchor stores, as well as big-box stores such as Home Depot and Walmart, have these features. In these instances, the driver/operator should account for this factor when known, as the result of previous experience at similar structures or preplanning activities. In these cases, it may be a better decision to use the rear or a different side of the structure to obtain access to the roof. When this is not possible, a straight ladder may be used to safely climb down to the flat roof deck, and then this ladder should be secured. Some modern aerial platforms are designed so that this ladder may be mounted securely to the platform.

Use of the Aerial to Position Members for Ventilation

To practice positioning the aerial device for use in ventilation, the driver/operator should select a location that is free of hazards and any obstructions. When the aerial apparatus is positioned and stabilized at a given location with simulated fireground conditions, the driver/operator should follow the steps in **SKILL DRILL 15-5** to practice positioning the aerial device for use in ventilation.

1. Drive to the location, select an appropriate place, and position the apparatus as best possible to utilize the aerial device to achieve the assigned ventilation task. Stabilize the apparatus per the manufacturer's instructions and your department's policy. **(STEP 1)**

SKILL DRILL 15-5 Using the Aerial Device for Ventilation
NFPA 1002, 6.2.3, 6.2.3(B)

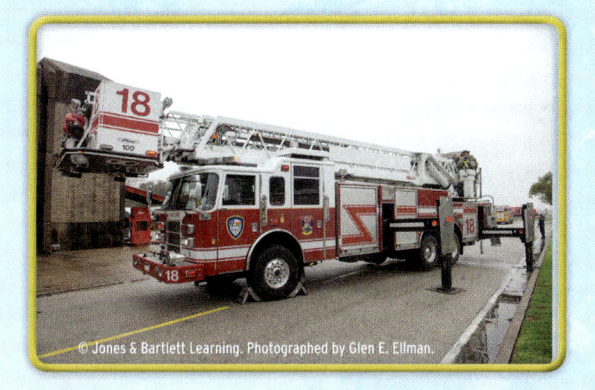

1. Drive to the location, select an appropriate place, and position the apparatus as best possible to utilize the aerial device to achieve the assigned ventilation task. Stabilize the apparatus.

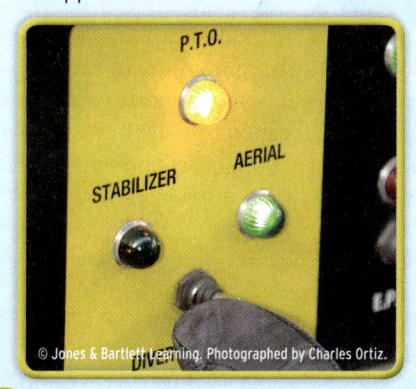

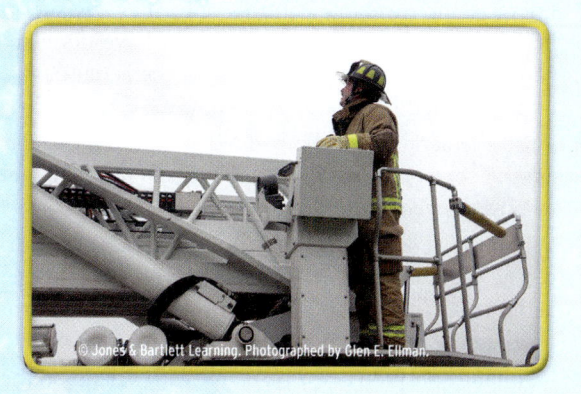

2. Access the turntable and look up and around for overhead hazards, such as electrical wires or obstructions, and for surface obstacles, such as light poles and signs.

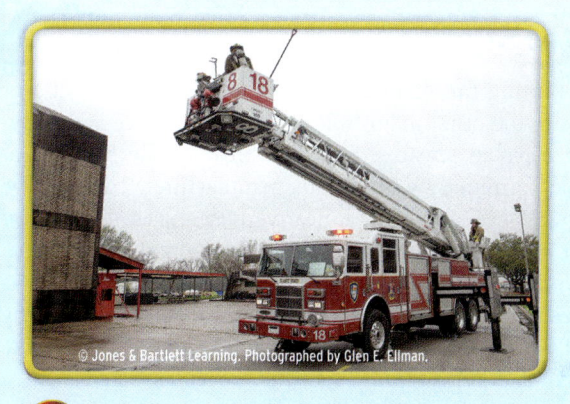

3. Energize the turntable controls only after any members who are to occupy the platform have done so, and their position and readiness for the aerial device to be operated have been verified.

4. Raise the aerial from the bedded position and operate the controls to raise, rotate, and extend the aerial toward the ventilation location.

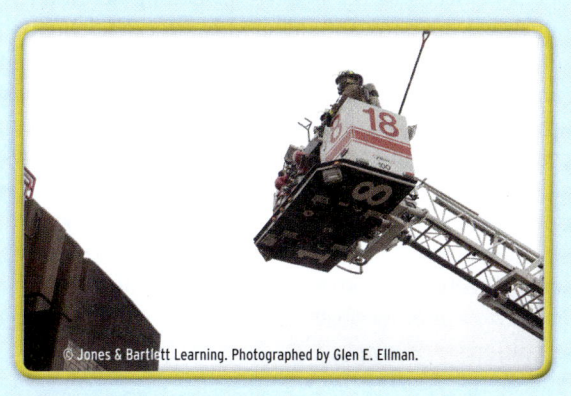

5. When the aerial tip or platform is within 10 ft (3 m) of the ventilation objective, transfer control of the aerial to a crew member at the tip or in the platform for the final positioning.

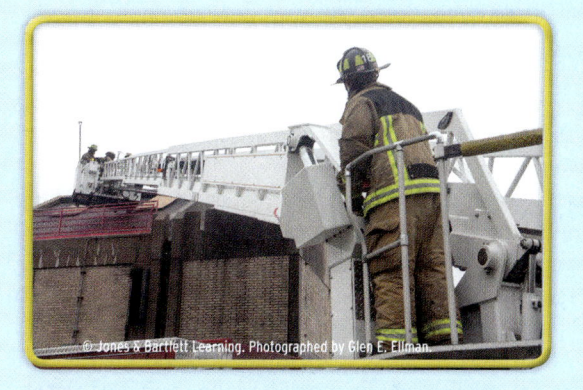

6. Maintain a position at the turntable with a hand on the control and eyes on the tip/platform observing for hazards and listening for needs of the tip/platform members.

2. Access the turntable and look up and around for overhead hazards, such as electrical wires or obstructions, and surface obstacles, such as light poles and signs. **(STEP 2)**

3. Energize the turntable controls only after any members who are to occupy the platform have done so, and their position and readiness for the aerial device to be operated have been verified. **(STEP 3)**

4. Raise the aerial from the bedded position and operate the controls to raise, rotate, and extend the aerial toward the ventilation location. **(STEP 4)**

5. When the aerial tip or platform is within 10 ft (3 m) of the ventilation objective, transfer control of the aerial to a crew member at the tip or in the platform for the final positioning. **(STEP 5)**

6. Maintain a position at the turntable with a hand on the control and eyes on the tip/platform observing for hazards and listening for needs of the tip/platform members. If necessary, use the turntable controls to override the actions of the tip/platform operator. **(STEP 6)**

FIGURE 15-35 Ensure any positioning pins for waterways are properly set.

Elevated Streams

Besides placing fire fighters into high positions for rescue or ventilation, the other major role of the aerial device is deployment of elevated streams. Elevated streams may be used at any angle permitted by the aerial's manufacturer. This may be below grade level as well as at near-vertical angles. The driver/operator must know at which vertical/horizontal and longitudinal/lateral angles use of the aerial device for this purpose is permitted, as well as when aerial loads must be reduced during elevated stream operations.

Aerial ladders may or may not be constructed with a prepiped waterway and tip-mounted master stream. The latter is most common, but portable ladder pipes are still used and preferred by some departments. The prepiped master stream offers the advantage of quicker deployment, but the disadvantage of potentially being in the way or becoming damaged during some operations.

Elevated Stream Positioning

During elevated stream operations, reach has two components:
- Reach of the stream from the nozzle
- Reach of the aerial

For the water to reach its objective, both of these components must be considered. The reach of the water stream will vary depending on the type of stream, the stream pattern, and the pressure at the nozzle. For straight and solid streams, an 80–100 psi (550–700 kPa) nozzle pressure can achieve a reach of more than 100 ft (30 m). For streams launched from the aerial, the reach will never be more than the apparatus' design. Rarely are elevated streams operated at elevations greater than 75 degrees. In many cases, the best results are produced when the stream is as low and close to the fire as possible.

Some aerial ladders with a prepiped waterway are designed to allow the master stream to be pinned to either the tip of the fly section or the section below it. This is usually accomplished by means of a manual pin. In this configuration, it is essential that the pin is properly set **FIGURE 15-35**. If it is not, one or more safety issues may develop. First, if the pin is not set at all, the waterway may separate from the ladder and become a projectile that could strike and injure or even kill a fire fighter or other person. Second, if two or more pins are used and they are set in conflicting locations (such as one pin set for the fly's tip and a second set for the midsection of the ladder), twisting of the ladder may occur, resulting in damage that could disable the aerial.

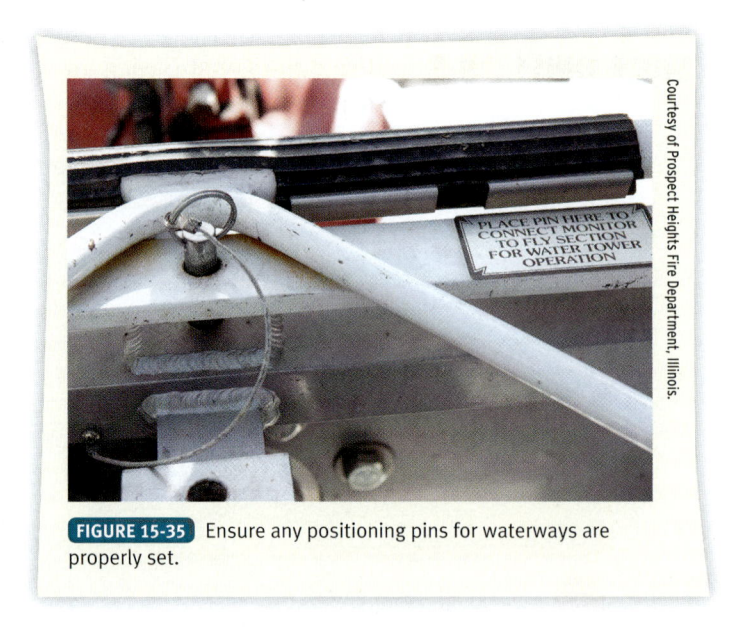

No matter what the positioning of the aerial apparatus, the reach of the fully extended aerial is roughly twice the vehicle length. Approximately 7 to 9 ft (2 to 3 m) of the rated length is attributable to the chassis and turntable. With many elevated stream operations, however, some of this "length" is lost from the aerial **FIGURE 15-36**. Also, as the aerial becomes more horizontal, some reach of the aerial is lost due to the setback of the turntable's centerline due to the needs of the stabilizers.

When the aerial apparatus was originally set up for rescue but later needs to be used for providing an elevated stream, the driver/operator should modify it and do his or her best under the circumstances. When elevated streams are required immediately upon arrival, the need for victim rescues via aerial apparatus is usually not required later in the operation. However, the need for access to upper levels should always be considered. The primary considerations related to elevated stream operations are ensuring adequate separation from the fire and staying out of the collapse zone. Other considerations include wind direction and speed, the presence of ice or snow, overhead wires or other obstructions and hazards, and the roadway conditions.

Operating Under Adverse Environmental Conditions

Two types of adverse conditions that may present to the driver/operator of an aerial apparatus are fire and weather. Anytime the aerial is exposed to high winds and/or ice and snow, the load on the aerial may have to be reduced. This factor becomes

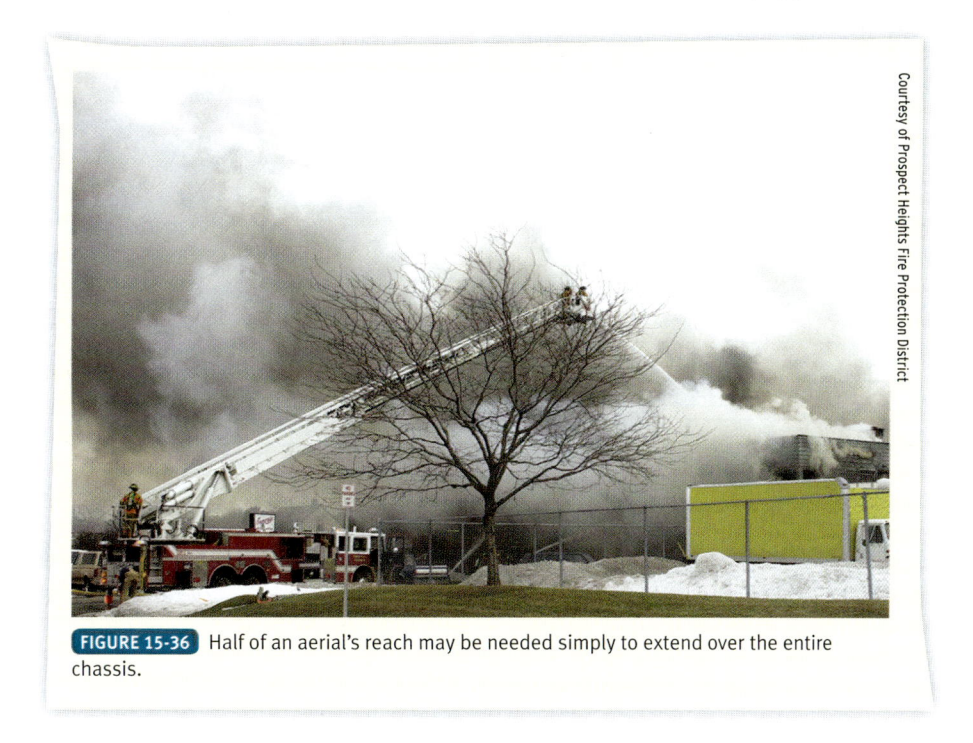

FIGURE 15-36 Half of an aerial's reach may be needed simply to extend over the entire chassis.

Courtesy of Prospect Heights Fire Protection District

an even more pronounced consideration when elevated streams are deployed. Consult the operator's manual as well as the placards that are usually posted at the turntable pedestal. To maximize stability and load-bearing capacity of the aerial, operate the aerial extended over the cab or off the rear, maintaining the aerial's force in-line with the chassis and maximizing the load distribution onto all stabilizers as equally as possible **FIGURE 15-37**. When ice and snow begin to accumulate on the aerial, the driver/operator should periodically maneuver the aerial to prevent its build-up.

The modern aerial's elevated stream is usually operable using remote controls. When faced with heavy fire conditions that impinge on the aerial, the IC, the safety officer, and the aerial company officer should all determine if the tip or platform should be unstaffed to maximize fire fighter safety. Many aerial platforms will include a sprinkler or spray nozzle located underneath that can be operated to keep the basket cool.

■ Stream Types

Elevated streams can be either solid or fog patterns. Solid streams or solid-bore nozzles come in a variety of sizes **TABLE 15-1**. Tip sizes generally range in 1/8-inch (3-mm) diameter increments from a 1⅜-inch (35-mm) tip up to a 2¼-inch (57-mm) tip, with the 1½-, 1¾, and 2-inch (38-, 45-, and 50-mm) sizes being most

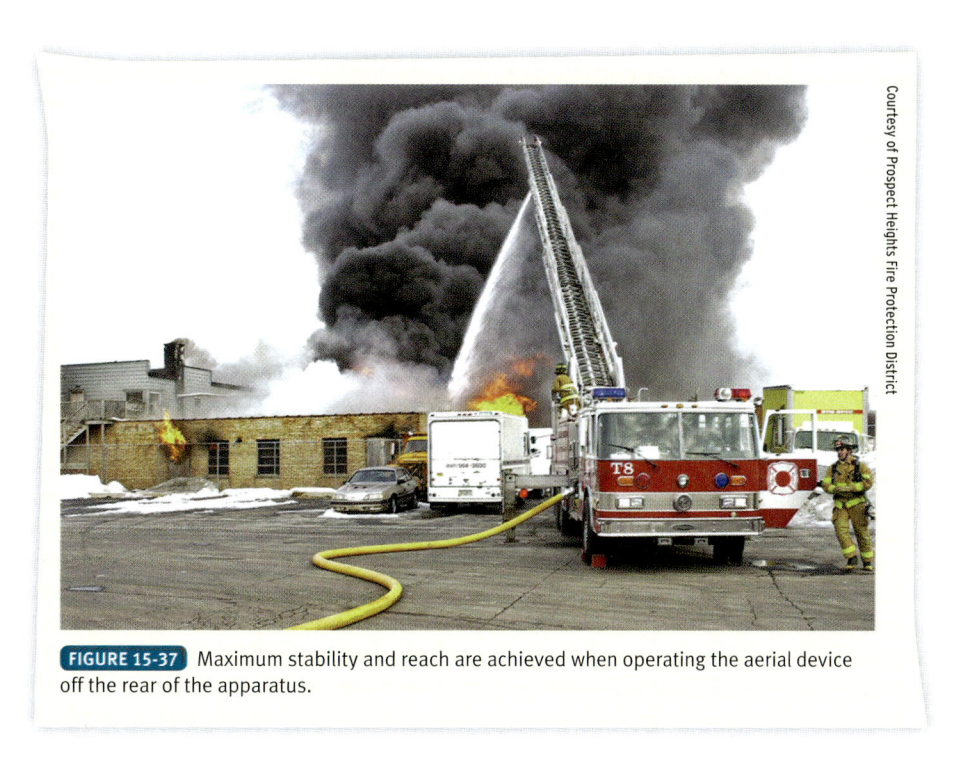

FIGURE 15-37 Maximum stability and reach are achieved when operating the aerial device off the rear of the apparatus.

Courtesy of Prospect Heights Fire Protection District

Fire Apparatus Driver/Operator

TABLE 15-1	Solid-Bore Nozzle Sizes and Flows	
Tip size	Gallons per minute (L/min) with an 80 psi (560 kPa) nozzle pressure (approximate)	Gallons per minute (L/min) with a 100 psi (700 kPa) nozzle pressure (approximate)
1⅜ inch (35 mm)	500 (2000)	550 (2200)
1½ inch (38 mm)	600 (2400)	670 (2680)
1¾ inch (44 mm)	800 (3200)	900 (3600)
2 inch (51 mm)	1000 (4000)	1200 (4800)
2¼ inch (57 mm)	1350 (5400)	1500 (6000)

popular. There are three types of fog nozzles—fixed-gallonage fog nozzles, adjustable-gallonage fog nozzles, or automatic-adjusting fog nozzles—and they generally will flow between 500 and 1250 gpm (2000 and 5000 L/min) depending on the model and manufacturer. Regardless of the tip size used, the manufacturer must construct the aerial based on a design that can safely experience the desired maximum gpm (L/min) flow with a master stream capable of producing that flow. While a certain nozzle may be capable of a higher flow, the aerial driver/operator cannot permit the aerial's rated design to be exceeded. The aerial driver/operator must, in all circumstances, ensure the safe operation of the aerial and its fire fighters.

Solid-bore nozzles and fog nozzles have different operating characteristics, as discussed elsewhere in this text. The driver/operator must understand the advantages and disadvantages of each as well as know exactly which nozzles he or she has on the assigned aerial. Maximum penetration and reach are desirable qualities for an elevated stream. Also important is the elevated stream's ability to resist breaking up due to the effect of wind. While straight and solid streams will have better reach and, therefore, better penetration, the greater coverage of a fog pattern is sometimes desired. In particular, exposure protection and cooling operations during a hazardous materials incident are two times when a fog pattern may be of benefit. However, whenever a fog pattern is used, the effective reach of the elevated stream is diminished significantly. Driver/operators must train with the nozzles they have and are expected to have a full understanding of the reach, penetration, and coverage achievable with those devices.

The driver/operator can use engineering calculations to deliver an approximate flow. The calculation method depends on the driver/operator having accurate data such as hose diameter and lengths; friction loss for any appliances, a prepiped waterway, and the master stream device; and an accurate height for the master stream's operating position. Provided accurate data are available and used, the calculations of the driver/operator should be fairly accurate. Being accurate is the key to ensuring the desired flow.

On modern aerial apparatus with a prepiped waterway, using a flow meter is the best way to ensure the desired flow is delivered. Combining pressure gauges with a flow meter will allow for the most accurate flow delivery **FIGURE 15-38**. On aerial platforms, it may be desirable to have flow meter displays

FIGURE 15-38 A flow meter with pressure gauge.

located both at the turntable and in the platform basket. If the aerial is equipped with a pump, a flow meter display should also be available at the pump panel.

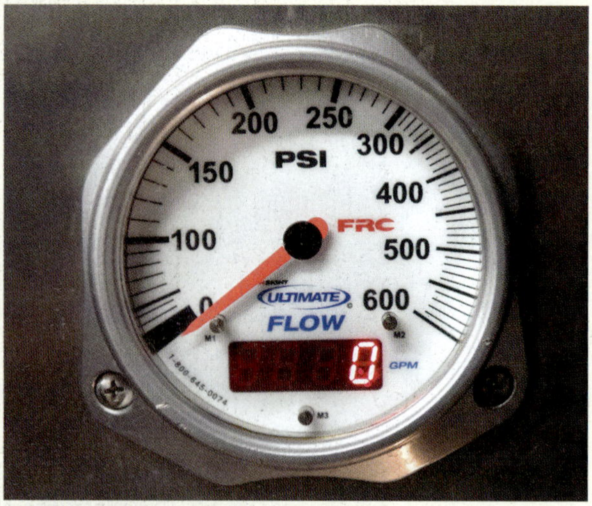

■ Water Supply

Water supply for the aerial must be of sufficient pressure and volume. The IC, the aerial company officer, and the driver/operator must ensure the action plan is understood by all. This includes giving clear orders for whether a pump will directly supply the aerial or, if the apparatus is so equipped, the aerial's pump; the size of hoselines to be used must also be identified. If the aerial is equipped with its own pump that will be used to supply the elevated stream, then the aerial may secure its own water source or be supplied via relay pumper. If the aerial's pump will not be used or the aerial lacks its own pump, then the supplying pumper must directly feed the waterway or ladder pipe.

■ Stream Application

While it is more commonly used for defensive operations, the elevated stream can also be used offensively. When operating in offensive mode, the objective is to stop the forward progress of the fire and ensure its extinguishment. If hand lines are of an insufficient flow or quantity, the elevated stream may be next choice for providing the necessary flow. Elevated streams can easily produce flows two to four times that of a large hand line **FIGURE 15-39**. The elevated stream may be a better choice than a pumper's deck gun for this purpose, because it can move horizontally across the fire building and get up close to windows and doors.

Whenever an elevated stream is flowed into a building, a large dead load is imposed on the structure. A flow of 1000 gpm (4000 L/min) equals 4 tons (4000 kg) of water weight being added every minute. The driver/operator should monitor this load and report to the company officer any signs of potential collapse, including failure of the applied water to drain from windows, doors, or balconies.

The driver/operator must exercise care to avoid applying the exterior stream into areas within a structure where

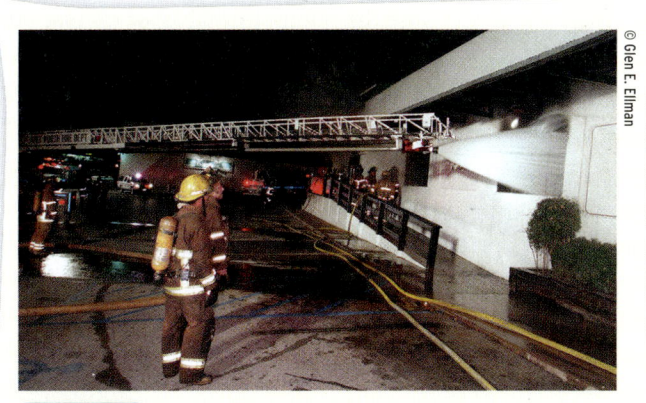

FIGURE 15-39 Use of an elevated stream at grade level to achieve high flows and maneuverability.

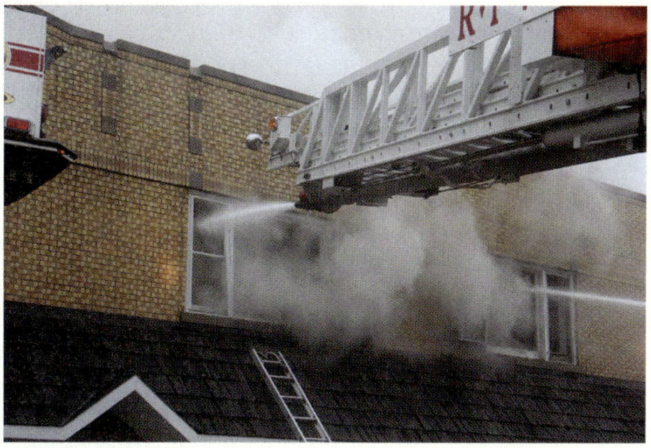

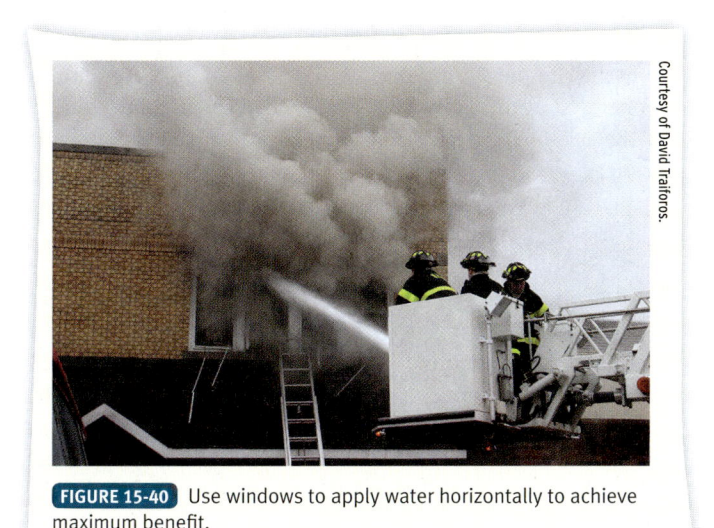

FIGURE 15-41 When possible, maneuver the aerial instead of the nozzle to keep the stream in line with the aerial.

companies are also located. Doing so can injure or kill those fire fighters due to blunt force trauma from the stream, any collapsed building materials struck by the stream, and heat or steam. Also to be avoided is placing the elevated stream into openings in the building intended for ventilation. Doing so prevents the heat and smoke from escaping and may drive these fire components down onto any companies working in the building's interior.

Applying water from the aerial is not restricted to just streams targeted directly at open flames. In some cases, the aerial may be moved up to windows or other wall openings while staying out of the collapse zone and the effects of heavy fire; the stream may then be sent through the window and toward the ceiling to bounce water onto the fire. Nevertheless, if possible, a direct attack with the elevated stream will have the best results. When horizontal application of the stream onto the fire is possible, better results can be achieved **FIGURE 15-40**. Vertical streams directed downward onto the fire may be less effective due to the deterioration of the stream from wind and/or heat in the fire's thermal column.

As the elevated stream is operated and the fire is extinguished, it will become necessary to maneuver the stream to reach other fire locations. When possible, move the ladder or platform horizontally before adjusting the master stream device itself **FIGURE 15-41**. It is best to keep the nozzle reaction as in line with the ladder as possible. Best practices include keeping the stream's angle relative to the ladder's beams within 15 degrees whenever possible. The more perpendicular the force to the beams, the less equally the beams are loaded. While many aerial manufacturers specify that streams may be operated at angles of even 90 degrees, it is wise to avoid doing so when possible.

Exposure Protection

The driver/operator must be versed in the Incident Command System and able to identify exposure buildings using the proper terminology. When the aerial company is ordered to protect a specific exposure, all considerations that arise when positioning the apparatus at the fire building must also be taken into account, with particular consideration given to the collapse zone. The direction and effect of wind on both the ladder and the potential fire spread must be evaluated. Building separation and construction will aid in the risk–benefit evaluation. The aerial apparatus should not be positioned in a location where it will be exposed to fire and from which both the fire fighters and the apparatus cannot reposition themselves.

When ordered to protect the exposure, the aerial company should direct the water from the elevated stream onto the exposure and not the fire. In this situation, resist the urge to put the water on the fire. The goal is to keep the fuel (the exposure) below its ignition temperature so it will not burn. The exposure protection stream must be maneuvered so the entire surface of the structure exposed to fire is cooled.

When faced with a fire at a large structure, the IC may elect to use fire attack and exposure protection simultaneously but in different areas. For example, with heavy fire on the Delta side of a big-box store, the IC might deploy elevated streams for protection of the Delta exposure while ordering other companies to attack the main body of fire from the Alpha or Bravo side. Such a strategic decision is perfectly acceptable provided the two groups do not operate in the same location.

FIGURE 15-40 Use windows to apply water horizontally to achieve maximum benefit.

Other Considerations

When operating a platform's nozzle over a fire or near an exposure, it is best to turn on the platform's sprinkler. This is done using the valve control located in the platform. Open the valve fully, never partially, as a partially open valve may close itself. Before retracting a charged waterway, it is best to uncharge it (shut off the supply of water to it), keep the nozzle valve open, and open the drain. Since no liquid (water included) can be compressed, opening valves and drains will allow water in the waterway to be discharged. Even with the use of a relief valve, closed drains and valves can allow the water to build up in the waterway, causing damage to the seals (which may cost several hundred dollars to repair) or to the pipes (which may bend from the pressure and cost several hundred dollars to repair).

Use of the Aerial to Deploy an Elevated Stream

To practice using the aerial to deploy an elevated stream, the driver/operator should select a location that is free of hazards and any obstructions. When the aerial apparatus is positioned and stabilized at a given location with simulated fireground conditions, the driver/operator should follow the steps in **SKILL DRILL 15-6** to practice using the aerial device to deploy an elevated stream.

1. Drive to the location, select an appropriate place, and position the apparatus as best as possible to utilize the aerial device to deploy an elevated stream. Stabilize the apparatus per the manufacturer's instructions and your department's policy. (**STEP 1**)
2. Secure the water supply for an elevated stream from a pumper assigned to supply it or a hydrant located near the aerial's operating position. To use a hydrant, the aerial itself must be equipped with a fire pump and have a separate pump operator assigned.
3. If required, affix the ladder pipe and hose to the end of the aerial's fly section and secure them per the manufacturer's instructions and your department's policy. This step should generally be performed by the company members and not the driver/operator.
4. Access the turntable and look up and around for any overhead hazards, such as electrical wires or obstructions, and surface obstacles, such as light poles and signs. (**STEP 2**)
5. Energize the turntable controls only after any members who are to occupy the platform have done so, and their position and readiness for the aerial device to be operated have been verified.
6. Raise the aerial from the bedded position and operate the controls to raise, rotate, and extend the aerial toward the location where the elevated stream is to be applied. (**STEP 3**)
7. When in an appropriate location and after any members at the tip or in the platform acknowledge they are ready, charge the elevated stream in a manner so as to not cause water hammer or extreme reaction of the aerial device. Manipulate the nozzle and aerial as needed to achieve the desired application of the water stream. (**STEP 4**)
8. Open and close the pump, turntable, or tip/platform valves slowly to avoid water hammer or extreme reaction of aerial device. When possible, keep the stream direction in line with the length of the aerial device. Avoid operating the stream perpendicular to the aerial device if possible, and never exceed the load limits as specified by the aerial's manufacturer for operating under excessive personnel, wind, snow, or ice loads.
9. Maintain a position at the turntable with a hand on the control and eyes on the tip/platform observing for hazards and listening for needs of the tip/platform members. If necessary, use the turntable controls to override the actions of the tip/platform operator. (**STEP 5**)
10. When the elevated stream is no longer needed, reduce the pressure at the supplying pump and close off the supply valve, rather than closing the valve at the tip/platform. This will reduce nozzle reaction and water hammer and facilitate the draining of the waterway or hose. In cold weather, this procedure will reduce the potential of the waterway freezing. (**STEP 6**)

Use of the Aerial Device's Emergency Power or Operations Feature

In the event that the aerial is raised and operating and experiences a failure of its controls or power supply, it will be necessary to switch to the emergency system. These systems generally rely on an electrically operated pump and/or a manual hand-crank as a means to operate the aerial and lower it from a raised position. Each manufacturer will use a specific procedure and system, and the driver/operator must know the requirements for each specific aerial apparatus. Two aerials produced by the same manufacturer (e.g., an elevated platform and a straight ladder) or two aerials manufactured years apart may have entirely different emergency operating systems. Often an emergency hydraulic pump that uses 12-volt power from the chassis cannot operate indefinitely without sustaining damage. In these cases, a brief period of use may require that the hydraulic pump undergo a period of cooling before it can be operated again. However, should there be a failure requiring the use of the emergency system, consider the following questions:

- Can any personnel occupying the aerial tip or platform remain in that location without risk?
- Should any elevated stream be terminated to reduce load and force on the aerial? Can this be done without significant damage occurring to the aerial apparatus or the fire structure?
- How much time do you have before the aerial must be lowered? Fire threatening the aerial apparatus presents challenges that do not exist when the failure occurs during training behind the fire station and the aerial can be cordoned off to await arrival of an emergency vehicle technician.

SKILL DRILL 15-6: Using the Aerial Device to Deploy an Elevated Stream
NFPA 1002, 6.2.5, 6.2.5(B)

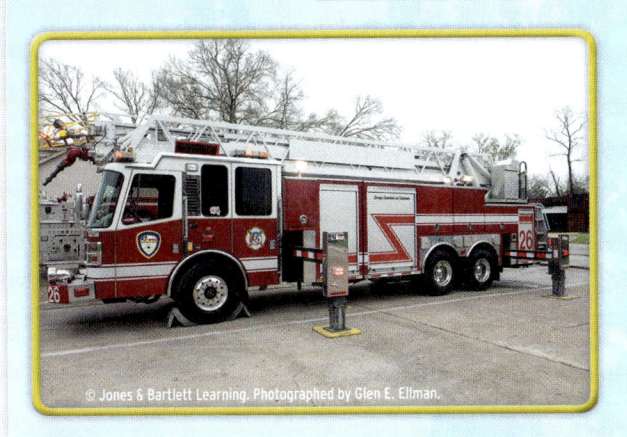

1. Position the apparatus as best as possible to utilize the aerial device to deploy an elevated stream and stabilize the apparatus.

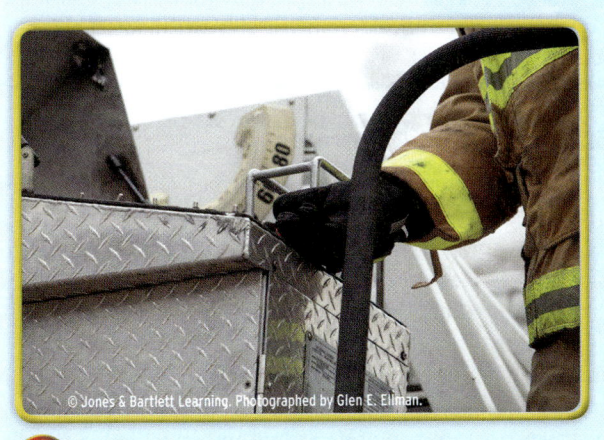

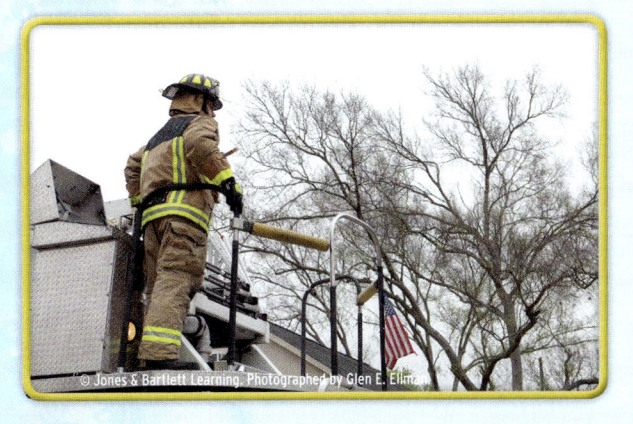

2. Access the turntable and look up and around for overhead hazards, such as electrical wires or obstructions, and for surface obstacles, such as light poles and signs.

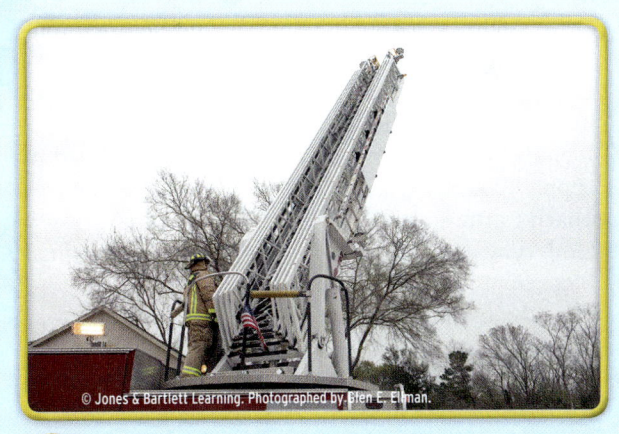

3. Raise the aerial from the bedded position and operate the controls to raise, rotate, and extend the aerial toward the location where the elevated stream is to be applied.

4. Charge the elevated stream in a manner so as to not cause water hammer or extreme reaction of the aerial device, and manipulate the nozzle and aerial as needed to achieve the desired application of the water stream.

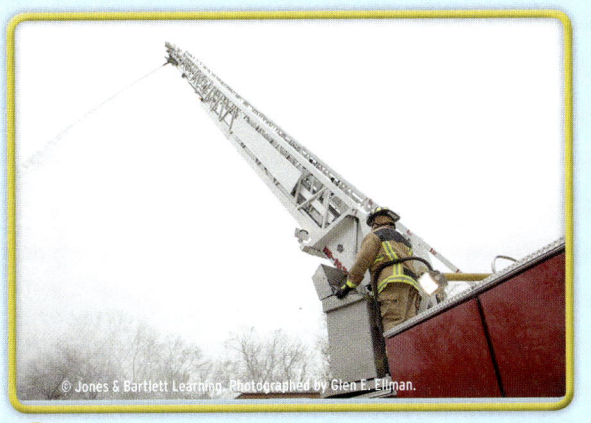

5. Maintain a position at the turntable with a hand on the control and eyes on the tip/platform observing for hazards and listening for needs of the tip/platform members.

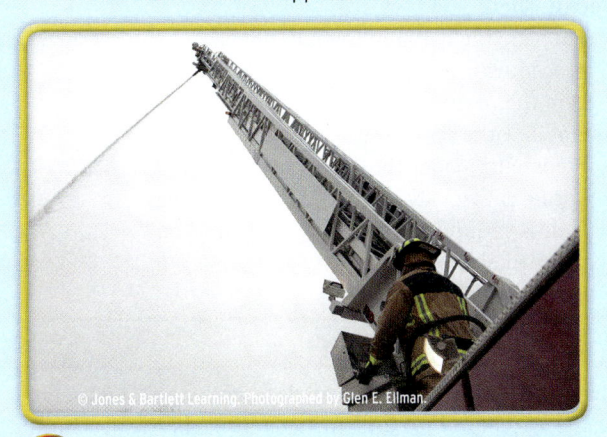

6. When the elevated stream is no longer needed, reduce the pressure at the supplying pump and close off the supply valve, rather than closing the valve at the tip/platform.

© LiquidLibrary

Key Points for the Driver/Operator

As the assigned driver/operator, consider the following:

Before dispatch:
- Know your aerial's operator's manual thoroughly, including stabilization requirements and load limitations.
- Perform and complete a thorough check of the aerial during each shift worked or at least weekly if on call.
- Practice, practice, practice positioning, stabilizing, and maneuvering the aerial at a variety of structures in your area.

Upon dispatch:
- Recall your previous knowledge of and experiences at the structure, including not just fires but also emergency medical services (EMS) and service calls. These can aid in decision making.
- Understand the nature and other dispatch information that can aid in making positioning decisions.
- Use preplan information to confirm the structure and occupancy type.

En route:
- Drive safely. Be part of the solution and not the problem. An aerial that never arrives is useless.
- Listen to the two-way radio traffic to gain insight and information about the nature of the incident.
- Identify possible water supplies that may be needed to supply an elevated stream.

On approach to the scene:
- Slow down and drive slowly as you enter the final block approaching the scene.
- Note the building type and occupancy. Is it what was expected?
- What is the separation between the building and the roadway or parking lot? This includes landscapes, hardscapes, and parked vehicles.
- Note the terrain, environmental conditions, fire and smoke conditions, and victim locations that may impact final positioning.

Once positioned:
- Energize the aerial following the manufacturer's in-cab procedures.
- Don the required PPE.
- Stabilize the apparatus.
- Prepare to maneuver the aerial device as required.
- Locate previously identified water supplies.
- Unless required otherwise, maintain your position at the turntable controls.

Skill Building

Training in operating the aerial needs to go far beyond merely setting the apparatus up and maneuvering the device in an open space behind the fire station or in a parking lot. Positioning at actual structures and maneuvering the aerial ladder or platform around structural features or obstacles is a must. There are several ways to accomplish this kind of skill building.

■ Positioning and Setup

Seek out the permission of property owners to bring the aerial to their property and set it up to check what can be reached and which issues with accessibility arise. Suitable surfaces that will allow access for the apparatus should be verified. It may be easier to start with buildings owned by the governing body or other governmental agencies that can provide access on days they are not open for business. Schools, for example, usually have winter and spring breaks as well as summer time when the fire department could operate without disturbing students. At these residential, commercial, industrial, and institutional structures, actually position the apparatus, stabilize it, and maneuver the ladder near the structure. In some cases, it may be possible only to position and stabilize the aerial apparatus without disturbing the occupants or their business functions, but that is better than doing nothing.

> **DRIVER/OPERATOR Tip**
>
> Positioning should include all sides as well as corners where sweep and scrub activities can be practiced. Use good public relations skills to avoid embarrassing occupants on upper floors.

■ Stabilizing the Apparatus

Seek out parking lots and roadways free of regular traffic and use that have differences in lateral and longitudinal grades. Use these areas to practice stabilizing the apparatus when side-to-side or front-to rear (or both) grades are present. These operations may also require the use of cribbing blocks to build up the area under one or more stabilizers. Other challenges that should be practiced include stabilizing the aerial apparatus where there is no road shoulder, a poor shoulder, or unimproved surfaces. An instructor or company officer can find suitable locations to challenge the driver/operator under supervision.

■ Operation of Aerial Controls

To build proficiency with the aerial's turntable controls, there are several options for practicing:

1. With the aerial properly stabilized in an open area free of overhead hazards, securely tie a rope to the tip or platform. At the other end of the rope, secure either a traffic cone or a small, lightweight object. Space out one or more other traffic cones or other targets such as old tires, plastic barrels, or similar objects that the operator can set the load into. Then simply practice smoothly maneuvering the controls to raise, extend, rotate, and lower the load into the target. For new operators, controls can be operated individually with a focus on achieving a smooth and jerk-free technique. As skill is developed, maneuvers should be combined and speed developed to produce a perfect technique that results in rapid, efficient, and smooth results.
2. If the fire station, training tower, or other structure owned by the governing body has multiple roof or wall levels, the aerial can be properly stabilized in an area

free of overhead hazards. Then the operator can trace the outline of the walls and roof, maintaining a safe and uniform distance from the structure while smoothly maneuvering the controls to raise, extend, rotate, and lower the tip or platform. Start by operating each control individually; then, as skill is developed, combine the various maneuvers. However, when working in close proximity to a structure, a safe operation—not speed—is the objective. This same evolution can be used for building proficiency with the tip or platform controls as well as the turntable controls.

3. One often-overlooked but essential skill related to rear-mount ladders or platforms is the ability to raise the unextended aerial up completely vertical, rotate it 180 degrees, and then lower it while extending it to an objective. When roadways or driveways are narrow or tree-lined, this skill may be vital to a successful operation. A narrow path is not necessary to practice this skill. Many locations, such as a parking lot or space behind a fire station, will be suitable for this evolution.

■ Maneuver to Multiple Windows/Targets

Training towers or actual structures where the fire department has permission for training should be used to practice maneuvering the aerial ladder or platform. The driver/operator should be given orders to maneuver from the bedded position to a specific window. Upon successful completion, the driver/operator should be directed to move to a different window—one that is not simply adjacent, but rather will require the aerial to be rotated, retracted or lowered, and/or raised or lowered. An evolution may include rebedding the aerial or lowering its tip or platform to the ground each time. As competence is developed, maneuvering around obstacles, overhangs, and other encumbrances can be incorporated into the training.

■ Maneuver to the Roof

Through the use of a variety of structures, most of the same positioning, stabilizing, and maneuvering skill development exercises can be applied to both flat and pitched roof operations. Any structure with a roof will allow for practice with setting the ladder tip or platform to the roof. Both flat and pitched roofs should be used during such training. Key considerations include making sure that the driver/operator and the fire fighter at the tip/platform communicate via radio or intercom, that the controls are feathered to prevent the aerial from striking the parapet or roof, and that changes in the load when fire fighters get on or off the tip or platform have been accounted for so as to minimize the risk of deflection.

■ Flow Water into a Training Tower

If a training tower is available, the operator can practice applying an elevated stream to a building. First, ensure the structure is unoccupied. Before flowing water, make sure all doors are open and any scuppers or drains are not blocked, so that water can exit the training tower rather than overloading structural members. It is best to use the smallest flow possible, as the technique will be the same whether the flow is 200 gpm (800 L/min) or more than 1000 gpm (4000 L/min). A 1- to 1¼-inch (25- to 32-mm) tip can be used if a solid-bore stream is desired. For a fog stream, a 200 to 300 gpm (800 to 1200 L/min) fog nozzle can be used. Remember to remove these nozzles when training is completed to ensure the aerial is battle-ready for an actual fire. Skills that can be practiced include charging the master stream device to avoid water hammer and shock loads, maneuvering the master stream device itself using its controls or remote controls, and maneuvering the aerial to keep the stream reaction/nozzle force in line with the aerial versus perpendicular to the ladder or platform.

■ Combining Multiple Skills

Additional skills that the driver/operator should practice include the following:

- Rapidly bringing the aerial tip or platform with a simulated victim and a fire fighter to the ground so the victim can be offloaded by other responders, and then returning the aerial to ferry another victim.
- Positioning the aerial for flat roof access when there is a tall parapet, which will require the use of a ground ladder either affixed to the aerial tip or platform or resting against the top of the parapet wall. This technique must be planned and trained on before fire fighters and a driver/operator attempt it at an actual emergency.

An Example of Skills in Action

On December 24, 2006, at approximately 10:00 hours, the Prospect Heights (Illinois) Fire District dispatched fire fighters to a reported fire in a condominium complex. The complex consisted of several three-story wood-frame buildings arranged in connected groups of four. Each building had 24 units. A flat roof of lightweight construction and a Mansard façade for the third floor were part of the design.

Upon arrival of the first engine company, it reported smoke showing **FIGURE 15-42**. The company officer entered to make a complete size-up and discovered a second-floor fire extending from the lobby **FIGURE 15-43**. As he upgraded the alarm and ordered his company to stretch a hand line, the second engine and the tower ladder arrived. The second engine was positioned with the first engine in a courtyard, while the tower ladder proceeded to the rear, where it could access the roof and several units, including the D-side exposure should the need arise.

Because of the configuration and construction of the structure, the fire spread rapidly. Before the first hoseline could contain the fire, it had spread from the original second-floor unit to the unit next door, to the two units directly above, and into the roof. Simultaneous with this, turbulent smoke began to push out from the entire Mansard façade and more than a dozen third-floor occupants presented on both the A- and C-side balconies with the smoke pushing out behind them.

To control fire progress, the IC had the tower ladder apply its master stream onto all visible fire, while the engine companies held their positions in the stairwell. The officer assigned the aerial driver/operator to secure a water supply from the hydrant near the apparatus and pump the waterway. He also ordered one of the skilled and proficient fire fighters who was a backup driver/operator to operate the platform's turntable

392 Fire Apparatus Driver/Operator

FIGURE 15-42 Fire conditions upon arrival of the aerial company.

FIGURE 15-44 Use of an elevated stream to control a large volume of fire.

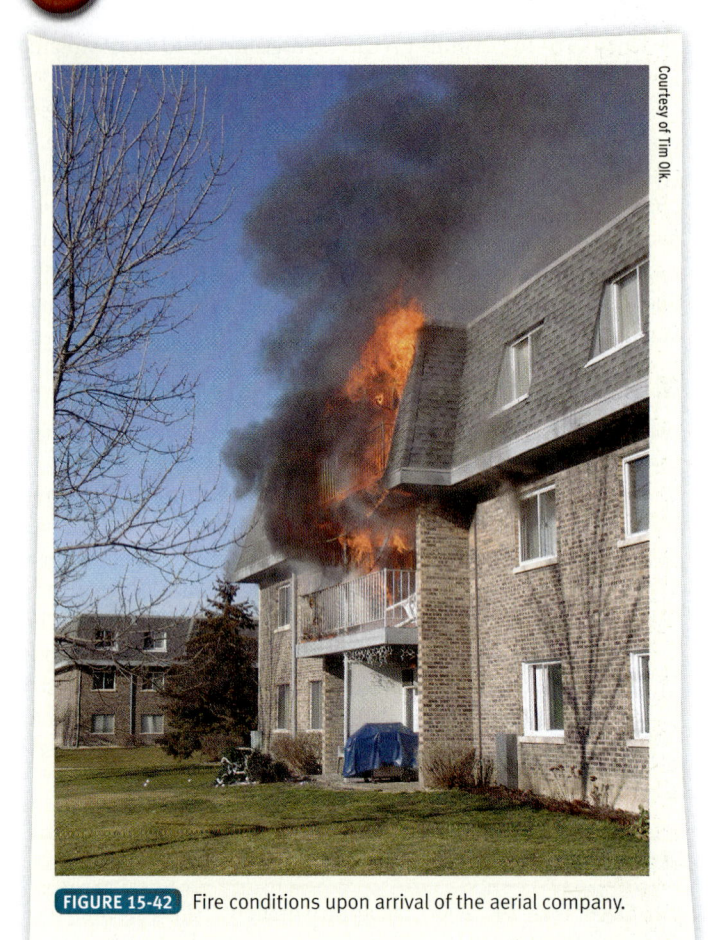

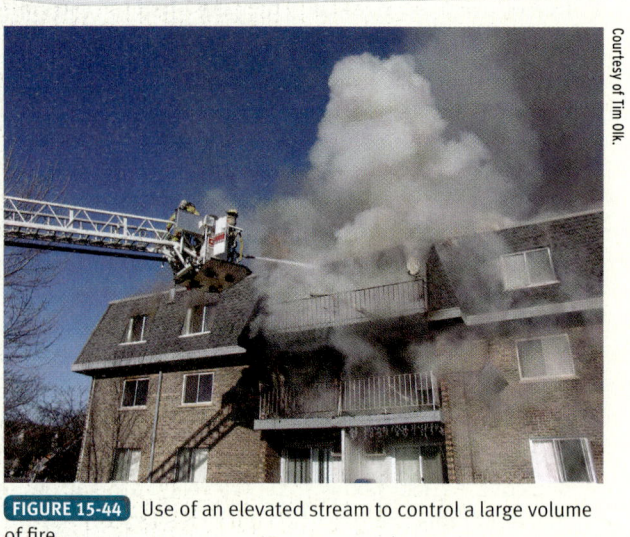

controls. Then he and the other fire fighter staffed the platform basket to maneuver the master stream into the fire units and the Mansard and roof truss space **FIGURE 15-44** . Teamwork, clearly assigned duties, and past training and experience allowed for the application of the elevated stream in a timely manner that controlled the fire enough to stop its forward progress, permit the rescue of those trapped occupants, and enable the engine companies to advance their hoselines into position for final extinguishment, search, and overhaul. While the tower ladder applied its stream, the second-arriving aerial ladder company deployed its aerial to the third floor; this company's fire fighters

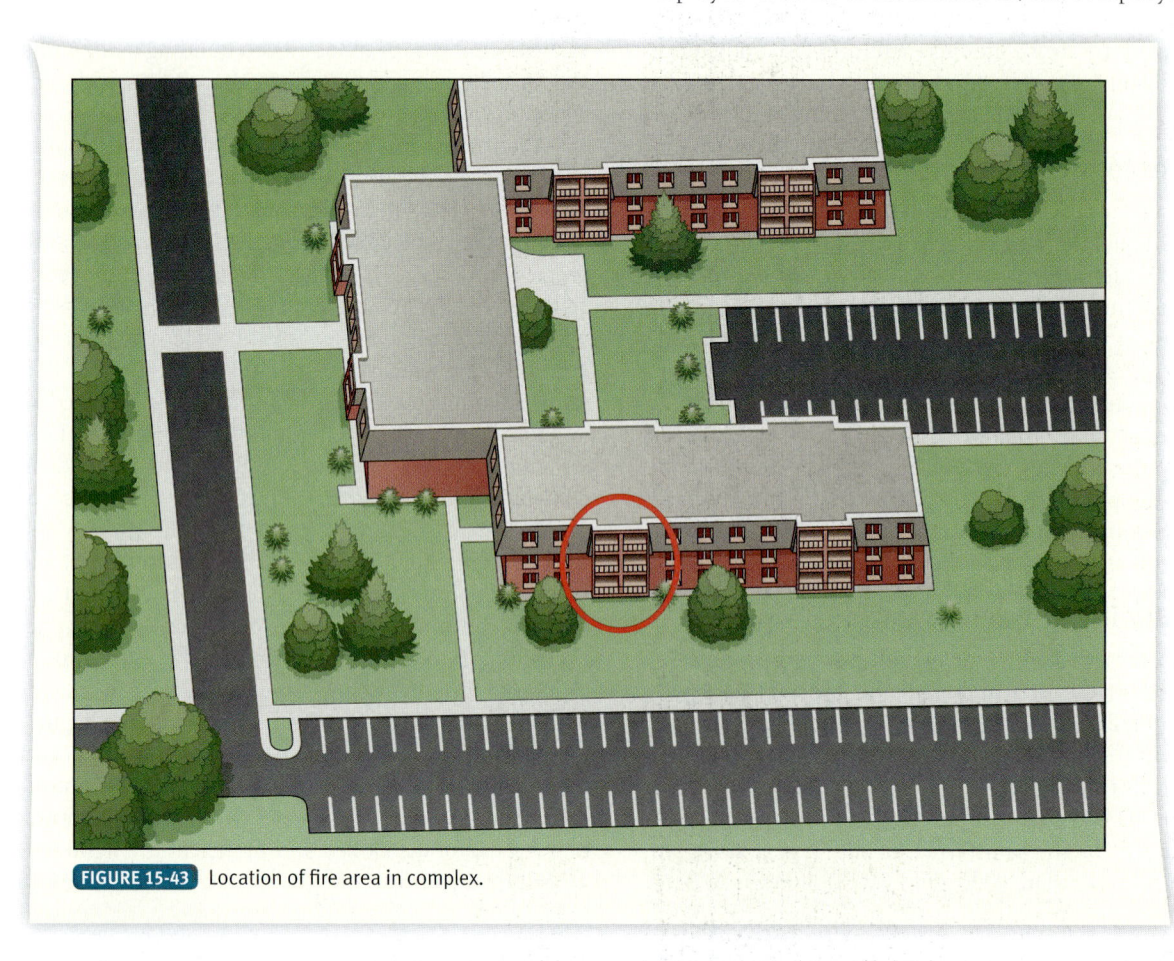

FIGURE 15-43 Location of fire area in complex.

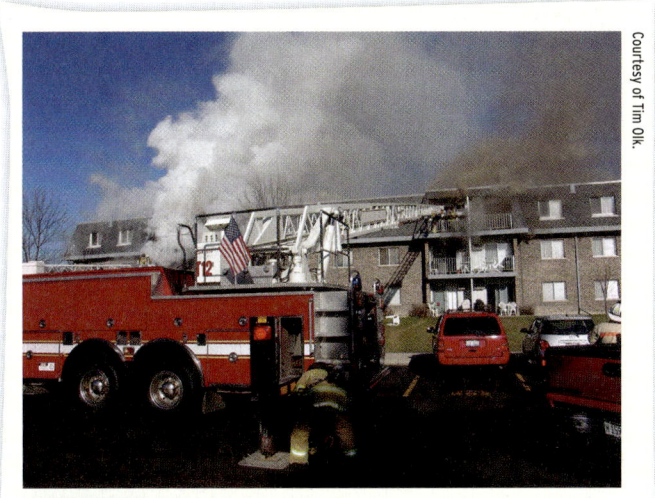

CHAPTER 15 Apparatus Equipped with an Aerial Device   393

FIGURE 15-45 The second aerial was positioned for search and rescue of the third floor—a placement that would also permit roof operations if required.
Courtesy of Tim Olk.

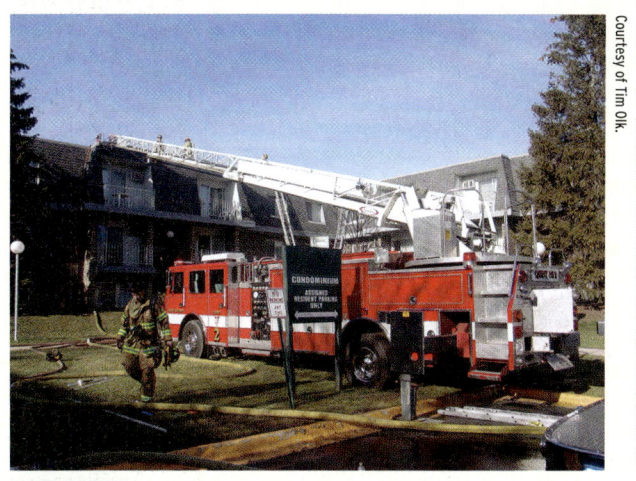

FIGURE 15-46 The third aerial positioned to ensure access and stability—note that the stabilizers are on firm ground.
Courtesy of Tim Olk.

assisted the threatened occupants and then performed a primary search **FIGURE 15-45**.

The third aerial was ordered to begin roof ventilation of the D exposure from the A side. Because of the setback of the structure from the parking lot, the driver/operator had to position the apparatus over the sidewalk to reach the roof **FIGURE 15-46**. Due to his training and experience, this occurred in short order and without delay. The fourth and fifth aerial apparatus were also ordered to positions where the D side of the fire building connected to the D exposure. The driver/operators of these aerials—a ladder and a platform—were able to position their apparatus for maximum reach and properly stabilize them while keeping a traffic lane open through which additional companies could access the scene **FIGURE 15-47**.

DRIVER/OPERATOR Tip

When faced with a rapidly spreading fire and multiple rescues needed on upper floors, it is imperative that you are well practiced, so other companies can count on you!

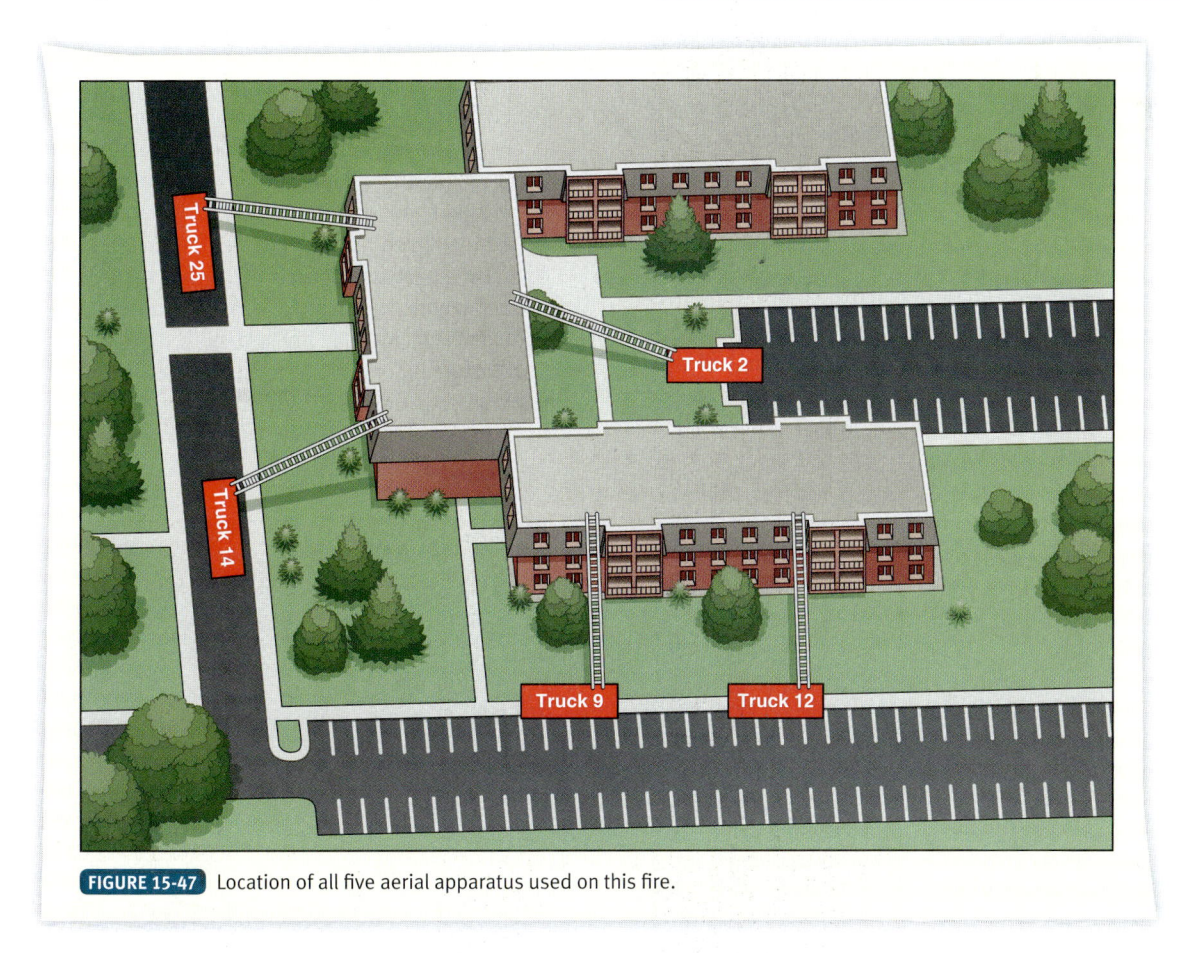

FIGURE 15-47 Location of all five aerial apparatus used on this fire.

Wrap-Up

Chief Concepts

- The aerial apparatus should be an effective tool, not just an expensive taxi.
- The driver/operator should use the aerial apparatus to support the tactical priorities, in the following order: (1) rescue, (2) exposure protection, (3) ventilation, and (4) application of an elevated stream.
- There are three types of aerial apparatus: the straight ladder, the elevated platform, and the articulating platform. Straight ladders and elevated platforms are the most commonly encountered units.
- Most aerial ladders are of truss construction, meaning that the driver/operator must understand how the load of the ladder itself applies compression and tension to the truss. The driver/operator must also understand how resting any portion of the aerial's truss against a structure can reverse this compression and tension, leading to damage or device failure.
- The chassis powertrain supplies energy to the hydraulic and electrical systems used to operate the aerial device. It is essential that the driver/operator understands the functioning and operation of each of these systems.
- Safe and effective aerial operations starts with effective stabilization. Each aerial uses one or more types of stabilizers to achieve this goal. The driver/operator must know which type(s) are used on his or her apparatus and how to properly use them to achieve full stabilization of the apparatus prior to operating the aerial device.
- Knowing the effective reach of the aerial device is key to positioning the apparatus and performing setup.
- Positioning factors include, at a minimum, the tactical priority of the incident and any rescue profile; the structure type, occupancy, and features; the terrain characteristics and surface features as well as overhead obstructions and hazards; the collapse zone, if applicable; and the effective sweep or scrub area for the aerial.
- Stabilization begins with properly executing in-cab procedures, activating and deploying the stabilizers, and finally setting the stabilizers in a full- or short-jacked manner to achieve the needed stabilization.
- If uneven grades are encountered or short-jacking is required, then the driver/operator must completely understand and adhere to the operational limitations required for safe continued operation of the aerial apparatus.
- To safely operate the aerial device, the driver/operator must identify and avoid risks such as overhead electrical wires, excessive heat or flame exposure, and overloading of the aerial in any manner with fire fighters or civilians.
- Proper PPE must be worn by all members operating on the aerial. This includes fall protection.
- An aerial apparatus should never be used as a crane.
- When using the aerial apparatus to deliver an elevated stream, the driver/operator must compensate per the manufacturer's recommendation to reduce load.
- When presented with excessive winds or the build-up of ice or snow on the aerial device, the driver/operator must compensate per the manufacturer's recommendation to reduce load.
- To prevent damage to the apparatus, the driver/operator must take deflection of the aerial ladder or boom into account when maneuvering it.
- When conducting a rescue via the aerial device, victims should be approached from above and in the order of priority commensurate with the conditions encountered.
- The driver/operator, in consultation with the company officer, should consider the risk–benefit tradeoff of having victims attempt to climb down the aerial ladder versus lowering the tip or platform and then repositioning it if additional victims are present.
- When using the aerial device to support fire fighters performing ventilation, the driver/operator must ensure there is adequate egress from roofs and approach the work area from an upwind direction.
- When using the aerial device for an elevated stream operation, factors such as permitted load on the aerial, nozzle reaction, freezing weather, exposures, collapse zone, and reach of the fire stream must all be considered.
- The water supply must be adequate for the fire stream gpm flow desired. Either direct pumping into the waterway or the use of the aerial's own pump or an adjacent engine company may be necessary to ensure an adequate flow.

Hot Terms

articulating platform An aerial device consisting of two or more booms connected at midsection by a hinge or swivel and equipped with an area where two to four fire fighters can stand and perform work.

big-box A large, free-standing commercial structure generally in excess of 100,000 square feet of floor space.

collapse zone A distance away from a structure equal to or greater than 1.5 times its height.

deflection The downward movement of an aerial device boom or ladder caused by its extension or the imposition of load such as fire fighters or victims climbing on the ladder or into the platform.

downriggers Mechanical devices, usually hydraulically powered, that exert downward force onto the ground and distribute the aerial apparatus' load over a large surface area, effectively stabilizing the vehicle so as to permit its aerial device to be raised, extended, and rotated without collapse.

elevated platform An extendable boom or ladder equipped with an area where two to four fire fighters can stand and perform work. Includes tower ladders and ladder towers.

full-jacking The complete extension and setting of all stabilizers on an aerial apparatus.

jacks Mechanical devices, usually hydraulically powered, that exert downward force onto the ground and distribute the aerial apparatus' load over a large surface area, effectively stabilizing the vehicle so as to permit its aerial device to be raised, extended, and rotated without collapse.

outriggers Mechanical devices, usually hydraulically powered, that exert downward force onto the ground and distribute the aerial apparatus' load over a large surface area, effectively stabilizing the vehicle so as to permit its aerial device to be raised, extended, and rotated without collapse.

physical rescue An act that requires multiple fire fighters to move a victim onto and off of an aerial device when the victim is unable to do so alone.

power take-off (PTO) A gear of a motor or transmission used to supply mechanical power, which is then used to operate an aerial device.

rescue profile The experience-based determination of victim survivability and the ability of fire fighters to attempt a rescue when all facts and circumstances are considered.

scrub or sweep area The total area of a one or more walls of a building, both width and height, that can be effectively reached by an extended aerial device without repositioning the chassis.

setback The distance between the wall of a building and an improved surface (such as a road or parking lot) from which an aerial device can be positioned and operate.

short-jacking The complete extension and setting of the stabilizers on one side of an aerial apparatus, while the opposite-side stabilizers are not completely extended outward before they are set down to stabilize the apparatus.

stabilizers Mechanical devices, usually hydraulically powered, that exert downward force onto the ground and distribute the aerial apparatus' load over a large surface area, effectively stabilizing the vehicle so as to permit its aerial device to be raised, extended, and rotated without collapse.

straight ladder An extendable aerial device without a work platform; usually made of truss construction and equipped with ladder rungs for climbing.

strip mall A commercial structure usually of a single story with a common façade and attic and multiple occupancies.

Wrap-Up, continued

References

National Fire Protection Association (NFPA) 1002, *Standard for Fire Apparatus Driver/Operator Professional Qualifications.* 2014. http://www.nfpa.org/codes-and-standards/document-information-pages?mode=code&code=1002. Accessed March 27, 2014.

National Fire Protection Association (NFPA) 1071, *Standard for Emergency Vehicle Technicians Professional Qualifications.* 2016. http://www.nfpa.org/codes-and-standards/document-information-pages?mode=code&code=1071. Accessed December 30, 2014.

National Fire Protection Association (NFPA) 1901, *Standard for Automotive Fire Apparatus.* 2009. http://www.nfpa.org/codes-and-standards/document-information-pages?mode=code&code=1901. Accessed March 27, 2014.

National Fire Protection Association (NFPA) 1911, *Standard for the Inspection, Maintenance, Testing, and Retirement of In-Service Automotive Fire Apparatus.* 2012. http://www.nfpa.org/codes-and-standards/document-information-pages?mode=code&code=1911. Accessed December 18, 2014.

National Fire Protection Association (NFPA) 1983, *Standard on Life Safety Rope and Equipment for Emergency Services.* 2012. http://www.nfpa.org/codes-and-standards/document-information-pages?mode=code&code=1983. Accessed December 30, 2014.

U.S. Fire Administration/Technical Report Series. *Aerial Ladder Collapse Incidents.* USFA-TR-081/April 1996. https://www.usfa.fema.gov/downloads/pdf/publications/tr-081.pdf. Accessed August 14, 2014.

DRIVER/OPERATOR in action

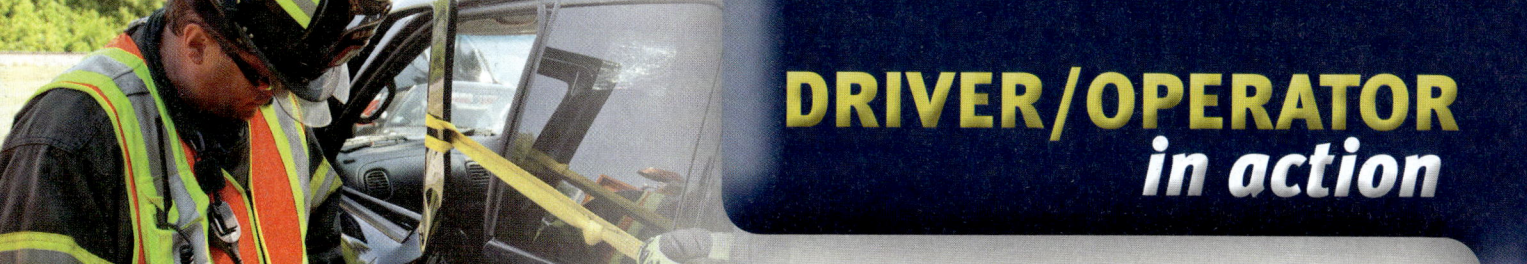

You are assigned as the driver/operator of your company's aerial apparatus for a multiple-company evolution at the training center. Your company officer briefs you that upon arrival, the IC will assign the aerial to deploy its elevated stream into the upper-floor windows of the training tower; that an engine company will be assigned to supply the aerial's waterway. As you depart for this drill, you should be prepared to answer several questions:

1. Which surface hazard may be present where you need to position at the training center?
   A. Storm water manhole
   B. Overhead power wires
   C. Large-diameter hoselines
   D. Other participating fire apparatus

2. Which gpm (L/min) flow will the supply pumper need to send to your aerial if you are using a 2-inch (50-mm) solid-stream nozzle?
   A. 500 (2000)
   B. 750 (3000)
   C. 1000 (4000)
   D. 1250 (5000)

3. How will you estimate elevation of the stream so the pump operator can calculate the necessary pump discharge pressure?
   A. Complete length of aerial extension
   B. Use a graph or table located at the turntable controls
   C. Estimate height using past experience
   D. Mathematical calculation using angle of elevation

4. When using an elevated stream, the number of members occupying the aerial's tip or platform must be reduced based on which information?
   A. Length of the aerial device
   B. Total gpm (L/min) being flowed
   C. General weather conditions
   D. Data published by the aerial apparatus' manufacturer

5. If the stabilizers on one side of the aerial apparatus cannot be fully extended but can be otherwise deployed, which operation(s) can be performed?
   A. All operations
   B. No operations
   C. Only operations on the fully extended side of the aerial apparatus
   D. Only those operations directly over the cab or straight off the rear of the chassis

6. When the evolution is complete, the water supply to the elevated stream should first be shut down at which location?
   A. The fire hydrant being used
   B. The supplying fire pump
   C. The base of the waterway
   D. The master stream nozzle

Driving Apparatus Equipped with a Tiller

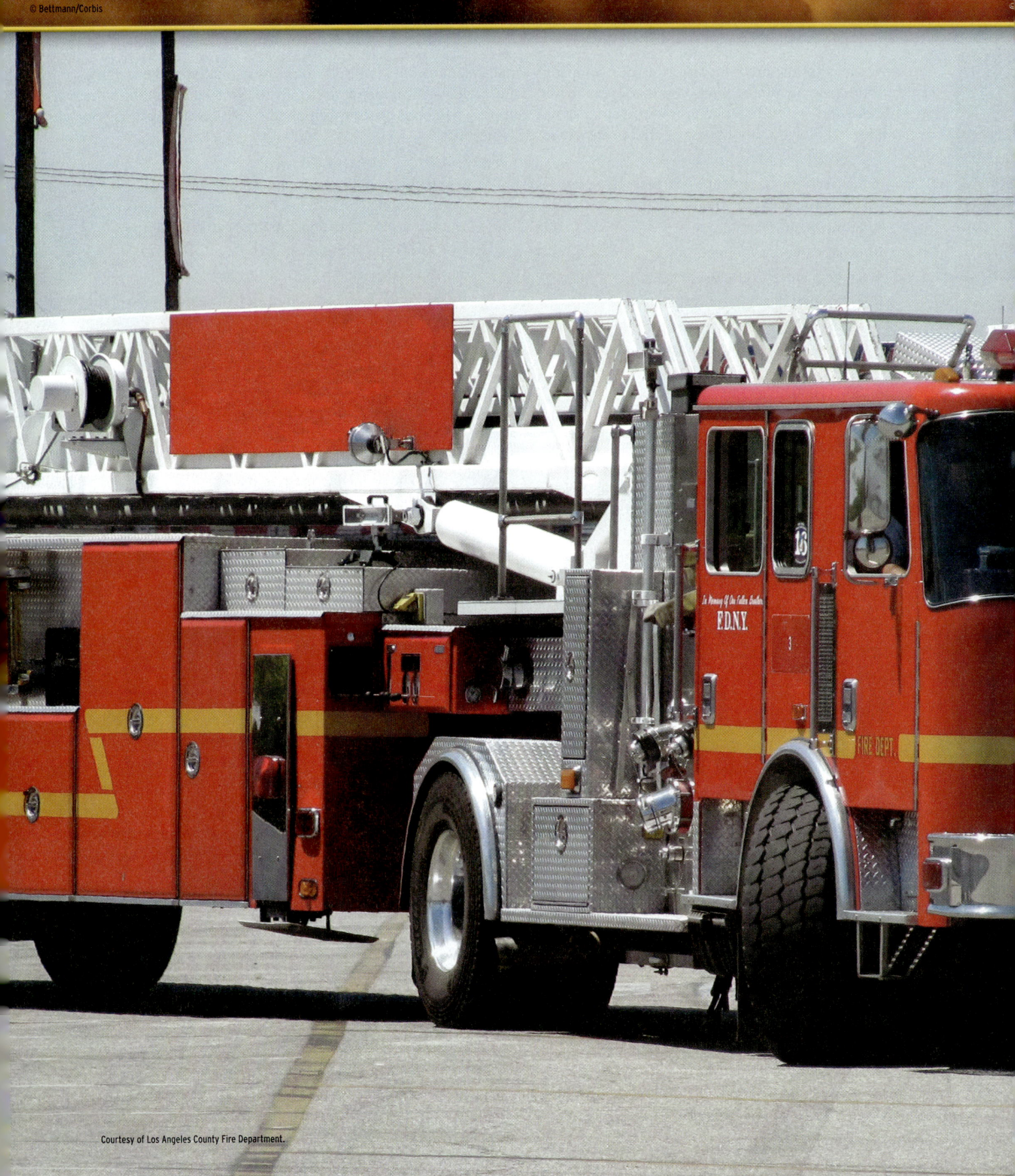

CHAPTER 16

Knowledge Objectives

After studying this chapter, you will be able to:

- Describe the principles of tiller operation. (NFPA 1002, 7.1, 7.2.2(A) ; p 406–407)
- Describe the methods of communication with the tiller apparatus driver. (NFPA 1002, 7.2.2(A) ; p 401–403)
- Describe the effects on vehicle control of general steering reactions, night driving, and negotiating intersections. (NFPA 1002, 7.2.2(A) ; p 400–401, 403–410, 412)
- Describe the manufacturer operation limitations for tiller aerial devices. (NFPA 1002, 7.2.1(A) ; p 406)
- Describe the capabilities and limitations of tiller aerial devices related to reach tip load, angle of inclination, and angle from chassis axis. (NFPA 1002, 7.2.1(A) ; p 414–416)
- Describe the use of a tiller aerial device. (NFPA 1002, 7.2.3(A) ; p 413–416)

Skills Objectives

After studying this chapter, you will be able to:

- Demonstrate the ability to determine the correct position for the tiller. (NFPA 1002, 7.2.1, 7.2.2, 7.2.3, 7.2.3(B) ; p 406, 414–416)
- Demonstrate the ability to maneuver the tiller into the correct position. (NFPA 1002, 7.2.1(B), 7.2.2 ; p 406, 414–416)
- Demonstrate the ability to avoid obstacles to tiller operations. (7.2.1(B), 7.2.3(B) ; p 400–401, 403–410, 412)
- Demonstrate the ability to operate the communication system between the tiller operator's position and the driver's compartment. (NFPA 1002, 7.2.2(B) ; p 401–403)
- Demonstrate the ability to maintain control of the tiller while accelerating, decelerating, and turning. (NFPA 1002, 7.2.2(B) ; p 400–401, 403–406)
- Demonstrate the ability to operate the vehicle during nonemergency conditions. (NFPA 1002, 7.2.2, 7.2.2(B) ; p 407–410, 412–413)
- Demonstrate the ability to operate under adverse environmental or driving surface conditions. (NFPA 1002, 7.2.2(B) ; p 406, 415–416)
- Demonstrate backing up a vehicle from a roadway into restricted spaces on both the right and left sides of the vehicle, given a fire apparatus, a spotter, and restricted spaces 12 ft (3.7 m) in width, requiring 90-degree right-hand and left-hand turns from the roadway, so that the vehicle is parked within the restricted areas without having to stop and pull forward and without striking obstructions. (NFPA 1002, 4.3.2, 7.2.1, 7.2.2 ; p 404–405, 407–408)
- Demonstrate the ability to maneuver a vehicle around obstructions on a roadway while moving forward and in reverse, given a fire apparatus, a spotter for backing, and a roadway with obstructions, so that the vehicle is maneuvered through the obstructions without stopping to change the direction of travel and without striking the obstructions. (NFPA 1002, 4.3.3, 7.2.1(B) ; p 407, 409)
- Demonstrate the ability to turn a fire apparatus 180 degrees within a confined space, given a fire apparatus, a spotter for backing up, and an area in which the vehicle cannot perform a U-turn without stopping and backing up, so that the vehicle is turned 180 degrees without striking obstructions within the given space. (NFPA 1002, 4.3.4, 7.2.1, 7.2.1(B), 7.2.2 ; p 407, 409)
- Demonstrate the ability to maneuver a fire apparatus in areas with restricted horizontal and vertical clearances, given a fire apparatus and a course that requires the operator to move through areas of restricted horizontal and vertical clearances, so that the operator accurately judges the ability of the vehicle to pass through the openings and so that no obstructions are struck. (NFPA 1002, 4.3.5, 7.2.1(B) ; p 407, 409)
- Demonstrate the ability to use mirrors and judge vehicle clearance. (NFPA 1002, 4.3.2(B), 4.3.3(B), 4.3.4(B), 4.3.5(B) ; p 404–405)

You Are the Driver/Operator

You are the driver/operator of an apparatus equipped with a tiller. A new fire fighter has been assigned to be your tiller operator. The new fire fighter advises you that he has been trained by another shift for this role. Your fire officer has asked you to ensure the new fire fighter is properly trained in the tiller operator position.

1. Should you just rely on the new fire fighter's word or should you test the new tiller operator?
2. Which questions might you ask the new tiller operator?
3. Which skills might you want to test the new tiller operator on?

Introduction

Of all the apparatus in the fire service, the rig that has the most interesting configuration is the tractor-drawn tiller aerial. This aerial apparatus has the unique feature of requiring two drivers to operate the vehicle so that it can get from the firehouse to the incident and back again safely. This concept has been around for many years.

As buildings expanded upward in cities across the United States during the 1800s, the fire service found it necessary to develop ever-longer ladders. To get these ladders to and from incidents, longer-frame apparatus were designed as transport vehicles. The sheer length of these apparatus made it difficult to maneuver them through cities' narrow streets and around tight corners. Allowing the rear wheels to turn and having a driver in the rear to steer these wheels gave the longer vehicles a reduced turning radius, which allowed the extended apparatus to negotiate the challenges inherent in the city environment.

Today's modern tiller aerial follows the same principles as those vehicles of yesteryear. The tiller aerial is a tractor-drawn vehicle with two operators. The driver of the tractor—that is, the **driver/operator**—is responsible for operating this vehicle like any other vehicle. The driver/operator must get the vehicle to all incidents while following all road laws and maintaining control of the vehicle. The **tiller operator** (also referred to as the trailer operator or tillerman) assists the driver/operator by controlling the trailer. With the assistance of the tiller operator controlling the path of the trailer, the driver/operator can maneuver the vehicle in and out of traffic and around tight corners.

The layouts of many city streets can create tricky challenges for emergency response drivers as they seek to get the apparatus from the firehouse to the incident. For example, traffic patterns along the streets and traffic arteries will likely affect the response. Major traffic thoroughfares may become congested during prime commuting hours, necessitating that fire apparatus weave in and out of traffic or take alternative routes. Traffic islands placed down the middle of some major traffic arteries may safely separate cars and vehicles traveling in opposite directions, but present obstacles to fire apparatus.

Pedestrian safety is an important issue in every U.S. city. Traffic-claiming devices are often deployed that provide changes in street alignment—for example, barriers, sidewalk bump-outs, speed bumps, and other physical measures that are designed to reduce traffic speed or reroute traffic volume **FIGURE 16-1**. Public transit passenger islands in the middle of the street make it easier for people to board and exit public transit vehicles **FIGURE 16-2**. While such mechanisms may certainly protect pedestrians, they also affect how fire apparatus respond to incidents and influence how drivers may position apparatus on the fireground.

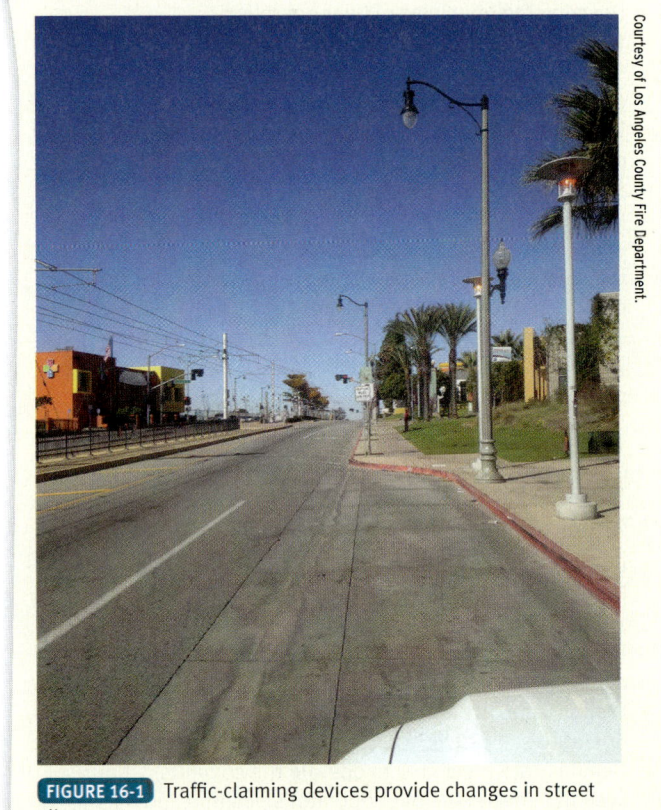

FIGURE 16-1 Traffic-claiming devices provide changes in street alignment.

Safe Driving

The number one priority when driving emergency vehicles—or any vehicle (personal or business), for that matter—is safety. As an apparatus operator, you are responsible for getting your

FIGURE 16-2 Public transit passenger islands.

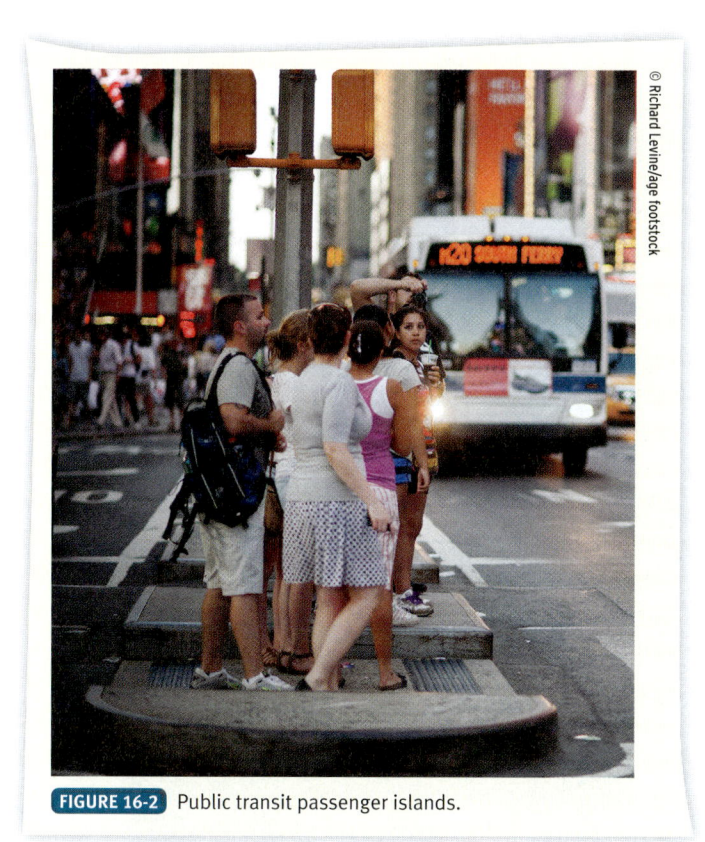

crew to the incident safely. Reckless and aggressive driving to an incident will put your crew, pedestrians, and other vehicles at risk, with dangerous consequences in the balance. Moreover, the driver/operator's inability to get the crew safely to an incident will prevent the crew from doing the tasks required to mitigate the situation, whether it is a fire call or any other emergency. Failure to get a truck company to the fire scene means other companies may have to operate on the scene with limited ability to force entry, search, rescue victims, ventilate a structure, or ladder a building.

En Route

Rapid response is essential for effective handling of emergencies, including limiting property damage and saving lives. Given the potentially variable role played by traffic conditions in the response, the ability to drive fast should not be considered a skill that will get the company to the incident more quickly.

Many factors will determine the rate of speed at which the apparatus will travel. Traffic congestion, weather, road conditions, apparatus condition, and experience of the driver/operator and tillerman are all factors that will affect the speed at which the apparatus responds. Thus, the driver/operator must weigh all of these variables when determining the appropriate driving speed—a speed that is reasonable and proper for the existing conditions, even if the law permits the vehicle to respond at a higher speed than you are driving.

As part of the quest to eliminate the mentality that "greater speed is the fastest way to an incident," crews must be educated that the most efficient way to an incident is getting on the rig and getting out the firehouse in a timely manner. That is the best way to save time when responding to an emergency.

> **DRIVER/OPERATOR Tip**
>
> Driving in heavy traffic can be a very stressful experience. The driver/operator must be cognizant of everything that is happening around the rig. Making a lane change in heavy traffic with a fire apparatus can really test the driver/operator's driving skills. An experienced tiller operator can assist the driver/operator with a lane change in heavy traffic.

Turning at Intersections

En route to an emergency, the most dangerous place—and the most likely place for an accident to occur—is the intersection. The operator must use caution as the apparatus approaches busy and blind intersections. Be mindful that the thought process and actions to safely stop a large fire apparatus will require more time and distance. The two most difficult maneuvers are (1) right-hand turns from a dedicated right-hand turn lane with a vehicle to your left and (2) traveling through an intersection from the opposite side and continuing through to the correct right-hand side **FIGURE 16-3**.

Modern cars are insulated against outside noise, bicyclists often ride with headsets, and pedestrians routinely cross streets while texting or talking on the phones. Consequently, fire apparatus driver/operators must be on the lookout for other people and vehicles that are oblivious to their presence and always be prepared to stop as they approach the intersection. If the intersection has a red light, the driver/operator must bring the apparatus to a complete stop and ensure that the intersection is clear or cross traffic has stopped before proceeding with the rig through the intersection.

Major intersections will have multiple lanes with cross-traffic traveling in opposite directions. In such a setting, the driver/operator must bring the apparatus to a complete stop. Look both ways. Once automobile drivers in the closest lane yield to the apparatus, the driver/operator can proceed into the intersection slowly. If the car in one lane yields to the fire rig, the driver/operator should not expect all cars in the other lanes to automatically yield. In addition, the driver/operator must continue to observe all lanes as the truck proceeds through the major intersection.

Communications

The driver/operator must rely on the tiller operator to safely operate the apparatus, and the tillerman must know what the driver/operator is doing so as to assist the driver/operator maintain control of the apparatus. Thus, good **communication** is essential between the two drivers, and the driver/operator and the tillerman should always follow their department's standard operating procedures/standard operating guidelines (SOPs/SOGs).

In older apparatus, a buzzer system was set up in the cab of the tractor and the tiller box. A simple tap of a button created a sound/signal that allowed the driver and the tiller

FIGURE 16-3 Taking a right-hand turn from a dedicated right-hand turn lane with a vehicle to the left during normal driving conditions. During an emergency, the fire apparatus would be in the center of the roadway and the car would be yielding to the right.

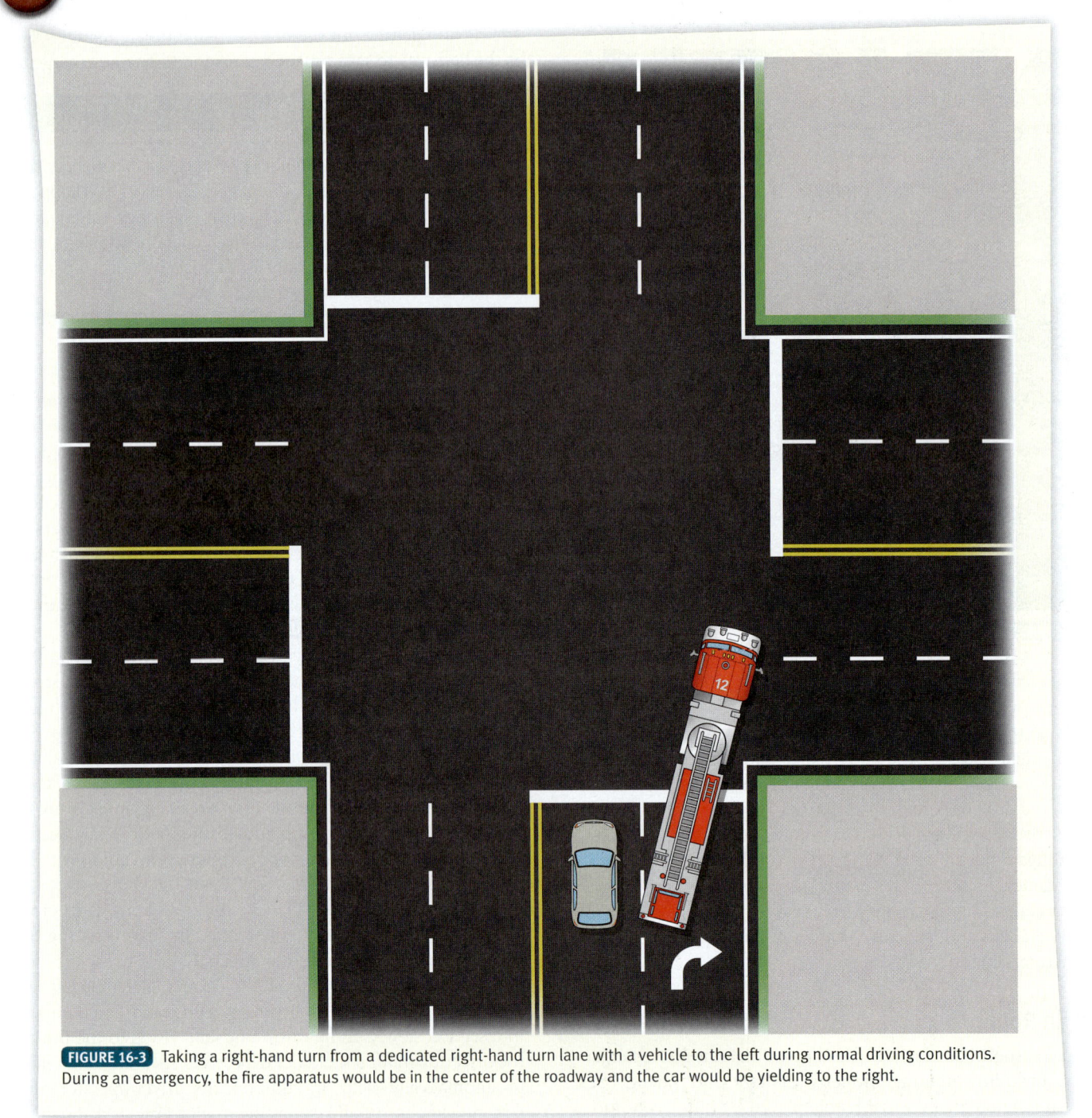

operator to communicate with each other. Communication was kept simple, given the rudimentary nature of this system. A series of codes was instituted so that the driver/operator and the tillerman were able to communicate the essential information. The signal system was as follows:

- One sound: stop
- Two sounds: go
- Three sounds: reverse

This signal could originate from either the driver/operator or the tiller operator. Whoever received the signal acknowledged it by sending back the same signal. The only signal that did not require an acknowledgment was the one-buzz "stop" signal sent from the tiller operator. When the driver/operator heard one buzz, he or she was expected to automatically stop the rig.

In all tiller-equipped apparatus (old and new), a turn signal indicator is also installed in the tiller box. Thus, the tiller operator is always aware if the driver/operator is turning left or right.

On modern apparatus or refurbished older rigs, headsets are installed for each riding position on the rig. All fire fighters assigned to that rig for the shift should have access to a headset. Such equipment allows all fire fighters to communicate with one another while they are on the apparatus.

Over many years, the roaring noise of the apparatus engine and high-pitched sound of the siren have damaged the hearing of many fire fighters. The headsets, however, both give the fire fighters the ability to communicate in a noisy environment and protect their hearing. For these reasons, headsets must be used at all times when fire fighters are riding in the apparatus.

> **Safety Tip**
>
> The driver/operator must communicate with the tillerman to make sure the tiller is ready to go. Confirm that there is a response from the tillerman before driving off; otherwise, the driver/operator could easily put the rig in drive and take off without a fire fighter in the tiller box.

> **DRIVER/OPERATOR Tip**
>
> To execute a lane change, the driver/operator and the tiller operator can communicate both with turn signals and via headsets. Once the lane to which the driver/operator wishes to change over is clear, the tiller operator can adjust the trailer steering wheel to slide the tractor over to the clear lane. Swinging the trailer over first will prevent automobile traffic from coming up on the side of the apparatus and allow the driver/operator to safely move the rig over and complete the lane change.

Vehicle Control

The driver/operator and the tiller operator must work as a team to keep the tractor-drawn aerial under control. As a general rule, the driver/operator is responsible for the tractor portion of the apparatus, while the tiller operator is responsible for the trailer end. To ensure that both the driver/operator and the tillerman operate as one cohesive unit, effective communication between the two is of utmost importance.

The driver/operator has the responsibility of getting the crew to the incident safely and quickly. He or she must possess knowledge of the response area, determine the route, and dictate the speed of the vehicle based on the road conditions, weather, vehicle traffic, and road laws.

Driving a fire apparatus is both challenging and nerve wracking. The stress level is further intensified when driving in an urban environment. Whether driving on a major traffic artery with multiple traffic lanes or on narrow streets with traffic traveling in opposite directions, the driver must keep the vehicle within the lane. Keeping the vehicle within the width of a traffic lane might seem like a daunting task considering the width of the fire apparatus. When the vehicle is going straight, the driver/operator should position the vehicle so that it is hugging the lane divider on the driver's side. This tactic will give the driver/operator the confidence that the vehicle is within the traffic lane as it travels through the streets. The driver/operator must still maintain awareness of everything around the vehicle during any movement.

■ Traveling Forward

The tillerman's responsibility is to keep the trailer in-line with the tractor when the tractor is going straight. To assist with this task, a small beacon, which should be centrally located, can be installed on roof of the tractor **FIGURE 16-4**. The tiller operator can use this beacon as a point of reference to help align the trailer with the cab. From the tiller cab, the tiller operator can

FIGURE 16-4 The small beacon (yellow lights) on the roof of the tractor as seen from the tiller operator's position.

look straight down the middle of the bedded aerial ladder. If the middle of the ladder is aligned with the beacon, the tiller operator will know that the tractor is in-line with the trailer. When the tractor is going straight and the trailer is properly aligned, very little steering is required from the tiller operator. The inability of the tiller operator to keep the trailer in-line with the tractor moving forward will create a wider width for the apparatus.

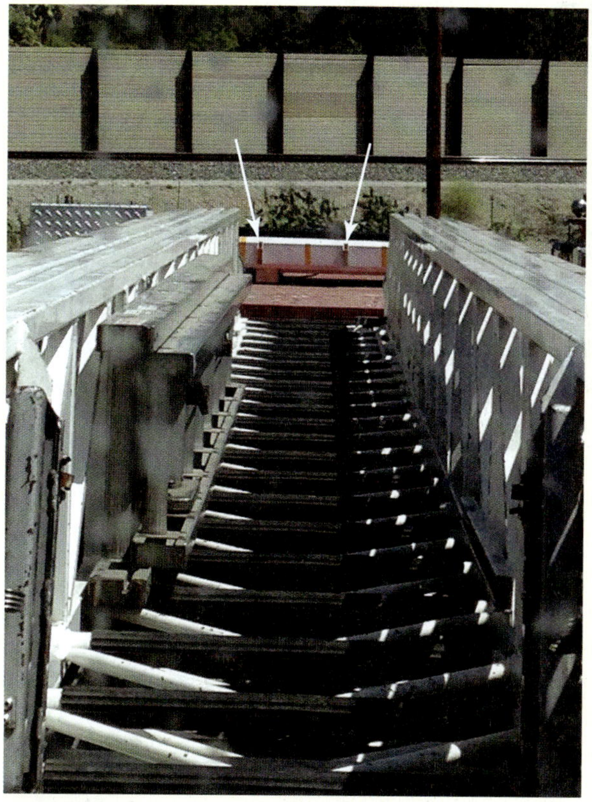

> **DRIVER/OPERATOR Tip**
>
> The tiller operator should check the position of the trailer wheels before climbing up to the tiller compartment. If the wheels are not aligned properly, the tiller operator must adjust the wheels as the apparatus begins to move. Otherwise, the trailer will sway once the truck begins to move and possibly hit objects as the truck is leaving the firehouse.

In addition to keeping the trailer aligned with the forward-moving tractor, the tiller operator is responsible for noticing obstructions on both sides of the trailer, anticipating upcoming traffic conditions, and maintaining awareness of situations behind the rear of the trailer. The tillerman can also communicate with the driver/operator to stop or slow down, if in doubt about any situation.

FIGURE 16-5 When making a right-hand turn from a dedicated right-hand turn lane, the driver/operator must pull out far enough for the tillerman's trailer wheels to clear the corner.

FIGURE 16-6 Turning the tiller.

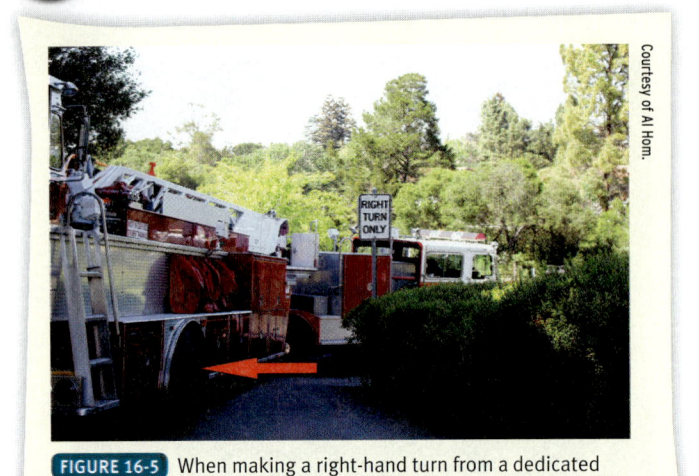

Mistakes that tiller operators may make include **over-steering**, **under-steering**, and **over-tillering**. When the tractor and the trailer are in-line and going straight, the tiller operator should simply hold onto the wheel and keep the trailer straight. The tillerman can make the trailer swing out to the right or left by turning the steering wheel to the right or left, respectively.

Procedures for Negotiating Intersections

During the turns (specifically, right-hand turns), the driver/operator can assist the tiller operator by making a wide turn. This maneuver will limit the distance the tillerman is required to swing out to clear the corner and complete the turn. Where the streets are wide enough, the tillerman may not be required to turn the wheel if the driver/operator makes a wide and safe turn **FIGURE 16-5**.

When the streets are narrow or parked cars reduce the width of a street, the driver/operator and the tiller operator must work as a team to make a safe and complete turn. If the apparatus is approaching the fire block and must turn right at the approaching intersection, the driver/operator can communicate his or her intentions to the tiller operator as the apparatus nears the intersection via the headset and the turn signal. The driver/operator will assist the tiller operator by driving out into the intersection as far as possible to safely make the turn. This maneuver eliminates the need for the driver/operator to cut the corner. As the driver/operator makes the right turn, the tiller operator swings the tractor out left by turning the wheels in the opposite direction of the driver to avoid the curb, objects on the sidewalk, or parked cars **FIGURE 16-6**. Allowing enough room for the **overhang** to clear both sides of the trailer, the tillerman must also look left to ensure that the vehicle does not swing too far left and strike any object. Once the truck is halfway into the turn, the tiller operator begins to turn the steering wheel in the opposite direction to bring the trailer back in-line with the tractor. If the tiller operator waits until the apparatus has completed the turn before turning the wheel back to its in-line position, the trailer will hit objects on the sidewalk or parked cars in adjacent lanes.

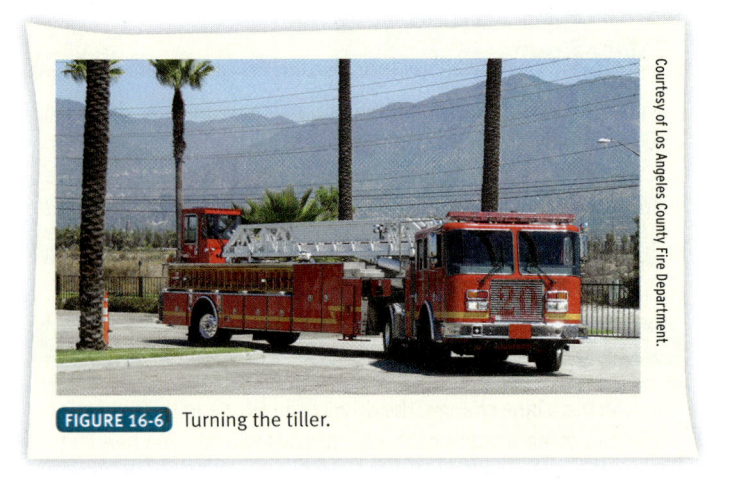

Backing Up

A driver/operator of a fire apparatus will make some moves with his or her vehicle that are taken for granted in this role—but that civilians will never make in a lifetime with their personal vehicles. Among those moves are putting the apparatus in reverse and backing it into the firehouse many times during a shift and backing an apparatus straight down an entire city block.

At the firehouse, the driver/operator pulls the apparatus past the apparatus bay that stores the ladder truck, with the entire apparatus moving past the firehouse doors. The tiller operator swings the trailer out and angles it toward the firehouse to create a shorter turning radius for the truck as it is backing in. Once the entire apparatus is past the truck bay doors and the trailer is angled properly, the driver/operator puts the apparatus in reverse and begins backing into the firehouse **FIGURE 16-7**. During this maneuver, the tiller operator looks left and right and behind to control the trailer and guide the trailer portion into the firehouse. Once the rear of the trailer and tiller box has cleared the sides of the apparatus door, the tiller operator can look up and locate the center of the apparatus door. The top of this door should be marked with a vertical line in the middle. The tiller operator should line up the middle of the bedded aerial ladder with that vertical line as the driver is

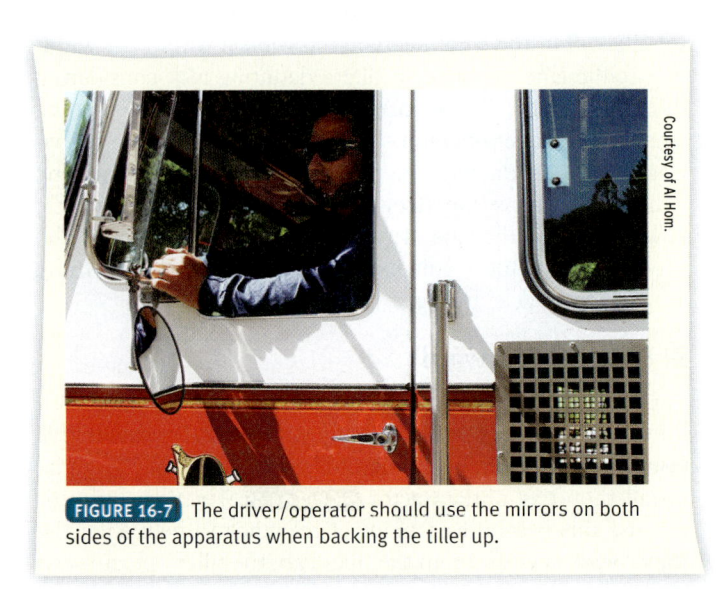

FIGURE 16-7 The driver/operator should use the mirrors on both sides of the apparatus when backing the tiller up.

backing the apparatus into the firehouse. This will help ensure that the trailer comes in straight to the firehouse.

> **Safety Tip**
>
> When backing the apparatus, the driver/operator should use the mirrors on both the driver side and the officer side. The driver/operator should not turn his or her head to look backward.

The driver/operator focuses on backing the tractor and aligning the dual wheels with the common targets (painted guidelines on the sidewalk and apparatus floor). Experienced driver/operators and tiller operators will have predetermined targets or markers in the firehouse that help them back the apparatus and assist the driver/operator in determining where to safely stop the rig.

Some situations may warrant backing the apparatus down a city block. For the aerial apparatus, this will usually occur when the incident is over and the truck is packed up and ready to go home. The incident could be down a dead-end street, for example, or other apparatus remaining on the scene may have blocked the truck from going forward.

When it comes to backing a tractor-drawn aerial down a city block, the responsibilities are reversed. In this scenario, the tiller operator takes the lead in backing up the truck. While the driver/operator still controls the speed of the apparatus, it is the tillerman who issues the orders.

Backing the tiller apparatus offers the tiller operator a very unique experience. The tiller operator's ability to control the steering wheel will determine the path of travel as the apparatus is moving backward. If the tiller operator turns the steering wheel to the right, the trailer of the apparatus going backward will begin to veer left, and vice versa.

One technique used by many tiller operators to help control the path of travel as the apparatus backs up relies on the positioning of the hands on the steering wheel. The operator uses the bottom half of the wheel as a point of reference. With the palm of the hands face up, the tiller operator holds the wheel at the 4 o'clock and 8 o'clock positions. As the operator holds onto the wheel, he or she points the thumbs in an outward position. As the rig moves in reverse, the tiller operator controls the path of travel for the trailer by letting the steering wheel slide through the hands. With this technique, the operator does not use hand-over-hand steering. The thumbs can be used as a reference point to control the direction the apparatus is backing up. When the steering wheel is moved in the direction in which the thumb is pointed, the trailer will move in the same direction **FIGURE 16-8**.

As the apparatus begins to back up, it is the tiller operator who gives the clearance signal, communicates with the driver/operator regarding any oncoming obstructions, and dictates the speed by telling the driver/operator, "Come on," "Slow down," or "STOP." As the apparatus backs down the street, the tillerman controls the trailer by steering—while being careful not to over-steer—the trailer, thereby ensuring that it remains on the correct course.

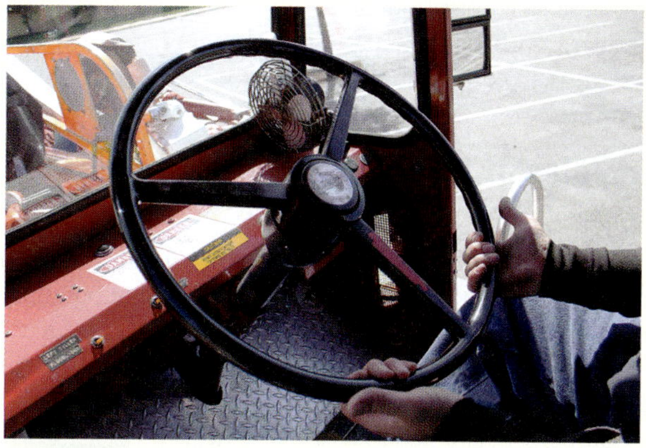

FIGURE 16-8 Steering the tiller.

> **DRIVER/OPERATOR Tip**
>
> An easy way for the tiller operator to keep track of the direction in which the trailer is traveling is to place his or her hands at the bottom of the wheel with the thumbs pointed outward. When the wheel is turned in the direction in which the left thumb is pointing, the trailer will swing left. When the wheel is turned in the direction in which the right thumb is pointing, the trailer will swing right.

When backing down a city street, if the apparatus is approaching an intersection, the tiller operator should communicate with the driver/operator about his or her intentions when they reach the intersection. Specifically, the tillerman should instruct the driver/operator if the apparatus will go straight through the intersection, turn left, or turn right.

The front-end driver/operator concentrates on the tractor as the tiller apparatus is backing down the street. The driver/operator focuses on the dual-wheel axle (driver side) of the tractor and uses the driver-side and officer-side mirrors to ensure the truck is backing down the street in the proper manner.

Anytime the apparatus is backing up, the officer and fire fighters who are not driving or tillering should work as spotters and walk alongside the moving rig.

■ Braking

The driver/operator should always be ready to stop the truck to avoid hitting an object. Be aware that a tillered apparatus is limited to a total weight of 80,000 pounds, similar to an 18-wheeler truck. An 18-wheeler, however, has at least five braking axles, while a tillered apparatus has only three braking axles, and the rear trailer axle is limited to 60 percent braking capacity because it is a turning axle.

■ Night Driving

Always attempt to keep the trailer in-line by using truck landmarks, such as the lights on the air-conditioning unit. Driving in a darkened atmosphere provides less visibility, so good communication between the driver/operator and the tillerman is crucial to safe operation. To aid in night driving, ensure that the trailer's curb lights and/or ground lights are used, if the apparatus is so equipped.

Principles of Tiller Operation

One of the many tasks that a truck company must conduct on the fireground is laddering the fire building. To utilize the aerial ladder, the truck must be parked in front of the fire building. In many older large cities, the driver/operator must maneuver the truck down narrow streets, make turns around tight corners, and weave the apparatus in and out of heavy traffic to get the truck properly positioned so as to raise the aerial **FIGURE 16-9**.

The tiller aerial ladder truck is equivalent in size to a semi big-rig or an 18-wheeler truck, but the semi big-rig has only one driver. For an 18-wheeler to make turns around a corner, its driver must take the rig far into the intersection and make as wide a turn as possible. When the driver of an 18-wheeler has to make a delivery in a big city, he or she will most often travel the city's main streets, which are wide enough to handle long vehicles.

This luxury is not afforded to emergency vehicles. Put simply, fire apparatus must have the ability to enter streets of all widths. In addition, fire apparatus driver/operators will encounter everyday challenges such as traffic islands, public transit platforms, temporary street repair/construction sites, rush-hour traffic, and events that require periodic street closures. These conditions are just some of the factors that may make it difficult for the fire apparatus to reach the incident and be positioned in front of the fire building.

The tiller operator sits in the rear tiller compartment (the tiller box) of the trailer, which is perched on top of the trailer behind the bedded aerial ladder. The tillerman's ability to control and steer the trailer—by keeping it in-line with the tractor or by having it swing right or left—enables the driver/operator to weave in and out of heavy traffic, negotiate narrow streets, and make tight turns.

■ Manufacturer Limitations

All manufacturers list the limitations of their equipment regarding turning, braking, and weight limitations. Be sure that you read and follow all manufacturer-specified limitations and recommendations prior to operating the apparatus, and know the maximum rotations of the tiller steering wheel and the different apparatus' turning radii. The number of steering wheel rotations in an apparatus may vary from 2 to 2½ to 3 full rotations from year to year and from manufacturer to manufacturer.

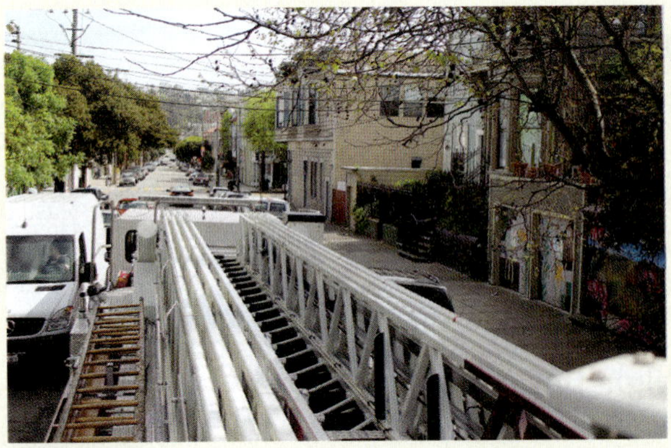

■ Maneuvering in Adverse Weather

Operating a tillered apparatus in adverse weather takes additional skill and knowledge. In such a setting, the secondary braking systems should be shut off or placed into the lowest setting. The tiller axle braking is reduced to 60 percent capacity, but when roads are wet or slick, this apparatus can still lose traction, causing a skid or slide, especially when negotiating corners. Given these risks, speed should be reduced in adverse weather and the driver/operator should always allow for additional time when stopping, due to the tiller's lack of braking systems.

Responsibilities

Before the shift starts, the officer must assign a driver/operator and a tiller operator for the entire shift. The driver/operator will be responsible for the tractor portion of the aerial truck, and the tiller operator will be responsible for the trailer (the body and the tiller section) of the truck.

The ladder truck must be inspected at the beginning of every shift. The driver/operator should check the tractor for passenger compartment cleanliness, fuel, emergency lights, head lights, rear lights, and air pressure. The driver/operator should then raise the cab and check the engine compartment for fluid levels, hoses, belts, and cleanliness. The driver/operator is also responsible for checking the tools and equipment stored in the tractor compartments. In addition, he or she should walk around the rig to check the tires and look for any new body damage.

The driver/operator of the tractor also serves as the aerial ladder operator. Once the tractor has been checked, the driver/operator will visually inspect the aerial ladder, checking the fly sections and the bedded section first, and then inspecting the rungs, the beams, and the braces for any structural damage. The driver/operator must ensure that the lights at the tip of the aerial and the intercom system on the aerial ladder, which allows a fire fighter at the tip of an extended aerial to communicate with the operator at the turntable, are in good working condition. When the driver/operator raises and extends the aerial during the daily inspection, he or she should also check the movements of the pulley, cables, and reel to ensure that they move freely and that there is no damage **FIGURE 16-10**. Additional items that the driver/operator inspects and other tests that he or she performs include the following:

- Visual ladder inspection
- Fifth-wheel bearing clearance
- Timed operational test
- Hydraulic pressure test
- Visual inspection of power take-off (PTO) and lines

The daily inspection is also a great time for new members of the department to learn about the operations of the aerial and practice how to operate the aerial ladder proficiently in a smooth

FIGURE 16-9 The tiller driving down a narrow street.
Courtesy of Al Hom.

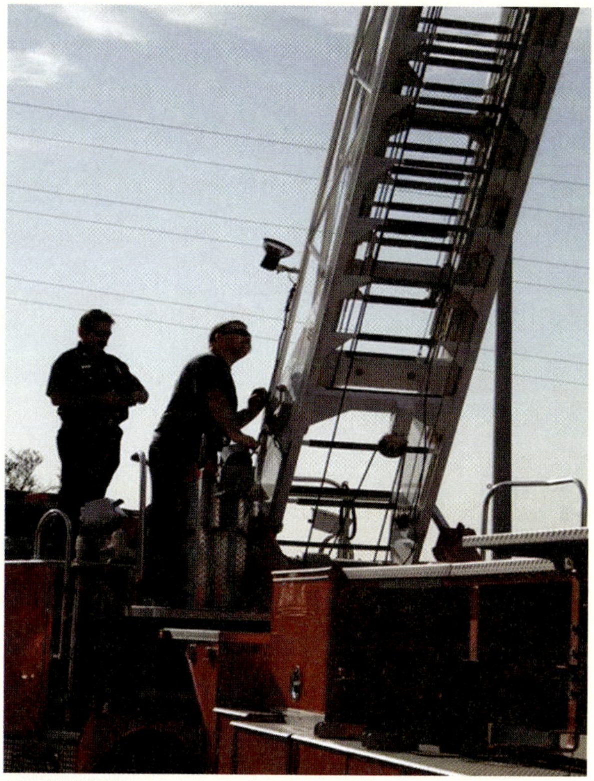

FIGURE 16-10 The driver/operator inspecting the aerial.
Courtesy of Los Angeles County Fire Department.

and efficient manner. Skills to practice include raising the ladder to specific targets and applying a feather touch at the control levers to eliminate sudden jerky movements of the aerial ladder.

The tiller operator is responsible for the trailer. At the beginning of the shift, the tiller operator should check the inventory and readiness of all the equipment situated in the trailer compartments.

New Driver/Operators

Becoming a good apparatus driver/operator and tiller operator does not happen overnight. Rather, this process takes time and patience. Before a fire fighter can get behind the wheel of an aerial ladder truck, he or she should attend an orientation class that explains the dynamics of operating a fire apparatus and a hands-on driving class that allows the fire fighter to drive a tiller apparatus around a driving obstacle course. This course includes several stations that are set with orange plastic cones.

One station is designed to allow the driver/operator to drive the apparatus in the forward direction down a lane. Once the apparatus reaches the end of the lane, the driver/operator will put the tractor in reverse, and the driver/operator and the tiller operator will back the rig back down the straight lane.

At the serpentine station, the driver/operator and the tillerman must weave the apparatus in and around a set of cones that are spaced evenly apart. The driver/operator and tillerman go forward and serpentine the truck around the cones. When they come to an end, the driver/operator puts the rig in reverse and then the truck moves backward around the cones.

Lastly, cones can be set up to simulate a ladder truck backing into a firehouse. The rig can come in from the right or the left, and the driver/operator and the tiller operator can practice backing into a simulated firehouse.

Once the fire fighters get a feel for driving and tillering the apparatus, it is time to take the information learned in lectures and the controlled obstacle course and apply it onto the streets.

Practical Driving Exercises

The best time for new fire fighters to gain street experience operating both ends of the tiller apparatus is during company drills, which can be set up by the officer. To assist the fire fighter in learning how to drive the tiller apparatus, the officer can take the company to a quiet street with no traffic or a huge outside parking lot, set up some cones, and have the driver/operator and the tiller operator practice serpentine moves going forward and backward. Cones can also be set to have the apparatus go forward and backward in a straight line. Additional practical driving exercises include the alley dock, the serpentine course, the confined-space turnaround, diminishing clearance, the straight-line drive, the lane change, straight-in parking, and crossover backing.

■ Alley Dock

The alley dock driving exercise tests the driver/operator and tiller/operator's ability to maneuver the apparatus backward from a nonrestricted area into a restricted area such as an alley, a dock, or the firehouse. This exercise exemplifies the difficulties involved in backing up the apparatus without striking walls or boundaries and being able to bring the apparatus to a stop near the rear wall. Boundary lines created for this exercise should simulate driving the apparatus forward on a street, stopping, and then backing it up into a driveway or alley **FIGURE 16-11**. The apparatus should be driven beyond the target area, stopped, then put into reverse and backed up until it is stopped at the rear boundary line. Backup guides and spotters should be utilized during this drill.

■ Serpentine Course

The serpentine driving exercise tests the driver/operator and tiller/operator's ability to maneuver the apparatus around obstacles from left to right. The tiller operator is required to maneuver the apparatus in one continuous motion around set cones while moving forward and then stop the apparatus just beyond the last marker **FIGURE 16-12**. Once the apparatus is stopped at this position, it should then be put into reverse and backed up around the cones until it is just beyond the last marker. Backup guides and spotters should be utilized during this drill.

■ Confined-Space Turnaround

The confined-space turnaround exercise measures the driver/operator and tiller operator's ability to turn the apparatus around in a restricted area, such as a cul-de-sac, without striking any obstacles. To set up this exercise with cones, establish a 50-ft (15-m) lane that is 12 ft (3.7 m) wide. Then, designate the cul-de-sac at one end with a diameter that is the length

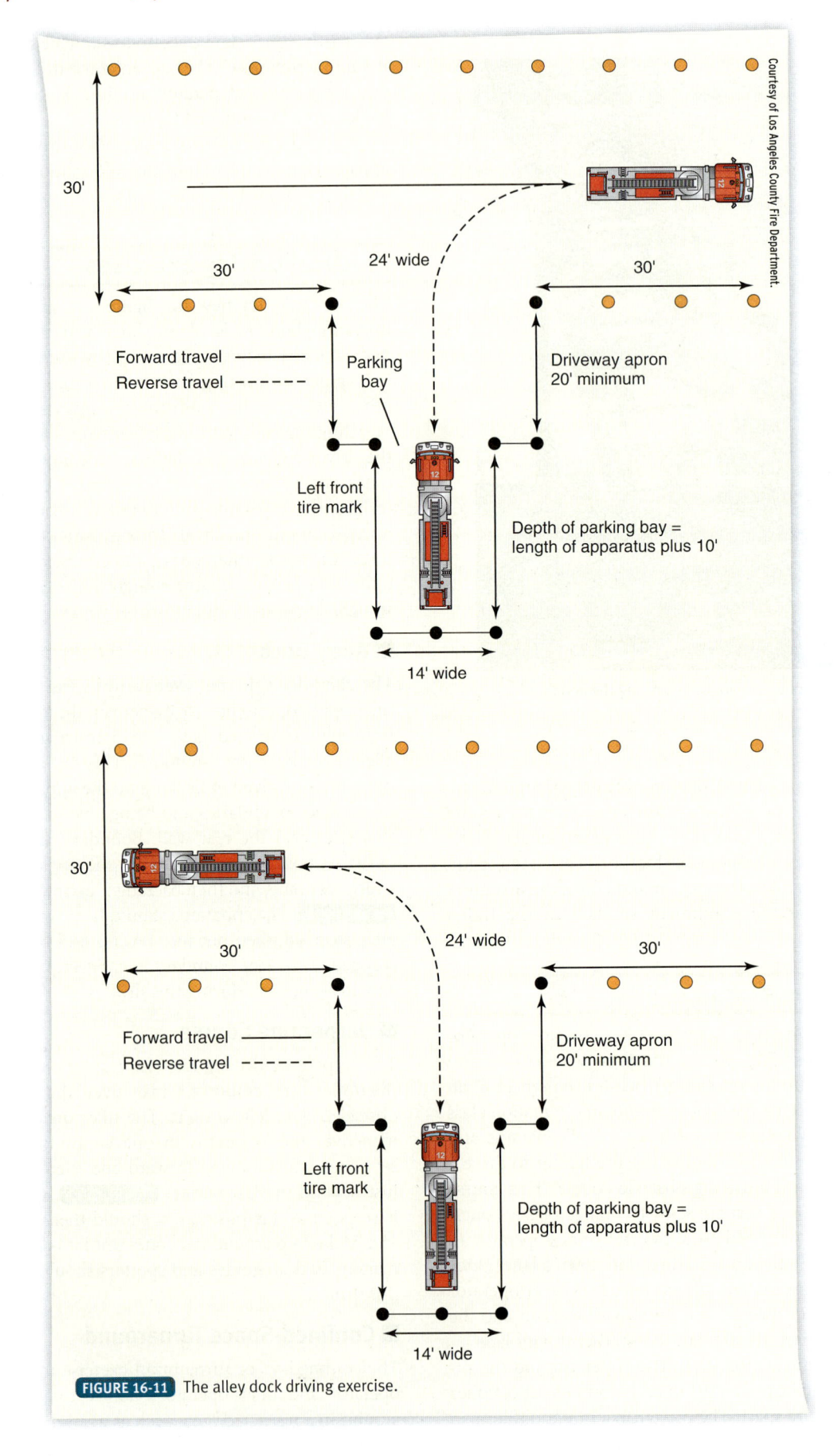

408 Fire Apparatus Driver/Operator

FIGURE 16-11 The alley dock driving exercise.

CHAPTER 16 Driving Apparatus Equipped with a Tiller 409

FIGURE 16-12 The serpentine driving exercise.

FIGURE 16-13 The confined-space turnaround exercise.

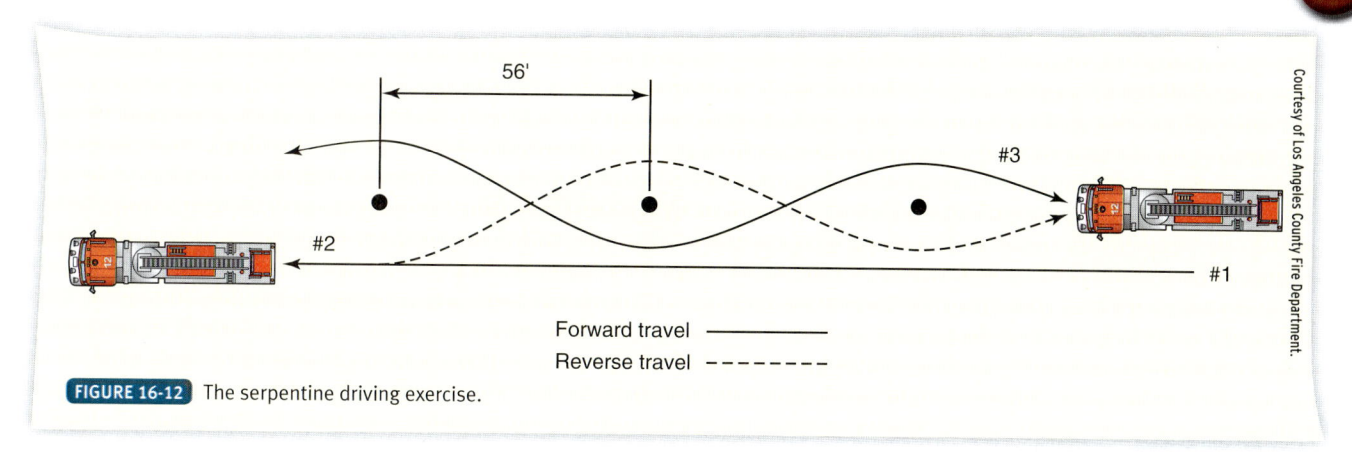

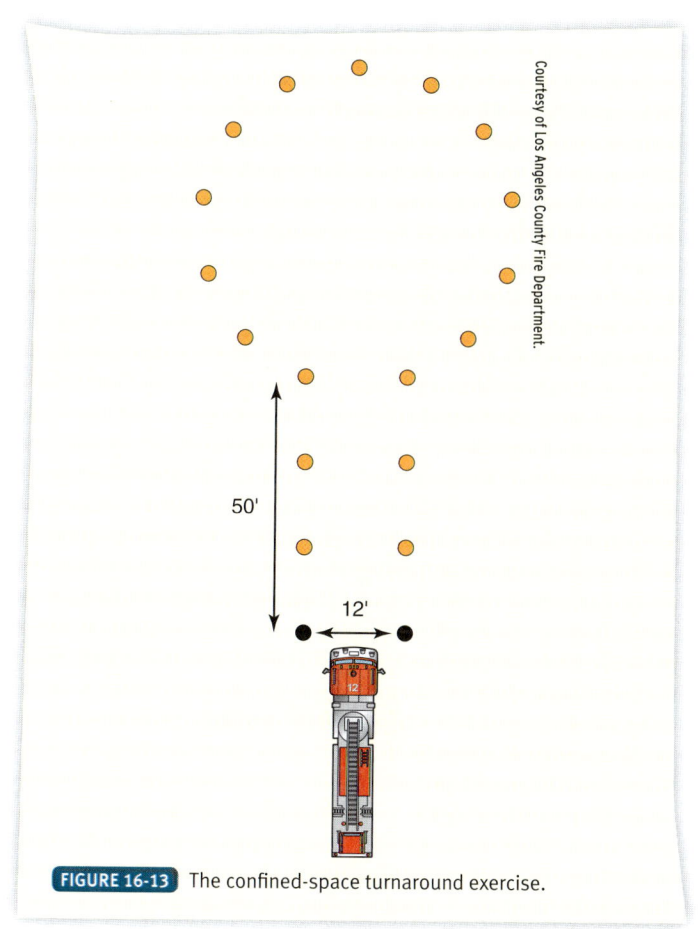

of the apparatus being used plus two times its width. The driver/operator and tiller operator will enter into the cul-de-sac through the 12-ft (3.7-m)-wide lane, turn the apparatus 180 degrees, and then return through the lane in one continuous maneuver **FIGURE 16-13**.

■ Diminishing Clearance

The exercise demonstrating diminishing clearance teaches the driver/operator and tiller operator about depth perception and the handling characteristics of a tillered apparatus. In this exercise, the driver/operator must maneuver the apparatus in a diminishing straight line without touching the set cones; thus, it measures a driver/operator's ability to judge distances from the wheel to the object while steering the apparatus in a diminishing straight line **FIGURE 16-14**. At the instructor's signal, the driver/operator and tiller operator then back the apparatus out of the lane without touching the markers. Backup guides and spotters should be utilized during this drill.

■ Straight-Line Drive

The straight-line drive exercise demonstrates to the driver/operator and tiller operator the braking characteristics of the apparatus. The driver/operator and the tiller operator first drive forward between two rows of markers, then maneuver the apparatus through this lane without touching the markers, and finally stop the tillered apparatus within 6 inches (15 cm) of the set cones **FIGURE 16-15**. At the instructor's signal, the driver/

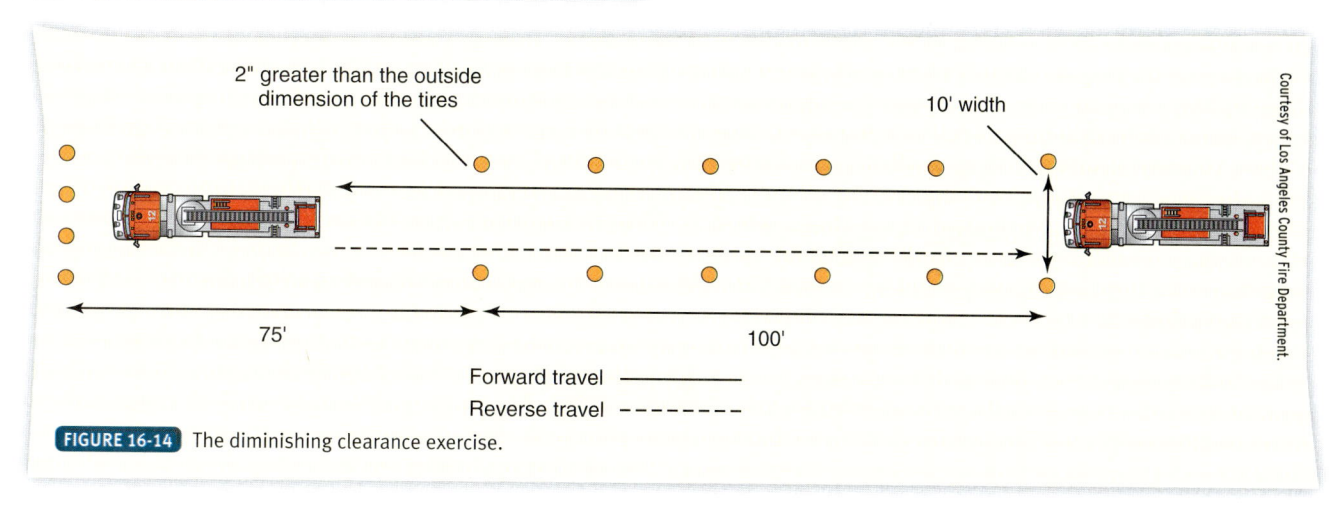

FIGURE 16-14 The diminishing clearance exercise.

FIGURE 16-15 The straight-line drive exercise.

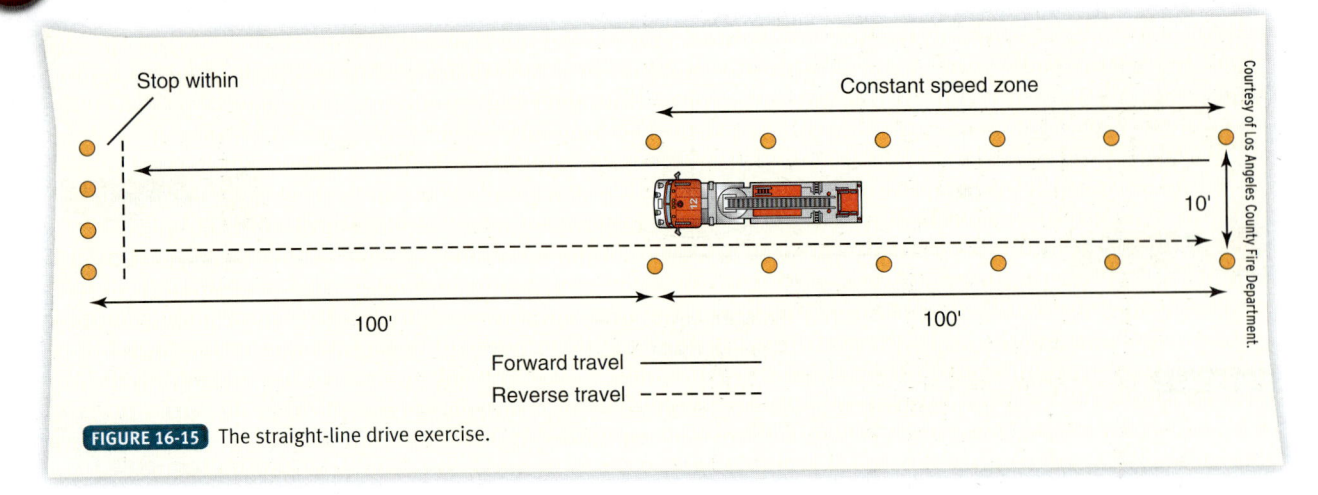

operator and the tiller operator then back the apparatus out of the lane in a straight line without touching the markers. Backup guides and spotters should be utilized during this drill.

■ Lane Change

The offset alley (lane change) exercise is a test of the driver/operator and tiller operator's ability to quickly change lane positions—a need that may arise due to changing traffic conditions. In this exercise, the driver/operator and the tiller operator maneuver the apparatus forward through the lanes in a continuous motion without touching any markers, and then stop the apparatus after it has cleared all the markers **FIGURE 16-16**. At the instructor's signal, they then back the apparatus through the lanes in one continuous motion without touching any markers, stopping the apparatus once all the markers have been cleared. Backup guides and spotters should be utilized during this drill.

■ Straight-In Parking

The straight-in (parallel parking) exercise allows the driver/operator and tiller operator to demonstrate their ability to park the apparatus safely in sites with limited space. The driver/operator and the tiller operator drive forward into the parking space using the "crabbing" technique, which requires a lateral movement of the vehicle, stopping the apparatus at the forward cones of the marked parking space **FIGURE 16-17**. They

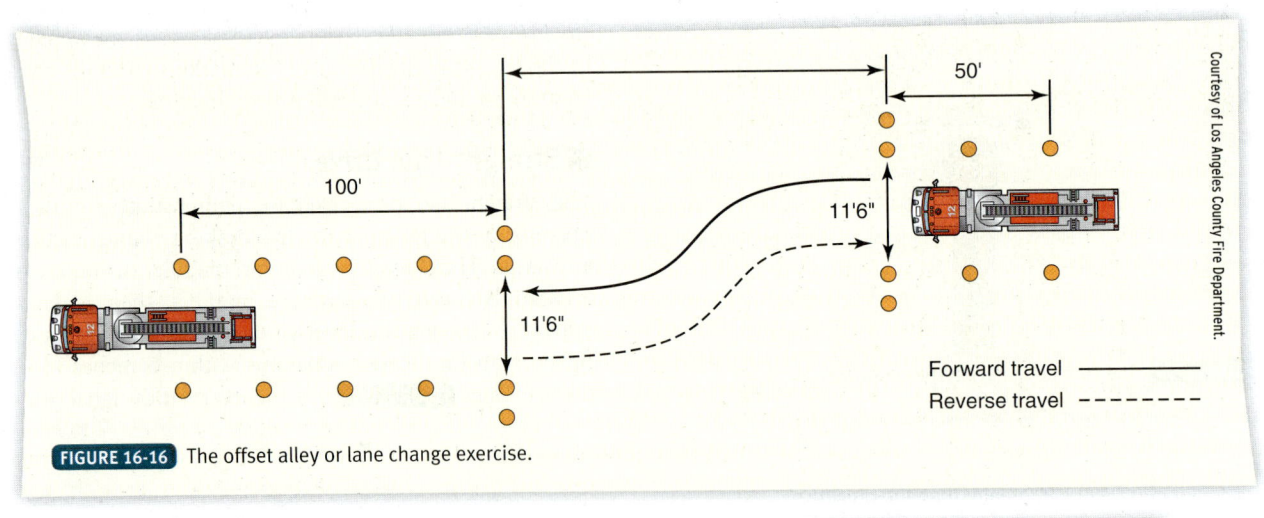

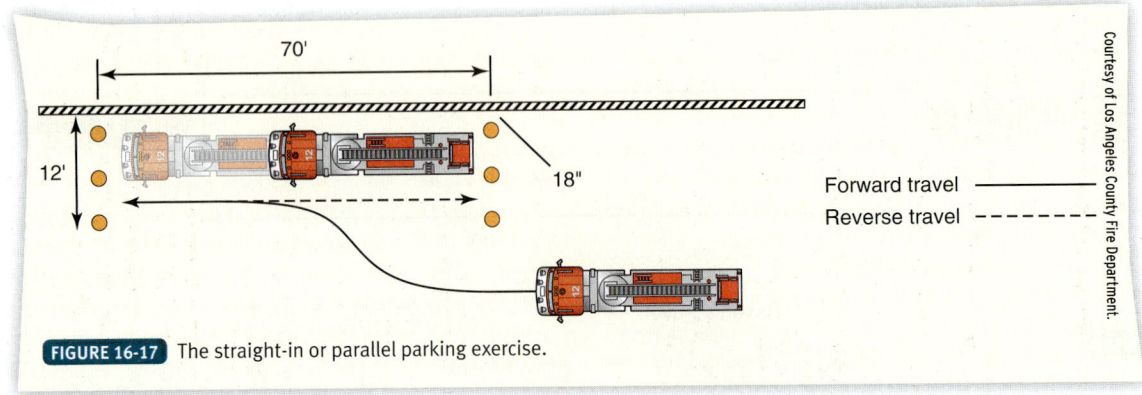

FIGURE 16-16 The offset alley or lane change exercise.

FIGURE 16-17 The straight-in or parallel parking exercise.

VOICES
OF EXPERIENCE

There is perhaps no other activity in the fire service that catches the interest of an observer more quickly than the work of a tiller operator. When a ladder truck responds to an alarm, the sight of the ladder truck maneuvering in and out of traffic with the tillerman negotiating turns that appear impossible always thrills the public. There is, however, more to the tiller operator's job than steering and maneuvering the trailer of a ladder truck. The responsibility of driving a tractor-drawn trailer is shared between the apparatus driver/operator and the tiller operator. The driver/operator is assigned the operation of the tractor, and the tillerman has the responsibility for lateral control of the trailer. It is important that the driver/operator and tiller operator are in good communication at all times.

I cannot tell you how many times I have pulled up to a fire, only to have my tillerman jump out of his seat to start putting up ground ladders or grabbing a saw and go to work without notifying me. Then, when I need to move the apparatus to a more advantageous location or different assignment—perhaps to the rear of the fire structure—I now have no one to help me move the truck. More than once has a tiller truck started moving without a tillerman in the seat. Remember, if the truck is already running, the deadman's switch does not have to be engaged to get the apparatus to move. I then find myself in the position of trying to find my tillerman or call him on the radio to return to the truck.

I have, therefore, come up with a simple solution that avoids me driving the truck down the road without a tillerman and taking out a row of parked cars in the process. Our agreement is that the tiller operator does not remove his headset or get out of the tillerbox until I have set the Maxi (parking) brake. By my setting the parking brake, I am telling the tillerman he can go to work, and if I need him, it is then my responsibility to get him to assist me with moving the truck.

Tim McIntyre
Engineer/Apparatus Operator
Los Angeles County Fire Department
Los Angeles, California

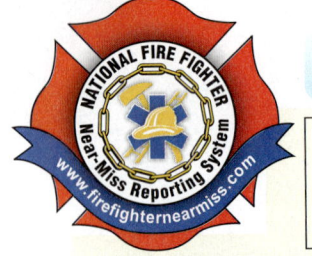

Near-Miss REPORT

Report Number: 07-0000681

Synopsis: Tiller cab hits downed powerline causing serious injuries to tillerman.

Event Description: A hurricane had just passed, and our station was on damage assessment, checking buildings that were damaged. Our response on this incident was routine. The engine and a tiller ladder truck were returning back to the station after our response. We were working on our 32nd hour of duty. The ladder, which had two drivers (one driver/operator and one tillerman) and a captain, was heading northbound at a speed of about 25 mph (40 km/h) and traveling in the left lane of a four-lane road. As the ladder approached the station, a police car pulled in front of them and stated that their tiller driver was in the street eight blocks south. The driver and the captain got into the squad car and went to the scene where they saw the tillerman in the street with critical injuries and a tiller cab that was demolished. The tiller driver suffered multiple traumatic injuries. It was determined that a low hanging power line hooked the tiller cab and tore it off the truck. The driver/operator of the ladder had no indication that anything was wrong. The ladder truck was a 100-ft (30-m) tiller drawn truck.

Lessons Learned: The tiller cab of this truck offered little protection to the person in the cab. It was hard to see a power line hanging low, but maybe it could have been recognized. A rain lip on the roof of the cab caught the power line and that should be redesigned.

---

then back the apparatus in one continuous motion to align the apparatus along the curb line. The apparatus should be within 18 inches (46 cm) of the curb when parked.

■ Crossover Backing

The crossover backing exercise is the reverse of the serpentine driving maneuver.

The Learning Curve

New fire fighters can drive or tiller the apparatus when the company is out of the firehouse during nonemergency situations. For example, they can operate the apparatus when the company must leave the firehouse for inspections, meal shopping, drills, and area orientation. New fire fighters may also drive or tiller the apparatus back to the firehouse after responding to emergencies. There should be a period of time during every shift where the apparatus should leave the firehouse and conduct area orientation.

Training the tiller operator proceeds over time and requires practice and hands-on repetition. Initial tiller operating requires a veteran operator to assist the new fire fighter who is learning the job of tillering the ladder truck. An effective aid that will allow a seasoned tiller operator to assist the new fire fighter is a seat attached just outside the tiller compartment **FIGURE 16-18**. While sitting on the outside seat, the seasoned fire fighter can offer guidance, valuable information, and assistance to the novice operator at all times.

The best way to prepare for the challenge of apparatus placement is to know your assigned district or neighborhood and become familiar with the obstacles that can affect rig placement. Familiarize yourself with the nuances of your area, get accustomed to the narrow streets, learn where the alleys are, and know which streets come to a dead end. As you survey the buildings in the area, identify those structures that you think would be extremely difficult and challenging

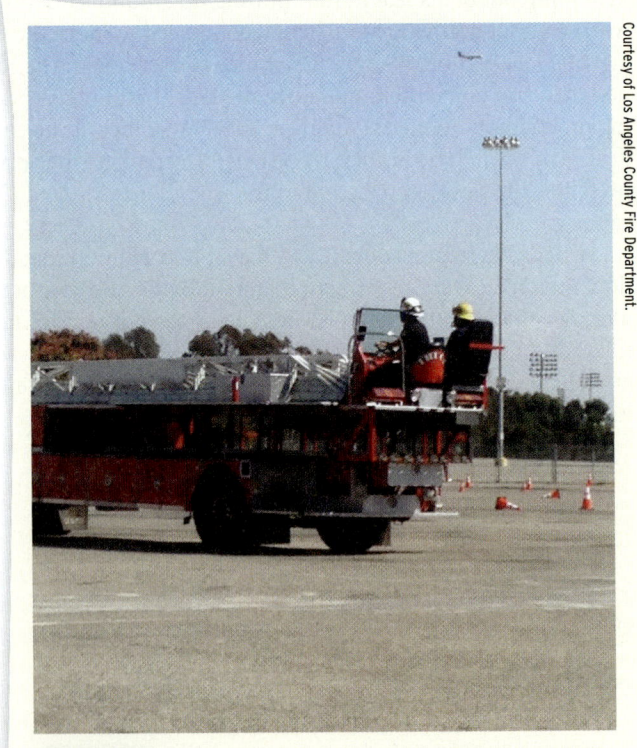

FIGURE 16-18 A seat attached just outside the tiller compartment allows a seasoned operator to assist the new fire fighter.

to approach if they were to catch on fire. If you are part of an urban fire department, take note of vacant buildings, buildings that involve plenty of police activity, and overcrowded apartment buildings. Whether you are a newly assigned driver/operator or a seasoned veteran, ask the officer to make it part of the crew's daily routine to take the rig out of the firehouse and explore the surrounding area.

Take advantage of the so-called routine dispatches. For a residential fire alarm, many fire departments will engage in a modified response and send an engine company and truck company to investigate. More times than not, the call will turn out to be a false alarm or nothing serious. However, companies must still treat it as a structure fire call until the cause of the alarm has been determined. Such responses offer great opportunities for driver/operators to familiarize themselves with apparatus placement, for several reasons. First, these dispatched companies would usually be the first-due companies at the incident address. Second, this is not a full assignment; therefore, driver/operators do not have to worry about other responding rigs. Once on the scene, position the rigs as if your company is the first-arriving group at a working fire. If the site is a larger building, the engine and truck drivers should locate and note the standpipes, fire escapes, and entryways. In addition, the truck operator should become familiar with obstacles that might potentially affect the use of the aerial device at this address.

Building inspections offer another opportunity to familiarize yourself with good apparatus placement. Check for any obstacles that might hinder engine and truck operations. Discuss where the apparatus would be positioned if a fire call were to come in. Many times the truck crew will discuss how the building should be laddered during the inspection, and engine companies can take this opportunity to discuss hose leads.

Never assume that you know where you are going—make sure you know the street, the cross streets, and the address of the incident before leaving the firehouse. Ask the officer for verification and order of other apparatus responding to the scene. Knowledge of the street and cross streets will assist in determining the quickest route to the scene. Also, the route that is selected will offer the opportunity to anticipate the direction from which other responding rigs are coming. It is important that drivers understand where other rigs are responding from. Not only does the direction of the responding rigs help determine placement of the apparatus, but it also allows safety issues to be considered. Drivers can anticipate where other apparatus may be approaching certain intersections, as rigs oftentimes will converge within seconds upon the same intersections while responding to the incident.

At the beginning of each shift, discuss neighborhood happenings—such as neighborhood block parties, parades, and street festivals—that are occurring during the shift and may affect the response time or route. If streets are closed, preplan the company's response around those street closures.

When the Alarm Sounds

When the alarm comes in, everybody goes! The crews suits up and everybody gets onboard the apparatus, strapping on their seat belts and donning their headsets. **Teamwork** between the driver/operator and the tiller operator begins with the driver/operator communicating with the tiller operator. The tiller operator must be secure and ready in the tiller box for the rig to start. Specifically, the tiller operator must typically press a button (the "dead man switch") in the tiller compartment before the driver/operator can start the apparatus. This switch is installed in newer tiller apparatus so that the driver/operator cannot start the apparatus and drive off without the tiller operator.

The driver/operator looks around the cab, making sure that everyone is onboard, and then advises the tiller operator that everyone is ready to go. The driver/operator must know the preplanned route, the cross street for the reported incident, the responding companies from other firehouses, and traffic patterns. The tiller operator must also know the response route so that he or she can anticipate any turns that the driver/operator may make to get to the incident. Getting on the rig quickly and getting out of the firehouse as rapidly as possible is the quickest and fastest way to get to an incident.

As the rig is responding to the call, the driver/operator must obey all traffic laws, operate the vehicle within safe speed limits, and always expect the unexpected. Many civilian drivers will pull aside and let emergency vehicles pass; however, many civilian drivers are now preoccupied while they are driving their personal vehicles. Not only are newer cars are better insulated against outside noise, but drivers may have their radios turned up, be talking on their cell phones, or be texting. Given these distractions, it is very easy for civilian drivers to miss seeing fire apparatus responding with lights and sirens.

When the apparatus approaches an intersection against a stop sign or red light, the driver/operator must bring the rig to a complete stop before it can enter the intersection. After checking that the intersection is clear and that cross traffic has come to a stop, the driver/operator can proceed through the intersection. When the tiller approaches a major intersection with multiple traffic lanes crossing in both directions, the driver/operator must ensure that traffic in all lanes has come to a stop.

Approaching the Incident

In most cases, the engine company is the first company to show up on the scene. Listen for the initial report and size-up of the first-due engine company. As the ladder truck approaches the fire block, observe the actions of the engine crew. The truck crew might not see any fire or smoke, but if the engine crew is pulling hoselines for deployment, it is a good sign that the call will be upgraded to a working structure fire and everybody will be going to work.

The most important thing that the apparatus driver/operator of the ladder company can do is to *slow down* and approach the fire block in a controlled manner. This will allow the driver/operator, officer, and crew to size up the situation **FIGURE 16-19**. It is important that the driver/operator know the street address and recognize that odd- and even-numbered buildings are on opposite sides of the street. Street-related factors that can affect the placement of the aerial apparatus include overhead obstructions, other fire apparatus already on the scene, narrow

FIGURE 16-19 Scene size-up.

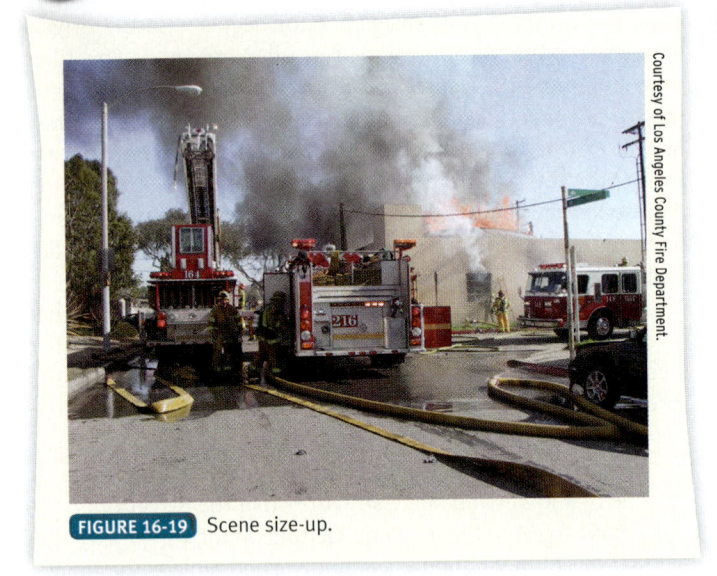

streets, and parked cars. When approaching, the driver/operator may be asked, or may decide him- or herself, to hold in a location just outside the fire area until given direction by the on-scene incident commander (IC) due to the many positioning factors with regard to this type of apparatus.

Maneuvering and Positioning a Tiller Apparatus

Driver/operators and officers should take into account all the information at their disposal when determining the best placement for the apparatus and utilization of the aerial ladder. The initial positioning effort should be considered the only opportunity for placement of the apparatus, because in most situations there will not be a chance to make any major adjustments.

Many factors must be considered in regard to aerial ladder placement. The ladder truck must be placed in front of the incident building if the crew is to have any opportunity to utilize the aerial device. At all fire incidents, engine drivers and ladder truck driver/operators must work as a team to get all apparatus positioned appropriately so that all the equipment, tools, and crews can be utilized. If the first-due truck company is parked down the block and away from the fire building, that positioning renders the aerial ladder useless, and the crew must carry all tools and ground ladders to the scene. A ladder truck that is improperly positioned can also hamper the placement of other responding units.

As the driver/operator brings the apparatus into the fire block, the tiller operator sitting in the tiller box will have the best vision for the placement of the aerial. In many cases, it is the tiller operator who can determine if the aerial ladder can clear any overhead obstructions **FIGURE 16-20**. Good communications and an excellent working relationship between the driver/operator and the tillerman will pay big dividends in positioning the apparatus.

In many older neighborhoods, overhead wires and power lines are still a common sight. As intimidating as these wires might seem to the apparatus driver/operator, there is always the chance that the aerial device can still be deployed. As the driver/operator approaches the fire block, observe the side on which the utility poles are situated. Older cities that still have

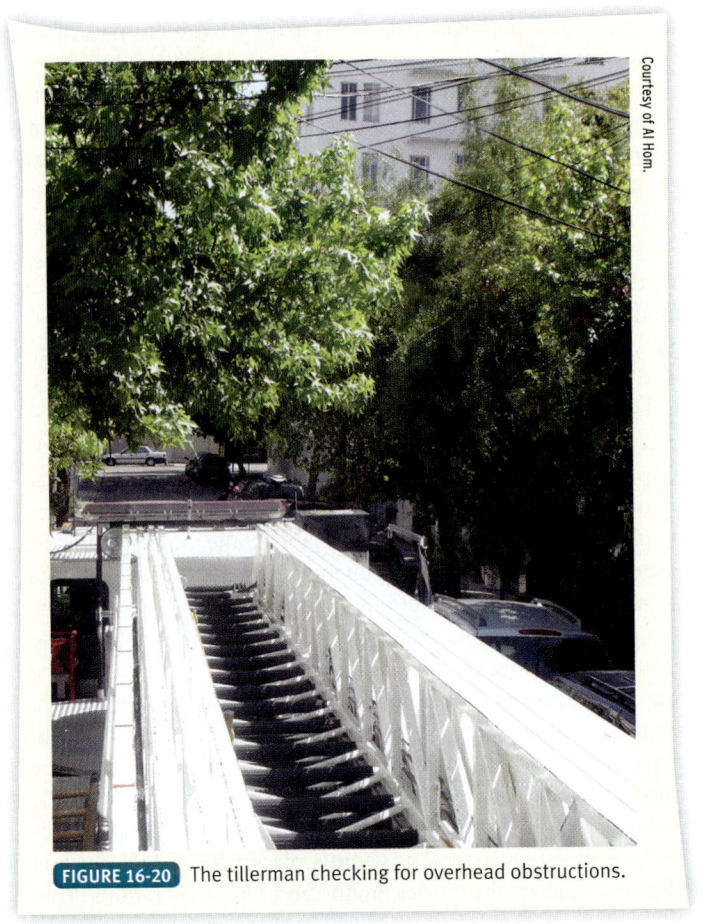

FIGURE 16-20 The tillerman checking for overhead obstructions.

overhead wires usually place the utility poles on only one side of the street. On the side where the poles are located, many high-voltage wires will be attached to the poles and run parallel along the front of the houses. These wires will prevent the aerial from being deployed to the houses situated on that side of the street; however, the houses across the street are another story. Because there are no utility poles on the opposite side of the street, wires will be strung across the street from those existing power poles with the wires attached to those houses at different angles. From the viewpoint of the apparatus driver/operator, these buildings may be laddered, with the aerial device deployed between the wires.

Such overhead wires will also force the driver/operator to rotate the aerial device underneath the wires to get the ladder in position before it can be raised and extended. Because the ladder must be rotated at a low angle of inclination to get below the wires, the ideal distance that the apparatus should be placed away from the building is approximately 25 to 30 ft (8 to 9 m). This distance should allow a fully retracted ladder to be freely rotated. Once the aerial device is rotated under the wires and reaches a position where the wires are no longer a factor, the ladder can then be raised and extended.

Benefit of the Aerial Ladder

Getting the aerial ladder to the incident and properly positioned for use can provide many benefits on the fireground. The aerial device can be used for providing extra egress or rescue and is also a major benefit when it comes to staffing and deployment of the crew. It takes only one fire fighter to deploy the aerial on the fireground, freeing up other members of the truck crew to accomplish other tasks on the fireground.

Tactics May Determine the Placement

The IC, based on the chosen tactics and strategy, may dictate where the ladder truck is to be placed and how the aerial is to be utilized.

What is the strategy? The answer to that question depends on the specific conditions encountered. Is the building fully involved upon arrival, such that fire fighters are unable to enter the building and make an aggressive attack? In this case, the strategy will be defensive and the tactics will focus on proper placement of the tiller apparatus so that the aerial ladder can be used as a ladder pipe to deliver a high volume of water to put out the fire. When positioning the apparatus, the officer will consider keeping the truck away from the building in case of potential collapse. As a general rule, the collapse zone should be 1½ times the height of the building; therefore the apparatus should be positioned 45 ft (14 m) away from a 30-ft (9-m)-high building if the strategy is defensive.

When the strategy is offensive, many tactical decisions must be made. Is there an immediate rescue need? Generally, the first-due truck company should ladder the fire building. Some of its main objectives would be to provide forcible entry, search, and ventilation, so as to make operations easier for the members inside. However, if there are civilians at a window or on the fire escape who need to be removed and ground ladders are not sufficient to reach them, the aerial apparatus may be utilized to affect a rescue.

Where no immediate rescue effort is required, the size of the building's frontage may affect the aerial placement. For taller buildings, the apparatus must be placed closer to the building to allow the ladder to achieve its maximum reach. By comparison, the apparatus may be parked farther away from a shorter building to deploy the aerial. This tactic will enable the first-due engine and other arriving companies good access to the front of the fire building.

The smoke, heat, and fire from the incident building could cause a dangerous exposure to the ladder and the crew members climbing the ladder. With isolated buildings, survey all sides of the structure and ladder the side least affected by the fire. This maneuver will enable the crew to safely climb the ladder to the roof of the fire building and proceed to the area to do their job. In an older, more congested city, many homes are attached to their neighbors at their sides and share a common height. If this is the case, place the aerial so that it reaches the roof of one of the adjoining buildings; the crew can then walk across the connected roofs to get to the roof of the fire building.

Conditions Are Never Ideal

No amount of words can stress the importance of getting the aerial truck placed properly and utilizing the aerial ladder if needed. These measures will allow the crew to accomplish the objectives of the truck company and make operations for the

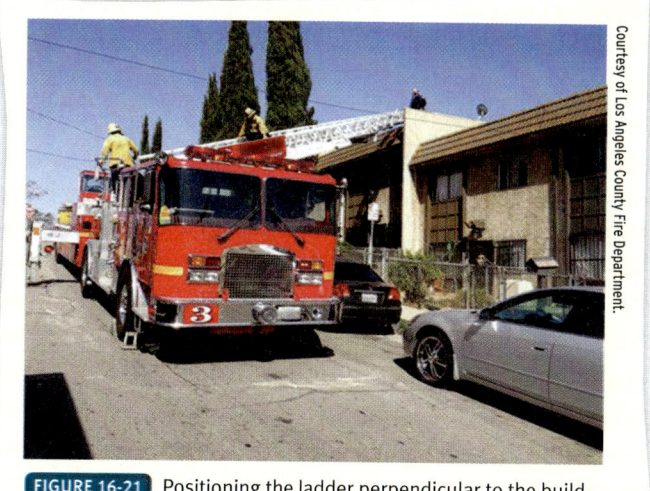

FIGURE 16-21 Positioning the ladder perpendicular to the building at a low angle.

engine company much easier. In contrast, a misplaced truck can render the aerial ladder useless, block other incoming companies, and hamper the entire operations on the fireground.

Under ideal conditions—no overhead obstructions and wide streets—the apparatus should be placed approximately 30 ft (9 m) away from the building. This will allow the driver/operator to rotate the aerial ladder into a position so that the ladder is perpendicular to the building at a low angle **FIGURE 16-21**. Such positioning allows the driver/operator to place the ladder into the windows of lower floors, as well as raise the aerial to windows located on the upper floors **FIGURE 16-22**.

The fireground, however, rarely presents ideal conditions, so fire crews oftentimes must become creative. Overhead obstructions, for instance, may hinder aerial operations. A good example would be a small business complex where the offices and businesses facing the street have obstructions that complicate the laddering process. However, the back of the complex might have a customer parking lot where the driver/operator can bring the apparatus so that the aerial can be utilized.

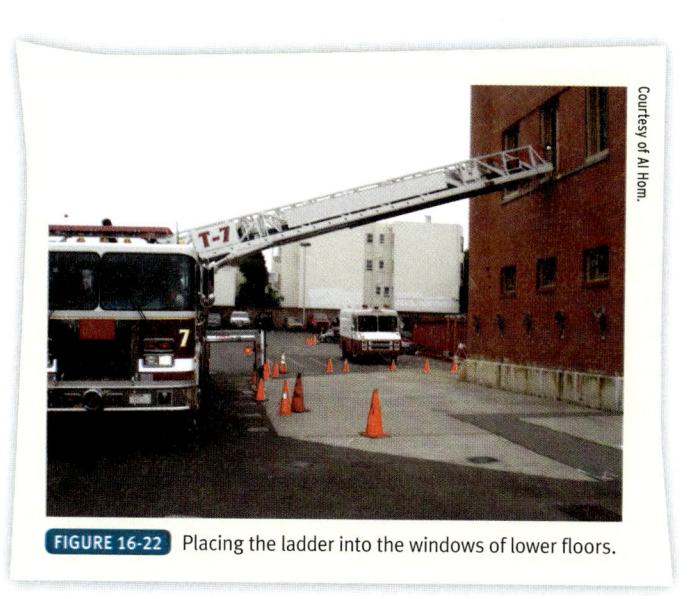

FIGURE 16-22 Placing the ladder into the windows of lower floors.

Other instances may also require creative ladder deployment. Suppose that the ladder truck proceeds down a narrow street to the incident and pulls up directly behind the engine. The driver/operator observes overhead wires strung across the street, which means the aerial must be rotated at a low angle of inclination. However, if the ladder were to be rotated toward the fire building, a tree on the sidewalk would obstruct the ladder from rotating into a perpendicular position facing the fire building. In this instance, the driver/operator can simply rotate the aerial ladder away from the fire building, bring the ladder around over the cab, and then position it to be raised and extended.

In some situations, the truck may be the first apparatus on the scene. If there is room to deploy the aerial, the driver/operator should immediately position the apparatus and deploy the aerial while also leaving room for the incoming engine company. If there is no room to deploy the aerial device, the driver/operator should consider placing the apparatus away from the building while leaving room for the incoming units and not blocking any hydrants. In addition, incoming units must consider the placement of the apparatus and not park close to the rear of the truck company. Parking close to the rear of the ladder truck will prevent the crew from removing any ground ladders that may be needed **FIGURE 16-23**.

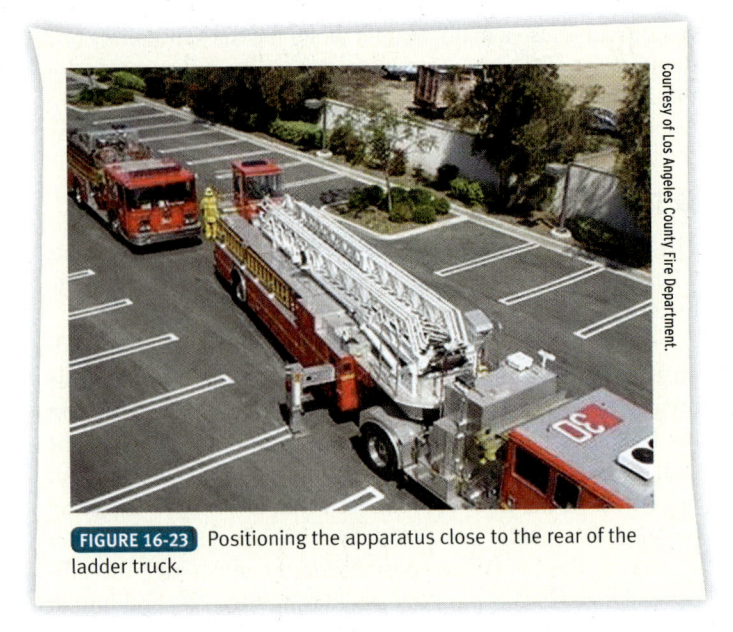

FIGURE 16-23 Positioning the apparatus close to the rear of the ladder truck.

Courtesy of Los Angeles County Fire Department.

Wrap-Up

Chief Concepts

- Proper driver/operator and tiller operator signaling include audio communications, using turn signals, and using the beeper.
- Smooth coordinated tillering operations are required when making a right-hand turn from a dedicated right-hand turn lane, backing up, maneuvering the apparatus around obstacles from left to right, and performing a confined space turn-around.
- Maneuvering the direction of the tiller wheels include planning your turn ahead of time and being set up for the turn in advance.
- The tiller operator should always maintain the trailer portion of the apparatus in-line with the tractor unless involved in a driving maneuver.
- It is important for the tiller operator to quickly bring the trailer back in-line after making turns to avoid over-steering.
- It is also important for the tiller operator to avoid over-tillering or any rough and jerky movements from unnecessarily turning the steering wheel.
- The tiller operator needs to be continuously aware of the trailer overhang when making turns. The overhang of the trailer can work like a pendulum and strike objects if not careful.
- The tiller operator skill of negotiating right-handed turns from a dedicated right turn lane is difficult but can be mastered with practice.
- The qualifications and certifications for tiller operator are determined by your department.

Hot Terms

communication The verbal coordination that occurs between the driver/operator controlling the tractor portion of the apparatus and the tiller operator who is responsible for control of the trailer portion of the apparatus. It is important that the driver/operator and tiller operator are in good communication at all times.

driver/operator A person having satisfactorily completed the requirements of driver/operator as specified in National Fire Protection Association (NFPA) 1002, *Standard Fire Apparatus Driver/Operator Professional Qualifications*.

over-steering Allowing the trailer to swing out or move past an in-line position after a turn is completed.

over-tillering The occurrence when the tiller operator turns the steering wheel unnecessarily.

overhang The portion of the trailer that extends from the center of the trailer wheels (pivot point) to the rear of the trailer. It is important to allow enough room for the overhang to clear both sides of the trailer.

teamwork The driver/operator and tiller operator of a tractor trailer ladder truck have a dual responsibility unique among fire department apparatus drivers. Both must work together and coordinate their actions to ensure the safe and efficient operation of the tractor and trailer as a unit.

tiller operator The tiller operator has the responsibility for lateral control of the trailer portion of the apparatus.

under-steering Not turning the steering wheel sufficiently while making a sharp turn and cutting a corner.

Wrap-Up, continued

References

Los Angeles County Fire Department, Tiller Operator Instruction Lesson Plan. California State Fire Training for Apparatus Driver/Operator Tiller Truck.

National Fire Protection Association (NFPA) 1002, *Standard for Fire Apparatus Driver/Operator Professional Qualifications.* 2014. http://www.nfpa.org/codes-and-standards/document-information-pages?mode=code&code=1002. Accessed March 27, 2014.

DRIVER/OPERATOR
in action

You are the tiller operator responding to an emergency call. You are approaching an intersection from the opposing lanes of traffic. You must be aware of oncoming traffic, and the vehicle already at the intersection stopped.

1. When entering the intersection, in which direction may you have to turn your wheels?
   A. To your right
   B. Hold the wheel tight
   C. To your left
   D. Quickly right, then left slowly

2. When in the intersection, what is it called if you go past the center point of the tractor?
   A. Over-steering
   B. Under-steering
   C. Over-tillering
   D. Under-tillering

3. When exiting the intersection, in which direction may you have to turn your wheels?
   A. To your left
   B. To your right
   C. Do not turn wheels
   D. To left slowly, then right quickly

4. How can you be sure not to over-steer?
   A. Hum the steering song
   B. Don't steer
   C. Close eyes
   D. Count your turns

5. If you are going to strike a vehicle or object, what should you do?
   A. Tell the apparatus operator to stop
   B. Say "whoa"
   C. Strike it then leave a note
   D. Try not to cause much damage

Operating Apparatus Equipped with a Tiller

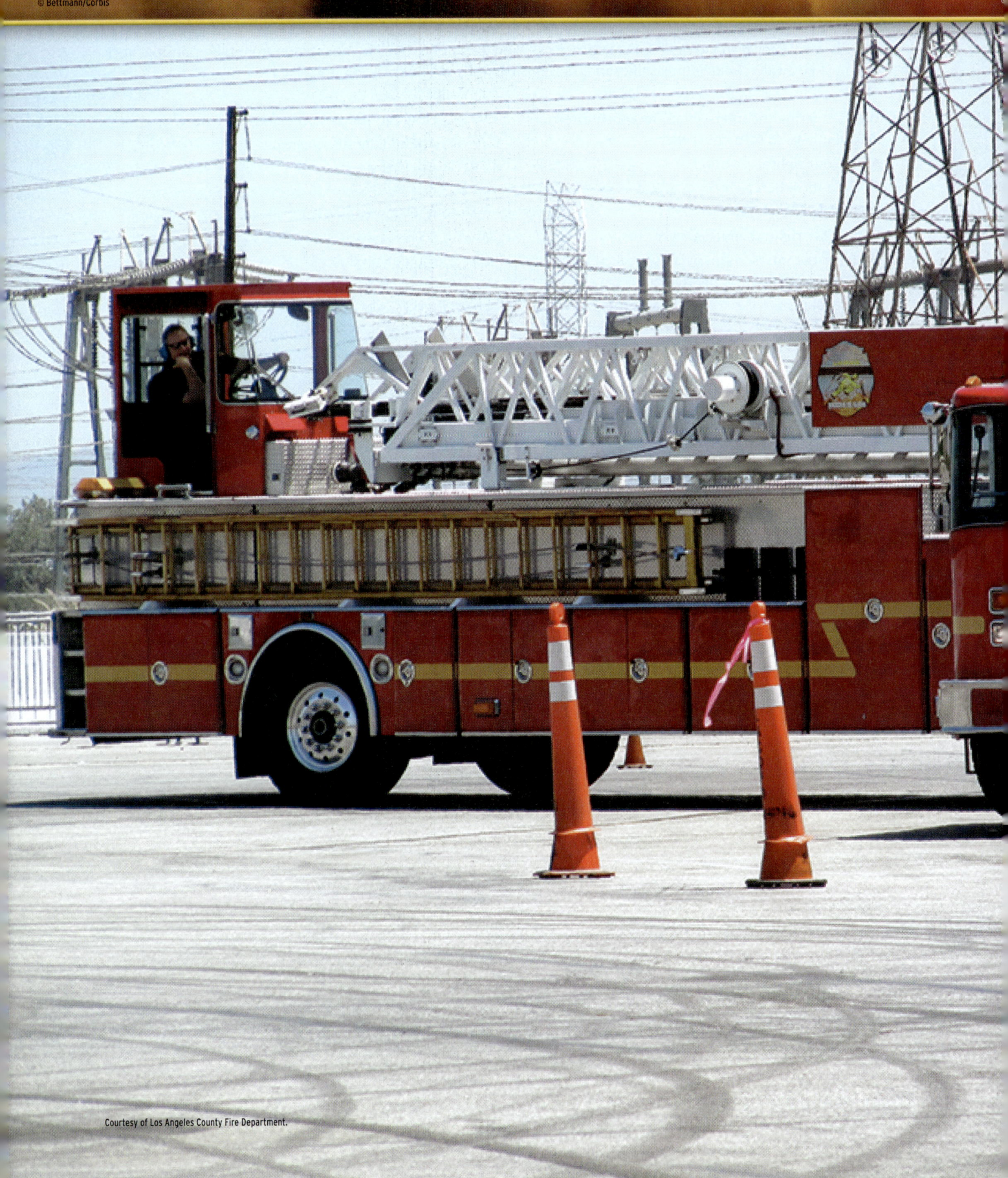

CHAPTER 17

Knowledge Objectives

After studying this chapter you will be able to:

- Understand the operation of the tiller apparatus' cable systems (if applicable), the aerial device hydraulic systems, the slides and rollers, the stabilizing systems, aerial device safety systems, the breathing air systems, and the communication systems. (NFPA 1002, 6.1.1(1), 6.1.1(2), 6.1.1(3), 6.1.1(4), 6.1.1(5), 6.1.1(6), 6.1.1(7), 6.1.1(A); p 422–429)
- Describe the capabilities and limitations of tiller aerial devices related to reach tip load, angle of inclination, and angle from chassis axis. (NFPA 1002, 7.2.1(A); p 423–425, 427–428)
- Describe the principles of tiller operation. (NFPA 1002, 7.1, 7.2.2(A); p 422–425, 427–429)

Skills Objectives

After studying this chapter, you will be able to:

- Perform routine tests, inspections, and service of the tiller apparatus' cable systems (if applicable), the aerial device hydraulic systems, the slides and rollers, the stabilizing systems, aerial device safety systems, the breathing air systems, and the communication systems. (NFPA 1002, 6.1.1(1), 6.1.1(2), 6.1.1(3), 6.1.1(4), 6.1.1(5), 6.1.1(6), 6.1.1(7), 6.1.1(B); p 422–429)
- Determine the correct position for the tiller, maneuver the tiller into the correct position, and avoid obstacles to operations. (NFPA 1002, 7.2.1, 7.2.1(B), 7.2.3, 7.2.3(B); p 423–425, 427–429)

Additional NFPA Standards

- NFPA 1500, *Standard on Fire Department Occupational Safety and Health Program*
- NFPA 1911, *Standard for the Inspection, Maintenance, Testing, and Retirement of In-Service Automotive Fire Apparatus*
- NFPA 1914, *Standard for Testing Fire Department Aerial Devices*

You Are the Driver/Operator

You are the driver/operator of an aerial apparatus responding to an incident. When arriving at the incident, you must position your apparatus for correct aerial device deployment.

1. How do you determine the correct angle?
2. How do you determine the correct length?
3. How do you determine the correct height?

Introduction

When identifying the capabilities and limitations of a tiller, in relation to its reach, tip load, angle of inclination, and angle from chassis axis, it is important to understand the effects of topography, ground, and weather conditions for safe deployment of the aerial. Specific variables that need to be taken into consideration include the following:

- Aerial device hydraulic systems
- Hydraulic pressure relief systems
- Gauges and controls
- Cable systems
- Communications systems
- Electrical systems
- Emergency operating systems
- Locking systems
- Manual rotation and lowering systems
- Stabilizing systems
- Aerial device safety systems
- System overrides and the hazards of using overrides
- Safe operational limitations of the given aerial device
- Safety procedures specific to the device
- Operations near electrical hazards and overhead obstructions

Safety Tips Before Aerial Deployment

Consider these few simple, yet important, tasks before putting the aerial to work. When you come to a complete stop and the apparatus is properly positioned, put the rig in neutral. Always set the parking brakes. On the tiller aerial, two brakes must be applied: the parking brake and the trailer brake. With newer apparatus, the aerial will not operate unless both of these brakes are set. Engage the aerial power and power take-off (PTO) switch; a light will come on indicating that both switches are properly set and the aerial is ready to be deployed.

■ Positioning the Tiller

To determine the best placement and maneuver the tiller apparatus into the correct position, it is important to avoid any obstacles to operations. Engagement of your decision-making skills for **apparatus placement** begins before you are en route to a fire. Upon arriving at the scene, the driver/operator must make sure there is sufficient room for the apparatus' jack extension and then determine where the fire is in relationship to the fire structure. The jacks are used for side-to-side stabilization while using the aerial ladder and apply forces toward the **torque box**, increasing the overall footprint of the apparatus. The climbing angle of the aerial must be considered as well. If you can see the spot where you want the aerial to extend from your seat, you should be successful. The bed of the aerial ladder is at roughly the same height as the engineer's head, and its axis is located above the dual axles. The driver/operator should position the dual axles on the spot from which he or she views the ladder extending.

■ Transferring Power

The process of transferring the power from the vehicle's engine to the hydraulic system to operate the apparatus' stabilization devices begins when the driver/operator first turns the batteries to "both" and then turns the ignition to "on." Next, the driver/operator depresses both starter buttons while the tillerman operates the foot switch. If no tillerman is present, the driver/operator should turn batteries to "both," turn the ignition to "on," and then turn the aerial ladder power on. After these steps are taken, the driver/operator can exit the truck and start the apparatus by the remote start.

■ Stabilization Requirements

The next step is for the driver/operator to get out of the rig and stabilize the apparatus so that it is safe to raise the aerial ladder. Always chock the wheels, with one set of chocks being placed on each side of the apparatus. For the tractor-trailer aerial apparatus, place the chocks both ahead of and behind the front steering axle. Restraining the front axle will provide additional friction to prevent movement of the apparatus on the outrigger system, which is particularly important when operating on hilly terrain.

The driver/operator can then fully extend the outriggers, which will provide added stability to prevent the apparatus from tipping over when the aerial device is raised and rotated. In many cases, the manufacturer provides a switching system that will prevent movement of the aerial ladder unless the outriggers are deployed. Under most situations, the stabilizing

CHAPTER 17 Operating Apparatus Equipped with a Tiller 423

FIGURE 17-1 Place the stabilizing plates under the outriggers.

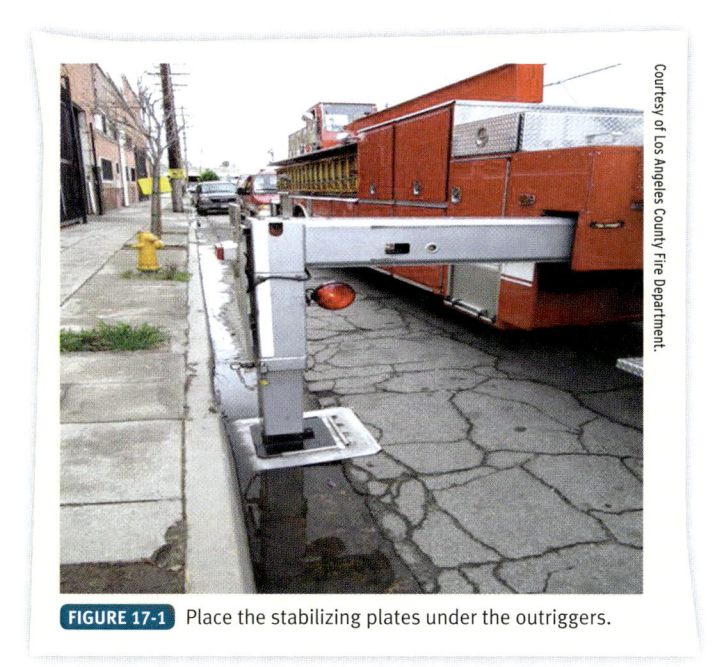

plates should be placed under the outriggers——this is especially important when the apparatus is positioned on a sidewalk **FIGURE 17-1**. The stabilizing plates will provide a greater surface-to-ground contact to stabilize the apparatus. Finally, insert the outrigger pin to prevent potential collapse of the outrigger leg. It is not recommended to use the outrigger pads on hills, as doing so can increase the risk of the apparatus sliding down the hill. In addition, do not set the outrigger jacks over a manhole cover or a storm drain. The driver/operator should always take into account the durability of the surface upon which the apparatus is positioned.

Be aware of what is happening around the turntable before the aerial is raised and rotated. Tools, impediments, or personnel must be clear of the area around the aerial and the turntable as the ladder is being raised and rotated **FIGURE 17-2**. Always keep within the operating limits recommended by the manufacturer.

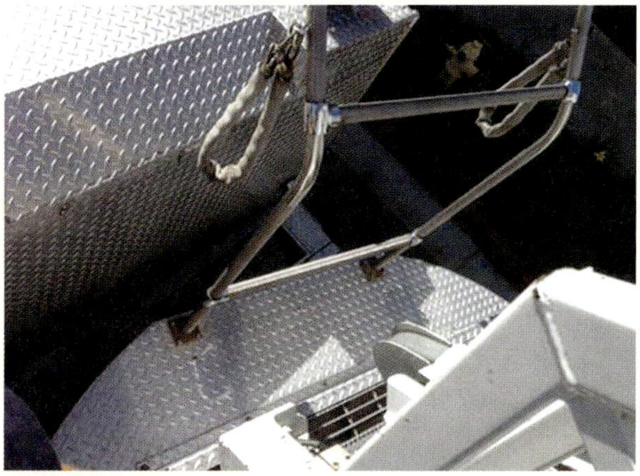

FIGURE 17-2 Clear the area around the aerial and turntable of tools, impediments, or personnel.

Raise, Rotate, Extend, and More

Once the apparatus is properly placed and stabilized, the aerial ladder is ready to be utilized. There are three steps for the deployment of the aerial ladder:

1. Raise the ladder from the cradle so that the ladder is angled.
2. Rotate the aerial so that the tip of the aerial is facing in the general direction of the intended target.
3. Extend the aerial toward its intended target.

Under ideal conditions, these evolutions are done one at a time and in proper operating sequence. Do not try to raise, rotate, and extend the device simultaneously, as this can lead to confusion and will not hasten the deployment of the aerial.

■ Raising the Aerial

Raising the aerial ladder in a timely manner with minimal sway is the responsibility of the driver/operator. As the driver/operator checks the apparatus and aerial ladder at the beginning of the shift, he or she should take this opportunity to practice ladder placement. Pick a target, such as a window or roof of a building, and practice raising and placing the aerial ladder to that target. The aerial driver/operator can overcome the challenges inherent in deploying such a device with hands-on practice and by becoming familiar with the equipment. The driver/operator should look for shortcuts that will help and aid in raising the aerial ladder accurately.

To eliminate miscalculations, the driver/operator can take advantage of some simple tips when placing the aerial to the target with a minimal amount of movement. For smooth, continuous aerial ladder movement and final positioning, the retracted aerial should be raised from the cradle to an angle where the driver/operator can rotate the ladder to a perpendicular position facing the building. From this position, the driver/operator can make adjustments to the angle of the aerial—adjustments intended to align the retracted ladder with the target. Once the correct alignment has been determined, he or she can extend the aerial to a closer proximity over the target. With the ladder over the target, the driver/operator can then bring it toward the object in a smooth and controlled manner.

To assist in raising and accurately placing the aerial ladder, the driver/operator could select a section of the ladder—such as the tip—and use it as a reference point. When the driver/operator arrives at an incident where the aerial will be required, he or she should select the area where the aerial will be placed and then utilize the reference point when positioning the rig by aiming it to the area where the ladder must be finally placed.

As an example, if the apparatus is parked and the driver/operator has orders to raise the aerial ladder to the roof, he or she should raise the ladder from the bedded position to an angle that will clear the roof. Next, the driver/operator rotates the ladder toward the building and then visually aligns the tip of the aerial to the intended target, keeping in mind that the aerial should be extended over the edge of the roof. Once the aerial is extended over the roof, the driver/operator slowly lowers the aerial so that the bottom of the ladder (the beam) is 3 to 6 inches (77 to 150 mm) above the roof edge.

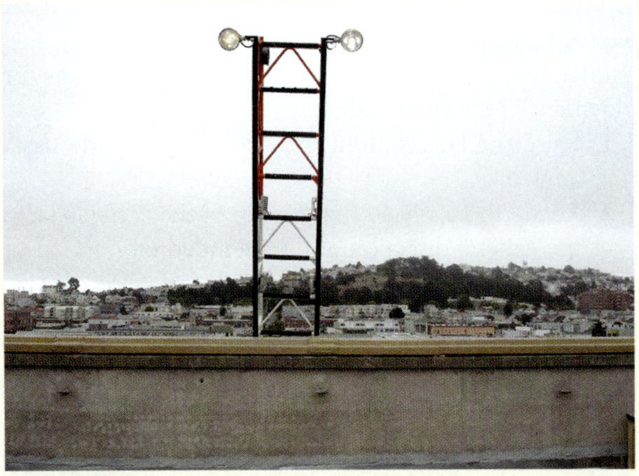

FIGURE 17-3 The aerial should extend three to six rungs over the edge of the roof.

Courtesy of Al Horn.

As a general rule, when raising the aerial ladder to the roof, the aerial should extend three to six rungs over the edge of the roof **FIGURE 17-3**. The fire fighter climbing the aerial ladder can then safely dismount the aerial onto the roof by holding onto the rail of the aerial while stepping off. Also, as the fire fighter exits the roof, he or she can grab the rail of the aerial ladder and safely step onto the aerial to begin the descent. A ladder that is extended over the roof line will also be more visible to the crew on the roof, enabling them to quickly locate this exit route should conditions begin to deteriorate. On older apparatus, it may be necessary to relocate the tiller operator's control station; on some apparatus it is necessary to flip the whole station to one side, while on others, you may only have to remove the steering column.

DRIVER/OPERATOR Tip

Depth perception is a major issue when it comes to raising the aerial ladder. There are two common miscalculations that driver/operators make: (1) placing the ladder well above the target and (2) extending the ladder well short of the target. These common errors will force the driver/operator to make time-consuming adjustments to get the aerial properly deployed.

■ Placing the Aerial

When the aerial is raised to rescue a victim from a window, the aerial ladder should be extended to the window so that the rung at the tip of the aerial is just below the windowsill. Do not extend the aerial into the window; doing so will compromise the space provided by the window opening and make it difficult to get on and off the aerial. When conducting firefighting operations, such as ventilation practices or firefighting from the ladder, the aerial should be raised and placed above the window and to the upwind side.

When the aerial ladder is raised to the roof, it should extend three to six rungs over the roof. At that point, however, the aerial driver/operator must still make minor adjustments. Align the rungs so that footing for the climb up the aerial will be safer for the fire fighters. Also, the ladder must be lowered to the roof so that fire fighters can safely step off the aerial. The driver/operator should lower the ladder gradually and smoothly so that it is 3 to 6 inches (77 to 150 mm) above the roof line. This movement will prevent the driver/operator from having the aerial come in hard contact with the edge of the roof and putting unnecessary strain or damage to the aerial ladder.

Obstructions may cause the driver/operator to deviate and make adjustments during some of the evolutions. For example, the driver/operator may raise the ladder out of the bed and then be forced to rotate it under an overhead wire before being able to get the tip of the ladder positioned facing the building; however, the ladder may still need to be raised so that its incline angle can reach the roof before the ladder can be extended. In this instance, the theory of raising the aerial will basically remain the same.

Always be aware of overhead obstructions as the aerial is being deployed. Keep the aerial device at least 10 ft (3 m) away from any overhead wires, which allows for ladder sway, rock, or sag when operating near power lines and cables. If the aerial should contact any power lines, personnel should remain on the apparatus until the power is shut off or the aerial is freed from contact.

The driver/operator should always consider the stability of any structure that the ladder is placed against. For windows and fire escapes, the rung at the tip of the ladder should be placed flush to the windowsill or the top railing of the fire escape. Do not extend the aerial into the window or past the top railing of the fire escape, as this tactic will compromise the opening and diminish the space that the window or fire escape provides if members or civilians need a quick bailout.

Placement of the apparatus so that the rotated aerial ladder is perpendicular toward the building provides the driver/operator with the opportunity to position the ladder as squarely as possible against the building. Placing the aerial at an angle toward the building causes one beam of the ladder to contact the building first. As the climbing member's weight subsequently approaches the tip, the ladder will twist until the other beam also rests on the edge of the roof. This twisting can weaken all sections of the ladder, leading to significant damage to the aerial ladder **FIGURE 17-4**.

If the fire building is situated on a steep hill, place the apparatus in a position such that the aerial ladder, which should be pointing uphill, will be rotated at an angle—approximately 45 degrees from the center line of the vehicle. The driver/operator can then extend the aerial, causing the ladder to be at an angle with the windowsill or the edge of the roof, which in turn will reduce the side tilt of the ladder under a heavy load **FIGURE 17-5**.

■ Climbing the Aerial

Climbing the aerial ladder can be physically taxing. This task becomes much more difficult when one considers that the fire fighters will be wearing full personal protective equipment (PPE) and carrying tools. Among the tools required to be carried up the aerial are power saws, axes, ceiling hooks, and forcible entry tools. Once the fire fighters step off the aerial, they are expected to go to work. If the fire is on the top floor, the fire fighters must cut a hole in the roof and help ventilate the fire

CHAPTER 17 Operating Apparatus Equipped with a Tiller 425

FIGURE 17-4 As the fire fighter approaches the tip of the aerial, the added weight can cause an improperly positioned ladder to twist.

FIGURE 17-6 Hand tools may be stored in the top fly section near the tip of the aerial.

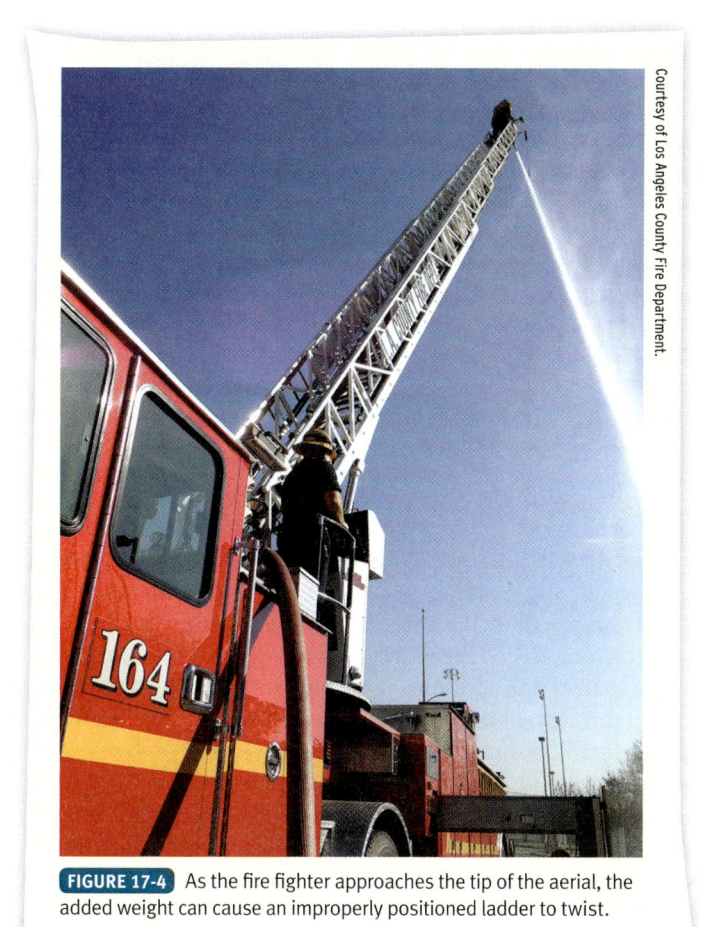

floor directly below them. If they are on the roof of a multistory building but the fire is several floors below them, they may be required to make forcible entry through common openings such as a penthouse door. In major cities, in areas where houses are side-by-side, fire fighters on the roof can walk to the back of the building, look over the edge, and advise the incident commander (IC) of any situation happening in the rear of the building.

To make it easy for fire fighters climbing the aerial, some hand tools can be stored in the top fly section near the tip of the aerial **FIGURE 17-6**. The aerial is then raised and extended to its desired location, and the fire fighters can climb the aerial. Once they get close to the tip of the aerial, some hand tools will await them as they get ready to get off the aerial.

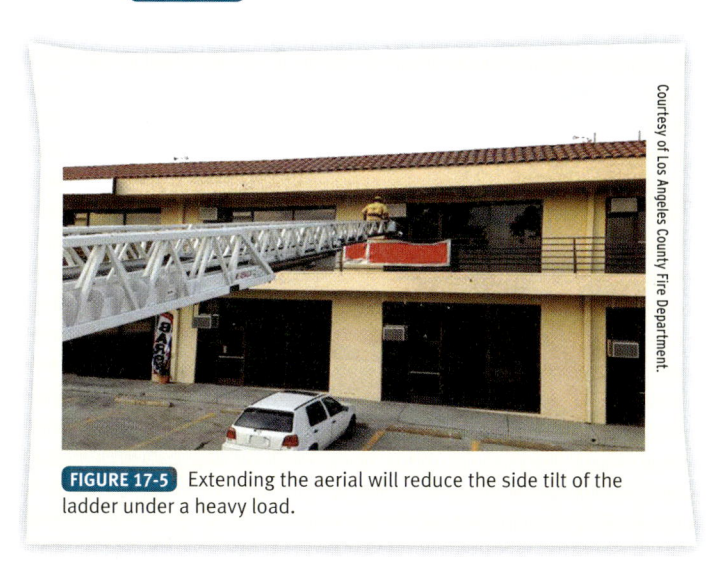

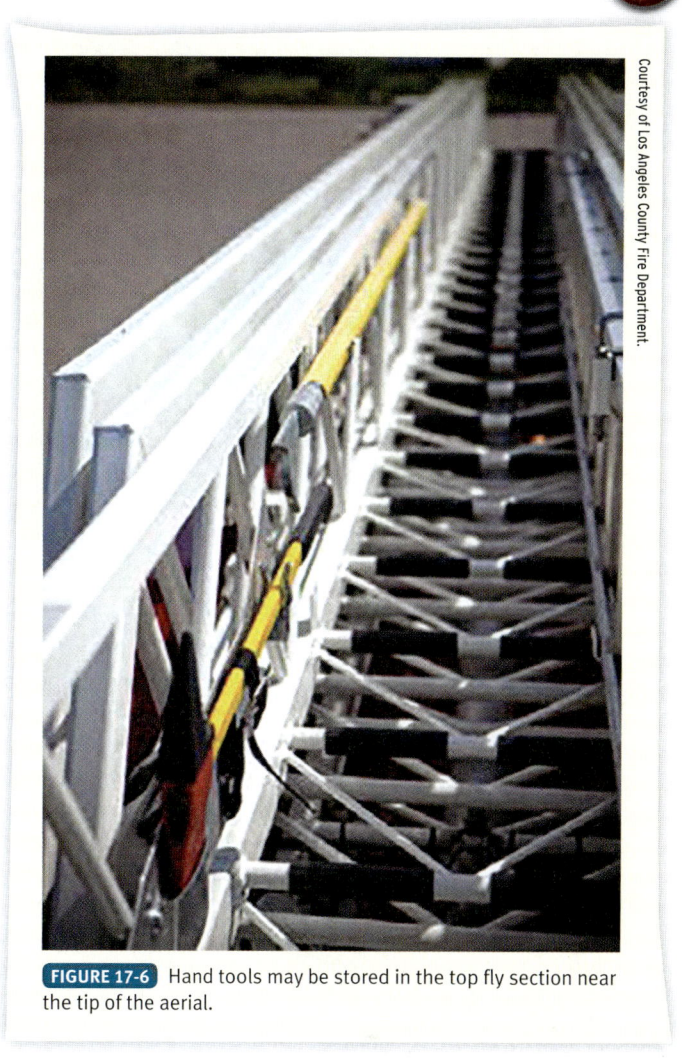

■ Ladder in Place

Once the aerial ladder is in position, the driver/operator must stay near the turntable. Under most situations, this ladder should never be moved. The driver/operator should be aware of which members climbed the aerial ladder, when they did so, and where they are positioned. If ordered to move the aerial, the driver/operator must inform the IC that the aerial was utilized, and the crew must be notified via radio that the ladder is being moved.

With the driver/operator standing on the turntable, he or she can be utilized to carry any additional tools or equipment when needed to the upper floors or roof. Avoid rotating the ladder when fire fighters are on it, except to remove them from serious exposure or for an extreme rescue effort. Never extend or retract the ladder while members are climbing, and always align the rungs when the aerial is extended to the roof. Allow for a safe distance between members when multiple people are climbing the aerial.

■ Aerial Ladder Supporting Weight

Sometimes the aerial may be required to support extra weight over an extended period of time, such as in defensive operations.

FIGURE 17-5 Extending the aerial will reduce the side tilt of the ladder under a heavy load.

VOICES
OF EXPERIENCE

An old British army adage known as the "seven Ps" or "proper pre-planning prevents a piss-poor performance" is one that many in the fire department have adopted as their own when preplanning buildings and other target hazards, such as considering what specific truck company functions might be required. Ideal apparatus placement might be different for roof access versus water tower operations, and the seven Ps have helped me on more than one occasion. As an engineer/apparatus operator, we plan our routes of travel throughout our district, which allows us to get to the scene of an incident in the most timely manner.

Recently, I was working overtime and driving the engine at one of my old assignments. The crew I was working with that day were all newer to the station, but they were aware that I had previously been assigned there. On more than one occasion, we responded to the correct location of a scene in the most direct manner without having to look anything up on the map. One early evening, we were headed to a structure fire in a neighboring company's district, when one of the fire fighters in the jump seat said, "wouldn't it be great if we beat them to their own fire," and I responded, "we will." And lo and behold, we did.

After the fire when we were headed back to the station, the crew was commenting on how we had beat the other company in, how surprised they were at the route we took, and the fact that I wasn't driving any faster than normal. I told them that during that time of day, I always take a certain street because it is less congested and cuts through our district at an angle, unlike any other street in the jurisdiction. I will then always turn a block earlier than the street the call was on and approach the location from the backside, which allows us to bypass the congested traffic of a shopping mall and grocery store. I then told them that if everyone assigned to the call leaves from their stations, you will always beat them in to that part of the district if you take that route.

Preplanning is done on buildings for apparatus placement, ladder placement, and hydrant connections, as well as many other tactical decisions. Preplanning is used by all of us daily, without us even realizing it. Even on your day off, you will plan your route so that you are not crisscrossing the city to get your errands done.

Tim McIntyre
Engineer/Apparatus Operator
Los Angeles County Fire Department
Los Angeles, California

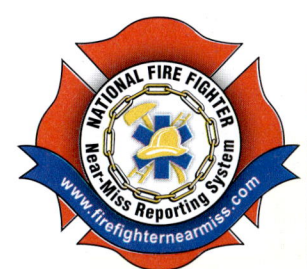

Near-Miss REPORT

Report Number: 07-0000776

Synopsis: Aerial stabilizer narrowly misses fire fighter.

Event Description: Our fire company was dispatched to a report of smoke in a fast food restaurant. We responded with a six-person truck company on an automatic aid call to one of our neighboring fire departments. Upon arrival on the scene, the incident commander ordered our company to raise the aerial to the roof of the structure. A probationary fire fighter was laying out the ground plates. The operator yelled to the fire fighter that he was going to lower the stabilizers. The fire fighter did not hear him and was still bent over positioning the plate as the operator was engaging the stabilizers. Another fire fighter from our company saw what was happening and yelled at the fire fighter to get out of there.

Lessons Learned: The biggest lesson that was learned is to constantly pay attention and be aware of your surroundings. My suggestion to prevent a similar event would be to stress that more attention be paid at the scene of an incident and better recruit orientation.

When the aerial ladder is used as a ladder pipe, it must support the weight of water running up the ladder via a preconnected waterway or hoselines lying on the aerial between the rails and secured to the rungs. The aerial ladder should be set to an incline of 70 to 75 degrees—at this angle, it will be in the most stable position to support the additional weight on the ladder. Always be aware of shock loading.

■ Using the Aerial in a Defensive Strategy

When a defensive fireground strategy is employed, the aerial ladder becomes an invaluable tool. Modern aerial ladders come preconnected with a waterway that can deliver an elevated master stream and knock down heavy fire in a time-efficient manner. Older aerial ladders or departments that want their aerial ladders designed without the preconnected waterway must set up a ladder pipe system that will deliver massive amounts of water at an elevated level.

Although this is an antiquated method of delivering a master stream, setting up the ladder pipe can take very little time. The ladder needs to be raised slightly out of the bed and rotated slightly off-center so that the crew can stand on the surface area of the bedded aerial. A nozzle is hooked up to the tip of the aerial ladder, and 2½- or 3-inch (65- or 77-mm) hoselines are then connected to this nozzle. The length of hose should equal 100 ft (30 m). The hoselines are laid on top of the rungs and straight down the middle of the bedded ladder. The excess length lies on the ground on the side of the rig opposite the fire building. The end coupling of the large line is connected to the outlet of the Siamese coupling. An outside source (engine company) then supplies water to the ladder pipe.

With this setup, the driver/operator can raise, rotate, and extend the ladder pipe to its desired position so that a master stream can be delivered to knock down heavy fire. The master stream should be positioned so that water is delivered through a window or side opening to push the fire up and out of the fire-involved building. Do not position the ladder pipe above the roof and aim the stream at fire coming through the roof.

When setting up the ladder pipe, attach guide wires to the tip of the nozzle and the handle of the nozzle **FIGURE 17-7**,

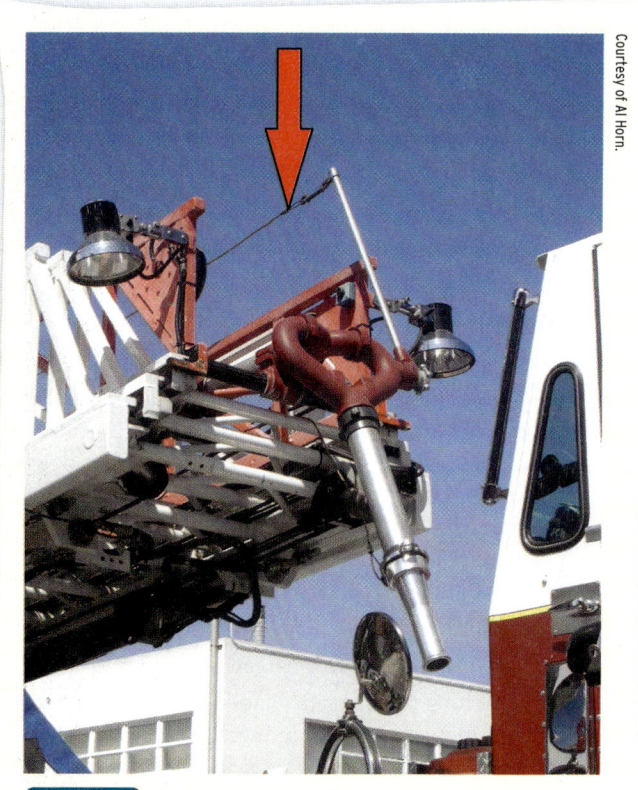

FIGURE 17-7 Guide wires are attached to the tip of the nozzle and the handle of the nozzle when setting up the ladder pipe.

letting the wire attached to the tip of the nozzle drop straight down once the ladder is in position. The wire attached to the handle stretches down the middle of the aerial, just like the hose attached to the nozzle. Fire fighters on the ground can grab the wires and control the vertical movement of the nozzle tip, which eliminates the need to put a fire fighter at the tip of the ladder where he or she may be exposed to heat and smoke. The aerial driver/operator can control the horizontal movement of the water stream by rotating the aerial left or right.

■ Operating the Aerial Under Adverse Conditions

The driver/operator needs to be able to operate the aerial in high winds, low temperatures, and exposure to fire, and if the aerial device experiences a mechanical or power failure. It is important for the driver/operator to know the limits of the aerial for wind, as high winds will limit the extension capabilities of the aerial. Also, in the event of a mechanical or power failure, the driver/operator should be familiar with and understand how to operate the apparatus' emergency power unit and/or its manual cranks and valves. During both normal and adverse conditions, some of the forces that act on the aerial device include personnel, portable equipment, water, and nozzle reaction. The weight of the aerial device includes the structure itself and all materials, components, mechanisms, and equipment that are permanently fastened to the aerial. The total amount of weight includes all personnel and equipment that can be safely supported on the outermost rung of an aerial ladder or on the platform of an elevated platform with the waterway uncharged. Dynamic loads to the aerial may also occur—for example, from striking the aerial or any collisions or other impacts that might occur from any nozzle reaction, or when the aerial is used in windy conditions, as a crane, or in any rescue effort.

> **Safety Tip**
>
> The driver/operator should follow all manufacturer's recommendations regarding operation of the aerial apparatus during adverse weather conditions and increased wind speeds.

■ Lowering the Aerial

In order to lower an aerial device using the emergency operating system on older lightweight aerials without holding valves, so that the device is lowered to its bedded position, the driver/operator should follow the steps in **SKILL DRILL 17-1**. This operation is intended to retract, rotate, and lower the aerial device in the event of engine failure or when it is imperative to bed the ladder to prevent damage to or loss of the device.

1. Ensure the in-cab aerial setup is in operation.
2. Ensure the battery is on and the ignition switch is on.
3. Switch from normal to emergency mode.
   - Switching to emergency mode will allow power to the emergency power unit (EPU).
   - The EPU is an engine starter motor that, when activated, will provide a few minutes of hydraulic power.
   - Once the EPU is activated by operating the aerial controls, it should remain on for no longer than 2 minutes continuously and then be given the appropriate rest.
4. At the pedestal, ensure the throttle switch is on.
5. To activate the EPU, choose the "raise," "extend," "left," or "right" mode.
6. Raise the ladder out of the target area if necessary.
7. Extend the ladder enough to release the device that holds the ladder in place on older lightweight aerials, which is also referred to as "dogs."
8. Release the dogs.
9. Open the extension bypass valve and allow the ladder to drift down slowly.
10. Close the valve when the ladder is fully retracted.
11. To rotate the ladder over the bed, unlock the rotation brake, open the hand-rotation valve, and install the hand-crank.
12. Give the hand-rotation valve 2 turns.
13. Rotate the ladder to line up with the bed.
14. Open the lowering freefall valve.
15. Operate the lowering lever to get the desired reaction.
16. Use the hand-crank to guide the ladder into the bed.
17. Once the ladder is lowered into the bed, close the lowering freefall valve.
18. Close the hand-rotation valve and lock the rotation brake.
19. Remove the hand-crank.
20. Turn off the throttle switch at the pedestal.
21. Ensure the hold-down locks engage.
22. Return the controls to normal operating mode.

Aerial Rescue Strategies and Tactics

Aerial rescues can require laddering a window, a balcony, or a fire escape to rescue a victim. Timing is a must, and you need to be aware of victims attempting to jump onto the aerial tip causing a dynamic shock load and damaging the aerial. It may be best to have a fire fighter at the tip of the aerial before it arrives to rescue a victim. Care must also be taken not to strike any objects on the building, causing damage to the aerial. These skills and maneuvers can be a challenge for any driver/operator and should be practiced before a real incident happens.

■ Positioning the Aerial for Rescue

Laddering windows for rescue should be accomplished by placing the fly section of the ladder below the windowsill, which allows the rescuer to pull nonambulatory victims onto the ladder. Always consider your ladder load limits before victim entry onto the ladder. Spotting the aerial perpendicularly to the target eliminates any potential fall space when rescuing victims, and spotting at an angle allows the driver/operator to see and reach two sides of the building easily. Balconies should be laddered to allow easy access on and off of the fly section of the aerial device. A typical balcony rail height is roughly 4 ft (1.2 m), which can create difficulties for victims and fire fighters as they try to climb on the ladder; in such scenarios, use of a 14-ft (4-m) roof ladder can aid victims in making the transition onto the aerial. Fire escapes are similar to balconies, with the exception that they include a stairwell leading from floor to floor. The driver/operator should take advantage of the fire escape stairwell to make easier transitions on and off the aerial ladder.

Controversy persists about how best to "enter in" with the aerial ladder when victims are in need of rescue. Extending the aerial into the target space is the worst option, because the victims then need to jump to the ladder. Lowering the aerial into the target space, therefore, is the driver/operator's best option.

If a fire fighter is ordered to "ride" the fly section up, the driver/operator needs to know the safe extension before that fire fighter is at risk of getting pinched. Extending the aerial past the base section's sixth rung, or 55 ft (17 m), will keep the tip of the fly section clear. Good communication between the driver/operator and the crew at the tip is important and can include either voice box, hand-held radio, or hand signals.

Shift Change

At shift changes, apparatus driver/operators should always pass information about happenings from the previous shift to the next shift. This information should include the following points:
- If there was a fire on the previous shift
- Which tools were used
- If the aerial was used
- Which tools need to be checked and cleaned
- Which tools and equipment were left on the fireground or are missing

If the apparatus was dispatched to a working fire, exchange information on how the rig was positioned, whether any challenges were encountered when laddering the building, and what the crew accomplished at the fire. Determine whether the apparatus needs fuel or whether any other fluids need to be topped off. Point out anything that occurred during the previous shift that had not occurred before, such as the crew noticing oil on the apparatus floor as the rig was parked, or anything unusual about the apparatus, such as differences in engine noise, braking capabilities, aerial operations, or chassis damage.

■ Aerial Ladder Testing

In addition to the daily inspections that the driver/operator and crew conduct on the aerial ladder, a stringent and more detailed inspection of the aerial ladder must be conducted on a periodic basis. National Fire Protection Association (NFPA) 1911, *Standard for the Inspection, Maintenance, Testing, and Retirement of In-Service Automotive Fire Apparatus*, identifies the standards and requirements for testing of aerial ladders on an annual basis. During the **aerial ladder inspection**, certified mechanical technicians will review service records and previous inspections in addition to the manufacturer's specification and performance requirements. The technicians will visually inspect and test all parts of the aerial ladder, including the stabilizers, turntable, control levers, and overrides. An operations test will be performed to determine whether the aerial ladder can meet elevation, rotation, and extension time requirements, and a strength test will be performed in which the aerial ladder is extended to its maximum reach at zero degrees. At this position, a weight will be added to the tip of the aerial ladder.

Summary

Placement of apparatus, in regard to truck company operations, simply refers to how and where an apparatus is placed at the scene. Virtually all fire incidents require apparatus in some way, and the success of most fireground operations depends, either directly or indirectly, on the effective placement of fire apparatus. An important concept to remember is that there is a direct relationship between apparatus placement and function. Incorrect placement can slow or hinder operations, and truck company placement cannot be addressed specifically without discussing engine company placement. Ideally, operations involving truck company placement and engine company placement will be complementary.

Wrap-Up

Chief Concepts

- Understand the construction of your apparatus and its limitations prior to use. Due to forces created by elevation and rotation, torsional or twisting movement is present in all aerial devices. The top of the base section is where the majority of twisting action occurs, which may also be referred to as "Euler" buckling and can lead to collapse.
- Apparatus placement, in regard to truck company operations, refers to how and where an apparatus is placed at the scene. Incorrect placement can slow or hinder operations. Truck company placement cannot be addressed specifically without discussing engine company placement, as the two must coordinate placement of apparatus. Once an aerial truck is placed at an incident, it is usually there for the duration. Because of its increased size and other apparatus placed around it, the tiller may not be able to be moved.
- Jack operations are used for side-to-side stabilization while using the aerial ladder. The jack applies forces toward the torque box and increases the overall foot print of the apparatus.
- All ladder operations, including all aerial elevations and angles of operation, should be operated within the manufacturer's recommended limits. These limits need to be adhered to during unsupported and ladder pipe operations.
- Controversial discussion persists regarding how best to "enter in" with the aerial ladder when victims are in need of rescue. Extending the aerial into the target space is the worst option, due to the victim needing to jump to the ladder. Lowering the aerial into the target space, therefore, is the driver/operator's best option.
- Safety systems are located strategically on the aerial ladder and the H-jack equipment as a safety mechanism to prevent driver/operators from doing something potentially dangerous. These safety systems can be bypassed by the manual override procedures under certain circumstances and with the proper knowledge.

Hot Terms

aerial ladder inspection With the ladder in bedded position, the aerial is tested by raising it to 60 degrees, rotating it 90 degrees to the left or right, and then fully extending it within 60 seconds while utilizing fast idle.

apparatus placement In regard to truck company operations, apparatus placement refers to how and where an apparatus is placed at the scene. Virtually all fire incidents require and utilize the support from apparatus in some way. The success of most fireground operations often depends, directly or indirectly, on the effective placement of fire apparatus.

torque box A welded structural steel pedestal plate that supports the turntable, outriggers, trailer, and gooseneck as one integral unit, the torque box structure transfers all of the aerial loads to the outriggers.

References

Los Angeles County Fire Department, Manuals. California State Fire Training for Apparatus Driver/Operator Tiller-Truck.

National Fire Protection Association (NFPA) 1002, *Standard for Fire Apparatus Driver/Operator Professional Qualifications*. 2014. http://www.nfpa.org/codes-and-standards/document-information-pages?mode=code&code=1002. Accessed March 27, 2014.

National Fire Protection Association (NFPA) 1911, *Standard for the Inspection, Maintenance, Testing, and Retirement of In-Service Automotive Fire Apparatus*. 2012. http://www.nfpa.org/codes-and-standards/document-information-pages?mode=code&code=1911. Accessed December 18, 2014.

DRIVER/OPERATOR
in action

While spotting for roof access during an incident, you are manning the basket of a midmounted 100-ft (30-m) basket aerial apparatus. You have five personnel getting into the basket and only three ladder belts.

1. What is the NFPA standard for operating from an aerial device?
   - **A.** All personnel should wear ladder belts.
   - **B.** The captain does not have to wear a ladder belt.
   - **C.** You might need your axe.
   - **D.** No snacks on the aerial.

2. Which of the five members should wear a ladder belt?
   - **A.** The new fire fighter
   - **B.** The driver/operator
   - **C.** Anyone on the aerial
   - **D.** The cook for the day

3. Should someone always be at the pedestal when the aerial is operated?
   - **A.** No
   - **B.** Yes
   - **C.** Only if more than one person is on the aerial
   - **D.** Unless they are pumping a line

4. How many members can be in the basket at one time?
   - **A.** One
   - **B.** Two
   - **C.** Five
   - **D.** Depends on load limits and the number of belts available

5. Why should you train as if your life depends on it?
   - **A.** Because it does
   - **B.** So you can go home at night
   - **C.** Because you might have a family
   - **D.** So you get stronger

Testing, Maintaining, and Troubleshooting Aerial and Tiller Apparatus

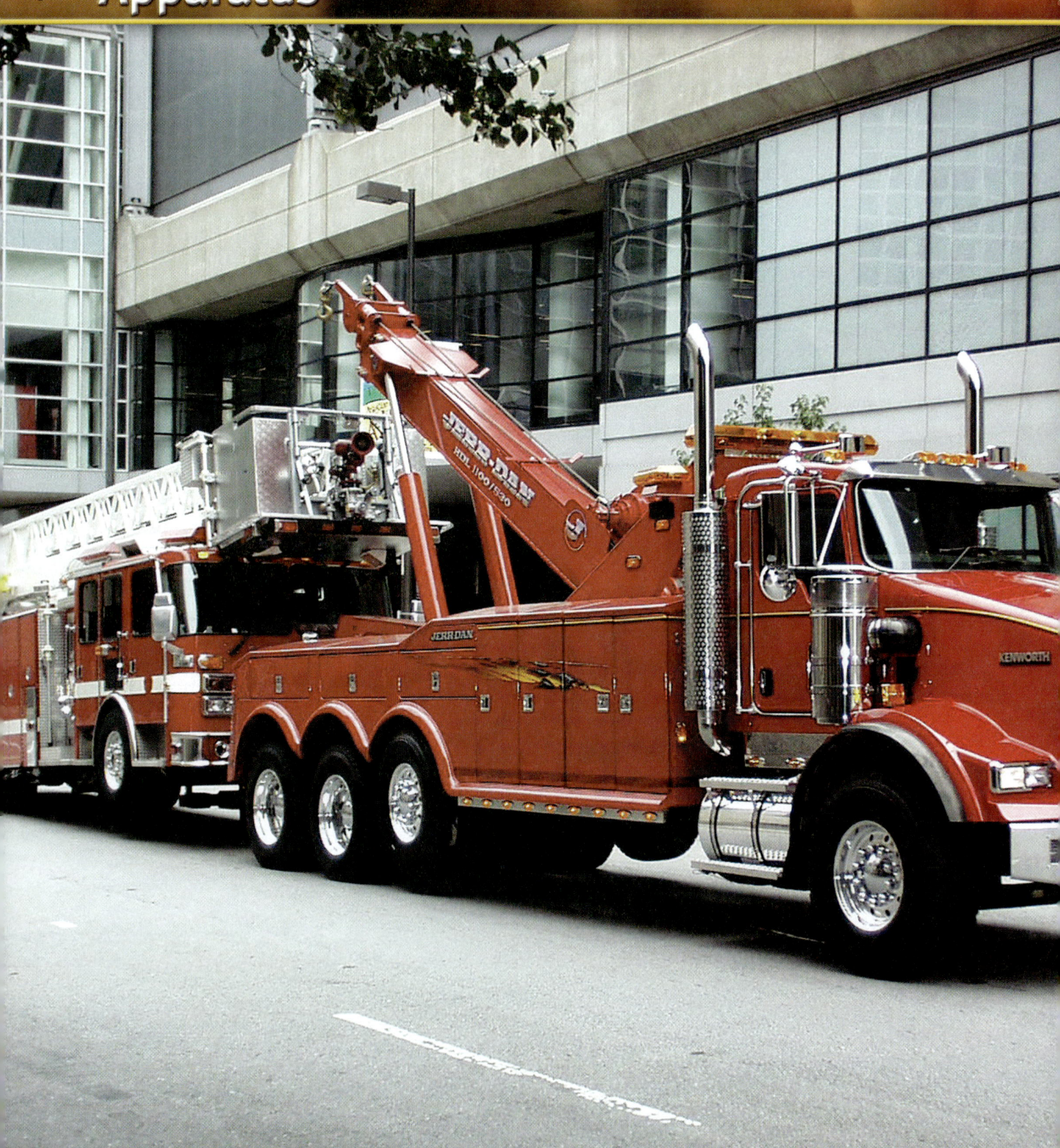

CHAPTER 18

Knowledge Objectives

After studying this chapter you will be able to:

- Describe the routine tests, inspections, and servicing functions, for a given fire department's aerial apparatus and tiller apparatus. (NFPA 1002, 6.1.1(A)); p 434–460)
- Describe the routine tests, inspections, and servicing functions, for a given fire department's aerial apparatus and tiller apparatus, according to the manufacturer's specifications and requirements, and the policies and procedures of the jurisdiction. (NFPA 1002, 6.1.1(A)); p 434–460)
- Describe the aerial device inspection requirements and process for cable systems (if applicable). (NFPA 1002, 6.1.1(1)); p 436–437)
- Describe the aerial device inspection requirements and process for aerial device hydraulic systems. (NFPA 1002, 6.1.1(2)); p 436–440)
- Describe the aerial device inspection requirements and process for slides and rollers. (NFPA 1002, 6.1.1(3)); p 456)
- Describe the aerial device inspection requirements and process for stabilizing systems. (NFPA 1002, 6.1.1(4)); p 457)
- Describe the aerial device inspection requirements and process for aerial device safety systems. (NFPA 1002, 6.1.1(5)); p 452, 454–458)
- Describe the aerial device inspection requirements and process for breathing air systems. (NFPA 1002, 6.1.1(6)); p 438, 457)
- Describe the aerial device inspection requirements and process for communication systems. (NFPA 1002, 6.1.1(7)); p 457)
- Perform the aerial device inspection for aerial device safety systems. (NFPA 1002, 6.1.1(5)); p 452, 454–458)
- Perform the aerial device inspection for breathing air systems. (NFPA 1002, 6.1.1(6)); p 438, 457)
- Perform the aerial device inspection for communication systems. (NFPA 1002, 6.1.1(7)); p 457)
- Demonstrate the ability to recognize system problems and correct any deficiencies noted according to policies and procedures. (NFPA 1002, 6.1.1(B)); p 458–460)

Additional NFPA Standards

- NFPA 1071, *Standard for Emergency Vehicle Technician Professional Qualifications*
- NFPA 1901, *Standard for Automotive Fire Apparatus*
- NFPA 1911, *Standard for the Inspection, Maintenance, Testing, and Retirement of In-Service Automotive Fire Apparatus*

Skills Objectives

After studying this chapter, you will be able to:

- Perform the routine tests, inspections, and servicing functions, for a given fire department's aerial apparatus and tiller apparatus. (NFPA 1002, 6.1.1(B)); p 452, 454–460)
- Perform the aerial device inspection for cable systems (if applicable). (NFPA 1002, 6.1.1(1)); p 436–437)
- Perform the aerial device inspection for aerial device hydraulic systems. (NFPA 1002, 6.1.1(2)); p 436–440)
- Perform the aerial device inspection for slides and rollers. (NFPA 1002, 6.1.1(3)); p 456)
- Perform the aerial device inspection for stabilizing systems. (NFPA 1002, 6.1.1(4)); p 457)

You Are the Driver/Operator

Today is the first day that you will be serving as the primary driver/operator on your department's aerial apparatus, and it is also the day that a full operational and maintenance check is performed weekly by the primary driver/operator. You pull the apparatus out to the area where the operational checks take place and begin. After checking the fluids and doing your walk-around, you begin to operate the unit. The unit runs as expected, but as you are rotating the device, it becomes sluggish and moves at erratic speeds. The unit seems to be operating more slowly in all functions, and you contact maintenance for assistance. The maintenance personnel advise you to record your findings and report them back to their department, and they will show the unit as out of service pending the results of their own investigation.

1. Which safety procedures would you ensure are in place before you begin to check the device?
2. Which part of the rotation unit might potentially be malfunctioning?
3. What are some of the reasons that you would remove the device from service?

Visual Inspection

You begin any tour of duty or shift with virtually the same routine—an inspection of the apparatus. The objective of this segment is to teach personnel who operate aerial devices how and what to look for. Key aspects of the **visual inspection** are discussed next.

■ The 360-Degree Walk-Around

The first thing that should happen whenever any drill or when another shift turns over any type of apparatus is to perform a 360-degree walk-around inspection. This inspection is your first look at the condition of the vehicle and can give you some good instant indicators of potential problems before you take custody of the rig. Remember that you—and you alone—will be responsible for the safe and efficient operations of any apparatus once you are designated as the primary driver/operator.

It is not uncommon to find problems with any unit upon the initial look. Just as in firefighting tactics, in which a good officer will recognize the condition of the fireground, it is extremely important for the driver/operator to know the condition of the rig at any time.

The 360-degree walk-around provides you with that initial size-up. Most inspections should start at the driver's door and continue with a quick cursory look at the apparatus. During this step, you should make mental notes or annotate a check sheet to describe what you observe and plan for any corrections. These corrections will either be performed by the primary driver/operator or referred to the technician at the shop who maintains your rigs.

This nice, slow look at the unit includes the following elements:

- Check that the apparatus is clean.
- Check that all the tools are on the rig and stowed where they belong.
- Check for any visible leaks or fluids under the unit or coming from anywhere on the truck's system.
- Thump all of the tires and remember that you will check them later with a pressure gauge.
- Check that all the compartments are shut.
- Check that all the outriggers are properly stowed and that all the chocks and ground plates are in their holders.
- Check that all the ground ladders are safely secured in their racks and that the doors to the ladder compartment are secured.
- Check that the truck is plugged into the shore line power to keep the batteries and the accessories on the rig charged. What does the LED bar graph or indicator show regarding battery condition?
- Look up, and see if anything seems out of place on the aerial itself. This status will be double-checked in more detail later, but the initial review should identify items like leaves or tree limbs in the aerial itself. Many driver/operators have been quite surprised by what they find in the aerial after an early morning run.
- Check for any broken lenses or glass from the previous night's run that no one noticed while refitting the truck. Remember, it is better to ask the driver coming off duty what happened than have to explain it later.
- Once you get back to your 360-degree walk-around starting point, check with the last shift's driver/operator regarding which runs the crew had, if the members used the aerial apparatus on the last shift, and if so, which actions they performed and how long the apparatus was used.

A good 360-degree walk-around is relatively easy to do if you have an understanding of the device you are operating. You should quickly recognize when equipment is not in its proper place, and then you should investigate the problem further. Just as putting on your personal protective equipment (PPE) becomes second nature to fire fighters, so you must become an expert on your equipment so that you can readily identify what you need to do and process other information while your muscle memory gets the job done.

Before discussing the ways to check out and service your aerial, it is necessary to break down the inspection into several smaller pieces, so that the function of each component in the system is understood.

Operational and Equipment Checklists

Each fire department's standard operating procedures (SOPs) or standard operating guidelines (SOGs) are different, and career departments often operate differently than volunteer companies. Nevertheless, there should be designated procedures and qualified personnel responsible for operations, testing, and maintenance of aerial devices. Aerial apparatus are manufactured by multiple companies, and all of these **original equipment manufacturers (OEMs)** have different requirements for their products. At a minimum, the OEM recommendations should be followed, and most OEMs have set time-based standards for specific items to be checked on the devices. In particular, the standards are usually linked to the 10-, 50-, 100-, 200-, and 400-hour times located on the aerial hour meter. These meters are usually found in the driver's compartment close to the switches that activate the aerial power and **power take-off (PTO)** unit **FIGURE 18-1**. Depending on the manufacturer, the apparatus may also have an additional hour meter on the **turntable** at the control station.

An aerial checklist will identify the specific items that need to be checked, and a great deal of controversy is always associated with how much should be checked. Departmental SOPs are written based on many items that come into play. For example, some stations have to move their apparatus to a safer test area based on issues such as access and overhead electric lines. In addition, it is not always practical to check a device every day. Volunteer companies might have meeting days and apparatus check days based on the availability of personnel. One department may test its unit only once per week, whereas other departments will mandate a daily full check of the apparatus. Of course, in the middle of a rescue while utilizing your apparatus is not the time to have doubts about your unit: if you checked it, you would have confidence that it will perform appropriately.

To ensure that every possible mechanical item is at least visually inspected, the following points are some of the basic items that should appear on your checklist.

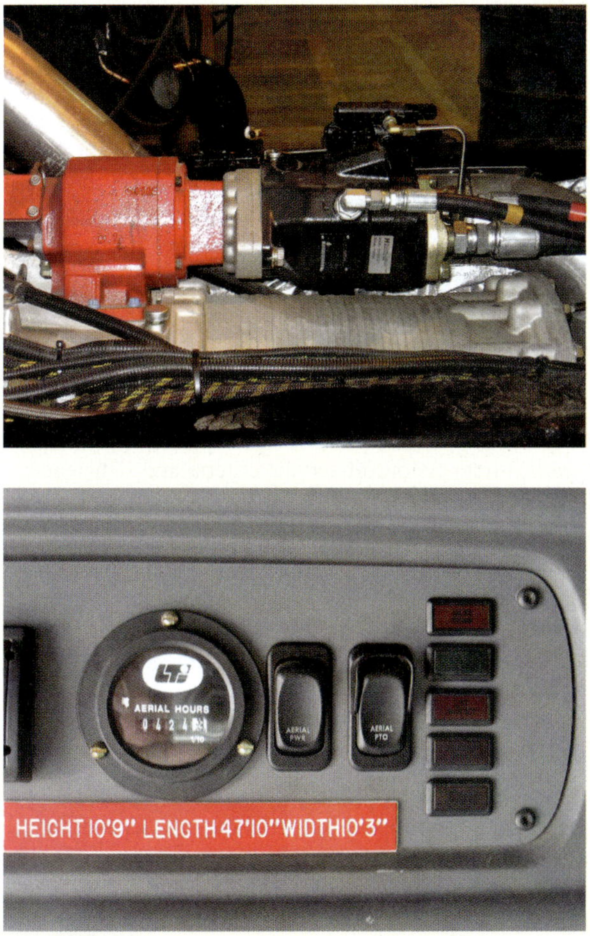

■ Aerial Device Hydraulic Fluid

Driver/operators should be familiar with the location of the hydraulic reservoir. Hydraulics can be found in numerous locations in the apparatus, including the following:

- Under the aerial ladder
- In the center of the truck under access doors
- On the tractor of the tiller-drawn aerial
- Mounted integral to the cradle
- Located above the pump module on **quints**

Hydraulic reservoirs have to be checked at least weekly, according to your department's SOPs, the manufacturer's recommendations, and designated procedures. Make sure that the fluids are at the proper levels at the beginning of every shift. Many manufacturers have supplied sight glasses and visual marks to alert the driver/operator that the level is incorrect. These sight glasses can also show milky or cloudy hydraulic oils and be a good indicator of the need to take a unit out of service or be evaluated by a technician. The levels on the sight gauge are marked because when an aerial operates, the oil in the system gets hot and can expand. For that reason, you should never fill an aerial hydraulic tank above the recommended FULL line. If this occurs, a driver/operator should seek assistance from the maintenance section and enlist the **emergency vehicle technician (EVT)** as referred to in National Fire Protection Association (NFPA) 1071, *Standard for Emergency Vehicle Technician Professional Qualifications*, in rectifying the situation. On the visual inspection, the driver/operator should return to the sight gauge once the aerial has been operated during checkout. Note whether a significant drop in the level has occurred and look for leaks. Driver/operators should also observe the sight gauge after operations to determine whether any metallic-like particles are floating in the fluid. This can easily be accomplished by shining a flashlight into the sight glass **FIGURE 18-2**.

Filling the hydraulic oil unit should be done after the unit's current oil supply reaches ambient temperature, while being cognizant to not overfill the unit. Overfull units will boil out hydraulic oil and create an environmental issue that must be mitigated. Make sure that you use the right hydraulic oil or a recommended brand and **viscosity**. Oil compatibility charts are always supplied by the manufacturer, along with the unit's owner's manual **FIGURE 18-3**. Whenever you have any doubts about the appropriate type of oil, always double-check the manufacturer's information. Introduction of the wrong type of oil can

FIGURE 18-1 **A.** A power take-off (PTO) unit. **B.** The aerial hour meter.

FIGURE 18-2 Shining a flashlight into the aerial reservoir sight glass.

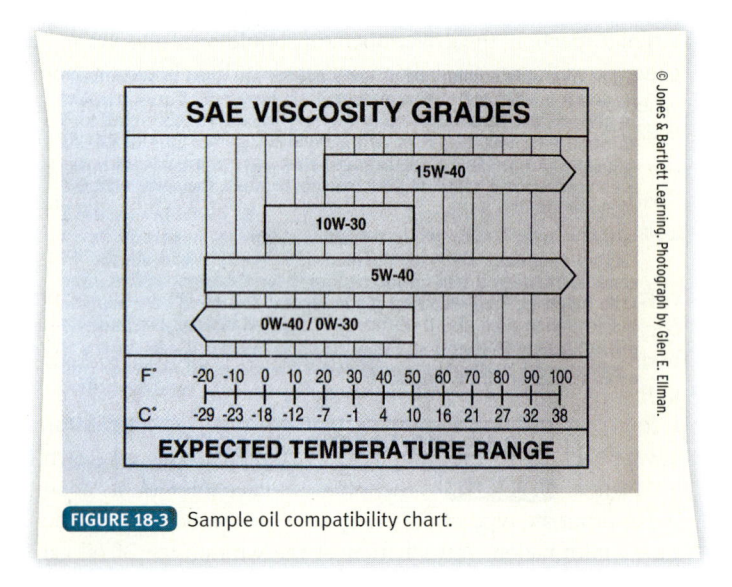

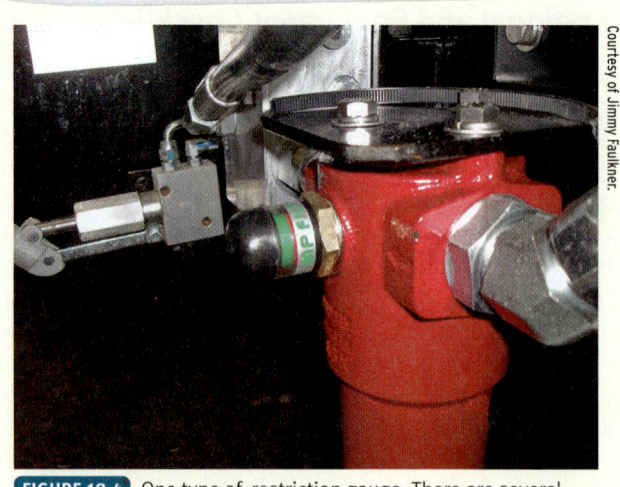

FIGURE 18-4 One type of restriction gauge. There are several different types of indicators used on the filter restriction. Others include a simple indicator light.

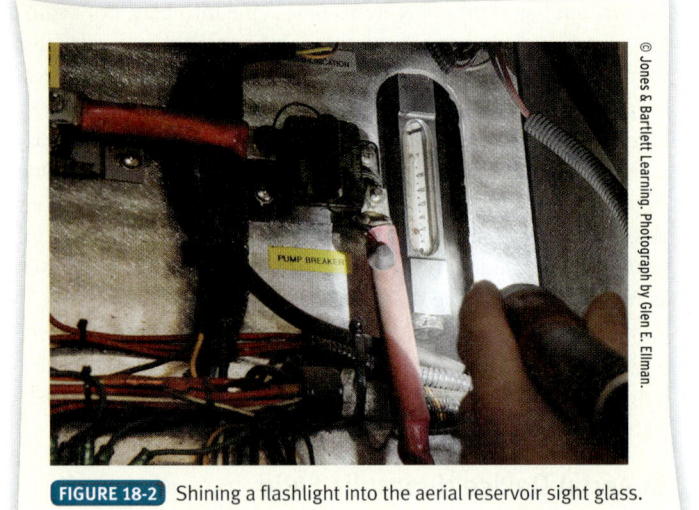

require the unit to be taken out of service and possibly damage pumps and components, which has expensive ramifications.

If the reservoir is equipped with a filter minder or restriction gauge, it needs to be checked as well. Verify that the arrow or gauge pointer is in the green zone. The reservoir contains an integral filter that cleans the oil of particles as small as 10 microns. A micron is approximately the size of a human hair, so the filter needs to be kept clean. If the gauge is showing red, it is time to notify the EVT of the need for filter replacement **FIGURE 18-4**.

■ Stabilizer Systems

While doing the visual inspection, the driver/operator should examine each stabilizer. Some units have four stabilizers, and some smaller have only two. Some of the larger tower devices also have a front stabilizer under or as part of the front bumper. The driver/operator should assess whether the footplates attached to the aerial are fully retracted. This is a good time to shake the plate to check that the attached hardware, which actually holds the plate to the jack itself, is tight. Look on the plate for any evidence of hydraulic oil leaking from the cylinder, and observe whether the plates have experienced any impact damage. Road potholes and railroad crossings are often responsible for tearing off or damaging these plates. Crossing railroad tracks shortens the **angle of approach**, the **angle of departure**, and the break over angles—that bump you heard during the last call might possibly have been an outrigger plate or a low-hanging piece of apparatus under the truck hitting the track as the apparatus passed over it.

Be sure that the outrigger beams or under-slung stabilizers are fully retracted on the unit. If you have already engaged the PTO, the outrigger lights should be on. When you perform the operational check and actually operate the beam or stabilizer handle, you will need to listen and feel the truck. If you retract the beam, stabilizer, or outrigger jack and it moves up, clicks, or bangs, then you need to have it checked by a qualified person. Any movement of any component in this scenario indicates that some drift has occurred, and some hydraulic components may need resetting.

The National Fire Protection Association (NFPA) mandates certain items in NFPA 1911, *Standard for the Inspection, Maintenance, Testing, and Retirement of In-Service Automotive Fire Apparatus*, under its out-of-service criteria and deficiencies list in chapters 6.10.1 and 6.10.2 **FIGURE 18-5**. All driver/operators should be able to identify these items or know where to reference them. In most cases, these out-of-service criteria are included in the departmental SOPs; in any event, they are the best guidelines available. Common sense plays a big part in instances such that "When in doubt, take it out of service" is the safe play.

■ Extension Retraction and Hoist Cables

On the visual and walk-around inspection, it is difficult to see all of the aerial cables. Instead, they are best observed while operating the unit and positioning the aerial over the back of the truck or on the side, in the case of a mid-mount apparatus. The driver/operator can then safely lower the aerial below the 0-degree grade and actually get a better view of the cables and control wires. Obvious fail items would include the following:

- Frayed cables
- Dry cables (cables should be lubed and not dry)

FIGURE 18-3 Sample oil compatibility chart.

Aerial Device Systems
• The following deficiencies of the aerial device and its systems shall cause the aerial device to be taken out of service:
   (1) Power take-off (PTO) that will not engage
   (2) Stabilizer system that is not operational
   (3) Aerial device that is not operational
   (4) Hydraulic system components that are not operational
   (5) Cable sheaves that are not operational
   (6) Cables that are frayed
   (7) Base and section rails that show ironing beyond the manufacturer's recommendations
   (8) Aerial device that is structurally deformed
   (9) Torque box fasteners that are broken or missing
   (10) Turntable fasteners that are broken or missing

• If there are deficiencies of the following systems or components, a qualified technician shall conduct an out-of-service evaluation and make a written report, including recommendations to the AHJ:
   (1) Hydraulic relief valve
   (2) Hydraulic system components
   (3) Emergency hydraulic system
   (4) Visual and audible alarm systems
   (5) Aerial lighting system
   (6) Aerial intercom system
   (7) Labels or warning signs
   (8) Aerial water delivery system

FIGURE 18-5 Out-of-service criteria and deficiencies chart.

Safety Tip
It is imperative that stretching out an aerial behind the vehicle be done in a protected area. Cones or closed course areas will keep individuals from running into a device that is deployed low to the ground. In any circumstance, aerials should never be operated without properly setting outriggers and plates.

Safety Tip
Never extend or retract a 0-degree-set ladder during checkout with someone on the ladder.

The Turntable and Its Components

The visual and walk-around inspection also includes the turntable and its components **FIGURE 18-6**. The checklist for the turntable should consist of the following items:

- Safety chains or protective guards are in place to keep fire fighters from falling off the turntable.
- Turntable handrails are secure.
- Because all components on the turntable deck are subject to impact damage from low-hanging branches, evidence of impact on any component should be reported immediately for evaluation.
- The turntable control box is secured and control door covers, safety devices, and lighting are functional.
- The dead man's switch is functional.
- There is no evidence of hydraulic leaks from any area on the turntable.
- Indicator lights for the cradle alignment and rung alignment are functional.
- If the PTO is engaged and there are no outriggers deployed or set, nothing should move when the operator attempts to raise the aerial by depressing the dead man's switch. If there is any motion at all, the safety aerial interlock is not functioning and needs to be serviced. Make sure that the ladder is nested in the cradle and take the apparatus to be serviced immediately.

- Sagging cables during extension and retraction
- Loose clevis pins and bolts on the end of the cables
- Flexible cable protector or Igus track is binding or not flowing smoothly
- Excessive squealing while moving the cables
- Jerking motions
- Uneven sheave wheels (pulleys) that are binding while the ladder is moving
- The ladder jerking from side to side while extending
- Abrasion wear on the winch drum for older ladders with winch-style hoist systems for ladder extension and retraction
- Check roller and roller assemblies
- Loose or missing slide blocks

These checks can be part of the operational check, and the checklist should have a space to document any abnormal action that is experienced. It is easier to look at an aerial that is stretched out while standing underneath it, and you can reach up and perform many of the checks at this point. You can then get up on the aerial device and walk out to the tip to get a topside view.

This is also a good time to check for loose rung covers as well as proper side and lower roller operations. While up on the ladder itself, check the security of the mounted tools on the tip. Roof ladders, axes, and pike poles on the fly section can come loose; if they get between the ladder sections, they can cause significant damage. Check the condition of the mounting hardware and annotate the checklist if replacement straps or pins need to be replaced.

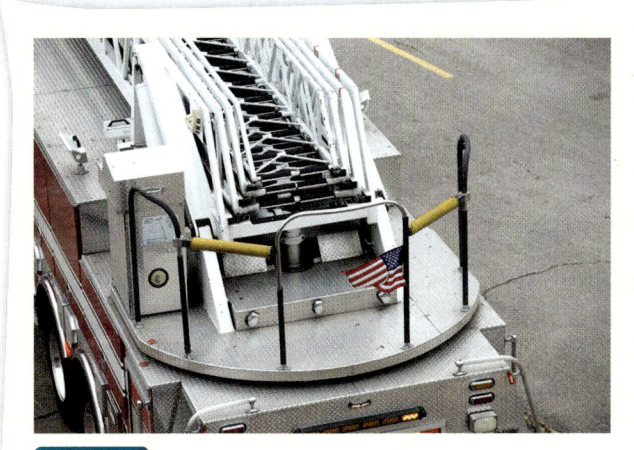

FIGURE 18-6 The turntable.

Turntable Control Pedestal

The turntable control pedestal is where all of the aerial hydraulic and electrical controls are installed. The movement of the aerial is managed from this position by the aerial operator. The following controls are found at the pedestal:

- **Raise and lower control handle:** Used to lift the ladder from the cradle and place it into operation. This handle is connected to the **double-acting lifting cylinders**, which utilize hydraulics to lift and hold the ladder up or bring it down smoothly under power.
- **Extend and retract control handle:** Used to extend the ladder sections through the action of hydraulic cylinders connected to cables under the ladder. These cables are connected to both the cylinder and the ladder; by utilizing the pulleys, they can extend, retract, and hold the ladder in place.
- **Rotation control handle:** Connected to a hydraulic motor that can be reversed by the position of the handle and that is connected through a rotation gear box and brake, which allows the turntable to rotate. When the rotation control handle is used, a brake that holds the turntable in position at all times is released hydraulically and allows the motor to turn the gear box and move the turntable with a large rotating gear called the bull gear **FIGURE 18-7**.
- **Dead man's switch:** Installed on the turntable and meant to ensure that an operator is always at the pedestal. The operator at the turntable must stand on this guarded foot switch; otherwise, a blocking solenoid does not open. This solenoid is an electrohydraulic device that either blocks or allows free flow of hydraulic oil to the controls. When the solenoid is closed, there is no oil and, therefore, no movement of the device. This is generally the same valve, called a diverter valve, that is enabled once the outriggers or stabilizers are properly set and is an additional safety interlock. The dead man's switch allows operation of the aerial device only when certain parameters are safely met.
- **Master power switch:** Completely disconnects all electricity at the control box and acts as a safety measure while personnel are working on the aerial. It is used to stop operations in a dangerous environment.
- **Nozzle controls:** Electric switches placed on the panel of the control box that direct the stream of the nozzle and monitor movement on the tip or in the platform. The driver/operator can select electric momentary toggle switches for left or right and up and down movement and either fog or straight stream. Another control at the tip or in the platform basket allows the personnel working on the tip to direct the nozzle from that vantage point as well. In some cases, platforms have two nozzles, and a separate control is installed for the second nozzle both at the pedestal and at the tip.
- **Hydraulic pressure gauge:** Shows that the hydraulic system is producing sufficient pressure.
- **Rung alignment indicator light:** Shows that all of the ladder rungs in the section are aligned so that they are easier to climb. As the ladder extends and retracts, the rungs will stack, a condition that is indicated with this light. In most instances, the driver/operator sets the ladder to the job and location it is needed and then tries to align the rungs for ease of climbing.
- **Cradle alignment light:** Shows when the ladder is in the best position to be lowered into the cradle. An arrow or some type of reflective indicator is also mounted directly to the turntable and the body to give the driver/operator a reference point for setting the ladder into the cradle, but this light keeps the driver/operator from missing the cradle, in which case the ladder might crush lights or air-conditioning units on the roof of the apparatus. It is always best to use these aids, but to prevent damage it is also important to verify placement visually with your eyes on the ladder and the cradle.
- **Fast idle switch:** A momentary toggle switch that sends a signal to the engine to speed up to a predetermined revolutions per minute (rpm) level, usually in the range of 1000 to 1500 rpm. This speeds up the hydraulic pump and allows more oil to flow at a higher pressure, in turn allowing faster and more powerful movement of the device. To disengage the unit, the driver/operator must again depress the toggle to idle the engine down.
- **Air minder or air gauge alarm:** Some devices have **Grade D air** cylinders installed on the ladder, and these permanently attached cylinders must provide at least 400 cubic feet of air. Air is piped to the ladder tip or platform so that fire fighters can couple in with a hose while at the tip. This setup allows them to keep their individual self-contained breathing apparatus (SCBA) air intact in case of emergency when working above the fire for long periods. The air gauge alarm tells the driver/operator when air is low, just like a SCBA buzz alert, by using buzzers or bells and a visual "air remaining" psi (kPa) readout.
- **Platform leveling switch:** Used with platforms that have hydraulic leveling cylinders attached to the platforms. This switch can help correct leveling problems and is generally used by maintenance personnel to set levels of the platform itself. It is not found on straight stick aerial devices.

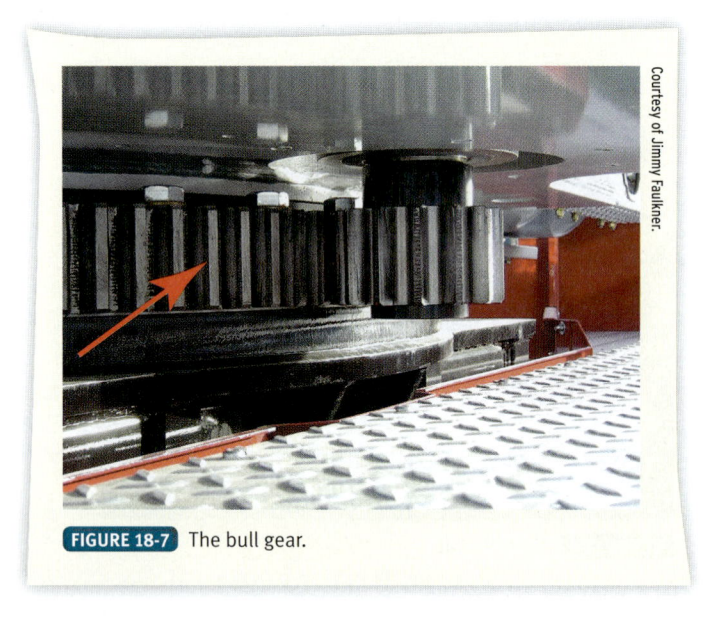

FIGURE 18-7 The bull gear.

CHAPTER 18 Testing, Maintaining, and Troubleshooting Aerial and Tiller Apparatus

- **Cab or obstruction alarms:** Buzzers or lights that tell the driver/operator when the apparatus is at an angle in which the ladder can damage the truck. These alarms are generally found on midmount aerials and are intended to keep driver/operators from lowering the ladder into the cab when working off the front of the unit. They are also found on other types of aerials that have special toolboxes or body configurations in which contact can occur by lowering the device in certain positions.

> **Safety Tip**
> Obstruction alarms are designed to prevent contact of the ladder with the truck only. They do not warn of impending contact with buildings, overhead wires, or other structures at the fire scene.

- **Short-set indicator lights:** Used in a scenario in which the full extension of one of the outriggers was prohibited. This visual indicator is a warning light only. Short-set outriggers are commonly used in apparatus that must operate in larger cities with narrow streets. In such an environment, the driver/operator is forced to deploy the outriggers to the side facing the fire. He or she then deploys or extends the outriggers on the opposite side as far as possible, but not to full extension. This causes the **outrigger interlock** to illuminate this light. At the same time, an additional set of electric-over-hydraulic valves called the **rotation interlock** come into play. This system consists of two valves that can stop the aerial from rotating. The rotational switch(es) automatically ensure that the aerial cannot rotate to the short side, thereby preventing a ladder rollover failure. The driver/operator must use another manual guard toggle override switch on the pedestal in such a scenario **FIGURE 18-8**. This switch ensures the driver/operator is aware of the possibly dangerous conditions in which the apparatus is operating.

FIGURE 18-8 Manual guard toggle override switch.
Courtesy of Jimmy Faulkner.

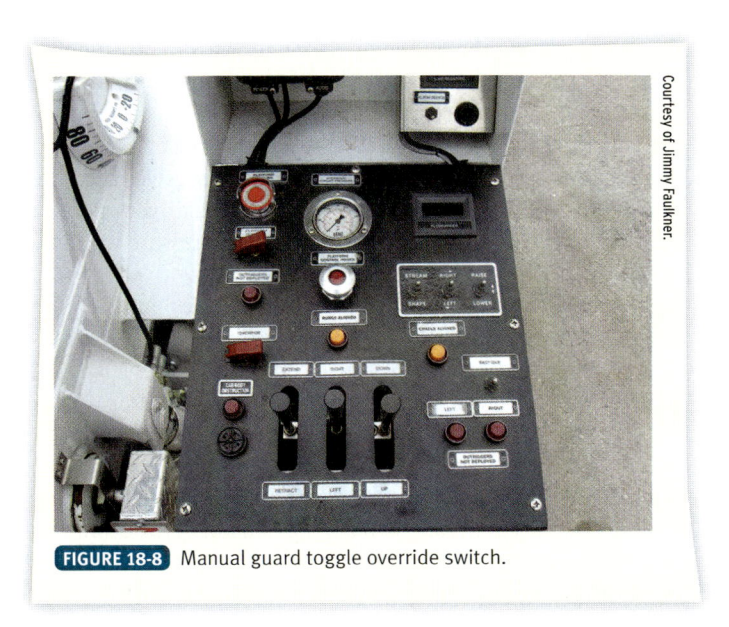

- **Outrigger override switch:** A guarded momentary toggle switch, along with the dead man's foot switch, that must be operated to perform any movement with the aerial device. This additional safety measure is intended to make the driver/operator think and ensure that he or she does not attempt to go over to the short-set side. This switch must be depressed and held while any movement control is initiated. The aerial, if all systems are functioning properly, will then be stopped from rotating over the short-set side by the rotation interlock. In some cases, the ladder will not move to the unsafe side once locked down, but can be recovered to the safe side using the override. Some aerials require a reset from a different location than the pedestal, while some will allow the operator to rotate back to the no-short-jacked side with no additional intervention.

> **Safety Tip**
> An override means you are circumventing an installed safety system. Any mishap while operating the override places all of the responsibility on the driver/operator. Always make every attempt to operate without short-setting your device.

> **Safety Tip**
> Whenever a fire fighter is on the ladder or in the tower, there should always be an operator at the turntable. Controls at the turntable can be used to override the operations performed by fire fighters at the tip or platform, and the operator at the turntable can stop any dangerous movement of the device.

- **Controls in the platform:** The same motion controls are installed in the platform that are found on the turntable pedestal. While some of the older aerial platforms still use hydraulic lines and controls between the basket and the pedestal, newer apparatus have controls that are electrically operated and send an electric or **multiplexed** signal to the valves on the truck below. These controls act much like a dimmer switch: the more that you engage them or turn them up, the more power that is sent down to the valves. An electromagnet receives the power from the upper controller and translates it into movement of the control handle. A plunger installed on both sides of the valve pulls or pushes the valve spool. The spool valve is the part of the hydraulic valve that allows hydraulic fluid to move through the system; this fluid movement controls the operations that raise, lower, extend, retract, and rotate the tip. Monitor controls as well as the air alarms and intercom systems are also found in the platform, as are a fast idle switch and obstruction warning lights.

- **Aerial communication and intercom:** A two-way speaker and volume controller that allows the fire fighter at the tip to communicate by voice-operated transmission (VOX) or open mic to the driver/operator at ground level or at the turntable. The bottom unit, which requires a push-to-talk (PTT) button to operate, allows communication to go from the ground to the tip.

Ladder Components and Classifications

According to NFPA 1901, *Standard for Automotive Fire Apparatus*, an aerial device is an aerial ladder, elevating platform, or water tower that is a self-supporting, turntable-mounted, power-operated ladder of two or more sections permanently attached to a self-propelled automotive fire apparatus that is designed to position personnel and handling materials and provide discharge water and a continuous egress route from an elevated position to the ground FIGURE 18-9.

■ Ladder Sections

The bottom section of the ladder is referred to as the base section, and the outermost ladder is called the fly section. Because most ladders have more than the two sections required by NFPA 1901, the other sections are called midsections. If there are just three sections of ladder, the middle section is simply referred to as the midsection. If there are two sections between the base and the fly sections, making it a four-section ladder, the inner sections are referred to as the inner-mid and the outer-mid sections FIGURE 18-10.

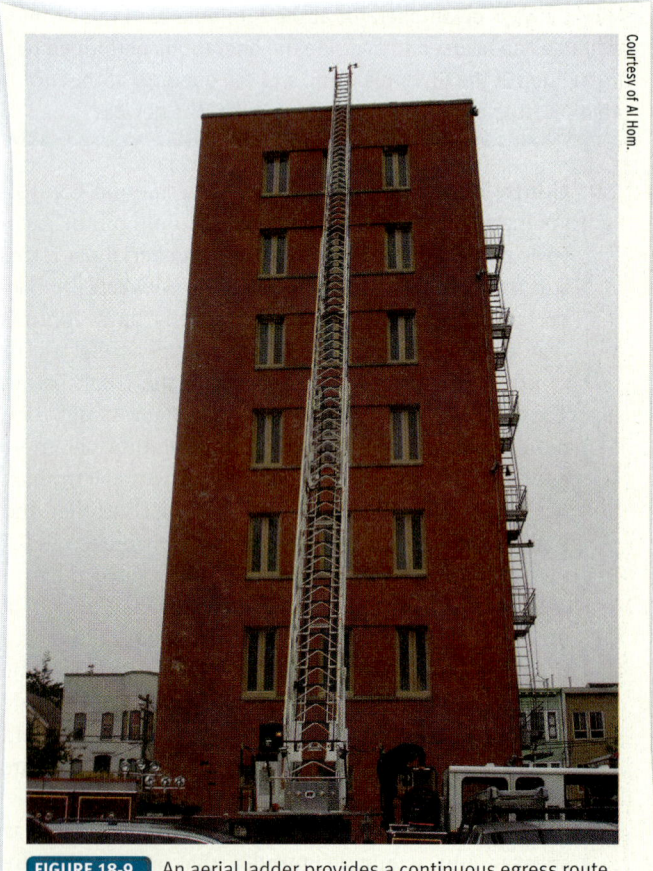

FIGURE 18-9 An aerial ladder provides a continuous egress route from an elevated position to the ground.

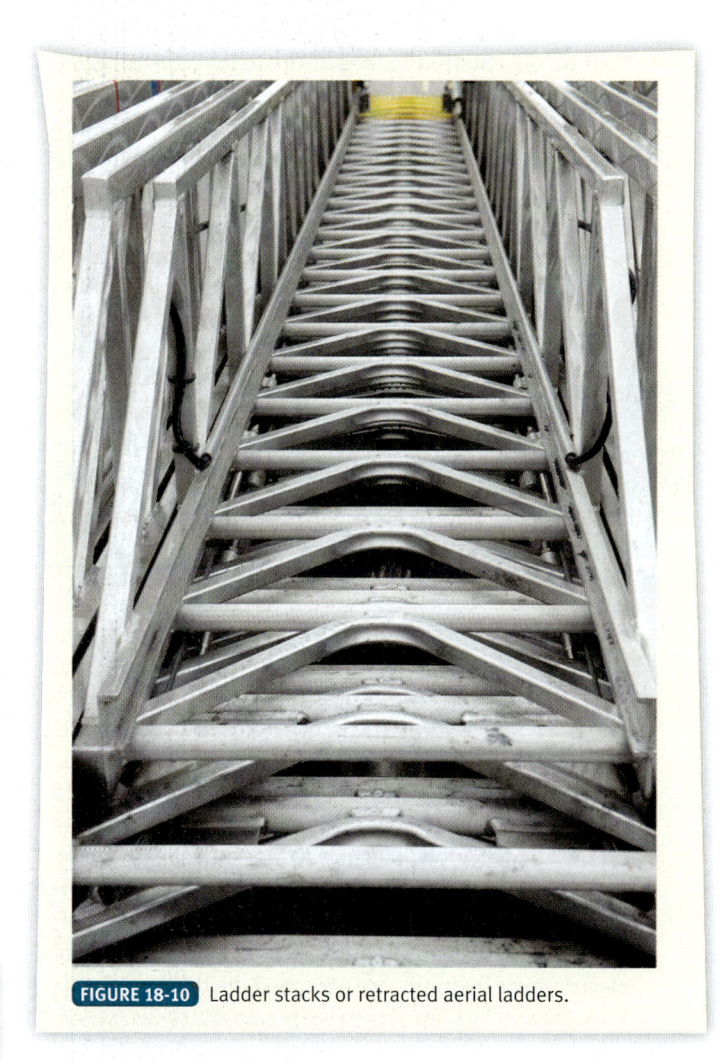

FIGURE 18-10 Ladder stacks or retracted aerial ladders.

■ Lift Cylinders

The lift cylinders are the largest and most powerful hydraulic system on the aerial apparatus. These double-acting cylinders are used to raise and lower the aerial through the application of hydraulics. They also have **pilot-operated check (POC) valves** that will hold the cylinders in the position requested. To open the POC, the hydraulic oil overpowers the spring that keeps the check valve closed. The lift cylinders use hydraulic fluid that is pumped from the PTO pump and through a valve body into the cylinders. A POC is installed in the cylinder, and it opens and allows fluid to pass only when it receives pressure from a valve being selected and operated. If the driver/operator pulls back on the raise handle, the hydraulic pressure will flow into the cylinder block and open up the POC.

At that point, the fluid can flow into the cylinder on the bottom of the cylinder. The fluid forces a piston in the cylinder to be pushed upward. This piston has a chrome-plated ram attached to it inside the cylinder, which exits the top (or in some cases the bottom) of the lift cylinder. The ram is connected to the ladder by a device called the lift cylinder clevis. Note that there are two lift cylinders that receive fluid during this process, and both fill and push the ram out of the cylinders. This action causes the ladder to raise and pivot upward. The ladder is pushed up either by utilizing separate pins on each side of the ladder or by engaging a lifting cradle that attaches to the ladder where the lift cylinders push it upward. The ladder pivots on a set of pins or a long pin at the base section called the **heel pins**.

The lift is timed so that both cylinders raise and lift together and the ladder rises evenly. If the ladder lifts on only one side or the other, the aerial apparatus should be referred to the maintenance EVT for service. Once the ladder is set to the desired height or topped out, the driver/operator releases the raise valve handle. At this point, there is no hydraulic pressure to move the ladder, so it stops. Likewise, the POC does not receive any hydraulic pressure, so it closes. The loss of pilot pressure turns the valve into a check valve. The fluid, which is compressed and trapped in the lift cylinders, cannot escape and so holds the ladder up.

When lowering the ladder, the same chain of events happens, only in reverse. The driver/operator engages the lower valve and both POC valves open. The valve for the raise opens and allows the fluid to escape from the bottom of the cylinder. At the same time, the lower POC allows the valve to let hydraulic fluid into the upper part of the cylinder; it pushes the ram back down. The fluid in the lower unit acts as a buffer and prevents it from slamming down.

In the past, many ladders relied on single-action cylinders, which used hydraulic pressure to force the ladder up using the same ram and lift yokes or clevises; when the aerial was lowered, the weight of the ladder itself was relied upon to push the fluid out. When the driver/operator engaged the lower valve, it simply let the captured fluid out of the cylinder, and the work was done by weight and gravity. The same types of cylinders are used on cab lifts today. Hydraulics are used to lift the cab and move the cylinder, but the weight of the cab is used to force the fluid out.

The advantage of the double-acting cylinder is that it allows the driver/operator to configure the unit to fly below the 0-degree grade and still have enough power to lift the aerial back up. The fluid on both sides of the cylinder acts as a shock absorber. In the single-acting cylinder, once the ladder went below zero-degree grade, it was sometimes difficult to raise it back up. The double-acting cylinder also allows for smooth synchronous operations and enables the driver/operator to **feather** the controls and perform movements of the ladder without jerking and getting the units into a bind.

■ Rotation Controls

The rotation controls have several hydraulic and moving parts that are required for rotating the aerial. Once the operator has selected the direction of the rotation, either left or right, by operating the handle, several things happen in the rotation system. Hydraulic fluid enters a valve block or manifold that is called the motion controller. The fluid opens POC valves that allow the fluid to move one direction or another into a hydraulic motor that supplies the energy to rotate the aerial. This motor is connected into a rotation brake—a friction-style set of plates that are always locked in the stop position. When the operator engages the rotation control and sends fluid to the motor, the motion controller allows fluid from a POC to go to this brake. This fluid is then used to force the brake open.

At the point, the motor can turn, and it rotates a shaft that is connected to a rotation gear box commonly called the swing drive. This gear box multiplies the motor energy and causes the bull gear to turn. The entire turntable is mounted on a large bearing that allows the ladder to rotate and support the ladder in any position. The ladder turntable bearing has teeth that mesh into the bull gear, which rotates and thereby causes the turntable to move to the left or right, as dictated by the driver/operator.

Some aerial devices that have a long reach or heavy sections will utilize two rotation gears. According to engineers, this arrangement reduces **backlash**—that is, side-to-side motion of the aerial turntable. The use of the two rotation gears provides a more positive control and allows the manufacturer to use smaller swing drives in constructing the aerial apparatus.

■ Waterway and Associated Plumbing

The minimum flow on an aerial device, per NFPA standards, is 1000 gpm (4000 L/min). To provide this flow, a ladder is equipped with its own waterway system. Such a system consists of two or more pipes that become progressively smaller as they telescope out of each other. There can be one large pipe attached under the ladder or two smaller pipes, one down each side of the ladder. For example, in a four-section ladder, four pipes are required. If the base or bottom pipe has a 4½-inch (114-mm) inside diameter (ID), the next pipe would have a 4-inch (100-mm) ID, the pipe after that would have a 3½-inch (90-mm) ID, and the final or fly pipe on the waterway would have a 3-inch (77-mm) ID. The waterways are sized to the flow that the fire department wants to project from the ladder. Some aerials can flow 2000 gpm (8000 L/min) or better, depending on the water supply and pumping capacity.

The waterway system starts with a feeder or intake pipe that is found in the rear of the device—usually a 4-inch (100-mm) National Standard Thread (NST) connection or larger. This pipe is connected to the waterway through plumbing under the turntable and flows up through the middle of the **hydroelectric swivel** **FIGURE 18-11**. If the aerial is a quint-type device, this pipe will also be connected to a valve from the fire pump and be able to supply the waterway without the rear connection being utilized. The rear connection is capped in this evolution, and there is a pressure gauge right next to it from which the operator can read the pressure from the pump or the pressure when using it alone as an intake to flow to the tip.

> **Safety Tip**
>
> Never attempt to remove the rear inlet cap while flowing water from the fire pump up the ladder pipe.

■ The Hydroelectric Swivel

The hydroelectric swivel allows the ladder to turn while the waterway stays connected. In the middle of the device is a water passage with **victaulic connections** on both the top and the bottom of the swivel. This pipe connects the lower

FIGURE 18-11 The hydroelectric swivel.

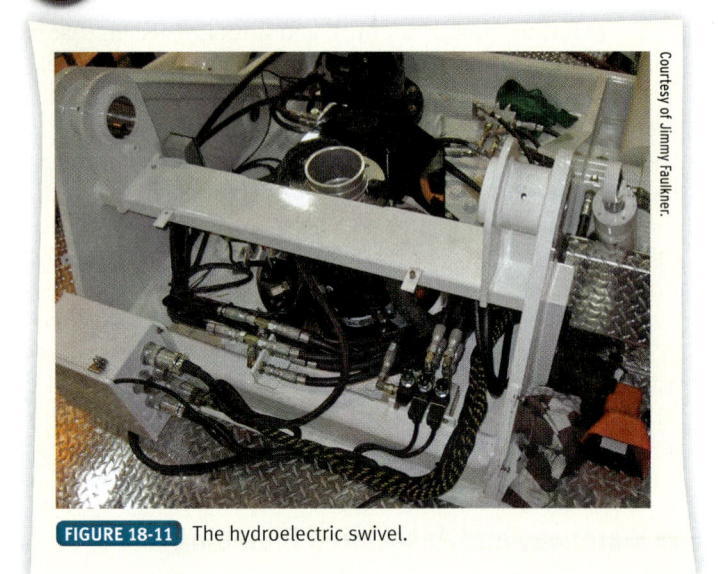

plumbing to the aerial waterway pipe; that is, it allows water to flow up from the bottom through the swivel and then through the waterway, coming out the monitor at the tip or platform.

The swivel has passageways that allow hydraulic oil to be introduced at the bottom and come out the top. It also has wires from the electric controls and circuits that enter the swivel at the bottom and exit the top. This wiring uses a combination of **collector rings** that are installed inside the swivel and that allow the unit to rotate or swivel. The lower set of wires touches the collector rings at the 9 o'clock position, and the wires that exit the top connect to the collector rings at the 3 o'clock position. The only thing that moves is the center core. This unit includes three cavities: one for water through the middle, one for hydraulics in the core, and one for electric power with the collector rings that makes contact with the brushes connected to the wiring harnesses.

The Ladder Section

As the driver/operator, you need to be familiar with the basic nomenclature of the pieces of a ladder section. The base rails are the bottom part of the ladder that holds the rungs—all of the section's bottom rails are called base rails. The rungs are the actual stepping surface that is used to climb the ladder. At a minimum, the rungs have an outer diameter (OD) of 1¼ inches (32 mm) around and should be capable of supporting 250 pounds (113 kg) at the center of each rung. This rationale of weight limit comes from the NFPA, which assumes that the average fire fighter wearing full PPE represents 250 pounds (114 kg) of load. The rung has to be able to support two fire fighters or a fire fighter and a victim. Rungs must also provide some sort of nonslip surface. To meet this requirement, some manufacturers provide rubber rung covers that are wrapped around and attached to each rung. Other manufacturers that utilize aluminum rungs in their ladders will actually make grip ridges when the ladder rung is **extruded**.

K braces are stiffening members of the lower rung and base rail assembly. They attach at the base rails on both sides and at the rung in the middle, and make the rung look like the letter "K." The uprights and diagonals are the vertical tubes that rise at 90 degrees from the base rail and give the handrail its bracing and attaching points. Uprights go straight up and attach to the handrails, and diagonals go from the uprights at the base to the next upright, attaching to the handrail at 45 degrees.

The handrails are the rails that fire fighters hold onto while climbing each section of the ladder. They need to be at least 1-inch (2.5-cm) tubing and must rise at least 12 inches (30.5 cm) from the base rail. The width between the handrails at the top must be at least 18 inches (45.7 cm) and is sometimes called the "top rail."

Also found in the fly section of the aerial, for availability to roof crews, are ladder-mounted accessories. This equipment can include axes, pike poles, short ladders, and roof ladders.

Platform Controls

Controls located at the platform are the same as those found at the turntable control. All functions of the platform controls can be overridden by the turntable operator from the lower control station. There is a master disconnect on the platform and, in some cases, a basket-leveling valve. The communications speaker is mounted, so PTT is not needed to operate the intercom; this arrangement allows the driver/operator to "fly" the basket using both hands so that multiple operations can be performed at the same time. The control station can be mounted anywhere in the platform, and some manufacturers installed movable options. The platform has breathing air hookups and places to store additional tools and handlines to deploy to upper floors when necessary.

A valve is also provided that taps into the waterway pipe in the platform. It protrudes through the protective cover installed under the platform and will spray up to 75 gpm (300 L/min) for cooling under the platform in case of impinging fire. This valve is operated by personnel in the platform manually.

Two-man gates minimum for egress in and out of the platform are required. Electric or manual controls for single or dual monitors are included in the controls, with an additional discharge valve with hose threads provided to allow the platform to act like a standpipe connection when raised to an upper floor.

Tiller Trucks

Tiller trucks are simply tractor-trailer aerial apparatus. They are more maneuverable than straight-chassis trucks because they bend in the middle and have the advantage of rear steering. The rear driver or **tillerman** sits in a cab mounted on the back of the trailer behind the ladder tip. The aerial ladder is attached to the trailer, and the tillerman sits in the tiller cab, high above the street, looking straight down the aerial through the handrails at the back of the cab **FIGURE 18-12**.

The Tillerman

The tillerman has an unobstructed view, and his or her job is to steer the back of the trailer. This tiller operator accomplishes

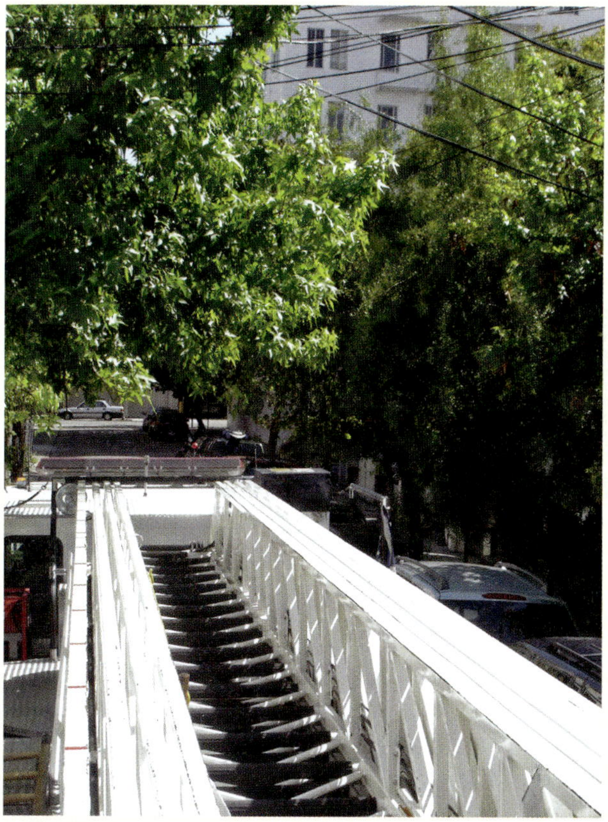

CHAPTER 18 Testing, Maintaining, and Troubleshooting Aerial and Tiller Apparatus

FIGURE 18-12 The tillerman's view. *Courtesy of Al Hom.*

this by turning the wheel in the opposite direction that the front driver/operator does, which causes the whole unit to pivot instead of tracking like a trailer. In this way, the tillerman is able to adjust the track of the trailer. This member has an intercom or headset that he or she uses to communicate with the front driver/operator and his or her own controls for heating and air conditioning. An electric buzzer foot switch is provided in the event of headset failure, through which the tiller operator can signal the driver with one buzz for "stop" and two buzzes for "go." The tillerman also has a safety or dead man's switch on the floor that he or she must press so that the front driver/operator can start the truck, thereby preventing the front driver/operator from leaving the firehouse without a tiller operator.

A dash-mounted gauge called the rudder control indicator informs the tillerman of the position of the rear wheels—either centered, left, or right. This gauge has a pointer that indicates the orientation looking right down the middle of the ladder. A tracking light is mounted on the back of the truck cab that is visible to the tiller cab; the tillerman uses this light as a centering guide to keep the tiller straight.

The tillerman plays a major role in capitalizing on the versatility of the tractor-drawn aerial. Driving and maneuvering a tiller take a lot of practice and coordination, especially when backing up a unit that bends in the middle. Experienced crews are able to back these units up and maneuver sideways and around tight corners with ease.

Aerial Device Operations

Operational inspection of aerial devices should include operating the apparatus at least once every work period so that the driver/operator is fully prepared during an emergency. Your department's SOPS will stipulate how often full inspections should occur (e.g., daily, weekly, or monthly) and the documentation that goes along with the inspections (e.g., daily, weekly, or monthly).

The most important consideration in aerial operations is proper setup and good ground to work from. Whenever you set up an aerial, whether it is for training, operational checks, or firefighting, you need a good base. A good driver/operator must be very quick in making the initial size-up or deciding on the placement of the aerial device. This is especially true in a firefighting scenario, because the fireground is constantly changing. In the 2 minutes it takes to set up the vehicle, many things can happen—other apparatus may position themselves on the fireground and deploy hoselines around the aerial device. A bad setup, such that the aerial cannot be fully utilized, can result in the loss of the device from a tactical perspective and potentially jeopardize the entire firefighting operation.

■ Placement and Foundation

Whenever you are setting up the aerial and for whatever purpose, it is important to be sure that the terrain and the ground are correct for placement of the apparatus. A driver/operator has to be aware of many conditions that affect the aerial placement and range of operations. Whenever possible, you will want to avoid setting up the aerial in certain areas, and you must be wary of some obstacles that can give you trouble even in a safe setup. In some cases, the most dangerous spot is the approach in front of the fire station. Obstacles, dangerous terrain, and situations to be aware of when setting up an aerial include the following:

- Manhole covers. Never set the apparatus close to them, and never set an aerial on a manhole cover.
- Newly constructed streets where the blacktop has not hardened and the base has not compressed under the asphalt level.
- Drains and sewer pipe openings. These areas are sometimes undermined by water flowing around them and have large subterranean hollow spots that the aerial's outriggers effectively punch holes in.
- Overhead electric lines anywhere in the 360-degree rotation range of the aerial device. When responding to an incident, both the driver/operator and the fire officer need to look up for wires crossing the roadway prior to entering a street or fireground. Aerial apparatus need to stay at least 10 to 15 ft (3 to 4.6 m) away from any potentially energized lines. Energized lines can also fall from the fire building and become entangled in the aerial, in which case they can immediately ground through the outrigger plates.
- Sidewalks. Never set outriggers on sidewalks. Sidewalks are not designed to support 60,000-lb (27,300 kg) vehicles.

- Training and testing sites. The best place to test and train with the aerial is on a controlled site like a fire department training center or a large parking lot with no overhead obstructions.

Other placement considerations include the following:
- Always try to get the turntable in the best position for scrubbing the building and utilizing the maximum reach of the device.
- Know the weight limits and horizontal reach of the device and confirm them through trial and practice during training.
- Know the position of the cab control's outrigger and aerial controls, so that these actions are committed to muscle memory.
- Practice the same way every time with your crew.
- Understand that you must be able to set up the aerial apparatus alone if the situation dictates.

Cab and Predeployment Procedures

Before committing your unit, make sure that you are not in the collapse zone and that there is room for companies to pass you or lay lines whenever possible. Treat any setup, either real or training, as a test of your placement decision. Preplan your district's target hazards and look for landmarks that you can refer to during a real incident.

> **DRIVER/OPERATOR Tip**
>
> Situational awareness is a skill that the driver/operator must constantly practice to learn to notice everything. Every time you train, do it like your life or a crew member's life depends on your actions.

The aerial is most effective when deployed off the rear of the apparatus, because you can get maximum reach of the device with maximum stability. Unfortunately, in most instances, you will be working off the side from the street. Very seldom will you achieve the ideal setup location or geography. Try to get the center of the turntable in line with the target, so that you can raise, rotate, and extend the aerial with maximum efficiency **FIGURE 18-13**.

Before doing anything, set the spring brakes and put the truck transmission shifter into neutral. Engage the aerial PTO and/or the aerial power switch. Utilizing some old-school double-check logic, always put one hand on the brake knob and the other hand on the door latch or knob when leaving the cab. If you commit this practice to muscle memory, the truck will never roll away inadvertently. This failsafe system can be employed anytime you exit a vehicle and is a good habit to teach your rookies. Be sure to close the cab door after exiting—high winds or other fire equipment that need to pass are very unforgiving when large fire truck doors stick into the roadway.

Know the location of the chocks and put them both under the front wheels. Walk with a sense of urgency and get to the back of the unit. There, you should open the doors to the outriggers and make sure the diverter valve or switch is in the outrigger position. Ease over to the officer's side to start deploying the system. As you exited the apparatus from the driver's side, you should have done your assessment of that side of the apparatus as you walked toward the rear; starting at the officer's (off) side gives you the opportunity to take a last look and confirm that all is well before you set and plant the outriggers.

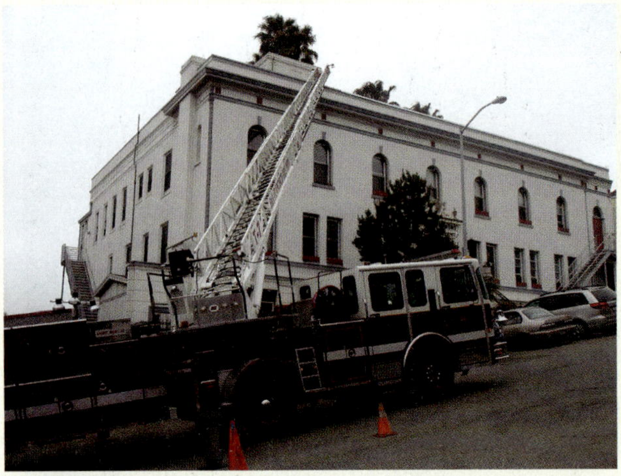

In the worst-case scenario, you may have to set up the device alone. Your officer and crew may be making a 360-degree walk-around or getting the assignment, leaving you to set up the apparatus correctly without help.

FIGURE 18-13 Effective apparatus placement.

Outrigger Types and Deployment

Depending on the type of apparatus, there are several different styles and deployment procedures for outriggers. Outrigger styles include H-style jacks, modified H-style jacks, underslung jacks, and X-style jacks.

H-Style Jacks

The H-style jack stabilizing system will have a handle or switch for the jack beam and one for the outriggers jack at the rear in a control box or panel **FIGURE 18-14**. Such a system has two major moving parts: the **beam** and the jack cylinder. The beam is connected to a hydraulic ram located inside a steel-reinforced tube. The beam tubes are placed horizontally in the **torque box** and are housed in a larger tube that allows the beam to slide in and out as the hydraulic cylinder extends and retracts the beam. The jacks are connected to the end of the beam; they lower the jack down or raise the jack up using a hydraulic cylinder inside the jack. These systems are controlled from the valves actuated at the rear by the driver/operator. On smaller devices, the H-style system may include a set of beams and jacks at the rear of the apparatus. With larger and heavier aerials, it may include one set at the front of the unit and one set at the rear on each side, for a total of four.

Modified H-Style Jacks

A modified H-style jack system uses a beam and a jack system just like the H-style system, but instead of orienting the jack at

Courtesy of Jimmy Faulkner.

FIGURE 18-14 An H-style jack.

Courtesy of Jimmy Faulkner.

FIGURE 18-16 Under-slung jacks.

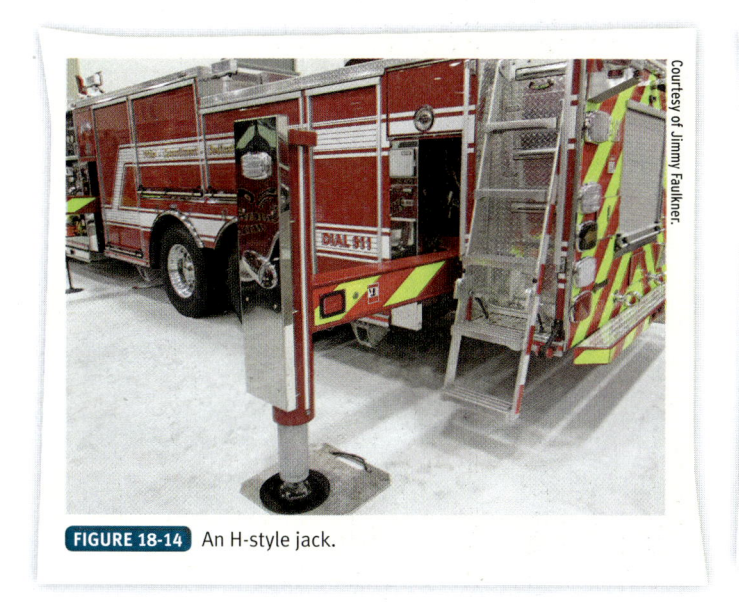

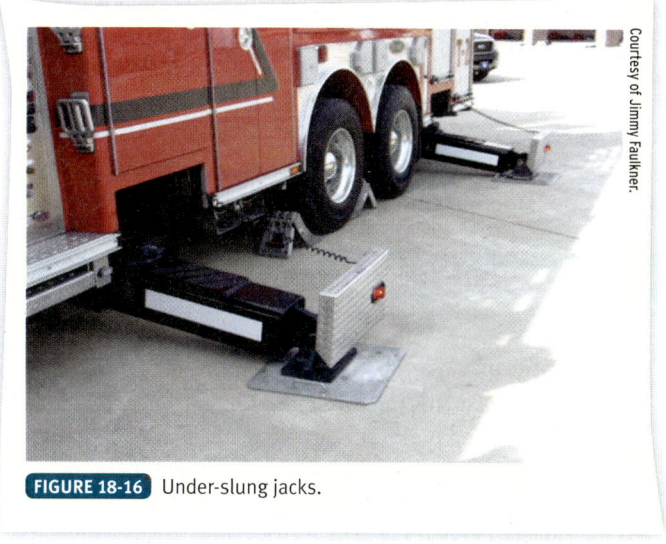

90 degrees, the jack is mounted to the beam at a slight angle FIGURE 18-15. The deployment of this jack increases the footprint and jack spread and thereby provides for more stability. A third control system adds a third motion to the truck setup. The beams are still encased in a slightly larger tube, but the tube has a pivot, which allows the system to apply downward pressure on the beam, and the pivot action sets the truck up further. An additional hydraulic cylinder forces the beam to push down on a separate control as well. The front system of the jacks in this setup is also angled, but the jacks just go down at an angle with no beam to move. A modified H-style jack system gives more of a triangular base than a square base for the unit, and it allows the apparatus to realize some degree of versatility on the street.

Under-Slung Jacks

Another type of system consists of under-slung jacks, which are mounted lower and under the torque box FIGURE 18-16. Such a system is deployed by extending both beams on one side of the unit until they are fully extended. The driver/operator can pause and set jack ground plates under the unit and then return to the control. At this point, both beams will be pushed to the ground by a hydraulic cylinder activated by the driver/operator. These beams are also able to pivot and raise the truck using the downward force of the hydraulic cylinders.

X-Style or A Frame Jacks

In the past, X-style jack systems were commonly found on smaller aerial apparatus and some boom-type systems FIGURE 18-17. With this setup, the jack is installed in an almost 45-degree orientation at the rear of the truck and attached to the torque box. Such systems utilize inner and outer tubes, called a **jack box**; the inner jacks boxes are moved by one hydraulic cylinder inside the jack box. To set the unit, the driver/operator holds the handle for either side jack until the truck is level.

Fast Idle Control

Each control station will have a fast idle switch, which tells the diesel to idle up to 1000 to 1500 rpm to supply hydraulic

Courtesy of Jimmy Faulkner.

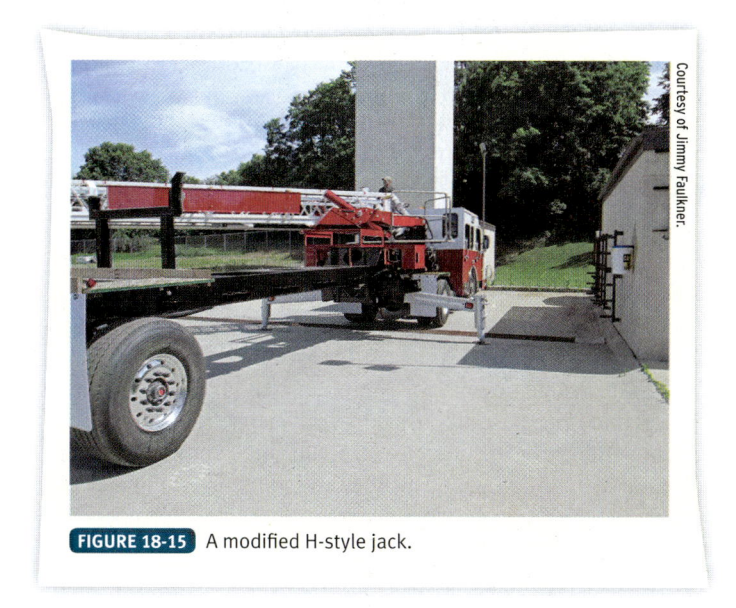

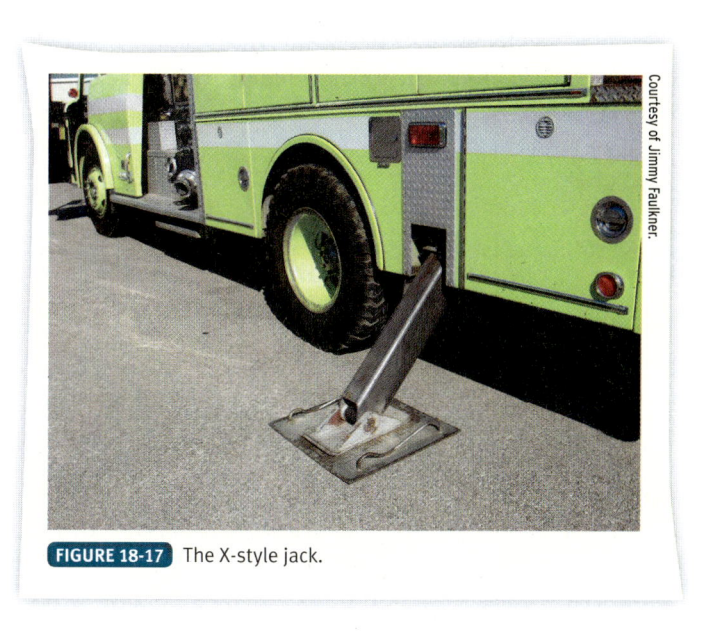

FIGURE 18-15 A modified H-style jack.

Courtesy of Jimmy Faulkner.

FIGURE 18-17 The X-style jack.

volume and pressure. This momentary switch should be utilized for outrigger deployment. The hydraulics will work at idle speed, but will operate more efficiently at fast idle settings. To deactivate the fast idle control, the driver/operator toggles the momentary switch. On some devices, the movement of any outrigger or aerial control handle activates the high idle; once it is released, the high idle switch disengages.

DRIVER/OPERATOR Tip

If an aerial apparatus has a fire pump, the fast idle switch will be disabled by the pump interlock. The movement and speed of the aerial depend on the throttle setting that the pump requires to pump the needed pressure. This relationship protects handlines that are operating from the unit from suddenly being overpressured when the high idle control is activated. Otherwise, the high idle power and speed might exceed the pressure that a handline needs and injure a fire fighter.

■ Deploying the Outriggers

Once the driver/operator is ready to deploy the apparatus' jacks (in this example, H-style jacks will be utilized), the high idle switch should be engaged. Remember that when deploying units with four jacks, it is imperative to watch the moving part as it extends and goes to the ground. The front beams should be extended first, which will trigger the green deployed lights to become illuminated. This signal provides a clear indicator to the driver/operator to then extend the rear beams, which will in turn illuminate the extended lights. Whenever anything on the outriggers that operates hydraulically is moving, an audible signal is produced as well. This signal alerts the crew members that they need to be aware of the movement and stay clear of the deployment zone. While the beams are extending, it is possible for someone to get between them and a fixed object and be easily crushed by the hydraulic system's power. The driver/operator should be watching the beam's deployment, and he or she should stop the part's movement immediately if anyone is in danger by simply releasing the control switch.

When both beams are out, the driver/operator then places the auxiliary ground or footplates under the attached jack plates **FIGURE 18-18**.

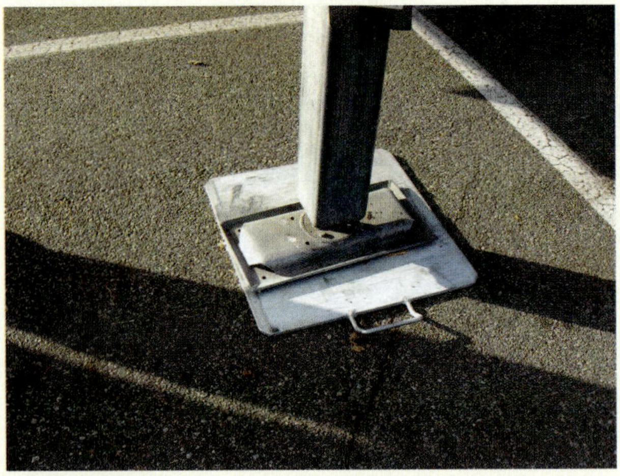

FIGURE 18-18 Footplates under the attached jack plates.

Safety Tip

Never set any aerial without the ground plates in use.

Once the ground plates are under the unit's jacks, the driver/operator can begin to lower the jacks and raise the device. Again, the driver/operator needs to keep an eye on the jacks as they are going down to ensure that no tools, hose, or personnel are trapped under the jacks. The jacks will raise a 77,000-pound (35,000-kg) vehicle off the ground, so crushing anything under the jacks may have catastrophic results. Using the control handles, set the jacks such that they raise the beams and touch the top of their beam tubes. The goal is to just barely lift the truck about 1 inch (25 mm) or so—you can see it or feel it by holding on to the truck. This is done with both jacks. Next, repeat the same sequence on the other side, again just barely getting the jacks to lift the unit.

Find the level gauge and get ready to set the truck to the green zone by operating the handles and lifting the truck one side at a time. If there are two sets of jacks on one side, you will want to use both handles simultaneously. Lift the truck until the level indicator is slightly past level. Then go to the other side and do the same action. There are three colors on the level gauge:

- The green zone shows that the apparatus is between 0 and 3.5 degrees, which indicates that you will be able to use 100 percent of the ladder's capacity.
- The yellow zone indicates that the apparatus is between 3.5 and 6.0 degrees, which limits the use of the ladder's capacity to 50 percent.
- The red zone indicates that the apparatus is exceeding safe limits. In this case, you should not continue operations until a better setup can be accomplished. In all cases, always refer to the OEM recommendations for safe sets and fly zones.

In a perfect world, the driver/operator will set up the apparatus so that the truck's leveling ball shows zero degrees in the green zone. Be sure that the outrigger controls show all green lights before turning off the fast idle.

■ Outrigger Safety Devices

On every function of the outrigger controls, there is a green light to indicate that the driver/operator has safely and successfully deployed that part of the device. A green light is illuminated when the beams are all the way out, and another indicator signals that the jacks have sufficient load on them to support the truck. The beams down light is illuminated when the unit has been planted and has sufficient support. If any of these lights are not lit, you have either missed a step, not sufficiently extended a beam or jack, or not loaded or lifted the truck up enough.

Sometimes, such as when there is a short street or a parked car in the way, it is not possible to extend a beam all the way out. This scenario and setup, called a **short-set**, limits the use of the device. The beam extended light will not illuminate, and the safety or outrigger interlock will not allow the ladder to operate without a manual override. The ladder will be limited to extending on the long-set side only. The short-set side may potentially fail to support the ladder on the short side and could cause a ladder rollover.

Once the truck is leveled, you can prepare to climb the access ladder to the turntable. Before climbing up, if the device has safety pins in the jack, make sure they are installed. Take a last look to ensure that the jacks are not sinking; if the jacks are sinking, reevaluate the situation for safety. Finally, turn off the fast idle control and shut the outrigger control station doors.

Safety Tip

Avoid short-setting the apparatus whenever possible to realize full, safe use and range of the device. If you do have to short-set the apparatus, remember the adage, "The long side is the strong side," which indicates that the short-set side has to be the side away from the fire.

Operating the Aerial Device

There are many manufacturers, types, and classifications of aerial devices. Apparatus are broadly classified into the following groups:

- Aerial ladder apparatus, which include aerial ladders
- Elevating platforms
- Telescoping aerial platforms, which include both aerial ladder platforms and articulating aerial platforms
- Water towers

For the most part, all aerial apparatus operate in basically the same manner. Moreover, the aerial device, whether it is a two-piece telescoping squirt-type device or a four- or five-section ladder, will generally have the same operating control characteristics. After successfully deploying the outriggers, the driver/operator makes his or her way to the turntable or to the driver/operator's control station. Some apparatus have a pump panel–mounted control; in such a case, initial operations will begin from there.

Safety Tip

Any operations involving the pump panel should be done from a step so that the driver/operator is **NEVER** in contact with the ground. This rule applies **anytime** the operation takes place here and will keep the driver/operator from becoming the route-to-ground if the device accidentally comes in contact with high-voltage lines during operations. This scenario has caused many serious injuries to fire fighters during morning checkout or at firefighting operations.

To do anything with the device, it must be raised from the cradle or bed. The ladder will then need to be rotated to the direction of the fire or the rescue, and extended to the fire floor or operating area to deploy aerial fire streams or provide egress.

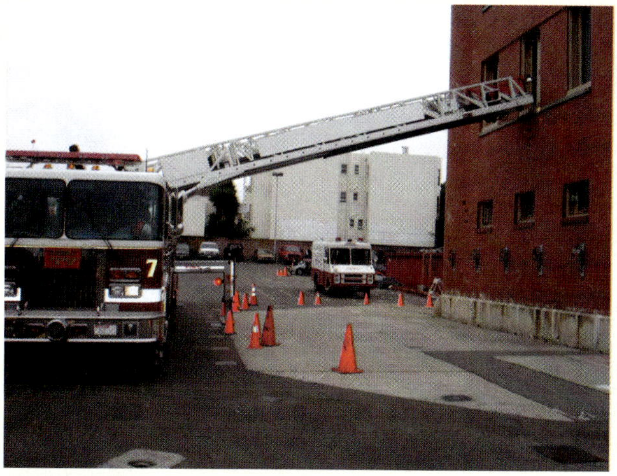

FIGURE 18-19 Horizontal reach.

Before any crew member performs any operations involving the aerial device, he or she must be very familiar with a number of factors that apply to any aerial device.

Aerial Device Working Height

Driver/operators must be familiar with the working height of the aerial device. The working height of the unit is measured from the ground to the highest ladder rung at full elevation. Ladders are built with anywhere from 75 to 135 ft (23 to 41 m) of vertical height and can operate at up to 75 degrees of elevation. **Horizontal height** is measured from the heel pin or centerline of the truck to the outermost reach of the ladder itself. The horizontal reach is less than the vertical or working height of the unit, because the height of the truck is lost as the ladder pivots down. For example, if a ladder is 103 ft (31 m) tall, subtracting the height of the truck from the total working height of the ladder will provide a good approximation of the horizontal reach **FIGURE 18-19**.

Angles of Operation

Ladder trucks are capable of operating at different angles. The age of the truck will dictate which angles are safe for climbing and delivering water supplies. Newer aerial apparatus are capable of operating at full capacity while in angles ranging from −10 degrees to +75 degrees. These angles are displayed on the unit in the form of angle indicators, either manual or electronic (on a mounted LED screen), so the driver/operator (or driver/operators in the case of a pump panel control) can easily see them **FIGURE 18-20**. As the ladder is raised or lowered, the angle shown on the indicator will increase or decrease. This is done with an electronic angle readout, a glass tube and ball-type indicator, or a simple pendulum-style pointer with a chart.

When an aerial device is in the cradled or horizontal position, the angle is considered to be zero degrees. It is also considered zero degrees when the ladder is in use horizontally, facing directly off the rear of the device.

Newer aerial devices with more powerful hydraulic systems are capable of lowering the ladder below zero degrees to a

FIGURE 18-20 Manual angle indicator.

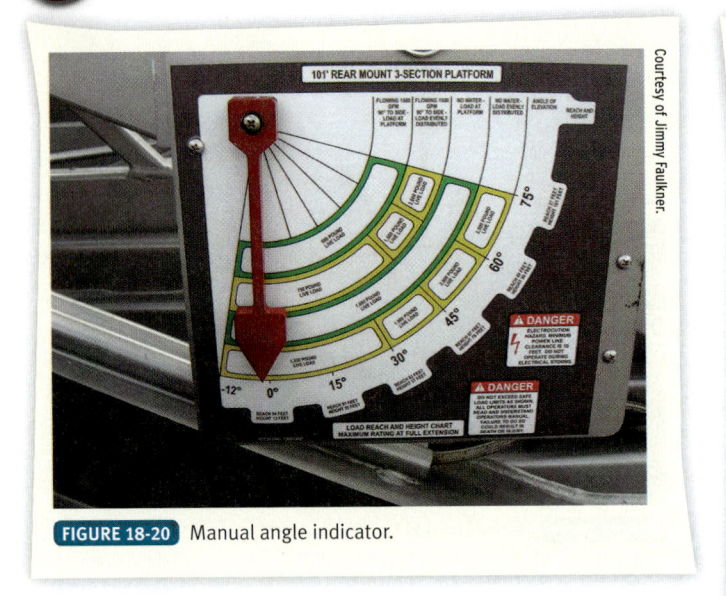

negative or below-horizontal angle. These types of maneuvers are usually performed at 90 degrees off the side over the outriggers or directly over the back of the apparatus. Attempting to lower the aerial device below zero degrees in any other areas creates the risk of striking the truck body. In most cases, the obstruction alarm will alert the driver/operator in such a scenario before damage is done. Some obstruction alarms actually lock out the control function as well, thereby preventing the aerial from crushing part of the truck.

Safety Tip

When working below zero degrees or off the rear of the apparatus, do not let the ladder tip touch flowing or moving water, such as a creek or river. Remember: the farther a fire fighter walks out on a horizontally placed ladder, the more it will deflect down. Monitors can be crushed on the ground, and in a water rescue scenario, the ladder might potentially be torn off.

DRIVER/OPERATOR Tip

Driver/operators must not rely on alarms to alert them to hazardous situations. The working parameters of the unit should be memorized and its operating limitations respected and practiced frequently. During actual firefighting operations, audible and visual alarms may not always be detected.

■ Load Charts

Load charts are the most important charts carried on the aerial apparatus **FIGURE 18-21**. The load chart provides the aerial device's safety parameters and includes the following information:
- Tip load, or how many fire fighters and what weight can be carried on the outermost rung of the ladder
- Number of fire fighters or distribution on each ladder section
- Working height

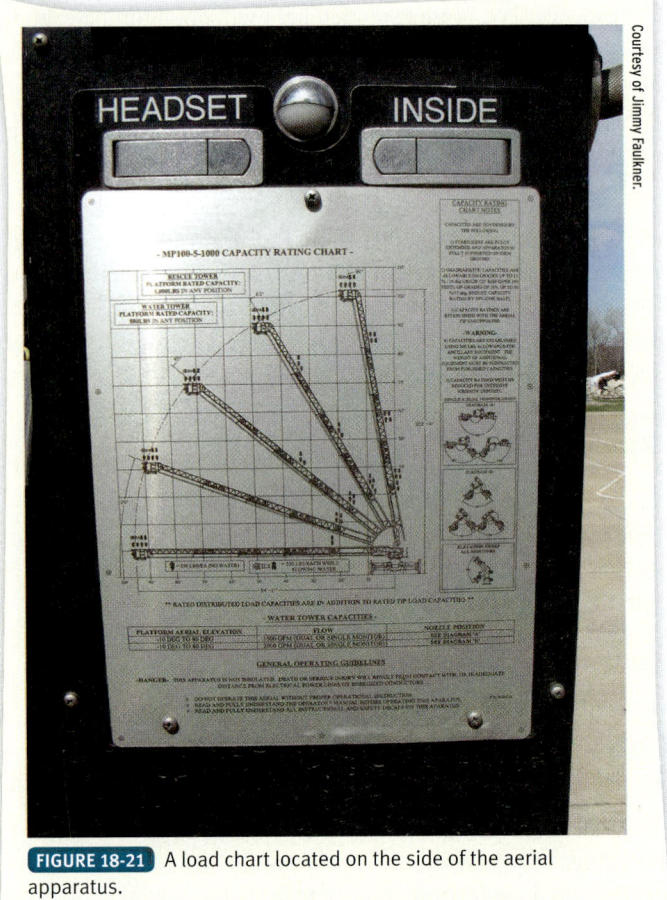

FIGURE 18-21 A load chart located on the side of the aerial apparatus.

- Horizontal reach
- Flow characteristics and gpm (L/min) capabilities
- Flow capabilities and personnel limitations when working the ladder dry (with no water flowing) and when discharging water
- Nozzle capabilities and ranges
- Icing warnings

Raising the Device

If all safety systems have been addressed and checks and balances have been accomplished, the driver/operator can now raise the ladder from the cradle. To do so, the driver/operator opens the console cover and quickly checks for any unsafe indicators, such as those signaling a short-set or outrigger not deployed. If they show an unsafe condition and the driver/operator did not intentionally short-set for the operation, it is best to go back down and find out what is wrong.

After ensuring that all is safe and properly deployed, the driver/operator steps on the dead man's switch at the floor of the turntable. In most cases, you will hear a "klunk" that indicates the hydraulic pressure has been delivered to the control bank. You will also notice a rise in pressure on the hydraulic gauge. Before moving anything, make one last 360-degree scan. Look at the controls, look up for wires, and confirm that no one is on the ladder prior to its movement. To raise the ladder gently and slowly, pull the raise handle back. To lower the aerial, you would push this handle forward. Some aerials will rise without the fast idle control being engaged. If you raise the aerial gently for the first 2 ft (610 mm), any inadvertent movement on the controls that you make, on purpose or by accident, will be slow. Many a beacon and cradle have been damaged by pulling the aerial out too fast and letting go of a control. Once the aerial is clear of any possible obstructions, you can engage the fast idle switch and raise the aerial to the desired angle. This is a skill that needs practice, practice, and practice. Your situational awareness must be set on high during this operation, because you need to watch the aerial tip and be aware of potential hazards—especially when you begin the rotation part of the evolution. When you are a new driver/operator, you need to always operate in this fashion: **raise–rotate–extend**.

New driver/operators need to be able to gauge the relationship between the speed of the device and the amount of control action they input. Every device is different and will react differently with fast idle settings. You can actually use the fast idle settings to increase the device's speed or to slow it down to a barely moving action with a little hand-to-control coordination. Good driver/operators can raise and rotate an aerial at the same time, and better driver/operators can do all three functions (raise, rotate, and extend) and be on target for a window for rescue every time. Your skill level is directly proportional to your training time and your mentor's patience with you when you are new. Learn to watch the tip of the aerial when it moves. Muscle memory will enable you to simultaneously use the controls and your eyes to watch movement and the periphery areas into which the device is moving. Remember, the moving part is what you must watch, no matter what it is. The control in your hand will not do anything unless you provide input.

Rotation

More accidents happen during the rotation phase than during any other operation of aerial devices. Whenever possible, you want to rotate to the side of the turntable control or pedestal. This direction provides you with an unobstructed view of the movements both when raising and rotating the ladder. It is not always possible to work in this way, but it increases the odds of not hitting something. Utilize the ladder tip lights whenever possible to visualize wires and to get an idea of where the aerial tip will set once you extend the ladder. When rotating the device, look at the tip. The direction in which you want the tip to move is the direction in which you move the handle. To rotate the device left or counterclockwise, pull the handle toward you; to rotate the device right or clockwise, push the handle away. The rotation speed is directly proportional to how much you push the handle forward, and it will be a little more sluggish on rotation when the ladder is at full extension.

DRIVER/OPERATOR Tip

Never just release the rotation control or any other control handle when the movement is complete. Slowly stop the movement by feathering out the control.

As part of safe operations, the driver/operator must ensure that no one is attempting to climb up to or get on the turntable while it is rotating. The power required to move the aerial is quite substantial and is very unforgiving to human limbs placed in the wrong areas. In addition, the driver/operator must power around and slowdown in smooth movements; otherwise, the ladder will backlash. In such a case, the ladder stops moving and bounces back and forth from the bull gear mesh on the turntable bearings. The longer the ladder is extended, the more pronounced the backlash will be.

Safety Tip

Under no circumstances should you reverse directions with the controls under power to stop the aerial. This will cause severe whipping of the aerial and possibly catastrophic damage to the unit.

Extension and Retraction

Once the driver/operator has raised the aerial to the angle of the intended target and has rotated it to get to the target, the aerial must be extended to provide the necessary reach. Most aerial devices are 35 to 40 ft (11 to 12 m) long when they are not extended and all sections are bottomed out in the fully retracted position. To extend the ladder, the driver/operator pushes the control handle forward. The double-acting or double-ram cylinders then move, causing the ladder to stretch out. A series of cables in sheave wheels multiply the movements of the cylinders, which translates to cables actually pulling the aerial out or back in. The speed of extension depends on the slow or fast idle speed and the control handle input from the driver/operator. The control allows the hydraulic fluid to enter slowly or rapidly, thus moving the cylinder and causing the ram to extend or retract, which causes the corresponding action of the ladder sections.

Extension and retraction require that devices have either an indicator gauge or a set of numbers on the handrails. These indicators tell the driver/operator how much ladder is left to reach the target. They provide a reference for cross-checking with the load chart. This information is important during operations: the farther out the ladder's extension, the less its carrying capability.

During extension, the driver/operator has to be cognizant of a few things. The tips of aerial ladders have different lights installed to illuminate the scene, but they do not always fit into windows—which can be a problem. The monitor on the fly section may stick out farther than the fly section itself and, therefore, get in the way in a rescue situation. The monitor is locked to the fly pipe by a pin or lever. This pin has two positions, and the outer most position is commonly referred to as the **water tower position**. Some aerial devices are capable of locking the monitor back at the outer midsection, which allows the fly section to have a clear bottom without a waterway or monitor that might interfere with ladder placement. Most departments run their waterways in this fashion, which is called the **rescue position**. The rationale is that if a company must move quickly for a rescue, fire fighters do not want the waterway impeding them from getting closer to the building. Keeping the monitor out from under the fly section also allows for crews' quick deployment to roofs and over cornices for ventilation.

During the initial setup of an aerial device into rescue position, a fire fighter has to run down the ladder while it is cradled, make the monitor lock movement, and then get off the ladder. Because a crew member must physically shift the monitor from the water tower position to the rescue position, this step takes valuable time. In a water tower operation, it is often not that time-critical, because lines must be laid to the apparatus (which also takes time). Tiller trucks have an advantage in this situation, because the tillerman can shift the water monitor to the rescue or water tower position before he or she exits the trailer.

DRIVER/OPERATOR Tip

Movable waterways on an aerial device should never be shifted unless the ladder is in the cradle and bedded, to prevent waterway locks from failing.

When extending or retracting the aerial, it is best to have a ground spotter assist the operator. If ladder sections connect or smash into buildings, the device will be rendered useless in an evolution and an expensive repair will be necessary. The hydraulic systems on modern aerials are equipped with a relief valve system, but any contact can bend or warp the device in an instant.

Safety Tip

At no time should an aerial device be extended or retracted with personnel on the ladder.

Discharging Water and Waterway Safeties

Suppose that when your company arrives on the scene, the incident commander (IC) advises your officer that he wants your aerial to provide an elevated stream. Your setup is complete, and the water tower mode of the monitor has been manually selected and locked in. Some monitors contain a gate valve on the waterway that can block off the monitor flow, with a small 2½-inch (65-mm) valve being mounted for standpipe use. Make sure that the monitor valve is open fully. If your department uses electric fog or stream nozzles, you can get ready to raise the aerial device. If your department uses straight-bore nozzles, you will need to select the proper size of smooth-bore tip based on the water supply. If the chosen nozzle is not the standard device on the monitor, install it on the ladder monitor before it comes out of the cradle.

Raise, rotate, and extend the aerial to the area where you will operate the stream. The water supply should be connected to the aerial, and the driver/operator should be in contact with the engine and advise that operator to flow the pipe slowly and on command. Do not allow the waterways to be charged unless the pipe is directed to a target. The flow from a 100-ft (30-m) aerial with a smooth-bore tip can hit people operating at the fire and cause serious injury if the stream is not directed into the fire. It is also a good idea to leave fog or stream nozzles in the fog position at all times. Then, if someone charges the pipe before the stream is directed to its intended target, fire fighters will simply get wet—rather than pounded into the ground by a straight stream aimed the wrong way.

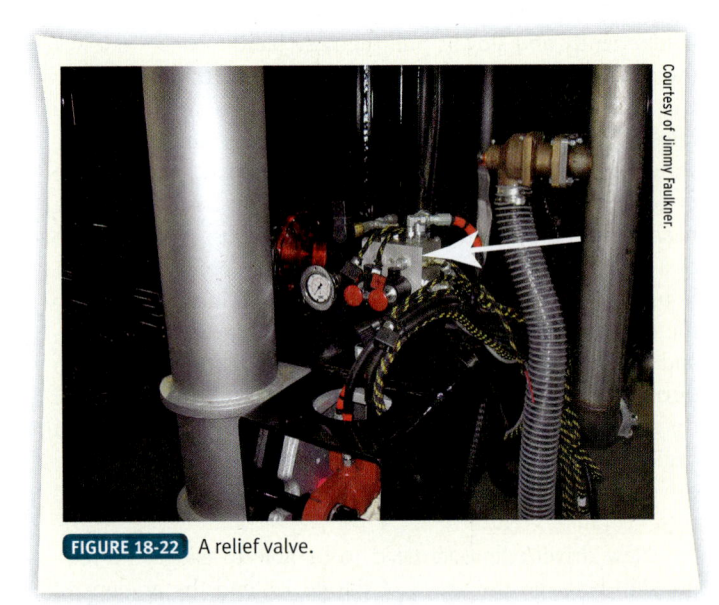

Friction loss and nozzle pressure require that the engine apparatus driver/operator know what the elevation is as well as what gpm (L/min) rate is needed. If an engineer over-pumps the aerial, a spring-loaded relief valve on the waterway pipe under the unit will vent the excess water to the ground. It operates based on the same principle as the suction-side relief on the engine apparatus. Such valves can be set by driver/operators or maintenance personnel to pressures slightly above the worst-case scenario flows. On tower ladders and platforms, another spring-loaded relief valve is located under the platform and works in the same fashion **FIGURE 18-22**.

FIGURE 18-22 A relief valve.

On platforms flowing water, basket personnel must pay special attention to those streams. The platform driver/operators should have a valve open all of the time, because if basket personnel move the platform or try to retract it, a pipe rupture may occur. Remember that water is noncompressible, and a 96-ft (29-m) column of water cannot get any smaller. Once you begin to retract a ladder or platform, the water needs a place to vent. Water should always be flowing during the fire operations. Platforms may move into a variety of positions during the fire as a result of commands issued by the basket operator. Once aerial streams are no longer needed, there is a drain at the bottom that can be opened that allows the pipe to drain **FIGURE 18-23**.

The retraction of the ladder will not cause a problem in a tower or ladder if the tip valves stay open. When retracting the device, if someone forgets to pull the drain, the water simply pushes out of the nozzles and vents. The problem usually occurs when the tip is shut down in the platform or on

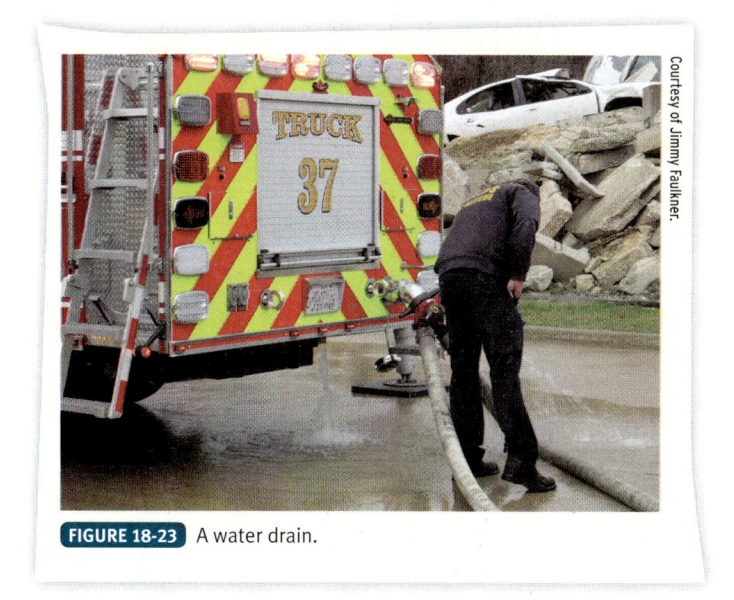

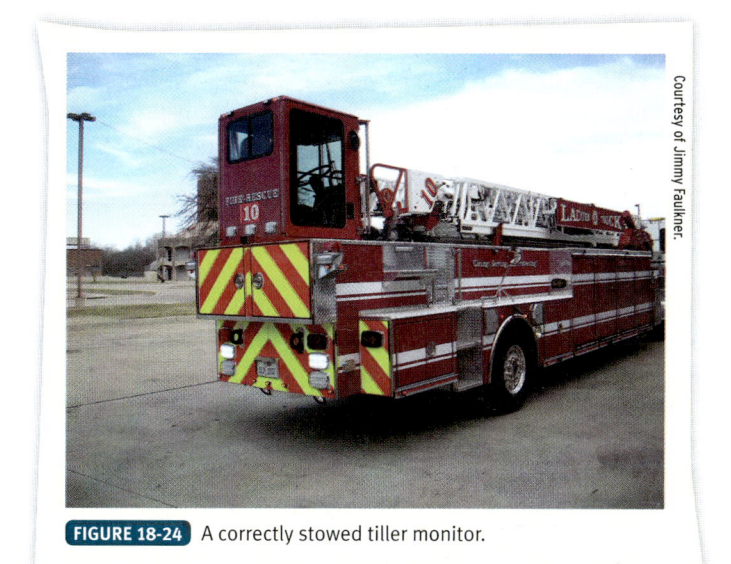

FIGURE 18-23 A water drain.

FIGURE 18-24 A correctly stowed tiller monitor.

Cradling Up and Going Home

Once training, operational checks, or firefighting is complete, it is time to put the device away.

The retraction and stowing of the aerial device is the opposite of deployment. First, the driver/operator engages the fast idle control, remembering the dead man's switch. Second, after the waterway has been drained and the monitor has been stowed back into its nested position by pulling the retract handle back, the aerial device can be retracted. When the ladder sections get close to being fully retracted, the driver/operator should ease off the retract control, which will slow the hydraulic flow down and slow the retraction. Try not to bang the ladders into their nested positions, as this action is rough on the **ladder stops**. If you hold the handle until the ladders stop moving downward, you will see the hydraulic gauge rise, which indicates that the hydraulic relief valve is working and the ladders are fully retracted. Watch the control cables, the igus track, and the ladder itself for abnormal movements, shaking, or misalignment, and report any such problems to a maintenance EVT. Again, doing a 360-degree scan, rotate the ladder slowly until it aligns with the cradle. A cradle alignment light and an additional mark somewhere on the turntable may used for reference **FIGURE 18-25**.

> **Safety Tip**
>
> Do not get in the habit of resting your hand on the handrail of the ladder. During retraction, the ladders can crush your hand between sections. Be sure anyone on the turntable is clear of any moving parts.

The next function is the lowering of the aerial. Before you attempt to lower the device, walk around the apparatus and confirm that the monitor is properly nested or stowed and that no one has left any equipment under the ladder. Lower the ladder by pushing the control handle forward, and control the speed of the hydraulics by varying how much input you use. Once the ladder pipes in an effort to turn the device into a standpipe connection. In such a scenario, a handline is connected to the 2½-inch (65-mm) connection and flows water for firefighting or mop-up purposes. The handline is usually shut off at this valve for ladder retraction. If no one remembers that the monitors are shut down when the ladder retracts, the water may blow out one or more components of the waterway when it cannot compress the water in the pipe.

After water operations are complete, make sure that the monitor is in its proper stowed position **FIGURE 18-24**. Many a fire truck cab has been harpooned by a nozzle that is facing down and not in its nested position. This is also true of stream shapers added to monitors. On tiller trucks, there is very little space between the cradled ladder and the tiller cab, so be careful not to leave extensions like stream shapers on the monitors where they can crash into the tiller cab.

FIGURE 18-25 A cradle alignment light.

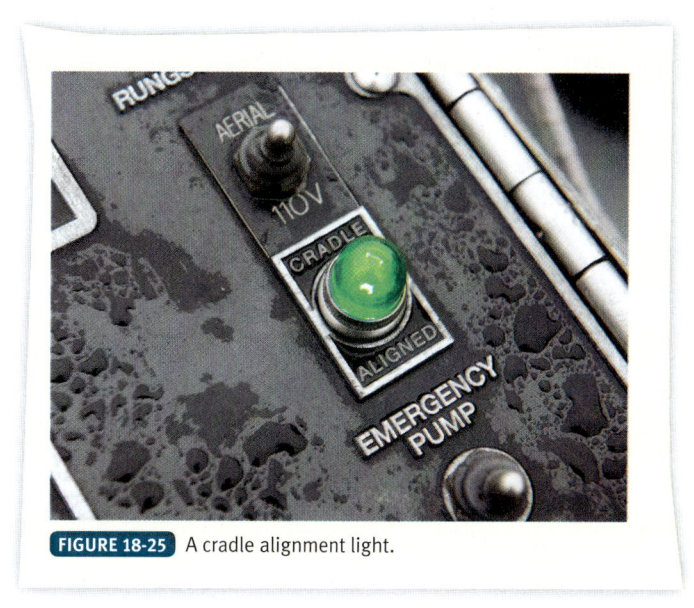

ladder gets close to the cradle, double-check the alignment lights and marks and then disengage the fast idle control. It is generally safer to lower into the cradle while the unit is operating on regular idle speed. This option makes the control very slow and gives you more margins to correct any errors while lowering the aerial.

Although the lights may indicate that the aerial is properly aligned, use your eyes to place the fly section of the ladder into the cradle. At slow idle speeds, this is relatively easy to do. If you are significantly off the mark either left or right, raise the aerial above the cradle a foot or so and reset the ladder. Do not try to move the aerial left or right when it is almost down in the cradle—you could rotate the ladder so that it climbs over the cradle ears and possibly damages the aerial and the truck's cab. It is better to reset the ladder than to risk the alternatives.

Before leaving the turntable, power down the ladder into the cradle so that the holding valves keep it locked down. When driving down the road, an aerial that is not set into the cradle properly will bounce. This road damage can be significant and can literally jar the teeth of the fire fighters riding in the cab. Finally, close the pedestal cover and secure it, remove the safety chains, and exit the ladder turntable by backing down the ladder.

■ Storing Outriggers

Once you have left the turntable, it is time to pick up the outriggers or stabilizers. This is done in the opposite order of setup. If the jacks have pins to hold them in case of emergency, pull them out before you retract a jack. Remember that there are both inner and outer jack boxes. The inner box is less durable than the outer box and is made of lighter steel. This box basically keeps the jack aligned, protects the ram, and provides a place to put the safety pins.

The jack's hydraulic cylinders use the same power to retract up as they do to lift the truck when pushing down. If the jack can lift a 70,000-lb (31,750-kg) truck off the ground, you can imagine what it does to the pin and the jack box when it retracts with the same power. Before engaging any controls, always look around the truck for anything under it or resting on it. A ladder, hose, or nozzle can easily be crushed if the driver/operator does not see them under the unit.

Because the outrigger storage procedure is the reverse of setup, the last item deployed—either the jack cylinder or the beam plant cylinders—will be picked up first. If the unit is high off the ground or high on one side due to ground topography, let the unit down evenly. Pull up the beams first and then unload the weight off the jacks. During all of these actions, an audible alarm will be sounding. The rest of the crew, in an effort to help, may want to come in and pick up the ground footplates, but keep everyone away from the beams and jacks until everything is nested in the body. If a driver/operator is tired after a fire, he or she may engage a handle and fail to look at the beams while they are moving. A fire fighter bent over picking up a ground plate can easily be pulled into the body by a retracting beam cylinder and killed. Do not pick up the ground plates or chocks until the doors to the outrigger controls are closed, with the buzzer silent and the fast idle off. Only then is it safe to pick up and stow the ground plates and chocks. Not surprisingly, the locations of most storage mounts for the ground plates are conveniently close to the outriggers **FIGURE 18-26**.

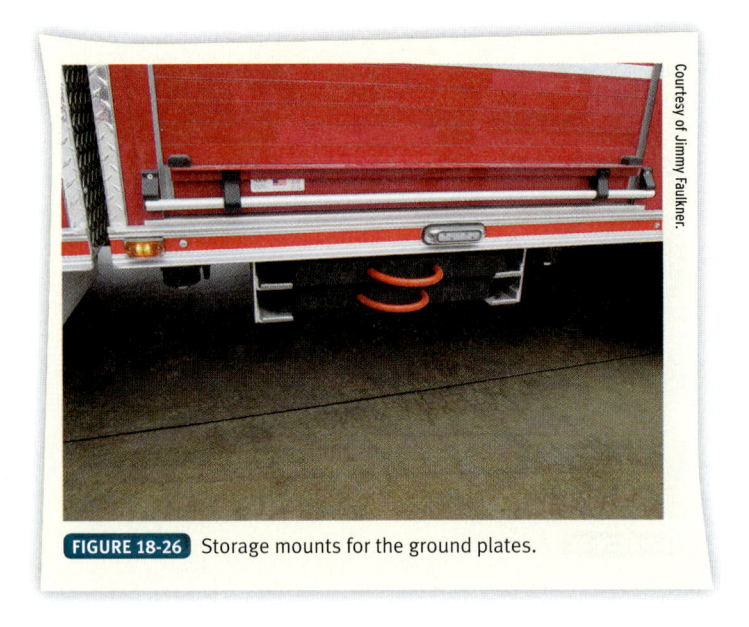

FIGURE 18-26 Storage mounts for the ground plates.

Finally, make a last lap around the truck to verify that everything is stowed, that the outriggers and beams are up and nested, and that all of the doors are closed. You can then return to the truck's cab and disengage the PTO. Once you are sure that the entire crew is safely onboard with seat belts on, you can release the parking brake and drive back home.

Apparatus Testing

Various components of aerial devices are checked and tested because in the normal scope and operations of the device, these components can be stressed or overworked. NFPA 1911 specifies the criteria for annual and **nondestructive testing (NDT)** and indicates which types of testing are required—different types of aerial apparatus are tested with procedures that best indicate failures in a specific component. Several types of testing devices and methods are used on aerial devices for both the annual tests and the preservice tests.

NDT seeks to test an aerial component without physically altering, disassembling, or damaging the unit **FIGURE 18-27**. The

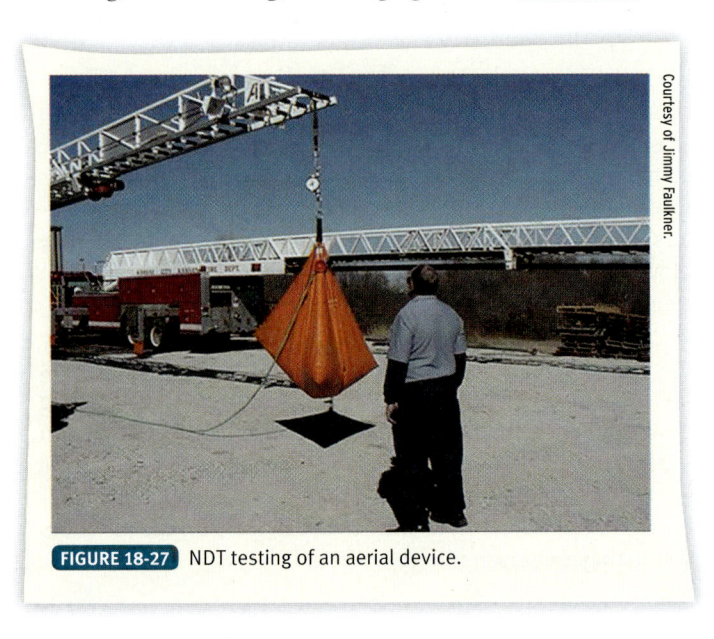

FIGURE 18-27 NDT testing of an aerial device.

VOICES OF EXPERIENCE

During service at a local service facility, two factory representatives began working on a tower ladder. The work was being performed on a gravel driveway and there had been recent rains. The outriggers were set, but the ground plates were not utilized by the factory personnel. The tower ladder was raised and extended about 40 ft (12 m). The ladder was then rotated to the side so that the cables could be checked.

Both of the factory representatives were on the ground, and one was working on the left front of the truck. This worker noticed that the truck was beginning to rise off the ground on his side and shouted a warning. The other worker immediately noticed that the outrigger was sinking into the gravel, and the weight of the ladder over the right side was beginning to tip the apparatus. He quickly went to the turntable and very slowly retracted the ladder, which allowed the truck to settle back on the ground. His quick thinking averted a potentially disastrous rollover. He then safely rotated the ladder back over the center of the apparatus and returned it to the cradle so that the truck could be moved to safer ground.

When asked why they did not use the ground plates, the workers stated that the pad they used at the factory was 18 inches (46 cm) thick, and they never used the pads because there was no reason to worry about the possibility of the ground having problems. The lesson learned here is that no matter who you are or where you set the ladder, you should always use the jack ground pads because you never know how stable your ground is—with or without concrete.

Jimmy Faulkner
Dallas Fire Rescue
Dallas, Texas

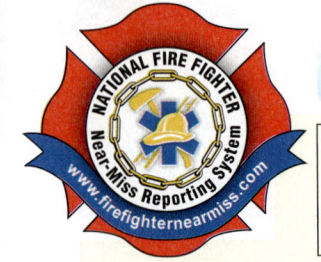

Near-Miss REPORT

Report Number: 10-0001201

Synopsis: Aerial ladder outrigger fails during inspection.

Event Description: The following is a description of the failure of our department's aerial ladder apparatus resulting in the collapse of the ladder during routine maintenance and inspection.

We have a 100-ft (30-m) tiller aerial apparatus with A-frame outriggers manufactured in 2007. The ladder is rated at 250 pounds (113 kg) at the tip at 0 degrees elevation with full extension.

We were training on the procedures included in our 10-hour inspection of the aerial ladder. We had the ladder deployed at approximately 15 degrees of elevation, 100-inch (3-m) extension, and approximately 70 degrees of right rotation with both outriggers fully extended. I was inspecting the ladder visually and manually walking out the ladder for signs of damage and was five rungs from the tip when I heard a loud pop and the ladder free fell for approximately 15–20 ft (5–6 m). My fall slowed and then sprung back upwards coming to rest about 10 ft (3 m) from the ground. The ladder never went all the way to the ground. The driver's side outrigger, on the same side the ladder was deployed, had failed. The top of the jack box had peeled open on the top on both sides allowing the outrigger to go flat to the ground resulting in the ladder falling. The outriggers had no previous damaging incidents and had been recently inspected by the manufacturer. The ladder truck was taken out of service and left in the place of the incident until the Battalion Chief and department administrative personnel, as well as fleet maintenance personnel, could be brought in to inspect and document.

Lessons Learned: Both our department and the manufacturer's investigation have found no fault in the operation of the ladder for the failure. Instead, the investigations have lead all parties to believe that the failure was caused by a combination of incomplete welds as well as a prepressurization condition in the outrigger at the time of initial service testing, causing damage that slowly progressed leading to eventual catastrophic failure. The prepressurization was a result of "over shimming" by the factory of the jack that extends from the jack box. The oversized shims were inserted and then the covers ratcheted down with eight ½-inch (13-mm) bolts, bowing the top plate of the jack box and creating stress points in both the outboard top corners of the outrigger jack box. These stress points were then exacerbated by loading with the extension of ladder during normal use. Signs to look for on your ladder that may indicate a prefailure condition:

- Binding of A-frame outriggers after deployment upon retraction.
- Bowing of the top plate of the jack box.
- Cracking of the paint on the outboard top corners of the A-frame jack box.
- Signs of rust inside the jack box, specifically in the top corner seams.

Adding nondestructive weld testing (magnetic particle, X-ray, ultrasonic, etc.) to your annual inspection of the ladder is highly recommended.

---

interval for NDT testing is usually every 5 years, but many departments elect to test their units every year. Because ladders are subjected to road damage on the device while they are in transit, departments with severe duty cycles on aerial apparatus will do complete tests on them on a frequent basis. Testing is also done whenever there is any flame contact to the aerial or some sort of structural damage is inflicted on the device (e.g., a road accident bends the sections of the ladder, the ladder is smashed into a structure during firefighting operations). These tests are usually performed by a professional third-party testing company that must be certified by a Level II NDT technician as referenced in NFPA 1911.

In any instance where a testing entity is working on an aerial apparatus and performing tests, it is incumbent on the department to provide a driver/operator who is familiar with that device. Before testing begins, a suitable location must be established to perform that testing. The area chosen should be free of any overhead wires and should have a good solid surface area. Some of the tests exert high stress loads on the ground and can pose a problem if a surface failure occurs FIGURE 18-28. The ladder will need to be rotated 360 degrees for one of the tests, so the testing location also needs to be an open area that can be protected from any traffic coming into the test area. Tests are performed utilizing weights as well; therefore the area needs to be secured should a ladder

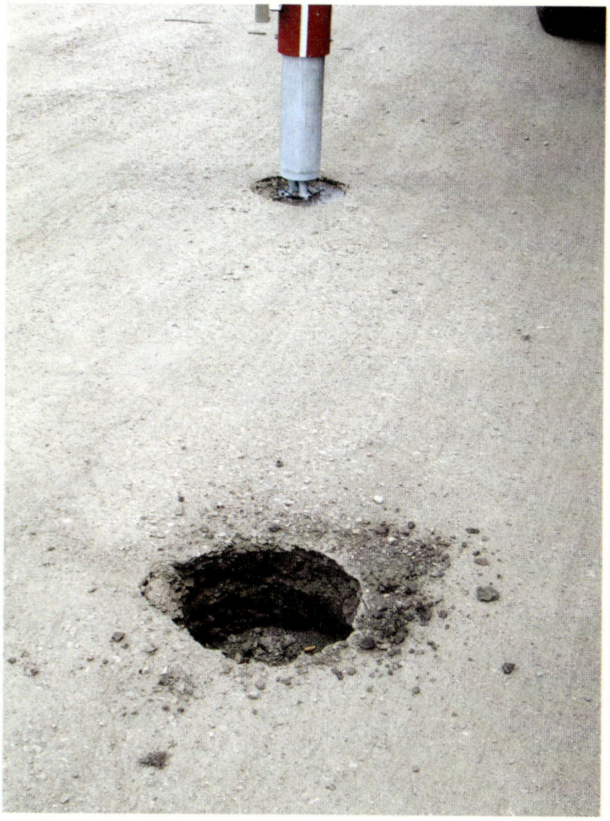

CHAPTER 18 Testing, Maintaining, and Troubleshooting Aerial and Tiller Apparatus

FIGURE 18-28 Failure to use groundplates can be catastrophic.

FIGURE 18-29 A mag yoke.

failure occur. Depending on the type of aerial or the component being tested, additional testing devices and procedures—including magnetic particle testing, acoustic testing, ultrasonic testing, or dye penetrant testing—may be utilized.

> **Safety Tip**
> Under no circumstances should an aerial device be tested over a building or with personnel under the unit.

Magnetic Particle Testing

Magnetic particle testing is used on steel aerial apparatus. It relies on a magnetic current that is applied through a device called a mag yoke **FIGURE 18-29**. The test is performed by using a small amount of steel particles that are puffed onto the area being tested by a small snuffer that mimics a small bulb syringe. The metal particles will be pulled into any flaw or <u>discontinuity</u> by the magnetic (eddy) current produced by the mag yoke when the Level II NDT technician presses the appropriate button. This steel powder is attracted to open spaces, which allows weld cracks to be found. Each crack is then marked with a soap stone or grease pencil, and the flawed weld can be inspected and corrected by rewelding it. Sometimes during the annual inspection, there will be an indication of a crack that proves to be only a flaw in the paint. The EVT will clean out the weld in such a case, and the tester can recheck the area with the mag yoke to verify that it is sound.

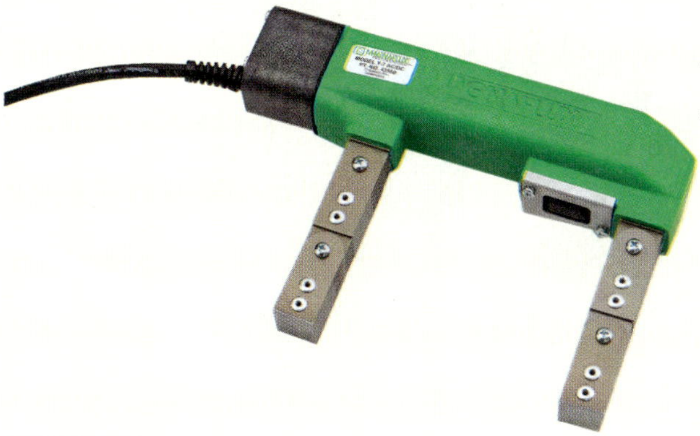

Acoustic Testing

Acoustic testing utilizes sound waves to test a material for thickness. In aerial device testing, the sound waves travel through the ladder, and the return signal is translated to determine the density of the test site. This technique is also used to test aluminum ladders by assessing their conductivity.

■ Ultrasonic Testing

Ultrasonic testing also uses sound waves, but it relies on a scope that, via a display signature, indicates if there are defects in the material. This testing technique is used on bolts, ladder pins, sheave wheel pins, and ladder base rails. Areas that cannot be seen are the prime candidates for this type of test.

■ Dye Penetrant Testing

Dye penetrant testing is used to reveal surface defects only. A colored dye is applied to the area of suspected deficiency, and a developer is subsequently applied. It causes the dye to bleed to the surface and provides a visual indicator of the flaw **FIGURE 18-30**. Dye penetrant testing is primarily used for testing aluminum ladders.

■ Additional Testing

Additional testing done by the third-party tester per NFPA 1911 can occur on any of the following:
- Turntable bolts and attaching hardware
- Rotation bearing mounting bolts
- Torque box mounting to the frame
- Tractor mounts
- Suspension
- Rotation gear and bearings

These tests are needed because when a unit is put together, all attaching bolts are torqued to the proper setting. A technician will check whether these torque values are within the tolerance limits by taking a torque wrench and testing each bolt.

FIGURE 18-30 Dye penetrant testing.

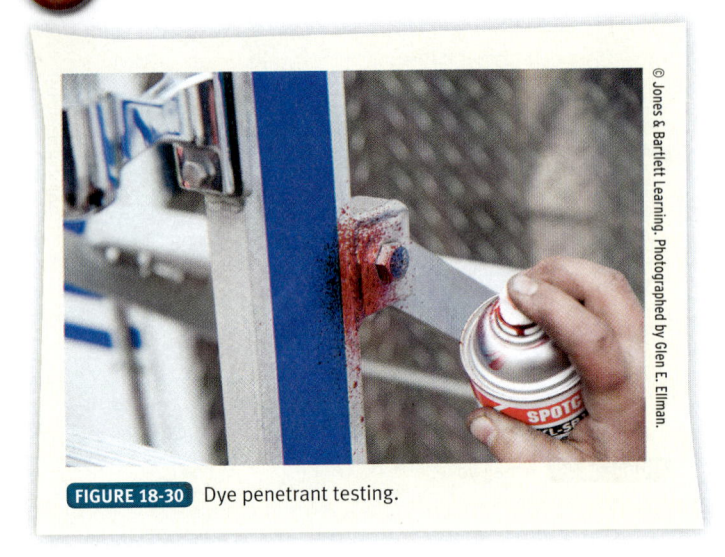

The torque wrench is set to the foot-pounds value and will click at that setting. If the bolt moves or if the torque wrench does not click, the bolts may potentially be loose or stretched. Bolts may become loose as a result of road travel, but can also be stressed by improper operation.

For example, if the driver/operator puts the outriggers out and does not apply forces to them equally, the body, torque box, and frame bolts are put in a bind and may become stretched. The test criteria are intended to prevent a bolt failure. Once the bolt is initially installed and set to its proper torque level, there is no way to know if it is stretched or loose; therefore, if testing indicates that a bolt is possibly loose or stretched, it needs to be replaced.

Testing of Structural Components

The structural components of aerial devices, from the ladder rung covers to the electrical control cables, are also examined by a third party testing company that will test the components and note any deficiencies. The EVT will then make the repairs. Leaks are located and corrected, and items such as rollers, slide pads, and cables are adjusted due to wear or abuse. Visual inspections and indicators are used to identify hydraulic internal leakage or holding valve failures. Structural components tested include the following items:

- The rotation swivel and all lines and connections are checked for leaks, and smooth operations of the swivel should be the norm. There should be no dead spots in the swivel in which control or electrical function is compromised, and water should not be leaking through the hydroelectric swivel.
- Elevation, extension, and rotation locks should be functional, with no external leakage. Testing is done by placing dial indicators on the cylinders and measuring any movement when there is no hydraulic power to the cylinder. These tests check the holding valves or POC to ensure that they are set to the proper **crack pressure** and that there is no internal leakage in the cylinder. On manual systems, the lock bars and stops should hold the ladder up and be free of deviations, cracks, or loose control cables or levers.
- PTOs and hydraulic components are checked for proper pressures, relief valve settings, and the ability to flow the rated gpm (L/min) for the system. Leaks are noted and classified, and the PTO shaft (if applicable) is checked for U-joint function and lubrication. All of the hydraulic controls are checked for leakage and smooth operation. If electric-over-hydraulic controls are used, the electric valves are checked for full open and close functioning. The manual valves, overrides, and diverter valve are checked as well. The operating controls at all stations are checked. In the case of a platform, the lower controls are checked to ensure that they can override all of the tip controls. The dead man's switch is usually checked at this time as well.
- The overrides for the rotation and the short-set outriggers are checked. Any short-set outrigger should prohibit any aerial functions from occurring if the short-set or outrigger override is not engaged. Cradle switches are checked for the transfer of the hydraulic power to the lower and upper systems.
- The hydraulic reservoir is checked for metallic particles, and a sample is drawn for analysis. This test will show if there are any particles from valve bodies or rubber O-rings present, which might potentially cause the water infiltration system to fail. The tester also notes when the high and return filters were changed.

DRIVER/OPERATOR Tip

Some older aerial devices include filters in the turntable under the ladder. They should be checked at every preventive maintenance check or annual inspection. Remove and replace all filters at these tests that show discrepancies.

- The auxiliary hydraulic pump is checked at this time. This pump is normally a 12-volt motor with a small hydraulic pump that can lower the ladder in the event that the engine or PTO fails. It works very slowly and has limited power, because it is designed simply to assist in cradling a disabled ladder and raising the outriggers. The pump has its own separate feeder line from the reservoir and is protected by a check valve. It is never used to set the aerial device. Some aerial apparatus use a 120-volt motor attached to the pump for this purpose. To accomplish this task requires an outside power supply from a generator or house plug. The auxiliary hydraulic pump is sometimes referred to as the **emergency power unit (EPU)**. A switch to activate this pump is mounted at each control station. Use of this device may also require manual movement of the aerial or outrigger hydraulic solenoid valve if no power is available from the truck system **FIGURE 18-31**.

CHAPTER 18 Testing, Maintaining, and Troubleshooting Aerial and Tiller Apparatus

FIGURE 18-31 Override solenoid.

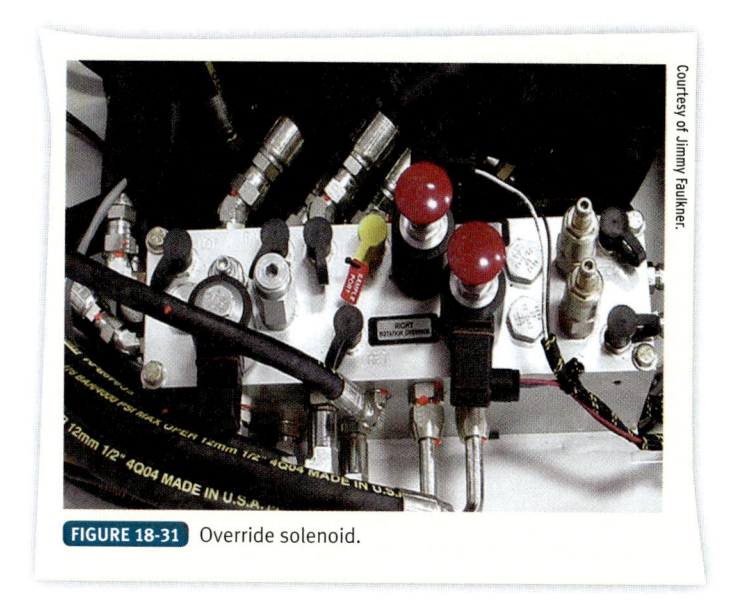

■ Testing Throttle Controls and Communication Systems

Throttle controls and communication systems are checked for the proper rpm settings by operating all of the switches for fast idle speed at any operating station. The communications system is then tested for PTT mode and hands-free or VOX operation at all control stations **FIGURE 18-32**.

Some of the specific controls tested are as follows:
- Interlocks. The tester will try all of the interlocks to verify that they are functional.
- The transmission/aerial interlock, which keeps the PTO from being engaged unless the transmission is in neutral and the parking brake is set.
- The engine speed interlock, which keeps the throttle from shifting to fast idle speed unless the parking brake is set and the truck is in neutral. This interlock is intended to prevent a runaway vehicle when the driver/operator has the transmission in gear and the parking brake set. At 1500 rpm, the truck's engine can overpower the spring brakes, allowing the truck to move without a driver. There have been several fatalities connected to incidents of this nature.

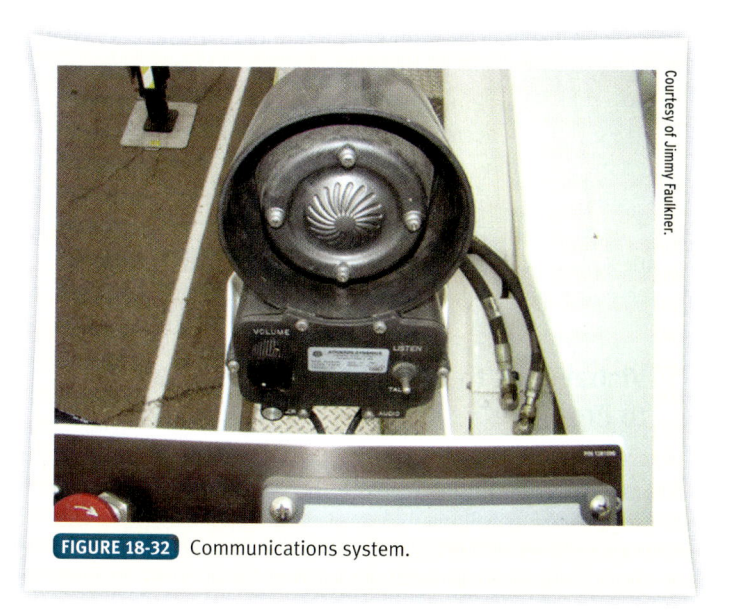

> **Safety Tip**
>
> On an aerial with a fire pump, an additional interlock allows the throttle control to be raised by the pump driver/operator at the pump panel but will not allow the fast idle speed to be set. A fast idle at 1500 rpm, if engaged in this scenario, can cause a runaway handline and serious injury to fire fighters. Aerial operations can utilize the engine rpm only to produce the desired pump pressure and hydraulic pressure.

- Breathing air systems. These systems are checked for leaks and proper pressures to the regulators at the aerial device's tip. The tester also notes the last time the cylinders were hydrostatically tested to OEM standards.

■ Stabilizer Inspections and Tests

Third-party testing is also performed on all components of the outriggers, stabilizers, and jack systems. The stabilizer checklist and corrections that will be made are outlined here:
- Stabilizers are checked for leaks and damaged parts.
- Hoses are checked for rubbing, chaffing, and leaks at the fittings.
- All stabilizer pads must be in place and all attaching hardware intact.
- Inner and outer jack boxes should have no deformations, and pin holes (where supplied) should be rounded and not damaged. Pins should be straight and secured to the outrigger.
- Footplates or auxiliary pads should be provided for each outrigger.
- The mounting of the stabilizers to the body and the torque box are checked for cracks and deformities.
- Any and all accessible bolts are checked for proper torque and replaced when a discrepancy is noted.
- The switches that indicate short-set and jacks and beams deployed are checked for proper operation, and the appropriate interlocks should function correctly.
- Cylinders are checked for internal leakage, and holding valves or POC valves are checked for drift. Pins can be placed in the outriggers per the manufacturer's recommendation, but they should be inserted at a sufficient distance that the operator can use the dial indicators for measurements. Drift is not measured with jack boxes setting on the safety pins.

■ Stability and Load Test

The ladder is tested for stability and load capacity and should be capable of sustaining a static load of 1½ times the **rated capacity** in every operational position. In this testing step, a water bag or container is suspended from a fully extended ladder. Weight is gradually added by filling the bag with water and measuring it with a scale until the ladder's rated capacity is being applied. The

FIGURE 18-32 Communications system.

rated capacity information can be found on the load chart that is supplied with every apparatus. During testing, the weight is never more than 3 ft (0.9 m) off the ground, and the assessment is performed in several positions. For example, one test will be at full extension and full elevation off the rear, and one test at the horizontal full extension of zero degrees off the rear. This test is conducted for 5 minutes and the ladder is observed from a safe position for flaws or potential failures.

> **Safety Tip**
>
> At no time during stability and load testing should any personnel be under the ladder or attempt to rotate the ladder. All testing with weights should be done with ground-speed winds blowing at less than 10 mph (16 km/h).

■ Time Trial Test

The time trial test allows the tester to see whether adequate hydraulic flow and control functions are operating on the device. It requires that the device be on level ground, with all outriggers or stabilizers properly set and footplates in use. The tester instructs the designated driver/operator to raise the ladder to full elevation. The operator must then rotate the device to 90 degrees on a predetermined side that is free of obstructions and personnel on the ground. Once this is accomplished, the driver/operator must then fully extend the ladder or boom. These tasks are best done by a driver/operator who is familiar with the unit and its controls. The timing starts when the ladder lifts from the cradle and stops when all three functions have been completed and the extension of the upper section stops. This test also acquaints the driver/operator with the operating times needed to deploy the aerial device during actual firefighting operations. The time specified for each type of aerial will differ based on its weight and extension length and can be found in NFPA 1911.

■ Water System Inspection and Test

The aerial waterway is first inspected for visual signs of damage, rust, corrosion, or other defects, and then a water supply is attached and pressurized. The waterway is filled with water and all air is removed from the piping. Once the ladder is full of water and reaches the maximum rated working pressure per NFPA 1911, the ladder is raised, extended, and rotated 360 degrees while charged. Leaks are noted in waterway seals, plumbing and drains, all piping, and the hydroelectric swivel. These leaks are then documented and repaired by the EVT.

> **Safety Tip**
>
> Failure to remove all air from the piping can cause catastrophic failure of a component and potentially severe injuries to anyone in the test area. Always refer to the standard and OEM manuals for precise operating procedures for each type of aerial. The water system inspection and test should be done only after careful review of these procedures.

> **Safety Tip**
>
> Under no circumstances should any aerial device be retracted without some drain at the ground or nozzle at the tip being open. Water is essentially noncompressible: it takes 30,000 psi (206,850 kPa) to compress water by just 1 percent. Water should always be drained prior to retracting the aerial device after the water system inspection and test is complete. The systems relief valve cannot relieve all of the pressure from this compressing action. Component failure, such as blown waterway seals, blown gaskets, or waterway piping structural rupture, is a certain outcome if water is not drained and can cause serious injury.

Troubleshooting Aerial Problems During Tests and Checkouts

It is not possible to provide an all-inclusive list that will cover all types and manufacturers of all aerial devices. For this reason, it is recommended that all potential driver/operators of your aerial and tiller truck devices review the device-specific information provided by the OEM. An in-depth troubleshooting guide must be included with all aerial devices delivered today, per NFPA 1901; that is, all manufacturers are required to provide specific and detailed instructions on troubleshooting and repairs for their units. The manufacturer's recommendation is just the minimum acceptable program—the **authority having jurisdiction (AHJ)** may implement more stringent inspections based on its operations, weather conditions, and personnel.

When problems with aerial apparatus develop that exceed the capabilities of the on-shift personnel, the appropriate EVT on the maintenance staff should be contacted. EVTs are governed by NFPA 1911; this standard also spells out the skill levels regarding who is qualified to perform repairs. Although many departments have qualified personnel on staff at their firehouses, there will inevitably be a time when resolution of a problem exceeds the skill level of a driver/operator. In such a case, you should locate the OEM service personnel locally or contact the manufacturer by telephone and ask for assistance. The OEM will readily advise you if you are attempting repairs that will require special tools, skills, or certifications (e.g., welding on aerial devices). Ask the manufacturer to provide any directions for repairs in an e-mail or in writing, as very important details can get lost in verbal directions. The manufacturer should be more than happy to comply with this request, as it protects both you and the OEM. **TABLE 18-1** shows some common problems that may require troubleshooting.

■ Visual Cues to Alert the Driver/Operator to Problems

There are often visual cues that the driver/operator can recognize that indicate problems with the aerial apparatus. Some of these cues are as follows:

- **Erratic or jerking ladder movements:** May indicate problems with the ladder slide, pads, or rollers on

TABLE 18-1	Troubleshooting Common Problems with Aerial Apparatus
Aerial Problem	**Potential Reasons for Problems**
PTO will not engage	–PTO switch is not engaged. –Truck's transmission is in drive and not in neutral. –Parking brake is not set. –Aerial power switch is not engaged. –Failure of electrical system component; refer to EVT at maintenance.
PTO will not make hydraulic pressure	–Failure of interlock or solenoid; refer to EVT at maintenance. –Failure of PTO drive gear; refer to EVT at maintenance. –No hydraulic oil is going to the pump. Check the reservoir for the pump for proper position of valves and proper fluid levels. –Hydraulic pump failure; refer to EVT.
Fast idle is inoperative	–Truck is in pump gear and fast idle is locked out by pump interlock. –Electrical issue with switch or connection. Check at another location; if this fails, refer to EVT.
Outriggers will not extend	–No hydraulics to valve bank. Check for proper position of manual diverter valve. –Ladder possibly raised in cradle. –Using the wrong handle position. –Interlocks inoperative. Check whether electric blocking solenoid valves are improperly set. –Electrical issues with switches or wires; refer to EVT.
Jacks will not operate	–Short-set interlock may be engaged and requires the driver/operator to override it. –Ladder may be out of cradle. Reset the truck and raise the jacks evenly. –The driver/operator is moving the control in the wrong direction. –Hydraulic or electrical malfunction; refer to EVT.
Green indicator lights not illuminated	–Beam not extended fully. –Jack not properly planted or insufficient weight distribution on jacks. –Beam down has insufficient plant psi (kPa). –Tiller fifth wheel locks are not set. –The driver/operator intentionally short-set the apparatus. –Pendant control not activated or loose connection. –Bad bulbs. –Loose connections or interlock problem; refer to EVT.
Aerial will not raise	–Master on pedestal not turned on. –The driver/operator is not using the dead man's switch. –Short-set requires an override on all functions. –Manual or electric diverter is not in aerial mode. –The driver/operator did not verify "all green" on the lights for jacks and beams before going topside to the pedestal. –Light jack or tiller locks are shutting down the system. Reset the problem lock. –Low hydraulic fluid. –The driver/operator is operating the handle in the wrong direction. –Malfunction in the aerial hydraulic blocking solenoid; refer to EVT. –POC check or holding valve failure; refer to EVT. –Malfunction in wiring or connections on electric-over-hydraulic controls; refer to EVT.
Ladder will not rotate	–Dead man switch is not depressed. –Override is not being used for short-set. –Short-set condition. Long-side operations only. –An interlock problem is blocking the hydraulics to the swing drive. –Failure or insufficient hydraulic oil to the swing brake or the swing drive motor. –Possible POC check valve failure; refer to EVT. –Bull gear or turntable bearing failure; refer to EVT.
Ladder will not extend or retract	–Dead man switch is not depressed. –Override is not being used for short-set. –The driver/operator is operating the handle in the wrong position. –Insufficient hydraulic oil or POC valve malfunction. Refer to EVT. –Malfunction in wiring or connections on the electric-over-hydraulic controls; refer to EVT.
Tip ladder controls inoperative	–Dead man's switch at the turntable is inoperative or not depressed. –Dead man's switch at the tip is inoperative or not depressed. –The turntable driver/operator is not overriding on a short-set. (**Note:** This is an extremely risky scenario.) –The driver/operator is operating the handle in the wrong position. –Insufficient hydraulic oil or POC valve malfunction; refer to EVT. –Malfunction in wiring or connections on the electric-over-hydraulic controls; refer to EVT.
Platform controls inoperable	–Master switch at the pedestal or in the platform is not engaged. –Dead man's switch is not depressed. –Pedestal controls are engaged and overriding the platform controls. –Malfunction in wiring or connections on the electric-over-hydraulic controls; refer to EVT.

extension and retraction. A simple fix may be required, such as lubrication, or the problem could involve a more serious situation such as severe misalignment of a slide pad. Ladder movements should be smooth and synchronous. Ladders that bounce back and forth can indicate loose cables or a timing issue with the cylinders. In all instances, these problems should be referred to the EVT.

- **Noises:** Growling, popping, and loud squeals from sheave wheels and ladders are cause for concern. Try to locate the area producing the noise and point it out to maintenance staff.
- **Dragging sounds from the waterway:** Usually a simple lubrication issue that requires the seals to be greased and the actual waterway pipe to be cleaned and lubricated.
- **Any fluid leakage:** Requires immediate action for maintenance.
- **Intermittent control functions on rotation:** May indicate a problem in the hydroelectric swivel. There will be dead spots where the contacts are burned, shorted, or loose, and the unit may become unmovable if it stops at a dead spot.
- **Cracks or rusty spots:** Any crack should be immediately referred to the EVT. It indicates a situation where stress has been put on the unit, and it needs repairs by a certified technician and a certified welder. In cases of rust coming from a ladder section, usually there has been some water infiltration into the rails or rungs of the ladder. This needs to be corrected immediately and the ladder components retested for thickness. In some cases, the rust "bleed" shows on the outside only after major degradation on the inside of the rails has occurred.
- **Ladder does not stop moving when control is released:** May indicate any number of problems, but requires immediate attention. The source might be a holding valve that stays open or a valve control with debris in the spools. The weight of the ladder coming down may have pushed the fluid out so that the valve closes more slowly. Stray voltage might also potentially keep an electrohydraulic control open when it is released. Control functions should stop whenever the handles are released, and all handles are designed to return to neutral center.
- **Outrigger beams making noise on extension and retraction:** Most beams ride steel-to-steel as they extend from the aerial device. The beams are heavy, and they will make some scraping noises. Silicone or graphite sprays can dampen the noise and make things move more smoothly.

DRIVER/OPERATOR Tip

When the outrigger beams are making noise, the worst thing you can do is to spread grease on the bottom of the beams to stop the noise. When the beam is not supported by the jack, it rides back into the truck and scrapes itself on the beams opening in the bed. If you put large amounts of grease here, the outer box will act like a squeegee. It will scrape off all of the grease and leave it in a big ball right where the outrigger switches for deployment are mounted; the lever arms that operate the indicator lights will then get stuck, and there will be no safe set and no lights.

- **Sagging extension and retraction cables:** Usually involves an easy adjustment, but requires the unit to be stretched out and all of the cables to be retimed to pull evenly. Cable adjustment is also needed if the driver/operator notices that the ladder cocks to one side or the other at full extension. These adjustments need to be performed by an EVT or qualified person.
- **Tree limb damage:** Ladder apparatus are taller than engines, and sometimes the driver/operator needs to drive down a street under less than ideal conditions. Even so, it is important to slow down and look—any damage to the ladder fly section should be found on the 360-degree walk-around visual and operational inspection that the driver/operator completes on every shift. Damage to the ladder fly section is the major reason why most manufacturers have changed their apparatus to utilize a removable fly section at the tip. It is easier to replace 2 ft (61 cm) of extension than a complete fly section.
- **Loose ladder cradles:** These problems are not as prevalent today as they were in the past. Many OEMs have developed a shock mount or flex in the cradle that keeps it from being so rigid and prone to failure. When the ladder is up, take a minute to shake the cradle and see if it moves. The visual clue of a failure is a loose cradle pad on the base rail or a half-moon scrape area on the ladder base rail. This needs to be reported immediately.

For the driver/operator, it is important to know how to describe and recognize any system problems and how to correct any deficiencies noted according to the policies and procedures for the fire department's aerial and tiller apparatus. Recognizing a specific problem and correcting a specific deficiency could potentially be integrated into any of the driver/operator's specific inspections for that particular part of the apparatus.

Wrap-Up

Chief Concepts

- A 360-degree walk-around should be done for aerial apparatus at the beginning of each shift.
- Driver/operators of aerial apparatus need to be familiar with all of the key points to check on each type of aerial they operate.
- Aerial driver/operators should be familiar with the operating characteristics of the device and be able to recognize any difference in normal operations.
- Driver/operators should be familiar with the aerial device parts and be able to properly identify areas that need attention, either by the driver/operator or, when necessary, through referral to an EVT.
- Driver/operators must be familiar with out-of-service criteria and, when given the time and latitude, be able to properly access a situation regarding maintenance issues.
- Driver/operators should perform operational checks in a safe area.
- Driver/operators should be familiar with the pressure and load characteristics of their devices and should be able to read and understand load charts.
- Driver/operators should know the minimum times allowed to deploy the device and recognize which causes might potentially slow the device operational times down.
- Driver/operators need to know which types of fluids the device uses and where and when fluids need to be added.
- Driver/operators should be able to lower the aerial device and stow it after any system failure, and should also be aware of the function and location of system overrides and know when to use them.

Hot Terms

angle of approach The smallest angle made between the road surface and a line drawn from the front point of ground contact of the front tire to any projection of the apparatus in front of the front axle. An angle of at least 8 degrees will be maintained on a fully loaded apparatus.

angle of departure The smallest angle made between the road surface and a line drawn from the rear point of ground contact of the rear tire to any projection of the apparatus behind the rear axle.

authority having jurisdiction (AHJ) An organization, office, or individual responsible for enforcing the requirements of a code or standard or for approving equipment, materials, an installation, or procedure.

backlash In the case of the aerial device, the motion that occurs when rotating the aerial, and when the bull gear and turntable bearing have play in the gear spacing. The aerial will rock slightly back and forth if there is excessive end-play or backlash.

beam The horizontal component of an H-style jack or outrigger system. The jack is welded to the end of the beam.

collector rings The electric bands inside the swivel that allow two-way contact with wires going from the top of the swivel and wires exiting from the bottom. The ring is internal to the swivel, and it has two contacts points for electric transfer.

crack pressure The pressure at which a pressure-operated valve begins to pass fluid.

discontinuity A welding term used to indicate that inspectors have found a flaw or uneven weld. It is corrected by a certified welder with permission and instructions from the OEM.

double-acting lifting cylinder A cylinder in which fluid pressure can be applied to the movable piston rod in either direction.

emergency power unit (EPU) A device that makes hydraulic power from an auxiliary source pump installed on the aerial. This pump is intended for emergency cradling of the device only.

emergency vehicle technician (EVT) An individual who performs inspections, maintenance, and operational checks on emergency response vehicles and who, by possession of a recognized certificate, professional standing, or skill, has acquired the knowledge, training, and experience and has demonstrated the ability to deal with issues related to the subject matter, the work, or the project.

extruded A descriptor for a part that is forced through a mold very similar to a cookie press. In extrusion, steel or aluminum is pushed through a dye and comes out in a predetermined shape. Most aluminum ladder rungs are produced through this process.

feather To operate the controls of a hydraulic device by slowly and smoothly opening and closing the valves; it comes from the expression "as smooth as a feather."

Grade D air An air quality content measurement for breathing air supplied to self-contained breathing apparatus.

heel pins Slang term for the pivot pins that attach the ladder base rail to the turntable and allow the ladder a pivot point when raised and lowered.

horizontal height The span from the heel pin or centerline of the truck to the outermost reach of the aerial ladder. The horizontal reach is less than the vertical or working height of the unit.

Wrap-Up, continued

hydroelectric swivel A common rotation point in the aerial where hydro/water and hydraulic fluids can be transferred from the lower system through a rotating aerial. The electrical system as well as a straight-through water pipe is included in the unit. Also called simply the "swivel."

jack box The vertical piece welded to the beam that houses the actual jack or outrigger cylinder. The outer jack box is welded to the beam, and a movable inner jack box that is slightly smaller than the outer box moves up and down when the stabilizer jacks are set.

ladder stops The parts of the aerial device that allow each section to stop and keep from over-retracting or over-extending the unit; usually a steel bar or a bolt that is adjustable and will stop the ladder's movement.

multiplexed A system that uses digital communications via a communication wire to turn systems on and off. Such a system eliminates extensive wiring in the vehicle and can be programmed to enact interlocks and safety shutdowns when certain parameters programmed into the system are met.

nondestructive testing (NDT) One of several methods used to inspect a structural component without physically altering or damaging the material.

original equipment manufacturer (OEM) The manufacturer of the device or apparatus.

outrigger interlock The system that prevents ladder operations from occurring until the outriggers are properly set. The device must be fully and correctly deployed before the outrigger interlock will allow the aerial system to energize. In a short-set scenario, the outrigger interlock interfaces with the rotation interlock; initiating any ladder movement requires the driver/operator to override the short-set outriggers.

pilot-operated check (POC) valve A hydraulic spring-operated valve; also referred to as a holding valve. It keeps fluid locked in a cylinder until the hydraulic pilot pressure releases the spring check and fluid can pass through and move the cylinder. When the pilot pressure is released, the check spring part of the valve closes and locks the fluid in, holding the cylinder in place.

power take-off (PTO) A small gear case that uses an internal gear connected to the main transmission to take power from the main transmission and transmit it, when engaged, to an auxiliary system such as a hydraulic pump for a generator or an aerial device.

quint Firefighting equipment that can perform the five major functions of fire apparatus: carrying hose, carrying water, carrying ladders, pumping water, and providing aerial and water tower operations.

raise–rotate–extend The recommended sequence to operate an aerial device.

rated capacity The total amount of weight that can be supported at the outermost rung of an aerial ladder or on an elevated platform with an uncharged waterway.

rescue position The position of the movable monitor when it is pinned or latched to the outer midsection of the aerial device. It allows a clean bottom for ladder placement into windows or over roof ledges or cornices. The monitor and the waterway pipe are essentially out of the way. Most departments leave their monitors in this position in case they must immediately begin to remove victims from a fire when they arrive on scene. If the fire goes to a water tower or defensive operation, there is time to reset the monitor position.

rotation interlock A device that interfaces with the outrigger interlock after a short-set signal is received. The driver/operator uses an override switch to move the aerial, and an indicator light at the pedestal indicates which side is short-set. The driver/operator will be able to move the aerial to the fully deployed side in a 180-degree arc on the properly set side. If the driver/operator attempts to maneuver the aerial so that it crosses the centerline of the truck at the front or the rear, the rotation interlock will shut down the rotation hydraulic circuit to prevent a potential ladder rollover. The driver/operator can then go back to the properly set side. If the driver/operator cannot move the aerial in some circumstances, another manual control valve must be pushed to return the aerial to the safe side.

short-set A situation in which the aerial is intentionally or unintentionally set without all of the outriggers, beams, and jacks deployed to their maximum reach. This setup is used when streets or obstructions limit the space available so that the device cannot fully extend a beam or jack setup. The driver/operator is then forced to override all ladder actions and is limited to operations over the side that is fully and correctly deployed.

tillerman The driver who operates the rear of a tractor-drawn aerial.

torque box The subframe of the aerial device that is mounted to the chassis frame members. Those members house or support the outrigger beams and jacks, and the turntable assembly is mounted to the torque box. Some manufacturers incorporate the torque box as the actual chassis frame, in which case they attach running gear underneath it and weld the front axles and frames directly to the torque box.

turntable A structural component that connects the aerial device to the chassis and stabilization system through a rotating bearing that permits 360-degree continuous rotation of the aerial device.

victaulic connection Also referred to as a Gruvlok; a device used to attach two pipes together using a rubber doughnut-like gasket that goes over both pieces of pipe. A two-piece, half-moon clamp that surrounds the gasket is then placed over the rubber sealing gasket. The pipes are grooved circumferentially, and the clamp halves fit into the grooves. Two bolts are used to hold the clamps together; they are designed to allow any size of piping to be easily disassembled and reassembled on water systems.

viscosity Resistance to flow.

visual inspection Inspection by eye without recourse to any optical devices, except prescription eyeglasses.

water tower position The position where a movable monitor is set to extend to the ladders full extension. It is pinned or latched to the fly section for maximum elevation of the waterway and monitor.

References

National Fire Protection Association (NFPA) 1002, *Standard for Fire Apparatus Driver/Operator Professional Qualifications*. 2014. http://www.nfpa.org/codes-and-standards/document-information-pages?mode=code&code=1002. Accessed March 27, 2014.

National Fire Protection Association (NFPA) 1071, *Standard for Emergency Vehicle Technician Professional Qualifications*. 2016. http://www.nfpa.org/codes-and-standards/document-information-pages?mode=code&code=1071. Accessed March 27, 2015.

National Fire Protection Association (NFPA) 1901, *Standard for Automotive Fire Apparatus*. 2009. http://www.nfpa.org/codes-and-standards/document-information-pages?mode=code&code=1901. Accessed March 27, 2014.

National Fire Protection Association (NFPA) 1911, *Standard for the Inspection, Maintenance, Testing, and Retirement of In-Service Automotive Fire Apparatus*. 2012. http://www.nfpa.org/codes-and-standards/document-information-pages?mode=code&code=1911. Accessed December 18, 2014.

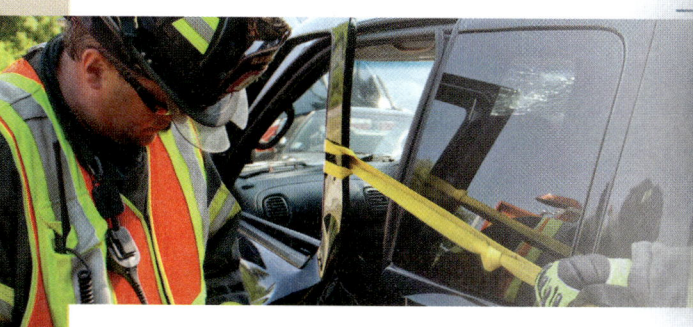

DRIVER/OPERATOR in action

After successfully completing several courses with the manufacturer of your department's apparatus, you have been named to the apparatus committee. This committee has been charged with the implementation of an aggressive maintenance program. You have been assigned the task of instructing young and old fire fighters and engineers on the proper way to effectively and safely check out the apparatus according to the manufacturer's recommendations. Your job is to develop the timetables for maintenance and a plan for coordination with the shop's emergency vehicle technicians to ensure that all of the needed service and repairs are completed to industry standards. All of the reference materials from the NFPA and OEM manuals have been put at your disposal. You immediately see a difference in the condition of the equipment based on the better understanding of the systems by the driver/operators.

1. If a hydraulic cylinder fails to stay in one position and slowly creeps down, this failure is called:
   A. Drop.
   B. Drift.
   C. Bleed-by.
   D. Release.

2. The component in the aerial system that keeps the aerial device from being raised when the outriggers are not set is the:
   A. Aerial block.
   B. Aerial interlock.
   C. Safety lock.
   D. Safety control block.

3. Fluids in all aerial apparatus should be checked as recommended by the manufacturer, and driver/operators should add fluids after fluid compatibility has been confirmed. These fluids are added directly into the:
   A. Power take-off.
   B. Cylinders.
   C. Reservoir.
   D. Hydroelectric swivel.

4. The electric system that allows a driver/operator to raise the ladder even when the outriggers are short-set is the
   A. Safety block.
   B. Override.
   C. Bypass.
   D. Disengagement circuit.

5. The amount of weight that can be carried on the tip of the ladder or in the basket is found at the control station on the:
   A. Load chart.
   B. Calculation table.
   C. Payload gauge.
   D. Indicator panel.

Performance Testing

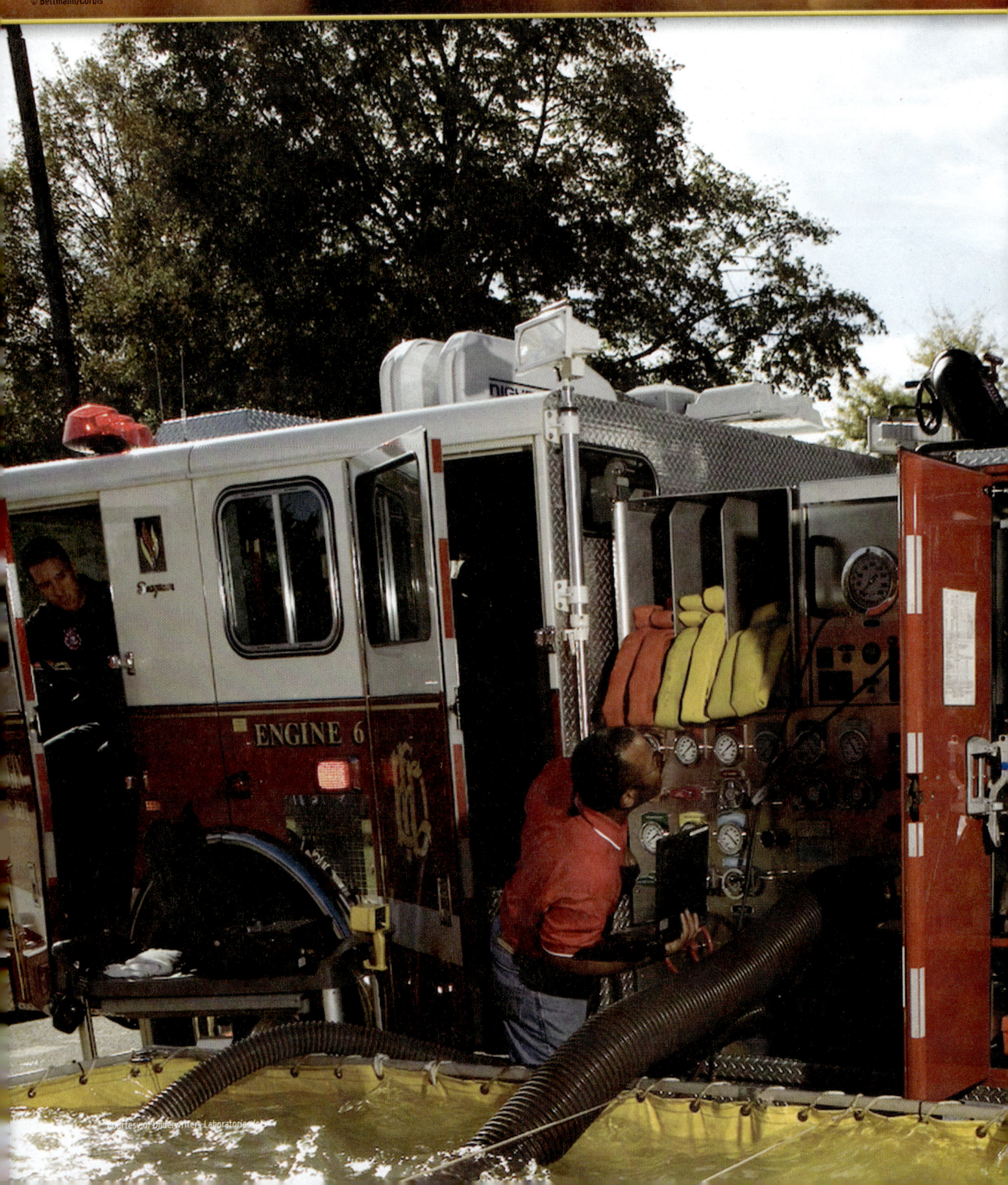

CHAPTER 19

Knowledge Objectives

After studying this chapter, you will be able to:

- Describe and understand the requirements for the performance tests and inspections on the apparatus' batteries, braking systems, cooling systems, electrical systems, fuel systems, hydraulic fluid systems, oil, tires, steering system, and fan belts, given the policies and procedures of a department's jurisdiction. (NFPA 1002, 4.2.1, 4.2.1(1), 4.2.1(2), 4.2.1(3), 4.2.1(4), 4.2.1(5), 4.2.1(6), 4.2.1(7), 4.2.1(8), 4.2.1(9), 4.2.1(10), 4.2.1(11), 4.2.1(A) ; p 467–504)
- Describe and understand the requirements for the performance tests and inspections on the apparatus' pumping and foam systems, given the policies and procedures of a department's jurisdiction. (NFPA 1002, 5.1.1, 5.1.1(2), 5.1.1(3), 5.1.1(A) , p 471–476, 481–504)
- Describe and understand the requirements for the performance tests and inspections on the apparatus' aerial systems, given the policies and procedures of a department's jurisdiction. (NFPA 1002, 6.1.1, 6.1.1(2), 6.1.1(5), 6.1.1(A) , p 471, 474–476)
- Describe the criteria for rerating fire pumps. (p 504)

Skills Objectives

After studying this chapter, you will be able to:

- Perform battery visual and operational inspection. (NFPA 1002, 4.2.1(1), 4.2.1(B) ; p 468–469)
- Perform braking system visual and operational inspection. (NFPA 1002, 4.2.1(2), 4.2.1(B) ; p 467–468)
- Perform electrical system visual and operational inspection. (NFPA 1002, 4.2.1(4), 4.2.1(B) ; p 468–471)
- Perform operational, visual inspection, and performance testing of low-voltage electrical system. (NFPA 1002, 4.2.1(4), 4.2.1(B) ; p 468–471)
- Perform operational, visual inspection, and performance testing of the pumping system. (NFPA 1002, 5.1.1(2), 5.1.1(B), 10.1.1(2), 10.1.1(B) ; p 471, 481–489, 491–500)
- Perform operational, visual inspection, and performance testing of aerial devices. (NFPA 1002, 6.1.1, 6.1.1(B) ; p 471, 474–476)
- Perform operational, visual inspection, and performance testing of the foam system. (NFPA 1002, 5.1.1(1), 5.1.1(3), 5.1.1(B), 10.1.1(1), 10.1.1(4), 10.1.1(B) ; p 471–474)
- Perform operational, visual inspection, and performance testing of compressed-air foam systems (CAFS). (NFPA 1002, 5.1.1(1), 5.1.1(3), 5.1.1(B), 10.1.1(1), 10.1.1(4), 10.1.1(B) ; p 473–474)
- Perform operational, visual inspection, and performance testing of line voltage electrical systems. (NFPA 1002, 4.2.1(4), 4.2.1(B) ; p 474–475)
- Perform operational, visual inspection, and performance testing of breathing air compressor systems. (NFPA 1002, 6.1.1(6), 6.1.1(B) ; p 475–476)
- Perform the no-load governed engine speed test, the pump shift indicator test, and the pump engine control interlock test. (NFPA 1002, 5.1.1(2), 5.1.1(B), 10.1.1(2), 10.1.1(B) ; p 480–484)
- Perform a gauge meter test, a flow meter test, a tank-to-pump flow test, a vacuum test, and an internal relief valve test. (NFPA 1002, 5.1.1(2), 5.1.1(B), 10.1.1(2), 10.1.1(B) ; p 481, 483, 485–491, 500–501)
- Perform a priming system test, pressure control tests, and pumping and overload tests for fire pumps. (NFPA 1002, 5.1.1(2), 5.1.1(B), 10.1.1(2), 10.1.1(B) ; p 491–493, 495–504)

Additional NFPA Standards

- NFPA 1071, *Standard for Emergency Vehicle Technician Professional Qualifications*
- NFPA 1901, *Standard for Automotive Fire Apparatus*
- NFPA 1911, *Standard for the Inspection, Maintenance, Testing, and Retirement of In-Service Automotive Fire Apparatus*
- NFPA 1989, *Standard on Breathing Air Quality for Emergency Services Respiratory Protection*

You Are the Driver/Operator

As a newly promoted driver/operator, you are assigned to a station and need to do a vehicle inspection as required by NFPA 1002 and NFPA 1911, and perform a battery visual and operational inspection.

1. What do you need to inspect on the batteries?
2. Which equipment will you need to perform the inspection?
3. What should you do if you find any defects or deficiencies related to the batteries on the fire apparatus prior to testing?

Introduction

As a newly promoted driver/operator, when you are assigned to an apparatus, one of your first duties is to do an inspection on the vehicle. To complete the inspection, you will need to gather your department's daily/weekly inspection form—an example of which can be found in the appendices of National Fire Protection Association (NFPA) 1911, *Standard for the Inspection, Maintenance, Testing, and Retirement of In-Service Automotive Fire Apparatus*, Figure C.3(a). The form used in your department may be set up slightly differently, but it should contain all the pertinent checks as listed in this standard (see Appendix A, *Daily/Weekly Inspection Check Sheet*, of this text book for a list of pertinent checks). The NFPA 1911 inspection form is just an example, however, and is the minimum standard. Your department's own checklist may have been set up specifically for your emergency vehicle type.

You should first become familiar with all the information on the daily/weekly checklist, then fill in the required information on the top of the worksheet. The initial section to work on, according to the daily/weekly form, may be the engine. On some vehicles, you may have to raise the cab to complete this part of the inspection. Be sure to follow the manufacturer's instructions. As the driver/operator, you should document any deficiencies found and report them to either the **authority having jurisdiction (AHJ)** or the specific person taking care of such deficiencies in your department. (The AHJ is an organization, office, or individual responsible for enforcing the requirements of a code or standard, or for approving equipment, materials, an installation, or a procedure.) Further evaluation may need to be performed by a qualified emergency vehicle technician (EVT).

Safety Tip

The driver/operator should always refer to the department's standard operating procedures/standard operating guidelines (SOPs/SOGs), local and state safety guidelines, as well as safety precautions included in the manufacturer's operating manual. During the inspection, the driver/operator should wear the appropriate personal protection equipment (PPE) while doing performance testing—this may include helmet, gloves, eye protection, and/or hearing protection—depending on what test is being performed.

Most fire departments have a specific policy or procedure to follow for apparatus that are out of service or have deficiencies.

Performance Testing

Once a fire apparatus has been accepted and placed in service, it must be properly inspected, operated, maintained, and tested over its entire useful lifetime. On certain fire apparatus (any emergency vehicle with a pump of 250 gpm or larger [1000 L/min]), the pumping system is designed to deliver a certain amount of water at a desired pressure, and the hoselines and nozzles used are based on the pump's design. Failure of a fire pump to deliver the required amount of water at a certain pressure will impair the company's fire suppression ability and diminish the safety of fire fighters, possibly leading to injury and increased property damage.

DRIVER/OPERATOR Tip

Note that performance testing is typically performed by a qualified EVT Level 2 technician as defined by NFPA 1071, *Standard for Emergency Vehicle Technician Professional Qualifications*. The driver/operator should assist or participate in the visual and operational inspection. The next revision of NFPA 1002, *Standard for Fire Apparatus Driver/Operator Professional Qualifications*, and NFPA 1911, *Standard for the Inspection, Maintenance, Testing, and Retirement of In-Service Automotive Fire Apparatus* will help clarify the driver/operator duties to be "visual and operational inspection" only, and the "performance testing" shall be performed by a qualified EVT.

■ Weight Verification Test

The weight verification test, as well as the braking system test, the parking brake system test, and the road test, require that the fire apparatus be fully loaded with all the items that are typically onboard while the apparatus is in service. The fuel tank, foam tank(s) (if so equipped), water tank, drinking water coolers, ice chests, and portable equipment fuel containers should all be filled. Find a location with certified truck scales—typically a truck stop—and weigh the front axle, the rear axle (single or tandem), and the entire apparatus. Then, using the fire department's weight form or using the one provided in NFPA

1911 [see NFPA 1911, Figure 16.2.4 and Table A.16.2.4(3)], you will need to do the following:

1. Record the axle weight ratings shown on the rating plate of the apparatus on line A.
2. Record the weight data obtained when the apparatus is weighed on line B.
3. Determine the personnel allowance by multiplying the number of riding positions in the driving and crew compartment by 200 lb (90 kg), and record that value on line C.
4. Determine other weight that might be added, including any items normally carried on the fire apparatus when it is in service but missing during the weighing, such as personal clothing and additional equipment that might be transported during the response to certain incidents, and enter those values on line D.
5. Add lines B, C, and D for each column and record the value on line E.
6. Subtract line E from line A and record the value on line F.

Now that you have completed the weight verification test, you can proceed to test the braking system. First, you will need to find a location that is safe for performing a braking test. The procedure for the braking test then proceeds as follows:

1. Lay out a course that is 12 ft (3.7 m) wide with start and stop lines; the stop line should show the stopping distance for the specific type of vehicle (see NFPA1911, Table 16.3.3).
2. Approach the start line with the vehicle being tested centered in the course and traveling at a speed of 20 mph (32 km/h).
3. Apply the service brake firmly as the vehicle's front bumper crosses the start line.
4. Observe whether the vehicle comes to a smooth stop within the prescribed distance without pulling to the right or left beyond limits (across the sides of the course boundaries).
   - Fire apparatus that weighs 10,000 lb (4540 kg) or less should stop within 25 ft (7.5 m).
   - Fire apparatus that weighs more than 10,000 lb (4540 kg), except a truck tractor, should stop within 35 ft (10.5 m).
   - Combination vehicles and truck tractors that weigh more than 10,000 lb (4540 kg) should stop within 40 ft (12 m).

Once the braking test is completed, you may proceed to the parking brake system. The parking brake system needs to be able to hold the fully loaded fire apparatus on a grade of 20 percent or, alternatively, the steepest grade in the fire department's jurisdiction if a grade of 20 percent is not available. Again, extreme caution needs to be exercised when testing the parking brake. The fire apparatus should be stopped while facing uphill, the parking brake applied, and the transmission put in neutral. Observe any movement after the parking brake has been applied. Next, do the same thing with the fire apparatus facing downhill and note any movement.

Road Test

After the parking brake test, you may proceed to the road test, again making sure to operate in a safe location and manner.

The test must be conducted on dry, level, paved roads that are in good condition. The engine should not be operated in excess of the maximum governed speed.

1. Find a safe location where you can accelerate up to 50 mph (80 km/h) at a minimum.
2. Observe and record the following while driving at least 1 mile (1.6 km) at a safe speed for the conditions and making turns of 90 degrees to both left and right:
   - Improper transmission shifting
   - Driveline and vehicle vibrations
   - Drifting and pulling during acceleration or braking
   - Abnormal noise
   - Resistance to steering recovery after a 90-degree turn.

Any deficiencies should be reported and investigated by a qualified EVT. Remember that the reason performance testing is done is to determine the current condition of the fire apparatus and to compare those results to the performance when the apparatus was new. The goal is for the apparatus to be able to perform at its full capacity when necessary and to be a safe vehicle to drive and operate under severe conditions.

Testing Low-Voltage Electrical Systems

More detailed and specialized performance testing includes the performance testing of the apparatus' low-voltage electrical systems, which includes the batteries, the starter system, and the charging system, as detailed in NFPA 1911, Chapter 17.

Batteries

To test the condition of the batteries, you will need some common hand tools as well as some specialized tools, including a digital volt-ohm meter (DVOM) **FIGURE 19-1** and another type of meter. Instruction manuals should be available for the two common types of meters utilized—a conductivity tester and a battery load tester—and you should become familiar with whichever device your department has prior to using it. Follow the manufacturer's recommendation when using these instruments, always wear safety glasses, and avoid any type of spark when batteries are involved.

Before testing the batteries, perform a good visual inspection. Check for any swelling, deformation, cracks, or other deficiencies. Such flaws may indicate that the batteries have

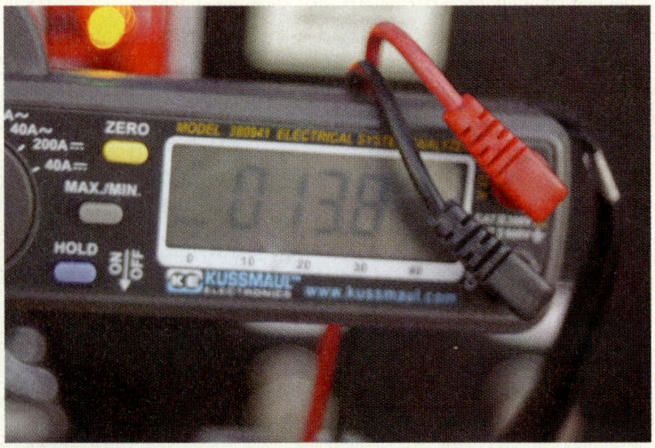

FIGURE 19-1 A digital volt-ohm meter.

been overcharged or frozen and internally damaged. The batteries should be cleaned of any accumulated dirt or corrosion, and the connections should be checked to ensure they are clean and tight. Batteries that are not sealed should be checked to verify that the cells have the proper electrolyte level, and distilled water added if necessary. Exercise caution to ensure no sparks are created in or around the batteries, as the gases emitted by the batteries are very volatile and may cause injury to personnel in the area. Sealed batteries should be inspected to verify that any electrolyte level indicator indicates the presence of sufficient electrolyte.

Conductivity testing is preferred to load testing, because it does not stress the battery, gives a more accurate indication of the state of health of the battery, and provides values that can be recorded and tracked for trend analysis. To test the batteries, you must disconnect each one. Use caution when doing so, and make certain you identify each cable and wire so that they may be reinstalled in the proper location. This type of test is typically performed by the EVT or someone specially trained.

Safety Tip

Exercise caution when testing batteries to ensure that no sparks are created, as the gases emitted by the batteries are very volatile and may cause injury to personnel in the area.

If you are using an electronic battery conductivity tester, follow the steps in **SKILL DRILL 19-1**, and always remember to use caution and follow the test instruments' directions.

1. Test the battery terminal voltage with a DVOM or the tester. If the terminal voltage is less than 12.4 volts for a 12-volt battery or less than 6.2 volts for a 6-volt battery, then the battery will need to be fully charged before proceeding.
2. Turn off the fire apparatus and remove any charger.
3. Disconnect all battery cables from the battery to be tested.
4. Connect the tester to the battery to be tested, making the connection to the lead pad of the battery post or terminal and not to a battery cable. It is very important to have a solid connection and to make contact with the lead pad. A poor connection may result in incorrect readings.
5. Perform the test in accordance with the instructions provided by the tester manufacturer.
6. Record the cold cranking amperage (CCA) value reported in the apparatus maintenance records for trend analysis.
7. If the measured CCA of the battery is less than 80 percent of the original CCA rating of the battery, which can be found marked on the top or side of the battery, the battery has failed.

If a battery conductivity tester is not available, the battery can be tested with a load tester by following the steps in **SKILL DRILL 19-2**.

1. If the battery terminal voltage is less than 12.6 volts for a 12-volt battery or less than 6.3 volts for a 6-volt

TABLE 19-1	Voltage for a Battery to Pass the Load Test		
Battery Temperature °F (°C)	**Voltage (V)**	
	12-Volt Battery	6-Volt Battery
80 (27)	9.70	4.85
70 (21)	9.60	4.80
60 (16)	9.50	4.75
50 (10)	9.40	4.70
40 (4)	9.30	4.65
30 (−1)	9.10	4.55
20 (−7)	8.90	4.45
10 (−12)	8.70	4.35
0 (−18)	8.50	4.25

Source: NFPA 1911, Table 17.3.2.2.1.

battery, you will need to fully charge the battery before proceeding.
2. Turn off the fire apparatus and remove any charger.
3. Disconnect all battery cables from the battery to be tested.
4. Connect a load tester to the battery to be tested.
5. Connect a DVOM that has a ±0.5 percent direct current (DC) voltage accuracy or better if the load tester being used has no voltmeter.
6. Adjust the current load of the load tester to one-half the CCA rating for the battery being tested.
7. Measure and record the temperature of the battery.
8. Apply the load for 15 seconds. **Note:** It is important to remove the load after 15 seconds, as serious damage or injury could result if this time period is extended.
9. Record the battery terminal voltage at the end of the 15 seconds.
10. Discontinue the load test.
11. If the voltage was less than the value noted in NFPA 1911, Table 17.3.2.2.1, the battery has failed **TABLE 19-1**.

If you are performing a load test and the battery fails, you have the opportunity to do some further testing. Using a DVOM, observe the battery voltage for 15 minutes with no load. Typically, the battery voltage will recover and rise with no load on it. If the voltage fails to reach 12.45 volts for a 12-volt battery or 6.23 volts for a 6-volt battery, the battery should be fully recharged and the test repeated once. If the voltage recovers and reaches 12.45 volts for a 12-volt battery or 6.23 volts for a 6-volt battery, the battery has failed. Should battery replacement be necessary, it is recommended that all batteries on the apparatus be replaced as a group by a qualified EVT.

Starter System

The starter wiring is another part of the low-voltage electrical system that requires testing. To perform this testing, you will need some specialized tools and knowledge of the proper use of a DVOM and/or other electrical test meters, as well as some knowledge of basic electrical theory and the procedure to perform voltage drop tests. First, perform a good visual inspection of the wiring from the battery to the starter, checking for corrosion, loose connections, worn insulation, or potential chafing points. With a DVOM or a starter electrical tester, check the voltage drop in the positive (+) wiring between the positive post on the starter (not the wire or connector) and the positive (+) battery terminal (not the wire or connector).

To perform the voltage drop test, place the DVOM in the DC voltage setting. Put one electrical test lead on the positive (+) battery terminal and one electrical test lead on the positive (+) input post on the starter, and measure the voltage. Then, while exercising caution, measure the voltage with the engine cranking. This test is then repeated on the negative side of the low-voltage electrical system. Place one test lead on the case of the starter (not the engine block or frame) and the other test lead on the negative (−) battery terminal (not the wire or connector), and record the voltage. Then, record the voltage with the engine cranking. The voltage drop in each side of the wiring, both positive (+) and negative (−), should not exceed 0.2 volt for a 12-volt nominal system or 0.4 volt for a 24-volt nominal system. Document the voltage drop on the positive (+) and negative (−) side of the system, and compare your results to past results. Report any condition that may cause concern, and have it investigated by a certified EVT.

■ Charging System

Now that you have ensured that the starting system is in good condition, the testing moves systematically to the charging system. Once again, you will need one or more good DVOMs with a ±0.5 percent or better DC voltage accuracy and an ammeter capable of measuring the full output of the alternator with a ±3 percent or better DC current accuracy, or an alternator electrical tester and/or a carbon pile tester. You will also need to be familiar with the manufacturer's recommendation regarding use of the test equipment, and should always follow the alternator manufacturer's safety and test recommendations.

Attach the DVOM set to DC voltage or the alternator electrical tester electrical test lead at the positive (+) output post of the alternator (not the wire or connector) and the other electrical test lead to the positive (+) battery terminal (not the wire or connector) for the voltage drop test. If a second electrical tester is available, connect the alternator's negative (−) lead for the voltage drop to be measured from the alternator's case or the negative (−) output post of the alternator (not the wire or connector) to the negative (−) battery terminal (not the wire or connector). While exercising caution, start the engine. The alternator is then tested as described in **SKILL DRILL 19-3**:

1. Start the test with the engine temperature below 100°F (38°C).
2. Increase the engine speed to 75 percent of the maximum governed engine speed.
3. Turn on enough electrical loads on the apparatus for the total draw to exceed the alternator output, adding load at the battery if necessary. If necessary, the load can be increased using an electrical carbon pile tester. The goal is to determine the maximum output for the alternator.
4. Record the maximum alternator current (amps) and the voltage drop in the positive (+) and negative (−) alternator leads.
5. Stop the test and turn off the loads.
6. If the alternator output current (amps) does not reach at least 80 percent of its rated output current (as identified on the nameplate), the test has failed.
7. If the voltage drop exceeds 0.2 volt for a 12-volt nominal system or 0.4 volt for a 24-volt nominal system in either alternator lead, the test has failed.

■ Regulator Test

The regulator test is performed with fully charged batteries. Connect the DVOM and measure the voltage at the battery terminals. Also, document the temperature of the regulator. Temperature is important to regulator and alternator performance: As temperature increases, performance will decrease.

The regulator should be tested twice. The first test is run with all the loads that can be turned off, off and with the engine at idle speed. First, start the engine and allow the engine to idle, turning all lights, fans, air conditioners, and electrical loads off. Measure and record the voltage at the battery terminals. For the second test, raise the engine rpm to one-half of the rated engine speed. You can find the engine's rated rpm on the pump certification paperwork or the tag on the pump panel. Turn on sufficient loads so that the alternator produces a minimum of one-half of its rated capacity. Document the voltage measurement at the battery terminals and the temperature of the regulator. Compare your readings to those in listed in NFPA 1911, Table 17.6.6 **TABLE 19-2**. If the voltage is less than that listed in the table, the test has failed. Document the test results and report your findings to the AHJ. In case of a failing test, a qualified EVT should evaluate the condition of the charging system and recommend necessary corrective action.

TABLE 19-2 Voltage Range for a Battery to Pass the Regulator Test

Regulator Temperature °F (°C)	12-Volt Nominal System	Voltage (V) 24-Volt Nominal System	42-Volt Nominal System
200 (93)	13.6–14.2	27.2–28.4	40.8–42.6
150 (66)	13.7–14.3	27.4–28.6	41.1–42.9
100 (38)	13.8–14.4	27.6–28.8	41.4–43.2
50 (10)	14.0–14.9	28.0–29.8	42.0–44.7
0 (−18)	14.2–15.5	28.4–31.0	42.6–46.5

Source: NFPA 1911, Table 17.6.6.

Battery Charger/Conditioner Test

If the apparatus is equipped with a battery charger or conditioner, you should also test it. You will need a good DVOM capable of testing voltage and current (amps). With the apparatus turned off and electrical loads that exceed the rated output of the charger/conditioner turned on, the output of the battery charger/conditioner should be at least 80 percent of the rated output of the battery charger/conditioner. You can normally find the output rating of the battery charger/conditioner on a tag located on the battery charger/conditioner.

First, check the battery voltage with a DVOM or battery electrical tester to make sure the battery is fully charged. Then, with the DVOM, place the tester in the DC voltage position, the negative (−) or black test lead on the negative (+) post of the battery charger/conditioner, and the red test lead on the positive terminal of the battery charger/conditioner. Check the voltage of the battery charger/conditioner to make sure it is at least 13.8 volts for a 12-volt nominal system, 27.6 volts for a 24-volt nominal system, or 41.4 volts for a 42-volt system. Follow the manufacturer's instructions for inspection of the battery charger/conditioner.

Total Continuous Electrical Load Test

The total continuous electrical load test is normally conducted during the pump performance test by an EVT, but the test procedure is described here so that you can determine how to best test your own system. The voltage measurements for this test should be made with a voltmeter with a resolution of 0.01 volt or better and a good-quality DVOM.

Advance the engine speed (rpm) to at least 50 percent of the governed speed of the engine. Turn on all loads that make up the total continuous electrical load, *except* loads associated with the following components:

- Aerial hydraulic pump
- Foam pump
- Hydraulic-driven equipment
- Winch
- Windshield wipers
- Four-way hazard flashers
- Compressed-air foam system (CAFS) compressor

The first step is to measure the battery voltage at the battery terminals and document it. The apparatus then needs to be operated for at least 20 minutes, with the throttle engine speed being 50 percent of the governed engine speed and, if the apparatus is equipped with an automatic electrical load management system, with load shedding as permitted by the system. Check the voltage at completion of the test. If the voltage drop exceeds 0.05 volt from the beginning to the end of the test, the test is considered a failure. Document your findings, and report any failures to the AHJ and/or EVT.

Solenoid and Relay Test

Next to be tested are the electrical solenoids and relays that control the power to motors, or loads of 50 amperes or more, which include the following:

- Starter motor
- Primer motor
- Aerial emergency power source
- Cab tilt hydraulic pump
- Hydraulic or electric ladder equipment racks
- Battery or master load disconnects
- Mechanical sirens

For these tests, you will need a good-quality DVOM with a resolution of 0.01 volt or better. These voltage drop tests are similar to the tests that were performed for the starter and the alternator. Begin by attaching the voltmeter test leads from the input power stud to the point between the contacts and the motor load, making sure that the DVOM is set to read DC voltage. Next, activate the load and record the voltage across the power connections. The number displayed on the DVOM will be the voltage drop for that particular solenoid or relay. If, for example, you had a 12-volt system and were testing the primer motor relay, you would locate the relay, place the DVOM electrical test leads on the incoming and outgoing sides of the solenoid, set the DVOM to DC voltage, activate the primer, and then note the voltage difference between the posts on the solenoid. The result would be the voltage drop in that solenoid. If the voltage drop exceeded 0.3 volt, the test would be considered to have failed.

Any excessive voltage drop across a power relay or solenoid indicates a problem with the component and, if not repaired, will often lead to a failure of the device by which it is controlled. Consequently, any deficiencies should be documented and reported in writing to the AHJ and a qualified EVT for evaluation and repair.

Foam Proportioning Systems

Performance testing of foam proportioning systems, if the apparatus is so equipped, is described in NFPA 1911, Chapter 20; a good form to document your results can be found in NFPA 1911, Appendix 1911-94, Figure C.3(g). The test that is performed determines whether the foam proportioning system is capable of delivering foam solution at a concentrate setting established for the agent(s) used—specifically Class A foam, Class B foam, and or any other agent that may be used, such as an emulsifier. At a minimum, the foam system should be tested annually.

First, the entire foam system should be given a good visual inspection. The foam system should be operated at the proportioning ratio specified by the AHJ and at the water flow and pressure for the agent(s) employed. Thus, if you have Class A foam, which is mixed at a ratio of 0.1 to 1 percent, and you use a 1¾-inch (45-mm) discharge hose, you would flow that discharge at the normal flow rate, pressure, and percentage. If you are using Class B foam, aqueous film-forming foam (AFFF), or alcohol-resistant aqueous film-forming foam (AR-AFFF), which is typically mixed at a ratio of 1, 3, or 6 percent, you would operate the system at the normal flow rate, pressure, and percentage normally used for that foam. The system should be tested for accuracy, and one of the following four methods used:

1. Substitute water for the foam concentrate
2. Measure the foam concentrate pump's output directly
3. Determine the foam percentage with a refractometer
4. Determine the foam percentage with a conductivity meter

One of the most commonly used foam systems today is the electronic direct-injection system, as exemplified by the FoamPro, FRC, Hale, or Class One, Pierce Husky, and Waterous systems. It is a fairly simple process to follow the manufacturer's instructions to measure the concentrate output of the foam pump on these systems. Of course, it is always important to be familiar with the manufacturer's information, as some of these systems may produce foam injection pressures in excess of 450 psi (3150 kPa).

To test an electronic direct-injection system, typically you will use a calibrated container, such as a 5-gallon (20-L) bucket. Mark the bucket in 1-gallon increments. Locate the injection pump and the flush/calibration/inject/valve on the discharge side of the pump. Position the calibrated container under the flush/calibrate/inject hose. Following the manufacturer's instructions, put the foam system in the manual mode of operation and/or the calibrate mode. Start the system and watch the display, making sure the amount of concentrate discharged is the amount displayed on the control head. When this step is complete, make any adjustments necessary and retest the system if changes were made. Make sure that the system is put back into normal operation mode and that the flush/calibrate/inject valve is switched back to the inject position. Remember, too, that if you use more than one type of solution, each type needs to be tested separately. Document your calibration procedure and results; you may find the form in NFPA 1911 helpful for this purpose.

You may use whichever of the four methods that will best meet your needs to determine the accuracy and performance of the apparatus foam system.

Test Method 1: Substitute Water for the Foam Concentrate

The foam system is operated at the water flow rates at which the system is to be tested. Suppose you have foam on one 1¾-inch (45-mm) hoseline discharge and you typically discharge 125 gpm (500 L/min). In this test method, water is used as a substitute for the foam concentrate. This water is drawn from a calibrated tank instead of foam concentrate from the concentrate tank. The volume of water drawn from the calibrated tank divided by the volume of water pumped over the same time period multiplied by 100 represents the percentage of foam that the foam proportioner is producing. Therefore, if you are discharging 150 gpm (568 L/min) with the foam proportioner set at 1 percent, and you flow for 5 minutes, in theory you flowed 750 gallons (3000 L) of water; thus the amount of water (foam concentrate) drawn from the calibrated tank should be 7.5 gallons (30 L). This 7.5 gallons divided by 750 gallons (45 mm) of water equals 0.01; 0.01 multiplied by 100 equals 1 percent. Because the foam proportioner was set to discharge a 1 percent solution, the foam system is accurate at that percentage.

For this test, you should use the percentage rate and flow rates commonly used for your type foam and your department's typical operation.

Test Method 2: Measure the Foam Concentrate Pump's Output Directly

With some direct-injection systems, it is possible to directly measure the foam concentrate pump's output. With the foam system operating at a given water flow rate, and using either foam concentrate or water as a substitute for foam concentrate, the output of the foam concentrate pump is measured by diverting that output into a calibrated container for direct measurement over a measured period of time. An alternative is to measure the foam concentrate flow or water substitute with a calibrated meter.

Test Method 3: Determine the Foam Percentage with a Refractometer

A refractometer is used to measure the refractive index of a foam solution sample. First, a base calibration curve is prepared using the same water and foam concentrate that will be used with the system to be tested. Three known foam solution samples are needed:
1. The nominal intended percentage
2. The nominal intended percentage plus 1 percent
3. The nominal intended percentage minus 1 percent

If the nominal intended percent is 1 percent or less, the following three samples should be obtained:
1. The nominal intended percentage
2. The nominal intended percentage plus 0.3 percent
3. The nominal intended percentage minus 0.3 percent

The required amount of water is placed in a 100-mL or larger graduated cylinder, leaving space for the foam concentrate. A 10-mL pipette or 10-cc syringe is used to carefully add the required amount of foam concentrate to the water. Each measured foam solution is then poured from the graduated cylinder into a 100-mL or larger plastic bottle, and the bottle is marked to indicate the percentage of solution it contains. The bottle is capped and thoroughly shaken to mix the foam solution.

An alternative method for making the three foam solution samples is to use a very accurate scale. The density of the foam concentrate needs to be known and can be found on the product data sheet or the Material Safety Data Sheet (MSDS) for the foam concentrate. For example, to make a 100-mL sample of a 3 percent foam solution using a foam concentrate with a density of 1.04, 97 g of water is measured into a beaker and 3.12 g of foam concentrate is added to the beaker (1.04 × 3 g = 3.12 g).

After the foam solution samples are thoroughly mixed, a refractive index reading is taken of each sample. To do so, place a few drops of the solution on the refractometer prism, close the cover plate, and observe the scale reading at the dark field intersection. Because the refractometer is a temperature-compensated device, it could take 10 to 20 seconds for the sample to be read properly. It is important to take all refractometer readings at an ambient temperature of 50°F (10°C) or above.

Using standard graph paper, the refractive index readings are then plotted on one axis and the percentage of concentration on the other. This curve serves as the known baseline for the test series. The solution samples should be set aside in the event the measurements need to be rechecked.

Foam solution samples are then collected from the proportioner system, making certain that the samples are taken at an adequate distance downstream from the foam proportioner being tested to allow for complete mixing of the water and the foam concentrate. Refractive index readings of the samples are taken and compared to the plotted curve to determine the percentage of foam.

This method might not be accurate for AFFF, alcohol-resistant foam, or certain other types of foam that typically exhibit very low refractive index readings. Also, the refractometer method should not be used when testing foam percentages of 1 percent or lower, because the accuracy for determining the percentage of foam concentrate in a solution when using a refractometer is ±0.1 percent, at best. For this reason, test method 4, the conductivity method, might be preferable where AFFF, alcohol-resistant foam, or 1 percent or less foam (Class A) is to be tested.

Test Method 4: Determine the Foam Percentage with a Conductivity Meter

The conductivity test method is based on changes in electrical conductivity as foam concentrate is added to water. Conductivity is a very accurate method, provided there are substantial changes in conductivity as foam concentrate is added to the water in relatively low percentages. Because saltwater and brackish water are very conductive, this method might not be suitable where these waters are used to produce foam because of the small conductivity changes as foam concentrate is added. If saltwater or brackish water is used, it is necessary to make foam solutions in advance to determine whether adequate changes in conductivity can be detected. This method also cannot be used if the water has more total solids than the foam concentrate.

Three variations of the conductivity method can be used to determine the foam percentage during testing:

- **Direct-reading conductivity method.** A sample of the water to be used in the test is put in a 100-mL or larger container. The conductivity meter head is immersed in the water sample, and the meter display is set at zero. If the direct-reading foam solution conductivity meter is mounted in a discharge line, the meter should be set at zero with plain water flowing. If the manufacturer of the conductivity meter does not indicate that the percentage of foam solution can be read directly for the foam concentrate being used, a calibration curve needs to be developed. This calibration curve might show that the direct meter readings are correct for the foam concentrate being used, or it might indicate that the calibration curve needs to be used when the foam concentrate is tested.

  The foam proportioner system is then operated, and a sample of the foam solution produced by the system is collected using a 100-mL or larger container. The conductivity meter head is immersed in the foam solution sample, and the percentage of the foam solution is read on the meter display. If the conductivity meter is mounted in a discharge line, the percentage of the foam solution is read on the meter display, while foam solution is being discharged.

- **Conductivity comparison method.** A sample of the water to be used in the test is put in a 100-mL or larger container. Using a conductivity meter reading given in units of microsiemens per centimeter (µS/cm), the conductivity value of the water sample is determined. The foam proportioning system is operated, and a sample of the foam solution produced by the system is collected in a 100-mL or larger container. Using the conductivity meter, the conductivity value of the foam solution sample is determined. The conductivity value of the water sample is subtracted from the conductivity value of the foam solution sample, and the result is divided by 500 to obtain the percentage of foam concentrate in the solution.

  Percent foam
  $$= \frac{\text{Conductivity of foam solution} - \text{Conductivity of water}}{500}$$

  Note that the divisor is 500 only if the conductivity meter units are microsiemens per centimeter (µS/cm). Other units of conductivity can be used, but the value of the divisor (500) will need to be adjusted in such a case.

- **Conductivity calibration curve method.** A baseline calibration curve is prepared using the water and foam concentrate from the system to be tested. Three known foam solution samples are made using the procedure described in test method 3. After the foam solution samples are thoroughly mixed, the conductivity of each solution is measured using a conductivity meter. Care should be taken to ensure that the proper procedures are used for taking readings and that the meter is switched to the correct conductivity range. Most synthetic-based foams used with freshwater result in foam solution conductivity readings of less than 2000 µS/cm. By comparison, protein-based foams used with freshwater generally produce conductivity readings in excess of 2000 µS/cm. Because of the temperature-compensation feature of the conductivity meter, it could take a short time to obtain a consistent reading. Once the solution samples have been measured and recorded, the bottles should be set aside as control sample references. The conductivity readings are then plotted on standard graph paper. It is more convenient to place the foam solution percentage on the horizontal axis and the conductivity readings on the vertical axis. A straight line should be drawn that approximates the connection of all three points. While it might not be possible to connect all three points with a straight line, they should be very close to the line. If not, the conductivity measurements should be repeated, and, if necessary, new control sample solutions should be prepared and used until all three points plot in a nearly straight line. This plot serves as the known baseline (calibration) curve to be used for the test series.

- Once this curve has been plotted, foam solution samples are collected from the proportioner system. The conductivity of the test samples is measured, and the percentage of foam solution is determined from the base curve. Foam solution samples that have been allowed to drain from expanded foam should not be used, because they can produce misleading conductivity readings [see NFPA 1911, Figure C.3(g); the Foam Proportioning System Performance Test].

■ Performance Testing of Compressed-Air Foam Systems

If the apparatus is equipped with a compressed-air foam system (CAFS), a test should be performed to determine if that system is capable of delivering the manufacturer's maximum recommended airflow at rated pressures. First, a visual and operational inspection of the complete CAFS is performed. You will need a good-quality calibrated airflow meter in conjunction with standard cubic feet per minute (SCFM) flow or a fixed-orifice flow meter in conjunction with various sizes of orifices to test the flow volume in SCFM. You may find the CAFS Compressor Performance Test Form in NFPA 1911, Annex C Figure C.3(h).

The test procedure should follow these steps:

1. Run the compressed air system at the CAFS manufacturer's recommended maximum airflow at 125 psi (875 kPa) for 20 minutes. **Note:** Make sure the water pump is engaged and circulating enough water to cool the air compressor. Most systems use pump water flow to keep the air compressor cool. If you do not cool the pump properly, it may overheat or an air compressor sump fire may occur, damaging the compressor. To ensure that the compressor does not overheat, it may be a good idea to flush the cooler prior to performing this test.
2. Record the airflow, air pressure, and compressor temperature at start-up and in 5-minute increments.
3. Record the maximum air pressure developed by the compressed air system.
4. Connect a 100-ft (30-m) 1½-inch (38-mm) or smaller hoseline to the CAFS discharge, and stretch it out on level ground.
5. Secure the nozzle end of the hoseline to a stationary object with a rope, with straps, or in some other manner, so that when the nozzle is opened (no faster than 3 seconds and no slower than 10 seconds), the operator is protected from nozzle movement. **Note:** Remember that air is compressible, but water is not. Tremendous amounts of energy may be stored in the end of the hose, and kickback or nozzle reaction force may be severe.
6. Engage the water pump and establish a pump pressure of 125 psi (875 kPa), but do not charge the hoseline with water. You will be recirculating the water or otherwise moving water to ensure that the pump or air compressor does not overheat.
7. Circulate pump water through the water tank or otherwise discharge water to maintain the pump temperature within the manufacturer's recommendations.
8. Ensure that air pressure and water pressure are within ±10 percent of the original set point.
9. Fill the hoseline with compressed air.
10. Slowly (no faster than 3 seconds and no slower than 10 seconds) open the nozzle until it is no more than one-fourth open.
11. Ensure that the air pressure and water pressure are within ±10 percent of the original set point.
12. Close the nozzle.
13. Continue to operate the air and water system for 5 minutes.
14. Check whether the water pressure and air pressure remain within ±10 percent of the original set point.

If the CAFS does not maintain the water pressure and air pressure within ±10 percent of the original set point, or if the air compressor temperature exceeds the manufacturer's limit during the test, the test should be stopped and considered a failure. Record your results and report any deficiencies. Further evaluation or repairs should be performed by a qualified EVT.

■ Performance Testing of Line Voltage Electrical Systems

The same general considerations hold true for the line voltage electrical system as for all the rest of the major fire apparatus systems. Performance testing should be conducted at least annually, unless otherwise noted, and whenever major repairs or modifications to the line voltage electrical system or any component of this system have been made. Caution needs to be exercised when testing line voltage systems, as serious injury may result.

The line voltage electrical system test includes the following elements:

1. Power source testing
   - The line voltage power source should be tested annually except when the full load test described in item 5 is performed (full 60-minute test).
   - The power source should be tested using the electrical loads normally carried on the apparatus connected simultaneously, up to the limit specified.
   - The total connected load applied should not exceed the continuous rating as specified on the power source specifications label, or the power source nameplate rating if there is no power source specification label.
   - The power source should be run for a minimum of 10 minutes under the test load.
   - The voltage, frequency, and load should be measured and recorded at the following times:
     • At the beginning of the test under no load conditions
     • After the test load has been applied
     • After 10 minutes under test load
     • At the end of the test when the test load has been removed
     • The voltage and frequency should be within the limits specified by NFPA 1901, *Standard for Automotive Fire Apparatus*, at the time the apparatus was built.
2. Receptacle wiring
   - You will want to make sure that all loads are disconnected while doing continuity testing. The polarity of the wiring, the ground continuity, and the neutral bonding or isolation of all 120-volt outlets should be tested, including receptacles on the body, cord reels, and aerial device.
   - If the neutral conductor is bonded to the vehicle frame, the testing should be done with a tester that verifies that the hot and neutral wires are connected to the correct receptacle pins and that the ground is connected. Inexpensive receptacle testers with lights to indicate correct or problem wiring are available from any hardware store or home center. Many also include a button for testing ground-fault circuit interrupters (GFCIs) as needed for the testing in NFPA 1911, 22.5.2. Testing can also be done with the power off using a continuity tester to the hot and neutral buses in the circuit breaker panel for the hot

and neutral wires and to the body for the protective ground wire. Testing of twist lock or other special receptacles may require the use of an adapter.

- If the neutral conductor is not bonded to the vehicle frame, the testing should be done with the power off, using a continuity tester or ohmmeter to verify that both of the current carrying conductors are isolated from the vehicle body and frame, and that the protective ground is connected to the vehicle body and frame. With an isolated system, the three light testers will, and should, indicate an open ground. To maintain the safety of the isolated system, it is important to verify the isolation between the current-carrying conductors and the body. This test detects faults that do not cause other indications.
- Any receptacles that can be powered both from an onboard power source and from a shore line should be tested both ways. Receptacles supplied from a shore line should always have a bonded neutral conductor when being powered from the shore line; they should have an isolated neutral conductor when powered from the onboard source if the onboard system is isolated. If the transfer switch operation is powered from the onboard power source, the testing must be done with a three-light tester, which should indicate an open ground.
- Duplex receptacles should be tested in each receptacle.

3. GFCI testing
   - If the wiring system or any appliances on the apparatus incorporate GFCIs, their operation should be checked.
   - All GFCIs shall be checked, whether they are integrated into receptacles or circuit breakers or are separate devices.
   - The operational check should verify that the integrated test button trips the GFCI, that the reset button restores the GFCI, and that the GFCI trips when a ground fault is simulated with an external tester.

4. Line voltage equipment testing
   - All line voltage equipment on the apparatus should be run for a minimum of 10 minutes.
   - The testing should include, but not be limited to, light towers, permanently wired lights, electric motors, fixed wired appliances, receptacles (each individual receptacle if they are present in multiples), fixed cords, and cord reels, each loaded to at least 50 percent of the rating of the circuit breaker for that circuit.
   - All equipment should operate properly without arcing, failure, or excessive heating.

5. Full load test of the power source, which shall be performed at least every 5 years

Performance Testing of Breathing-Air Compressor Systems

If the apparatus is supplied with a breathing-air compressor system, that system should be tested annually by the manufacturer or the manufacturer's authorized representative to verify that the system still meets the manufacturer's requirements for the system when it was new. Note that this test needs to be performed by the manufacturer or authorized representative; the fire department only needs to do the air quality test. To perform the latter test, you follow the manufacturer's recommendation and take an air quality sample, send it to the testing lab, and document the results. The goal is to make sure that the quality of the clean compressed air meets NFPA 1989, *Standard on Breathing Air Quality for Emergency Services Respiratory Protection*, and is a Grade D breathing air. The air quality records should be maintained for the life of the apparatus.

The original acceptance test and the certification test by a third party may require more than 3 hours of pumping time and 4 hours of testing time for the fire apparatus. By comparison, annual performance testing may consist of 45 minutes of pumping time and several other pump performance tests. Annual pump service testing should be performed by personnel who are qualified in accordance with NFPA 1071. Today, performance testing can be done by agencies other than Underwriters Laboratories (UL), Factory Mutual, or American Testing. The critical point is that the fire apparatus must be periodically (annually or whenever a major repair has been made that may affect the performance of the pump per NFPA 1911) tested by an NFPA 1071–compliant EVT.

Low-voltage electrical system, pump, aerial device, foam proportioning, CAFS, line voltage electrical system, and breathing-air compressor performance tests are conducted after a fire apparatus has been put into service to determine if its performance continues to meet the predetermined specifications or standards. Performance testing of all of these systems is an integral and vital part of fire apparatus safety and maintenance. Imagine arriving on the scene of a multiple-alarm fire, laying hose, hooking up to the hydrant, and starting to pump water—only to have the pump fail after 10 minutes. One question that might be asked in this scenario is whether the pump failure could have been prevented by annual performance testing.

The Insurance Services Office (ISO) reports that fire continues to be the leading cause of loss cited in conjunction with personal and commercial property insurance policies. The ISO also reports that there is a definite correlation between improved fire protection and compliance with the NFPA standards. During the annual performance testing of fire pumps, the ISO Fire Suppression Rating Schedule assigns the highest point total to fire apparatus pumps.

NFPA 1911 calls for annual **performance testing** or **service testing** of fire apparatus pumps. Fire pumps are water pumps that have a **rated capacity** of 250 gpm (1000 L/min) or greater at 150 psi (1000 kPa) net pump pressure and that are mounted on a fire apparatus and used for firefighting purposes. Fire pumps that are placed in service should be tested each year to determine whether they are still capable of achieving their designed performance.

The performance tests for fire pumps do not just test the pump; rather, they test the entire pumping system—the engine, transmission, and pump, plus related accessories and devices used in operating the pumping system. You might consider the annual performance tests of fire pumps to be a "stress test" for the fire apparatus: To pass, the fire apparatus must deliver its original design flow and pressure; must show no signs of overheating, loss of power, or over-acceleration; and must not exhibit any other major defects.

NFPA 1911 regulates the actual conduct of performance testing of fire pumps. It states that such a test is to be conducted annually for all fire apparatus that have a fire pump with 250 gpm (1000 L/min) or larger capacity or if the pump and/or engine on the fire apparatus has been repaired or modified. Note that this test is not the same as a new apparatus acceptance or third-party test, which is conducted by an independent agency for the manufacturer and requires approximately 3 hours of pumping time and 4 hours of testing time. The annual performance test generally follows the same test procedure but involves shorter pumping times. In addition to the annual performance test, NFPA 1911 calls for a fire pump test to be conducted whenever major repairs or modifications have been made to the pump or any component of the fire apparatus used in pump operations.

Fire Apparatus Requirements

Engine-driven accessories should not be functionally disconnected or otherwise rendered inoperative during the annual performance test. If the chassis engine drives the pump, all headlights, running lights, warning lights, and air conditioners, if provided, should continue to operate during the pumping portion of this test. This would be the total continuous electrical load as defined in NFPA 1901 and NFPA 1911. If fire apparatus is built to the 1996 or later editions of NFPA 1901, and if the apparatus is equipped with a fixed power source (such as a hydraulic generator) driven by the same engine that drives the fire pump, the power source should run at a minimum of 50 percent of its rated capacity throughout the pumping portion of the pump test. The following devices are permitted to be turned off (or at least not operated) during the pump performance test:

- Aerial hydraulic pump
- Foam pump
- Hydraulic-driven equipment (other than a hydraulic-driven line voltage generator, which must be operated at least 50 percent of its rated capacity throughout the pumping portion of the pump test; see NFPA 1911, 1996 and later)
- Winch
- Windshield wipers
- Four-way hazard flashers
- CAFS compressor

If any electrical loads are connected through an automatic electrical load management system, then that system should be permitted to automatically disconnect those loads during the course of the test.

When operating a pump, it is important that the engine temperature is kept within the proper range; neither a cold engine nor an excessively hot engine will give as good service as one that is run at the proper temperature. The oil pressure on the engine should be watched to confirm that the engine is being lubricated properly. The transmission temperature should be monitored for overheating. Any unusual vibration of the engine or the pump, or any leak in the pump casing or connections, should be noted and managed. Centrifugal pumps are not self-priming, so they could lose their prime if a leak in the suction lines occurs.

When conducting performance tests on fire pumps, the fire apparatus should use the side intakes, if possible. Note that this does not include emergency vehicles with a rear- or front-mount pump; their intake suction must be used. Although not always preferred, front- or rear-mount intakes on midship-mounted pumps may be used in conjunction with side intake suction(s) for all pumps that provide flows of 1500 gpm (6000 L/min) or greater. All other intakes should remain in the closed position and be properly capped. Storz fittings are not recommended and should be removed prior to testing; they may be replaced with steamer caps during the performance test.

In case of any fire/apparatus failure, time should be allotted to make the necessary repairs where applicable. **Failure** is defined as a cessation of proper functioning or performance. Other defects in the performance of the engine or the pump should be documented as well, and minor defects should be corrected immediately if possible. If such repairs cannot be done on site, then the fire apparatus should be rescheduled for testing at a later date.

■ Environmental Requirements

Before beginning any performance tests on fire apparatus pumps, the following environmental conditions must be determined and recorded prior to and immediately after the pump performance testing:

- Ambient air temperature
- Water temperature
- Atmospheric pressure

NFPA 1911 specifies that tests must be conducted when the ambient air temperature is between 0°F and 110°F (−18°C and 43°C). **Ambient air temperature** is the temperature of the surrounding environment and usually refers to the temperature of the air in which a structure is situated or a device operates. The water temperature should be between 35°F and 90°F (1.7°C and 32°C), and the air pressure (atmospheric pressure) at 29 in. Hg (736.6 mm Hg or 98.6 kPa) or greater (corrected to sea level).

People who regularly conduct pump tests know that those extremes are of little help if the goal is to maximize pump performance. For example, hot air temperatures can cause the engine cooling fan to run more frequently, which increases the parasitic power loss. Cold air temperatures can affect battery power. Although no one makes a specific recommendation, days with moderate temperatures are generally better choices for conducting performance tests than very hot or cold ones.

Water temperature extremes are even more important. Warm water, usually defined as water at a temperature greater than 90°F (32°C), is more likely to cavitate inside the pump and may result in a loss of as much as 500 gpm (2000 L/min) in the flow rate. It is particularly important that the water supply be non-aerated and that its temperature not exceed 90°F (32°C) when you are conducting tests at a test pit, where repeated circulation of the water through the pump can increase water temperatures over time. At the other end of the scale, cold water is more likely to freeze and foul test equipment, especially if the air temperature is also low. The general recommendation is to ensure a water temperature in the range of 35°F to 90°F (1.7°C to 29°C), with about 60°F (16°C) being ideal. If these criteria are not met, the pump performance could be affected dramatically.

Atmospheric pressure (sometimes called air pressure or barometric pressure) is also important. High atmospheric pressure pushes harder on the surface of the water being drafted and makes it easier to lift; low atmospheric pressure makes it harder to lift the water. Conducting the performance test on a day when a high-pressure system is parked over your test site will give the best results.

To correct local atmospheric pressure readings to sea level, add 1 in. Hg (25 mm Hg or 3.4 kPa) for every 1000 ft (300 m) of elevation at the site. If the resulting corrected reading is less than 29 in. Hg (736.6 mm Hg or 98.6 kPa) or if the atmospheric pressure readings are falling steadily, then postpone your test to a more favorable day.

If any environmental conditions are not within the specified limits, the test should be delayed until they are satisfactory. Otherwise, the results will need to be confirmed by another test at a later date.

■ Test Site

The test site should be located along an improved roadway or on solid ground where the water is from 4 to 8 ft (1.2 to 2.4 m) below grade. It should be possible to reach the water from the pump intake with not more than 20 ft (6 m) of hard suction hose with the strainer submerged at least 2 ft (0.6 m) and with no humps in the hose.

DRIVER/OPERATOR Tip

The test site should be flat. A sloped test site will steal power from the motor and is not compliant with NFPA 1911.

The water should be at least 4 ft (1.2 m) deep where the strainer is located to provide clearance below the strainer and sufficient depth above it. A poor test site can result in as much as 150 to 500 gpm (600 to 2000 L/min) of lost flow rate. In some cases, a bad site can even force you to stop the test and start over **FIGURE 19-2**.

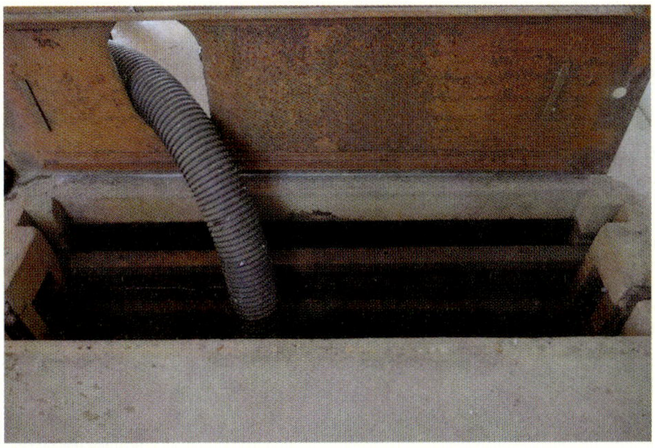

FIGURE 19-2 A good test site is safe and will give accurate results for the fire apparatus' performance.

All tests requiring the flowing of water should be conducted whenever possible with the pump drafting. If it is impractical to provide all of the specified conditions, the AHJ may authorize tests under other conditions.

When a suitable site for drafting is not available, the chosen site must provide a level area for stationing the fire apparatus, a source of hydrant water with sufficient flow, and an area that is suitable for discharging water. Both the elevation of site and the lift should be recorded. The lift is the vertical height that water must be raised during a drafting operation, as measured from the surface of a static source of water to the centerline of the pump intake. Depending on the rated capacity (gpm or L/min) of the pump that you are testing, a specific suction arrangement, diameter of suction hose, maximum number of suction lines, and maximum allowable lift will be required. You should consult NFPA 1911, Table 18.5.1.1.1, for the required suction hose size, number of suction lines, and lift for fire pumps.

The maximum lift is the greatest difference in elevation at which the fire apparatus can draft the required quantity of water under the established physical characteristics of operation. These characteristics will take into account the following considerations:

- The design of the pump
- The adequacy of the engine
- The condition of the pump and the engine
- The size and condition of the suction hose and strainers
- The elevation of the pumping site above sea level
- The atmospheric conditions
- The temperature of the water

The theoretical values of lift and maximum lift must be reduced by the entrance and friction losses in the suction hose equipment to obtain the actual or measurable lift. The vacuum (i.e., negative pressure) on the intake side of a pump is measured in inches or millimeters of mercury. A vacuum of 1 in. Hg is equal to a negative pressure of 03.49 psi; that is, 1 in. Hg = 0.49 psi. A positive pressure of 0.49 psi (3.4 kPa) at the bottom of a 1-inch (645-mm) container will support a column of water that is 1.13 ft (0.034 m) high; therefore, a negative pressure of 0.49 psi (3.4 kPa) at the top of the container will support the same column of water. Thus, a reading of 16 in. Hg (406 mm Hg) on a vacuum gauge will be equivalent to approximately 8 psi (55 kPa).

The proper way to calculate suction loss, as described in NFPA 1901 and 1911, Table 8.5.1.1, is to add the height of lift from the top surface of the water to the center of the intake, divide by 2.3 to get the corrected suction loss, and then use this value to calculate net pressure. Measurement of water pressure is based on the following relationships:

- 1 cubic ft (0.03 m^3) of water weighs 62.5 lb (28 kg)
- The surface area of 1 cubic ft (0.03 m^3) of water is 144 sq. inches (92903 mm^2)
- A column of water 1 sq. inch (645 mm^2) exerts a pressure of 0.434 psi (3 kPa)
- 62.5 lb (28 kg) = 0.434 psi (3 kPa) with a surface area of 144 sq. inches (92903 mm^2)
- 1 psi (7 kPa) of water pressure equals a 1 sq. inch (645 mm^2) column of water that is 2.3 ft (700 mm) high

This information is required to determine net pump pressure for the test. Some fire departments use a rule of thumb;

however, that is not the proper way to conduct such testing. <u>Net pump pressure (NPP)</u> is defined as the sum of the discharge pressure and the suction lift converted to psi or kPa when pumping at draft, or the difference between the discharge pressure and the intake pressure when pumping from a hydrant or other source of water under pressure.

Fire departments that want to achieve the best performance from their pumps should consider several other factors when conducting performance tests. For example, they should select a test site with an adequate source of clear, fresh water. Saltwater is denser than freshwater and should not be used in these periodic tests for two reasons: (1) it reduces performance, and (2) it accelerates the corrosion process within the apparatus' pump and piping. Muddy water also should be avoided because it often contains hidden debris and can clog the pump, valves, fittings, and gauge lines. It will also accelerate pump impeller and wear ring wear and decrease pump life.

Make sure that the water source is configured to allow good performance and easy accessibility. Water sources should be located where the fire apparatus can be parked on a level, hard surface. The fire apparatus should be positioned such that a 20-ft (6-m) length of hard suction hose can be connected to the pump inlet with the strainer submerged according to the NFPA 1911 requirements. It is preferable that suction and discharge hoses be placed on the opposite side of the operator for safety reasons. Operating on a side slope can result in air pockets forming within the plumbing that might reduce performance. Operating on soft soil on a side slope can result in a dangerous tip-over condition and should also be avoided. Operating with the strainer too close to the surface of the water or in water that is too shallow can result in air entrainment and cavitation caused by formation of a whirlpool.

Another option in conducting any performance testing is to use a properly designed pump test pit **FIGURE 19-3**. Hale Products' *Pump Test Pit Design Recommendations* publication suggests using a pit that is 13 to 15 ft (4 to 5 m) deep and approximately 2½ to 3 times longer than it is wide. For example, if the pit is 10 ft (3 m) wide, it should be 25 to 30 ft (7 to 9 m) long. A 10-ft (3-m) wide by 30-ft (9-m) long by 15-ft (5-m) deep pit would have a total volume of 4500 ft^3 (135 m^3). Multiply cubic feet by 7.5 to determine gallons. In this case, the pit has a total capacity of 33,750 gal (135,000 L), of which about 30,000 gal (120,000 L) is usable after allowing for partial fill. This would be sufficient to test pumps up to 3000 gpm (12,000 L/min) using the recommended 10 gal (40 L) of pit capacity for every 1 gpm (4 L/min) of pump flow. The water should be drafted from one end of the pit and discharged back into the other end. Hale Products recommends that several removable baffles be placed within the pit between the two ends to control turbulence and help reduce aeration of the water.

As mentioned earlier, the usable capacity of the test pit should be at least 10 gal (40 L) for every 1 gpm (4 L/min) of the pump. For example, a pump flowing water at a rate of 1500 gpm (6000 L/min) would require a pit with a usable capacity of at least 15,000 gal (60,000 L). Pits with less capacity can result in air entrapment and excessive water temperature rise, which can lead to loss of suction, cavitation, and significantly reduced pump performance.

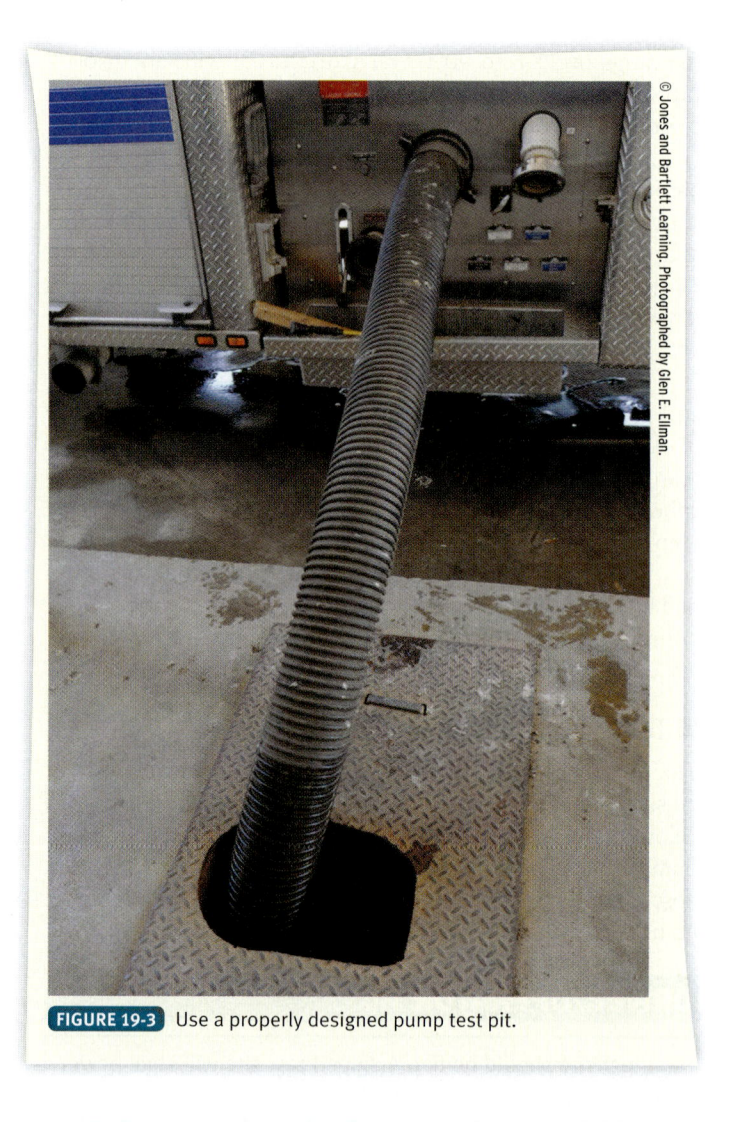

FIGURE 19-3 Use a properly designed pump test pit.

DRIVER/OPERATOR Safety

Because of the significant pressure being applied when conducting pump testing, nozzles should be used with a portable or mounted monitor. Hand-held nozzles should never be used during performance tests.

Safety Tip

Ground monitors should be secured to a fixed object to prevent movement during the performance test.

Equipment Requirements

Prior to conducting performance (service) tests on fire apparatus, the AHJ must ensure that the proper equipment is available and in satisfactory working condition. The following is a list of equipment that will be needed during the testing period:

- One 0–400 psi (0–2800 kPa) test gauge marked in 5-psi (35-kPa) increments ±5 percent accuracy and with a 3½-inch (90-mm) diameter (QC-Test Kit)

- One 0–30 in. Hg (0–762 mm Hg) vacuum gauge marked in 0.5-inch (13-mm) increments and with a 3½-inch (90-mm) diameter (QC-Test Kit)
- One or two 0–160 psi (0–1120 kPa), 2½-inch (65-mm) diameter test gauges
- One or two Pitot gauges, preferably the fix-mounted type or a hand-held unit with knife edge and air chamber
- One or more flowmeters (optional) in lieu of the Pitot gauges
- Assorted smooth-bore testing nozzles of appropriate diameter (size) for the required flow (gpm or L/min) for the various test points
- Measuring equipment to measure engine speed, which is accurate to within ±50 rpm of actual speed
- Suction hoses of appropriate sizes (diameter) and lengths with the appropriate type of strainer(s)
- One or more mallets to be used for tightening hard suction connections
- One or two deluge appliances with stream straighteners
- Numerous lengths of 2½-inch (65-mm) or 3-inch (77-mm) hoses according to the recommended hose layouts
- A minimum of two wheel chocks
- Assorted wrenches and Allen keys
- Roll of plumber's tape or tape measure
- Assorted spanner wrenches
- Hydrant wrench
- Calculator

Always keep the gauges used for testing purposes separate from the fire apparatus' gauges **FIGURE 19-4**. The test gauges should themselves be regularly tested and calibrated within 60 days prior to the tests for accuracy. They are also used to inspect the fire apparatus' gauges to see if they are in within acceptable ranges.

FIGURE 19-4 Keep testing gauges separate from the fire apparatus' gauges.

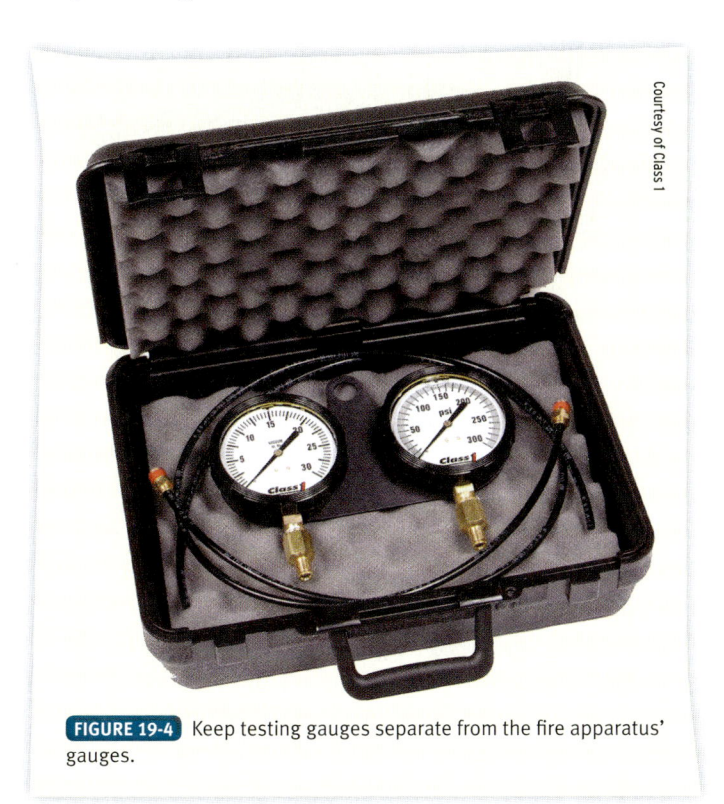

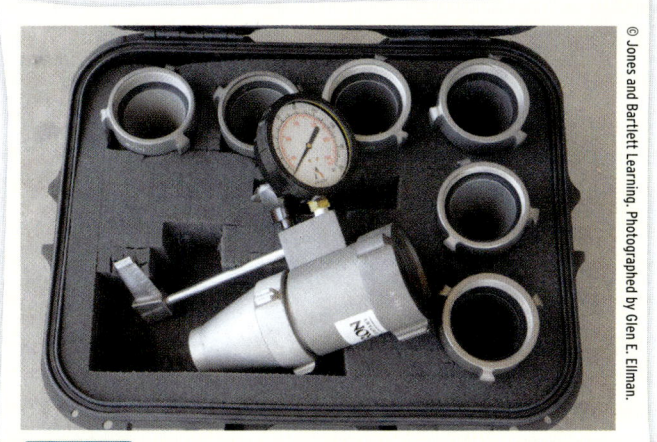

FIGURE 19-5 Testing nozzles with affixed Pitot tubes and gauges is recommended, and should be conducted whenever possible with secured portable or mounted monitors.

Nozzles that are suitable for testing usually can be found among the regular equipment of a fire department. However, the actual coefficient of discharge of each nozzle should be known; otherwise, the test results reported could be erroneous. The actual coefficient of discharge needs to be determined by a test conducted by a competent person using equipment such as volumetric tanks or calibrated flowmeters. Testing nozzles with affixed Pitot tubes and gauges is recommended, and should be conducted with secured portable or mounted monitors **FIGURE 19-5**.

The size of the nozzle is usually chosen to give the desired discharge at a nozzle pressure between 60 psi and 70 psi (420 kPa and 490 kPa). This pressure is neither so high that the Pitot gauge becomes difficult to handle in the stream, nor so low that the normal inaccuracies of a gauge that is used at low pressure would come into play. Nozzle (Pitot) pressures less than 50 psi (350 kPa) or greater than 100 psi (70,690 kPa) should be avoided. The nozzle should always be used in conjunction with a securely placed monitor, and a test should never be conducted while any person holds the nozzle. Failure to abide by this recommendation can lead to serious injury.

Only smooth-bore nozzles should be used. Care should be taken that washers or gaskets do not protrude into the nozzle, because a perfectly smooth waterway is essential during the test. Nozzle tips of 1½ inches (38 mm) to 2¼ inches (57 mm) in diameter are desired for use during various capacity and pressure tests. These tips should be free of nicks and scratches to ensure a smooth stream. Tips should be inspected, preferably prior to being attached and made ready for the test, to ensure that there is no mistake about the size of the tip being used. Use of a stream straightener is beneficial in testing applications.

A Pitot tube with an air chamber and pressure gauge is necessary for determining the velocity pressure of the water at the nozzle. The Pitot tube should be kept free of dirt and the air chamber free of water. Any water that accumulates in the air chamber should be removed after each test. The knife edges will inevitably get battered in service, but need to be kept sharp to reduce as much as possible the spray caused by inserting the Pitot tube into the stream. To ensure accurate and consistent readings,

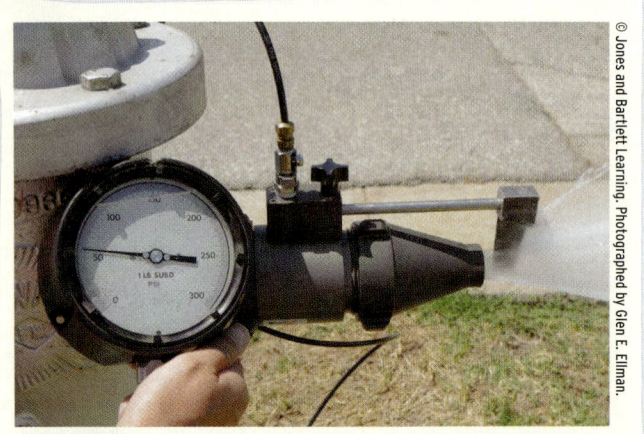

FIGURE 19-6 To ensure accurate and consistent readings, Pitot tubes should be fixed in the center of the stream, with the end of the tube located away from the end of the nozzle by a distance that is equal to half of the nozzle diameter.

Pitot tubes should be fixed in the center of the stream, with the end of the tube located away from the end of the nozzle by a distance that is equal to half of the nozzle diameter **FIGURE 19-6**.

No-Load Governed Engine Speed Test

The first performance test checks the governed engine speed. If the engine speed is not within ±50 rpm of the governed speed when the fire apparatus was brand new, this problem must be corrected before proceeding with the additional pump tests. This step is important because failure to have the proper governed engine speed will invalidate the results of the subsequent tests. You can check this speed while you are preparing the fire apparatus prior to the day of testing. Failure to operate at the correct governed speed during the performance tests is one of the most common problems that you will encounter.

To get the maximum rpm from the engine, put the transmission in neutral and run the engine up to the governed engine speed; make sure it stays there once the engine has reached normal operating temperature. At no time should you allow the engine to exceed its rated no-load governed speed. Check the air cleaner restriction and fuel filter restrictions, pressure (if the apparatus is equipped with such gauges), and replace the filter elements if necessary to avoid power loss. Check the fan belt and adjust the tension to provide adequate engine cooling during the pump performance test. Likewise, check the alternator belt tension (most of today's emergency vehicles have an auto tensioning system, in which case you simply do a visual inspection of the system and belt condition) and the battery charge to ensure that they will provide enough electrical power to allow up to 45 seconds of uninterrupted primer operation during the vacuum and priming device tests.

Readings should be compared to the documentation created when the fire apparatus was new. This information is listed on the original acceptance form(s) and should also be found on or near the pump panel on the UL plate **FIGURE 19-7**.

To conduct the no-load governed engine speed test, follow the steps in **SKILL DRILL 19-4**:

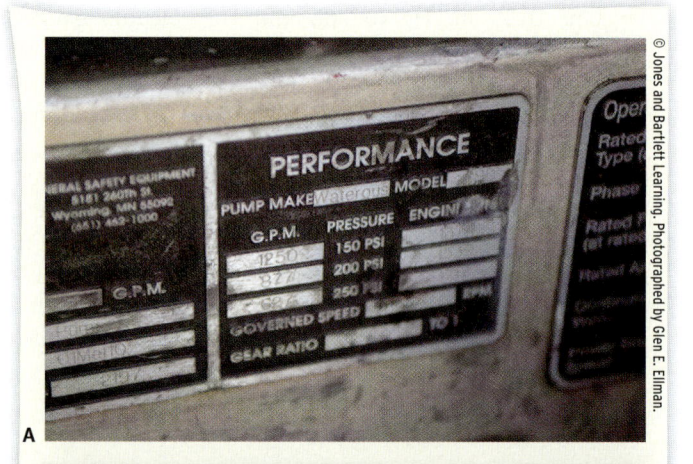

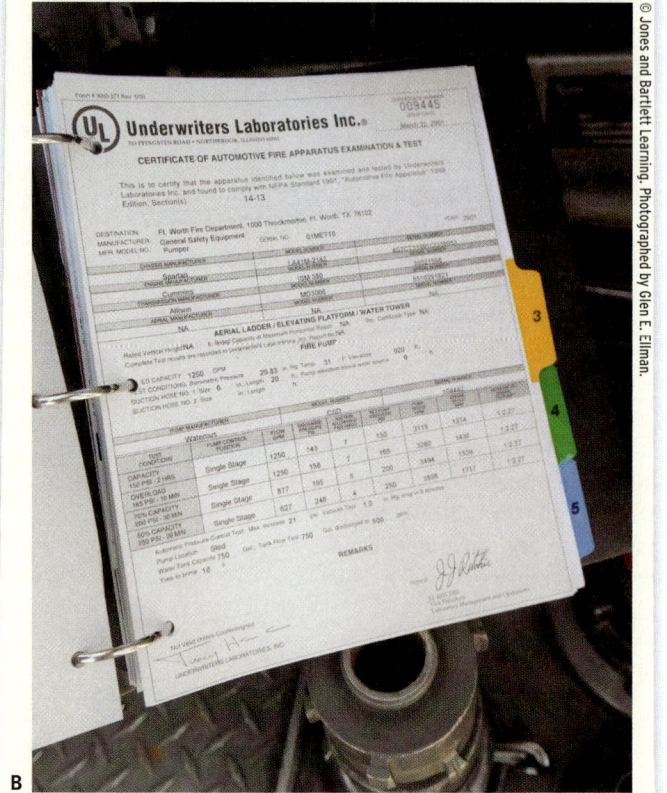

FIGURE 19-7 The no-load governed engine speed can be found on or near the pump panel on the third-party testing plate. **A.** UL plate. **B.** UL Certificate of Automotive Fire Apparatus Examination and Test.

1. With the assistance of another person, turn off all accessories powered by the engine, including headlights, emergency lights, siren activation switch, radio, and air conditioning. Place the drive train in neutral, or in park if the apparatus has an automatic transmission with a park position. (**STEP 1**)
2. Increase the engine speed (rpm) slowly, until the maximum governed engine speed is obtained. (**STEP 2**)
3. Record the readings from the tachometer inside the cab and the tachometer on the pump panel. Note any discrepancies between each tachometer.
4. Record all data on the performance test form. (**STEP 3**)

CHAPTER 19 Performance Testing

SKILL DRILL 19-4 Conducting the No-Load Governed Engine Speed Test
NFPA 1002, 5.1.1

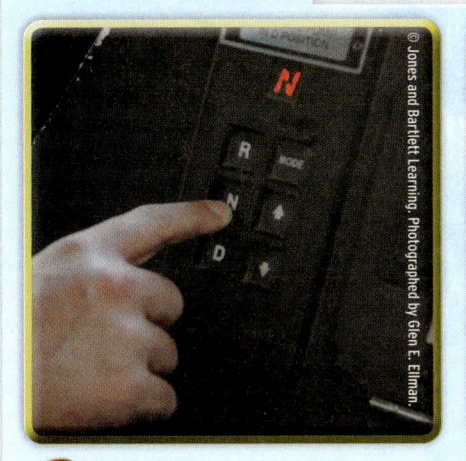

1 With the assistance of another person, turn off all accessories powered by the engine, including headlights, emergency lights, siren activation switch, radio, and air conditioning. Place the drive train in neutral or park (if so equipped) if the apparatus has an automatic transmission.

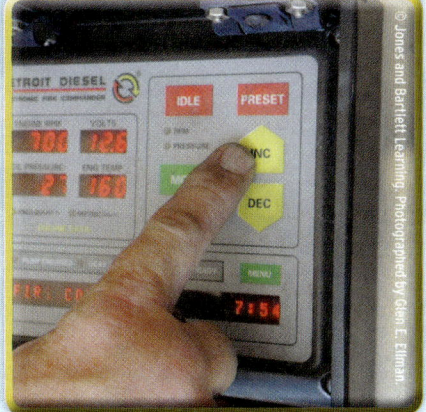

2 Increase the engine speed (rpm) slowly, until the maximum governed engine speed is obtained.

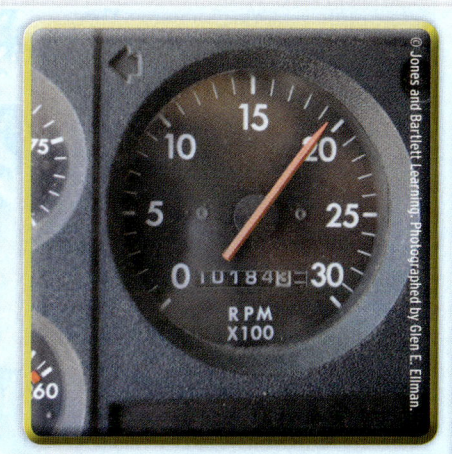

3 Record the readings from the tachometer inside the cab and the tachometer on the pump panel. Note any discrepancies between each tachometer. Record all data on the performance test form.

Safety Tip

Ensure that the wheel chocks have been placed correctly prior to conducting the no-load governed engine speed test. Also verify that the air brake has been engaged.

Intake Relief Valve System Test

If the fire apparatus is equipped with an intake relief valve system or a combination intake/discharge system, an intake relief valve system test must be conducted to ensure that the system is operating in accordance with the manufacturer's specifications. A relief valve is a device that allows the fluids to bypass the main circuit, thereby limiting the pressure in a system. One strategy for conducting this test is to use a second pumper to supply water to the emergency vehicle being tested. With this setup, pressure from the supply pump should be increased until the receiving pumper's intake relief valve system opens a dump valve. The pressure at which the system opens, dumps, or otherwise starts to operate should be recorded and reviewed against current operating procedures and the system adjusted accordingly. Record all data from this test on the performance test form.

Pump Shift Indicator Test

A test of the pump shift indicators seeks to verify that the pump shift indicators in the cab of the fire apparatus and on the driver/operator's panel indicate the correct pump status when the pump is shifted from road mode to pump mode. Pump shift controls might include electrical, pneumatic, or mechanical components working individually or in combination to shift the pump drive system into and out of pump mode **FIGURE 19-8**. Some pumps have manual backup shift controls available as well. Pump shift indicators in the cab and on the driver/operator's pump panel on split shaft power take-off (PTO) pump drive systems typically require an electromechanical device, such as a switch mounted on the pump transmission, to sense pump shift status.

To perform the pump shift indicator test; follow the steps in **SKILL DRILL 19-5**:

1. Place the transmission in the neutral position. (**STEP 1**)
2. Engage the parking brake. (**STEP 2**)
3. Engage the pump shift. After the pump shift has been engaged, engage the transmission in the drive position. In a manual transmission, shift it into the highest gear or the indicated over-the-road gear. Note that some transmissions have an overdrive capability and generally pump while in direct drive, not overdrive. (**STEP 3**)

FIGURE 19-8 Pump shift controls might include electrical, pneumatic, or mechanical components working individually or in combination to shift the pump drive system into and out of pump mode.

FIGURE 19-9 The interlock system on the pump panel.

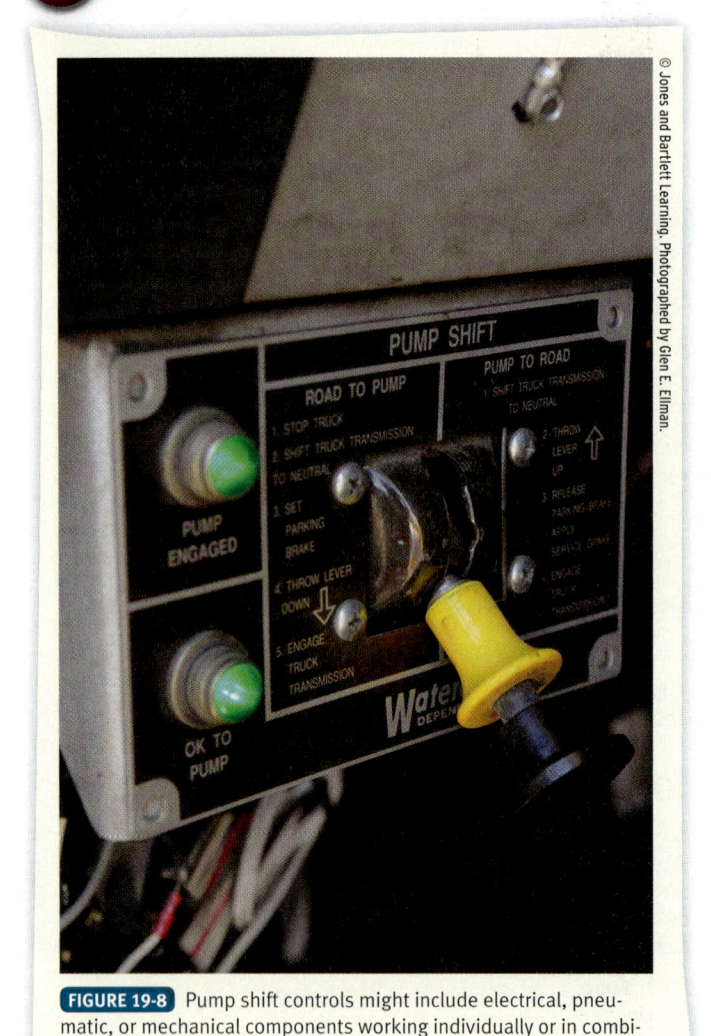

④ A green indicator light should come on inside the cab and on the pump panel labeled "Pump engaged" or "Okay to pump," indicating that the pump has been successfully engaged.

⑤ Record the information on the performance test form. (**STEP ④**)

Pump Engine Control Interlock Test

Beginning with the 1991 edition of NFPA 1901, fire apparatus equipped with electronic or electric engine throttle controls were required to include an interlock system to prevent engine speed advancement, except in three conditions: (1) when the chassis transmission is in neutral with the parking brake engaged; (2) when the parking brake is engaged, the fire pump is engaged, and the chassis transmission is in pumping gear; or (3) when the fire apparatus is in the "Okay to pump" mode. This test is intended to inspect the proper operation of the interlock system **FIGURE 19-9**.

While the NFPA 1911 standard requires testing of the interlock in only two configurations, there are various combinations in which the chassis, transmission gear, parking brake, and pump shift in the driving compartment can be arranged. The engine speed control should also be adjustable at the driver/operator's panel when that combination is employed. You may wish to test whether the engine speed control is capable of being advanced in other configurations.

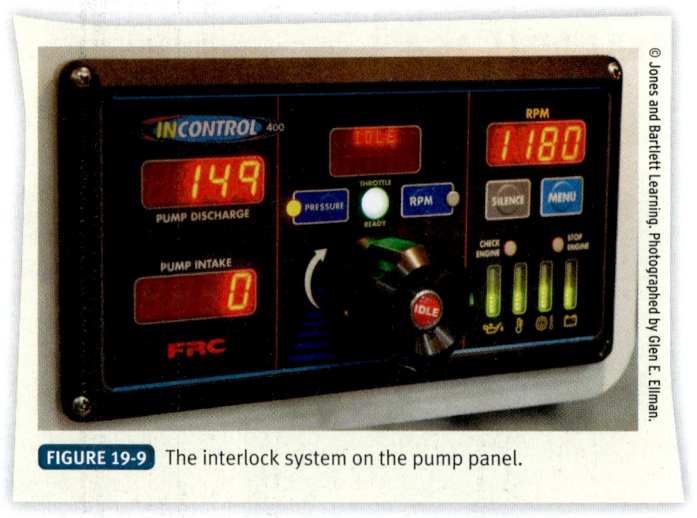

Three tables in NFPA 1911 specify the different pump configurations. Table 18.7.4.1, Stationary Pump Driven Through Split Shaft Power Take-Off (PTO), is the most common configuration and is described in Skill Drill 19-6. However, you may also encounter a pump driven by a side-mounted PTO as described in NFPA 1911, Table 18.7.4.2, Stationary Pump Driven Through Transmission Mounted PTO Front-of-Engine Crankshaft PTO or Engine Flywheel PTO (REPTO Style), or you may have an emergency vehicle with pump and roll capabilities as described in NFPA 1911, Table 18.7.4.3, Stationary and Pump and Roll Pump.

To perform the pump engine control interlock test, follow the steps in **SKILL DRILL 19-6**:

① With the fire apparatus running, the pump gear in road mode with the transmission gear in the neutral position, and the parking brake engaged, you should be able to advance the interlock system (throttle) located at the pump panel. (**STEP ①**) This will include all three configurations noted previously.

② With the fire apparatus running, the pump gear in road mode with the transmission gear in the neutral position, and the parking brake disengaged, you should not be able to advance the interlock system (throttle) located at the pump panel. (**STEP ②**) This will include all three configurations noted previously.

③ With the fire apparatus running, the pump gear engaged ("Pump engaged" or "Okay to pump"), the parking brake engaged, and the transmission in pump gear, you should be able to advance the interlock system (throttle) located at the pump panel. (**STEP ③**) For other configurations, see NFPA 1911, Table 18.7.4.2, or see NFPA 1911, Table 18.7.4.3, for emergency vehicles with pump and roll capabilities.

④ With the fire apparatus running, the pump gear engaged ("Pump engaged" or "Okay to pump"), the parking brake disengaged, and the transmission in pump gear, you should not be able to advance the interlock system (throttle) located at the pump panel.

CHAPTER 19 Performance Testing 483

SKILL DRILL 19-5 Performing the Pump Shift Indicator Test
NFPA 1002, 5.1.1

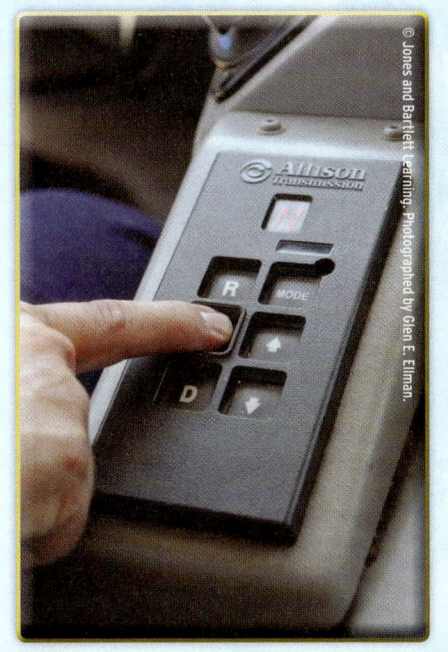

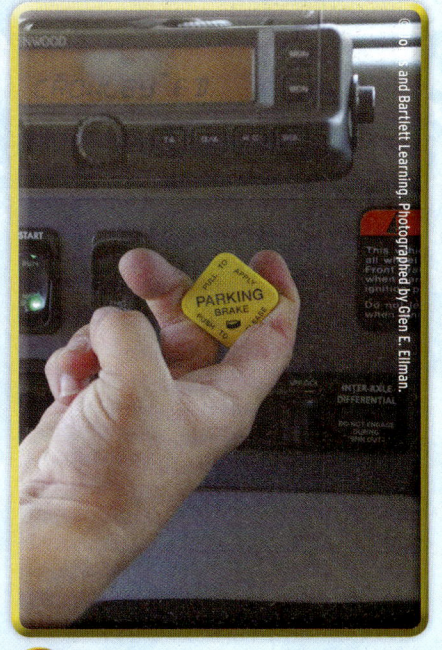

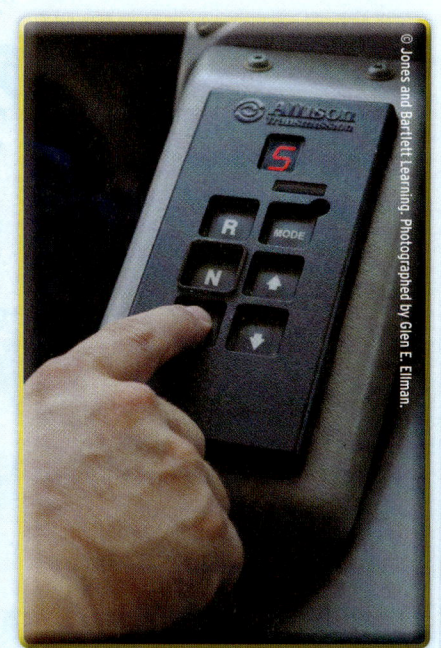

1 Place the transmission in the neutral position.

2 Engage the parking brake.

3 Engage the pump shift. After the pump shift has been engaged, engage the transmission in the drive position. In a manual transmission, shift it into the direct drive or pumping gear specified by the manufacturer gear. (Some emergency vehicles have overdrive transmissions, in which case they will normally pump in direct drive. Some vehicles may pump in a lower range.)

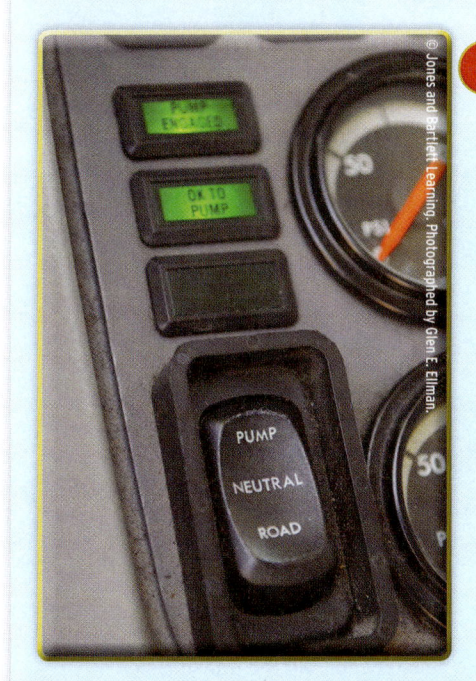

4 An indicator light should come on inside the cab and on the pump panel labeled "Pump engaged" and or "Okay to pump," indicating that the pump has been successfully engaged. Record the information on the performance test form.

Caution: During this portion of the pumping test, the wheels shall be chocked properly to ensure the apparatus does not move or roll, causing injury to personnel or property.

5 Record all information on the performance test form. **(STEP 4)**

Gauge and Flow Meter Test

Discharge pressure gauges can be checked quickly against test gauges to determine their accuracy. Individual discharge lines with gauges should be capped and the discharge valve opened slightly. The test gauge, the master discharge gauge,

SKILL DRILL 19-6: Performing the Pump Engine Control Interlock Test
NFPA 1002, 5.1.1

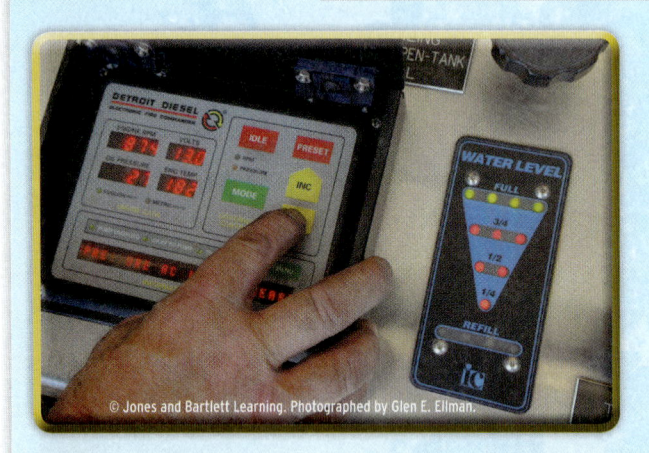

1. With the fire apparatus running, the pump gear in road mode with the transmission gear in the neutral position, and the parking brake engaged, you should be able to advance the throttle located at the pump panel.

2. With the fire apparatus running, the pump gear in road mode with the transmission gear in the neutral position, and the parking brake disengaged, you should not be able to advance the throttle located at the pump panel.

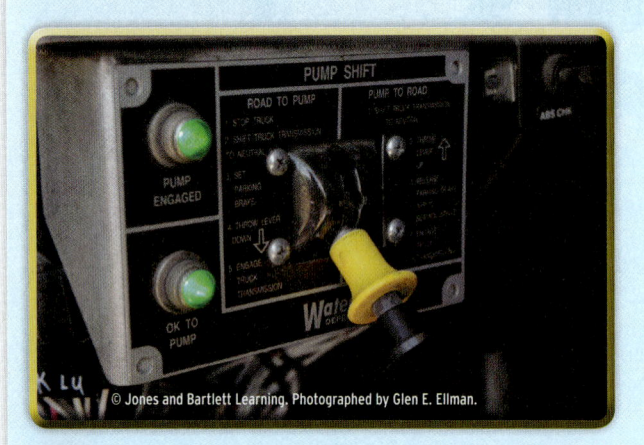

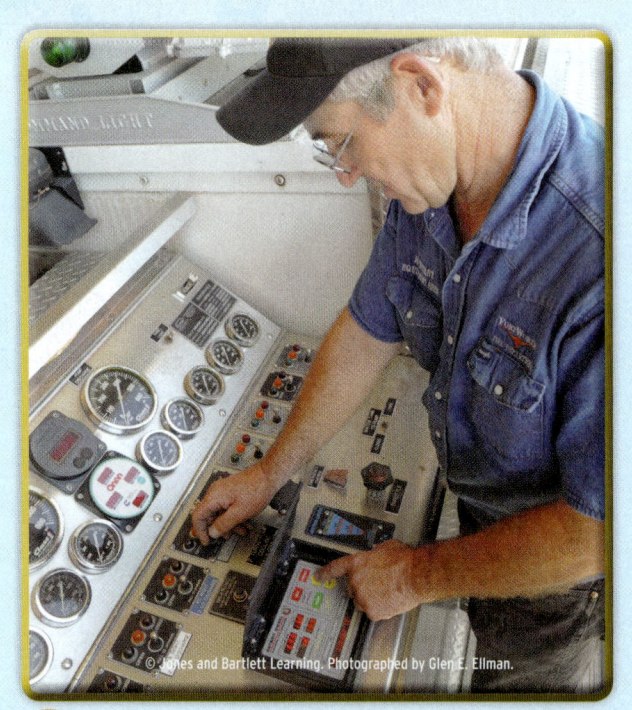

3. With the fire apparatus running, the pump gear engaged ("Pump engaged" or "Okay to pump"), the parking brake engaged, and the transmission in pump gear, you should be able to advance the interlock system (throttle) located at the pump panel.

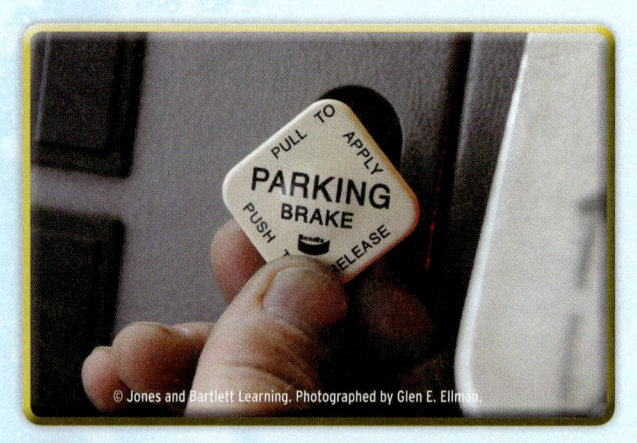

4. With the fire apparatus running, the pump gear engaged ("Pump engaged" or "Okay to pump"), the parking brake disengaged, and the transmission in pump gear, you should not be able to advance the interlock system (throttle) located at the pump panel. **Caution:** During this portion of the pumping test, the wheels shall be chocked properly to ensure the apparatus does not move or roll, causing injury to personnel or property. Record all information on the performance test form.

and all discharge gauges should display the same reading. The test gauges are attached to the testing ports located on the pump panel.

Each water pressure gauge or flow meter must be checked for accuracy. Pressure gauges should be checked at a minimum of three points, including 150 psi (1000 kPa), 200 psi (1350 kPa), and 250 psi (1700 kPa). Any gauge that is off by more than 10 psi (70 kPa) must be recalibrated, repaired, or replaced.

Follow the steps in **SKILL DRILL 19-7** to perform a gauge test:

1. Connect the pressure test gauge (Si-Span QC Test kit) to the pressure testing port connection located on the pump panel. Do not connect the vacuum gauge at this time. (**STEP 1**)
2. Engage the pump on the fire apparatus.
3. Ensure that all discharges with gauges, including any preconnected lines, have been capped and that all discharge bleeder valves are in the closed position. (**STEP 2**)
4. Ensure that the relief valve and governor have been turned off or set in the highest position. (**STEP 3**)
5. Open all discharge valves. Note that discharge valves do not need to be in the fully opened position. (**STEP 4**)
6. Slowly increase the pump throttle until the test pressure gauge is at 150 psi (1000 kPa). Inspect all discharge gauges and the master compound gauge to verify that they are at 150 psi (1000 kPa). (**STEP 5**)
7. Increase the pump throttle until the test pressure gauge is at 200 psi (1350 kPa). Inspect all discharge gauges and the master compound gauge to verify that they are at 200 psi (1350 kPa). (**STEP 6**)
8. Increase the pump throttle until the test pressure gauge is at 250 psi (1700 kPa). Inspect all discharge gauges and the master compound gauge to verify that they are at 250 psi (1700 kPa).
9. Decrease the pump throttle to idle and check the pump water temperature. If necessary, recirculate the pump water.
10. Note any discrepancies and record the information on the performance test form. (**STEP 7**)

DRIVER/OPERATOR Safety

Ensure that all discharges have been capped and are on securely before beginning the gauge meter test. Keep any personnel from standing in front of any discharge valves, as the pressures exerted on these valves during this test are extremely high and serious injury could occur in case of an unexpected discharge.

Flow meters (flow minders) need to be checked individually, using a hose stream sent through a smooth-bore tip and a Pitot tube to measure actual flow. Each flow meter must be checked for accuracy during the test. The correct flows are listed in NFPA 1911, Table 18.7.13.1, Flow-Measuring Points for Flow Meter. Any flow meter whose accuracy is off by more than 10 percent must be recalibrated, repaired, or replaced **FIGURE 19-10**. Depending on the type of device, most

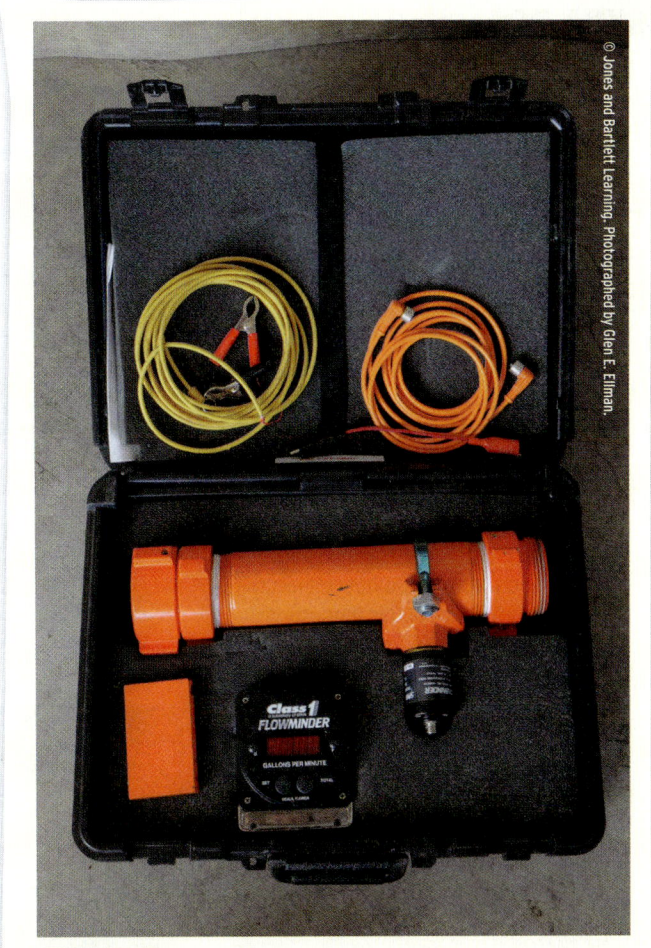

FIGURE 19-10 Any flow meter whose accuracy is off by more than 10 percent must be recalibrated, repaired, or replaced.

flow meters can be recalibrated using either a small (eyeglass) screwdriver or a magnet during this test. Always follow the manufacturer's recommendations when recalibrating any flow meter.

To perform a flow meter test, follow the steps in **SKILL DRILL 19-8**:

1. Connect the supply line to the intake valve on the fire apparatus. (**STEP 1**)
2. Connect hoselines and nozzles that are suitable for discharging water at the anticipated flow rate to one or more of the discharge outlets. (**STEP 2**)
3. Connect the flow meter to the nozzle or portable monitor. (**STEP 3**)
4. Connect the hoseline to the flow meter. (**STEP 4**)
5. Put the fire apparatus into pump mode. (**STEP 5**)
6. Make sure that the discharge valves leading to the hoselines and nozzles are fully opened.
7. Adjust the engine throttle until the maximum consistent pressure reading on the Pitot gauge or the test flow on a flow meter is obtained for that specific pipe size.
8. Record the information on the performance test form. (**STEP 6**)

SKILL DRILL 19-7 Performing a Gauge Test
NFPA 1002, 5.1.1

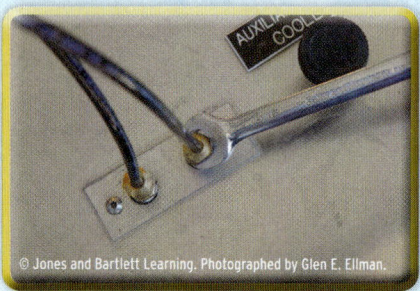

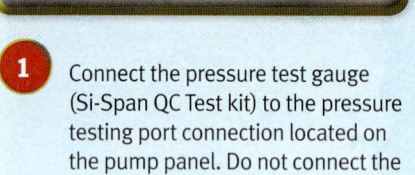

1 Connect the pressure test gauge (Si-Span QC Test kit) to the pressure testing port connection located on the pump panel. Do not connect the vacuum gauge at this time.

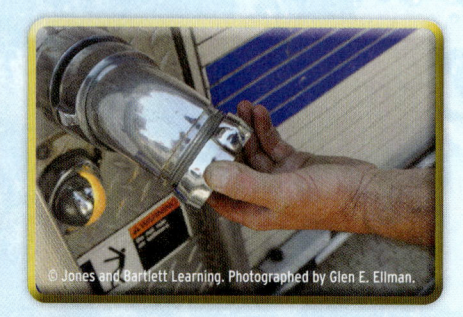

2 Engage the pump on the fire apparatus. Ensure that all discharge gauges, including any preconnected lines, have been capped and that all discharge bleeder valves are in the closed position.

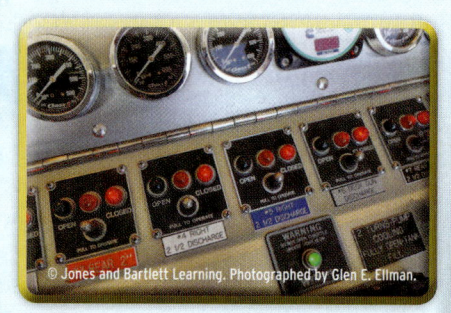

3 Ensure that the relief valve and governor have been turned off or set in the highest position.

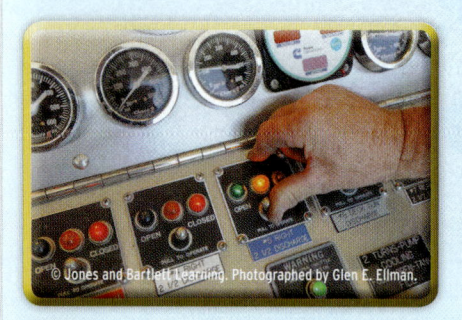

4 Open all discharge valves. Note that discharge valves do not need to be in the fully opened position. It is advisable to slightly open the tank to pump or recirculation line to keep from overheating the pump during the gauge test.

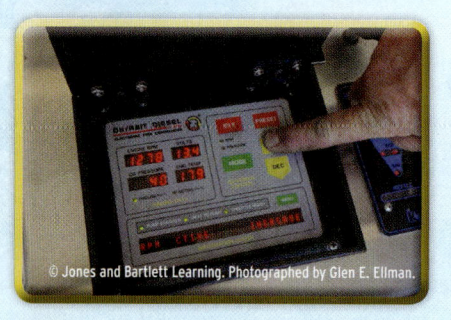

5 Slowly increase the pump throttle until the test pressure gauge is at 150 psi (1000 kPa). Inspect all discharge gauges and the master compound gauge to verify that they are at 150 psi (1000 kPa).

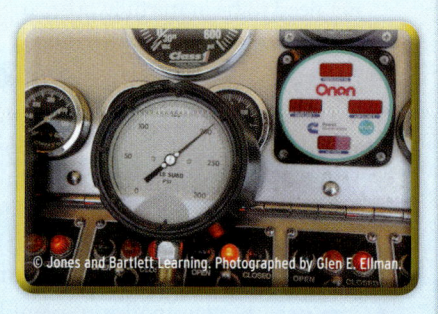

6 Increase the pump throttle until the test pressure gauge is at 200 psi (1350 kPa). Inspect all discharge gauges and the master compound gauge to verify that they are at 200 psi (1350 kPa).

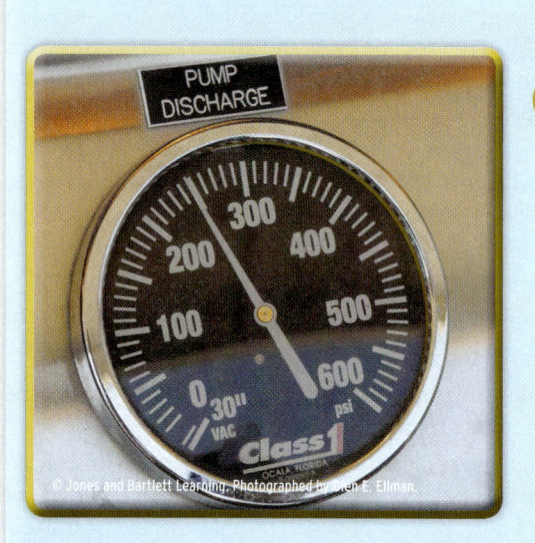

7 Increase the pump throttle until the test pressure gauge is at 250 psi (1700 kPa). Inspect all discharge gauges and master compound gauge to verify that they are at 250 psi (1700 kPa). Decrease the pump throttle to idle and check the pump water temperature. If necessary, recirculate the pump water. Note any discrepancies and record the information on the performance test form.

© LiquidLibrary

CHAPTER 19 Performance Testing   487

SKILL DRILL 19-8 Performing a Flow Meter Test
NFPA 1002, 5.1.1

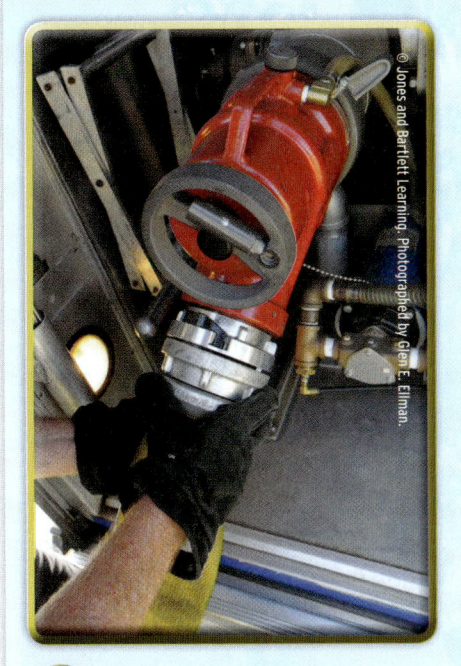

1 Connect the supply line to the intake valve on the apparatus.

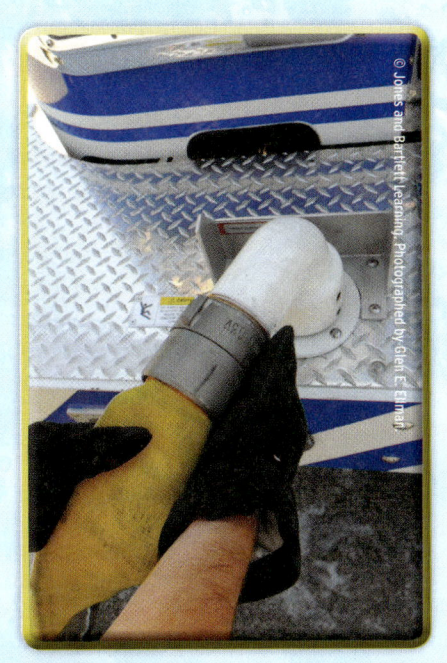

2 Connect hoselines and nozzles that are suitable for discharging water at the anticipated flow rate to one or more of the discharge outlets.

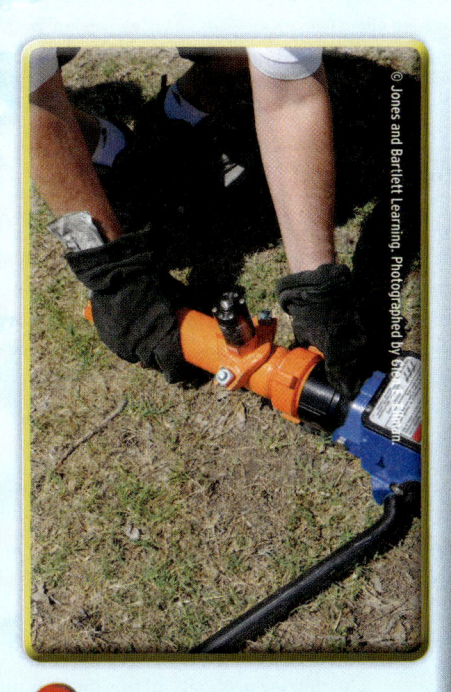

3 Connect the flow meter to the nozzle or portable monitor.

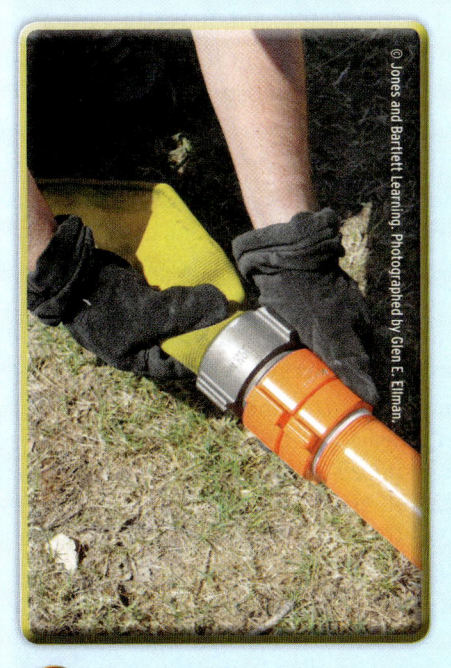

4 Connect the hoseline to the flow meter.

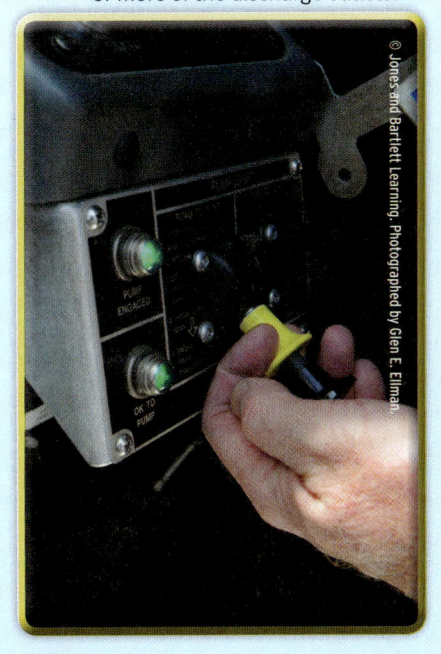

5 Put the fire apparatus into pump mode.

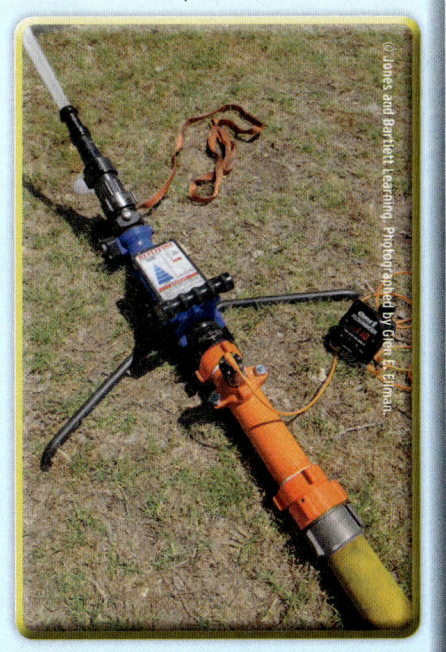

6 Make sure that the discharge valves leading to the hoselines and nozzles are fully opened. Adjust the engine throttle until the maximum consistent pressure reading on the Pitot gauge or the test flow on a flow meter is obtained for that specific pipe size. Record the information on the performance test form.

> **Safety Tip**
>
> During the tank-to-pump test, if you suspect that the pump is beginning to run away, reduce the engine throttle quickly and close the appropriate discharge. This will prevent any unnecessary increase in pump temperature and cavitation.

Tank-to-Pump Flow Test

The flow rate should be compared with the rate designated by the manufacturer when the fire apparatus was new or with the rate established in previous testing. Rates less than the rate when the fire apparatus was new or as established in previous testing indicate problems in the tank-to-pump line tank, tank-to-pump swing check valve, or possibly tank baffles.

If the fire apparatus is equipped with a water tank, the tank-to-pump flow rate must be checked using the steps in **SKILL DRILL 19-9**:

1. Connect the supply line to the intake valve on the fire apparatus. Fill the water tank until it overflows. (**STEP 1**)
2. Close all intakes to the pump. (**STEP 2**)
3. Close the tank fill and bypass cooling line. (**STEP 3**)
4. Connect hoselines and nozzles that are suitable for discharging water at the anticipated flow rate to one or more of the discharge outlets. (**STEP 4**)
5. Make sure that the tank-to-pump valves and discharge valves leading to the hoselines and nozzles are fully opened. (**STEP 5**)
6. Adjust the engine throttle until the maximum consistent pressure reading on the discharge pressure gauge, Pitot gauge, or flow meter is obtained.
7. Close the discharge valves, and refill the water tank by opening the tank fill valve. The bypass line may be opened temporarily, if needed, to keep the water temperature in the pump within acceptable limits. (**STEP 6**)
8. Fully reopen the discharge valves, and take a Pitot reading or other flow measurement while the water is being discharged. If necessary, adjust the engine throttle to maintain the discharge pressure. Caution needs to be exercised, as it is very easy to run low on water and cavitate the pump, causing damage and or harm to both equipment and or personnel. Terminate the tank flow test if the pump speed (rpm) increases without an increase in discharge pressure. Generally, as soon as a decrease of 10 psi (70 kPa) is seen on this test, the pump is starting to cavitate, and you should begin reducing the rpm level.
9. Record the flow rate on the performance test form. (**STEP 7**)

Vacuum Test

The fire apparatus' pump must be able to develop a vacuum of 22 in. Hg (559 mm Hg), unless the altitude is greater than 2000 ft (600 m); in the latter case, the vacuum attained is permitted to be less than 22 in. Hg (559 mm Hg) by 1 inch (25 mm) for each 1000 ft (300 m) of altitude above 2000 ft (600 m). The vacuum (i.e., reduction in atmospheric pressure) inside a pump or suction hose should not drop in excess of 10 in. Hg (254 mm Hg) in 5 minutes.

The vacuum test is basically a test of the priming system—specifically, the tightness of the pump, including its valves and fittings. It is not a test of the pump's ability to maintain a vacuum while pumping water. Remember to use the required vacuum based on your elevation above sea level, as noted in the NFPA 1911. Leaking valves, gaskets, and improperly adjusted pump packing are three of the biggest sources of problems on this test, so preparation of the apparatus is important. If the primer device fails to produce a vacuum of at least 22 in. Hg (559 mm Hg) at sea level, the reason for this discrepancy must be determined and corrected prior to conducting any further testing.

To perform a vacuum test, follow the steps in **SKILL DRILL 19-10**:

1. Drain the pump, all discharges, discharge drains, and intakes of water. (**STEP 1**)
2. Inspect the priming oil reservoir (if the apparatus is so equipped). Most primers today are oil-less or even air-type primers to reduce oil discharge to the ground. If applicable, replace the fluid as recommended by the pump manufacturer. (**STEP 2**)
3. Install the vacuum-testing gauge (Si-Span QC Test kit) in the vacuum testing port connection located on the pump panel. (**STEP 3**)
4. Remove any Storz fittings and piston intake valves on the intakes, and replace them with steamer caps. (**STEP 4**)
5. Inspect all intake screens, and replace any damaged or corroded screens as necessary. (**STEP 5**)
6. Make sure that all intake valves are open and either capped or plugged.
7. Remove the caps on all discharges, and close all discharge valves, all drains, and the pump drain. (**STEP 6**)
8. With the fire apparatus running, operate the primer device in accordance with the manufacturer's instructions.
9. Ensure that the recirculating, engine or auxiliary cooling, and tank-to-fill valves are all closed.
10. With the fire apparatus running and all intakes valves open and capped (Step 6) and all discharge valves closed and uncapped (Step 7), confirm that a vacuum of at least 22 in. Hg (559 mm Hg)—unless the altitude is 2000 ft (600 m) or higher—is developed using the priming device. (**STEP 7**)
11. Reduce the engine speed, turn off the fire apparatus engine, and listen for any air leaks. The vacuum should not drop more than 10 in. Hg (254 mm Hg) in 5 minutes. Do not use the primer after the 5-minute test period has begun.
12. Do not operate the engine at any speed greater than the governed speed during this test.
13. Close all intake valves, remove all caps and/or plugs from each valved intake, and repeat test Steps 2 through 6. By conducting a second vacuum test with

CHAPTER 19 Performance Testing 489

SKILL DRILL 19-9
Testing the Tank-to-Pump Rate
NFPA 1002, 5.1.1

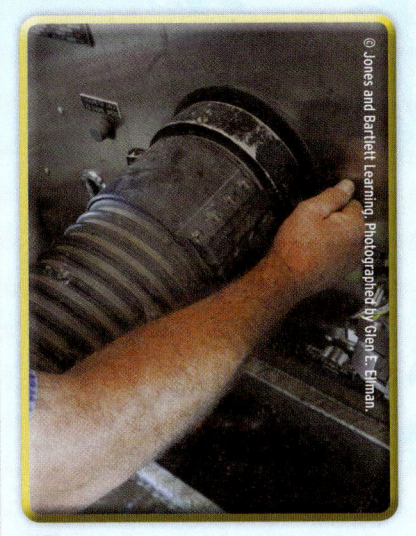

1 Connect the supply line to the intake valve on the fire apparatus. Fill the water tank until it overflows.

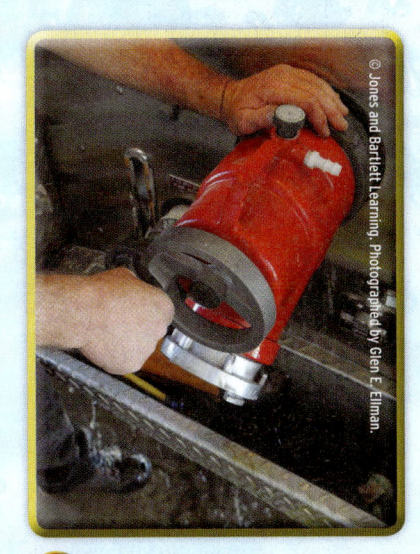

2 Close all intakes to the pump.

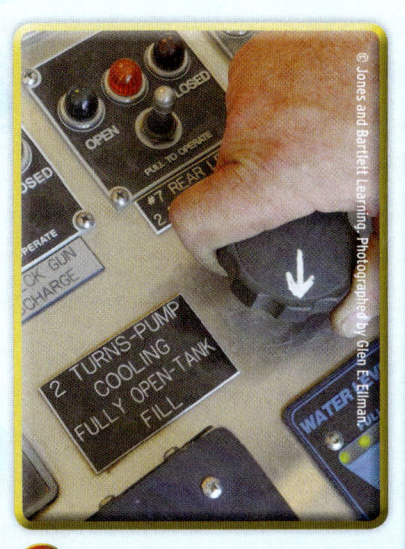

3 Close the tank fill and bypass cooling line.

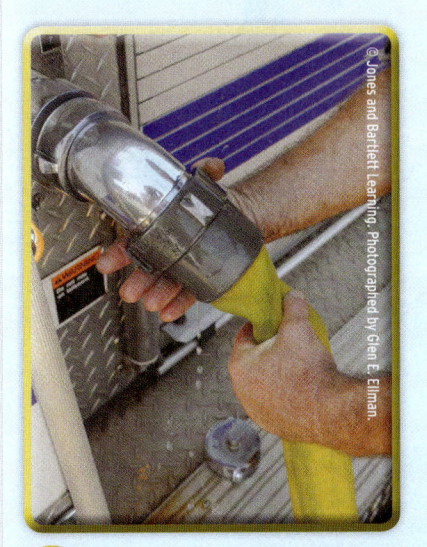

4 Connect hoselines and nozzles that are suitable for discharging water at the anticipated flow rate to one or more of the discharge outlets.

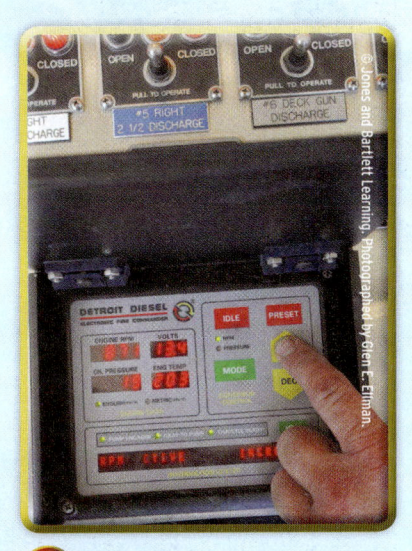

5 Make sure that the tank-to-pump valves and discharge valves leading to the hoselines and nozzles are fully opened.

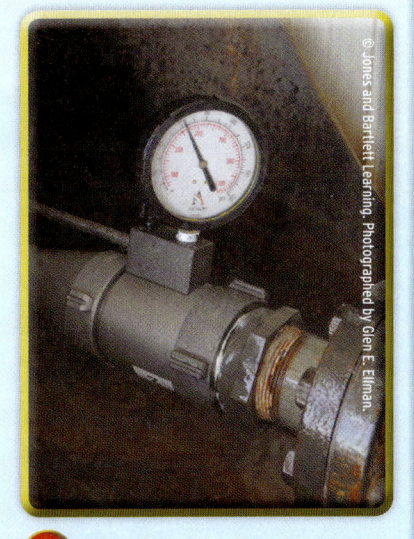

6 Adjust the engine throttle until the maximum consistent pressure reading on the discharge pressure gauge, Pitot gauge, or flow meter is obtained. Close the discharge valves, and refill the water tank by opening the intake valve and the tank fill valve. The bypass line may be opened temporarily, if needed, to keep the water temperature in the pump within acceptable limits. Close the intake valve and tank fill valve prior to step 7.

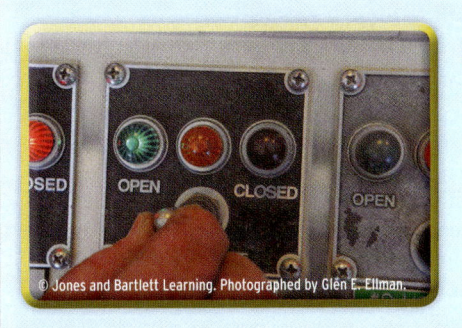

7 Fully reopen the discharge valves, and take a Pitot reading or other flow measurement while the water is being discharged. If necessary, adjust the engine throttle to maintain the discharge pressure. Record the flow rate on the performance test form.

SKILL DRILL 19-10 Performing a Vacuum Test
NFPA 1002, 5.1.1

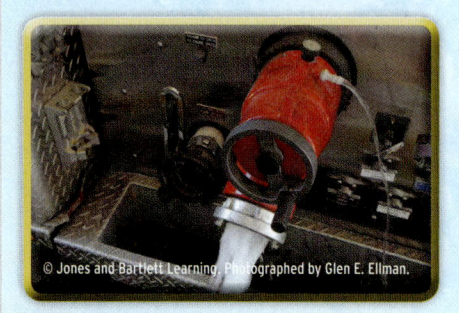

1. Drain the pump, all discharges, discharge drains, and intakes of water.

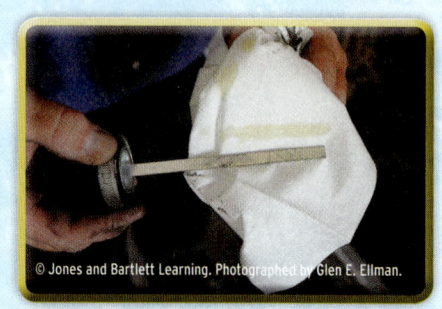

2. Inspect the priming oil reservoir. If the apparatus is equipped with one, recognize that most primers today are oil-less and or even air-type primers to reduce oil discharge to the ground. If applicable, replace the fluid as recommended by the pump manufacturer.

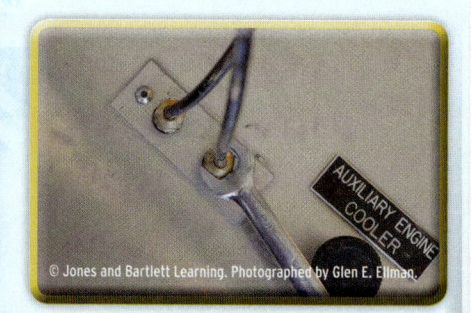

3. Install the vacuum-testing gauge (Si-Span QC Test kit) in the vacuum testing port connection located on the pump panel.

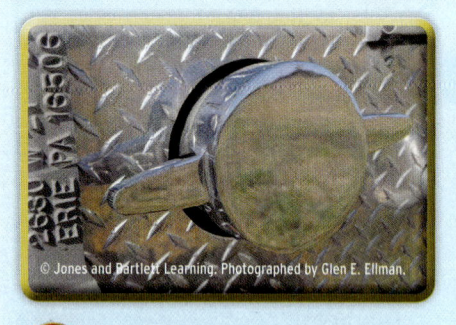

4. Remove any Storz fittings and piston intake valves on the intakes, and replace them with steamer caps.

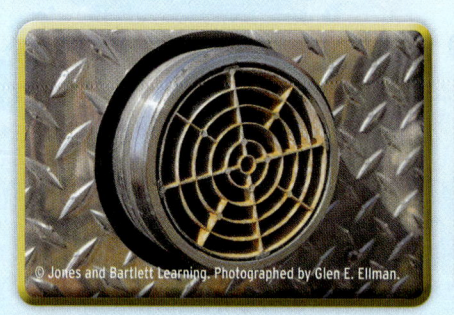

5. Inspect all intake screens, and replace any damaged or corroded screens as necessary.

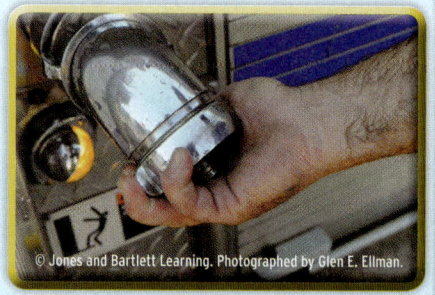

6. Make sure that all intake valves are open and either capped or plugged. Remove caps on all discharges, and close all discharge valves, all drains, and the pump drain.

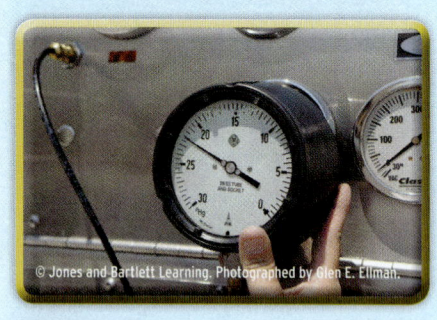

7. With the fire apparatus running, operate the primer device in accordance with the manufacturer's instructions. Ensure that the recirculating, engine or auxiliary cooling, and tank-to-fill valves are all closed. With the vehicle running and all intake valves open and capped or plugged and all discharge valves closed and uncapped, confirm that a vacuum of 22 in. Hg (559 mm Hg) or higher is developed using the priming device.

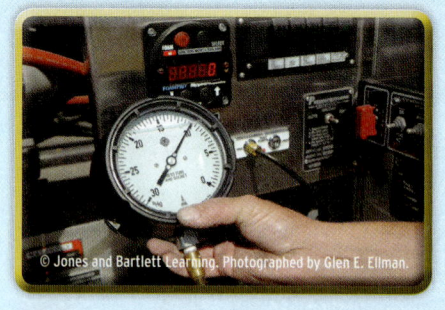

8. Reduce the engine speed, turn off the apparatus engine, and listen for any air leaks. The vacuum should not drop more than 10 in. Hg (254 mm Hg) in 5 minutes. Do not use the primer after the 5-minute test period has begun. Do not operate the engine at any speed greater than the governed speed during this test. Close all intake valves, remove all caps and/or plugs from each valve intake, and repeat the vacuum test. Record all data on the performance test form.

© LiquidLibrary

the valves closed on the intakes so equipped and the caps or plugs removed on those intakes, a leaking intake valve can be detected.

14. Record all data on the performance test form. **(STEP 8)**

> **Safety Tip**
>
> Prior to activating any device, you and the crew should ensure that you have hearing protection on. Most priming devices can produce high decibels that can be harmful to the ears.

Priming System Test

At the start of the priming test, pay attention to the ease with which the pump can develop a vacuum. Before starting the priming process, close all discharges, drains, and water tank valves and petcocks; make sure that the gaskets in the suction line hose(s) are in place and free of foreign matter; close all intake valves; and tighten all intake caps and couplings.

For pumps that operate at less than 1500 gpm (6000 L/min), the priming device should be able to create the necessary vacuum in 30 seconds to lift water 10 ft (3 m) through 20 ft (6 m) of suction hose of the appropriate size. The priming device on pumps that operate at 1500 gpm (6000 L/min) or more should be able to accomplish this task in 45 seconds. An additional 15 seconds might be needed when the pump system includes an auxiliary 4-inch (100-mm) or larger intake pipe having a volume of 1 ft^3 (0.03 m^3) or more.

Operate the controls as necessary to develop pressure, and then open one discharge valve to permit the flow of water. If the pump fails to pull a draft in a specific amount of time, note the cause and make any adjustments and/or repairs as necessary.

To perform a priming system test, follow the steps in **SKILL DRILL 19-11**:

1. Attach suction hose(s) to the appropriate intake(s), and spot the fire apparatus. Place suction lines a minimum of 2 ft (0.6 m) below the surface of the water; this should eliminate any whirlpools that might otherwise lead to cavitation.
2. Attach the appropriate length of hoses, flow meters, and Pitot gauges with testing nozzles to the fire apparatus and deluge sets based on the fire apparatus' rated capacity.
3. Make sure all testing gauges and Pitot gauges are in positions where you can see them clearly. To prevent injury, make sure that all testing nozzles and appliances are secured. **(STEP 1)**
4. Make sure the pump has been drained of all its water. Close and cap any intake valves and the pump drain. **(STEP 2)**
5. Ensure that all discharge drains, valves, and engine and pump recirculating lines are in the closed position. **(STEP 3)**
6. Put the fire apparatus in pump mode. **(STEP 4)**
7. Slowly increase the pump throttle until a speed of 800 to 1200 rpm has been achieved. Always follow the manufacturer's recommendations for pump speed.
8. Activate the priming mechanism, noting the starting time and the time after the prime is obtained. The starting time is defined as the instant when the priming device begins to operate.
9. The pump is considered primed when water under pressure has entered a discharge hose or discharges onto the ground beneath the fire apparatus.
10. Record the time to prime on the performance test form. **(STEP 5)**

Pumping Test Requirements

NFPA 1911 requires that if the pump is driven by the engine of the fire apparatus, then engine-driven accessories should not be functionally disconnected or otherwise rendered inoperable during the pumping tests. If the chassis engine drives the pump, all headlights, running lights, warning lights, and air conditioners should be operating during the pumping portion of this test.

Other equipment normally driven by the engine, such as the air compressor, engine fan, and power-steering pump, must remain in normal operation. Check for air system leaks, improper operation of the air compressor unloader, improper activation of the fan clutch, and other potential sources of power loss. During the pumping test, the pump should not be stopped except when discharges are closed to permit changing the hose layout or nozzle diameter. It is recommended that you continue to flow water from a discharge outlet when changing testing nozzles, as this action prevents the pump from overheating. The engine compartment should remain closed during the pumping test unless the fire apparatus was designed to meet an older standard that permitted testing with the compartment open.

When testing a pump at elevations up to 2000 ft (600 m), use 20 ft (6 m) of suction hose of the appropriate size for the rated capacity of the pump. A suction strainer and hose that will allow flow with total friction and entrance loss not greater than that specified should be used as well. When multiple suction lines are deployed, all suction lines are not required to be the same size. The number, length, and condition of suction hoses, as well as the altitude, water temperature, atmospheric pressure, and lift, are all factors that will affect the apparatus' performance while pumping from draft.

The discharge table for smooth-bore nozzles can be found in NFPA 1911, Appendix Table B.3, which lists nozzle psi and nozzle diameter **TABLE 19-3**. The test site should be arranged to meet those requirements. In addition, all gauges and flow measurement devices must be inspected and calibrated 60 days prior to conducting the pump test.

Pump Performance Test

In testing the pump, three variable factors come into play: pump speed, net pump pressure, and pump discharge rate. A change in any one of these factors will cause a change in at least one of the other factors. For example, any change in engine speed

SKILL DRILL 19-11 Performing a Priming System Test
NFPA 1002, 5.1.1

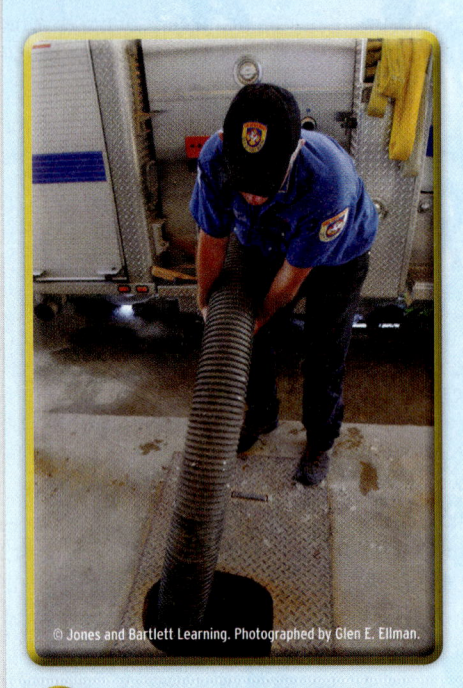

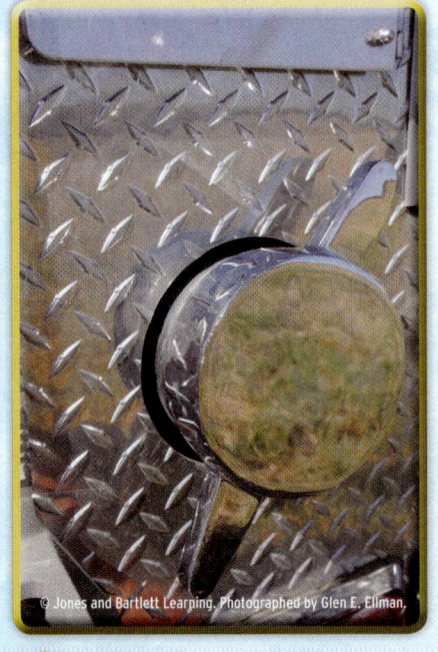

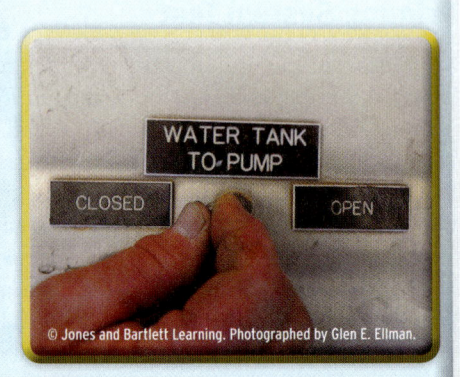

1. Attach suction hose(s) to the appropriate intake(s), and spot the apparatus. Place suction lines a minimum of 2 ft (0.6 m) below the surface of the water; this should eliminate any whirlpools that might otherwise lead to cavitation. Attach the appropriate length of hoses, flow meters, and Pitot gauges with testing nozzles to the apparatus and deluge sets based on the apparatus' rated capacity. Make sure all testing gauges and Pitot gauges are in positions where the operator can see them clearly. To prevent injury, make sure that all testing nozzles and appliances are secured.

2. Make sure the pump has been drained of all its water. Close and cap any intake valves and pump drain.

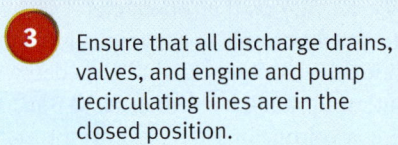

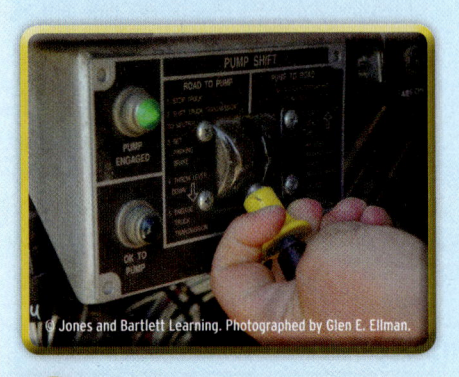

3. Ensure that all discharge drains, valves, and engine and pump recirculating lines are in the closed position.

4. Put the fire apparatus in pump mode.

5. Slowly increase the pump throttle until a speed of 800 to 1200 rpm has been achieved. Always follow the manufacturer's recommendations for pump speed. Activate the priming mechanism, noting the starting time and the time after the prime is obtained. The starting time is defined as the instant when the priming device begins to operate. The pump is considered primed when water under pressure has entered a discharge hose or discharges onto the ground beneath the fire apparatus. Record the time to prime on the performance test form.

TABLE 19-3 Test Data for Pumps

Pump's Rated Capacity (gpm)	Nozzle Size (inches)	Nozzle Pressure (psi)	Flow (gpm)	Pump Pressure (psi)	Proportion of Capacity (%)
500	1½	58	508	150	100
	1½ 4	58	351	200	70
	1	72	251	250	50
750	1¾	68	750	150	100
	1½	62	525	200	70
	1¼	66	375	250	50
1000	2	72	1008	150	100
	1¾	0	704	200	70
	1½	58	508	250	50
1250	2¼	70	1260	150	100
	1⅞	70	875	200	70
	1⅝	64	627	250	50
1500	Two: 1¾	68*	750*	150	100
	2	78	1050	200	70
	1¾	68	750	250	50
1750	Two: 1⅞	70*	875*	150	100
	2¼	67	1233	200	70
	1⅞	70	875	250	50
2000	Two: 2	71*	1001*	150	100
	Two: 1⅝	80*	700*	200	70
	2	72	1008	250	50

* Indicates each separate nozzle pressure and flow.

changes the pump speed; any change in hose layout or valve position changes the pump pressure; and any change in the nozzle tip changes the discharge rate. Managing these variables is the only way to reach the standard test condition desired.

During the pump performance test, the pump should be operated at reduced capacity and pressure for several minutes to allow the engine and transmission to warm up gradually. The pump speed should then be increased until the desired pressure at the pump is reached. If the desired pressure is not attained, one or more lengths of hose might have to be added, a smaller nozzle used, or a discharge valve throttled. When the desired pressure is obtained at the pump, the Pitot gauge should be read to see if the required amount of water is being delivered. If the discharge is not as great as desired and it is believed that the pump will deliver a greater quantity of water, the discharge can be increased by further speeding up the pump. If speeding up the pump increases the pump pressure by more than 5 psi (35 kPa) or 10 psi (70 kPa), a length of hose should be taken out, a discharge valve should be opened slightly, or a larger nozzle should be used. Remember that the ideal Pitot pressure reading should be 60 to 70 psi (420 to 490 kPa), with a minimum of 50 psi (350 kPa) or maximum of 100 psi (700 kPa) Pitot pressure. Select a nozzle size to obtain the correct flow with the desired Pitot pressure.

A speed reading should be taken at the same time that the pressure readings are obtained. Counting the revolutions for 1 minute generally ensures that readings will be sufficiently accurate **FIGURE 19-11**. Note that pump speed readings are no longer required, and most pump manufacturers no longer include the pump counter as standard equipment. Most offer it as an option, however, because it is no longer a required part of the NFPA 1901 or NFPA 1911 test. The engine rpm is still required.

To achieve the maximum pump performance, check the suction screen on the pump inlet and remove any accumulated debris. Check the priming device fluid level (if supplied) and add more fluid if necessary. If the pump has packing seals, check and adjust the packing as required to minimize vacuum losses. Check for and replace cracked or missing suction and discharge hose and cap gaskets. Make sure that the hard suction hoses and suction strainer are free of soda cans, polishing rags, and other obstructions. You will need one 20-ft (6.1-m) length of hard suction hose or two 10-ft (3-m) lengths of hard suction hose to conduct the tests. Pumps with rated capacities of 1500 gpm (6000 L/min) and greater may require more than two 10-ft (3-m) lengths of hose. The hose suction diameter, number of suction lines, and maximum lift for fire pumps are specified in NFPA 1911, Table 18.5.1.1.2(a, b, c, d), or in NFPA 1901, Table 16.2.4.1.(a) **TABLE 19-4**.

In general, hard suction hoses with smooth interiors produce lower friction losses than do more flexible suction hoses with spiral-corrugated interiors. Basket-type suction strainers usually have lower entrance losses than do barrel-type strainers

VOICES OF EXPERIENCE

In early February 2001, I was promoted to driver/operator. On my first day in this role, I began dealing with the effects of a snowstorm. Everything was shut down. Despite the weather, we had a structure fire that night on the south side of the city. Obviously nervous and driving in the snow, I took my time driving the apparatus and was extra-careful.

Upon arrival, we found a two-story house with fire coming from the Alpha side out the front door. I stopped where we thought a hydrant should be according to our hydrant maps. I dropped off a fire fighter and continued on past the house, so the captain could get a good look at the other three sides of the structure. Unfortunately, the hydrant was not there. Luckily, however, the fire fighter quickly discovered its actual location.

The captain performed a size-up and called for additional engines. A member of our crew immediately pulled a 1¾-inch (45-mm) attack hoseline to start a defensive operation until the rest of the crews could arrive on scene. Before our attack line could be charged, the captain noticed that a live electrical line had fallen onto the attack line, due to the snow and ice. Immediately, we stopped the operation. We pulled another attack line out and put it in place.

When the second attack line was charged and operating, a crew member aimed it toward the fire coming out of the front door. The nozzle reaction pushed him backward on the snow and ice.

When the other engines arrived on scene, two fire fighters entered the building to extinguish the fire so that a primary search could be started. During the quick primary search, an unconscious male victim was found next to the door. The fire fighters immediately started CPR, but to no avail; the victim passed away.

That was a day to remember. Snow, ice, finding a hydrant, live electric lines down on the attack line, a house destroyed, and a death: Many things happened that were not normal, but many things could have happened to make the situation even worse. The main thing to remember is that you always need to be ready to adapt and overcome any situation that might be handed to you. If I did not have confidence in my abilities and the department did not have confidence in me, then the situation that night could have easily become much worse.

Todd Dettman
Rocky Mount Fire Department
Rocky Mount, North Carolina

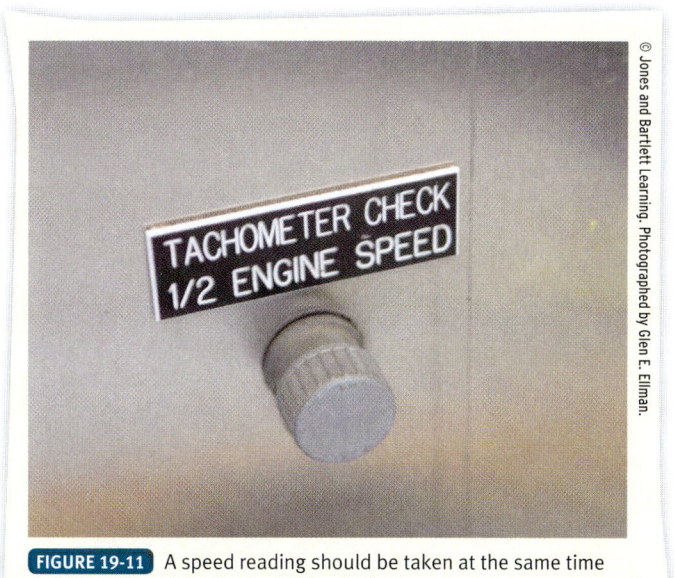

and are recommended for use with 1500 gpm (6000 L/min) or greater pumps. Float-type suction strainers should not be used during the pump performance test because the NFPA standard requires the strainer to be submerged at least 2 ft (0.6 m) below the surface of the water.

Testing a pump at draft is preferable to testing it from a hydrant, because the true performance of the pump is easier to evaluate while pumping from a draft. All fire pump manufacturers build and test pumps from draft; in turn, to evaluate the condition of a pump, it needs to be compared to the original test conditions or conditions as close to them as possible. If no suitable drafting locations are available, however, testing a pump from a hydrant is acceptable. Note that safety concerns arise when using a hydrant or positive-pressure water supply for this purpose. See the NFPA 1911 cautions and review the NPP definition, should this be a necessary alternative during your testing.

Discharge pressure is the water pressure on the discharge manifold of the fire pump at the point of gauge attachment. Gauge readings of this parameter reflect the pressure necessary

FIGURE 19-11 A speed reading should be taken at the same time that the pressure readings are obtained.

TABLE 19-4 Hose Suction Size, Number of Suction Lines, and Lift for Fire Pumps

Rated Capacity (gpm)	(L/min) (m)	Maximum Suction Hose Size (inches)	(mm)	Maximum Number of Suction Lines	Maximum Lift (ft)	(m)
250	1000	3	77	1	10	3
300	1200	3	77	1	10	3
350	1400	4	100	1	10	3
500	2000	4	100	1	10	3
750	3000	4.5	110	1	10	3
1000	4000	6	150	1	10	3
1250	5000	6	150	1	10	3
1500	6000	6	150	2	10	3
1750	7000	6	150	2	8	2.4
2000	8000	6	150	2	6	1.8
2000	8000	8	200	1	6	1.8
2250	9000	6	150	3	6	1.8
2250	9000	8	200	1	6	1.8
2500	10000	6	150	3	6	1.8
2500	10000	8	200	1	6	1.8
3000	12000	6	150	4	6	1.8
3000	12000	8	200	2	6	1.8
3500	14000	6	150	4	6	1.8
3500	14000	8	200	2	6	1.8
4000	16000	6	150	4	6	1.8
4000	16000	8	200	2	6	1.8
4500	18000	6	150	4	6	1.8
4500	18000	8	200	2	6	1.8
5000	20000	6	150	4	6	1.8
5000	20000	8	200	2	6	1.8

Reproduced with permission from NFPA's 1911, *Inspection, Maintenance, Testing, and Retirement of In-Service Automotive Fire Apparatus*, Copyright © 2012, National Fire Protection Association. This reprinted material is not the complete and official position of the NFPA on the referenced subject, which is represented only by the standard in its entirety.

for the pump to perform at the required NPP, which is the sum of the discharge pressure and the suction lift converted to psi or kPa when pumping at draft, or the difference between the discharge pressure and the suction lift converted to psi or kPa when pumping at draft, or the difference between the discharge pressure and the intake pressure when pumping at a hydrant or other source of water under positive pressure. For example, if the intake pressure gauge reads 30 psi (210 kPa) and the test requires a 150 psi (1000 kPa) net pump pressure, the discharge pressure gauge should read 180 psi (1210 kPa). When testing a pump from a hydrant (not recommended unless a suitable drafting location is not available), the intake hose should be of a size and length that will allow the necessary amount of water to reach the pump with a minimum intake gauge pressure of 20 psi (140 kPa) while flowing at the rated capacity.

Intake pressure is the pressure on the intake passageway of the pump at the point of gauge attachment. Only the strainer (screen) at the pump intake connection will be required to test this component of the pump's performance.

Taking this into consideration, suppose you are doing the 100 percent capacity test at 150 psi (1000 kPa) NPP and the intake gauge shows a pressure of 20 psi (140 kPa). You would add the 20 psi (140 kPa) intake pressure to the 150 psi (1000 kPa) discharge pressure, and it would be necessary to operate the pump at 170 psi (1190 kPa) to achieve the goal of 150 psi (1000 kPa) NPP.

Now suppose that during the 70 percent test at 200 psi (1350 kPa) NPP, you obtain an intake reading of 30 psi (210 kPa); such a pressure might be necessary because you are now reducing the gpm (L/min) flow to 70 percent. You would now have to add that 30 psi (210 kPa) to the 200 psi (1350 kPa), requiring pump operation to be at 230 psi (1560 kPa) to produce the required 200 psi (1350 kPa) NPP.

The 50 percent test at 250 psi (1700 kPa) NPP might produce another increase in inlet pressure, as you are again reducing the gpm (L/min) output. In this case, it would be reasonable to expect a 40 psi (280 kPa) reading at the inlet. Add 40 psi (280 kPa) to the 250 psi (1700 kPa) test pressure, and you would have to operate the pump at 290 psi (1980 kPa) to achieve the 250 psi (1700 kPa) NPP.

Most fire apparatus are rated for operations at elevations up to 2000 ft (600 m). Engine and pump performance may be reduced at higher elevations. If your location is more than 2000 ft (600 m) above sea level, contact your fire apparatus manufacturer for a corrected pump rating before you attempt to conduct the pump test.

The pumping test should last for at least 45 minutes in duration. Allow the pump, transmission, and engine to warm up for approximately 10 minutes prior to beginning such a test. The pump should not be throttled down except when discharges are closed to permit changing the hose or a nozzle, or to change the position of a transfer valve **FIGURE 19-12**.

If the pump is a two-stage, parallel/series-type pump, the test at 100 percent capacity should be run with the pump in volume/parallel mode; the test at 70 percent capacity can be run with the pump in either pressure/series or volume/parallel mode (as indicated on the third party testing plate); and

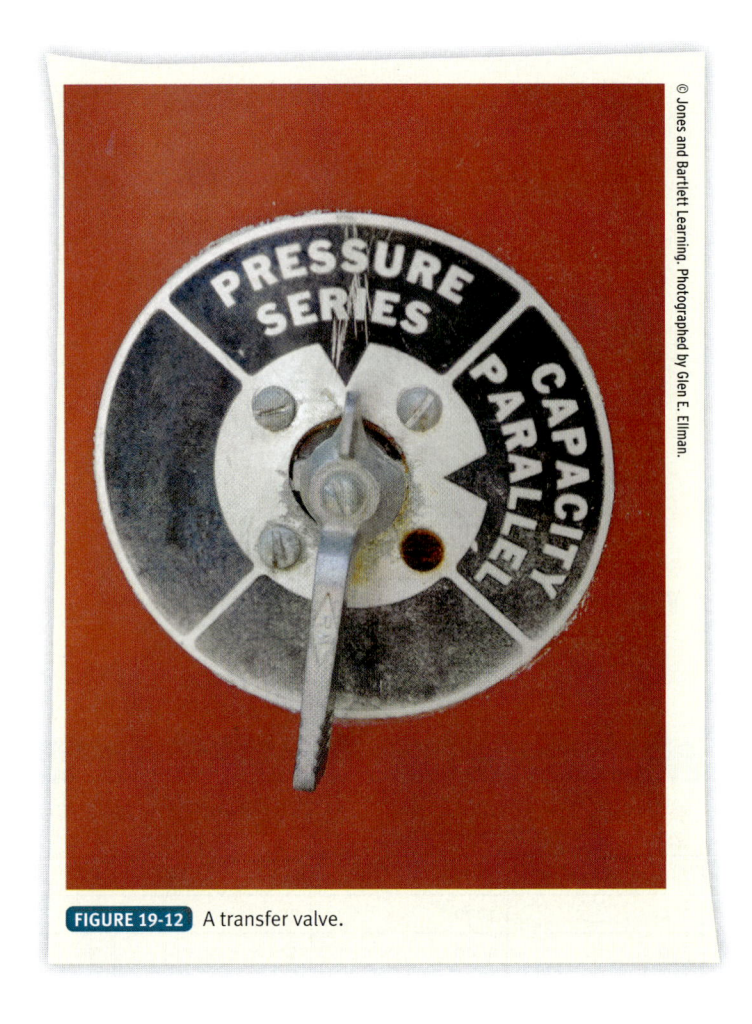

FIGURE 19-12 A transfer valve.

the test at 50 percent capacity should be run with the pump in pressure/series mode. The engine should not be throttled down except when the hose, a nozzle, or the position of the transfer valve is being changed.

A complete set of readings should be taken and recorded a minimum of five times during the 20-minute test for 100 percent rated capacity, a minimum of two times during the overload test, and a minimum of three times during each of the 10-minute tests for 70 percent capacity and 50 percent capacity. Document the time, pump speed counter (rpm), pump speed (rpm), pump tachometer, pump intake test gauge (in. Hg or mm Hg), apparatus pump discharge, testing gauge pump discharge, nozzle Pitot readings, and flow meter(s) readings. During each testing period, record the engine water temperature, engine oil pressure (psi or kPa), transmission oil temperature, and voltage on the performance test form.

If the fire pump flow or pressure readings vary by more than 5 percent during a particular test, the reason for the fluctuation should be determined, the cause corrected, and the test continued or repeated. If a pump counter speed shaft (rpm) is not provided, the engine speed can be read with a phototachometer or strobe light off a rotating element. More typically, today's electronic engines and electronic pump governor controls have a very accurate tachometer that may be utilized to document engine speed.

The pump should be subjected to a pumping test consisting of the following tasks:

- Twenty minutes pumping at 100 percent of the rated capacity at 150 psi (1000 kPa), net pump pressure. Readings should be taken a minimum of five times. For a two-stage parallel/series-type pump, the test at 100 percent of capacity must be run with the pump in volume/parallel mode.
- Ten minutes pumping at 70 percent of the rated capacity at 200 psi (1350 kPa), net pump pressure. Readings should be taken a minimum of three times. For a two-stage parallel/series-type pump, the test at 70 percent of capacity can be run with the pump in either series/pressure or volume/parallel mode.
- Ten minutes pumping at 50 percent of the rated capacity at 250 psi (1700 kPa), net pump pressure. Readings should be taken a minimum of three times. For a two-stage parallel/series-type pump, the test at 50 percent of capacity can be run with the pump in series/pressure mode.

Capacity Test/150 psi (1000 kPa) Test (100 Percent Test)

The capacity test is conducted within several minutes after the priming test has been successfully completed. This sequence is intended to ensure that the engine, pump, and transmission have had an adequate amount of time to warm up. Inspect the fire apparatus gauges—that is, engine water temperature, engine oil pressure, transmission temperature, and pump temperature, if applicable—to see if they are within their normal operating ranges prior to subjecting the fire apparatus to any further testing.

To perform a capacity test or 150 psi (1000 kPa) test, follow the steps in **SKILL DRILL 19-12**:

1. Ensure that the appropriate hoselines and deluge appliances are fixed and secured, and that testing nozzles, Pitot gauges, and flow meters are all attached. **(STEP 1)**
2. After opening the discharge valves to the appropriate hose layout, gradually increase the engine speed until the net pump pressure of 150 psi (1000 kPa) is achieved. Remember that NPP is defined as the sum of the discharge pressure and the suction lift converted to psi or kPa when pumping at draft, or the difference between the discharge pressure and the intake pressure when pumping from a hydrant or other source of water under pressure. To find suction pressure, add feet of lift to the value in the "ft. water" column [Table 18.5.1.1.(c) in NFPA 1911 or Table 16.2.4.1(b) in NFPA 1901, friction loss in inch pounds per 20 ft of hard suction] and divide by 2.3. For example, suppose you have a 1500 gpm (6000 L/min) pump, 150 psi (1000 kPa) NPP, 100 percent test with 5-ft (1.5-m) lift using a 6-inch (150-mm) suction hose. Pressure correction 5 ft (1.5 m) lift + 7.6 (1.4) suction hose loss divided by 2.3 (0.1) = 5.47 lb (29 kPa). While pumping from draft, you would be allowed to subtract the suction hose entrance loss of 5.47 psi (rounded to 5.5 psi) from 150 psi [29 kPa (rounded to 30 kPa) from 1000 kPa]; thus you would want the pump discharge pressure to be 144.5 psi (970 kPa). The corrected value would be 150 psi (1000 kPa) NPP. **(STEP 2)**
3. Check the nozzle pressures with the Pitot gauges [60 to 70 psi (420 to 490 kPa), with 50 psi (350 kPa) minimum and 100 psi (700 kPa) maximum], and check the flow rates if using flow meters. If the pressure is too high, gate down the appropriate valves and readjust the engine speed to the correct net pump pressure. If the flow is too low, gate open the appropriate valves and increase the engine speed to the correct net pump pressure. **(STEP 3)**
4. Begin testing once the current water flows and net pump pressure are obtained.
5. The following readings should be made and recorded every 5 minutes during the 20-minute test. **(STEP 4)**
   a. Time
   b. Pump counter (rpm; if used) or pump speed (rpm; based on the specific type of pump manufacturer's correlation)
   c. Engine tachometer
   d. Engine temperature
   e. Oil pressure
   f. Voltage
   g. Automatic transmission temperature (if equipped)
   h. Pump intake (vacuum) apparatus gauge
   i. Pump intake (vacuum) test gauge
   j. Pump master discharge apparatus gauge
   k. Pump discharge test gauge
   l. Pitot gauges and/or flow meter readings

Overload Test/165 psi (1150 kPa) Test

If the pump has a rated capacity of 750 gpm (3000 L/min) or greater, the fire apparatus must be subjected to an overload test consisting of pumping the rated capacity at 165 psi (1150 kPa) net pump pressure for at least 5 minutes without exceeding the maximum no-load governed speed. The overload test should be performed immediately following the test of pumping the rated capacity at 150 psi (1000 kPa) net pump pressure. The pumping tests should not be started until the pump pressure and the discharge quantity are satisfactory.

To perform an overload test, follow the steps in **SKILL DRILL 19-13**:

1. Gradually increase the throttle speed to reach a net pump pressure of 165 psi (1100 kPa).
2. Check the nozzle pressures with the Pitot gauges [60 to 70 psi (420 to 490 kPa), with 50 psi (350 kPa) minimum and 100 psi (700 kPa) maximum], and check the flow rates if using flow meters. If the pressure is too high, gate down the appropriate valves and readjust the engine speed to the correct net pump pressure. If the flow is too low, gate open the appropriate valves and increase the engine speed to the correct net pump pressure.
3. Begin testing once the current water flows and net pump pressure are obtained.

SKILL DRILL 19-12 Performing a Capacity Test [150 psi (1000 kPa) Test]
NFPA 1002, 5.1.1

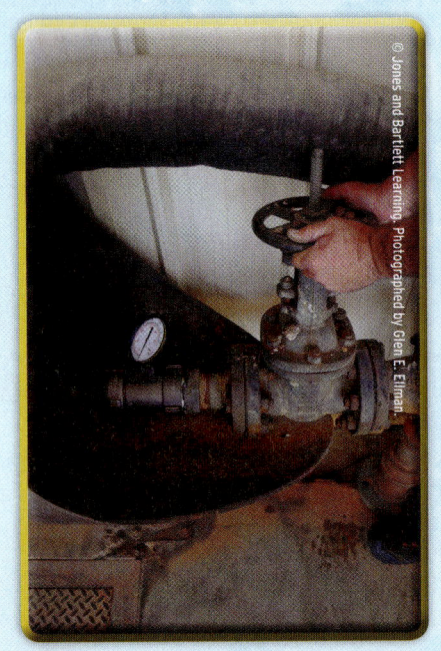

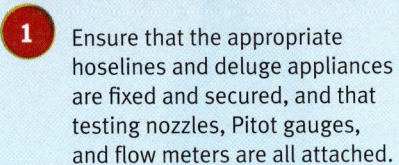

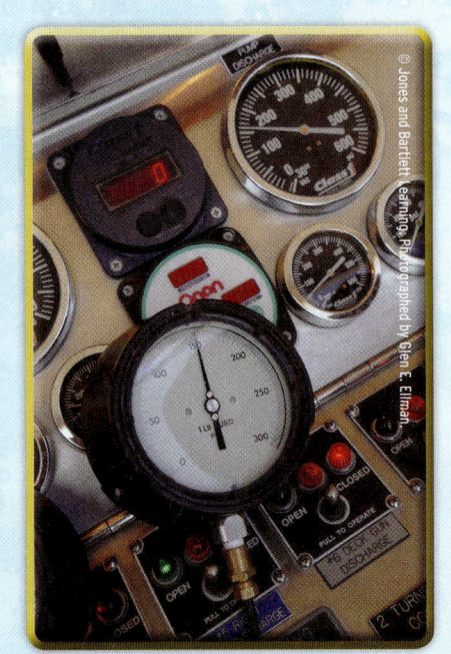

1. Ensure that the appropriate hoselines and deluge appliances are fixed and secured, and that testing nozzles, Pitot gauges, and flow meters are all attached.

2. After opening the discharge valves to the appropriate hose layout, gradually increase the engine speed until the net pump pressure of 150 psi (1000 kPa) is achieved. The NPP is defined as the sum of the discharge pressure and the suction lift converted to psi or kPa when pumping at draft, or the difference between the discharge pressure and the intake pressure when pumping from a hydrant or other source of water under pressure.

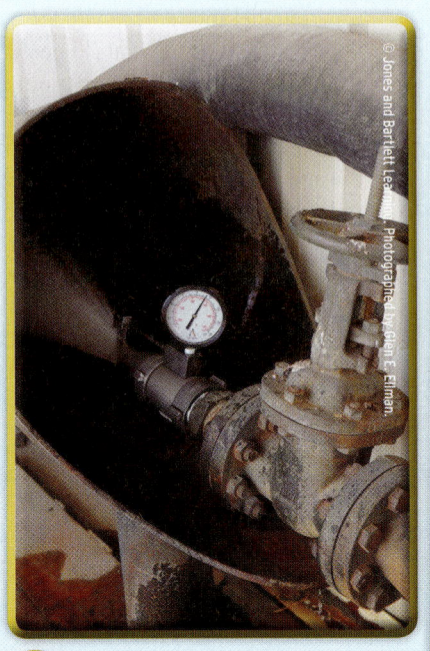

3. Check the nozzle pressures with the Pitot gauges, and check the flow rates if using flow meters. If the pressure is too high, close the appropriate valves and readjust the engine speed to the correct net pump pressure. If the flow is too low, open the appropriate valves and increase the engine speed to the correct net pump pressure.

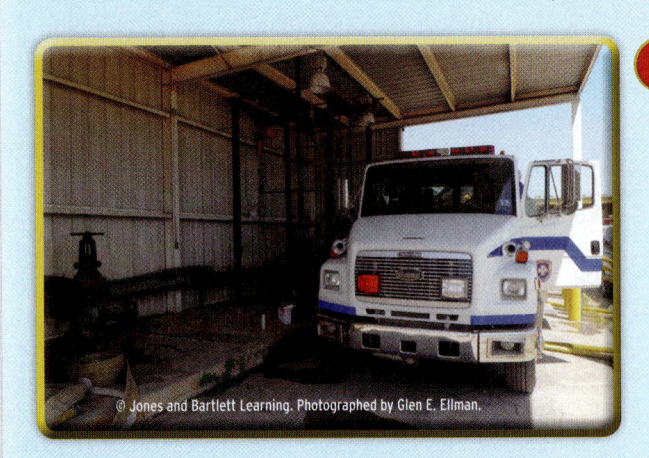

4. Begin testing once the current flows and net pump pressure are obtained. The following readings should be made and recorded every 5 minutes during the 20-minute test:
   a. Time
   b. Pump counter (rpm; if used) or pump speed (rpm; based on the specific type of pump -manufacturer's correlation)
   c. Engine tachometer
   d. Engine temperature
   e. Oil pressure
   f. Voltage
   g. Automatic transmission temperature (if equipped)
   h. Pump intake (vacuum) apparatus gauge
   i. Pump intake (vacuum) test gauge
   j. Pump master discharge apparatus gauge
   k. Pump discharge test gauge
   l. Pitot gauges and/or flow meter readings

CHAPTER 19 Performance Testing

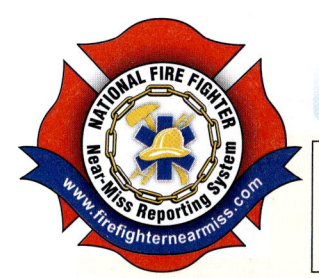

Near-Miss REPORT

Report Number: 05-0000581

Synopsis: Coupling fails during test of 5-inch (127-mm) hose, striking fire fighter.

Event Description: While conducting the annual testing of a 5-inch (127-mm) supply hose at 300 psi (2068 kPa), a coupling failed and the hose rapidly struck a fire fighter from behind, spinning him upside down and slamming his head and back into the concrete. No permanent injuries were sustained; however, there was lost time at work. The fire fighter was approximately 35 ft (11 m) away from the hose/coupling/pumper discharge at the time of failure.

Lessons Learned: Be aware of the absolute power in a 5-inch (127-mm) supply hose under testing pressures! Do not stand close enough to be struck if a failure does occur. This could have been a disabling or even fatal event. Also, wear full personal protective equipment (PPE) while testing hose. The fire fighter was not at the time.

---

4 The following readings should be made and recorded at least two times during this 5-minute test:
  a. Time
  b. Pump counter (rpm; if used) or pump speed (rpm; based on the specific type of pump manufacturer's correlation)
  c. Engine tachometer
  d. Engine temperature
  e. Oil pressure
  f. Voltage
  g. Automatic transmission temperature (if equipped)
  h. Pump intake (vacuum) apparatus gauge
  i. Pump intake (vacuum) test gauge
  j. Pump master discharge apparatus gauge
  k. Pump discharge test gauge
  l. Pitot gauges and/or flow meter readings

5 Reduce the pump speed to make any necessary nozzle tip changes.

■ 200 psi (1350 kPa) Test (70 Percent Test)

The 200 psi (1350 kPa) test is conducted immediately after the 165 psi (1150 kPa) overload test. There should be no delay in time between these tests unless a testing nozzle tip change is made.

To perform the 200 psi (1350 kPa) test, follow the steps in **SKILL DRILL 19-14**:

1 Use the same test procedures as for the capacity test, except use the proper nozzle sizes and hose layout to flow 70 percent of the pump's rated capacity.

2 For a two-stage pump, check the third-party test placard located on the pump operator's panel or the previous performance test sheets to see if the test should be run in volume/parallel or pressure/series mode.

3 After opening the discharge valves to the appropriate hose layout and testing nozzles, gradually increase the engine speed until the net pump pressure of 200 psi (1350 kPa) is achieved.

4 Check the nozzle pressures with the Pitot gauges, and check the flow rates if using flow meters. If the pressure is too high, gate down the appropriate valves and readjust the engine speed to the correct net pump pressure. If the flow is too low, gate open the appropriate valves and increase the engine speed to the correct net pump pressure.

5 Begin testing once the current flows and net pump pressure are obtained.

6 Run the test for 10 minutes, and check and record the following readings at a minimum of three intervals during this test:
  a. Time
  b. Pump counter (rpm; if used) or pump speed (rpm; based on the specific type of pump manufacturer's correlation)
  c. Engine tachometer
  d. Engine temperature
  e. Oil pressure
  f. Voltage
  g. Automatic transmission temperature (if equipped)
  h. Pump intake (vacuum) apparatus gauge
  i. Pump intake (vacuum) test gauge
  j. Pump master discharge apparatus gauge
  k. Pump discharge test gauge
  l. Pitot gauges and/or flow meter readings

7 Reduce the pump speed to make any necessary nozzle tip changes.

■ 250 psi (1700 kPa) Test (50 Percent Test)

The 250 psi (1700 kPa) test is conducted immediately after the 200 psi (1350 kPa) test. There should be no delay in time between these tests unless a testing nozzle tip change is made.

To perform the 250 psi (1700 kPa) test, follow the steps in **SKILL DRILL 19-15**:

1. Use the same test procedures as for the capacity test, except use proper nozzle sizes to flow 50 percent of the pump's rated capacity.
2. For a two-stage pump, the test should be run in pressure/series mode. This requires you to reduce the engine speed to idle and then change the transfer valve to pressure/series mode (if you have not already done so).
3. After opening the discharge valves to the appropriate hose layout, gradually increase the engine speed until a net pump pressure of 250 psi (1700 kPa) is achieved.
4. Check the nozzle pressures with the Pitot gauges, and check the flow rates if using flow meters. If the pressure is too high, gate down the appropriate valves and readjust the engine speed to the correct net pump pressure. If the flow is too low, gate open the appropriate valves and increase the engine speed to the correct net pump pressure.
5. Begin testing once the current flows and the net pump pressure are obtained.
6. Run the test for 10 minutes, and check and record the following readings at a minimum of three intervals during this test:
    a. Time
    b. Pump counter (rpm; if used) or pump speed (rpm; based on the specific type of pump manufacturer's correlation)
    c. Engine tachometer
    d. Engine temperature
    e. Oil pressure
    f. Voltage
    g. Automatic transmission temperature (if equipped)
    h. Pump intake (vacuum) apparatus gauge
    i. Pump intake (vacuum) test gauge
    j. Pump master discharge apparatus gauge
    k. Pump discharge test gauge
    l. Pitot gauges and/or flow meter readings
7. Reduce the pump speed to make any necessary nozzle tip change.

Pressure Control Test

The pressure control device—a relief valve or pressure governor located on the pump panel—should be tested at 150 psi (1000 kPa), 90 psi (630 kPa), and 250 psi (1700 kPa) intervals. Care should be taken to perform the pressure control test using net pump pressure and pressure rise readings. Some pressure control systems might not operate correctly if the hydrant pressure is too high; consult the system manufacturer's manual for further information **FIGURE 19-13** and **FIGURE 19-14**.

Closing all discharges in less than 3 seconds could cause instantaneous pressure rises, such that the pressure control device might not be able to respond rapidly enough to avoid damage to the pumping system. Taking more than 10 seconds to close the discharges is not a reasonable test of the pressure control device's response capability. Controlling closure of the discharges can be performed manually or otherwise.

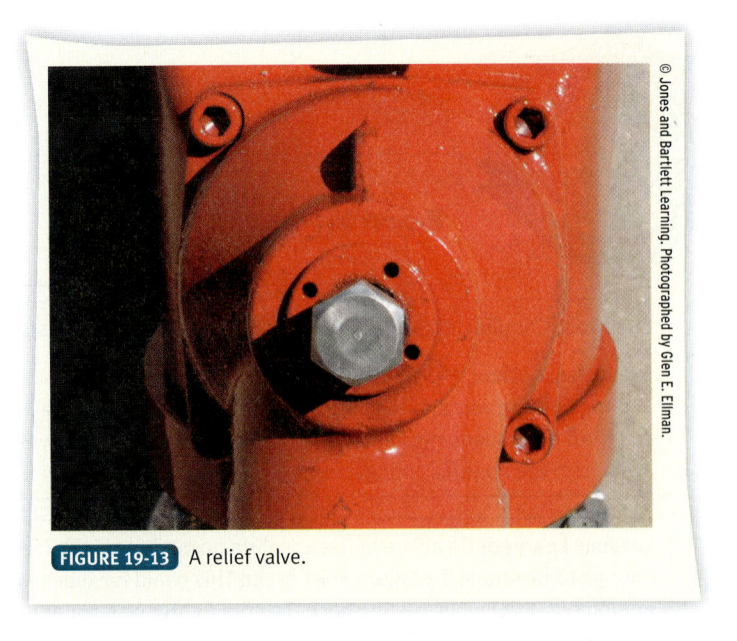

To perform a pressure control test, follow the steps in **SKILL DRILL 19-16**:

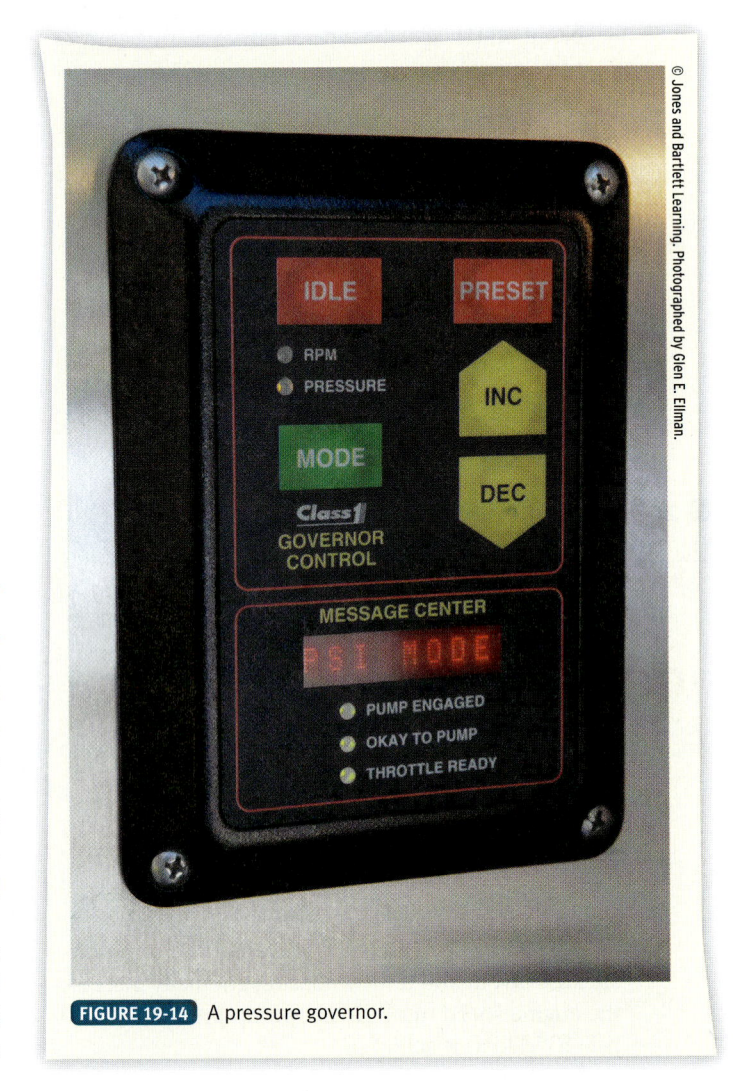

FIGURE 19-13 A relief valve.

FIGURE 19-14 A pressure governor.

1. The pump should be delivering a flow at the rated capacity at a net pump pressure of 150 psi (1000 kPa).
2. The pressure control device should be set in accordance with the manufacturer's instructions to maintain a discharge at a net pump pressure of 150 psi (1000 kPa).
3. All discharge valves should be closed no more rapidly than in 3 seconds and no more slowly than in 10 seconds. The rise in discharge pressure must not exceed 30 psi (210 kPa). (**STEP 1**)
4. The original conditions of pumping the rated capacity at a net pump pressure of 150 psi (1000 kPa) should be reestablished. The discharge pressure should be reduced to a net pressure of 90 psi (630 kPa) by throttling back the engine fuel supply with no change to the discharge valve setting, hose, or nozzles. (**STEP 2**)
5. The pressure control device should be set in accordance with the manufacturer's instructions to maintain a discharge at a net pump pressure of 90 psi (630 kPa). (**STEP 3**)
6. All discharge valves should be closed no more rapidly than in 3 seconds and no more slowly than in 10 seconds. The rise in discharge pressure must not exceed 30 psi (210 kPa). (**STEP 4**)
7. Reduce the engine speed and make the necessary adjustments to the hose layout and nozzle tip size for the 250 psi (1700 kPa) test. (**STEP 5**)
8. The pump should be delivering 50 percent of the rated capacity at a net pump pressure of 250 psi (1700 kPa).
9. The pressure control device should be set in accordance with the manufacturer's instructions to maintain a discharge at a net pump pressure of 250 psi (1700 kPa). (**STEP 6**)
10. All discharge valves should be closed no more rapidly than in 3 seconds and no more slowly than in 10 seconds. The rise in discharge pressure must not exceed 30 psi (210 kPa).
11. Record all data—including the rise in pressure at 150 psi (1000 kPa), 90 psi (630 kPa), and 250 psi (1700 kPa)—on the performance test form. (**STEP 7**)

Remember, for a relief valve to function properly, there must always exist a pressure differential of 70 to 90 psi (490 to 630 kPa) or greater between the intake manifold and the discharge header of the pump. The excess flow [gpm (L/min)] must have somewhere to go.

Post Performance Testing

After conducting all of the performance tests, it is recommended that you reduce the engine speed of the fire apparatus to idle. This will allow the engine, pump, and transmission to cool down for approximately 10 minutes. After the cool-down period, you can turn off all the engine-driven accessories that were turned on during the testing period. After about 5 minutes, the fire apparatus can be switched from pump mode back to road mode. It is very important to keep the fire apparatus running at idle engine speed to allow the engine turbo (if applicable) sufficient time to cool down. The pump and suction lines will still have a vacuum, so it will be necessary to open a discharge valve to remove the vacuum that was created inside the pump. Remove all testing equipment, hoses, hard suction hoses, and nozzles, and place the fire apparatus back in service.

It is always recommended when operating from a draft of a static water source to back-flush the pump and tank after pump testing. Back-flushing requires the fire apparatus to be attached to a clean water source, such as a hydrant; all discharge and intake valves and the pump are then flushed. The tank also should be drained of water and then refilled. If you are testing a Darley fire pump, back-flushing cannot be conducted by the standard method due to the Pitot valve located in the bottom of the discharge header. For a Darley pump, connect it to a high-volume water source and flush the system until all discharges are flowing clear.

The pumping system (i.e., engine, pump, and transmission) should exhibit no undue heating, loss of power, or other defect during the entire pump test. The average flow rate, discharge pressure, intake pressure, and engine speed should be calculated and recorded at the end of each phase of the performance test.

When the apparatus operates at or near full engine power while remaining stationary, the heat generated by its operation can raise the temperature of certain chassis and pumping system components above the level that can be touched without extreme discomfort or injury. However, as long as the fire apparatus can be operated and used satisfactorily for the required duration of the test under those conditions and the engine coolant temperature remains within the normal range, its performance should be considered acceptable.

Normal wear in the pumping system can require speeds greater than those required at the time of delivery for the pumping test. Such variances are acceptable as long as the fire apparatus passes the performance tests without exceeding the no-load governed engine speed.

Final Test Results

Just imagine taking all the time and effort to conduct good performance tests on your fire apparatus—and then not getting full credit for them. Unfortunately, this outcome happens far too frequently. If you do not record all test conditions, all readings, and all information about the fire apparatus being tested, then you will not receive full credit for the performance tests. Even worse, you will not be able to compare the most recent test results with previous ones, which might otherwise enable you to notice long-term changes that could indicate hidden problems. Also, if you do not keep records of the tests in a permanent file, ISO will not give you full credit on the next evaluation of your fire department.

NFPA 1911 contains a test data form to be used to record your annual performance tests. The test form found in NFPA 1911, Appendix C.3(c), can be used as is or can be modified to meet the fire department's needs. It contains headings and blank spaces to record all data from the test. You can photocopy this form and use it as a permanent record that will

SKILL DRILL 19-16   Performing a Pressure Control Test
NFPA 1002, 5.1.1

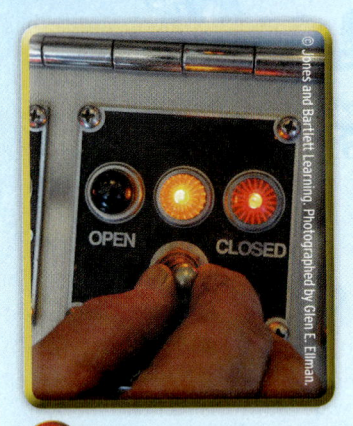

1. The pump should be delivering a flow at the rated capacity at a net pump pressure of 150 psi (1000 kPa). The pressure control device should be set in accordance with the manufacturer's instructions to maintain a discharge at a net pump pressure of 150 psi (1000 kPa). All discharge valves should be closed no more rapidly than in 3 seconds and no more slowly than in 10 seconds. The rise in discharge pressure must not exceed 30 psi (210 kPa).

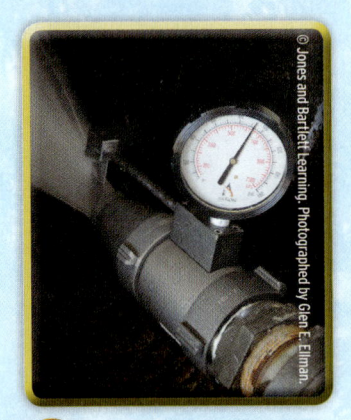

2. The original conditions of pumping the rated capacity at a net pump pressure of 150 psi (1000 kPa) should be reestablished. The discharge pressure should be reduced to a net pressure of 90 psi (630 kPa) by throttling back the engine fuel supply with no change to the discharge valve setting, hose, or nozzles.

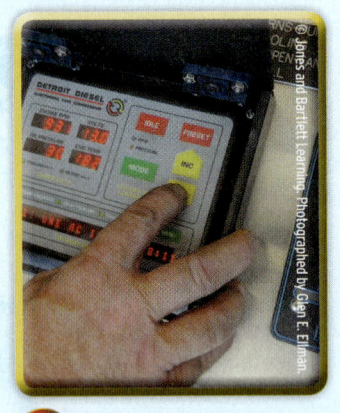

3. The pressure control device should be set in accordance with the manufacturer's instructions to maintain a discharge at a net pump pressure of 90 psi (630 kPa).

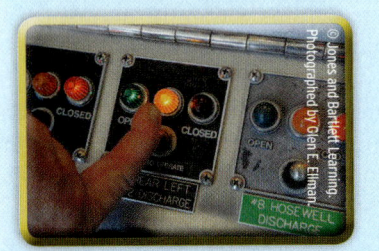

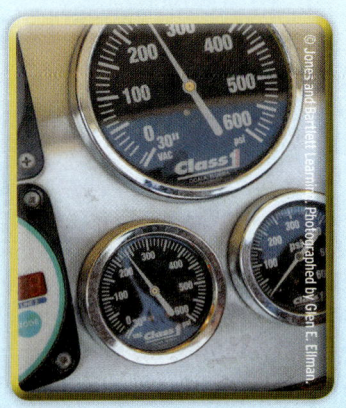

4. All discharge valves should be closed no more rapidly than in 3 seconds and no more slowly than in 10 seconds. The rise in discharge pressure must not exceed 30 psi (210 kPa).

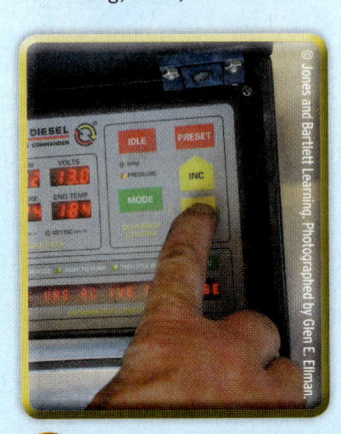

5. Reduce the engine speed and make the necessary adjustments in the hose layout and nozzle tip size for the 250 psi (1700 kPa) test.

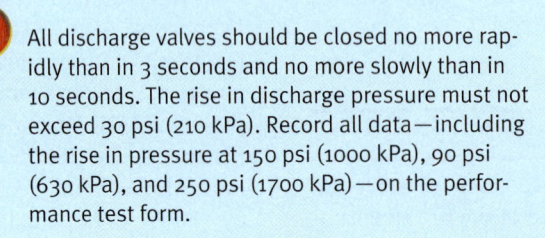

6. The pump should be delivering 50 percent of the rated capacity at a net pump pressure of 250 psi (1700 kPa). The pressure control device should be set in accordance with the manufacturer's instructions to maintain a discharge at a net pump pressure of 250 psi (1700 kPa).

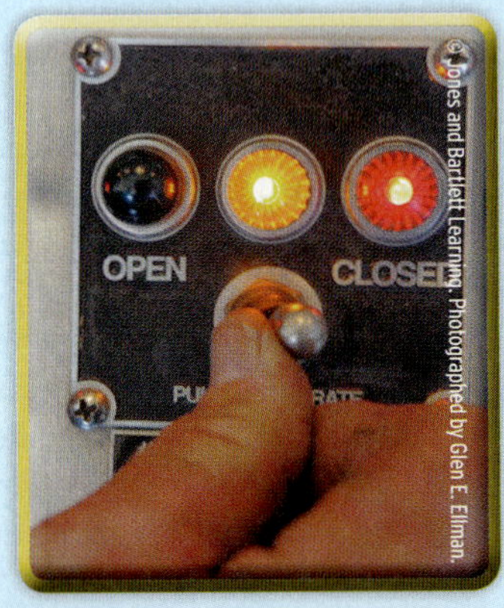

7. All discharge valves should be closed no more rapidly than in 3 seconds and no more slowly than in 10 seconds. The rise in discharge pressure must not exceed 30 psi (210 kPa). Record all data—including the rise in pressure at 150 psi (1000 kPa), 90 psi (630 kPa), and 250 psi (1700 kPa)—on the performance test form.

```
PUMP PERFORMANCE TEST
Apparatus number or designation _____
Manufacturer _____
Serial no. _____
Year manufactured _____
Model _____
Vehicle identification no. _____
Model _____
Model _____
Engine make _____
Pump make _____
Ratio to engine _____
Pump rated capacity _____ (gpm) (L/min)
                at _____ (psi) (kPa)
Speed check taken from _____
Test site location _____

Test performed from    ☐ Draft    ☐ Hydrant
Suction hose size _____ (in) (mm)
Length _____ (ft) (m)
```

FIGURE 19-15 Sample pump performance test form.

satisfy both NFPA and ISO requirements. The form has spaces for the vehicle information, the weather conditions at the start and end of the tests (both are needed), and the readings and results of all tests. As a reminder that some tests require you to take several readings, the form even has spaces to record the required number of readings, plus one extra space for any additional reading. Record information neatly, using pen instead of pencil, if possible. Be sure to fill in the Witnessed by and Date lines at the bottom of the first page to make the test form a more legally defensible document **FIGURE 19-15**.

Pump testing should be conducted once per year, every year. If you test your pumps less often, you will not be able to notice any serious trends, and you will not receive full credit for your irregular tests. For example, if the average time between the last three pump tests on an apparatus is three years, the ISO will give you only 50 percent of the test credit. If the average time between the last three tests is five years, you will get no credit, even if the vehicle passes the test.

If the test conditions are equivalent to those at the time of delivery of the fire apparatus and the speed of the engine increases by more than 10 percent of the original engine speed, the reason for this decrease in performance should be determined and the deficiency corrected. Where test conditions differ significantly from the original test conditions at the time of the apparatus' delivery, results should be compared with those from the previous year's test. The test conditions should be maintained as consistently as possible from one test period to the next.

Problem Solving

Most performance tests are conducted without incident. Nevertheless, trouble may develop during some tests, and an effort should be made to locate the source of trouble while the fire apparatus remains at the test site.

Failure to prime a centrifugal pump is a frequent source of trouble, with the usual reason for this failure being an air leak in the suction hose or pump. One way to trace this trouble is to remove all discharge hoselines, cap all discharge openings and the suction hose, and operate the priming mechanism in accordance with the manufacturer's recommendations. The intake gauge should be studied to determine the maximum vacuum that is developed; it should be at least 22 in. Hg (559 mm Hg) at altitudes of less than 1000 ft (300 m). The primer should then be stopped. If the vacuum drops 10 in. Hg (254 mm Hg) or more in less than 5 minutes, there is a leak in the suction hose or pump assembly; it could be in a valve, drain cock, piping, casing, or pump packing. You can also attempt to locate a leak by listening for air movement. Yet another method of checking for leaks is to connect the pump to a convenient hydrant, uncap the pump discharge outlets and close the valves, open the hydrant, and watch for water leaks. A leak can usually be corrected at the test site.

Two possible causes of failure of the pump to deliver the desired capacity, pressure, or both, are insufficient power and restrictions in the intake arrangement. Insufficient power is indicated by the inability of the engine to reach the required speed for the desired pumping condition.

Insufficient pressure when operating a centrifugal pump could result from pumping too much water for the available power and, in multistage pumps, pumping in the "volume" position instead of in the required "pressure" position. This problem can be checked by partially closing off all discharge valves until only a small flow is observed, then opening up the throttle until the desired pressure is reached, followed by slowly opening discharge valves and increasing the engine speed as necessary to maintain pressure until the desired capacity is obtained. An improperly adjusted or inoperative transfer valve can prevent the development of adequate pressure. Likewise, the pressure control system might be set too low or be defective.

Some possible causes of insufficient power are as follows:
- You might have failed to advance the throttle far enough or might be using the wrong transmission gear position.
- The engine might be in need of a tune-up.
- The grade of fuel might be improper for adequate combustion.
- Vaporization might be occurring in the fuel line.

Restriction in the intake arrangement is indicated if the pump speed is too high for the capacity and attained pressure levels. It could be the result of any one or a combination of the following conditions:
- A too-small suction hose
- A too-high altitude
- A too-high suction lift
- An incorrect strainer type
- An intake strainer that is clogged at the pump or at the end of the suction hose
- A collapsed or defective suction hose
- Aerated water or too-warm water [greater than 90°F (32°C)]
- Foreign material in the pump
- A pressure control device that is set too low or malfunctioning

An air leak in the suction hose connections or in the pump intake manifold also will result in excessive pump speed and eventually could cause loss of prime and complete cessation of flow.

Engine speed differences from the original pump test could be the result of any one or a combination of the following conditions:

- Operating the fire apparatus with the wrong transmission gear in use
- Stuck throttle control cable or electronic throttle control (TPS) malfunction
- Restrictions in the intake arrangements
- Suction hose under an insufficient depth of water
- Air leak on the intake side of the pump
- Changes in the environmental conditions
- Pump and/or engine wear
- High gear lockup not functioning (automatic transmission)

Every effort should be made to correct any problems that are found. Any portion of the performance tests that was deemed a failure should be redone to ensure that the problems have been corrected.

> **DRIVER/OPERATOR Tip**
>
> A hand-held tachometer is a useful tool to have at the pump site to verify the rpm of the motor and transmission, which can then be used to rule out transmission slipping if you exceed the 10 percent on rpm.

Rerating Fire Pumps

There are two conditions under which rerating a pump on a fire apparatus should be considered. The first condition is when the apparatus is delivered or repowered with an engine that is capable of supplying additional power beyond that needed by the pump, which warrants a larger capacity rating for the apparatus. This condition might require additional suction intakes or pump discharges to take full advantage of that capacity. The fire apparatus manufacturer and the pump manufacturer should be consulted as necessary to ensure that all components of the pumping system are adequate for the potential rerating.

The second condition warranting rerating is when the environment in which the engine or pump was initially delivered has changed, such that the engine can no longer achieve its original performance. This situation can occur when an engine or pump passed the original pump rating test with little or no reserve power and the apparatus is now operated by a department located at a higher elevation, or when the natural wear within the engine has reduced its power output over time.

A pump should never be considered for rerating if the engine is seriously worn or should undergo major restorative work. Likewise, the pump should not be considered for rerating if the testing results indicate that the pump has signs of wear or other problems. In these cases, there is a good chance that the pump will not pass the complete pump test.

If the AHJ wishes to rerate the pump, the pump should be subjected to the complete pumping test as specified in NFPA 1911, including having the test witnessed and certified by an accredited third-party testing organization. In such circumstances, problems with engine wear, pump wear, pump blockages, or other issues with the pump will worsen at an accelerated rate if they are not corrected, potentially resulting in catastrophic failure during an emergency incident. It might be necessary, for a variety of reasons, to continue to use the pump on an apparatus that does not meet its original rating until the pump can be repaired. This operational decision needs to be made on a case-by-case basis, depending on the specific deficiency of the pump and the apparatus that is available to replace the deficient fire apparatus while repairs are being made. Rerating the pump downward where such deficiencies are present merely creates a false sense of vehicle capability.

> **Safety Tip**
>
> - Whenever possible, park parallel to a sea wall, with the pump panel facing away from it if applicable.
> - Always use chaffing blocks and a salvage cover to prevent damage to suction hoses.
> - During testing, all personnel should wear the appropriate hearing protection. The noise level (decibels) produced by the apparatus is extremely significant during this process.
> - Pitot gauges should be fixed or secured to the testing nozzles. Use of hand-held Pitot gauges is not recommended when the apparatus is being operated at high pressures.
> - While taking nozzle Pitot gauge readings, personnel are required to wear helmets and safety glasses.
> - All appliances must be properly secured or affixed.
> - All hoselines, whenever applicable, should be attached to discharges that are away from the pump panel.
> - All fire apparatus must have wheel chocks and blocks in proper position during the test.

> **Safety Tip**
>
> Never conduct any performance tests on fire apparatus while you are alone; always have, at a minimum, one additional person with you. Ideally, the crew assigned to the fire apparatus will participate in its testing. They will likely know the history of the fire apparatus and be familiar with any defects or deficiencies concerning that apparatus.

Wrap-Up

Chief Concepts

- Failure of a fire pump to deliver the required amount of water at a certain pressure impairs the suppression ability and the safety of fire fighters, and may potentially lead to injury and increased property damage.
- Engine-driven accessories should not be functionally disconnected or otherwise rendered inoperative during performance testing.
- The first performance test is to check the governed engine speed.
- If the fire apparatus is equipped with an intake relief valve system or a combination intake/discharge system, an intake relief valve system test must be conducted to ensure that the system is operating in accordance with the manufacturer's specifications.
- A test of the pump shift indicators should verify that those indicators in the fire apparatus' cab and on the driver/operator's panel indicate correct pump status when the pump is shifted from road mode to pump mode.
- Beginning with the 1991 edition of NFPA 1901, fire apparatus equipped with electronic or electric engine throttle controls were required to include an interlock system to prevent engine speed advancement, except in three conditions: (1) the chassis transmission is in neutral with the parking brake engaged; (2) the parking brake is engaged, the fire pump is engaged, and the chassis transmission is in pumping gear; or (3) the fire apparatus is in the "Okay to pump" mode.
- Discharge pressure gauges can be checked quickly against test gauges for accuracy.
- Flow rates less than the rate when the fire apparatus was new or as established in previous testing indicate problems in the tank-to-pump line or tank.
- The vacuum test is basically a test of the priming system, including the tightness of the pump, plus its valves and fittings. It is not a test of the ability to maintain a vacuum while pumping water.
- At the beginning of the priming system test, attention should be paid to the ease with which the pump can develop a vacuum.
- In testing the pump, a change in any of three variable factors—pump speed, net pump pressure, and pump discharge rate—will cause a change in at least one of the other factors.
- The pressure control device—a relief valve or pressure governor located on the pump panel—should be tested at 150 psi, 90 psi, and 250 psi (1000, 630, and 1700 kPa) intervals. Care should be taken while performing the pressure control test to record the net pump pressure and net pressure rise readings.
- After conducting all of the performance tests, it is recommended to reduce the engine speed to idle.
- This will allow the engine, pump, and transmission to cool down for approximately 10 minutes.
- After the cool-down period, you can turn off all engine-driven accessories that were turned on during the testing period.
- There are two conditions under which rerating a pump on a fire apparatus should be considered.
  - The first condition is when the apparatus is delivered or repowered with an engine that is capable of supplying additional power beyond that needed by the pump, which warrants a larger capacity rating.
  - The second condition is when the environment in which the engine or pump was initially delivered has changed and the engine can no longer achieve its original performance—for example, when the engine or pump passed the original pump rating test with little or no reserve power and the apparatus is now operated by a department located at a higher elevation, or if the natural wear within the engine has reduced the power output.

Hot Terms

ambient air temperature The temperature of the surrounding medium. It typically refers to the temperature of the air in which a structure is situated or a device operates.

authority having jurisdiction (AHJ) An organization, office, or individual responsible for enforcing the requirements of a code or standard, or for approving equipment, materials, an installation, or a procedure.

discharge pressure The water pressure on the discharge manifold of the fire pump at the point of gauge attachment.

failure A cessation of proper functioning or performance.

intake pressure The pressure on the intake passageway of the pump at the point of gauge attachment.

net pump pressure (NPP) The sum of the discharge pressure and the suction lift converted to units of pounds per square inch (psi) or kilopascals (kPa) when pumping at draft, or the difference between the discharge pressure and the intake pressure when pumping at a hydrant or other source of water under positive pressure.

performance testing Tests conducted after a fire apparatus has been put into service to determine if its performance meets predetermined specifications or standards.

rated capacity (water pump) The flow rate to which the pump manufacturer certifies compliance of the pump when it is new.

service testing Tests conducted after a fire apparatus has been put into service to determine if its performance meets predetermined specifications or standards.

Wrap-Up, continued

References

Hale Products. *Pump Test Pit Design Recommendations*. n.d. http://www.haleproducts.com/_Downloads/hale/articles/Pump%20Test%20Pit%20Design.pdf. Accessed December 18, 2014.

National Fire Protection Association (NFPA) 1002, *Standard for Fire Apparatus Driver/Operator Professional Qualifications*. 2014. http://www.nfpa.org/codes-and-standards/document-information-pages?mode=code&code=1002. Accessed March 27, 2014.

National Fire Protection Association (NFPA) 1071, *Standard for Emergency Vehicle Technician Professional Qualifications*

National Fire Protection Association (NFPA) 1901, *Standard for Automotive Fire Apparatus*. 2009. http://www.nfpa.org/codes-and-standards/document-information-pages?mode=code&code=1901. Accessed March 27, 2014.

National Fire Protection Association (NFPA) 1911, *Standard for the Inspection, Maintenance, Testing, and Retirement of In-Service Automotive Fire Apparatus*. 2012. http://www.nfpa.org/codes-and-standards/document-information-pages?mode=code&code=1911. Accessed December 18, 2014.

National Fire Protection Association (NFPA) 1989, *Standard on Breathing Air Quality for Emergency Services Respiratory Protection*, 2013. http://www.nfpa.org/codes-and-standards/document-information-pages?mode=code&code=1989. Accessed December 18, 2014.

DRIVER/OPERATOR in action

It is that time of year again—time for the annual performance testing for your fire apparatus. Just like the daily inspection that you perform every morning, these tests ensure that your fire apparatus is working properly. The safety of your entire crew depends on the safety of your fire apparatus, so you take annual testing very seriously. Before driving out to the testing ground, you sit down to refresh your memory on a few points.

1. A test that is conducted on behalf of or by the purchaser at the time of delivery to determine compliance with the specifications for the fire apparatus is called a(n):
   A. Acceptance test.
   B. Underwriters Laboratory test.
   C. Annual performance test.
   D. Governed no-load test.

2. What is the water pressure on the discharge manifold of the fire pump at the point of gauge attachment called?
   A. Total discharge pressure
   B. Discharge pressure
   C. Intake pressure
   D. Net pump pressure

3. If the pump has a rated capacity of 750 gpm (3000 L/min) or greater, the apparatus must be subjected to an overload test.
   A. True
   B. False

4. For a two-stage, parallel/series-type pump, the test at 100 percent capacity, 150 psi (1000 kPa), should be run with the pump in which mode?
   A. Series mode
   B. Parallel mode
   C. Either series or parallel mode
   D. None of the above

5. When an apparatus is new and for the annual service test, the pump must be able to develop a vacuum of ____ unless the altitude is greater than 2000 ft (600 m).
   A. 10 in. Hg (254 mm Hg)
   B. 15 in. Hg (381 mm Hg)
   C. 20 in. Hg (508 mm Hg)
   D. 22 in. Hg (559 mm Hg)

Appendix A: Daily/Weekly Inspection Check Sheet

You should first become familiar with all the information on the daily/weekly check sheet. Fill in the required information at the top of the worksheet.

The first section to work on with the daily/weekly form may be the engine. On some vehicles, you may have to raise the cab to inspect the engine. Follow the manufacturer's instructions.

1. Check the engine oil and transmission level.
   a. Make sure the engine is "off." Locate the dipstick, which is typically found on the right or left side of the engine. Wipe the top of the dipstick and tube off to ensure that no dirt will fall into the dipstick tube when the stick is raised. Remove the dipstick and visually inspect the current oil level as marked on the stick. Most dipsticks will have a "Low" mark and a "Full" mark. The oil level should be noted and the condition of the oil inspected.
   b. Look for any discoloration, moisture, or milky look, indicating possible coolant contamination or water intrusion. Is the oil thinned out, indicating a possible fuel oil dilution challenge? Are there any shiny metal particles, indicating a possible internal engine challenge?
2. Note whether you have to add any oil, and do a visual inspection to identify any leaks. The National Fire Protection Association (NFPA) classifies leaks into three categories. According to NFPA 1911, *Standard for the Inspection, Maintenance, Testing, and Retirement of In-Service Automotive Fire Apparatus*, chapter 3.3.72, *leakage* is the escape of a gas or fluid from its intended containment, generally at a connection. Class 1 Liquid Leakage is the presence of liquid, as indicated by wetness or discoloration, that is not great enough to form drops. Class 2 Liquid Leakage is leakage of liquid great enough to form drops, but not enough to cause drops to fall from the item being inspected. Class 3 Liquid Leakage is leakage of liquid great enough to cause drops to fall from the item being inspected.
   a. Any Class 3 leakage should be noted and the vehicle taken out of service until it is remedied.
   b. Any Class 2 leakage in the fuel system should also cause the vehicle to be taken out of service.
3. Inspect the transmission fluid level by following the vehicle manufacturer's instructions. Most of today's emergency vehicles have an Allison automatic transmission, which is typically equipped with an electronic oil level sensor. It is recommended that these apparatus be inspected with the engine running, in neutral, at operating temperature on level ground, and at idle speed. Push the up and down arrow button on the shift pad the required number of times as described in the Allison operator's manual (either once or twice, depending on model year); the shift selector should display "OL." It will then go into a countdown mode to allow the fluid to drain into the sump. After the countdown is complete, the shift selector will display "OL OK" or "OL LO" for a low fluid level or "OL HI" for a high fluid level, followed by the amount low or high in quarts or liters.

   The electronic oil level inspection procedure is preferred over the dipstick. The dipstick method is not as accurate, because it does not take into account the fluid temperature and expansion that occurs with increasing temperature. It may be preferable to perform the transmission fluid level inspection after driving the vehicle, when it is up to operating temperature.
4. Check the engine coolant level. The engine should be cool during this inspection, and the level should be noted if it is low. Any Class 3 leakage or oil or fuel contamination should be noted and the vehicle taken out of service in such a case.
   a. Note the color of the coolant. Conventional-type ethylene glycol is typically a green, blue, or purple color; extended-life coolants, such as nitric organic acid technology (NOAT), typically have an orange or reddish color.
   b. If necessary, add more coolant. Most coolants today are permanent antifreeze types. Several types of coolants are available, however, and the correct type must be used for coolant top-off. Automotive antifreeze is generally *not* recommended for heavy-duty diesel engines. Do not mix different types of coolants in a cooling system, and do not use tap water in this system.
5. Check for integrity of the frame and suspension. Follow the vehicle manufacturer's instructions, and visually inspect the frame and suspension for any rust, loose bolts, or attaching hardware, cracks, or deformations. Note any defects found and check NFPA 1911, chapter 6, for "out of service" conditions and reporting requirements.
6. Check the power steering fluid. Follow the vehicle manufacturer's instructions. Check for proper level and visually inspect condition for discoloration and or unusual odors such as a burnt smell. Inspect for leakage. Any Class 3 leakage requires that the vehicle be taken out of service.

7. Outside the engine:
    a. Check for fluid leaks under the vehicle.
        i. Identify the fluid, color, and location of the leaks, as they are keys to what may be leaking.
        ii. Brown or dark fluid under the engine area may indicate a Class 3 leakage in the engine, placing the apparatus out of service.
        iii. Red coloration under the transmission may indicate a Class 3 leakage in the transmission, placing the apparatus out of service.
        iv. Brown or red fluid under the pump may indicate a Class 3 leakage in the pump transmission, placing the apparatus out of service.
        v. Dark, heavy-consistency fluid under the rear axle may indicate a differential leak, which is also a Class 3 leakage, placing the apparatus out of service.
    b. Check steering shafts and linkages.
        i. Do good visual inspections on the steering column slip joints and U-joints.
        ii. Do a visual inspection of the linkage under the vehicle. Are all pinch bolts, attaching nuts, and cotter keys in place and properly secured? Are the dust cover boots in good shape?
    c. Check wheels and lug nuts.
        i. Look at lug nuts for signs that they may be loose. Rust streaks may be a sign of loose lug retaining nuts.
    d. Check tire condition.
        i. Do good visual inspections looking for bulges, irregular wear, and tread depth. Note any unusual wear. Measure tread depth with a tire depth gauge. When inserted into the tire tread, the amount of tread left is indicated in increments of $1/32$ inch (0.8 mm). The NFPA 1911 and DOT out of service criteria specify a minimum depth on steer axles of $4/32$ inch (3.2 mm) and a minimum tread depth on drive axles of $2/32$ inch (1.6 mm).
        ii. Check tire date. Tire age can be determined by checking the DOT code found on either the inside or outside sidewall of each tire. The code begins with "DOT" and ends with a three-digit (through 1999) or four-digit (2000 and beyond) date code. The first two digits of the date code indicate the week of the year in which the tire was manufactured, and the last one or two digits identify the year of manufacture. For example, "DOT GJ HU234319" was manufactured in week 31 of 1999; "DOT BT FR872501" was manufactured in week 25 of 2001. Tires should be replaced every 7 years, or more frequently when the tread wear exceeds state or federal standards as determined by measurement with a tread depth gauge.
    e. Check tire air pressure.
        i. Tires should be at room temperature. Let them rest at this temperature for at least 30 minutes.
        ii. Use an accurate tire pressure gauge.
        iii. Inflate the tires to the proper pressure. Tire pressure needs to be the tire manufacturer's suggested pressure for the weight on the tire. The vehicle should be weighed every year to get accurate weight data. The tire pressure recommended by the apparatus manufacturer may be found on a label in the cab; however, this pressure was determined when the vehicle was manufactured and based on the weight of the vehicle when new.
        iv. The tire pressure on the sidewall of the tire is a maximum cold inflation pressure for that type of tire. Note the correct pressure for future daily/weekly checks. It is very important for safety reasons that the tire pressure be within 10 psi (70 kPa) of the recommended value. Low or high tire pressure can cause the vehicle to sway or maneuver dangerously.
        v. Check the tire manufacturer's date document, the DOT code, the 7 years' maximum, and the out of service criteria.
    f. Cab components:
        i. Check the seats and seat belts.
            1) Check for tears and frayed belts.
            2) Check latching mechanisms.
            3) If the cab is equipped with a seat belt warning system, check for its proper operation.
            4) If a seat belt is torn or has melted webbing, missing or broken buckles, or loose mountings, the following shall apply:
                a) If it is a seat other than the driver's seat, that seat shall be taken out of service.
                b) If it is at the driver's seat, the entire apparatus shall be taken out of service.
        ii. Start the engine and check all gauges.
            1) Do all gauges work properly? Does the volt and amp gauge indicate the alternator is charging properly? Do the air pressure gauges operate correctly?
            2) Check for proper operation of the ABS brake indicator.
                a) Does the ABS indicator illuminate on startup while it does a self-check and then go out?
        iii. Check the windshield wipers.
            1) Check for broken or missing windshield wipers.
            2) Check the condition of the windshield wiper blades.
        iv. Check the rear-view mirror adjustment and operation.
            1) Missing or broken rear-view mirrors that obstruct the driver/operator's view shall cause the apparatus to be taken out of service.
        v. Check the horn.
        vi. Check the steering shafts.
            1) Inspect all steering system components for structural integrity, security of mounting, leakage, and condition.
        vii. Check the cab glass and mirrors.

1) A cracked or broken windshield that obstructs the driver/operator's view shall cause the apparatus to be taken out of service.
g. Electrical components:
   i. Check battery voltage and charging system voltage.
      1) Test the batteries for storage and performance capabilities in accordance with the manufacturer's recommendation.
      2) Before testing them, carefully inspect the batteries.
      3) Clean the batteries of any accumulated dirt or corrosion, and check the connections to ensure that they are clean and tight.
      4) Inspect the batteries for cracks, swelling, deformation, or other physical defects.
      5) If the batteries are not sealed, verify that the cells have the proper electrolyte level, and add distilled water if necessary.
      6) If the batteries are sealed, verify that any electrolyte level indicator indicates sufficient electrolyte is present.
      7) With the shore power plugged in, check the battery charging system indicator light (if so equipped).
      8) In the operator's seat with the shore power disconnected (if so equipped) and power or ignition switch in the "on" position, check the volt gauge to make sure that it reads 12 volts (on 12-volt systems) or slightly higher.
      9) Start the vehicle and make sure the volt gauge goes up to 13 to 14 volts (on 12-volt systems).
      10) With the vehicle running, visually check the amp gauge. It should show a positive number, indicating that the alternator is charging. You may increase engine rpms slightly to help verify this operation if necessary.
   ii. Check the line voltage system (if so equipped).
      1) Inspect all power sources for security of mounting, condition, and fluid leakage.
      2) Inspect all line voltage appliances and controls, including but not limited to the following appliances and controls, for security of mounting and condition:
         a) Cord reels
         b) Extension cords
         c) Scene lights
         d) Circuit breaker boxes
         e) Switches
         f) Relays
         g) Receptacles
         h) Inlet devices
         i) Light towers
         j) Other line voltage devices on the apparatus not otherwise specified
   iii. Check all lights (ICC and warning).
      1) Inspect all fire apparatus lighting, including but not limited to the following, for security of mounting and deformation and for correct operation:
         a) Headlights
         b) Marker lights
         c) Clearance lights
         d) Turn signals and hazard lights
         e) Brake lights
         f) Dash lights
         g) Other fire apparatus lighting equipment on the apparatus not otherwise specified
h. Brakes:
   i. Check the air system for proper air pressure.
      1) Check the air pressure gauges on the dashboard. Most gauges today are electric, so you may need to have the battery switch and the ignition switch be in the "on" positions for the gauge to register the correct pressure.
      2) Inspect the "Low Air" warning system to ensure that it activates at the manufacturer's suggested pressure. With the engine power off and the ignition on, pump the brakes several times to use up the air in the system. Note when the "Low Air" alarm activates.
   ii. Check the parking brake.
      1) Inspect the parking brake for structural integrity, security of mounting, missing or broken parts, and wear.
      2) Inspect the parking brake controls and activating mechanism for structural integrity, security of mounting, and missing or broken parts.
      3) Operate the parking brake (air, hydraulic, or manual) to ensure that it holds the vehicle from movement. Use caution when performing this procedure; make sure that no one is around the vehicle in case it moves.
   iii. Check the hydraulic brake fluid level (if so equipped).
      1) If the fire apparatus has a hydraulic brake system, the components to be inspected and maintained shall include, but are not be limited to, the following:
         a) Pedal and linkage: Visual inspection to ensure that all linkage and attaching hardware is tight and in place.
         b) Brake switches: Visual inspection to ensure that all switches are in place and wires are intact.
         c) Master cylinder: Visual inspection to ensure there is no leakage. Class 2 leakage of hydraulic brake fluid is cause to take the apparatus out of service. Check the brake fluid level. If the master cylinder level is low, it suggests there is a leak somewhere in the system. This should be documented and further inspected by a qualified EVT.
         d) Brake booster: Visual inspection to ensure that all attaching hardware is intact and tight.
         e) Hydraulic lines: Visual inspection to ensure that all hydraulic lines are in place, clamps are in place, and no leakage is present.

Class 2 leakage is cause to take the apparatus out of service.
- f) Valves: Visual inspection of any brake valve that is visible to ensure that all attaching hardware is in place and tight and that no leaks are present. Class 2 leakage is cause to take the apparatus out of service.
- g) Wheel cylinders or calipers: Visual inspection, if possible, to ensure that attaching hardware is in place and tight, and no leaks are present. Class 2 leaks are cause to take the apparatus out of service. In most cases, the wheel cylinders and calipers will not be visible unless there is an inspection location on the braking system. In those cases, you should be aware of dampness or droplets of brake fluid dripping from the backing plate or brake assembly.
- h) Brake shoes or disc brake pads: Visual inspection to ensure adequate thickness. This thickness must meet the manufacturer's minimum requirement. Note that the brake shoes or pads may not be visible without removing wheels or other parts. Some systems, however, have an inspection slot location for visual inspection.
- i) Brake drums or rotors: Visual inspection should not find any cracks or bluing. Any deficiencies noted in the brake system should be noted and reported to the AHJ or the department's officer.
- j) Warning devices: Visual inspection to ensure that they illuminate properly. Most systems will illuminate when the system is powered on and then will go off.
- k) Mounting hardware: Visual inspection to ensure that all attaching hardware and or clamps are in place and tight.
- l) Fluid level and contamination: Fluid level and condition of fluid should be noted. A low fluid level indicates a leak. Note the color of the fluid and any discoloration. The fluid should not look burnt or milky. Any discoloration should be inspected by a qualified EVT.

i. Pump (if so equipped):
  i. Operate the pump; check the pump panel engine gauges.
  ii. Check the pump for pressure operation.
  iii. Check the discharge relief or pressure governor operation.
  iv. Check all pump drains.
  v. Check all discharge and intake valve operation.
  vi. Check the pump and tank for water leaks.
  vii. Check all valve bleeder/drain operation.
  viii. Check the primer pump operation.
  ix. Check the system vacuum for hold (leakage).
  x. Check the water tank level indicator.
  xi. Check the primer oil level (if applicable).
  xii. Check the transfer valve operation (if applicable).
  xiii. Check the booster reel operation (if applicable).
  xiv. Check all pump pressure gauge operations.
  xv. Check all cooler valves.
  xvi. Check for oil leaks in the pump area.
j. Aerial (if so equipped):
  i. Operate the aerial hydraulics.
  ii. Check the aerial outrigger operation.
  iii. Check the aerial operation.
  iv. Check the aerial hydraulic fluid level.
  v. Visually inspect the aerial structure.

Comments:
1. The driver/operator should document all deficiencies found and report them to the AHJ or the specific person taking care of such deficiencies in the fire department. Further evaluation may need to be performed by a qualified EVT. Most fire departments have a specific policy or procedure to follow for deficiencies or when taking an apparatus out of service.
2. The driver/operator should also inspect the following items and functionally test them for proper service in accordance with NFPA 1002, *Standard for Fire Apparatus Driver/Operator Professional Qualifications*, 5.1.1:
   a. Water tank and other extinguishing agent levels (if applicable):
      i. Do a visual inspection of the water tank and extinguishing agent tank.
      ii. Check for any leakage.
      iii. Check the tank levels. Standard practice is to keep tanks full. Check your fire department's standard operating procedure.
      iv. Check the tank level-indicating devices for proper operation. Note whether the level-indicating device is not functioning properly. An inspection should be performed to determine the cause and an "out of service" determination needs to be made and put in writing to the AHJ.
   b. Pumping systems:
      i. The driver/operator needs to understand the "out of service" criteria for the pumping system. The following deficiencies of the fire pump shall cause the pumping system to be taken out of service:
         1) Pump that will not engage
         2) Pump shift indicators in the cab and on the operator's panel that do not function properly
         3) Pressure control system that is not operational
         4) Pump transmission components that have a Class 3 leakage of fluid
         5) Pump operator's panel throttle that is not operational
         6) Pump operator's engine speed advancement interlock that is not operational
   c. Foam systems:
      i. If the apparatus is equipped with a foam proportioning system, inspect and maintain that system in accordance with the recommendations of the foam system manufacturer.
      ii. Inspect all components of the foam proportioning system for security of mounting, structural integrity, and leakage.

Appendix B: An Extract from NFPA 1002, *Standard for Fire Apparatus Driver/Operator Professional Qualifications*, 2014 Edition

Chapter 4 General Requirements

4.1 General. Prior to operating fire department vehicles, the fire apparatus driver/operator shall meet the job performance requirements defined in Sections 4.2 and 4.3.

4.2 Preventive Maintenance.

4.2.1* Perform routine tests, inspections, and servicing functions on the systems and components specified in the following list, given a fire department vehicle, its manufacturer's specifications, and policies and procedures of the jurisdiction, so that the operational status of the vehicle is verified:

(1) Battery(ies)
(2) Braking system
(3) Coolant system
(4) Electrical system
(5) Fuel
(6) Hydraulic fluids
(7) Oil
(8) Tires
(9) Steering system
(10) Belts
(11) Tools, appliances, and equipment

(A) Requisite Knowledge. Manufacturer specifications and requirements, policies, and procedures of the jurisdiction.

(B) Requisite Skills. The ability to use hand tools, recognize system problems, and correct any deficiency noted according to policies and procedures.

4.2.2 Document the routine tests, inspections, and servicing functions, given maintenance and inspection forms, so that all items are checked for operation and deficiencies are reported.

(A) Requisite Knowledge. Departmental requirements for documenting maintenance performed and the importance of keeping accurate records.

(B) Requisite Skills. The ability to use tools and equipment and complete all related departmental forms.

4.3 Driving/Operating.

4.3.1* Operate a fire apparatus, given a vehicle and a predetermined route on a public way that incorporates the maneuvers and features that the driver/operator is expected to encounter during normal operations, so that the vehicle is operated in compliance with all applicable state and local laws and departmental rules and regulations.

(A) Requisite Knowledge. The importance of donning passenger restraint devices and ensuring crew safety; the common causes of fire apparatus accidents and the recognition that drivers of fire apparatus are responsible for the safe and prudent operation of the vehicle under all conditions; the effects on vehicle control of liquid surge, braking reaction time, and load factors; effects of high center of gravity on roll-over potential, general steering reactions, speed, and centrifugal force; applicable laws and regulations; principles of skid avoidance, night driving, shifting, and gear patterns; negotiating intersections, railroad crossings, and bridges; weight and height limitations for both roads and bridges; identification and operation of automotive gauges; and operational limits.

(B) Requisite Skills. The ability to operate passenger restraint devices; maintain safe following distances; maintain control of the vehicle while accelerating, decelerating, and turning, given road, weather, and traffic conditions; operate under adverse environmental or driving surface conditions; and use automotive gauges and controls.

4.3.2* Back a vehicle from a roadway into restricted spaces on both the right and left sides of the vehicle, given a fire apparatus, a spotter, and restricted spaces 12 ft (3.7 m) in width, requiring 90-degree right-hand and left-hand turns from the roadway, so that the vehicle is parked within the restricted areas without having to stop and pull forward and without striking obstructions.

(A) Requisite Knowledge. Vehicle dimensions, turning characteristics, spotter signaling, and principles of safe vehicle operation.

(B) Requisite Skills. The ability to use mirrors and judge vehicle clearance.

4.3.3* Maneuver a vehicle around obstructions on a roadway while moving forward and in reverse, given a fire apparatus, a spotter for backing, and a roadway with obstructions, so that the vehicle is maneuvered through the obstructions without stopping to change the direction of travel and without striking the obstructions.

(A) Requisite Knowledge. Vehicle dimensions, turning characteristics, the effects of liquid surge, spotter signaling, and principles of safe vehicle operation.

(B) Requisite Skills. The ability to use mirrors and judge vehicle clearance.

4.3.4* Turn a fire apparatus 180 degrees within a confined space, given a fire apparatus, a spotter for backing up, and an area in which the vehicle cannot perform a U-turn without stopping and backing up, so that the vehicle is turned 180 degrees without striking obstructions within the given space.

(A) Requisite Knowledge. Vehicle dimensions, turning characteristics, the effects of liquid surge, spotter signaling, and principles of safe vehicle operation.

(B) Requisite Skills. The ability to use mirrors and judge vehicle clearance.

4.3.5* Maneuver a fire apparatus in areas with restricted horizontal and vertical clearances, given a fire apparatus and a course that requires the operator to move through areas of restricted horizontal and vertical clearances, so that the operator accurately judges the ability of the vehicle to pass through the openings and so that no obstructions are struck.

(A) Requisite Knowledge. Vehicle dimensions, turning characteristics, the effects of liquid surge, spotter signaling, and principles of safe vehicle operation.

(B) Requisite Skills. The ability to use mirrors and judge vehicle clearance.

4.3.6* Operate a vehicle using defensive driving techniques, given an assignment and a fire apparatus, so that control of the vehicle is maintained.

(A) Requisite Knowledge. The importance of donning passenger restraint devices and ensuring crew safety; the common causes of fire apparatus accidents and the recognition that drivers of fire apparatus are responsible for the safe and prudent operation of the vehicle under all conditions; the effects on vehicle control of liquid surge, braking reaction time, and load factors; the effects of high center of gravity on rollover potential, general steering reactions, speed, and centrifugal force; applicable laws and regulations; principles of skid avoidance, night driving, shifting, gear patterns; and automatic braking systems in wet and dry conditions; negotiation of intersections, railroad crossings, and bridges; weight and height limitations for both roads and bridges; identification and operation of automotive gauges; and operational limits.

(B) Requisite Skills. The ability to operate passenger restraint devices; maintain safe following distances; maintain control of the vehicle while accelerating, decelerating, and turning, given road, weather, and traffic conditions; operate under adverse environmental or driving surface conditions; and use automotive gauges and controls.

4.3.7* Operate all fixed systems and equipment on the vehicle not specifically addressed elsewhere in this standard, given systems and equipment, manufacturer's specifications and instructions, and departmental policies and procedures for the systems and equipment, so that each system or piece of equipment is operated in accordance with the applicable instructions and policies.

(A) Requisite Knowledge. Manufacturer's specifications and operating procedures, and policies and procedures of the jurisdiction.

(B) Requisite Skills. The ability to deploy, energize, and monitor the system or equipment and to recognize and correct system problems.

Chapter 5 Apparatus Equipped with Fire Pump

5.1* General. The requirements of Fire Fighter 1 as specified in NFPA 1001 (or the requirements of Advanced Exterior Industrial Fire Brigade Member or Interior Structural Fire Brigade Member as specified in NFPA 1081) and the job performance requirements defined in Sections 5.1 and 5.2 shall be met prior to qualifying as a fire department driver/operator — pumper.

5.1.1 Perform the routine tests, inspections, and servicing functions specified in the following list in addition to those in 4.2.1, given a fire department pumper, its manufacturer's specifications, and policies and procedures of the jurisdiction, so that the operational status of the pumper is verified:

(1) Water tank and other extinguishing agent levels (if applicable)
(2) Pumping systems
(3) Foam systems

(A) Requisite Knowledge. Manufacturer's specifications and requirements, and policies and procedures of the jurisdiction.

(B) Requisite Skills. The ability to use hand tools, recognize system problems, and correct any deficiency noted according to policies and procedures.

5.2 Operations.

5.2.1 Produce effective hand or master streams, given the sources specified in the following list, so that the pump is engaged, all pressure control and vehicle safety devices are set, the rated flow of the nozzle is achieved and maintained, and the apparatus is continuously monitored for potential problems:

(1) Internal tank
(2) *Pressurized source
(3) Static source
(4) Transfer from internal tank to external source

(A) Requisite Knowledge. Hydraulic calculations for friction loss and flow using both written formulas and estimation methods, safe operation of the pump, problems related to small-diameter or dead-end mains, low-pressure and private water supply systems, hydrant coding systems, and reliability of static sources.

(B) Requisite Skills. The ability to position a fire department pumper to operate at a fire hydrant and at a static water source, power transfer from vehicle engine to pump, draft, operate pumper pressure control systems, operate the volume/pressure transfer valve (multistage pumps only), operate auxiliary cooling systems, make the transition between internal and external water sources, and assemble hose lines, nozzles, valves, and appliances.

5.2.2 Pump a supply line of 2½ in. (65 mm) or larger, given a relay pumping evolution the length and size of the line and the desired flow and intake pressure, so that the correct pressure and flow are provided to the next pumper in the relay.

(A) Requisite Knowledge. Hydraulic calculations for friction loss and flow using both written formulas and estimation methods, safe operation of the pump, problems related to small-diameter or dead-end mains, low-pressure and private water supply systems, hydrant coding systems, and reliability of static sources.

(B) Requisite Skills. The ability to position a fire department pumper to operate at a fire hydrant and at a static water source, power transfer from vehicle engine to pump, draft, operate pumper pressure control systems, operate the volume/pressure transfer valve (multistage pumps only), operate auxiliary cooling systems, make the transition between internal and external water sources, and assemble hose lines, nozzles, valves, and appliances.

5.2.3 Produce a foam fire stream, given foam-producing equipment, so that properly proportioned foam is provided.

(A) Requisite Knowledge. Proportioning rates and concentrations, equipment assembly procedures, foam system limitations, and manufacturer's specifications.

(B) Requisite Skills. The ability to operate foam proportioning equipment and connect foam stream equipment.

5.2.4 Supply water to fire sprinkler and standpipe systems, given specific system information and a fire department pumper, so that water is supplied to the system at the correct volume and pressure.

(A) Requisite Knowledge. Calculation of pump discharge pressure; hose layouts; location of fire department connection; alternative supply procedures if fire department connection is not usable; operating principles of sprinkler systems as defined in NFPA 13, NFPA 13D, and NFPA 13R; fire department operations in sprinklered properties as defined in NFPA 13E; and operating principles of standpipe systems as defined in NFPA 14.

(B) Requisite Skills. The ability to position a fire department pumper to operate at a fire hydrant and at a static water source, power transfer from vehicle engine to pump, draft, operate pumper pressure control systems, operate the volume/pressure transfer valve (multistage pumps only), operate auxiliary cooling systems, make the transition between internal and external water sources, and assemble hose lines, nozzles, valves, and appliances.

■ Chapter 6 Apparatus Equipped with an Aerial Device

6.1* General. The requirements of Fire Fighter I as specified in NFPA 1001 (or the requirements of Advanced Exterior Industrial Fire Brigade Member or Interior Structural Fire Brigade Member as specified in NFPA 1081) and the job performance requirements defined in Sections 6.1 and 6.2 shall be met prior to qualifying as a fire department driver/operator — aerial.

6.1.1 Perform the routine tests, inspections, and servicing functions specified in the following list in addition to those specified in 4.2.1, given a fire department aerial apparatus, and policies and procedures of the jurisdiction, so that the operational readiness of the aerial apparatus is verified:

(1) Cable systems (if applicable)
(2) Aerial device hydraulic systems
(3) Slides and rollers
(4) Stabilizing systems
(5) Aerial device safety systems
(6) Breathing air systems
(7) Communication systems

(A) **Requisite Knowledge.** Manufacturer's specifications and requirements, and policies and procedures of the jurisdiction.

(B) **Requisite Skills.** The ability to use hand tools, recognize system problems, and correct any deficiency noted according to policies and procedures.

6.2 Operations.

6.2.1 Maneuver and position an aerial apparatus, given an aerial apparatus, an incident location, a situation description, and an assignment, so that the apparatus is positioned for correct aerial device deployment.

(A) **Requisite Knowledge.** Capabilities and limitations of aerial devices related to reach, tip load, angle of inclination, and angle from chassis axis; effects of topography, ground, and weather conditions on deployment; and use of the aerial device.

(B) **Requisite Skills.** The ability to determine a correct position for the apparatus, maneuver apparatus into that position, and avoid obstacles to operations.

6.2.2 Stabilize an aerial apparatus, given a positioned vehicle and the manufacturer's recommendations, so that power can be transferred to the aerial device hydraulic system and the device can be deployed.

(A) **Requisite Knowledge.** Aerial apparatus hydraulic systems, manufacturer's specifications for stabilization, stabilization requirements, and effects of topography and ground conditions on stabilization.

(B) **Requisite Skills.** The ability to transfer power from the vehicle's engine to the hydraulic system and operate vehicle stabilization devices.

6.2.3 Maneuver and position the aerial device from each control station, given an incident location, a situation description, and an assignment, so that the aerial device is positioned to accomplish the assignment.

(A) **Requisite Knowledge.** Aerial device hydraulic systems, hydraulic pressure relief systems, gauges and controls, cable systems, communications systems, electrical systems, emergency operating systems, locking systems, manual rotation and lowering systems, stabilizing systems, aerial device safety systems, system overrides and the hazards of using overrides, safe operational limitations of the given aerial device, safety procedures specific to the device, and operations near electrical hazards and overhead obstructions.

(B) **Requisite Skills.** The ability to raise, rotate, extend, and position to a specified location, as well as lock, unlock, retract, lower, and bed the aerial device.

6.2.4 Lower an aerial device using the emergency operating system, given an aerial device, so that the aerial device is lowered to its bedded position.

(A) **Requisite Knowledge.** Aerial device hydraulic systems, hydraulic pressure relief systems, gauges and controls, cable systems, communications systems, electrical systems, emergency operating systems, locking systems, manual rotation and lowering systems, stabilizing systems, aerial device safety systems, system overrides and the hazards of using overrides, safe operational limitations of the given aerial device, safety procedures specific to the device, and operations near electrical hazards and overhead obstructions.

(B) **Requisite Skills.** The ability to rotate and position to center, unlock, retract, lower, and bed the aerial device using the emergency operating system.

6.2.5 Deploy and operate an elevated master stream, given an aerial device, a master stream device, and a desired flow so that the stream is effective and the aerial and master stream devices are operated correctly.

(A) **Requisite Knowledge.** Nozzle reaction, range of operation, and weight limitations.

(B) **Requisite Skills.** The ability to connect a water supply to a master stream device and control an elevated nozzle manually or remotely.

■ Chapter 7 Apparatus Equipped with a Tiller

7.1* General. The requirements of Fire Fighter I as specified in NFPA 1001 and the job performance requirements defined in Chapter 6 and Section 7.2 shall be met prior to qualifying as a fire department driver/operator—tiller.

7.2 Operations.

7.2.1* Perform the practical driving exercises specified in 4.3.2 through 4.3.5 from the tiller position, given a qualified driver, a fire department aerial apparatus equipped with a tiller, and a spotter for backing up, so that each exercise is performed without striking the vehicle or obstructions.

(A) **Requisite Knowledge.** Capabilities and limitations of tiller aerial devices related to reach, tip load, angle of inclination, and angle from chassis axis; effects of topography, ground, and weather conditions on safe deployment; and use of a tiller aerial device.

(B) **Requisite Skills.** The ability to determine a correct position for the tiller, maneuver the tiller into that position, and avoid obstacles to operations.

7.2.2 Operate a fire department aerial apparatus equipped with a tiller from the tiller position over a predetermined route on a public way, using the maneuvers specified in 4.3.1, given a qualified driver, a fire department aerial apparatus equipped with a tiller, and a spotter for backing up, so that the vehicle is operated in compliance with all applicable state and local laws, departmental rules and regulations, and the requirements of NFPA 1500, Section 4.2.

(A) **Requisite Knowledge.** Principles of tiller operation, methods of communication with the driver, the effects on vehicle control of general steering reactions, night driving, negotiating intersections, and manufacturer operation limitations.

(B) Requisite Skills. The ability to operate the communication system between the tiller operator's position and the driver's compartment; operate passenger restraint devices; maintain control of the tiller while accelerating, decelerating, and turning; operate the vehicle during nonemergency conditions; and operate under adverse environmental or driving surface conditions.

7.2.3 Position a fire department aerial apparatus equipped with a tiller from the tiller position, given the apparatus operating instructions, an incident location, a situation description, and an assignment, so that the aerial device is positioned and stabilized to accomplish the assignment.

(A) Requisite Knowledge. Principles of positioning and stabilizing the aerial apparatus from the tiller position.

(B) Requisite Skills. The ability to determine a correct position for the tiller, maneuver the tiller into that position, and avoid obstacles to operations.

■ Chapter 10 Mobile Water Supply Apparatus

10.1 General. The job performance requirements defined in Sections 10.1 and 10.2 shall be met prior to qualifying as a fire department driver/operator—mobile water supply apparatus.

10.1.1 Perform routine tests, inspections, and servicing functions specified in the following list, in addition to those specified in 4.2.1, given a fire department mobile water supply apparatus, and policies and procedures of the jurisdiction, so that the operational readiness of the mobile water supply apparatus is verified:

(1) Water tank and other extinguishing agent levels (if applicable)
(2) Pumping system (if applicable)
(3) Rapid dump system (if applicable)
(4) Foam system (if applicable)

(A) Requisite Knowledge. Manufacturer's specifications and requirements, and policies and procedures of the jurisdiction.

(B) Requisite Skills. The ability to use hand tools, recognize system problems, and correct any deficiency noted according to policies and procedures.

10.2 Operations.

10.2.1* Maneuver and position a mobile water supply apparatus at a water shuttle fill site, given a fill site location and one or more supply hose, so that the apparatus is correctly positioned, supply hose are attached to the intake connections without having to stretch additional hose, and no objects are struck at the fill site.

(A) Requisite Knowledge. Local procedures for establishing a water shuttle fill site, method for marking the stopping position of the apparatus, and location of the water tank intakes on the apparatus.

(B) Requisite Skills. The ability to determine a correct position for the apparatus, maneuver apparatus into that position, and avoid obstacles to operations.

10.2.2* Maneuver and position a mobile water supply apparatus at a water shuttle dump site, given a dump site and a portable water tank, so that all of the water being discharged from the apparatus enters the portable tank and no objects are struck at the dump site.

(A) Requisite Knowledge. Local procedures for operating a water shuttle dump site and location of the water tank discharges on the apparatus.

(B) Requisite Skills. The ability to determine a correct position for the apparatus, maneuver apparatus into that position, avoid obstacles to operations, and operate the fire pump or rapid water dump system.

10.2.3* Establish a water shuttle dump site, given two or more portable water tanks, low-level strainers, water transfer equipment, fire hose, and a fire apparatus equipped with a fire pump, so that the tank being drafted from is kept full at all times, the tank being dumped into is emptied first, and the water is transferred efficiently from one tank to the next.

(A) Requisite Knowledge. Local procedures for establishing a water shuttle dump site and principles of water transfer between multiple portable water tanks.

(B) Requisite Skills. The ability to deploy portable water tanks, connect and operate water transfer equipment, and connect a strainer and suction hose to the fire pump.

Appendix C: NFPA 1002 Correlation Guide

NFPA 1002, *Standard for Fire Apparatus Driver/Operator Professional Qualifications*, 2014 Edition	Corresponding Chapters	Corresponding Pages
4.1	1, 2, 3	8–13, 26–28, 36–37
4.2	8	168–187
4.2.1	8, 19	168–187, 467–504
4.2.1(1)	8, 19	168–187, 467–504
4.2.1(2)	8, 19	168–187, 467–504
4.2.1(3)	8, 19	168–187, 467–504
4.2.1(4)	8, 19	168–187, 467–504
4.2.1(5)	8, 19	168–187, 467–504
4.2.1(6)	8, 19	168–187, 467–504
4.2.1(7)	8, 19	168–187, 467–504
4.2.1(8)	8, 19	168–187, 467–504
4.2.1(9)	8, 19	168–187, 467–504
4.2.1(10)	8, 19	168–187, 467–504
4.2.1(11)	8, 19	168–187, 467–504
4.2.1(A)	3, 8, 19	36–37, 168–187, 467–504
4.2.1(B)	8, 19	168–187, 467–471, 474–475
4.2.2	8	168–187
4.2.2(A)	8	169–172, 187
4.2.2(B)	8	168–187
4.3	9	194–199, 207, 209–210
4.3.1	9, 10	194–204, 207, 209–210, 219–225, 238–239
4.3.1(A)	9, 10	194–204, 207, 209–210, 219–225
4.3.1(B)	9, 10	194, 196–199, 207, 209–210, 238–239
4.3.2	9, 16	200–208, 404–405, 407–408
4.3.2(A)	9	200–204
4.3.2(B)	9, 16	205–208, 404–405
4.3.3	9, 16	200–204, 407, 409
4.3.3(A)	9	200–204
4.3.3(B)	9, 16	200–201, 404–405

NFPA 1002, *Standard for Fire Apparatus Driver/Operator Professional Qualifications*, 2014 Edition	Corresponding Chapters	Corresponding Pages
4.3.4	9, 16	200–204, 407, 409
4.3.4(A)	9	200–204
4.3.4(B)	9, 16	201–203, 404–405
4.3.5	9, 16	200–204, 407, 409
4.3.5(A)	9	200–204
4.3.5(B)	9, 16	203–204, 404–405
4.3.6	10	219–225, 238–239
4.3.6(A)	10	219–225
4.3.6(B)	10	238–239
4.3.7	6, 11	102–106, 246–250, 253–255, 257–274
4.3.7(A)	6, 11	102–109, 111–115, 246–250, 253–255, 257–272
4.3.7(B)	6, 11	105–106, 247–250, 254–255, 257–268, 271–274
5.1	1, 2, 3	8–13, 26–28, 37–38
5.1.1	6, 8, 19	105, 107–109, 111–115, 168–187, 471–476, 481–504
5.1.1(1)	8, 19	168–187, 471–474
5.1.1(2)	8, 19	168–187, 471–476, 480–504
5.1.1(3)	8, 14, 19	168–187, 327–350, 471–476, 481–504
5.1.1(A)	3, 8, 19	37–38, 168–187, 471–476, 481–504
5.1.1(B)	8, 19	168–187, 471–474, 480–504
5.2.1	7	121–147, 150–153, 156–162
5.2.1(1)	7, 11	121–127, 156–162, 246–250, 253–255, 257–274
5.2.1(2)	7, 11	121–127, 156–162, 246–250, 253–255, 257–274
5.2.1(3)	7, 11	121–127, 156–162, 246–250, 253–255, 257–274
5.2.1(4)	7, 11	121–127, 156–162, 246–250, 253–255, 257–274
5.2.1(A)	7, 11	121–127, 156–162, 246–250, 253–255, 257–274
5.2.1(B)	7, 11	124–147, 150–153, 158–162, 247–250, 254–255, 257–268, 271–274
5.2.2	13	312–321
5.2.2(A)	13	312–321
5.2.2(B)	13	312–321
5.2.3	14	327–350
5.2.3(A)	14	327–350
5.2.3(B)	14	334–343, 345–350
5.2.4	6, 7	105–106, 147, 149–155
5.2.4(A)	6, 7	105–106, 147, 149–155
5.2.4(B)	6, 7	105–106, 147, 149–155
6.1	3	42–44
6.1.1	8, 15, 19	168–187, 363, 471, 474–476
6.1.1(1)	8, 15, 17, 18	168–187, 363, 422–429, 436–437
6.1.1(2)	8, 15, 17, 18, 19	168–187, 359–360, 363, 422–429, 436–440, 471, 474–476

Fire Apparatus Driver/Operator

NFPA 1002, Standard for Fire Apparatus Driver/Operator Professional Qualifications, 2014 Edition	Corresponding Chapters	Corresponding Pages
6.1.1(3)	8, 15, 17, 18	168–187, 363, 422–429, 456
6.1.1(4)	8, 15, 17, 18	168–187, 363, 422–429, 457
6.1.1(5)	8, 15, 17, 18, 19	168–187, 363, 422–429, 452, 454–458, 471, 474–476
6.1.1(6)	8, 15, 17, 18, 19	168–187, 363, 422–429, 438, 457, 475–476
6.1.1(7)	8, 15, 17, 18	168–187, 363, 422–429, 457
6.1.1(A)	8, 15, 17, 18, 19	168–187, 363, 422–429, 434–460, 471, 474–476
6.1.1(B)	8, 15, 17, 18, 19	168–187, 363, 422–429, 452, 454–460, 471, 474–476
6.2.1	15	364–367
6.2.1(A)	3, 15	42–44, 363–367
6.2.1(B)	15	363–367
6.2.2	15	367–371
6.2.2(A)	15	359–360, 363–371
6.2.2(B)	15	367–371
6.2.3	15	364–367
6.2.3(A)	15	359–360, 364–367, 371–375, 377–380
6.2.3(B)	15	371–375, 377–384
6.2.4	15	388
6.2.4(A)	15	359–360, 388
6.2.4(B)	15	388
6.2.5	15	384–389
6.2.5(A)	15	384–389
6.2.5(B)	15	384–389
7.1	3, 16, 17	42–44, 406–407, 422–425, 427–429
7.2.1	16, 17	404–409, 414–416, 423–425, 427–429
7.2.1(A)	3, 16, 17	42–44, 406, 414–416, 423–425, 427–428
7.2.1(B)	16, 17	400–401, 403–410, 412, 414–416, 423–425, 427–429
7.2.2	16	404–410, 412–416
7.2.2(A)	16, 17	400–410, 412, 422–425, 427–429
7.2.2(B)	16	400–410, 412–413, 415–416
7.2.3	16, 17	406, 414–416, 423–425, 427–429
7.2.3(A)	16	413–416
7.2.3(B)	16, 17	400–401, 403–410, 412, 414–416, 423–425, 427–429
10.1	3	41–42
10.1.1	3, 8	41–42, 168–187
10.1.1(1)	8, 19	168–187, 471–474
10.1.1(2)	8, 19	168–187, 471, 480–504
10.1.1(3)	8	168–187
10.1.1(4)	3, 8, 19	46–47, 168–187, 471–474
10.1.1(A)	3, 8	46–47, 168–187

NFPA 1002, *Standard for Fire Apparatus Driver/Operator Professional Qualifications*, 2014 Edition	Corresponding Chapters	Corresponding Pages
10.1.1(B)	8, 19	168–187, 471–474, 480–504
10.2.1	12	280–298, 300–302
10.2.1(A)	12	280–298, 300–302
10.2.1(B)	12	290–296
10.2.2	12	287–298, 300–302
10.2.2(A)	12	287–298, 300–302
10.2.2(B)	12	290–296
10.2.3	12	302–306
10.2.3(A)	12	302–306
10.2.3(B)	12	302–306

Appendix D: Pro Board Assessment Methodology Matrices for NFPA 1002

NFPA 1002 - Driver/Operator Pump - 2014 Edition

IMPORTANT: The language from the standard on the AMMs is truncated. When completing the AMMs, the agency must refer to the NFPA standards for the complete text and a comprehensive statement of each Job Performance Requirement (JPR), Requisite Knowledge (RK), Requisite Skill (RS), and any applicable annex or explanatory information.

INSTRUCTIONS: Please review the instructions for filling out this Assessment Methodology Matrix at http://theproboard.org/AMM.htm. The submission of this form by an agency is affirmation that it is filled out in accordance with the instructions listed above.

AGENCY NAME:				DATE COMPILED:		
OBJECTIVE / JPR, RK, RS		**COGNITIVE**	**MANIPULATIVE**			
SECTION	ABBREVIATED TEXT	WRITTEN TEST	SKILLS STATION	PORTFOLIO	PROJECTS	OTHER
Chapter 4 General Requirements						
4.2.1	Perform routine tests					Chapter 8 (p 168–187), Chapter 19 (p 467–504)
4.2.1(A)	RK: Manufacturer specifications and requirements					Chapter 3 (p 36–37), Chapter 8 (p 168–187), Chapter 19 (p 467–504)
4.2.1(B)	RS: correct any deficiency					Chapter 8 (p 168–187), Chapter 19 (p 467–471, 474–475)
4.2.2	document routine tests, inspections, and servicing functions					Chapter 8 (p 168–187)
4.2.2(A)	RK: documenting maintenance					Chapter 8 (p 169–172, 187)
4.2.2(B)	RS: tools and equipment					Chapter 8 (p 168–187)
4.3.1	Operate a fire apparatus					Chapter 9 (p 194–204, 207, 209–210), Chapter 10 (p 219–225, 238–239)
4.3.1(A)	RK: importance of donning passenger restraint devices and ensuring crew safety					Chapter 9 (p 194–204, 207, 209–210), Chapter 10 (p 219–225)
4.3.1(B)	RS: ability to operate passenger restraint devices					Chapter 9 (p 194, 196–199, 207, 209–210), Chapter 10 (p 238–239)
4.3.2	Back a vehicle					Chapter 9 (p 200–208), Chapter 16 (p 404–405, 407–408)
4.3.2(A)	RK: principles of safe vehicle operation					Chapter 9 (p 200–204)
4.3.2(B)	RS: ability to use mirrors and judge vehicle clearance					Chapter 9 (p 205–208), Chapter 16 (p 404–405)
4.3.3	Maneuver a vehicle around obstructions					Chapter 9 (p 200–204), Chapter 16 (p 407, 409)
4.3.3(A)	RK: principles of safe vehicle operation					Chapter 9 (p 200–204)
4.3.3(B)	RS: ability to use mirrors and judge vehicle clearance					Chapter 9 (p 200–201), Chapter 16 (p 404–405)
4.3.4	Turn a fire department vehicle 180 degrees					Chapter 9 (p 200–204), Chapter 16 (p 407, 409)

SECTION	OBJECTIVE / JPR, RK, RS ABBREVIATED TEXT	COGNITIVE WRITTEN TEST	MANIPULATIVE SKILLS STATION	PORTFOLIO	PROJECTS	OTHER
4.3.4(A)	RK: principles of safe vehicle operation					Chapter 9 (p 200–204)
4.3.4(B)	RS: ability to use mirrors and judge vehicle clearance					Chapter 9 (p 200–203), Chapter 16 (p 404–405)
4.3.5	Maneuver a fire department vehicle in areas with restricted horizontal and vertical clearances					Chapter 9 (p 200–204), Chapter 16 (p 407, 409)
4.3.5(A)	RK: principles of safe vehicle operation					Chapter 9 (p 200–204)
4.3.5(B)	RS: ability to use mirrors and judge vehicle clearance					Chapter 9 (p 203–204), Chapter 16 (p 404–405)
4.3.6	defensive driving					Chapter 10 (p 219–225, 238–239)
4.3.6(A)	RK: importance of donning passenger restraint devices and ensuring crew safety					Chapter 10 (p 219–225)
4.3.6(B)	RS: ability to operate passenger restraint devices					Chapter 10 (p 238–239)
4.3.7	fixed systems and equipment					Chapter 6 (p 102–106), Chapter 11 (p 246–250, 253–255, 257–274)
4.3.7(A)	RK: Manufacturer specifications and operating procedures					Chapter 6 (p 102–109, 111–115), Chapter 11 (p 246–250, 253–255, 257–272)
4.3.7(B)	RS: recognize and correct system problems					Chapter 6 (p 105–106), Chapter 11 (p 247–250, 254–255, 257–268, 271–274)
Chapter 5 Apparatus Equipped with Fire Pump						
5.1	requirements of Fire Fighter I as specified in NFPA 1001 or Advanced Exterior Industrial Fire Brigade Member or Interior Structural Fire Brigade Member as specified in NFPA 1081					Chapter 1 (p 8–13), Chapter 2 (p 26–28), Chapter 3 (p 37–38)
5.1.1	routine tests, inspections, and servicing functions					Chapter 6 (p 105, 107–109, 111–115), Chapter 8 (p 168–187), Chapter 14 (p 327–350), Chapter 19 (p 471–476, 480–504)
5.1.1(A)	RK: Manufacturer specifications					Chapter 3 (p 37–38), Chapter 8 (p 168–187), Chapter 19 (p 471–476, 481–504)
5.1.1(B)	RS: ability to use hand tools, recognize system problems, and correct any deficiency noted					Chapter 8 (p 168–187), Chapter 19 (p 471–474, 480–504)
5.2.1	Produce effective hand or master streams					Chapter 7 (p 121–147, 150–153, 156–162), Chapter 11 (p 246–250, 253–255, 257–274)
5.2.1(A)	RK: Hydraulic calculations and safe operation of the pump					Chapter 7 (p 121–127, 156–162), Chapter 11 (p 246–250, 253–255, 257–274)
5.2.1(B)	RS: position a fire department pumper to operate					Chapter 7 (p 124–147, 150–153, 158–162), Chapter 11 (p 247–250, 254–255, 257–268, 271–274)
5.2.2	Pump a supply line of 2½ in. (65 mm) or larger					Chapter 13 (p 312–321)
5.2.2(A)	RK: Hydraulic calculations and, safe operation of the pump					Chapter 13 (p 312–321)
5.2.2(B)	RS: position a fire department pumper					Chapter 13 (p 312–321)
5.2.3	Produce a foam fire stream					Chapter 14 (p 327–350)
5.2.3(A)	RK: proportioning rates and concentrations					Chapter 14 (p 327–350)
5.2.3(B)	RS: ability to operate foam proportioning equipment					Chapter 14 (p 334–343, 345–350)

SECTION	OBJECTIVE / JPR, RK, RS — ABBREVIATED TEXT	COGNITIVE WRITTEN TEST	MANIPULATIVE SKILLS STATION	PORTFOLIO	PROJECTS	OTHER
5.2.4	Supply water to fire sprinkler and standpipe systems					Chapter 6 (p 105–106), Chapter 7 (p 147, 149–155)
5.2.4(A)	RK: operating principles of sprinkler systems					Chapter 6 (p 105–106), Chapter 7 (p 147, 149–155)
5.2.4(B)	RS: position a fire department pumper to operate at a fire hydrant and at a static water source					Chapter 6 (p 105–106), Chapter 7 (p 147, 149–155)
Chapter 6 Apparatus Equipped with an Aerial Device						
6.1	requirements of Fire Fighter I as specified in NFPA 1001 or Advanced Exterior Industrial Fire Brigade Member or Interior Structural Fire Brigade Member as specified in NFPA 1081					Chapter 3 (p 42–44)
6.1.1	Perform the routine tests, inspections, and servicing functions					Chapter 8 (p 168–187), Chapter 15 (p 359–360, 363), Chapter 17 (p 422–429), Chapter 18 (p 436–440, 452, 454–458), Chapter 19 (p 471, 474–476)
6.1.1(A)	RK: Manufacturer specifications and requirements					Chapter 8 (p 168–187), Chapter 15 (p 363), Chapter 17 (p 422–429), Chapter 18 (p 436–440, 452, 454–458), Chapter 19 (p 471, 474–476)
6.1.1(B)	RS: ability to use hand tools, recognize system problems					Chapter 8 (p 168–187), Chapter 15 (p 363), Chapter 17 (p 422–429), Chapter 18 (p 434–460), Chapter 19 (p 471, 474–476)
6.2.1	Maneuver and position an aerial apparatus					Chapter 15 (p 364–367)
6.2.1(A)	RK: Capabilities and limitations of aerial devices					Chapter 3 (p 42–44), Chapter 15 (p 363–367)
6.2.1(B)	RS: appropriate position for the apparatus					Chapter 15 (p 363–367)
6.2.2	Stabilize an aerial apparatus					Chapter 15 (p 367–371)
6.2.2(A)	RK: hydraulic systems					Chapter 15 (p 359–360, 363–371)
6.2.2(B)	RS: transfer power					Chapter 15 (p 367–371)
6.2.3	Maneuver and position the aerial					Chapter 15 (p 364–367)
6.2.3(A)	RK: Aerial device hydraulic systems					Chapter 15 (p 359–360, 364–367, 371–375, 377–380)
6.2.3(B)	RS: raise, rotate, extend, and position					Chapter 15 (p 371–375, 377–384)
6.2.4	Lower an aerial device					Chapter 15 (p 388)
6.2.4(A)	RK: Aerial device hydraulic systems					Chapter 15 (p 359–360, 388)
6.2.4(B)	RS: rotate and position					Chapter 15 (p 388)
6.2.5	Deploy and operate an elevated master stream					Chapter 15 (p 384–389)
6.2.5(A)	RK: Nozzle reaction, range of operation, and weight limitations					Chapter 15 (p 384–389)
6.2.5(B)	RS: connect a water supply to a master stream device					Chapter 15 (p 384–389)
Chapter 7 Apparatus Equipped with a Tiller						
7.1	requirements of Fire Fighter I and Chapter 6 of NFPA 1002, 2009 edition					Chapter 3 (p 42–44), Chapter 16 (p 406–407), Chapter 17 (p 422–425, 427–429)

Appendix D

SECTION	OBJECTIVE / JPR, RK, RS — ABBREVIATED TEXT	COGNITIVE WRITTEN TEST	MANIPULATIVE SKILLS STATION	PORTFOLIO	PROJECTS	OTHER
7.2.1	Perform the practical driving exercises specified in 4.3.2 through 4.3.5 from the tiller position					Chapter 16 (p 404–409, 414–416), Chapter 17 (p 423–425, 427–429)
7.2.1(A)	RK: Capabilities and limitations of tiller aerial devices					Chapter 3 (p 42–44), Chapter 16 (p 406, 414–416), Chapter 17 (p 423–425, 427–428)
7.2.1(B)	RS: ability to determine a correct position for the tiller					Chapter 16 (p 400–401, 403–410, 412, 414–416), Chapter 17 (p 423–425, 427–429)
7.2.2	operate from tiller position					Chapter 16 (p 404–410, 412–416)
7.2.2(A)	RK: principles of tiller operation					Chapter 16 (p 400–410, 412), Chapter 17 (p 422–425, 427–429)
7.2.2(B)	RS: operate communications systems					Chapter 16 (p 400–410, 412–413, 415–416)
7.2.3	position the aerial from tiller position					Chapter 16 (p 406, 414–416), Chapter 17 (p 423–425, 427–429)
7.2.3(A)	RK: principles of positioning and stabilizing aerial from tiller position					Chapter 16 (p 413–416)
7.2.3(B)	RS: determine correct position for the tiller					Chapter 16 (p 400–401, 403–410, 412, 414–416), Chapter 17 (p 423–425, 427–429)
Chapter 10 Mobile Water Supply Apparatus						
10.1.1	tests, inspections, and servicing functions					Chapter 3 (p 41–42, 46–47), Chapter 8 (p 168–187), Chapter 19 (p 471–474, 480–504)
10.1.1(A)	RK: specifications and requirements, policies, and procedures					Chapter 3 (p 46–47), Chapter 8 (p 168–187)
10.1.1(B)	RS: use hand tools					Chapter 8 (p 168–187), Chapter 19 (p 471–474, 480–504)
10.2.1	Maneuver and position a mobile water supply apparatus at a water shuttle fill site					Chapter 12 (p 280–298, 300–302)
10.2.1(A)	RK: establishing a water shuttle fill site					Chapter 12 (p 280–298, 300–302)
10.2.1(B)	RS: correct position for the apparatus					Chapter 12 (p 290–296)
10.2.2	Maneuver and position a mobile water supply apparatus at a water shuttle dump site					Chapter 12 (p 287–298, 300–302)
10.2.2(A)	RK: operating a water shuttle dump site					Chapter 12 (p 287–298, 300–302)
10.2.2(B)	RS: position for the apparatus					Chapter 12 (p 290–296)
10.2.3	Establish a water shuttle dump site					Chapter 12 (p 302–306)
10.2.3(A)	RK: water shuttle dump site					Chapter 12 (p 302–306)
10.2.3(B)	RS: portable water tanks					Chapter 12 (p 302–306)

Glossary

activity area The area of the incident scene where the work activity takes place; it may be stationary or may move as work progresses.

actuator A device that converts the fluid pressure in a hydraulic rescue tool system into a mechanical force.

adapter Any device that allows fire hose couplings to be safely interconnected with couplings of different sizes, threads, or mating surfaces, or that allows fire hose couplings to be safely connected to other appliances.

additive A liquid such as foam concentrates, emulsifiers, and hazardous vapor suppression liquids and foaming agents intended to be added to the water.

adjustable-gallonage fog nozzle A nozzle that allows the operator to select a desired flow from several settings.

advance warning area The section of highway where drivers are informed about an upcoming situation ahead.

aeration The process of introducing air into the foam solution, which expands and finishes the foam.

aerial device An aerial ladder, elevating platform, aerial ladder platform, or water tower that is designed to position personnel, handle materials, provide continuous egress, or discharge water.

aerial fire apparatus A vehicle equipped with an aerial ladder, elevating platform, or water tower that is designed and equipped to support firefighting and rescue operations by positioning personnel, handling materials, providing continuous egress, or discharging water at positions elevated from the ground.

aerial ladder A self-supporting, turntable-mounted, power-operated ladder of two or more sections permanently attached to a self-propelled automotive fire apparatus and designed to provide a continuous egress route from an elevated position to the ground.

aerial ladder inspection With the ladder in bedded position, the aerial is tested by raising it to 60 degrees, rotating it 90 degrees to the left or right, and then fully extending it within 60 seconds while utilizing fast idle.

air pressure gauges Gauges that identify the air pressure stored in the tanks or reservoirs of an apparatus equipped with a pneumatic braking system.

aircraft rescue and firefighting (ARFF) vehicle A vehicle intended to carry rescue and firefighting equipment for rescuing occupants and combating fires in aircraft at, or in the vicinity of, an airport.

ambient air temperature The temperature of the surrounding medium. It typically refers to the temperature of the air in which a structure is situated or a device operates.

ambulance A vehicle designed, equipped, and operated for the treatment and transport of ill and injured persons.

angle of approach The smallest angle made between the road surface and a line drawn from the front point of ground contact of the front tire to any projection of the apparatus in front of the front axle. An angle of at least 8 degrees will be maintained on a fully loaded apparatus.

angle of departure The smallest angle made between the road surface and a line drawn from the rear point of ground contact of the rear tire to any projection of the apparatus behind the rear axle.

anti-siphon hole A very small hole in the fitting on top of the primer oil reservoir or in the top of the loop on the lubrication line leading to the priming pump.

apparatus inspection form A document that identifies who performed the inspection and when the fire apparatus inspection was performed, identifies any equipment that is damaged and/or repaired, and details other preventive maintenance procedures performed on the apparatus.

apparatus placement In regard to truck company operations, apparatus placement refers to how and where an apparatus is placed at the scene. Virtually all fire incidents require and utilize the support from apparatus in some way. The success of most fireground operations often depends, directly or indirectly, on the effective placement of fire apparatus.

aqueous Pertaining to, related to, similar to, or dissolved in water.

aqueous film-forming foam (AFFF) A concentrated aqueous solution of fluorinated surfactant(s) and foam stabilizers that is capable of producing an aqueous fluorocarbon film on the surface of hydrocarbon fuels to suppress vaporization.

around-the-pump proportioning (AP) system A fire apparatus–mounted foam system that diverts a portion of the water pump's output from the discharge side of the pump and sends it through an eductor to discharge foam.

articulated booms An aerial device consisting of two or more folding boom sections whose extension and retraction modes are accomplished by adjusting the angle of the knuckle joints.

Glossary

articulating platform An aerial device consisting of two or more booms connected at midsection by a hinge or swivel and equipped with an area where two to four fire fighters can stand and perform work.

assessment center A series of simulation exercises for a promotional examination.

atmospheric pressure Pressure caused by the weight of the atmosphere; equal to 14.7 psi (101 kPa) at sea level.

attack hose (attack line) Hose designed to be used by trained fire fighters and fire brigade members to combat fires beyond the incipient stage.

attack pumper An engine from which attack lines have been pulled.

authority having jurisdiction (AHJ) An organization, office, or individual responsible for enforcing the requirements of a code or standard, or for approving equipment, materials, an installation, or a procedure.

automatic intake pressure relief device A device installed on the supply side of a valve to bleed off excessive pressure coming into the valve.

automatic load management system A system designed to protect the electrical system from needless damage while maintaining the operation of essential devices.

automatic-adjusting fog nozzle A nozzle that can deliver a wide range of water stream flows. It operates by means of an internal spring-loaded piston.

auxiliary appliance A standpipe and/or sprinkler system.

backlash In the case of the aerial device, the motion that occurs when rotating the aerial, and when the bull gear and turntable bearing have play in the gear spacing. The aerial will rock slightly back and forth if there is excessive end-play or backlash.

balanced-pressure system A fire apparatus–mounted foam system that uses a diaphragm-type pressure control valve to sense and balance the pressures in the foam concentrate and water lines to the proportioner.

ball valve A type of valve used on nozzles, gated wyes, and engine discharge gates. It consists of a ball with a hole in the middle of the ball.

bankshot (bankdown) method A method that applies the foam stream onto a nearby object, such as a wall, instead of directly at the fire.

batch mixing Pouring foam concentrate directly into the fire apparatus water tank, thereby mixing a large amount of foam at one time.

battery selector switch A switch used to disconnect all electrical power to the vehicle, thereby preventing discharge of the battery while the vehicle is not in use.

beam The horizontal component of an H-style jack or outrigger system. The jack is welded to the end of the beam.

big-box A large, free-standing commercial structure generally in excess of 100,000 square feet of floor space.

blind spots Areas around the fire apparatus that are not visible to the driver/operator.

booster hose (booster line) A noncollapsible hose that is used under positive pressure and that consists of an elastomeric or thermoplastic tube, a braided or spiraled reinforcement, and an outer protective cover.

booster line A rigid hose that is ¾ inches (20 mm) or 1 inches (25 mm) in diameter. Such a hose delivers water at a rate of only 30 to 60 gpm (115 to 225 L), but can do so at high pressures.

booster pump A water pump mounted on the fire apparatus in addition to a fire pump and used for firefighting either in conjunction with or independent of the fire pump.

brake fade Reduction in stopping power that can occur after repeated application of the brakes, especially in high-load or high-speed conditions.

braking distance The distance that the fire apparatus travels from the time the brakes are activated until the fire apparatus makes a complete stop.

Bresnan distributor nozzle A nozzle that can be placed in confined spaces. The nozzle spins, spreading water over a large area.

British thermal unit (Btu) The quantity of heat required to raise the temperature of one pound of water by 1°F at the pressure of 1 atmosphere and a temperature of 60°F. A British thermal unit is equal to 1055 joules, 1.055 kilojoules, and 252.15 calories.

bucket brigade An early effort at fire protection that used leather buckets filled with water to combat fires. In many communities, residents were required to place a bucket filled with water, typically on their front steps, at night in case of a fire in the community.

buffer space The lateral and/or longitudinal area that separates traffic flow from a work space or an unsafe area; it might also provide some recovery space for an errant vehicle.

burnback resistance The ability of a foam blanket to resist direct flame impingement.

butterfly valve A valve found on the large pump intake valve where the hard suction or soft sleeve hose connects to it.

bypass eductor A foam eductor that is mounted to the pump and can be used for application of either water or foam.

cavitation A condition caused by attempting to move water faster than it is being supplied to the pump.

cellar nozzle A nozzle used to fight fires in cellars and other inaccessible places.

centrifugal force The outward force that is exerted away from the center of rotation or the tendency for objects to be pulled outward when rotating around a center.

centrifugal pump A pump in which the pressure is developed principally by the action of centrifugal force.

changeover operation The process of transferring from use of the pumper's internal water tank to use of an external water source.

chart A document summarizing the typical handline and master stream calculations for the hoses, nozzles, and devices specific to the fire apparatus. It lists the most commonly used or reasonably expected hose lays.

chassis The basic operating motor vehicle, including the engine, frame, and other essential structural and mechanical parts, but exclusive of the body and all appurtenances for the accommodation of driver, property, passengers, appliances, or equipment related to other than control. Common usage might, but need not, include a cab (or cowl).

chemical foam Foam produced by mixing powders and water, where a chemical reaction of the materials creates the foam.

chemical wagon A small truck constructed with a large soda acid extinguisher and 50 ft (15 m) or more of small hose (booster line size).

Class A foam Foam intended for use on Class A fires.

Class B foam Foam intended for use on Class B fires.

Code 1 response Response in a fire apparatus in which no emergency lights or sirens are activated.

Code 2 response Response in a fire apparatus in which only the emergency lights are activated; no audible devices are activated.

Code 3 response Response in a fire apparatus in which both the emergency lights and the sirens are activated.

coefficient (C) A numerical measure that is a constant for a specified hose diameter.

collapse zone A distance away from a structure equal to or greater than 1.5 times its height.

collector rings The electric bands inside the swivel that allow two-way contact with wires going from the top of the swivel and wires exiting from the bottom. The ring is internal to the swivel, and it has two contacts points for electric transfer.

combination tool A powered rescue tool that is capable of at least spreading and cutting.

combustible liquid Any liquid that has a closed-cup flash point at or greater than 100°F (37.8°C) as determined by the test procedures and apparatus set forth in Section 4.4. Combustible liquids are classified according to Section 4.3.

command vehicle A vehicle that the fire chief uses to respond to the fire scene.

commercial driver's license A government-issued license that ensures the driver has met the requirements to operate certain types of commercial vehicles depending on the weight of the vehicle, the number of passengers, and the presence (or not) of any hazardous materials.

communication The verbal coordination that occurs between the driver/operator controlling the tractor portion of the apparatus and the tiller operator who is responsible for control of the trailer portion of the apparatus. It is important that the driver/operator and tiller operator are in good communication at all times.

communications center A building or portion of a building that is specifically configured for the primary purpose of providing emergency communications services or public safety answering point (PSAP) services to one or more public safety agencies under the authority or authorities having jurisdiction.

compressed-air foam system (CAFS) A foam system that combines compressed air and a foam solution to create firefighting foam.

concentration The percentage of foam chemical contained in a foam solution.

condensed Q method Fireground method used to quickly calculate friction loss in 3-inch (77-mm) to 5-inch (125-mm) hoselines.

control zones A series of areas at hazardous materials incidents that are designated based on safety concerns and the degree of hazard present.

corner safe areas Areas outside a building where two walls intersect; these areas are less likely to receive any damage during a building collapse.

crack pressure The pressure at which a pressure-operated valve begins to pass fluid.

critical rate of flow The essential flow, measured in gallons per minute, that is needed to overcome the heat generated by a fire.

critical speed Maximum speed that a fire apparatus can safely travel around a curve.

cutter A powered rescue tool with at least one movable blade that is used to cut, shear, or sever material.

deflection The downward movement of an aerial device boom or ladder caused by its extension or the imposition of load such as fire fighters or victims climbing on the ladder or into the platform.

dependable lift The height that a column of water can be lifted in a quantity considered sufficient to provide reliable fire flow.

dip stick A graduated instrument for measuring the depth or amount of fluid in a container, such as the level of oil in a crankcase.

discharge header The piping and valves on the discharge side of the pump.

discharge pressure The water pressure on the discharge manifold of the fire pump at the point of gauge attachment.

discharge pressure relief valve A device to control pressure by passing water from the discharge side of the pump back into the intake side of the pump.

discharge side The side of a pump where water is discharged from the pump.

discontinuity A welding term used to indicate that inspectors have found a flaw or uneven weld. It is corrected by a certified welder with permission and instructions from the OEM.

dispatch To send out emergency response resources promptly to an address or incident location for a specific purpose.

distributors Relatively small-diameter underground pipes that deliver water to local users within a neighborhood.

double-acting lifting cylinder A cylinder in which fluid pressure can be applied to the movable piston rod in either direction.

double-acting piston pump A positive-displacement pump that discharges water on both the upward and downward strokes of the piston.

double-female adapter A hose adapter that is used to join two male hose couplings.

double-male adapter A hose adapter that is used to join two female hose couplings.

downriggers Mechanical devices, usually hydraulically powered, that exert downward force onto the ground and distribute the aerial apparatus' load over a large surface area, effectively stabilizing the vehicle so as to permit its aerial device to be raised, extended, and rotated without collapse.

draft The pressure differential that causes water flow.

driver/operator A person having satisfactorily completed the requirements of driver/operator as specified in NFPA 1002, *Standard for Fire Apparatus Driver/Operator Professional Qualifications*.

dry hydrant An arrangement of pipes that is permanently connected to a water source other than a piped, pressurized water supply system; it provides a ready means of water supply for firefighting purposes, and takes advantage of the drafting (suction) capability of fire department pumpers.

dry-barrel hydrant The most common type of hydrant; it has a control valve below the frost line between the footpiece and the barrel. A drain is located at the bottom of the barrel above the control valve seat for proper drainage after operation.

due regard The care exercised by a reasonably prudent person under the same circumstances.

dump line A small-diameter hoseline that remains in the open position and flowing water during the entire drafting operation.

dump site A location where a fire apparatus can offload the water in its tank.

dump valve A large opening from the water tank of a mobile water supply apparatus that is used for unloading purposes.

duplex gauge A gauge at the pump panel that simultaneously monitors both the foam concentrate and water pressures.

eductor A device that uses the Venturi principle to siphon a liquid in a water stream. The pressure at the throat of the device is below atmospheric pressure, allowing liquid at atmospheric pressure to flow into the water stream.

electronic pump controller A device to control the engine and pump speed by means of a digital panel.

elevated platform An extendable boom or ladder equipped with an area where two to four fire fighters can stand and perform work. Includes tower ladders and ladder towers.

elevated water storage tower An above-ground water storage tank that is designed to maintain pressure on a water distribution system.

elevation gain The pressure gained when the nozzle is below the pump; it requires pressure to be subtracted from the discharge pressure.

elevation loss The pressure lost when the nozzle is above the pump; it requires pressure to be added to the discharge pressure to compensate for the loss.

elevation pressure (EP) In hydraulic calculations, the distance the nozzle is above or below the pump. The amount of pressure created by gravity.

emergency power unit (EPU) A device that makes hydraulic power from an auxiliary source pump installed on the aerial. This pump is intended for emergency cradling of the device only.

emergency vehicle technician (EVT) An individual who performs inspections, maintenance, and operational checks on emergency response vehicles and who, by possession of a recognized certificate, professional standing, or skill, has acquired the knowledge, training, and experience and has demonstrated the ability to deal with issues related to the subject matter, the work, or the project.

emitter A device that emits a visible flashing light at a specified frequency, thereby activating the receiver on a traffic signal.

exhaust primer A means of priming a centrifugal pump by using the fire apparatus' exhaust to create a vacuum and draw air and water from the pump.

extension ram A powered rescue tool with a piston or other type extender that generates extending forces or both extending and retracting forces.

extractor exhaust system A system used inside the fire apparatus bay that connects to the fire apparatus -tailpipe and draws its exhaust outside the building.

extruded A descriptor for a part that is forced through a mold very similar to a cookie press. In extrusion, steel or aluminum is pushed through a dye and comes out in a predetermined shape. Most aluminum ladder rungs are produced through this process.

failure A cessation of proper functioning or performance.

feather To operate the controls of a hydraulic device by slowly and smoothly opening and closing the valves; it comes from the expression "as smooth as a feather."

fill site A location where the fire apparatus can get water tanks filled.

film-forming fluoroprotein foam (FFFP) A protein-based foam concentrate incorporating fluorinated surfactants, which forms a foam capable of producing a vapor-suppressing, aqueous film on the surface of hydrocarbon fuels. This foam may have an acceptable level of compatibility with dry chemicals and may be suitable for use with those agents.

finished foam The homogeneous blanket of foam obtained by mixing water, foam concentrate, and air.

fire apparatus A fire department emergency vehicle used for rescue, fire suppression, or other specialized functions.

fire apparatus inspection An evaluation of the fire apparatus and its equipment that is intended to ensure its safe operation.

fire barrier A continuous membrane or a membrane with discontinuities created by protected openings with a specified fire protection rating. Such a membrane is designed and constructed with a specified fire resistance rating to limit the spread of fire, which also restricts the movement of smoke.

fire department connection (FDC) A connection through which the fire department can pump supplemental water into the sprinkler system, standpipe, or other system, thereby furnishing water for fire extinguishment to supplement existing water supplies.

fire department vehicle Any vehicle, including fire apparatus, operated by a fire department.

fire hook A tool used to pull down burning structures.

fire hose appliance A piece of hardware (excluding nozzles) generally intended for connection to fire hose to control or convey water.

fire plug A valve installed to control water accessed from wooden pipes.

fire pump A water pump with a rated capacity of 250 gpm (1000 L/min) or greater at 150 psi (1034 kPa) net pump pressure that is mounted on an fire apparatus and used for firefighting.

fire pump (fire apparatus) A device that provides for liquid flow and pressure and that is dedicated to fire protection.

fireground hydraulics Simpler fireground methods for performing hydraulic calculations.

fixed-gallonage fog nozzle A nozzle that delivers a set number of gallons per minute as per the nozzle's design, no matter what pressure is applied to the nozzle.

flammable liquid Any liquid that has a closed-cup flash point less than 100°F (37.8°C), as determined by the test procedures and apparatus set forth in Section 4.4, and a Reid vapor pressure that does not exceed an absolute pressure of 40 psi (276 kPa) at 100°F (37.8°C), as determined by ASTM D 323, Standard Test Method for Vapor Pressure of Petroleum Products (Reid Method). Flammable liquids are classified according to Section 4.3.

floodlights Lights that project a more diffuse light over a wide area.

flow meter A device for measuring volumetric flow rates of gases and liquids.

flow pressure Forward pressure at a discharge opening while water is flowing.

flow rate The volume of water moving through the nozzle measured in gallons per minute or liters per minute.

fluoroprotein foam (FP) A protein-based foam concentrate to which fluorochemical surfactants have been added. The resulting product has a measurable degree of compatibility with dry chemical extinguishing agents and an increased tolerance to contamination by fuel.

foam A stable aggregation of small bubbles of lower density than oil or water, which exhibits a tenacity for covering horizontal surfaces. Air foam is made by mixing air into a water solution containing a foam concentrate, by means of suitably designed equipment. It flows freely over a burning liquid surface and forms a tough, air-excluding, continuous blanket that seals volatile combustible vapors from access to air.

foam concentrate (foam liquid) A concentrated liquid foaming agent as received from the manufacturer.

foam heat exchanger A device that uses water as its cooling source and prevents the foam concentrate from overheating.

foam proportioner A device or method to add foam concentrate to water so as to make foam solution.

foam solution A homogeneous mixture of water and foam concentrate added in the proper proportions.

foam system A system provided on fire apparatus for the delivery of a proportioned foam and water mixture for use in fire extinguishment. The system includes a concentrate tank, a method for removing the concentrate from the tank, a foam-liquid proportioning system, and a method (e.g., handlines or fixed turret nozzles) of delivering the proportioned foam to the fire.

foam tetrahedron A geometric shape used to illustrate the four elements needed to produce finished foam: foam concentrate, water, air, and mechanical aeration.

fog-stream nozzle A nozzle that is placed at the end of a fire hose and separates water into fine droplets to aid in heat absorption.

forward lay A method of laying a supply line in which the line starts at the water source and ends at the attack pumper.

four-way hydrant valve A specialized type of valve that can be placed on a hydrant and is used in conjunction with a pumper to increase water pressure in relaying operations.

friction loss (FA) The reduction in pressure resulting from the water being in contact with the side of the hose. This contact requires force to overcome the drag that the wall of the hoses creates.

front mount An apparatus pump that is permanently mounted to the front bumper of the apparatus and is directly connected to the motor.

fuel gauge A gauge that indicates the amount of fuel in the fire apparatus' fuel tank.

fuel pick-up The absorption of the burning fuel into the foam itself.

fuel resistance A foam's ability to minimize fuel pick-up.

full-jacking The complete extension and setting of all stabilizers on an aerial apparatus.

gate valve A type of valve found on hydrants and sprinkler systems.

gated wye A valved device that splits a single hose into two separate hoses, allowing each hose to be turned on and off independently.

gating a valve Opening a valve just enough to deliver the desired pressure.

generator An engine-powered device that creates electricity.

global positioning system (GPS) A satellite-based radio navigation system consisting of three segments: space, control, and user.

Grade D air An air quality content measurement for breathing air supplied to self-contained breathing apparatus.

gravity-feed system A water distribution system that depends on gravity to provide the required pressure. The system storage is usually located at a higher elevation than the end users of the water.

hand lay A process in which the engine is positioned close to the fire scene and the driver/operator deploys the supply hose from the bed of the fire apparatus to the hydrant either alone or with very little assistance from other fire fighters.

hand pump A piston-driven, positive-displacement pump that is pushed up and down by fire fighters manning poles at the side of the pump.

handline nozzle A nozzle with a rated discharge of less than 350 gpm (1325 L/min).

hard suction hose A hose used for drafting water from static supplies (e.g., lakes, rivers, wells). It can also be used for supplying pumpers from a hydrant if designed for that purpose. The hose contains a semi-rigid or rigid reinforcement designed to prevent collapse of the hose under vacuum.

hardness The mineral content of the water; it usually consists of calcium and magnesium, but can also include iron, aluminum, and manganese.

heat of vaporization The energy required to transform a given quantity of a substance into a gas.

heel pins Slang term for the pivot pins that attach the ladder base rail to the turntable and allow the ladder a pivot point when raised and lowered.

high idle switch A switch that sets the apparatus engine to run at 900–1100 rpm.

high-expansion foam Any foam with an expansion ratio in the range of 200:1 to approximately 1000:1.

horizontal height The span from the heel pin or centerline of the truck to the outermost reach of the aerial ladder. The horizontal reach is less than the vertical or working height of the unit.

hose clamp A device used to compress a fire hose so as to stop water flow.

hose jacket A device used to stop a leak in a fire hose or to join hoses that have damaged couplings.

hydraulic reservoir A container that stores hydraulic fluid until it is needed in the system.

hydraulics The study of the characteristics and movement of water as they pertain to calculations for fire streams and fireground operations.

hydrocarbon A chemical substance consisting of only hydrogen and carbon atoms.

hydroelectric swivel A common rotation point in the aerial where hydro/water and hydraulic fluids can be transferred from the lower system through a rotating aerial. The electrical system as well as a straight-through water pipe is included in the unit. Also called simply the "swivel."

hydrolysis Decomposition of a chemical compound by reaction with water.

ignition switch A switch that engages operational power to the chassis of a motor vehicle.

impeller A metal rotating component that transfers energy from the fire apparatus' motor to discharge the incoming water from a pump.

impeller vanes Sections that divide the impeller.

incident space The area where the actual incident is located.

induction The use of an eductor to introduce a proportionate amount of foam concentrate into a stream of water flowing from a discharge.

initial attack fire apparatus Fire apparatus with a fire pump of at least 250 gpm (1000 L/min) capacity, water tank, and hose body, whose primary purpose is to initiate a fire suppression attack on structural, vehicular, or vegetation fires, and to support associated fire department operations.

injection system A foam system installed on a fire apparatus that meters out foam by pumping or injecting it into the fire stream.

intake pressure The pressure on the intake passageway of the pump at the point of gauge attachment.

intake side The side of a pump where water enters the pump.

intermediate traffic incident A traffic incident that affects the lanes of travel for 30 minutes to 2 hours.

inverter An appliance that converts 12-volt DC (direct current) from a vehicle's electrical system to 110-volt AC power.

jack box The vertical piece welded to the beam that houses the actual jack or outrigger cylinder. The outer jack box is welded to the beam, and a movable inner jack box that is slightly smaller than the outer box moves up and down when the stabilizer jacks are set.

jacks Mechanical devices, usually hydraulically powered, that exert downward force onto the ground and distribute the aerial apparatus' load over a large surface area, effectively stabilizing the vehicle so as to permit its aerial device to be raised, extended, and rotated without collapse.

jet siphon An appliance that connects a 1½- or 1¾-inch (38- or 45-mm) hose to a hard-sided hose coupling and creates a pathway for flowing water that is being forced through the hose by Venturi forces.

job aids A tool, device, or system used to assist a person with executing specific tasks.

junction box A device that attaches to an electrical cord to provide additional outlets.

kinetic energy The energy possessed by an object as a result of its motion.

knockdown speed and flow The time required for a foam blanket to spread out across a fuel surface.

ladder stops The parts of the aerial device that allow each section to stop and keep from over-retracting or overextending the unit; usually a steel bar or a bolt that is adjustable and will stop the ladder's movement.

ladder tower An aerial ladder with a work platform permanently attached to the end of the ladder.

large-diameter hose (LDH) A hose of 3½ inches (90 mm) size or larger.

Level I staging Initial staging of fire apparatus in which three or more units are dispatched to an emergency incident.

Level II staging Placement of all reserve resources in a central location until requested to the scene.

lift The vertical height that water must be raised during a drafting operation, measured from the surface of a static source of water to the center line of the pump intake.

liquid surge The force imposed upon a fire apparatus by the contents of a partially filled water or foam concentrate tank when the vehicle is accelerated, decelerated, or turned.

load monitor A component designed to prevent any additional electrical loads from exceeding the apparatus electrical system's capabilities.

load sequencer A component that activates electrical loads in a specific order to prevent overloading the electrical system.

load shedding A component that deactivates unnecessary electrical loads in order of necessity and thereby prevents damage to the electrical system.

low-expansion foam Any foam with an expansion ratio up to 20:1.

low-volume nozzle A nozzle that flows 40 gpm (150 L/min) or less.

major traffic incident A traffic incident that involves a fatal crash, a multiple-vehicle incident, a hazardous materials incident on the highway, or other disaster.

manifold An appliance that allows a large-diameter hoseline to be split into four or five medium-size hoselines.

manual throttle control A device to control the engine speed and pump speed.

master stream A portable or fixed firefighting appliance supplied by either hoselines or fixed piping that has the capability of flowing in excess of 350 gpm (1325 L/min) of water or a water-based extinguishing agent.

master stream device A large-capacity nozzle supplied by two or more hoselines of fixed piping that can flow 300 gpm (1135 L/min). These devices include deck guns and portable ground monitors.

master stream nozzle A nozzle with a rated discharge of 350 gpm (1325 L/min) or greater.

mechanical foam Foam produced by physical agitation of a mixture of water, air, and a foaming agent.

mechanical generator An electrically powered fan used to aerate certain types of foams.

medium-diameter hose (MDH) Hose with a diameter of 2½ inches (65 mm) or 3 inches (77 mm).

medium-expansion foam Any foam with an expansion ratio in the range of 20:1 to 200:1.

medium-size hose Hose that is 2½ or 3 inches (65 or 77 mm) in diameter.

metering device A device that controls the flow of foam concentrate into the eductor.

minor traffic incident A traffic incident that involves a minor crash and/or disabled vehicles.

miscellaneous equipment Portable tools and equipment carried on a fire apparatus, not including suction hose, fire hose, ground ladders, fixed power sources, hose reels, cord reels, breathing air systems, or other major equipment or components specified by the purchaser to be permanently mounted on the apparatus as received from the apparatus manufacturer.

miscible Readily mixes with water.

mobile data terminal (MDT) A computer that is located on the fire apparatus.

mobile foam fire apparatus Fire apparatus with a permanently mounted fire pump, foam proportioning system, and foam concentrate tank(s), whose primary purpose is use in the control and extinguishment of flammable and combustible liquid fires in storage tanks and other flammable liquid spills.

mobile water supply apparatus A vehicle designed primarily for transporting (pickup, transporting, and delivering) water to fire emergency scenes to be applied by other vehicles or pumping equipment. Also known as a tanker or tender.

motor vehicle accident (MVA) An incident that involves one vehicle colliding with another vehicle or another object and that may result in injury, property damage, and possibly death.

multiplexed A system that uses digital communications via a communication wire to turn systems on and off. Such a system eliminates extensive wiring in the vehicle and can be programmed to enact interlocks and safety shutdowns when certain parameters programmed into the system are met.

multiplexing Combining several different sensors or controls into one panel.

municipal water system A government-owned and -operated water distribution system that is designed to deliver potable water to end users for domestic, industrial, and fire protection purposes.

net pump discharge pressure (NPDP) The amount of pressure created by the pump after receiving pressure from a hydrant or another pump.

net pump pressure (NPP) The sum of the discharge pressure and the suction lift converted to units of pounds per square inch (psi) or kilopascals (kPa) when pumping at draft, or the difference between the discharge pressure and the intake pressure when pumping at a hydrant or other source of water under positive pressure.

nondestructive testing (NDT) One of several methods used to inspect a structural component without physically altering or damaging the material.

normal operating pressure The observed static pressure in a water distribution system during a period of normal demand.

nozzle A constricting appliance attached to the end of a fire hose or monitor to increase the water velocity and form a stream.

nozzle pressure (NP) The pressure required at the inlet of a nozzle to produce the desired water discharge characteristics.

nozzle shut-off A device that enables the fire fighter at the nozzle to start or stop the flow of water.

nurse tanker operation The process of supplying water to an attack engine directly by a supply engine.

oil pressure gauge A gauge that identifies the pressure of the lubricating oil in the fire apparatus engine.

oleophobic Oil hating; having the ability to shed hydrocarbon liquids.

original equipment manufacturer (OEM) The manufacturer of the device or apparatus.

outrigger interlock The system that prevents ladder operations from occurring until the outriggers are properly set. The device must be fully and correctly deployed before the outrigger interlock will allow the aerial system to energize. In a short-set scenario, the outrigger interlock interfaces with the rotation interlock; initiating any ladder movement requires the driver/operator to override the short-set outriggers.

outriggers Mechanical devices, usually hydraulically powered, that exert downward force onto the ground and distribute the aerial apparatus' load over a large surface area, effectively stabilizing the vehicle so as to permit its aerial device to be raised, extended, and rotated without collapse.

over-steering Allowing the trailer to swing out or move past an in-line position after a turn is completed.

over-tillering The occurrence when the tiller operator turns the steering wheel unnecessarily.

overhang The portion of the trailer that extends from the center of the trailer wheels (pivot point) to the rear of the trailer. It is important to allow enough room for the overhang to clear both sides of the trailer.

oxygenated Treated, combined, or infused with oxygen.

parallel/volume mode Positioning of a two-stage pump in which each impeller takes water in from the same intake area and discharges it to the same discharge area. This mode is used when pumping water at the rated capacity of the pump.

parking brake The main brake that prevents a fire apparatus from moving even when it is turned off and there is no one operating it.

performance testing Tests conducted after a fire apparatus has been put into service to determine if its performance meets predetermined specifications or standards.

physical rescue An act that requires multiple fire fighters to move a victim onto and off of an aerial device when the victim is unable to do so alone.

pick-up tube The tube from an in-line foam eductor that is placed in the foam bucket and draws foam concentrate into the eductor using the Venturi principle.

piercing nozzle A nozzle that can be driven through sheet metal or other material to deliver a water stream to that area.

pilot-operated check (POC) valve A hydraulic spring-operated valve; also referred to as a holding valve. It keeps fluid locked in a cylinder until the hydraulic pilot pressure releases the spring check and fluid can pass through and move the cylinder. When the pilot pressure is released, the check spring part of the valve closes and locks the fluid in, holding the cylinder in place.

piston intake valve (PIV) A large appliance that connects directly to the pump's intake and controls the amount of water that flows from a pressurized water source into the pump.

piston pump A positive-displacement pump that operates in an up-and-down action.

Pitot gauge A type of gauge that is used to measure the velocity pressure of water that is being discharged from an opening. It is used to determine the flow of water from a hydrant.

polar solvent A combustible liquid that mixes with the water contained in foam. Such solvents include non-petroleum-based fuels such as alcohol, lacquers, acetone, and acids.

polymer A naturally occurring or synthetic compound consisting of large molecules made up of a linked series of repeated simple monomers.

portable floating pump A small fire pump that is equipped with a flotation device and built-in strainer, capable of being carried by hand and flowing various quantities of water depending on its size.

portable master stream device A master stream device that may be removed from a fire apparatus, typically to be placed in service on the ground.

portable pump A type of pump that is typically carried by hand by two or more fire fighters to a water source and used to pump water from that source.

portable tank Any closed vessel having a liquid capacity in excess of 60 gal (240 L), but less than 1000 gal (4000 L), which is not intended for fixed installation.

positive-displacement pump A pump that is characterized by a method of producing flow by capturing a specific volume of fluid per pump revolution and reducing the fluid void by a mechanical means to displace the pumping fluid.

potential energy The energy that an object has stored up as a result of its position or condition. A raised weight and a coiled spring have potential energy.

power rescue tool A tool that receives power from the power unit component and generates energy used to perform one or more of the following functions: spreading, lifting, holding, crushing, pulling, or cutting.

power rescue tool system The combination of a reservoir, fluid, power unit, enclosed system, and an actuator used to operate a power rescue tool.

power steering system A system for reducing the steering effort on vehicles in which an external power source assists in turning the vehicle's wheels.

power take-off (PTO) A small gear case that uses an internal gear connected to the main transmission to take power from the main transmission and transmit it, when engaged, to an auxiliary system such as a hydraulic pump for a generator or an aerial device.

power take-off (PTO) unit A direct means of powering a pump with the fire apparatus' transmission and through a shaft directed to the gear case on the pump.

power unit A prime mover and the principal power output device used to power a rescue tool.

preincident plan A document developed by gathering general and detailed data, which is then used by responding personnel to determine the resources and actions necessary to mitigate anticipated emergencies at a specific facility.

prepiped elevated master stream An aerial ladder with a fixed waterway attached to the underside of the ladder, with a water inlet at the base supplying a master stream device at the tip.

pressure governor A device that controls the engine speed, which relates directly to the net pump pressure.

pressure-regulating valve (PRV) The type of valve found in a multistory building, which is designed to limit the pressure at a discharge so as to prevent excessive elevation pressures under both flowing (residual) and nonflowing (static) conditions.

preventive maintenance program A program designed to ensure that apparatus are capable of functioning as required and are maintained in working order.

primary feeder The largest-diameter pipe in a water distribution system, which carries the largest amount of water.

prime the pump To expel all air from a pump.

primer oil reservoir A small tank that holds the lubricant for the priming pump.

priming The process of removing air from a fire pump and replacing it with water.

private water system A privately owned water system that operates separately from the municipal water system.

proportioned Descriptor for a combination of foam concentrate and water used to form a foam solution.

protein foam Foam created from a concentrate that consists primarily of products from a protein hydrolysate, plus stabilizing additives and inhibitors to protect against freezing, to prevent corrosion of equipment and containers, to resist bacterial decomposition, to control viscosity, and to otherwise ensure readiness for use under emergency conditions.

pump discharge pressure (PDP) The pressure measured at the pump discharge needed to overcome friction and elevation loss while maintaining the desired nozzle pressure and delivering an adequate fire stream.

pump operator's panel The gauges, instruments, and controls necessary to operate the pump.

pump-mounted eductor An in-line eductor dedicated to the production of foam.

pumper fire apparatus Fire apparatus with a permanently mounted fire pump of at least 750 gpm (3000 L/min) capacity, water tank, and hose body, whose primary purpose is to combat structural and associated fires.

pumping element A rotating device such as a gear or vane encased in the pump casing of a rotary pump.

quint Fire apparatus with a permanently mounted fire pump, a water tank, a hose storage area, an aerial ladder or elevating platform with a permanently mounted waterway, and a complement of ground ladders.

radiator cap The pressure cap that is screwed onto the top of the radiator, and through which coolant is typically added.

raindown method A method of applying foam that directs the stream into the air above the fire and allows it to gently fall onto the surface.

raise–rotate–extend The recommended sequence to operate an aerial device.

rated capacity The total amount of weight that can be supported at the outermost rung of an aerial ladder or on an elevated platform with an uncharged waterway.

rated capacity (water pump) The flow rate to which the pump manufacturer certifies compliance of the pump when it is new.

ratio controller A device required for each foam outlet to proportion the correct amount of foam concentrate into the water stream over a wide range of flows and with minimal pressure loss.

reaction distance The distance that the fire apparatus travels after the driver/operator recognizes the hazard, removes his or her foot from the accelerator, and applies the brakes.

receiver A device placed on or near a traffic signal to recognize a signal from the emitter on an emergency vehicle and preempt the normal cycle of the traffic light.

reducer A device that connects two hoses with different couplings or threads together.

relay or hydrant valve A specialized type of valve that can be placed on a hydrant and is used in conjunction with a pumper to increase water pressure in relaying operations.

relay pumping operation The process of moving water from a water source through hose to the place where it will be needed.

relay valve A specialized type of valve that can be placed on a hydrant and is used in conjunction with a pumper to increase water pressure in relaying operations.

rescue position The position of the movable monitor when it is pinned or latched to the outer midsection of the aerial device. It allows a clean bottom for ladder placement into windows or over roof ledges or cornices. The monitor and the waterway pipe are essentially out of the way. Most departments leave their monitors in this position in case they must immediately begin to remove victims from a fire when they arrive on scene. If the fire goes to a water tower or defensive operation, there is time to reset the monitor position.

rescue profile The experience-based determination of victim survivability and the ability of fire fighters to attempt a rescue when all facts and circumstances are considered.

reservoir A water storage facility.

residual pressure The pressure that exists in the distribution system, measured at the residual hydrant at the time the flow readings are taken at the flow hydrant.

reverse lay A method of laying a supply line in which the line starts at the attack pumper and ends at the water source.

rotary gear pump A positive-displacement pump that uses two gears encased inside a pump casing to move water under pressure.

rotary pump A positive-displacement pump that operates in a circular motion.

rotary vane pump A positive-displacement pump characterized by the use of a single rotor with vanes that move with pump rotation to create a void and displace liquid.

rotation interlock A device that interfaces with the outrigger interlock after a short-set signal is received. The driver/operator uses an override switch to move the aerial, and an indicator light at the pedestal indicates which side is short-set. The driver/operator will be able to move the aerial to the fully deployed side in a 180-degree arc on the properly set side. If the driver/operator attempts to maneuver the aerial so that it crosses the centerline of the truck at the front or the rear, the rotation interlock will shut down the rotation hydraulic circuit to prevent a potential ladder rollover. The driver/operator can then go back to the properly set side. If the driver/operator cannot move the aerial in some circumstances, another manual control valve must be pushed to return the aerial to the safe side.

rotor A metal device that houses the vanes in a rotary vane pump.

scrub or sweep area The total area of a one or more walls of a building, both width and height, that can be effectively reached by an extended aerial device without repositioning the chassis.

secondary feeder A smaller-diameter pipe that connects the primary feeder to the distributors.

series/pressure mode Positioning of a two-stage pump in which the first impeller sends water into the second impeller's intake side and water is then discharged out the pump's discharge header, thereby creating more pressure with less flow.

service testing Tests conducted after a fire apparatus has been put into service to determine if its performance meets predetermined specifications or standards.

setback The distance between the wall of a building and an improved surface (such as a road or parking lot) from which an aerial device can be positioned and operate.

short-jacking The complete extension and setting of the stabilizers on one side of an aerial apparatus, while the opposite-side stabilizers are not completely extended outward before they are set down to stabilize the apparatus.

short-set A situation in which the aerial is intentionally or unintentionally set without all of the outriggers, beams, and jacks deployed to their maximum reach. This setup is used when streets or obstructions limit the space available so that the device cannot fully extend a beam or jack setup. The driver/operator is then forced to override all ladder actions and is limited to operations over the side that is fully and correctly deployed.

shut-off valve Any valve that can be used to shut down water flow to a water user or system.

Siamese connection A device that allows two hoses to be connected together and flow into a single hose.

single-acting piston pump A positive-displacement pump that discharges water only on the downward stroke of the piston.

single-stage pump A pump that has one impeller that takes the water in and discharges it out using only one impeller.

small-diameter hose (SDH) Hose with a diameter ranging from 1 inch (25 mm) to 2 inches (50 mm).

smooth-bore nozzle A nozzle that produces a straight stream that consists of a solid column of water.

smooth-bore tip A nozzle device that is a smooth tube and is used to deliver a solid column of water.

soft sleeve hose A large-diameter hose that is designed to be connected to the large port on a hydrant (steamer connection) and into the engine.

specific heat index The amount of heat energy required to raise the temperature of a substance. These values are determined experimentally and then made available in tabular form.

split hose bed A hose bed arranged such that either one or two supply lines can be laid out.

split hose lay A scenario in which the attack pumper lays a supply line from an intersection to the fire, and then the supply engine lays a supply line from the hose left by the attack pumper to the water source.

split lay A scenario in which the attack engine lays a supply line from an intersection to the fire, and the supply engine lays a supply line from the hose left by the attack engine to the water source.

spotlights Lights that project a narrow concentrated beam of light.

spotter A person who guides the driver/operator into the appropriate position while operating in a confined space or in reverse mode.

spreader A powered rescue tool that has at least one movable arm that opens to move material.

stabilizers Mechanical devices, usually hydraulically powered, that exert downward force onto the ground and distribute the aerial apparatus' load over a large surface area, effectively stabilizing the vehicle so as to permit its aerial device to be raised, extended, and rotated without collapse.

staging A specific function whereby resources are assembled in an area at or near the incident scene to await instructions or assignments.

staging area A prearranged, strategically placed area, where support response personnel, vehicles, and other equipment can be held in an organized state of readiness for use during an emergency.

staging area manager The person responsible for maintaining the operations of the staging area.

standpipe The vertical portion of the system piping that delivers the water supply for hose connections, and sprinklers on combined systems, vertically from floor to floor in a multistory building. Alternatively, the horizontal portion of the system piping that delivers the water supply for two or more hose connections, and sprinklers on combined systems, on a single level of a building.

standpipe riser The vertical portion of the system piping within a building that delivers the water supply for fire hose connections, and sprinklers on combined systems, vertically from floor to floor in a multistory building.

standpipe system An arrangement of piping, valves, hose connections, and allied equipment with the hose connections located in such a manner that water can be discharged in streams or spray patterns through attached hose and nozzles, for the purpose of extinguishing a fire and so protecting designated buildings, structures, or property in addition to providing occupant protection as required.

starter switch The switch that engages the starter motor for cranking.

static pressure The pressure in a water pipe when there is no water flowing.

static water source A water source such as a pond, river, stream, or other body of water that is not under pressure.

straight ladder An extendable aerial device without a work platform; usually made of truss construction and equipped with ladder rungs for climbing.

stressors Conditions that create excessive physical and mental pressures on a person's body; any type of stimulus that causes stress.

strip mall A commercial structure usually of a single story with a common façade and attic and multiple occupancies.

supply hose (supply line) Hose designed for the purpose of moving water between a pressurized water source and a pump that is supplying attack lines.

surface tension The elastic-like force at the surface of a liquid, which tends to minimize the surface area, causing drops to form.

sweep (roll-on) method A method of applying foam that involves sweeping the stream just in front of the target.

system check sequence A series of checks that an electrical system completes to ensure that all of the systems are functioning properly before the fire apparatus is started.

tactical benchmarks Objectives that are required to be completed during the operational phase of an incident.

tank fill A discharge directly into the on-board water tank.

tank-to-pump A pipe that leads from the apparatus water tank to the fire pump.

teamwork The driver/operator and tiller operator of a tractor trailer ladder truck have a dual responsibility unique among fire department apparatus drivers. Both must work together and coordinate their actions to ensure the safe and efficient operation of the tractor and trailer as a unit.

termination area The area where the normal flow of traffic resumes after a traffic incident.

theoretical hydraulics Scientific or more exact fireground calculations.

threaded hose coupling A type of coupling that requires a male fitting and a female fitting to be screwed together.

tiller operator The tiller operator has the responsibility for lateral control of the trailer portion of the apparatus.

tillerman The driver who operates the rear of a tractor-drawn aerial.

torque box A welded structural steel pedestal plate that supports the turntable, outriggers, trailer, and gooseneck as one integral unit, the torque box structure transfers all of the aerial loads to the outriggers. Some manufacturers incorporate the torque box as the actual chassis frame, in which case they attach running gear underneath it and weld the front axles and frames directly to the torque box.

total pressure loss (TPL) Combination of friction loss, elevation loss, and appliance loss.

total stopping distance The distance that it takes for the driver/operator to recognize a hazard, process the need to stop the fire apparatus, apply the brakes, and then come to a complete stop.

traffic control The direction or management of vehicle traffic such that scene safety is maintained and rescue operations can proceed without interruption.

traffic incident A natural disaster or other unplanned event that affects or impedes the normal flow of traffic.

traffic incident management area (TIMA) An area of highway where temporary traffic controls are imposed by authorized officials in response to an accident, natural disaster, hazardous materials spill, or other unplanned incident.

traffic signal preemption system A system that allows the normal operation of a traffic signal to be changed so as to assist emergency vehicles in responding to an emergency.

traffic space The portion of the highway where traffic is routed through the activity area of a traffic incident.

transfer case A gear box that transfers power, thereby enabling a fire apparatus' motor to operate a pump.

transfer valve An internal valve in a multistage pump that enables the user to change the mode of operation to either series/pressure or parallel/volume.

transition area The area where vehicles are redirected from their normal path and where lane changes and closures are made in a traffic incident.

triple-combination pumper A truck that carries water in a tank generally used for the booster line and commonly called the booster tank.

turbidity The amount of particulate matter suspended in water.

turntable A structural component that connects the aerial device to the chassis and stabilization system through a rotating bearing that permits 360-degree continuous rotation of the aerial device.

under-steering Not turning the steering wheel sufficiently while making a sharp turn and cutting a corner.

universal solvent A liquid substance capable of dissolving other substances, which does not result in the first substance changing its state when forming the solution.

vacuum Any pressure less than atmospheric pressure.

vane A small, movable, self-adjusting element inside a rotary vane pump.

vehicle data recorder (VDR) An apparatus-mounted recording system that notes what the fire apparatus was actually doing prior to a collision.

vehicle dynamics Vehicle construction and mechanical design characteristics that directly affect the handling, stability, maneuverability, functionality, and safeness of a vehicle.

vehicle intercom system A communication system that is permanently mounted inside the cab of the fire apparatus to allow fire fighters to communicate more effectively.

Venturi effect The creation of a low-pressure area in a chamber so as to allow air and water to be drawn in.

victaulic connection Also referred to as a Gruvlok; a device used to attach two pipes together using a rubber doughnut-like gasket that goes over both pieces of pipe. A two-piece, half-moon clamp that surrounds the gasket is then placed over the rubber sealing gasket. The pipes are grooved circumferentially, and the clamp halves fit into the grooves. Two bolts are used to hold the clamps together; they are designed to allow any size of piping to be easily disassembled and reassembled on water systems.

viscosity A measure of the resistance of a liquid to flow.

visual inspection Inspection by eye without recourse to any optical devices, except prescription eyeglasses.

voltage meter A device that registers the voltage of a battery system.

voltmeter A device that measures the voltage across a battery's terminals and gives an indication of the electrical condition of the battery.

volume The quantity of water flowing; usually measured in gallons (liters) per minute.

volute The part of the pump casing that gradually decreases in area, thereby creating pressure on the discharge side of a pump.

water additive An agent that, when added to water in proper quantities, suppresses, cools, mitigates fire and/or provides insulating properties for fuels exposed to radiant heat or direct flame impingement.

water flow The amount of water flowing through pipes, hoses, and fittings, usually expressed in gallons (liters) per minute (gpm or L/min).

water hammer The surge of pressure caused when a high-velocity flow of water is abruptly shut off. The pressure exerted by the flowing water against the closed system can be seven or more times that of the static pressure.

water main A generic term for any underground water pipe.

water pressure The application of force by one object against another. When water is forced through the distribution system, it creates water pressure.

water shuttle The process of moving water by using fire apparatus from a water source to a location where it can be used.

water supply A source of water that provides the flows (L/min) and pressures (kPa) required by a water-based fire protection system.

water thief A device that has a 2½-inch (65-mm) inlet and a 2½-inch (65-mm) outlet in addition to two 1½-inch (38-mm) outlets. It is used to supply many hoses from one source.

water tower position The position where a movable monitor is set to extend to the ladders full extension. It is pinned or latched to the fly section for maximum elevation of the waterway and monitor.

wet-barrel hydrant A hydrant used in areas that are not susceptible to freezing. The barrel of this type of hydrant is normally filled with water.

wetting agent A concentrate that when added to water reduces the surface tension and increases its ability to penetrate and spread.

wye A device used to split a single hose into two separate lines.

Index

NOTE: Page numbers followed by *f*, *t*, or *sd* indicate figures, tables, or skill drills, respectively.

A

A frame jacks (X-style jacks), 445, 445*f*
ABCDE mnemonic, 22
ABS. *See* Anti-lock braking systems (ABS)
Acoustic testing, aerial devices, 455–456, 456*f*
Activity areas, 236
Adapters
    characteristics, 107
    double couplings, 107–108, 108*f*
    for hydrant thread sizes, 5
    jet siphon, 304
    laying out hose with threaded couplings and, 252
Address of emergency scene, 218, 225–226, 226*f*
Adjustable-gallonage fog nozzles, 114
Advance warning areas, 236
Aeration, in foam solutions, 328, 341, 345
Aerial fire apparatus, 354–463. *See also* Aerial ladders; Elevated streams; Tiller aerial apparatus; Turntable
    angles of operation, 447–448, 448*f*
    classification of, 447
    cradling up and return to station, 451–452, 451–452*f*
    defined, 42–43, 42*f*
    deployment considerations, 357, 444–445, 444–445*f*
    described, 42–43, 42*f*, 43*t*, 44*t*
    discharging water and waterway safeties, 450–451, 450–451*f*
    emergency power with, 388
    equipment included on, 43*t*, 44*t*
    history, 356
    hydraulic and electrical systems, 359–360, 360*f*
    improvements in, 6–7, 7*f*
    key points for driver/operator, 390
    load charts, 448, 448*f*
    maintenance and inspection. *See* Aerial fire apparatus inspection and maintenance
    maneuvering safely, 378, 379*sd*
    operating the aerial device, 169*f*, 371–372, 372*f*, 447–448*f*, 447–450
    operational and equipment checklists, 435–440
    operations, 443–447, 444–446*f*
    overhead obstructions and, 229, 231, 231*f*
    platforms, 358–359, 358*f*, 438, 439, 442, 459*t*
    positioning, 228, 363–367, 364–366*f*, 378, 380–381, 382, 383*sd*, 384, 443–444
    preventive maintenance for, 168
    rescue operation using, 378, 380–382, 380*f*, 380*sd*, 381*f*
    rotation, 449
    safe practices with, 372–373, 373*f*, 374*f*, 375, 377–378, 377*f*
    setup, 367–368, 369*sd*, 370, 371*sd*
    skill building, 390–391
    skills in action, 391–393, 392–393*f*
    stabilization, 359, 360–362, 361*f*, 367–368, 369*sd*, 370, 371*sd*, 436, 437*f*, 457–458
    summary and review, 394–396, 461–463
    tactical priorities, 356–357
    testing, 452, 452*f*, 455–457*f*, 455–460, 459*t*
    troubleshooting, 458–460, 459*t*
    types, 358–359
    working height, 447, 447*f*
Aerial fire apparatus inspection and maintenance, 432–463
    aerial ladders, 440–442, 440*f*, 442*f*
    cradling up and return to station, 451–452, 451–452*f*
    discharging water and waterway safeties, 450–451, 450–451*f*
    ladder components and classifications, 440–442, 440*f*, 442*f*
    operating the aerial device, 169*f*, 447–448*f*, 447–450
    operational and equipment checklists, 435–440
    operations, 443–447, 444–446*f*
    storing outriggers, 452, 452*f*
    testing, 452, 452*f*, 455–457*f*, 455–460, 459*t*
    tiller trucks, 442–443, 443*f*
    troubleshooting, 458–460, 459*t*
    visual inspection, 434, 458, 460
Aerial hour meter, 435, 435*f*
Aerial ladders. *See also* Ladders; Tiller aerial apparatus
    classifications, 440–442, 440*f*, 442*f*
    climbing or riding safe practices, 377, 377–378*f*
    components, 440–442, 440*f*, 442*f*
    construction and capabilities, 358, 358*f*, 359*f*
    described, 42–43
    elevated stream positioning, 384
    evolution of, 6–7, 6–7*f*
    extension of, 436–437, 449–450
    history, 6, 6*f*
    hydroelectric swivel, 441–442
    inspection of, 359, 429, 440–442, 440*f*, 442*f*
    lift controls, 440–441
    lift cylinders, 440–441
    lowering, 451
    platform controls, 442
    for quints, 44, 44*f*
    raising, 448–450
    reach of, 362–363, 362*f*, 384, 444
    retraction of, 436–437, 449–450, 451, 451*f*, 458
    rotation controls, 441
    sections, 440, 440*f*, 442
    tiller apparatus and, 414–416, 415–416*f*
    tip positioning and operation, 380–381, 381*f*, 459
    troubleshooting movement of, 458, 459*t*, 460
    waterway system, 441–442, 442*f*
Aerial platforms, 358–359, 358*f*, 438, 439, 459*t*
AFFF. *See* Aqueous film-forming foam (AFFF)
Aherns-Fox fire apparatus, 80*f*
AHJ. *See* Authority having jurisdiction (AHJ)
Air bags/air curtains, cab, 10
Air brakes inspection, 178, 178*f*. *See also* Brakes

Index

Air gauge alarm, aerial device turntable, 438
Air minder, aerial device turntable, 438
Air pressure, 194, 477
Air supply units, 8
Air-aspirating foam nozzles, 345
Aircraft rescue and firefighting (ARFF) vehicle, 46
AL. *See* Appliance loss (AL) calculations
Alarms, limitations of, 448
Albuquerque Fire Department, fire boxes for, 219
Alcohol-resistant aqueous film-forming foam (AR-AFFF), 330*t*, 332, 332*f*, 333, 333*t*, 471
Alcohol-resistant film-forming fluoroprotein foams (AR-FFFP), 330*t*, 331
Alley dock exercise, 238, 239–240*sd*, 407, 411*f*
Alley lay, 252, 253*f*
Amber emergency lights, 11, 233
Ambient air temperature, 476
Ambulances, positioning at fire scene, 232
American LaFrance, 42
Angle of approach, aerial fire apparatus, 436
Angle of departure, aerial fire apparatus, 436
Angle or slope indicators, apparatus-mounted, 370, 370*f*
Angles of operation, aerial ladders, 436, 447, 448*f*
Angulo, Raul A., 182
Anti-lock braking systems (ABS), 10
Anti-siphon hole, 281, 283*f*
AP foam. *See* Around-the-pump (AP) foam proportioning system
Apartment complex addresses, 226, 226*f*
Apparatus inspection form, 171–172, 171*f*, 185, 186*sd*
Apparatus placement. *See* Fire apparatus positioning
Appliance loss (AL) calculations, 131, 135–136*f*, 135–139, 137*sd*, 139*sd*
Appliances. *See also* Fire hose appliances
    auxiliary, 231–232
    examples of, 135*f*
    for high-flow devices, friction loss calculations due to, 135*t*
    total pressure loss, 139–140, 141
Approaching the emergency scene, 225–226, 226*f*
Aqueous film-forming foam (AFFF), 326, 330*t*, 331, 332*f*, 471
Aqueous substances, 53
AR-AFFF. *See* Alcohol-resistant aqueous film-forming foam (AR-AFFF)
ARFF vehicle. *See* Aircraft rescue and firefighting (ARFF) vehicle
AR-FFFP. *See* Alcohol-resistant film-forming fluoroprotein foams (AR-FFFP)
Around-the-pump (AP) foam proportioning system, 337, 339, 339*sd*
Articulated booms, 8, 8*f*
Articulating platform, 356, 358*f*, 359
Aspirating foam nozzles, 331, 345
Assessment center, for driver/operator selection, 30
Assigned tactical radio frequency, 218
ATC. *See* Automatic traction control (ATC)
Atmospheric pressure, 280, 281*f*, 477
Attack hose/lines, 102, 102*f*, 103–104, 103*f*
Attack pumpers, 251, 301, 313, 313*f*

Attitude
    of driver/operator, 12, 29, 30
    toward safety, 19
A-type stabilizers, 360–361, 361*f*, 362
Authority having jurisdiction (AHJ), 458, 477, 478
Automatic intake pressure relief device, 86, 87*f*
Automatic load management system, 263–264
Automatic traction control (ATC), 10
Automatic transmission transfer case, 95–96, 95*f*
Automatic-adjusting fog nozzles, 114
Auxiliary appliances, engines and ladders, 231–232
Auxiliary brakes, 10

B

Backing procedures
    aerial apparatus, 404–405, 404*f*, 412
    basic procedure, 205–207, 205–207*f*, 208*sd*
    spotter's role, 12, 12*f*, 205–207, 205–207*f*
Backlash of aerial turntable, 441
Balanced-pressure foam proportioning systems, 340, 340*f*
Ball, blow-up, for portable tank operations, 305
Ball valves, 109, 109*f*
Baltimore, Great Fire of (1904), 5
Bankshot (bankdown) method for applying foam, 348, 349*sd*
Barometric pressure, 477
Barrel strainers, 289–290, 290*f*
Barron, Robert, 23
Batch mixing, of foam, 334, 334*f*, 335*sd*
Batteries
    inspection of, 176, 176*f*, 179, 180*f*
    low-voltage electrical system testing, 468–469, 468*f*, 469*sd*, 469*t*
    shutting down the fire apparatus, 209
Battery cables, safe removal of, 176, 176*f*
Battery charger/conditioner test, 471
Battery selector switch, 194
Belts, inspection of, 176
Big-box commercial structures, 366, 366*f*
Bleeder valves, pump intake connections, 86, 87*f*, 316, 317, 317*f*
Blind spots, 20, 221. *See also* Backing procedures
Blue emergency lights, 12, 233
Booster hose/lines, 7, 102, 104
Booster pumps, 7, 7*f*
Booster tanks, 7, 284, 287, 297
Bottoming out, chassis clearance and, 25
Brake pedal test, 178, 178*f*
Brakes. *See also* Parking brake
    air brakes inspection, 178, 178*f*
    anti-lock braking systems (ABS), 10
    auxiliary, 10
    compression, 224
    exhaust, 224
    faulty, near collision due to, 183

inspection of, 178–179, 178–179f
performance tests, 468
skidding and, 222
Braking, tiller apparatus, 405
Braking distance, 221
Breathing air system. *See also* Self-contained breathing apparatus (SCBA)
on aerial device, 185, 363
compressor system tests, 475–476
testing, 457
Bresnan distributor nozzles, 114, 114f
Bridges
as drafting sites, 287–288
as height obstacles, 223
British thermal units (Btu), 122
Btu. *See* British thermal units (Btu)
Bucket brigade, 4–5
Buffer space, 236
Building collapse incidents, 240
Building type and height, aerial device positioning, 365–366, 365–366f
Bull gear, 438, 438f
Burnback resistance, 330
Butterfly valves, 109, 109f
Bypass eductors, 336

C

C. *See* Coefficients; Coefficients (C)
Cab alarm, aerial device turntable, 439
Cab interior
aerial apparatus setup, 367
enclosed and with seatbelts, 8, 10
exiting considerations, 247, 248
fire department pumper, 76–77, 77f
fire pump procedures from, 246–248, 247–248f
inspection of, 176–177, 177f
safe design and crashworthiness testing, 10
Cable systems, aerial device, inspection of, 184
CAFS. *See* Compressed-air foam systems (CAFS)
Camera, rear-mounted, backing up fire apparatus and, 206, 207f
Cap gauge for fire hydrant testing, 66
Cap on discharge outlet, 88, 88f
Capacity test/150 psi test, 497, 498sd
Carries for rescuing victims, 381–382
Cascade units, 8
Cavitation, 296–297
CDL. *See* Commercial driver's license (CDL)
Cellar nozzles, 114, 114f
Centrifugal force, 81, 222–223
Centrifugal pumps
inspection of, 181, 181f
operational characteristics, 81, 83–84f, 83–86
priming, 76, 76f
Changeover operations, 246, 260–261, 263, 263f, 264sd

Charging system tests, 470, 470sd
Chassis, fire apparatus, 25, 39, 78
Chemical foams, 328
Chemical properties of water, 53–54, 53f
Chemical wagons, 7
Clapper valve, 257–258, 260f
Class 1 safety vest, 234
Class 2 safety vest, 234
Class 3 safety vest, 234
Class A foams, 329–330, 329f, 345–346, 347sd, 349
Class B foams
applying, 346, 348–349, 348sd, 349sd, 350sd
characteristics, 330–331, 331f
compatibility of, 349
types and properties of, 330t
Cleaning equipment, 25, 25f
Cleanliness, and apparatus maintenance, 174
Clear emergency lights, 233
Clearance, diminishing, exercise on, 203–204, 204sd
Clothing. *See also* Personal protective equipment (PPE)
reflective vests, 233–234
turnout gear, 200, 233–234
Code 1 response, 220
Code 2 response, 220
Code 3 response, 220
Coefficients (C)
friction loss, 127–128, 128t
for Siamese lines, 128t, 144–145, 145sd, 146sd, 146t
for standpipe risers, 149–150, 150t
Cold zones, at emergency medical scenes, 240
Collapse zone, apparatus positioning and, 230, 240sd, 364, 366
Collector rings, hydroelectric swivel, 442
Colors, for fire hydrants, 64, 65t
Combination load, 253
Combination (fog) nozzles, 122–123, 122–123f
Combination tools, hydraulic, 271, 272f
Combustible and flammable liquid incidents, 326
Command vehicles, 27, 27f, 232
Commercial driver's license (CDL), 27, 28f
Commercial structures, aerial device positioning, 364, 364–365f, 365–366, 366f
Communications. *See also* Radio communication
aerial device operation, 362, 386, 439–440, 457, 457f
for filling tankers, 301
inspection of aerial device, 185, 185f
for notifying on starting drafting water flow, 294
for nurse tanker operations, 306
skills in driver/operator selection, 29
with spotters, 205–206, 205–206f
testing of aerial apparatus controls, 457, 457f
tiller apparatus, 401–402, 429
vehicle intercom system, 20, 439–440
Communications center, 217
Compartment doors, 192, 196, 197, 197f, 207

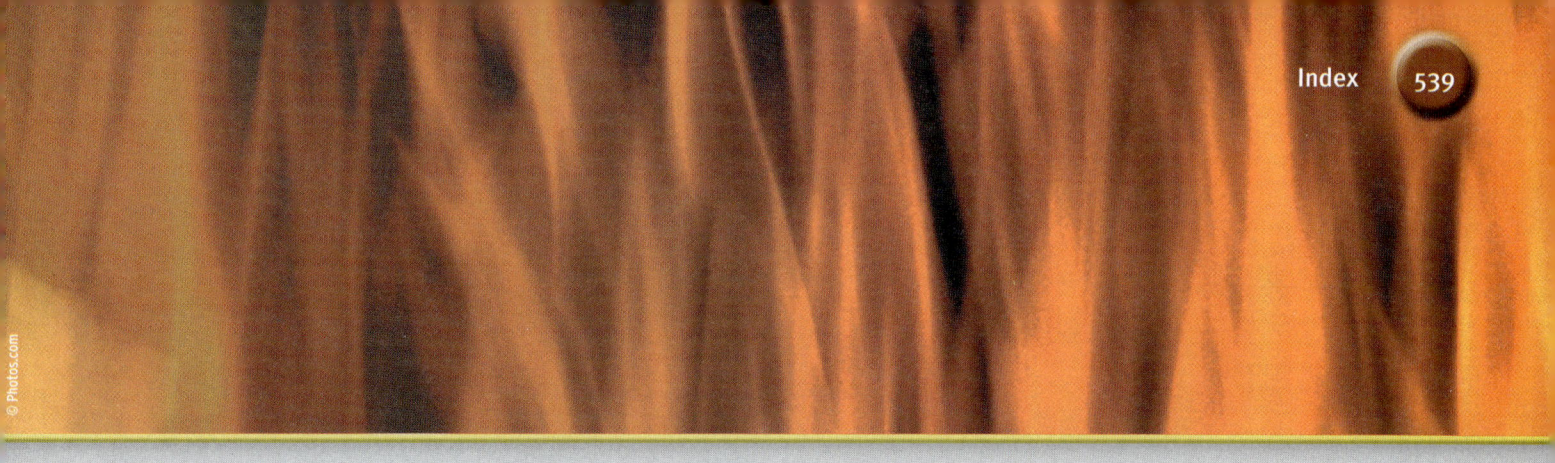

Index

Compressed-air foam systems (CAFS), 341–342, 341*f*, 343*sd*, 473–474
Compression brakes, 224
Compressors, 8, 475–476
Computers. *See* Technology
Concentrates, foam. *See* Foam concentrates
Condensed Q method, 160–162
Conductivity calibration curve percentage method, 473
Conductivity meter, foam percentage, 473
Conductivity testing, battery, 469
Confined-space turnaround exercise, 201–203, 202*sd*, 407, 409, 409*f*
Constant pressure relays, 316
Control valves
    for hydrants, 298, 298*f*
    water distribution system, 56
Control zones, at emergency medical scenes, 238, 240
Coolant level, inspection of, 175, 175*f*
Corner safe areas, apparatus positioning and, 230
Crack pressure setting for holding valves or POC, 456
Cradle alignment light, aerial device turntable, 438
Crew members. *See also* Clothing; Driver/operators
    for apparatus inspections, 169, 169*f*
    backing procedures and, 205–207, 205–207*f*, 208*sd*
    building confidence and efficiency, 18–19
    educating, 18, 20–21
    fire apparatus public appearances and, 196
    map reading by, 219
    monitoring fill site using a hydrant, 300
    notifying on starting drafting water flow, 294
    for relay pumping operations, 314
    responsibilities, 18
    safe equipment handling and, 19–20, 19–20*f*
    safety role of, 196–197, 203
    spotters, 12, 12*f*, 205–207, 205–207*f*, 208*sd*
    tiller operator, 400, 402–403, 406–407, 407*f*, 412–413, 442–443, 443*f*
    trust and team building among, 18–19, 21
Critical rate of flow, 122
Critical speed, for curves, 223
Crossover backing exercise, 412
Curbs, aerial device stabilizing on, 370, 370*f*, 371*sd*
Curved roadways, driving on, 222–223, 223*f*
Cutters, hydraulic, 271, 271*f*

D

Daily apparatus checks, 182
Daily engine inspection sheet, 171, 171*f*, 281, 282*f*
Dalmation dogs, 6
Dammed streams, as water source, 288, 288*f*
Dead man's switch, 438
Dead-end water mains, 56
DEF. *See* Diesel exhaust fluid (DEF) inspection
Defensive driving practices, 221–222

Deflection space, aerial device safe practices, 378
Dependable lift, 280
Dettman, Todd, 494
Diesel exhaust fluid (DEF) inspection, 176
Diesel-powered fire apparatus, 8, 8*f*
Digital volt-ohm meter (DVOM), 468, 468*f*, 469, 470, 471
Diminishing clearance exercise, 203–204, 204*sd*, 409, 409*f*
Dip stick, 170, 175
Direction of movement regulations, emergency vehicle flexibility with, 220
Directional arrows, fire apparatus, traffic control and, 233, 234*f*
Direct-reading conductivity foam percentage method, 473
Dirt and grease, fire apparatus inspections and, 173
Discharge header, 83
Discharge outlet connections, 87–88, 88*f*
Discharge pressure. *See also* Pump discharge pressure (PDP)
    for drafting operations, 293, 295–296*sd*, 296, 296*sd*
    flow meters (flow minders) test, 483, 485, 485*f*, 487*sd*
    gauge meter test of, 483, 485, 486*sd*
    for a standpipe, calculations, 149–150, 150*t*, 152–155*sd*
Discharge pressure gauge, master pump, 89, 89*f*
Discharge pressure relief valve, pump panel, 92, 93*f*
Discharge side of fire pumps
    centrifugal pump, 81, 83, 85, 86
    defined, 86
    discharge capacity, effect of lift on, 280, 281*f*
    outlet connections, 87–88, 88*f*
    positive-displacement pumps, 79, 80, 81
Discharge valves
    dangers of operating AP system while closed, 339
    filling hose line from drafting operation and, 293–294, 296*sd*
    flow meter test, 483, 485, 485*f*, 487*sd*
    gauge meter test of, 483, 485, 486*sd*
    pump, inspection of, 180
    of standpipe risers, 149, 149*f*
Discharges, inspection of, 180, 180*f*
Discontinuity in magnetic current, 455
Dispatch for emergency response, 217–218
Distance from vehicle ahead, 221
Distribution system, municipal water, 55–56, 55*f*, 56*f*
Distributors, 56
Double- versus single-action lift cylinders, 441
Double-acting lifting cylinders, turntable control pedestal, 438
Double-acting piston pumps, 80
Double-female adapters, 107, 108*f*, 252
Double-male adapters, 107, 108*f*, 252
Downriggers for stabilizing aerial apparatus, 360, 367
Drafting water, 280–297. *See also* Static water sources; Water supply
    complications during, 294, 296–297
    dump line, establishing, 293
    establishing pumping operations, 289–291, 290–291*f*, 292*sd*, 300
    inspection of priming system, 281, 282–283*f*
    mechanics of, 280, 281*f*
    preparing pump for, 293–294, 295*sd*

priming the pump for, 291, 293
producing water flow, 294–297, 296sd
in rural areas, 280
selecting site for, 284, 286–289, 287–288f
summary and review, 308–309
vacuum test of priming system, 284, 285sd
Drains and sewer pipe openings, aerial device positioning, 443
Drake, Christopher, 235
Driver/operators. See also Crew members; Training
driver's license requirements, 27, 28f
emergency vehicle response, 217f, 218f, 219
roles and responsibilities, 4, 18
safety role of, 9, 12, 12f, 196–197, 203
teams of experienced and inexperienced, 122
tillerman's roles and responsibilities, 406–407, 407f, 442–443, 443f
visibility for, 12, 12f
Driving emergency vehicles, 214–243
approaching emergency scene, 225–226
basic safety rules of, 220
bridges and overpasses, 223
defensive driving practices, 221–222
dispatch, 217–218
emergency medical scene positioning, 238, 239–240sd
fire apparatus positioning, 226–234
highways, 232–234
intersections, 223–225, 232–234, 237
laws concerning, 219–220
level of response, 220
maintaining control on hills, turns, and curves, 222–223
maps, 218–219
MUTCD, 234, 236–238
night driving, 223
passing vehicles, 220–221
pre-emergency vehicle response, 217–219
railroad crossings, 225
scene with no specific address, 225–226, 226f
special emergency scene positioning, 238, 240
summary and review, 241–242
360-degree inspection, 192, 193sd, 196
Driving exercises
alley dock exercise, 238, 239–240sd, 407, 411f
confined-space turnarounds, 201–203, 202sd, 407, 409, 409f
crossover backing exercise, 412
diminishing clearance exercise, 203–204, 204sd, 409, 409f
offset alley exercise, 410
parking exercise, tiller apparatus, 410, 410f, 412
serpentine maneuvers, 200–201, 201sd, 407, 409f
straight-line drive exercise, tiller apparatus, 410, 410f, 412
Driving fire apparatus, 190–213
backing procedures for, 12, 12f, 205–207, 205–207f, 208sd, 404–405, 404f, 412
defensive driving practices, 221–222
driving exercises, 200–204, 201–202sd, 204sd, 407, 408–410f, 409–410, 412

getting underway, 196–197, 198–199f
preparing to drive, 192–199, 193sd, 194f, 196–197f, 198–199sd
returning to the station, 204–210, 205–207f, 208sd, 209f, 211sd
safety role of driver/operator, 10–11, 26, 196–197, 203
securing the fire apparatus, 209, 209f
shutting down the fire apparatus, 207, 209, 209f, 210sd
starting the fire apparatus, 194, 196–197, 196f, 198–199sd
summary and review, 211–213
tanker safety, 302
tiller aerial apparatus, 407, 408–410f, 409–410, 412
tiller aerial apparatus safety, 400–401
Drop-down stabilizers, 361, 361f, 362
Dry hydrants, 68–69, 69f, 70f, 288, 288f
Dry penetrant testing, 455, 456f
Dry standpipe systems, 255
Dry-barrel fire hydrants, 61, 61f
Dual air brake system warning light and buzzer test, 178, 178f
Due regard, 22, 203, 220
Dump lines, 293, 304
Dump sites
offloading tankers for, 303
as static water source, 302
traffic flow within, 305, 305f
using portable tanks at, 302, 303–305, 304f
for water shuttle, 305–306
Dump valves, 302, 303, 304f
Dunn, Vincent, 230
Duplex gauge, 340, 340f
DVOM. See Digital volt-ohm meter (DVOM)
Dye penetrant testing, aerial devices, 455

E

Eductors, 281, 335–337, 336f, 338sd
Electric generators, 265–266, 265–266f, 267–268sd
Electrical system
line voltage electrical systems tests, 474–475
low-voltage electrical system testing, 468–471, 468f, 469sd, 469t, 470t
total continuous electrical load test, 471
Electromagnetic retarders, 224
Electronic direct-injection foam system, 471–472
Electronic Fire Commander, 93–94
Electronic pump controllers, pump panel, 93–94, 93f
Electronic stability control (ESC), 11
Elevated master streams, 145–147, 146f, 150–153sd, 384, 427
Elevated platforms, 358–359, 358f
Elevated streams
adverse environmental conditions, 384–385, 385f
aerial device use to deploy, 357, 388, 389sd, 427
application of stream, 386–387, 387f
exposure protection, 387
historical, 6
other considerations, 388

positioning and operation, 363, 384–388, 384f, 385f, 387f, 389sd
types, 385–386, 386t
water supply for, 386
Elevated water storage towers, 55, 55f
Elevation, extension and rotation locks, testing, 456
Elevation gain, 129
Elevation loss
calculations, 129–130, 129–130f
total pressure loss, 139–140, 141
Elevation pressure (EP)
calculations, 129–130, 134
fluid dynamics, 58–59
Emergency communications, 21. See also Communications
Emergency lights, 11–12, 197, 219, 233, 247
Emergency medical scene positioning, 238, 239–240sd
Emergency power, aerial device use of, 360, 388
Emergency power unit (EPU), 456
Emergency Vehicle Operations courses, 219
Emergency vehicle technician (EVT)
aerial device troubleshooting, 458
conductivity testing, 469
as hydraulic fluid troubleshooting resource, 435, 436
lift control problems, 441
as maintenance resource, 26, 26f
as troubleshooting resource, 458
weight verification reporting to, 468
Emergency vehicles, driving, 214–243
approaching emergency scene, 225–226
basic safety rules of, 220
bridges and overpasses, 223
defensive driving practices, 221–222
dispatch, 217–218
emergency medical scene positioning, 238, 239–240sd
fire apparatus positioning, 226–234
highways, 232–234
intersections, 223–225, 232–234, 237
laws concerning, 219–220
level of response, 220
maintaining control on hills, turns, and curves, 222–223
maps, 218–219
MUTCD, 234, 236–238
night driving, 223
passing vehicles, 220–221
pre-emergency vehicle response, 217–219
railroad crossings, 225
scene with no specific address, 225–226, 226f
special emergency scene positioning, 238, 240
summary and review, 241–242
360-degree inspection, 192, 193sd, 196
Emergency warning equipment inspection, 178, 187
Emitter, for traffic signal preemption, 224
Engine compartment inspection, 174–175f, 174–176, 176f
Engine coolant temperature gauges, pump panel, 91, 91f
Engine cooling devices, pump panel, 91, 91f

Engine oil level inspection, 170, 175
Engine oil pressure gauges, pump panel, 91, 92f
Engine speed interlock, testing, 457
Engine speed test, no-load governed, 480, 480f, 481sd
Engine tachometer, 90–91, 91f
Engine warm-up, 197
"Engineer" on steam fire pump, 5
Engines and ladders, positioning of, 229–232
auxiliary appliances, 231–232
exposures and, 230
fire conditions and, 230
overhead obstructions, 231, 231f
rescue potential and, 229–230
slope, 230
terrain and surface conditions, 230–231
water supply and, 230
wind conditions, 231, 231f
Environmental conditions
aerial device loading, 373, 375
elevated streams in adverse conditions, 384–385, 385f
requirements for performance tests, 476–477
stabilizer system checks due to rough roads, 436
tiller aerial apparatus operation in adverse conditions, 406, 428
EP. See Elevation pressure (EP)
EPU. See Emergency power unit (EPU)
Equipment for performance tests, 478–480, 479–480f.
See also Fire equipment
ESC. See Electronic stability control (ESC)
EVT. See Emergency vehicle technician (EVT)
Exhaust brakes, 224
Exhaust extractor system, 173, 209
Exhaust primer, 81
Exhaust system inspection, 174
Experience, importance for driver/operators, 12
Exposure protection
as aerial deployment priority, 357, 363
of apparatus at fire scenes, 230
elevated streams, 387
Extension ladders. See Aerial ladders
Extension ram, hydraulic, 272, 272f
Extension/retraction checklist, aerial device, 436–437
Exterior fire apparatus inspections, 173–174, 174f
Exterior functional control switches, inspection of, 177–178, 177f
Exterior mounted equipment, inspection, 187, 187f
Extinguishers, soda acid, 7
Extractor exhaust system, 172
Extrusion of ladder rungs, 442

F

Failure, of performance, 476
Fall protection, aerial device operation, 375, 377, 377f
Fast idle switch, aerial device turntable, 438, 459t
Fatal injuries to U.S. fire fighters, causes of (2012), 12, 12f, 232, 232t
Faulkner, Jimmy, 453

FDCs. *See* Fire department connections (FDCs)
Federal regulations for fire departments, 219
Female connections, 107, 108f, 252, 257
FFFP. *See* Film-forming fluoroprotein foam (FFFP)
50 percent test, 499–500
Fill sites, 298, 300–301, 306
Filling tankers, 87, 88f, 298, 301
Film-forming fluoroprotein foam (FFFP), 330t, 331, 333t. *See also* Alcohol-resistant film-forming fluoroprotein foams (AR-FFFP)
Finished foam, 328
Fire apparatus. *See also* Aerial fire apparatus; Fire apparatus inspection and maintenance; Fire apparatus positioning; Fire equipment; Pumper fire apparatus
    connecting to a water supply, 246–247, 287–288
    distance to hydrant from, 254
    effect on braking distance, 221
    engine speed, drafting water and, 294
    engine temperature during drafting operations, 296
    evolution of, 4–8, 10–3, 11–12f
    functions and limitations, 24–26, 25–26f
    modern, 12–13
    NFPA 1002 safety requirements, 26
    NFPA 1901 performance standards, 37
    performance test requirements, 476–480, 477–479f
    quint apparatus, 44, 44f, 44t, 45t, 435
    readiness, 169, 169f, 209, 209f
    safety considerations, 8, 10–12, 11–12f
    shutting down, 207, 209, 209f, 210sd
    skill building with, 29, 29f
    staging, 227–229, 228f, 229f, 235
    starting, 194, 196–197, 196f, 198–199sd
    traffic control devices on, 237
Fire apparatus, driving, 190–213
    backing procedures for, 12, 12f, 205–207, 205–207f, 208sd, 404–405, 404f, 412
    defensive driving practices, 221–222
    driving exercises, 200–204, 201–202sd, 204sd, 407, 408–410f, 409–410, 412
    getting underway, 196–197, 198–199f
    preparing to drive, 192–199, 193sd, 194f, 196–197f, 198–199sd
    returning to the station, 204–210, 205–207f, 208sd, 209f, 211sd
    safety role of driver/operator, 10–11, 26, 196–197, 203
    securing the fire apparatus, 209, 209f
    shutting down the fire apparatus, 207, 209, 209f, 210sd
    starting the fire apparatus, 194, 196–197, 196f, 198–199sd
    summary and review, 211–213
    tanker safety, 302
    tiller aerial apparatus safety, 400–401
Fire apparatus, evolution of, 2–15
    in current use, 8, 10–12, 11–12f
    early, 4–8, 4–8f
    modern, 12–13
    summary and review, 14–15

Fire apparatus, types of, 34–49
    aerial, 42–43, 42f, 43t, 44t
    initial attack, 38–40, 39f, 41
    mobile foam fire apparatus, 46, 46f, 46t, 47t
    mobile water supply apparatus, 41, 41f, 42t
    pumper fire apparatus, 37–38, 37f, 38t
    purchasing requirements, 36–37, 36f
    quint, 44, 44f, 44t, 45t
    special service, 44–45, 45f, 45t
    summary and review, 48–49
Fire apparatus inspection and maintenance, 168–189. *See also* Aerial fire apparatus inspection and maintenance
    aerial devices, 184–185, 184–185f
    apparatus inspection form, 171–172, 171f, 185, 186sd
    brakes, 178–179, 178–179f
    cab interior, 176–177, 177f
    completing forms for, 187
    driver/operators and, 25–26, 25–26f
    engine compartment, 174–175f, 174–176, 176f
    exterior, 173–174, 174f
    fire apparatus sections, 172–185
    general tools and equipment, 179–180, 179–180f
    positioning for, 172f
    preventive maintenance, 168
    priming system, 281
    procedures for, 169–170
    process and documentation, 171–172, 172f
    pumps, 180–181, 181f, 184
    review previous report on, 185, 186sd
    safety considerations, 187
    steps for inspection, 185, 186sd
    summary and review, 188–189
    360-degree, 192, 193sd, 196, 434
    tires, 22
    vehicle inspection, 467
    weekly, monthly, or other period inspection items, 187
Fire apparatus positioning, 226–234. *See also* Engines and ladders, positioning of
    aerial devices, 363–367, 364–366f
    ambulances, 232
    collapse zone and, 230, 240
    command vehicles, 232
    for drafting water, 289
    at emergency medical scenes, 238, 239–240sd
    engines and ladders, 229–232, 231f
    evaluating on approach, 226–227
    fire pump procedures and, 246–247
    at intersections or on highways, 232–234
    near railroad crossings, 238
    recognition of potential hazards, 226
    specialized emergency scenes, 238, 240
    specialized fire apparatus, 232
    staging, 227–229, 228f, 229f, 235
    tiller aerial apparatus, 414–416, 414f, 415–416f, 422–423, 428–429

Index

traffic incidents and, 234, 236–238
   for ventilation operations, 363, 382, 383sd, 384
   at working fire, 227
Fire crew. *See* Crew members
Fire department connections (FDCs), 227f
   connecting supply hose lines to, 257–258, 259sd
   locating, 255, 257, 258f
   purpose of, 255
   Siamese connections of, 144
   standpipe operations and, 147, 149–156
   types, 255
Fire department engines. *See* Fire apparatus
Fire departments
   on apparatus inspections, 169–170, 171–172, 172f
   emergency vehicle rules and regulations of, 219–220
   NFPA 1002 qualification to operate vehicles, 27, 27f
   volunteer, preventive maintenance programs, 168–169
Fire equipment
   on aerial fire apparatus, 43, 43t, 44t, 362–363, 435–440
   apparatus-mounted, operating, 264–266, 267–268sd, 269–272, 273–274sd
   in current use, 8, 10–12, 11–12f
   early, 4–8, 4–8f
   evolution of, 4–8, 4–8f
   functions and limitations, 24–26, 25–26f
   for initial attack fire apparatus, 39–40, 39t
   inspection of, 25–26, 25–26f, 178, 179–180, 179–180f, 187, 187f
   on mobile foam fire apparatus, 46, 46f, 46t, 47t
   for mobile water supply apparatus, 41, 42t
   modern, 12–13
   NFPA 1002 safety requirements, 26
   NFPA 1901 required storage on fire apparatus, 38, 39, 41, 43, 44, 46
   power equipment distribution, 269, 269–270f
   powered rescue tools, 270–272, 271–272f, 273–274sd
   on pumper fire apparatus, 38, 38t
   purchasing, safety and, 20
   on the quint, 44, 44t, 45t
   safe handling and storage of, 19–20, 20f, 187, 187f
   safety training and education on, 22
   secured, getting underway and, 196–197, 196–197f
   on special service fire apparatus, 45, 45t
Fire extinguishers, 22, 326, 328, 328f
Fire hooks, 4
Fire hose. *See* Hoses
Fire hose appliances. *See also* Hoses; Siamese connections; Valves; Wyes
   adapters, 5, 107–108, 108f, 252, 304
   defined, 105
   hose clamps, 108–109, 109f
   hose jackets, 108, 108f
   reducers, 108, 108f
   water thief, 107, 107f
Fire hose evolutions. *See* Supply line evolutions

Fire hydrants, 59, 61–68
   charging line from, 251
   colors for, 65t
   connecting Storz coupling soft sleeve hose to a pump from, 104–105, 106sd
   connectors on pumper fire apparatus, 38, 38t
   control valves for, 298, 298f
   coupling thread adapters, 5
   coupling thread standardization, 5
   determining additional water from, 161–162
   distance to fire apparatus from, 254
   dry, 68–69, 69f, 70f, 288, 288f
   dry-barrel, 61, 61f
   as fill sites, 300
   four-way valves for, 251, 251f
   hand lay to, 254–255, 254f, 257sd
   inspecting and maintaining, 62, 64–65, 64–66f
   locations, 62, 64–65, 219, 253
   operating source pumpers from, 313
   operation of, 61–62, 63sd
   positioning fire apparatus for soft suction hose to, 254
   relay valves, 109, 109f, 135f
   screw-type hydrant valve for, 298, 298f
   shutting down, 62, 64sd
   testing, 66–68, 66f, 67sd, 68, 68f
   types, 59, 61, 61f
   wet-barrel, 61, 61f
Fire officers, 173, 253–254
Fire plugs, 5. *See also* Fire hydrants
Fire pumps, 74–99. *See also* Discharge side of fire pumps; Portable pumps; Primer/priming pump; Priming the pump; Pump discharge pressure (PDP); *entries beginning with* Pump
   anatomy of, 86–88, 86–88f
   bleeder valves, pump intake connections, 86, 87f, 316, 317, 317f
   booster pumps, 7, 7f
   cab interior procedures, 246–248, 247–248f
   capacity ratings, 280
   centrifugal pumps, 76, 76f, 81, 83–84f, 83–86, 181, 181f
   connecting Storz coupling soft sleeve hose from hydrant to, 104–105, 106sd
   described, 77–79, 78f
   of different capacities, test data for, 493t
   discharge outlet connections, 87–88, 88f
   engaging, at fire ground, 248–249, 250sd
   engine control interlock test, 482–483, 482f, 484sd
   exterior of fire department pumper, 76, 77f
   fast idle switch and, 446
   fire apparatus positioning and, 246–247
   first mechanized, 5
   floating pumps, 288, 288f
   flow meters (flow minders) test, 483, 485, 485f, 487sd
   gauge meter test of, 483, 485, 486sd
   hand pumps, 5, 5f, 79
   harmful water characteristics, 54

hose suction size, number of suction lines, and lift for, 495t
in-cab procedures, 246–248, 247–248f
on initial attack fire apparatus, 39
inspection of, 180–181, 181f, 184
intake connections, 86–87, 86–88f
interior of fire department pumper, 76–77, 77f
lift effect on discharge capacity of, 280, 281f
monitoring, 261, 263, 263f, 264sd
municipal water distribution, 55
NFPA 20 definition, 79
NFPA 1901 definition, 39
NFPA 1911 on pump requirements and rating, 491, 493, 493t, 504
performance test form, 503, 503f
performance tests, 475–476, 491, 493, 493t, 495–500, 495f, 495t, 496f, 498sd
positive-displacement pumps, 79–81, 80–81f
power supplies for, 94–95f, 94–96
pressure control tests, 500–501, 500f, 502sd
preventive maintenance, 168, 168f
priming two-stage, 293
pump operator's panel, 76, 77f, 85, 88–94, 89–93f
pumping engine throttle, 93–94, 93f
for quints, 44, 44f
rerating, 504
safe positioning, 11–12
shift controls, 482f
shift indicator test, 481–482, 482f, 483sd
speed reading for, 493, 495f
summary and review, 97–99
temperature during drafting operations of, 296
test requirements, 491, 493t
types of, 79–86, 80–84f
vacuum test of, 284, 285sd, 488, 490sd, 491
water conditions and maintenance of, 54
water drafting operations, 289–291, 290–291f, 292sd, 293–294, 295sd, 300
Fire service hydraulic calculations, 156–160, 157f, 157t, 159sd
Fire station
backing into, 205–207, 205–207f, 208sd
returning to, 204–210, 205–207f, 208sd, 209f, 211sd
Fireground hydraulics
calculations, 156–160, 157f, 157t, 159sd
defined, 121
early protection in American cities, 5–7, 5–7f
Fireground operations, 244–277. *See also* Supply hose/lines;
Supply line evolutions
apparatus-mounted equipment, 264–266, 267–268sd, 269–272, 273–274sd
automatic load management system, 263–264
changeover operations, 246, 260–261, 263, 263f, 264sd
electric generators, 265–266, 265–266f, 267–268sd
fire pump operations, 246–249, 250sd
high idle switch, 263

internal water tank, 249
load sequencer, 263
load shedding, 263
monitoring the fire pump, 261, 263, 263f, 264sd
power equipment distribution, 269, 269–270f
powered rescue tools, 270–272, 271–272f, 273–274sd
pressurized water sources, 246, 249, 251–253
scene lighting equipment, 266, 266f, 269, 269f
standpipe/sprinkler connecting, 255, 257–258, 258f, 259sd, 260
static water source, 246, 247f
summary and review, 275–276
water source, securing, 253–255
Fires
Great Baltimore Fire (1904), 5
One Meridian Plaza, Philadelphia (1991), 154
protection in early American cities, 5–7, 5–7f
Fixed-gallonage fog nozzles, 114
FL. *See* Friction loss (FL) calculations
Flashlights, backing up fire apparatus and, 205, 207
Floating pumps, 288, 288f
Floating strainers, 290, 290f
Floodlights, 266
Flow meters (flow minders)
performance tests, 483, 485, 485f, 487sd
pump operator's panel, 90–91, 90f
Flow pressure, 59, 68, 122–123f, 122–124, 450. *See also* Pump discharge pressure (PDP)
Flow rate
calculations, 125–127, 125t, 126f, 126sd
fire pump capacity, 78, 85
Fluid dynamics for water, 56–58f, 56–59
Fluid levels, inspection of, 170, 174–176, 174f, 175f
Fluoroprotein foam (FP), 326, 330t, 331, 331f
Foam. *See also* Foam proportioning systems
applying, 345–346, 347–348sd, 348–349, 349sd, 350sd
characteristics, 326, 328–329
classifications, 329–333, 329f, 331–333f
compatibility, 349
expansion rates, 333–334
finished foam, 328
foam concentrates, 333, 333t
history of, 326–327
mobile foam fire apparatus, 46, 46f, 46t, 47t
nozzles for, 331, 342, 345
overview of, 327–328
storage supplies for, 345, 345f
summary and review, 351–353
tetrahedron components, 328, 328f
Foam blanket, 327f, 328, 329, 329f, 331f
Foam concentrate pump, 340–341
Foam concentrates, 327–328, 332, 333, 333t, 334, 472
Foam heat exchanger, 340
Foam proportioning systems

around-the-pump (AP), 337, 339, 339sd
balanced-pressure, 340, 340f
batch mixing, 334–335, 334f, 335sd
compressed-air foam, 341–342, 341f, 343sd, 473–474
eductors, 335–337, 336f, 338sd
injection, 340–341
for mechanical foam production, 326
metering devices, 336–337, 336f, 472–473
performance testing, 471–474
premixing, 335
Foam solution, 328, 341, 345
Foam supply tank inspection, 180
Foam tetrahedron, 328, 328f
Fog nozzles
foam use of, 345
nozzle pressure calculations, 122–123, 122–123f, 124, 124sd
protein foam caution, 330, 331, 331f
sizes and flows, 386
Fog-stream nozzles, 112, 112f, 114, 115sd
Fold-down stabilizers, 361, 361f, 362
Following distance, 221
Forward (hose) lay, 249, 251, 251f, 314, 314f
Four-way hydrant valves, 251, 251f
FP. See Fluoroprotein foam (FP)
Friction loss (FL) calculations, 127–147
aerial apparatus, 450
in appliances, 131, 135–136f, 135–139, 137sd, 139sd
coefficients, standard or metric, 128t
condensed Q calculation, 160–162
defined, 59
equations, 127–128, 156
GPM flowing calculation, 160, 160sd
hand method calculations, 158–160, 159sd
hydraulic calculators for, 158
in-line gauges for testing, 139sd
in multiple hose lines of different sizes and lengths, 128–129, 132–133sd
in relay pumping operations, 313, 314–316
in Siamese hose lines, 143–145, 144–146sd, 145sd, 146sd
in single hose lines, 130sd, 131sd
in standpipe operations, 149–150
subtract 10 calculation, 160, 160sd
total pressure loss and, 139–140, 141
in wyed hose lines, 140–143, 140–143sd
Front mount pumps, 94, 94f
Fuel cap inspection, 174
Fuel gauge, checking during starting procedure, 194
Fuel level
inspection of, 178
for power tools, 179
pump panel indicator, 92
Fuel pick-up, foam and, 329
Fuel resistance of foam, 329, 330t
Full-jacking, aerial device stabilizing, 368, 368f, 369sd

G

Gallons per minute (GPM) flowing method, 160
Galvanic corrosion, 54
Garrity, Charles, 82
Gasoline-powered fire apparatus, 6–7, 7f
Gate valves, 109, 109f
Gated ball valves, 254
Gated wyes, 105, 105f, 107, 135f
Gauge meter test of discharge pressure, 483, 485, 486sd
Generator, 265–266, 265–266f
GFCI, line voltage electrical systems tests, 475
Global positioning system (GPS), 219
GPM (gallons per minute) flowing method, 160, 160sd
GPS. See Global positioning system (GPS)
Grade D air cylinders, 438
Gravity-feed water distribution systems, 55, 55f
Great Baltimore Fire (1904), 5
Ground ladders on fire apparatus, 39, 42–43, 44, 290, 291f
Ground plates, 452, 452f, 453, 454–455, 455f

H

Hand lay to hydrant, 254–255, 254f, 257sd
Hand method calculations, 158–160, 159sd
Hand pumps, 5, 5f, 79
Hand signals, for backing fire apparatus, 205, 205–206f
Handline nozzles, 111
Handlines
aerial device operations, 357
charts of handline and master stream calculations, 157–158, 157f, 157t
selection, 156
Handrails, aerial ladders, 442
Hard suction hose, 105, 105f, 289, 290, 291, 293
Hardness, water, 54
Hayes, Daniel, 42
Hazardous materials incidents, 240
Hazards, recognizing emergency scene, 226, 227
Hearing protection, vacuum test of priming system and, 491
Heat of vaporization, 54
Heat resistance of foam, 329, 330t
Heel pins, 441
Height restrictions, for fire apparatus, 25
High idle switch, 263
High-expansion foam generators, 342, 345
High-expansion foams, 332–333, 333f, 334
High-pressure auxiliary pumps, 79
High-rise structures, 78, 129, 135f
High-visibility reflective vests, 233–234
Highways
emergency vehicle driving, 232–234
positioning fire apparatus on, 232–234, 237–238
Hills
driving up or down, 222
positioning at fire scene on, 230

Hoist cables checklist, aerial device, 436–437
Hook and ladder truck, 4, 6, 6f, 42f. *See also* Tiller aerial apparatus
Horizontal reach, aerial device, 447, 447f
Horizontal ventilation via windows, 382
Horse-drawn fire equipment and crew transportation, 5f, 6, 6f
Hose carts, 5, 5f
Hose clamps, 108–109, 109f
Hose jackets, 108, 108f
Hoses, 101–110. *See also* Fire hose appliances; Friction loss (FL) calculations; Large-diameter hose (LDH); Medium-diameter hose (MDH); Supply hose/lines; Supply line evolutions; *specific types of hoses*
   access to, positioning at fire scene and, 228
   aerial device operations, 357, 373
   attack hose/lines, 39, 102, 102f, 103–104, 103f
   booster hose/lines, 7, 102, 104
   connecting supply hose lines to FDCs, 257–258, 259sd
   discharge valves and drafting operation, 293–294, 296sd
   evolution of, 5
   for filling tankers, 301
   functions of, 102, 102f
   in-line pressure gauges for testing, 136f
   for mobile foam fire apparatus, 46
   for mobile water supply apparatus, 41
   NFPA 1901 requirements for, 38
   nozzle size and diameter of, 126–127
   for pumper fire apparatus, 38
   for quints, 44t
   size of, 102–103, 103f
   suction, 38, 78
   suction size, number of suction lines, and lift for fire pump, 495t
   supply hose/lines, 102–105, 102–105f, 104–105, 104–105f, 106sd
   types of, 103–105, 104–105f
Hot zones, at emergency medical scenes, 240
H-style jacks, 444–445, 445f
H-type stabilizers, 360, 361f, 362
Hydrants. *See* Fire hydrants
Hydraulic actuator, 271
Hydraulic combination tools, 271, 272f
Hydraulic cutters, 271, 271f
Hydraulic extension ram, 272, 272f
Hydraulic pressure gauge, 438
Hydraulic pump, 359, 456
Hydraulic reservoir, 270
Hydraulic solenoid valve, 456, 457f
Hydraulic spreaders, 271, 271f
Hydraulic system
   aerial devices, 184, 359–360, 360f, 435–436, 436f, 438
   engaging PTO-driven, 273–274sd
Hydraulics/hydraulic calculations, 121, 148, 158
Hydrocarbon combustible fuels, foam use on, 330
Hydroelectric swivel, 441–442, 442f

I

IC. *See* Incident commander (IC)
Ignition switch, 194, 209
Impeller, centrifugal pump, 81, 83f
Impeller vanes, 81, 83f
Incident commander (IC)
   on aerial device deployment and operation, 356, 357, 363, 364, 382, 385, 425
   cavitations and, 297
   Class B foam application and, 346
   drafting operations and, 284
   on duration of drafting operations, 294
   on emergency scene positioning, 240
   on fire apparatus placement, 231, 234
   on fire scene positioning, 227–228
   on relay pumping operations, 312, 313, 320, 321
   responsibility for uninterrupted water supply, 297
   on staging, 228–229
   on tanker operations, 301, 306
   on tiller apparatus positioning, 414, 415
   on water shuttle operations, 306
   water supply monitoring and, 301
Incident Management System (IMS), 227, 284, 306–307
Incident space, 236
Incontrol (electronic pump control mechanism), 94
Indicator lights, troubleshooting aerial device, 459t
Induction and eductor use, 335
Industrial structures, aerial device positioning, 366
Initial attack fire apparatus, 38–40, 39–40, 39t, 41
Injectors/injection systems, 340–341
In-line eductors, 335–337, 336f, 338sd
In-line pressure gauges, 136, 136f, 137sd, 138, 139sd, 149, 150
Inspections. *See also* Fire apparatus inspection and maintenance
   aerial devices, 184–185, 184–185f, 363
   fire equipment, 25–26, 25–26f, 179–180, 179–180f, 187, 187f
   job aids for, 21
   nozzles, 114, 115sd
   360-degree, 192, 193sd, 196, 434
   tiller aerial apparatus, 406–407, 407f
   work-safe environment and, 22
Insurance Services Office (ISO), 475
Intake connections, pump, 86–87, 86–88f
Intake pressure, 294, 496
Intake pressure gauge, master pump, 89, 89f
Intake relief valve system test, 481
Intake side of fire pumps
   centrifugal pump, 81, 83, 85, 86
   connections, 86–87, 86–88f
   defined, 86
   positive-displacement pumps, 79, 80, 81
Intakes, 296
Interior functional control switches, inspection of, 177
Interlocks, testing aerial device, 457
Intermediate traffic incidents, 234

Index

Internal water tanks, 249
Intersections
    emergency vehicle driving, 223–225, 232–234, 236–237
    tiller apparatus driving safety, 401, 402f, 404, 413
Inventory, fire apparatus, 25
Inverter, 265, 265f
ISO. *See* Insurance Services Office (ISO)

J

Jack beam, 444
Jack box, 445
Jack cylinder, 444
Jacks, 360, 361–362, 459t. *See also* Outriggers for stabilizing aerial apparatus
Jerking ladder movements, troubleshooting, 458, 460
Jet siphon, 304
Job aids for inspections, 21
Job performance requirements (JPR), 27, 29
JPR. *See* Job performance requirements (JPR)
Junction box, 270

K

K braces, aerial ladders, 442
Kinetic energy, 56
Knockdown speed and flow of foam, 330–331, 330t

L

Ladder belt, 375, 377
Ladder companies, setup position for, 231
Ladder hook truck, 6, 6f
Ladder stops, 451
Ladder wagons, horse-drawn, 6, 6f
Ladders. *See also* Aerial ladders; Engines' and ladders' positioning
    for drafting operations, 290–291, 291f
    early use in fire protection, 4
    fire apparatus positioning and, 228
    ground ladders, 39, 42–43, 44, 291f
    for initial attack fire apparatus, 39
    on pumper fire apparatus, 38, 38t
    for quints, 44, 44f
    tower ladders, 8, 8f
Lane changes, emergency vehicle driving, 220, 410, 410f
Lanterns, 266, 266f
Large-diameter hose (LDH)
    characteristics, 102
    to establish a fill site using a hydrant, 300
    hand lays using, 254, 254f
    pump intake connections, 86, 87f
    for relay pumping operations, 314
    as supply hose, 103, 230
Lateral acceleration alert device, 11
Laws, emergency vehicle, 219–220
LDH. *See* Large-diameter hose (LDH)
Leaks, checking for, 180, 180f

Leather fire buckets, 4, 4f
LED scene lights, 269
Length of hose, friction loss (FL) calculations, 128–129, 132sd
Level I staging, 228, 228f
Level II staging, 228–229, 229f, 232
Lift
    fire pump discharge capacity, effect on, 280, 281f
    height of, from water source, 284, 287–288
    hose suction size, number of suction lines, and fire pump, 495t
Lift controls, 440–441
Lift cylinders, 440–441
Lights
    aerial devices, 362, 438, 439, 459t
    apparatus-mounted, 266, 269, 269f
    cradle alignment light, aerial device turntable, 438
    emergency lights, 11–12, 197, 219, 233, 247
    flashlights, backing up fire apparatus and, 205, 207
    inspection of fire apparatus, 169, 178
    scene lighting equipment, 266, 266f, 269, 269f
    tower lights, 269, 269–270f
Lindroth, Ron, 40
Line voltage electrical systems tests, 474–475
Lines. *See* Hoses
Liquid surge, driving fire apparatus and, 222
Load on aerial device
    safe practices for, 372–373, 373f, 374f, 375, 424, 448, 448f
    testing, 457–458, 469, 475
Load sequencer, 263
Load shedding, 263
Location of emergency, 218, 225–226, 226f
Low-expansion foams, 334
Low-level strainers, 289–290, 290f, 296, 305
Low-voltage electrical system testing, 468–471, 468f, 469sd, 469t, 470t
Low-volume nozzles, 111

M

Mag yoke, 455
Magnetic particle testing, aerial devices, 455, 455f
Maintenance. *See* Fire apparatus inspection and maintenance
Major traffic incidents, 234
Male adapters, 107, 108f
Manhole covers, aerial device positioning, 443
Manifolds, 131, 135f, 298, 300, 314–315, 319, 319f
Manual guard override switch, aerial device turntable, 439, 439f
Manual on Uniform Traffic Devices for Streets and Highways (MUTCD), 11, 234, 236–238
Manual water drain valve, for air brake system, 179, 179f
Manufacturer documentation for fire apparatus operations, 169–170
Manufacturers of fire apparatus, 36–37, 36f
Maps, emergency vehicle response, 218–219, 218f
Master power switch, aerial device turntable, 438
Master pump discharge pressure gauges, 89, 89f
Master pump intake pressure gauges, 89, 89f

Master stream nozzles, 111, 122, 123f, 345
Master streams
    charts of handline and master stream calculations, 157f, 157t, 158
    defined, 131
    devices, 103, 103f, 107, 111, 144
    elevated, 145–147, 146f, 150–153sd, 384, 427
    prepiped elevated, 145–147, 150–151sd
    smooth-bore nozzles for, 111, 122, 123f
Mathematics, 118–165. *See also* Friction loss (FL) calculations
    appliance loss, 131, 135–136f, 135–139, 135f, 137sd, 139sd
    charts of handline and master stream calculations, 157f, 157t, 158
    "chunking" calculations for understanding, 139
    condensed Q calculation, 160–162
    elevated master streams, 145–147, 146f, 150–153sd
    elevation pressure, 129–130, 134
    fire service hydraulic calculations, 156–160, 157f, 157t, 159sd
    flow rate, 125–127, 125t, 126f, 126sd
    friction loss equation, 127–128
    hand method, 158–160, 159sd
    hydrant, determining additional water from, 161–162
    hydraulic calculators, 158
    introduction to, 121–122
    net pump discharge pressure, 155–156
    nozzle flow, 125–127, 125t, 126f, 126sd
    nozzle pressures, 122–123f, 122–124
    nozzle reaction, 124, 124sd
    prepiped elevated master streams, 145–147, 150–151sd
    preplanning discharge pressure for a standpipe, 153sd
    pressure-regulating valves, 151, 154
    pump discharge pressure, 122–123f, 122–127, 124sd, 125t, 126f, 126sd
    quantity of water available estimates, 286–287
    Siamese hose lines, 143–145, 144–145sd
    standpipe discharge pressure, 149–150, 150t, 152–155sd
    standpipe systems, 147, 149–156, 149f, 150–155sd
    subtract 10 method, 160, 160sd
    suction loss calculation, 477
    summary and review, 163–165
    theoretical hydraulic calculations, 156–160
    total pressure loss, 139–140, 141
    wyed hose lines, 140–143, 140–143sd
McGrail, David, 157
McIntyre, Tim, 411, 426
MDH. *See* Medium-diameter hose (MDH)
MDTs (mobile data terminals), 217, 217f, 219
Mechanical abilities of driver/operator, 29, 30
Mechanical foams, 328
Mechanical generators, 342, 342f
Medical qualifications of driver/operator, 28, 28f
Medium-diameter hose (MDH), 103, 103f, 298, 300, 314, 316, 319
Medium-expansion foam generators, 342, 345
Medium-expansions foams, 334
Members. *See* Crew members
Metric measurements

coefficients for multiple Siamese lines, 146t
coefficients for standpipe risers, 150t
in elevated master streams, 151sd, 153sd
elevation pressure (loss and gain), 134sd
friction loss coefficients, 128t
friction loss in multiple hose lines of different sizes and lengths, 131sd
friction loss in single hose lines, 131sd
of pump discharge pressure for a standpipe, 153sd, 155sd
of pump discharge pressure in wye scenario with equal lines, 141sd
of pump discharge pressure in wye scenario with unequal lines, 143sd
of Siamese hose FL by coefficient method, 145sd
of Siamese hose FL by percentage method, 146sd
of Siamese hose FL by split flow method, 144sd
smooth-bore handline nozzle flow, 126sd
for smooth-bore nozzles flows, 125t
of vacuum to water column and pressure, 280t
Minoia, Mario, 110
Minor traffic incidents, 234
Mirrors, fire apparatus, 177, 194, 194f, 196, 205f
Miscible fuels, 330
Mnemonics, crew training using, 22
Mobile data terminals (MDTs), 217, 217f, 219
Mobile foam fire apparatus, 46, 46f, 46t, 47t
Mobile water supply apparatus, 41, 41f, 42t, 52–53, 52f
Modified H-style jack system, 444–445, 445f
Moisture removal system, for air brakes, 179, 179f
Monthly fire apparatus inspections, 187
Motor vehicle accidents (MVA), 226, 234, 236–238
Motorists, reducing vision impairment of, 233
Moving water sources, estimating quantity of, 286–287
Multiple victims situation, rescue operation, 381
Multiple-connection standpipes, 258f
Multiplexing, 93, 439
Multistage pumps, 83–84, 83–85, 84f, 85–86, 86f
Multistory structures, 78, 129, 135f
Municipal water systems
    characteristics and sources for, 52, 54–56, 55f, 56f
    distribution system, 55–56, 55–56f, 55f, 56f
    treatment facilities, 55, 55f
MUTCD. *See* Manual on Uniform Traffic Devices for Streets and Highways (MUTCD)
MVA. *See* Motor vehicle accidents (MVA)

N

National Fallen Firefighters Foundation (NFFF), 203
National Fired Protection Association (NFPA). *See also* specific numbered standards at NFPA
    on ladder weight limits and dimensions, 442
    on waterway and associated plumbing, 441
National Institute for Occupational Safety and Health (NIOSH), 203
National Institute of Standards and Technology (NIST), 326

Index

NDT. *See* Nondestructive testing (NDT)
Near-Miss Reports
    aerial ladder outrigger fails inspection, 454
    aerial stabilizer narrowly missing fire fighter, 427
    attack team entry without proper water pressure, 156
    brake failure, 183
    close-call for traffic accident upon returning to station, 24
    cold weather freezes pumper, 260
    downed powerline injuries due to tiller cab contact, 412
    failed coupling during test strikes firefighter, 499
    fall from open cab in moving pumper, 10
    foam supply problem during incident, 346
    lack of communication in using aerial device, 377
    ladder truck slide into intersection on wet road, 237
    loss of water pressure during fire attack, 303
    missed pump operation step caused pump failure, 85
    on-scene fire apparatus collision, 200
    tanker slides off snowy road, 41
    unattended gated wye appliance strikes firefighter, 111
    water hammer results in burst hose, 319
    water hammer shears coupling, 65
Net pump discharge pressure (NPDP), 155–156
Net pump pressure (NPP) performance test, 477–478
Newly constructed roads, aerial device positioning, 443
Newsham, Richard, 5
NFFF. *See* National Fallen Firefighters Foundation (NFFF)
NFPA 11, *Standard for Low-, Medium-, and High-Expansion Foam,* 333–334
NFPA 13, *Standard for the Installation of Sprinkler Systems,* 151
NFPA 14, *Standard for the Installation of Standpipe and Hose Systems,* 151
NFPA 18A, *Standard on Water Additives for Fire Control and Vapor Mitigation,* 330
NFPA 20 *Standard for the Installation of Stationary Pumps for Fire Protection,* 79
NFPA 291, *Recommended Practice for Fire Flow Testing and Marking of Hydrants,* 64–65
NFPA 1002, *Standard for Fire Apparatus Driver/Operator Professional Qualifications*
    on backing up fire apparatus, 206–207, 238
    on confined-space turnarounds, 202
    on diminishing clearance exercise, 203
    driver/operator medical and physical requirements, 28, 28*f*
    driver/operator qualifications and requirements, 26–28, 26–28*f*, 29
    on seat belts, 19
    on serpentine driving exercise, 200
NFPA 1071, *Standard for Emergency Vehicle Technician Professional Qualifications*
    aerial device inspection, 363
    fire apparatus inspection and preventive maintenance, 169
    hydraulic fluid inspection, 435
    performance testing, 467
NFPA 1403, *Standard on Live Fire Training Evolutions,* 346
NFPA 1451, *Standard for a Fire and Emergency Service Vehicle Operations Training Program,* 28, 29*f*, 169
NFPA 1500, *Standard for Fire Department Occupational Safety and Health Program*
    driver/operator medical and physical requirements, 28, 28*f*
    on enclosed cab seating, 8, 10
    on seat belts, 10, 196
NFPA 1561, *Standard on Emergency Services Incident Management System,* 227
NFPA 1582, *Standard on Comprehensive Occupational Medical Program for Fire Departments,* 28, 28*f*
NFPA 1620, *Recommended Practice for Pre-incident Planning,* 232
NFPA 1901, *Standards for Automotive Fire Apparatus*
    on aerial fire apparatus, 42–43, 43*t*, 44*t*, 358, 359, 362, 440
    on air pressure discharge, 194
    capacity test/150 psi test, 497
    on enclosed cab seating, 8, 10
    on engine compartment maintenance, 174, 175
    on fire apparatus equipped with water tanks, 37
    as fire apparatus performance standards, 37
    on fire apparatus tests, 476, 477
    on fire pump flow meters, 91
    on fire pumps and pumping processes, 77, 78, 86, 89, 91, 284
    fluid chart, 175
    on initial attack fire apparatus, 39, 39*t*, 41
    on manufacturer documentation, 169–170
    on mobile foam fire apparatus, 46, 46*t*, 47*t*
    on mobile water supply apparatus, 41, 42*t*
    on monitoring of vehicle electrical system, 263
    on parking apparatus on slopes, 230
    on parking brake requirements, 194
    on performance test site, 477–478
    on power source testing, 474
    on pumper fire apparatus, 37–38, 78–79, 493
    on quints, 44, 44*t*, 45*t*
    on seat belts, 10, 196
    on special service fire apparatus, 44–45, 45*t*
    troubleshooting guide requirement, 458
    on vehicle data recorder (VDR), 11, 11*t*
    on vehicle height, 223
NFPA 1911, *Standard for the Inspection, Maintenance, Testing, and Retirement of In-Service Automotive Fire Apparatus*
    on aerial device inspection, 184, 359, 363, 429
    on annual testing of apparatus components, 452, 454, 455, 475–476
    on breathing-air compressor systems, 475–476
    on capacity test/150 psi test, 497
    on EVT as troubleshooting resource, 458
    on final test results, 501, 503
    on fire apparatus, 476, 477
    on fire pump certification test, 284
    on flow meters, 485
    on foam proportioning system testing, 472
    on pump engine control interlock test, 482

on pump performance test, 493
on pump test requirements, 491, 493t
on receptacle wiring tests, 474
on rerating fire pumps, 504
on stabilizer system visual inspection, 436
on test sites, 477–478
on time trial test for aerial devices, 458
on vehicle inspection, 467
on water system inspection and test, 458
on weight verification, 468
NFPA 1931, *Standard for Manufacturer's Design of Fire Department Ground Ladders*, 39
NFPA 1936, *Powered Rescue Tools*, 270
NFPA 1983, *Standard on Life Safety Rope and Equipment for Emergency Services*, 375
NFPA 1989, *Standard on Breathing Air Quality for Emergency Services Respiratory Protection*, 475
Nighttime
    driving during, 221, 223, 405–406
    identifying address/location during, 226
NIOSH. *See* National Institute for Occupational Safety and Health (NIOSH)
NIST. *See* National Institute of Standards and Technology (NIST)
No-load governed engine speed test, 480, 480f, 481sd
Nondestructive testing (NDT), 359, 363, 452, 452f, 454, 455
Nonmoving water sources, 286. *See also* Static water sources
Nozzle controls, aerial device turntable, 438
Nozzle pressure (NP), 59, 122–123f, 122–124, 450. *See also* Pump discharge pressure (PDP)
Nozzle shut-offs, 111
Nozzles, 111–116. *See also* Fog nozzles; Smooth-bore tips
    classifications, 111
    determining flow rate for, 125–127, 125t, 126f, 126sd
    fixed straight-stream, 4
    flow calculation, 125–127, 125t, 126f, 126sd
    fog-stream, 112, 112f, 114, 115sd
    function and types of, 111–114, 112f, 113sd, 114f, 115sd
    for hand pumps or leather hoses, 5
    hose diameter and size of, 126–127
    for initial attack fire apparatus, 39
    long pipe, 4
    maintenance and inspection, 114, 115sd
    master stream, 111, 122, 123f, 345
    for mobile water supply apparatus hoses, 41
    NFPA 1901 requirements for, 38
    for performance tests, 478, 479, 479f
    for pumper fire apparatus, 38
    for quints, 44t
    shut-offs, 111
    solid-bore sizes and flows, 386t
    standard nozzle pressure (SNP), 123–124
NP. *See* Nozzle pressure (NP)
NPDP. *See* Net pump discharge pressure (NPDP)
NPP. *See* Net pump pressure (NPP) performance test
Nurse tanker operations, 306

O

Obstruction alarm, aerial device turntable, 439
OEMs. *See* Original equipment manufacturers (OEMs)
Officer in charge (OIC), 20
Offset alley exercise, 410
OIC. *See* Officer in charge (OIC)
Oil pressure gauge, 196
Oil-less priming pump, inspection of, 181
Oleophobic quality of foam, 329
1½-inch (38-mm) attack hose, 103–104
One Meridian Plaza fire, Philadelphia (1991), 154
100 percent test, 497, 498sd
1¾-inch (45-mm) attack hose, 103–104
On-scene operations, 26
Operating manuals, 22, 25
Original equipment manufacturers (OEMs), 435, 458
Out-of-service criteria and deficiencies chart, aerial devices, 437f
Outrigger interlock, aerial device turntable, 439
Outrigger override switch, aerial device turntable, 439
Outriggers for stabilizing aerial apparatus
    deploying, 446, 446f
    positioning, 444
    safety devices, 446–447
    setup, 367
    short-set, 439, 446–447
    storing, 452, 452f
    tiller apparatus, 422–423
    troubleshooting, 459t, 460
    types, 360
    visual inspection, 436
Overhang, tiller apparatus driving, 404
Overhead obstructions, 231, 231f, 414, 424, 443, 460
Overload protection, stabilizing aerial devices, 362
Overload test/165 psi test, 497, 499
Overpasses, as height obstacles, 221, 223
Oversteering, tiller apparatus, 404
Over-tillering, tiller apparatus, 404
Oxygenated fuel additives, 331

P

Paper maps, 218f
Parallel/volume mode, of multistage pumps, 84, 84f, 85, 86
Parked fire apparatus, 227
Parking, 219–220, 233, 233f, 247, 247f
Parking brake
    performance tests, 468
    pump throttle and, 248
    shutting down the fire apparatus, 209
    starting the fire apparatus and, 194

Index

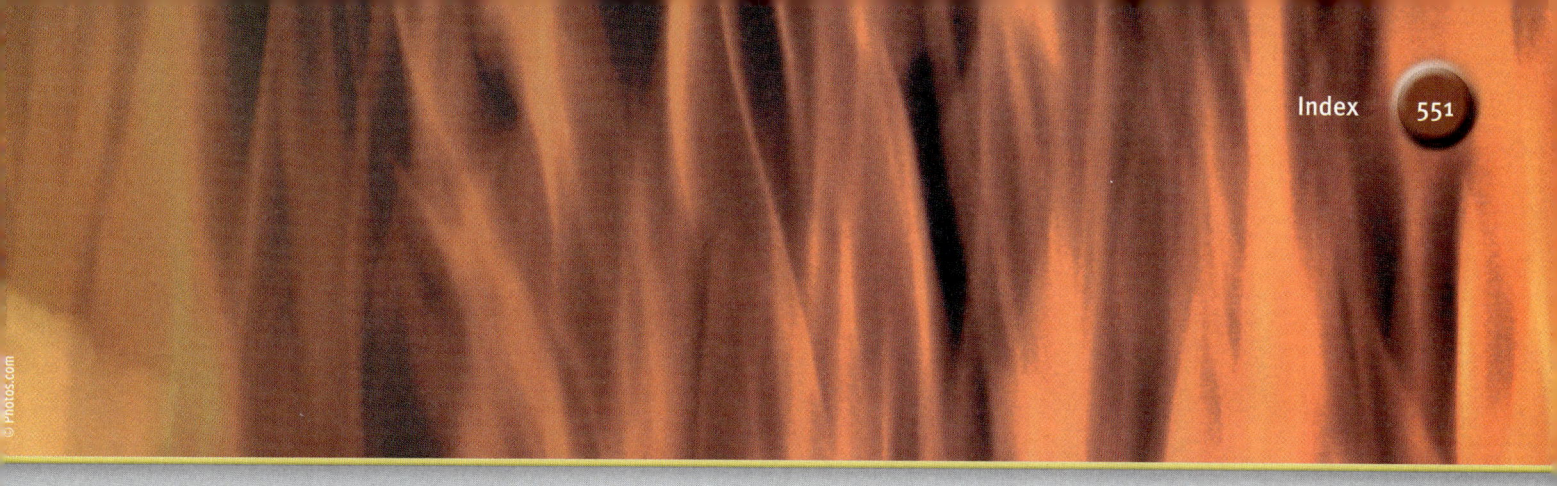

testing, 178–179, 179f
    traffic signal preemption systems and, 225
Parking exercise, tiller apparatus, 410, 410f, 412
PASS mnemonic, 22
Passing vehicles in emergency vehicle driving, 220–221
PDP. *See* Pump discharge pressure (PDP)
Percentage method (calculation), 144, 145, 146sd
Performance tests, 464–507
    aerial apparatus, 452, 452f, 455–457f, 455–460, 459t
    aerial fire apparatus, 457–458
    breathing-air compressor systems, 475–476
    capacity/150 psi (100 percent test), 497, 498sd
    environmental requirements for, 476–477
    equipment requirements, 478–480, 479–480f
    final results of, 501, 503, 503f
    fire apparatus requirements for, 476–480, 477–479f
    fire pump, 475–476, 491, 493, 493t, 495–500, 495f, 495t, 496f, 498sd
    flow meter, 483, 485, 485f, 487sd
    foam proportioning system testing, 471–474
    gauge test, 483, 485, 486sd
    intake relief valve system, 481
    line voltage electrical systems, 474–475
    no-load governed engine speed, 480, 480f, 481sd
    overload/165 psi, 497, 499
    post performance testing, 501, 503–504, 503f
    pressure control, 500–501, 500f, 502sd
    priming system, 491, 492f, 492sd
    problem solving, 503–504
    pump engine control interlock, 482–483, 482f, 484sd
    pump shift indicator, 481–182, 482f, 483sd
    pumping test requirements, 491, 493t
    rerating fire pumps, 504
    safety during, 478, 504
    summary and review, 505–507
    tank-to-pump flow, 488, 489sd
    test site, 477–478, 477–478f
    total continuous electrical load test, 471
    200 psi (70 percent), 499
    250 psi (50 percent), 499–500
    vacuum, 284, 285sd, 488, 490sd, 491
    vehicle, 467–471, 468f, 469sd, 469t, 470t
Periodic fire apparatus inspections, 187
Personal protective equipment (PPE), 11, 24, 170, 173, 196, 321, 375, 424
Petroleum-fueled fires, 327, 330
Physical properties of water, 53–54, 53f
Physical qualifications of driver/operator, 28, 28f, 30
Physical rescue, 364, 381–382
Pick-up tubes, 335, 345
Piercing nozzles, 114, 114f
Pilot-operated check (POC) valves, 440–441
Piston intake valve (PIV), 180
Piston pumps, 79–80, 80f

Pitot gauge(s)
    for fire hydrant testing, 66, 68, 68f, 69sd
    manual or threaded, 136f
    for testing appliance loss, 136, 136f, 137sd, 138sd
    and tubes, for performance tests, 479–480, 479–480f
Pitot pressure, 66
PIV. *See* Piston intake valve (PIV)
Platforms, aerial. *See* Aerial platforms
POC. *See* Pilot-operated check (POC) valves
Polar solvents, 329, 330, 331, 332, 332f, 333, 345
Police
    monitoring fill site using a hydrant, 300
    traffic control at MVAs and, 236
Poole, Todd, 40
Poor placement adjustments, aerial device positioning, 367
Portable generator, 265f
Portable lights, 266, 269f
Portable master stream devices, 144
Portable power units, 270, 271f
Portable pumps
    for accessibility to static water sources, 70, 70f, 288, 288f, 300–301
    floating, 288, 288f
    positive-displacement pumps as, 79
    for use in remote areas, 94, 94f
Portable tanks
    for drafting operations, 288, 290, 290f, 300
    source pumper considerations with, 304–305
    water shuttle operations, 302, 303–304, 304f
Positive-displacement pumps, 79–81, 80–81f
Potential energy, 56
Power equipment distribution, 269, 269–270f
Power rescue tool system, 270
Power source, line voltage electrical systems tests, 474
Power steering system inspection, 173, 174f, 176
Power supplies for fire pumps, 94–95f, 94–96
Power takeoff (PTO) units
    engaging, 265, 267–268sd
    fire pumps, 95, 95f
    hydraulic pump for aerial device, 359
    meters for, 435, 435f
    PTO-driven hydraulic system, 271, 273–274sd
    as rescue tool, 271
    troubleshooting, 459t
Power tools, inspection of, 179
Power transfer from tiller engine to hydraulics, 422
Powered rescue tools, 270–272, 271–272f, 273–274sd
PPE. *See* Personal protective equipment (PPE)
Preconnect lines, marking pressures for, 130
Pre-emergency vehicle response, 217–219
Preincident plans, 161, 232, 255. *See also* Preplanning
Premixing foam solutions, 335
Prepiped elevated master streams, 145–147, 150–151sd
Preplanning, 152–153sd, 286, 288, 298, 301. *See also* Preincident plans

Pressure control test, 500–501, 500f, 502sd
Pressure gauges, 89–90, 89f
Pressure governor, 92, 93f, 260, 261f, 500f
Pressure relief valve
　characteristics, 260, 261f
　performance test, 500–501, 500f, 502sd
　setting, 181
Pressure-regulating valves (PRV), 151, 154
Pressurized water sources, 246, 249, 251–253
Preventive maintenance program, 22, 25–26, 168
Primary feeders, municipal water systems, 56
Primer oil reservoir, 281, 283f
Primer valve, 284
Primer/priming pump
　inspection of, 181, 181f
　lubrication of, 281, 283f
　positive-displacement pumps as, 79
　primer control, pump panel, 92
　rotary pumps as, 80, 81
Priming the pump, 76
　drafting water operations, 281, 291, 294, 295sd, 297
　priming system test, 488, 491, 492f, 492sd
　vacuum test, 488
　for water drafting operations, 291, 293
Private water systems, 52, 52f
Problem solving
　in driver/operator selection, 29
　for performance tests, 503–504
Protective parking, 233, 233f
Protein foams, 326, 326f, 330–331, 331f
Prove-out sequence, 194
PRV. *See* Pressure-regulating valves (PRV)
PTO units. *See* Power takeoff (PTO) units
PTO-driven hydraulic system, 271, 273–274sd
Public response to emergency vehicles, 224–225
Pump discharge pressure (PDP)
　condensed Q method, 160–162
　defined, 121
　fire pump performance test, 495–496
　gauge, master pump, 89, 89f
　hand method calculations, 158–160, 159sd
　hydraulic calculations of, 121–127, 122–123f, 125t
　loss calculating, 122–123f, 122–124
　mathematics, 122–123f, 122–127, 124sd, 125t, 126f, 126sd, 156
　in prepiped elevated master streams, 147, 150–151sd
　relief valve, pump panel, 92, 93f
　in standpipe operations, 149–150, 152–155sd
　in wye scenario with equal lines, 140–141sd
　in wye scenario with unequal lines, 142–143sd
Pump engine control interlock test, 482–483, 482f, 483sd
Pump intake strainers, inspection of, 180–181, 181f
Pump operator's panel, 88–94, 89–93f
　described, 76, 77f, 88–89
　discharge pressure relief valve, 92, 93f
　electronic pump controllers, 93–94, 93f
　engine coolant temperature gauge, 91, 91f
　engine cooling devices, 91, 91f
　engine oil pressure gauge, 91, 92f
　engine tachometer, 90–91, 91f
　flow meters, 90–91, 90f
　fuel level indicator, 92
　master pump discharge pressure gauge, 89, 89f
　master pump intake pressure gauge, 89, 89f
　on multistage pump, 85
　NFPA 1901 required controls and instruments, 89
　pressure gauges, 89–90, 89f
　pressure governor, 92, 93f
　primer control, 92
　pump pressure control systems, 92–93, 93f
　voltmeter, 92, 92f
　water tank level indicator, 92, 92f
Pump panel, 77f, 85, 88–94, 89–93f
Pump pressure control systems, pump panel, 92–93, 93f
Pump seal, inspection of, 180, 180f
Pump shift control switch, 247–248, 248f
Pump shift indicator test, 481–182, 482f, 483sd
Pump test, 78
Pump test pits, 478, 478f
Pump transmission
　engaging, for drafting operations, 289
　switching from road transmission to, 247–248, 248f
Pump-and-gravity-feed water distribution system, 55–56
Pumper fire apparatus (pumpers), 37f. *See also* Fire pumps;
　Relay pumping operations
　attack pumpers, 251, 301, 313, 313f
　cab interior, 76–77, 77f
　described, 37–38, 38t
　exterior of fire department pumper, 76, 77f
　NFPA 1901 standards for, 37–38, 78–79, 493
　relay pumpers, 313, 313f
　source pumpers, 301, 302, 304–305, 312f, 313, 316
　triple-combination pumpers, 7, 7f
Pumping element, 80
Pumping engine throttle, 93–94, 93f
Pump-mounted eductors, 336
Pumps. *See* Fire pumps

Q
Q (quantity of water). *See* Water supply
Qualifications, importance for driver/operators, 12
Quarter-turn hydrant valve, 298, 298f
Quint fire apparatus, 44, 44f, 44t, 45t, 435

R
Radiator cap, safe removal of, 170, 175–176
Radio communication
　assigned tactical radio frequency, 218
　managing inside versus outside equipment, 247

Index

with spotters, 205, 206
   staging of fire apparatus and, 228
   tanker and water fill site, 301, 306
Railroad crossings, 225, 238
Raindown method for applying foam, 349, 350sd
Raise–rotate–extend process for aerial device operation, 449
Rate of flow, fire pumps, 77–78
Rated capacity, stability and load of aerial device, 457
Ratio controller, 340
Reaction distance, 221
Readiness, fire apparatus, 169, 169f, 209, 209f
Receptacle wiring, line voltage electrical systems tests, 474–475
Red emergency lights, 233
Red (stop) lights, emergency vehicle laws on, 220
Reducers, 108, 108f, 314
Reflective vests, ANSI-approved, 233–234
Refractometer, 472–473
Regulator tests, 470–471, 470t
Relay pumpers, 313, 313f
Relay pumping operations, 310–324, 312f
   attack pumper operation, 316–317, 317f
   calculated flow relay, 316
   calculating friction loss for, 315–316
   components, 312–313, 312–313f
   condensed Q method in, 161
   equipment for, 314
   joining an existing operation, 319–320, 320f
   personnel for, 314
   preparing for, 314–315
   pressure fluctuations in, 320
   relay pumper operation, 317
   safety for, 321
   shutting down, 320–321
   source pumper operation, 316
   summary and review, 322
   types, 316
   for uninterrupted water supply, 321
   water relay delivery options, 319, 319f
Relay test, 471
Relay (hydrant) valves, 109, 109f, 135f, 319–320, 320f
Relief valves, aerial device waterway system, 450, 450f
Repairs, fire departments' inspection of, 169
Rerating fire pumps, 504
Rescue operations
   positioning fire apparatus for, 229–230
   positioning of aerial apparatus for, 363, 367, 424
   tiller apparatus for, 415, 449–450
   using aerial apparatus for, 357, 378, 380–381, 380–382, 380f, 380sd, 381f
Rescue vehicle, NFPA 1002 qualification to operate, 27, 27f
Reservoirs, 54
Residential structures, aerial device positioning, 363, 364f, 365, 365f
Residential structures, floor spacing in, 129, 135f

Residual pressure, 59, 66, 67–68
Respiratory protection equipment. *See* Self-contained breathing apparatus (SCBA)
Restraints, 10. *See also* Seat belts
Retraction and stowing of aerial device, 436–437, 451, 451f, 458
Reverse (hose) lay, 251–252, 252f, 314, 315f
Reversing the fire apparatus, 205–207, 205–207f, 208sd
Rider positioning, assigned, 20
Right-of-way for fire apparatus, cautions on, 219, 224
Road surface condition, stopping and, 221
Road test, 468
Roll-on method for applying foam, 346, 348sd
Roof hooks, on pumper fire apparatus, 38, 38t
Rotary gear pumps, 80–81, 81f
Rotary pumps, 80–81, 81f
Rotary vane pumps, 80–81, 81f
Rotation controls, aerial turntable, 438, 438f, 460
Rotation interlock, aerial device turntable, 362, 370, 439
Rotation swivel, testing, 456
Rotors, in rotary pumps, 80–81
Rudder control indicator, tiller aerial apparatus, 443
Rung alignment indicator light, aerial device turntable, 438
Rungs of aerial ladder, specifications of, 442
Rural areas, finding address of fire in, 226
Rural water supplies, 68, 70, 70f

S

Safety. *See also* Near-Miss Reports
   adding fuel to power tools, 179
   aerial devices, 372–373, 373f, 374f, 375, 377–378, 377f, 428, 455
   aerial ladders, 377, 377–378f
   alcohol-resistant foams for alternative fuel incidents, 332
   appropriate use of foam concentrates, 332
   avoiding aerial ladder touching flowing water, 448
   avoiding maximizing aerial device capabilities, 375
   charging line from hydrant, 251
   with compressed-air foam systems, 342
   due regard, 22, 203, 220
   extending/retracting an aerial device, 437
   extension and retracting of aerial ladder, 450
   fire apparatus, 8, 10–12, 11–12f, 187
   during fire apparatus inspection, 170, 170f, 172
   fire apparatus public appearances and, 196
   fire fighter stance for forward hose lay, 251
   getting underway and, 196–197, 198–199f
   handline selection, 156
   ladder belt requirement for aerial devices, 377
   manning aerial device turntable, 439
   no nonessential conversation in cab, 21
   obstruction alarms for aerial devices, 439
   override switch caution, 439
   during performance testing, 478, 504
   positioning fire apparatus for drafting water, 287, 289

protecting driver/operator at the scene, 11
pump panel on aerial device, 447
for relay pumping operations, 321
retracting aerial ladder, 451
role of driver/operator, 19–20, 19–20f, 196–197, 203
rotation of aerial device, 449
seat belt issues, 196, 197
secured fire equipment, getting underway and, 196–197, 196–197f
short-setting the apparatus, 447
stability and load testing, 458
stabilizing apparatus, 370, 446
standards on, 9
teaching, 20
throttle control interlock for fire pump, 457
tiller apparatus operation, 422–423, 428
traffic incidents at fire scenes, 237
two crew members on a tanker, 301
vacuum test of priming system and, 491
water drain during aerial retraction, 458
water hammer and, 59
water shuttle operations, 301
waterway system for ladder, 441
wetting agent use in Class B foam application, 330
while driving apparatus, 10–11
work environment, maintaining, 19, 21–24
Safety and Survival on the Fireground (Dunn), 230
Safety equipment, training and education on, 22
Safety system of aerial devices, inspection of, 184–185
Salvage covers, for portable tanks, 288
Savannah, Georgia, first fully motorized fire department in, 7
SCBA. *See* Self-contained breathing apparatus (SCBA)
Scene lighting equipment, 266, 266f, 269, 269f
School bus loading/unloading, emergency vehicle laws on, 220
Scott-Uda ladders, 42
Screw-type hydrant valve, 298, 298f
Scrub area, 366
SDH. *See* Small-diameter hose (SDH)
Seagrave, 44
Seat belts
  driver/operator as first to buckle, 19f
  getting underway and, 196, 197
  importance as safety device, 19
  NFPA 1901 on warning devices for, 10
  safety issues, 196, 197
  supplemental restraint systems and, 10
Seats, fire apparatus, positioning for starting, 194
Secondary feeders, municipal water systems, 56
Self-contained breathing apparatus (SCBA)
  aerial device operations, 375
  as hazard in cab, 20, 196
  inspection of, 177, 177f, 179
  seat belt accommodation for, 19
  seat belts versus belts and straps of, 19, 19f, 177, 177f

Series/pressure mode, of multistage pump, 84–85, 84f, 85
Serpentine course exercise, 200–201, 201sd, 407, 409f
Serpentine maneuvers, 200–201, 201sd
Service manuals, 22
Service testing fire pumps, 475–476. *See also* Performance tests
Setback of structure from curb, 363, 365
70 percent test, 499
Short-jacking, aerial device stabilizing, 361, 367, 368, 368f, 370
Short-set outrigger, 439, 446–447
Shut-off valves, for water mains, 56, 56f
Shutting down the fire apparatus, 207, 209, 209f, 210sd
Siamese connections, 135f
  coefficients for, 128t, 144–145, 145sd, 146sd, 146t
  determining friction loss in, 143–145, 144–146sd
  in fire department connections, 257–258, 260f
  as fire hose appliance, 107, 107f
Sidewalks, aerial device positioning, 443
Single- versus double-action lift cylinders, 441
Single-acting piston pumps, 79–80, 79f, 80f
Single-stage pumps, 83, 84f
Sirens, 197, 203, 219, 220
Situational awareness, importance of, 444
Skids/skidding, 222
Slide rule hydraulic calculators, 158
Slides and rollers, aerial device, inspection of, 184, 185f
Slopes, positioning at fire scene on, 230
Small-diameter hose (SDH), 102, 103f
Smith, Drew, 376
Smooth-bore tips (nozzles)
  characteristics, 111–112, 112f
  for compressed-air foam systems, 345
  distributor type, 126f
  flow calculations, 124sd, 126sd
  handline, 122, 123f, 126sd
  maintenance and inspection, 113sd, 114
  master stream, 111, 122, 123f
  nozzle reaction, 124
  for performance tests, 479
  standard or metric flows by size or type, 125t
SNP. *See* Standard nozzle pressure (SNP)
Soda acid extinguishers, 7
Soft sleeve hose, 104–105, 104f, 106sd
Soft suction hose, 254, 254f
SOGs. *See* Standard operating guidelines (SOGs)
Solenoid test, 471
Solid-bore nozzle sizes and flows, 385–386, 386t
Solid-tip nozzles, 122, 158
Songer, Daryl, 148
SOPs. *See* Standard operating procedures (SOPs)
Source pumpers, 301, 302, 304–305, 312f, 313, 316
Special emergency scene positioning, 238, 240
Special service (specialized) fire apparatus, 44–45, 45f, 45t, 232
Specific heat index, 53
Speed limits, emergency vehicle driving, 220, 221, 401

Index

Speed of fire apparatus, stopping and, 221
Speed reading for fire pumps, 493, 495f
Split flow method (calculation), 144, 144sd
Split hose bed, 253
Split (hose) lay, 252–253, 253f, 314, 315f
Spotlights, 266
Spotters and spotting
 aerial device positioning, 364, 364–365f
 backing up the apparatus, 12, 12f
 reversing the fire apparatus, 205–207, 205–207f, 208sd
Spreaders, hydraulic, 271, 271f
Spring brake test, 178–179, 179f
Sprinkler systems, 232, 255, 257–258, 258f
Stabilization. *See also* Jacks; Outriggers
 aerial apparatus, 359, 360–362, 361f, 367–368, 369sd, 370, 371sd, 436, 437f, 457–458
 checklist for aerial devices, 436, 437f
 ground plates, 452, 452f, 453, 454–455, 455f
 inspection, 184, 184f, 457
 setup options, 368
 tiller apparatus, 422–423, 423f
Staging area, 228–229
Staging area manager, 228
Staging of fire apparatus, 227–229, 228f, 229f, 235
Standard measurements
 coefficients for multiple Siamese lines, 146t
 coefficients for standpipe risers, 150t
 in elevated master streams, 150sd, 152sd
 elevation pressure (loss and gain), 134sd
 friction loss coefficients, 128t
 friction loss in multiple hose lines of different sizes and lengths, 130sd
 of friction loss in Siamese hose by coefficient method, 145sd
 of friction loss in Siamese hose lines by percentage method, 146sd
 of friction loss in Siamese lines by split flow method, 144sd
 friction loss in single hose lines, 130sd
 hand method, 159sd
 of pump discharge pressure for standpipe, 152sd, 154sd
 of pump discharge pressure in wye scenario, 140sd, 142sd
 smooth-bore handline nozzle flow, 126sd
 for smooth-bore nozzles flows, 125t
 of vacuum to water column and pressure, 280t
Standard nozzle pressure (SNP), 123–124
Standard operating guidelines (SOGs)
 aerial device positioning, 363
 following and promoting compliance with, 19
 for operational, testing, and maintenance responsibilities, 435
 for vehicle inspection, 467
 for work-safe environments, 19
Standard operating procedures (SOPs)
 for aerial device positioning, 363
 for backing fire apparatus, 205
 for emergency communications, 21
 for emergency response, 218

following and promoting compliance with, 19, 22, 24, 28
 for operational, testing, and maintenance responsibilities, 435
 for positioning at fire scene, 227
 safety role of, 12
 for vehicle inspection, 467
 for work-safe environments, 19
Standards. *See under* NFPA
Standpipe risers, 149, 149f
Standpipe systems
 characteristics and calculations for, 147, 149–156, 149f, 150–155sd
 connection to, 255, 257–258, 258f, 259sd, 260
 discharge pressure calculations for, 152–154sd
 preincident plans on, 232
 pressure-regulating valves for, 151, 154
 water supply for, 149
Starter switch, 194
Starting the fire apparatus, preparing to drive, 194, 196–197, 198–199sd
State laws, on emergency vehicles, 219–220
Static pressure, of water, 58–59, 66, 67sd
Static water sources
 accessibility of, 287–289, 288f
 defined, 34
 determining reliability of, 284
 establishing a fill site from, 300–301
 establishing dump site operations from, 302
 estimating quantity, 286
 evaluating quality of, 287, 287f
 in fireground operations, 246, 247f
 operating source pumpers at, 302
 pump maintenance and conditions of, 54
 rural, 68, 68f, 70, 70f
Steam fire pumps (steamers), 5, 6f
Steam-powered pumps (steamers), 4–5, 5f, 6f, 80
Steering, during skids, 222
Steering wheel, free play in, 174, 174f
Stop (red) lights, emergency vehicle laws on, 220
Stop signs, emergency vehicle laws on, 220
Storz connections, 104, 106sd, 107
Straight ladders. *See* Aerial ladders
Straight roads, driving on, 221, 221f
Straight-in (parallel) parking exercise, tiller apparatus, 410, 412
Straight-line drive exercise, tiller apparatus, 410, 410f, 412
Strainers
 barrel, 289–290, 290f
 debris in, 297
 for drafting operations, 287, 287f, 289–290, 290f
 floating, 290, 290f
 low-level, 289–290, 290f, 296, 305
 pump intake, inspection of, 180–181, 181f
Stressors, 21
Strip mall structures, 365–366, 366f
Structural component testing, aerial devices, 456–457, 457f

Subtract 10 method (calculation), 160, 160sd
Suction hoses, 38, 78
Suction loss calculation, 477
Supplemental restraint systems, 10
Supply hose/lines
    bleeding, in relay pumper operations, 316, 317, 317f
    changeover operations, 246, 260–261, 263, 263f, 264sd
    described, 104–105, 104–105f, 106sd
    functions of, 102, 102f, 103f
    hand lay to hydrant, 254–255, 254f, 257sd
    to standpipe and sprinkler systems, 241–243, 242f, 243f, 245f, 246sd
    testing, 103
Supply line evolutions, 249, 251–252
    forward hose lay, 249, 251, 251f, 314, 314f
    four-way hydrant valve, 251, 251f
    objectives, 249
    reverse hose lay, 251–252, 252f, 314, 315f
    split hose lay, 252–253, 253f, 314, 315f
Supported versus unsupported aerial device positions, 372–373, 373f
Surface conditions, fire apparatus positioning and, 230–231
Surface tension, 53, 328
Suspension system inspection, 174
Sweep area, 366
Sweep (roll-on) method for applying foam, 346, 348sd
Synthetic detergent foams, 332–333, 333f
Synthetic foams, 331
System check sequence, fire apparatus and, 194

T

Tachometer
    engine, 90–91, 91f
    handheld, 504
Tactical benchmarks, 21
Tank fill valve, 87, 88f
Tankers, 87, 88f, 298, 300–302, 301, 303, 306. See also Water tanks
Tank-to-pump flow test, 488, 489sd
Tank-to-pump pipe, 86, 86f
Team building, 18–19, 21
Teamsters, 5, 6
Technology. See also specific systems and operations
    computer systems, battery cable removal and, 176, 176f
    electronic pump controllers, 93–94
    modern fire apparatus, 13
    vehicle data recorder (VDR), 11
    vehicle intercom system, 20, 439–440
Temperature
    engine and pump, during drafting operations, 296
    fire apparatus performance, 476–477
    weight of water and, 54
Tenders, 41, 41f. See also Tankers
Termination areas, 236

Terrain, fire apparatus positioning and, 230–231
Terrorism incidents, 240
Test sites, 454–455, 454f, 477–478, 477–478f
Testing. See Performance tests
Testing gauges, 478–480, 479–480f. See also Pitot gauge(s)
Theoretical hydraulics, 121, 156–160
Third-party testing, aerial devices, 455–456
Threaded hose couplings, 104
360-degree inspection, 192, 193sd, 196, 434
Three-second rule for following distance, 221
Three-stage pumps, 85
Throttle, pumping engine, 93–94, 93f
Throttle controls, aerial devices, 457
Tiller aerial apparatus, 398–431
    aerial ladder and, 414–416, 415–416f
    alarm, responding to, 413
    approaching the incident, 413–414, 414f
    climbing the aerial, 422, 424–425, 425f
    communications, 401–402, 429
    controlling the vehicle, 402–406, 403–405f
    in defensive strategy, 427–428, 427f
    defined, 42f, 358
    driving exercises, 407, 408–410f, 409–410, 412
    environmental conditions, 406, 428
    history, 400
    inspection of, 406–407, 407f
    learning curve for operating, 412–413, 412f
    loading considerations, 425, 427
    lowering the aerial, 428
    maintenance and inspection, 442–443, 443f
    positioning at scene, 414–416, 414f, 415–416f, 422–423, 428–429
    principles of operation, 406, 406f
    raising and placing the aerial, 423–424, 424f
    rescue strategies and tactics, 428–429
    responsibilities, 406–407, 407f
    safe driving, 400–401
    safe operation, 422–423
    stabilizing, 422–423, 423f
    summary and review, 417–418, 430
    training requirements, 407
    turntable monitoring, 425
Tiller operator (tillerman), 400, 402–403, 406–407, 407f, 412–413, 442–443, 443f
TIMA. See Traffic incident management area (TIMA)
Time trial test, aerial devices, 458
Tip of ladder, positioning and operation, 380–381, 381f, 459
Tires, inspection of, 22, 173
Tools
    for fire apparatus inspections, 169, 170f
    functions and limitations, 24–26, 25–26f
    inspection of, 179–180, 179–180f
    maintaining, 26
    promoting safety with, 19–20

Index

Top-mounted pump panels, for viewing scene, 11, 11*f*
Torque box, 422, 444
Total pressure loss (TPL), 139–140, 141
Total stopping distance, 221
Tower ladders, 8, 8*f*. *See also* Aerial fire apparatus
Tower lights, 269, 269–270*f*
TPL. *See* Total pressure loss (TPL)
Traction, automatic control (ATC), 10
Traffic
    direction of, emergency vehicle laws on, 220
    never trusting, 233
    into and out of dump sites, 305, 305*f*
Traffic control, 220, 233, 234, 234*f*, 236–238, 305
Traffic incident management area (TIMA), 234, 236
Traffic incidents, 226, 234, 234*f*, 236–238
Traffic signals
    emergency vehicle laws, 220
    preemption systems for, 225
Traffic space, 236
Trailer operator, 400, 402–403, 407, 412–413
Training and selection, driver/operators, 16–33.
    See also Driving exercises
    educating crew members, 18, 20–21
    for filling tankers, 298
    fire apparatus and equipment functions and limitations, 24–26, 25–26*f*
    fire apparatus and equipment inspections, 25–26, 25–26*f*
    with foam concentrates and foam systems, 327, 345
    importance for driver/operators, 219
    for joining an existing relay pumping operation, 320, 321
    leading by example, 22, 24
    maintaining safe work environment, 21–24
    mnemonics for exercises, 22
    NFPA 1002 requirements, 26–28, 26–28*f*
    roles and responsibilities, 18–21, 19–20*f*
    safety role of, 19–20, 19–20*f*, 26
    selection process, 29–30, 29–30*f*
    summary and review, 31–33
    tiller aerial apparatus requirements, 407
    trust and team building by, 18–19, 21
Transfer case, 95–96, 95*f*
Transfer valve, 84, 84*f*, 181, 260, 261*f*, 496, 496*f*
Transition areas, 236
Transmission, switching from "road" to "pump," 247–248, 248*f*.
    See also Pump transmission
Transmission fluid inspection, 176
Transmission retarders, 10, 224
Transmission/aerial interlock, testing, 457
Transmission-driven generator, 265, 267–268*sd*
Trench collapse incidents, 240
Triple-combination pumpers, 7, 7*f*
Trucks. *See* Aerial fire apparatus
Trust, team building and, 21
Turbidity, 54

Turnaround, confined-space, 201–203, 202*sd*, 407, 409, 409*f*
Turnout gear, 200, 233–234
Turntable, aerial apparatus
    control pedestal operation and maintenance, 438–439*f*, 438–440
    during cradling of device, 452
    filter check, 456
    hour meter, 435, 435*f*
    monitoring for tiller apparatus, 425
    operational and maintenance checklists, 437, 437*f*
    placement considerations, 444
    platform controls, 438, 439, 459*t*
    positioning and controls, 358, 366–367, 371, 423
    visual inspection checklist, 437, 437*f*
2½-inch (65-mm) attack hose, 104
250 psi test, 499–500
200 psi test, 499
Two-stage pumps, 83–84, 85–86, 86*f*, 293

U

UL. *See* Underwriters Laboratory (UL)
Ultrasonic testing, aerial devices, 455
Under-slung jacks, 445, 445*f*
Under-steering, tiller apparatus, 404
Underwriters Laboratory (UL), 78, 85, 480, 481*f*
Uneven grades, aerial device stabilizing on, 370, 370*f*, 371*sd*
Universal solvent, 53
Unsupported versus supported aerial device positions, 372–373, 373*f*
U.S. Fire Administration (USFA), 12, 358, 373
USFA. *See* U.S. Fire Administration (USFA)
Utility vehicle, NFPA 1002 qualification to operate, 27, 27*f*
U-turns, 222

V

Vacra, Jesse, 195
Vacuum
    for drafting operations, 280, 280*t*, 296, 297
    for dump line, 293
    fire pump test, 284, 285*sd*, 488, 490*sd*, 491
    priming a pump using, 81
    whirlpools while drafting water and, 296
Vacuum leaks, 284, 297
Valves, fire hose appliance, 109, 109*f*. *See also specific types*
Vanes, in rotary pumps, 80–81
Vapor suppression in foam application, 328, 330*t*, 331
VDR. *See* Vehicle data recorder (VDR)
Vehicle data recorder (VDR), 11
Vehicle dynamics, 25
Vehicle fires, 237, 237*f*
Vehicle intercom system, 20
Vehicle performance tests, 467–471
    battery charger/conditioner test, 471
    brake testing, 178–179, 178–179*f*, 468
    charging system, 470, 470*sd*

low-voltage electrical systems, 468–471, 468f, 469sd, 469t, 470t
  regulator, 470–471, 470t
  road test, 468
  starter system, 469–470
  weight verification test, 467–468
Velocity, of moving water sources, 286
Ventilation operations
  aerial deployment priority, 357
  positioning of aerial devices, 363, 382, 383sd, 384
Venturi effect/forces, 81, 281, 304, 336, 340
Vertical ventilation via rooftop operations, 382
Victaulic connections, 441–442
Violent scenes, response to, 235, 238, 240
Viscosity
  of hydraulic fluid, 435, 436f
  of protein foams, 330
Voices of Experience
  Angulo on fire apparatus inspections, 182
  Barron on driver/operator training and preparation, 23
  Carter on relay pumping operations, 318
  Dettman on adapting to the situation, 494
  Drake on staging near violent scene, 235
  Faulkner on consistent use of ground plates, 453
  Garrity on staying calm in emergencies, 82
  Lindroth on building fire service in Mexico, 40
  McIntyre on tiller operation, 411, 426
  Minoia on driver/operator safety role, 110
  Poole on uninterrupted water supply, 40
  Smith on aerial device operational safety, 376
  Songer on hydraulic calculations, 148
  Vacra on driving narrow city streets, 195
  Washington on water mains for water supply, 299
  Westhoff on efficiency in foam applications, 344
  Willis on securing water source, 256
  Winkler on "SAFETY" components, 9
Voltage
  battery charger/conditioner test, 471
  line voltage electrical systems tests, 474–475
  low-voltage electrical system testing, 468–471, 468f, 469sd, 469t, 470t
  starter system test, 469–470
  total continuous electrical load test, 471
Voltage meter inspection, 176
Voltmeter
  charging vehicle battery, 196, 196f
  fire pump operations, 92, 92f
  testing low-voltage electrical systems, 468, 468f, 469, 470
Volume, as measure of water flow or quantity, 55, 56, 59
Volume pumps, 85
Volute, 83

W

Warm zones, at emergency medical scenes, 240
Washington, Michael, 299
Washtubs, drafting water and, 300
Water, 50–73. See also Elevated streams; Foam; Water shuttle; Water sources; Water supply
  chemical properties of, 53–54, 53f
  flow and pressure, 55–59, 56–58f
  fluid dynamics, 56–58f, 56–59
  harmful characteristics of, 54
  municipal systems for, 52, 54–56, 55f, 56f
  NFPA 1901 on rate of delivery of, 37
  physical properties of, 53–54, 53f
  on pumper fire apparatus, 37–38, 37f
  rural supplies of, 68, 70, 70f
  securing source for, 253–256
  sources and supply, 52–53, 52f, 478
  summary and review, 71–73
  temperature and fire apparatus performance, 476–477
Water curtain nozzles, 114
Water flow, 56
Water flow monitor, 136f
Water hammer, 59, 65
Water mains, 55, 56
Water pressure, 55–59, 56–58f
Water pump for quints, 44, 44f
Water shuttle, 300–307
  described, 297–298
  dump site operations for, 302–306, 304–305f
  fill site operations for, 298, 300–301, 306
  filling tankers for, 301
  in Incident Management System, 306–307
  nurse tanker operations, 306
  offloading tankers for dump sites, 303, 304f, 306
  portable tanks, 302, 303–304, 304f
  safety for, 301
  summary and review, 308–309
  traffic flow within dump sites, 305–306, 305f
Water sources. See also Fire hydrants; Static water sources
  moving, 286–287
  pressurized, 249, 251–253
  quantity estimation, 286–287
  securing, 253–255
Water storage towers, 55, 55f
Water stream, early elevated water, 6
Water supply. See also Drafting water
  characteristics, 52–53, 52f
  connecting engine to, 252–253
  defined, 52
  for elevated streams, 386
  establishing uninterruptible source, 62
  filling tankers for, 87, 88f, 298, 301
  in Incident Management System, 284
  positioning at fire scene and, 230
  relay pumping operations for, 313, 314
  secondary or supplemental, thinking ahead for, 127
  static or dynamic, NPDP from, 156

tank inspection, 180
uninterrupted, 297
water shuttle for, 297–298, 300–307
Water supply officers, 122, 297, 301
Water system inspections, aerial devices, 458
Water tanks. *See also* Portable tanks; Tankers
in batch mixing of foam, 334–335, 334*f*
booster tanks, 7, 284, 287, 297
internal, 249
level indicator, 92, 92*f*
level indicator, pump panel, 92, 92*f*
NFPA 1901 rules on, 37
nurse tanker operations, 306
on pumper fire apparatus, 37, 78–79, 78*f*
tank-to-pump flow, 488, 489*sd*
Water thief, 107, 107*f*
Water tower position, aerial device, 449
Water treatment facilities, 55, 55*f*
Water-miscible fuels, 330
Waterway system and plumbing, aerial ladders
basic system, 442
monitoring and draining, 450, 451*f*
relief valve, 450, 450*f*
shifting of movable, 450
testing of, 458
troubleshooting, 460
Weekly fire apparatus inspections, 187
Weight restrictions, for fire apparatus, 25
Weight verification test, 467–468
Westhoff, Roger, 344
Wet standpipe systems, 255

Wet versus dry fire pumps, 180, 181
Wet-barrel fire hydrants, 61, 61*f*
Wheel alignment, tiller apparatus, 403
Wheel chocks
aerial device positioning, 444
aerial device stabilizing system inspection, 184, 422
air brake inspection, 178, 178*f*
no-load governed engine speed test, 481
parking at scene procedures, 248
for parking on slopes, 230
when working around fire apparatus, 284
Wheels and rims, inspection of, 174
Whirlpools, vacuum for drafting water and, 296
Willis, Brent, 256
Wind conditions, 231, 231*f*
Windows, inspection of, 177
Windshield wipers, inspection of, 177
Winkler, Dave, 9
Wivell, Abraham, 42
Work environment, maintaining safe, 19, 21–24
Working fire apparatus, 227. *See also* Fire apparatus positioning
Working height, aerial device, 447, 447*f*
Wyes
defined, 105, 107
as fire hose appliance, 105, 105*f*, 107, 140
friction loss (FL) calculations, 140–143, 140–143*sd*
gated, 105, 105*f*, 107

X

X-style jacks, 445, 445*f*
X-type stabilizers, 360–361, 361*f*